Enric Carreras • Carlo Dufour
Mohamad Mohty • Nicolaus Kröger
Editors

The EBMT Handbook

Hematopoietic Stem Cell Transplantation and Cellular Therapies

Editors
Enric Carreras
Spanish Bone Marrow Donor Registry
Josep Carreras Foundation
and Leukemia Research Institute
Catalunya, Barcelona
Spain

Mohamad Mohty
Department of Hematology
Pierre and Marie Curie University
Paris
France

Carlo Dufour
Hematology Unit
IRCCS Giannina Gaslini
Geneva
Switzerland

Nicolaus Kröger
Department of Stem Cell
Transplantation
University Medical Center
Hamburg-Eppend
Hamburg
Germany

https://doi.org/10.1007/978-3-030-02278-5

Preface

Hematopoietic stem cell transplantation has become a well-established life-saving treatment procedure for many patients with hematological malignancies, inborn errors, or bone marrow failure syndromes. Starting more than 60 years as an "ultima ratio" option, hematopoietic stem cell transplantation is now integrated as an essential part in many treatment concepts and protocols. The rapid development in the field with changing in transplant practices and the increasing numbers of long-term survivors require a continuous education for physician, nurses, and healthcare providers who are involved in stem cell transplantation and cellular therapies.

This new formatted EBMT Handbook, which is part of a broader EBMT educational strategy, addresses the most recent developments and innovations in stem cell transplantation and cellular therapy presented by more than 170 authors, known as experts and well-recognized authorities in the field. In more than 90 chapters, all types of stem cell and bone marrow transplantation including haplo-identical stem cell and cord blood transplantation, indication for transplantation, and management of complications as well as the new rapidly evolving field of cellular therapies are covered. Other important issues such as quality management and JACIE accreditation, stem cell collection, conditioning, donor selection, HLA typing, graft manipulation, ethical issues, psychological support, and quality of life are also properly addressed.

The aim of this new EBMT Handbook, which follows the long tradition of the *ESH-EBMT Handbook on Haematopoietic Stem Cell Transplantation*, is not to provide an in-depth knowledge like a textbook but rather to describe the state of practice to enhance the reader's knowledge and practice skills. Major key points are summarized at the end of each chapter.

The EBMT Board wants to express their great gratitude to the strong effort of the Working Party chairs and all authors in planning and writing the chapters and the tremendous work of the project leader Enric Carreras and the secretarial work of Marta Herrero Hoces from the Barcelona EBMT offices but also to Nathalie L'Horset-Poulain from Springer for her continuous support.

A heartfelt thanks goes to the Fondation José Carreras pour la lutte contre la leucémie, Geneve for the unconditioned educational grant, which permits the open-access publication as well as the printed version of this EBMT Handbook.

On behalf of the EBMT board, we hope this EBMT Handbook will be of help in your daily practice.

Barcelona, Spain	Enric Carreras
Geneva, Switzerland	Carlo Dufour
Paris, France	Mohamad Mohty
Hamburg, Germany	Nicolaus Kröger

Acknowledgment

This open-access and print edition have been possible thanks to the generous contribution of the Foundation José Carreras pour la lutte contre la leucémie, Genève.

Contents

Part III Methodology and Clinical Aspects

Part IV General Management of the Patient

Contributors

Miguel R. Abboud Department of Pediatrics and Adolescent Medicine, American University of Beirut Medical Center, Beirut, Lebanon

Alessandro Aiuti San Raffaele Telethon Institute for Gene Therapy (SR-TIGET)/Pediatric Immunohematology and Bone Marrow Transplantation Unit, IRCCS Ospedale San Raffaele, Vita-Salute San Raffaele University, Milan, Italy

Michael Albert Pediatric SCT Program, Dr. von Hauner University Children's Hospital, Ludwig-Maximilians Universität, Munich, Germany

Tobias Alexander Department of Rheumatology and Clinical Immunology, Charité – University Medicine Berlin, Berlin, Germany

Mahmoud Aljurf King Faisal Specialist Hospital and Research Centre, Riyadh, Saudi Arabia

Persis Amrolia Department of Bone Marrow Transplant, Great Ormond St Children's Hospital, London, UK

Emanuele Angelucci Department of Oncology and Hematology, IRCCS Ospedale Policlinico San Martino, Genova, Italy

Jane Apperley Centre for Haematology, Hammersmith Hospital, Imperial College London, London, UK

Diana Averbuch Pediatric Infectious Diseases, Hadassah Medical Center, Hebrew University, Jerusalem, Israel

Francis Ayuk Department of Stem Cell Transplantation, University Medical Center Hamburg-Eppendorf (UKE), Hamburg, Germany

Aleksandra Babic IOSI-Istituto Oncologico della Svizzera Italiana, OSG, Bellinzona, Switzerland

Andrea Bacigalupo Istituto di Ematologia, Fondazione Polclinico Universitario A. Gemelli, Universita' Cattolica del Sacro Cuore, Roma, Italy

Peter Bader Division for Stem Cell Transplantation and Immunology, University Hospital for Children and Adolescents, Goethe University Frankfurt am Main, Frankfurt, Germany

Adriana Balduzzi Outpatient Hematology and Transplant Department, Clinica Pediatrica, Università degli Studi di Milano Bicocca, Ospedale San Gerardo, Monza, Italy

Anna Barata Department of Hematology, Hospital de la Santa Creu i Sant Pau, Barcelona, Spain

Institut de Recerca Contra la Leucèmia Josep Carreras, Universitat Autònoma de Barcelona, Barcelona, Spain

Grzegorz W. Basak Department of Hematology, Oncology and Internal Medicine, Independent Public Central Clinical Hospital, Medical University of Warsaw, Warsaw, Poland

Annic Baumgartner Internal Medicine and Endcrinology/Diabetology/Clinical Nutrition and Metabolism, Medical University Clinic of Kantonsspital Aarau, University of Basel, Aarau, Switzerland

Tiene Bauters Pharmacy, Pediatric Hemato-Oncology and Stem Cell Transplantation, Ghent University Hospital, Ghent, Belgium

Ali Bazarbachi Bone Marrow Transplantation Program, Department of Internal Medicine, American University of Beirut Medical Center, Beirut, Lebanon

Alice Bertaina Division of Stem Cell Transplantation and Regenerative Medicine, Department of Pediatrics, School of Medicine, Stanford University, Stanford, CA, USA

Marc Bierings Pediatric Hematology and HSCT Division, Wilhelmina Kinderziekenhuis, Utrecht, The Netherlands

Joan Bladé Amyloidosis and Myeloma Unit, Department of Hematology, Hospital Clinic of Barcelona, IDIBAPS, Barcelona, Spain

Jaap Jan Boelens Laboratory of Translational Immunology, UMC, Utrecht, The Netherlands

Princess Maxima Center for Pediatric Oncology, Blood and Marrow Transplantation Program, Utrecht, The Netherlands

Attilio Bondanza Innovative Immunotherapies Unit, Division of Immunology, Transplantation and Infectious Diseases, University Vita-Salute San Raffaele and Ospedale San Raffaele Scientific Institute, Milan, Italy

Francesca Bonifazi Institute of Hematology "Seràgnoli", University Hospital S. Orsola-Malpighi, Bologna University, Bologna, Italy

Chiara Bonini Experimental Hematology Unit, Division of Immunology, Transplantation and Infectious Diseases, University Vita-Salute San Raffaele and Ospedale San Raffaele Scientific Institute, Milan, Italy

Benedetto Bruno Department of Oncology, AOU Città della Salute e della Scienza, University of Torino, Torino, Italy

Department of Molecular Biotechnology and Health Sciences, AOU Città della Salute e della Scienza, University of Torino, Torino, Italy

Jonathan Canaani Hematology and BMT Division, Chaim Sheba Medical Center, Tel-Hashomer, Israel

Barbara Cappelli Eurocord-Monacord, Centre Scientifique de Monaco, Monaco, Monaco

Enric Carreras Spanish Bone Marrow Donor Registry, Josep Carreras Foundation and Leukemia Research Institute, Barcelona, Catalunya, Spain

Hospital Clinic Barcelona, Barcelona University, Barcelona, Spain

Elio Castagnola Infectious Diseases Unit, Department of Pediatrics, Istituto Giannina Gaslini, Genoa, Italy

Simone Cesaro Pediatric Hematology Oncology, Azienda Ospedaliera Universitaria Integrata, Verona, Italy

Christian Chabannon Institut Paoli-Calmettes, Centre de Lutte Contre le Cancer, Marseille, France

Université d'Aix-Marseille, Marseille, France

Centre d'Investigations Cliniques en Biothérapie, Marseille, France

Yves Chalandon Department of Oncology, Hematology Division, Hôpitaux Universitaires de Genève, University of Geneva, Geneva, Switzerland

Shruti Chaturvedi Division of Hematology, Department of Medicine, Johns Hopkins Hospital, Baltimore, MD, USA

Fabio Ciceri IRCCS San Raffaele Scientific Institute, University Vita-Salute San Raffaele, Milan, Italy

Gordon Cook Haematology and Myeloma Studies, Leeds Cancer Centre, St James's University Hospital, Leeds, UK

Kenneth R. Cooke Pediatric Blood and Marrow Transplantation Program, Oncology Department, Sidney Kimmel Comprehensive Cancer Center, Johns Hopkins University School of Medicine, Baltimore, MD, USA

Jan J. Cornelissen Department of Hematology, Erasmus Medical Center Cancer Institute, Rotterdam, The Netherlands

Charles Craddock Centre for Clinical Haematology, Queen Elizabeth Hospital, Birmingham, UK

Jean-Hugues Dalle Department of Pediatric Hematology-Immunology, Hospital Robert-Debré, Assistance Publique-Hôpitaux de Paris, Paris Diderot University, Paris, France

Francesco Dazzi School of Cancer and Pharmacological Sciences, King's College London, London, UK

Rafael de la Cámara Department of Hematology, Hospital de la Princesa, Madrid, Spain

Cristina Díaz de Heredia Department of Pediatric Hematology and Oncology and HSCT Hospital Universitari Vall d'Hebron, Barcelona, Spain

Maribel Diaz-Ricart Hemostasis and Erythropathology, Hematopathology Section, Pathological Anatomy Department, CDB, Hospital Clinic, University of Barcelona, Barcelona, Spain

Sascha Dietrich Department of Hematology, University Hospital of Heidelberg, Heidelberg, Germany

Peter Dreger Abteilung Innere Medizin V, Universitätsklinikum Heidelberg, Heidelberg, Germany

Rafael F. Duarte Hospital Universitario Puerta de Hierro Majadahonda, Madrid, Spain

Carlo Dufour Hematology Unit, G. Gaslini Research Children Hospital, Genoa, Italy

Rémy Duléry Hematology Department, Hôpital Saint Antoine, AP-HP, Paris, France

Hermann Einsele Department of Internal Medicine II, Julius Maximilian University of Würzburg, Würzburg, Germany

Khaled El-Ghariani Department of Hematology, Sheffield Teaching Hospitals Trust and NHSBT, The University of Sheffield, Sheffield, UK

Irina Evseeva Anthony Nolan, London, UK

J. H. Frederik Falkenburg Department of Hematology, Leiden University Medical Center, Leiden, The Netherlands

Dominique Farge Unité Clinique de Médecine Interne, Maladies Auto-immunes et Pathologie Vasculaire, UF 04, Hôpital Saint-Louis, EA 3518, AP-HP Assistance Publique des Hôpitaux de Paris, Paris Denis Diderot University, Paris, France

Centre de Référence des Maladies auto-immunes systémiques Rares d'Ile-de-France (site constitutif), Filière FAI2R, Paris, France

Boris Fehse Research Department Cell and Gene Therapy, Department of Stem Cell Transplantation, University Medical Centre Hamburg-Eppendorf, Hamburg, Germany

Francesc Fernandez-Avilés Department of Hematology, Bone Marrow Transplantation Unit, Hospital Clínic de Barcelona, Universitat de Barcelona, Barcelona, Catalunya, Spain

Francesca Fioredda Hematology Unit, Istituto Giannina Gaslini, Genoa, Italy

Katharina Fleischhauer Institute for Experimental Cellular Therapy, University Hospital, Essen, Germany

Lydia Foeken Word Marrow Donor Association (WMDA), Leiden, The Netherlands

Andrew Gennery Paediatric Immunology + HSCT, Great North Children's Hospital, Newcastle University, Newcastle upon Tyne, UK

Binsah George Hematology and Stem Cell Transplantation Section, Division of Hematology/Oncology, Department of Medicine, Vanderbilt University Medical Center and Veterans Affairs Medical Center, Nashville, TN, USA

Khaled Ghanem BASMA Pediatric Oncology Unit, Al Bairouni Hospital, Damascus, Syria

Brenda E. S. Gibson Haematology Department, Royal Hospital for Children, University of Glasgow, Glasgow, UK

Sebastian Giebel Department of Bone Marrow Transplantation and Onco-Hematology, Maria Sklodowska-Curie Memorial Cancer Center and Institute of Oncology, Gliwice, Poland

Evgenia Glogova Studies and Statistics for Integrated Research and Projects, St. Anna Kinderkrebsforschung e.V., Vienna, Austria

Eliane Gluckman Department of Hematology, Hospital Saint Louis, University Paris-Diderot, Paris, France

Norbert Claude Gorin Department of Hematology and Cell Therapy, EBMT Paris Office, Hôpital Saint Antoine APHP, Paris, France

Paris Sorbonne University, Paris, France

Alois Gratwohl Hematology, Medical Faculty, University of Basel, Basel, Switzerland

Diana M. Greenfield Specialised Cancer Services, Sheffield Teaching Hospitals NHS Foundation Trust, University of Sheffield, Sheffield, UK

Hildegard Greinix Division of Hematology, Department of Internal Medicine, University Hospital Graz, Graz, Austria

Gonzalo Gutiérrez-García Department of Hematology, Bone Marrow Transplantation Unit, Hospital Clínic de Barcelona, Universitat de Barcelona, Barcelona, Catalunya, Spain

Rupert Handgretinger Department of Hematology/Oncology and General Pediatrics, Children's University Hospital, University of Tuebingen, Tuebingen, Germany

Shahrukh K. Hashmi Department of Adult Hematology, King Faisal Specialist Hospital and Research Center, Riyadh, Saudi Arabia

Mayo Clinic, Rochester, MN, USA

Shelley Hewerdine Data Management Lead, EBMT, London, UK

Britta Höchsmann Institute of Clinical Transfusion Medicine and Immunogenetics Ulm, German Red Cross Blood Transfusion Service Baden-Württemberg-Hessen and University Hospital Ulm, Ulm, Germany

Institute of Transfusion Medicine, University of Ulm, Ulm, Germany

Andrea Hoffmann Department of Orthopaedic Surgery, Laboratory of Biomechanics and Biomaterials, Hannover Medical School, Hannover, Germany

Ernst Holler Clinical and Experimental HSCT, Department of Internal Medicine 3 (Haematology/Oncology), University of Regensburg, Regensburg, Germany

Kai Hübel University of Cologne, Department of Internal Medicine, Cologne, Germany

Michael Hudecek Medizinische Klinik und Poliklinik II, Universitätsklinikum Würzburg, Würzburg, Germany

Simona Iacobelli Department of Biology, University of Rome Tor Vergata, Rome, Italy

EBMT, Leiden, The Netherlands

Heather Jim Department of Health Outcomes and Behavior, Moffitt Cancer Center, Tampa, FL, USA

Ulrike Koehl Institute of Clinical Immunology, University of Leipzig, Leipzig, Germany

Institute of Cellular Therapeutics, Hannover Medical School, Hannover, Germany

Fraunhofer Institute of Cellular Therapeutics and Immunology, Leipzig, Germany

Hans Joachim Kolb Department of Hematology-Oncology Immunology Infectious Diseases, Klinikum München-Schwabing, Munich, Germany

Sixten Körper Institute of Clinical Transfusion Medicine and Immunogenetics Ulm, German Red Cross Blood Transfusion Service Baden-Württemberg-Hessen and University Hospital Ulm, Ulm, Germany

Institute of Transfusion Medicine, University of Ulm, Ulm, Germany

Nicolaus Kröger Department of Stem Cell Transplantation, University Medical Center Hamburg-Eppendorf, Hamburg, Germany

Hermann Kreyenberg Division of Stem Cell Transplantation and Immunology, Center for Children and Adolescents, University Hospital Frankfurt, Frankfurt, Germany

Jürgen Kuball Department of Hematology, UMC, Utrecht, The Netherlands

Laboratory of Translational Immunology, UMC, Utrecht, The Netherlands

Princess Maxima Center for Pediatric Oncology, Blood and Marrow Transplantation Program, Utrecht, The Netherlands

Ruth Ladenstein Studies and Statistics for Integrated Research and Projects, St. Anna Children's Hospital, Department of Paediatrics and Children's Cancer Research Institute (CCRI), Medical University of Vienna, Vienna, Austria

Peter Lang Department of Hematology/Oncology and General Pediatrics, Children's University Hospital, University of Tuebingen, Tuebingen, Germany

Claudia Langebrake Department of Stem Cell Transplantation and Hospital Pharmacy, University Medical Centre Hamburg-Eppendorf, Hamburg, Germany

Arjan Lankester Department of Pediatrics, Stem Cell Transplantation Program, Willem-Alexander Children's Hospital, Leiden University Medical Center, Leiden, The Netherlands

Francesco Lanza Hematology and HSCT Unit, Department of Onco-Hematology, Hospital S. Maria delle Croci, Ravenna, Italy

Anita Lawitschka St. Anna Children's Hospital, Medical University Vienna, Vienna, Austria

Per Ljungman Department of Cellular Therapy and Allogeneic Stem Cell Transplantation, Karolinska University Hospital, Stockholm, Sweden

Division of Hematology, Department of Medicine Huddinge, Karolinska Institutet, Stockholm, Sweden

Franco Locatelli Department of Pediatric Hematology and Oncology, IRCCS Bambino Gesù Children's Hospital, Rome, Italy

Department of Pediatric Science, University of Pavia, Pavia, Italy

Department of Hematology, UMC, Utrecht, The Netherlands

Alejandro Madrigal Anthony Nolan, London, UK

UCL Cancer Institute, Royal Free Campus, London, UK

Johan A. Maertens Department of Haematology, University Hospital Gasthuisberg, Leuven, Belgium

David I. Marks Department of Haematology and BMT, Bristol Haematology and Oncology Centre, Bristol, UK

Carmen Martínez HSCT Unit, Department of Hematology, Institute of Hematology and Oncology, Hospital Clínic de Barcelona, Universitat de Barcelona, Barcelona, Spain

Rodrigo Martino Hospital de la Santa Creu I Sant Pau, Autonomous University of Barcelona, ES, Barcelona, Spain

Eoin McGrath European Society for Blood and Marrow Transplantation (EBMT), Barcelona, Spain

David Michonneau Hematology/Transplantation, AP/HP Hospital St Louis, Paris, France

University Paris VII, Denis Diderot, Paris, France

INSERM UMR 1160, Paris, France

Malgorzata Mikulska Division of Infectious Diseases, Department of Health Sciences (DISSAL), IRCCS Ospedale Policlinico San Martino, University of Genova, Genova, Italy

Monique Minnema Department of Hematology, UMC Utrecht Cancer Center, Utrecht, The Netherlands

Federica Minniti Mother and Child Department, Ospedale della Donna e del bambino, University of Verona, Verona, Italy

Mohamad Mohty Department of Clinical Hematology and Cellular Therapy, Hospital Saint-Antoine, Sorbonne University, Paris, France

Silvia Montoto Department of Haemato-Oncology, St. Bartholomew's and The Royal London NHS Trust, Queen Mary University of London, London, UK

Enrique Moreno Department of Psychology, Asleuval (Valencian Association of Leukemia), Valencia, Spain

John Murray Haematology and Transplant Unit, The Christie NHS Foundation Trust, Manchester, UK

Arnon Nagler Department of Medicine, Tel Aviv University, Tel-Hashomer, Israel

Hematology Division, BMT and Cord Blood Bank, Chaim Sheba Medical Center, Tel-Hashomer, Israel

Dietger W. Niederwieser University of Leipzig, Leipzig, Germany

Charlotte M. Niemeyer Department of Pediatrics and Adolescent Medicine, University Medical Center, Freiburg, Germany

Francesco Onida Department of Hematology, Fondazione IRCCS Ca' Granda Ospedale Maggiore Policlinico, University of Milan, Milan, Italy

Gert Ossenkoppele Department of Hematology, Universitaire Medische Centra, VU University Medical Center, Amsterdam, The Netherlands

Régis Peffault de Latour French Reference Center for Aplastic Anemia and Paroxysmal Nocturnal Hemoglobinuria, Saint-Louis Hospital, Paris, France

Assistance Publique–Hôpitaux de Paris, Saint-Louis Hospital, Paris, France

University Paris VII, Denis Diderot, Paris, France

Christina Peters Stem Cell Transplantation Unit, St. Anna Children's Hospital, Vienna, Austria

Alice Polomeni Service d'Hématologie clinique et thérapie cellulaire, Hôpital Saint Antoine - Assistance Publique-Hôpitaux de Paris, Paris, France

Sergio Querol Banc Sang i Teixits, Barcelona, Spain

Alessandro Rambaldi Department of Hematology-Oncology, Azienda Socio Sanitaria Territoriale Papa Giovanni XXIII, Bergamo, Università Statale di Milano, Milano, Italy

Walid Rasheed King Faisal Specialist Hospital and Research Centre, Riyadh, Saudi Arabia

Francesca Riccardi Consultant Hematology Unit, Hemato-Oncology and SCT Pole, Istituto Giannina Gaslini, Genoa, Italy

Antonio Risitano Department of Clinical Medicine and Surgery, Federico II University of Naples, Naples, Italy

Marie Robin Department of Hematology – Transplantation, Hôpital Saint-Louis, Assistance Publique Hôpitaux de Paris, Paris, France

Stephen Robinson Bristol Cancer Institute, University Hospital's Bristol, Bristol, UK

Vanderson Rocha Hospital de Clinicas, Hematology, Transfusion and Cell Therapy Service, University of São Paulo, Sao Paulo, Brazil

Churchill Hospital, NHS-BT, Oxford University, Oxford, UK

Montserrat Rovira HSCT Unit, Hematology Department, Hospital Clínic de Barcelona, University of Barcelona, Barcelona, Catalunya, Spain

BMT Unit, Haematology Department, IDIBAPS, Hospital Clinic, Josep Carreras Leukemia Research Institute (IJC), Barcelona, Spain

Carmen Ruiz de Elvira Registry Head, EBMT, London, UK

Tapani Ruutu Clinical Research Institute, Helsinki University Hospital, Helsinki, Finland

Riccardo Saccardi Department of Cellular Therapies and Transfusion Medicine, Careggi University Hospital, Florence, Italy

Nina Salooja Centre for Haematology, Imperial College, London, UK

Isabel Sánchez-Ortega Institut Català d'Oncologia Hospitalet, Barcelona, Spain

Jaime Sanz Department of Medicine, University Hospital La Fe, University of Valencia, Valencia, Spain

Instituto Carlos III, CIBERONC, Madrid, Spain

Miguel Á. Sanz Department of Hematology, University Hospital La Fe, University of Valencia, Valencia, Spain

Martin G. Sauer Pediatric Hematology, Oncology and Blood Cell Transplantation, Medizinische Hochschule Hannover, Hannover, Germany

Bipin N. Savani Hematology and Stem Cell Transplantation Section, Division of Hematology/Oncology, Department of Medicine, Vanderbilt University Medical Center and Veterans Affairs Medical Center, Nashville, TN, USA

Serena Scala San Raffaele Telethon Institute for Gene Therapy (SR-TIGET), IRCCS Ospedale San Raffaele, Milan, Italy

Johannes Schetelig Medical Clinic I, Department of Hematology, University Hospital Carl Gustav Carus, Technische Universität Dresden, Dresden, Germany

Christoph Schmid Klinikum Augsburg, University of Munich, Munich, Germany

Norbert Schmitz Department of Medicine A, Hematology, Oncology, Pneumonology and Hemostaseology, University Hospital Münster, Münster, Germany

Stefan Schönland Hematology, Oncology and Rheumatology, Internal Medicine, University of Heidelberg, Heidelberg, Germany

Hubert Schrezenmeier Institute of Clinical Transfusion Medicine and Immunogenetics Ulm, German Red Cross Blood Transfusion Service Baden-Württemberg-Hessen and University Hospital Ulm, Ulm, Germany

Institute of Transfusion Medicine, University of Ulm, Ulm, Germany

Philipp Schuetz Department of Endocrinology, Diabetes and Metabolism and Internal Medicine, Kantonsspital Aarau, University of Basel, Aarau, Switzerland

Ansgar Schulz Department of Pediatrics, University Medical Center Ulm, Ulm, Germany

Frank Schulz-Kindermann Pychooncological Outpatient Department, Institute of Medical Psychology, University Cancer Center Hamburg, University of Hamburg, Hamburg, Germany

Michael Schumm Department of Hematology/Oncology and General Pediatrics, Children's University Hospital, University of Tuebingen, Tuebingen, Germany

Basil Sharrack Academic Department of Neuroscience and Sheffield NIHR Translational Neuroscience BRC, Sheffield Teaching Hospitals, NHS Foundation Trust, University of Sheffield, Sheffield, UK

Avichai Shimoni Bone Marrow Transplantation, Chaim Sheba Medical Center, Tel-Aviv University, Tel Hashomer, Israel

Zeev Shoham Department of Obstetrics and Gynecology, Kaplan Medical Center, Rehovot, Israel

John A. Snowden Department of Haematology, Sheffield Teaching Hospitals NHS Foundation Trust, University of Sheffield, Sheffield, UK

Gérard Socié Hematology/Transplantation, AP/HP Hospital St Louis, Paris, France

University Paris VII, Denis Diderot, Paris, France

INSERM UMR 1160, Paris, France

Eric Spierings Laboratory for Translational Immunology, University Medical Center, Utrecht, The Netherlands

Matthias Stelljes Department of Medicine A, Hematology, Oncology, Pneumonology and Hemostaseology, University Hospital Münster, Münster, Germany

Rainer Storb Clinical Research Division, Fred Hutchinson Cancer Research Center and University of Washington, School of Medicine, Seattle, WA, USA

Brigitte Strahm Department of Pediatrics and Adolescent Medicine Division of Pediatric Hematology and Oncology, Medical Center Faculty of Medicine, University of Freiburg, Freiburg im Breisgau, Germany

Jan Styczynski Department of Pediatric Hematology and Oncology, Nicolaus Copernicus University Torun, Collegium Medicum, Bydgoszcz, Poland

Maria Suárez-Lledó HSCT Unit, Hematology Department, Hospital Clínic de Barcelona, University of Barcelona, Barcelona, Catalunya, Spain

Anna Sureda Hematology Department and Stem Cell Transplantation Program, Institut Català d'Oncologia – Hospitalet, Barcelona, Catalunya, Spain

André Tichelli Department of Hematology, University Hospital Basel, Basel, Switzerland

Antoine Toubert University Paris Diderot and Hopital Saint Louis, Paris, France

Luca Vago Unit of Immunogenetics, Leukemia Genomics and Immunobiology, Hematology and Bone Marrow Transplantation Unit, IRCCS San Raffaele Scientific Institute, Milano, Italy

David Valcárcel Department of Hematology, Vall d'Hebron Institute of Oncology (VHIO), University Hospital Vall d'Hebron, Barcelona, Spain

Jurjen Versluis Department of Hematology, Erasmus Medical Center Cancer Institute, Rotterdam, The Netherlands

Paul Veys Great Ormond Street Hospital (GOSH) for Children NHS Foundation Trust, and University College London GOSH Institute of Child Health, London, UK

Christof Weinstock Institute of Clinical Transfusion Medicine and Immunogenetics Ulm, German Red Cross Blood Transfusion Service Baden-Württemberg-Hessen and University Hospital Ulm, Ulm, Germany

Institute of Transfusion Medicine, University of Ulm, Ulm, Germany

Volker Witt Department of Pediatric Hematology and Oncology, St. Anna Kinderspital, Medical University Vienna, Vienna, Austria

Theo de Witte Tumor Immunology, Radboud Institute for Molecular Life Sciences, Radboud University Medical Center, Nijmegen, The Netherlands

Daniel Wolff Department of Internal Medicine III, University Hospital Regensburg, Regensburg, Germany

Liesbeth C. de Wreede Department of Biomedical Data Sciences, Leiden University Medical Center, Leiden, The Netherlands

DKMS Clinical Trials Unit, Dresden, Germany

Patrick Wuchter Institute of Transfusion Medicine and Immunology, German Red Cross Blood Service Baden-Württemberg – Hessen, Medical Faculty Mannheim, Heidelberg University, Mannheim, Germany

Robert Wynn Blood and Marrow Transplant Unit, Royal Manchester Children's Hospital, University of Manchester, Manchester, UK

Robert Zeiser Section for Tumor Immunology, Department of Hematology/Oncology, University Hospital Freiburg, University of Freiburg, Freiburg, Germany

About the Editors

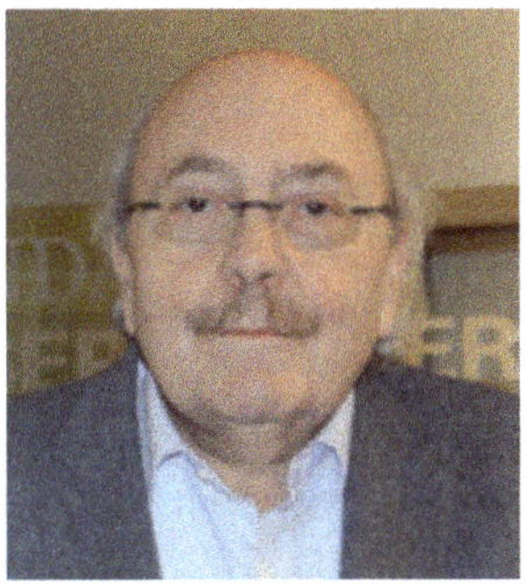

Enric Carreras is Director of the Spanish Bone Marrow Donors Registry at the Josep Carreras Foundation in Barcelona, Spain, since 2010. He obtained the degree in Medicine and Surgery (1975), becoming specialist in Internal Medicine and Hematology-Hemotherapy, and Doctor of Medicine (1984) in the University of Barcelona. From 1993 to 2010, he was Director of the HSCT Program at the Hospital Clínic in Barcelona.Along these years, his main clinical/research fields of interest have been focused in early complications and endothelial dysfunction after HSCT, HSCT in autoimmune diseases, and at-home HSCT. He is also founder of the Barcelona Endothelium Team at the Hospital Clinic campus of the Josep Carreras Leukemia Research Institute and the author of more than 180 peer-reviewed international publications mainly focused on HSCT. As member of the EBMT since 1980, he participated actively in the Chronic Leukemia Working Party, Autoimmune Diseases Working Party, and Late Complications Working Party. He was Chair of the EBMT/ESH training course in 12 editions and Chair of the EBMT Educational Committee. He is also editor of more than 12 books focused on hematology and HSCT, including the three last editions of the EBMT Handbook, and nominated Project Leader for the 2019 edition. In 2018, he was nominated Honorary Member of the EBMT.

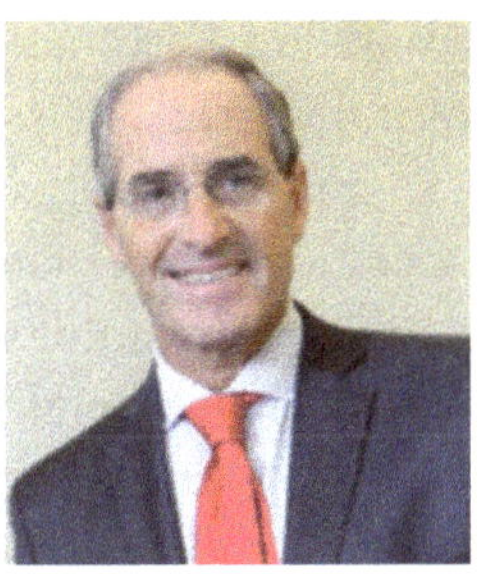

Carlo Dufour chairs, within in the G. Gaslini Children's Hospital, Genova, Italy, and coordinates the "Hemato-Oncology-SCT Pole and the Hematology Unit" where the national Registry of Neutropenia, the national Registry of Alps and related disorders, and the national Database of Fanconi Anemia have seats and where 75 clinical trials were or are still conducted. He authored or coauthored over 250 international publications and various hematology textbook chapters and co-edited a textbook called Congenital and Acquired Bone Marrow Failure. He acts as reviewer for top-ranking journals including The New England Journal of Medicine, Journal of Clinical Oncology, Leukemia, Clinical Immunology, and Blood. He serves as expert evaluator for different institutions including the French Registry for

Rare Diseases, the Fanconi Anemia Research Fund Inc. (USA), the Leukemia and Lymphoma Research Foundation (UK), and the American Society of Hematology Education Program. He is also Scientific Council Education Representative up to July 2018 and currently Chairman of the Working Party of the Severe Aplastic Anemia. He also serves as the Chairman of the Scientific Working Group on Granulocyte and Constitutional Marrow Failure Disorders of the European Hematology Association (EHA). In 2015 he received by the Fanconi Anemia Research Fund Inc. the discovery award for participating to the identification of gene FANCT.

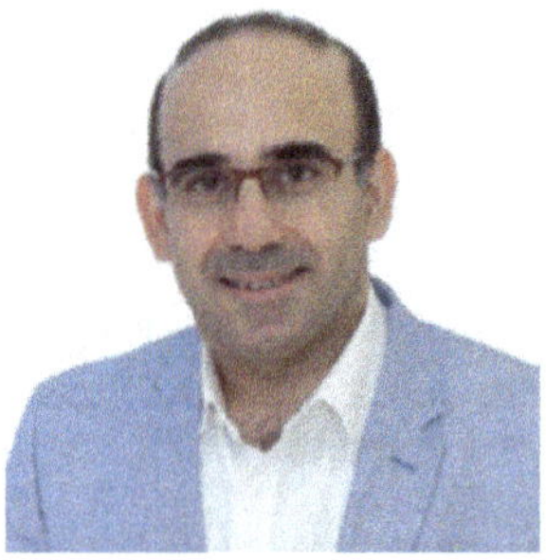

Mohamad Mohty is Professor of Hematology and Head of the Hematology and Cellular Therapy Department at Saint-Antoine Hospital and Sorbonne University (Paris, France).He has a special clinical focus on the development of reduced-toxicity conditioning regimens, immunotherapy, and different aspects of therapy of acute leukemia and multiple myeloma. He is Past-President of the European Society for Blood and Marrow Transplantation (EBMT), and the current Chairman of the Acute Leukemia Working Party of EBMT. He serves on the board of the EBMT and the "Intergroupe Francophone du Myelome" (IFM). He has published more than 550 peer-reviewed articles in the field of stem cell transplantation, leukemia, and myeloma in different hematology and immunology journals. He also serves as Editor-in-Chief of the journal Bone Marrow Transplantation.

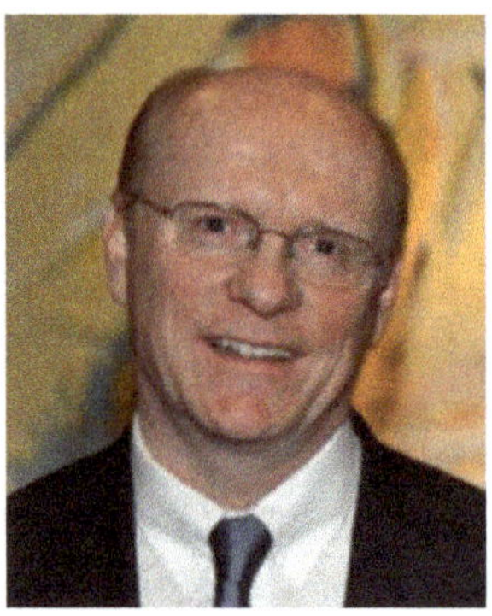

Nicolaus Kröger is Professor of Medicine and Medical Director of the Department of Stem Cell Transplantation at the University Medical Center Hamburg-Eppendorf, Germany. He is the President of the European Society for Blood and Marrow Transplantation (EBMT) and Chairman of the German Stem Cell Working Group (DAG-KBT) and Past Chair of the Chronic Malignancies Working Party and of the Scientific Council of EBMT.He is also member of the Scientific Program Committee and the Editorial Board of the European Hematology Association (EHA) and member of the Scientific Committee of the European School for Hematology (ESH).His research interests are on stem cell biology and stem cell transplantation, the detection and treatment of minimal residual disease by adoptive immunotherapy or novel drugs, the impact of NK-cell alloreactivity, optimizing the outcome with HLA-mismatched donor, improving conditioning regimen, and prevention and treatment of acute and chronic graft-versus-host disease.For his research he received several awards including the prestigious EBMT Van Bekkum Award in 2015.Prof. Kröger has published extensively in his area of expertise and has contributed to more than 550 publications in peer-reviewed journals such as The New England Journal of Medicine (NEJM), The Lancet, Journal of Clinical Oncology (JCO), Journal of the National Cancer Institute (JNCI), Proceedings of the National Academy of Sciences of the United States of America (PNAS), Blood, and Leukemia.

Abbreviations

AA	Aplastic anemia
Ab	Antibody
ADA	Adenosine deaminase
ADR	Adriamycin
ADV	Adenovirus
Ag	Antigen
aGVHD	Acute graft-versus-host disease
AID	Autoimmune disease
AIHA	Autoimmune hemolytic anemia
AKI	Acute kidney injury
AL	Amyloid light-chain
ALEM	Alemtuzumab
ALG	Antilymphocyte globulin
ALL	Acute lymphoblastic leukemia
Allo-BMT	Allogeneic BMT
Allo-HSCT	Allogeneic HSCT
AML	Acute myeloid leukemia
ANC	Absolute neutrophil count
APL	Acute promyelocytic leukemia
Ara-C	Cytosine arabinoside
ARDS	Acute or adult respiratory distress syndrome
ASBMT	American Society for Blood and Marrow Transplantation
ATG	Antithymocyte globulin
ATRA	All-trans-retinoic acid
AUC	Area under the curve
Auto-BMT	Autologous BMT
Auto-HSCT	Autologous HSCT
BAL	Bronchoalveolar lavage
BCNU	1,3-Bis(2-chloroethyl)-1-nitrosourea (carmustine)
BM	Bone marrow
BMDW	Bone Marrow Donors Worldwide
BMF	Bone marrow failure
BMI	Body mass index
BMT	Bone marrow transplantation
BO	Bronchiolitis obliterans
BOOP	Bronchiolitis obliterans organizing pneumonia
BOR	Bortezomib

BOS	Bronchiolitis obliterans syndrome
BSA	Body surface area
BU	Busulfan
BUN	Blood urea nitrogen
BW	Body weight
CAR	Chimeric antigen receptor
CB	Cord blood
CBT	Cord blood transplantation
CBU	Cord blood unit
CC	Complete chimerism
CCI	Charlson Comorbidity Index
CFU	Colony-forming unit
CGD	Chronic granulomatous disease
cGVHD	Chronic graft-versus-host disease
CHF	Congestive heart failure
CI	Comorbidity index
CIBMTR	Center for International Blood and Marrow Transplant Research
CKD	Chronic kidney disease
CLL	Chronic lymphoid/lymphocytic leukemia
CML	Chronic myeloid/myelogenous leukemia
CMML	Chronic myelomonocytic leukemia
CMV	Cytomegalovirus
CMV-IP	CMV-associated interstitial pneumonia
CNI	Calcineurin inhibitor
CNS	Central nervous system
COP	Cryptogenic organizing pneumonia
CR	Complete remission
CR1	First complete remission
CRS	Cytokine release syndrome
CSA	Cyclosporine A
CSF	Cerebrospinal fluid
CT	Computed tomography
CTN	Clinical Trials Network
CVC	Central venous catheter
CVD	Cardiovascular disease
CY	Cyclophosphamide
d	Days
DAH	Diffuse alveolar hemorrhage
DAMP	Damage-associated molecular pattern
DC	Dendritic cell
DEX	Dexamethasone
DFS	Disease-free survival
DIC	Disseminated intravascular coagulation
DLBCL	Diffuse large B-cell lymphoma
DLCL	Diffuse large cell lymphoma
DLCO	Diffusion capacity of the lung for carbon monoxide
DLI	Donor lymphocyte infusion

DLT	Dose-limiting toxicity
DM	Diabetes mellitus
DMSO	Dimethyl sulfoxide
DNA	Deoxyribonucleic acid
DSA	Donor-specific antibody
EBMT	European Society for Blood and Marrow Transplantation
EBNA	Epstein–Barr (virus) nuclear antigen
EBV	Epstein–Barr virus
ECG	Electrocardiogram
ECIL	European Conference on Infections in Leukemia
ECP	Extracorporeal photopheresis
EEG	Electroencephalogram
EFS	Event-free survival
ELISA	Enzyme-linked immunosorbent assay
ELN	European LeukemiaNet
EN	Enteral nutrition
EORTC	European Organisation for Research and Treatment of Cancer
EPO	Erythropoietin
ET	Essential thrombocythemia
EWOG	European Working Group
FA	Fanconi anemia
FACS	Fluorescence-activated cell sorter
FACT	Foundation for the Accreditation of Cellular Therapy
FDA	Food and Drug Administration
FEV1	Forced expiratory volume in 1 second
FFP	Fresh frozen plasma
FFS	Failure-free survival
FISH	Fluorescence in situ hybridization
FL	Follicular lymphoma
FLIPI	Follicular Lymphoma International Prognostic Index
FLU	Fludarabine
FVC	Forced vital capacity
G-CSF	Granulocyte colony-stimulating factor
GF	Graft failure
GFR	Glomerular filtration rate
GI	Gastrointestinal (tract)
GM	Galactomannan
GM-CSF	Granulocyte–macrophage colony stimulated factor
GNB	Gram-negative bacilli
GVH	Graft-versus-host
GVHD	Graft-versus-host disease
GVL	Graft-versus-leukemia
h	Hours
HAART	Highly active antiretroviral therapy
HADS	Hospital Anxiety and Depression Scale
hATG	Horse ATG
HAV	Hepatitis A virus
HBV	Hepatitis B virus

HC	Hemorrhagic cystitis
HCT-CI	HCT-Comorbidity Index
HCV	Hepatitis C virus
HDAC	High-dose Ara-C
HDT	High-dose therapy
HEPA	High-efficiency particulate air
HEV	Hepatitis E virus
HHV	Human herpesvirus
HIB	Haemophilus influenzae type B
HIV	Human immunodeficiency virus
HL	Hodgkin lymphoma
HLA	Human leukocyte antigen
HLH	Hemophagocytic lymphohistiocytosis
HPV	Human papillomavirus
HR	Hazard ratio
HRCT	High-resolution chest tomography
HRT	Hormone replacement therapy
HSC	Hematopoietic stem cell
HSCT	Hematopoietic stem cell transplantation
HSV	Herpes simplex virus
HTLV	Human T-cell lymphotropic virus
HU	Hydroxyurea
HUS	Hemolytic uremic syndrome
HVG	Host-versus-graft
IA	Invasive aspergillosis
IBW	Ideal body weight
ICU	Intensive care unit
IDM	Infectious disease markers
IFI	Invasive fungal infection
IFN	Interferon
Ig	Immunoglobulin
IgG	Immunoglobulin G
IL	Interleukin
IMID	Immunomodulatory drug
IND	Investigational new drug
INR	International normalized ratio
IP	Interstitial pneumonia
IPI	International Prognostic Index
IPS	Idiopathic pneumonia syndrome
IPSS	International Prognostic Scoring System
IRB	Institutional Review Board
IS	Immunosuppressive
IST	Immunosuppressive therapy
ITT	Intent-to-treat
IV	Intravenous
IVIg	Intravenous immunoglobulin
JACIE	Joint Accreditation Committee of ISCT-Europe and EBMT
JCV	JC virus

JMML	Juvenile myelomonocytic leukemia
KIR	Killer immunoglobulin-like receptor
KM	Kaplan–Meier
KPS	Karnofsky Performance Score
L-asp	L-asparaginase
LAF	Laminar air flow
LBL	Lymphoblastic lymphoma
LDH	Lactate dehydrogenase
LENA	Lenalidomide
LFS	Leukemia-free survival
LN	Lymph node
LPS	Lipopolysaccharide
LVEF	Left ventricular ejection fraction
M protein	Monoclonal protein
MA	Myeloablative
MAC	Myeloablative conditioning
MCL	Mantle cell lymphoma
MDS	Myelodysplastic syndrome
MEL	Melphalan
Mesna	Sodium 2-mercaptoethanesulfonate
methylPRD	Methylprednisolone
MF	Myelofibrosis
MFD	Matched family donor
MGUS	Monoclonal gammopathy of undetermined significance
MHC	Major histocompatibility complex
MIC	Minimum inhibitory concentration
min	Minutes
MIPI	Mantle Cell Prognostic Index
miRNA	Micro-RNA
MLC	Mixed leukocyte culture
MM	Multiple myeloma
MMF	Mycophenolate mofetil
MMRD	Mismatched related donor
MMSD	Mismatched sibling donor
MMUD	Mismatched unrelated donor
MoAb	Monoclonal antibody
MODS	Multiple-organ dysfunction syndrome
MOF	Multiorgan failure
MPN	Myeloproliferative neoplasm
MRC	Medical Research Council
MRD	Minimal residual disease
MRI	Magnetic resonance imaging
MRSA	Methicillin-resistant Staphylococcus aureus
MS	Multiple sclerosis
MSC	Mesenchymal stem cell
MSD	Matched sibling donor
MTX	Methotrexate
MUD	Matched unrelated donor

NAT	Nucleic acid amplification test
NC	Nucleated cell
NCI	National Cancer Institute
NGS	Next-generation sequencing
NHL	Non-Hodgkin lymphoma
NIH	National Institutes of Health
NIMA	Non-inherited maternal antigen
NK	Natural killer (cell)
NMA	Non-myeloablative
NMDP	National Marrow Donor Program
NRM	Non-relapse mortality
NSAID	Non-steroidal anti-inflammatory drug
OR	Odds ratio
OS	Overall survival
PAM	Pretransplant assessment of mortality
PB	Peripheral blood
PBSC	Peripheral blood stem cell
PBSCT	Peripheral blood HSCT
PCR	Polymerase chain reaction
PERDS	Peri-engraftment respiratory distress syndrome
PET	Positron emission tomography
PFS	Progression-free survival
PFT	Pulmonary function test
Ph	Philadelphia (chromosome)
PHQ-9	Patient Health Questionnaire-9
PICC	Peripherally inserted central venous catheter
PID	Primary immunodeficiency disease
PJP	Pneumocystis jirovecii pneumonia
PK	Pharmacokinetic
PMF	Primary myelofibrosis
PMN	Polymorphonuclear neutrophil
PN	Parenteral nutrition
PNH	Paroxysmal nocturnal hemoglobinuria
PO	Per os
POEMS	Polyneuropathy, organomegaly, endocrinopathy, M protein, skin changes
PR	Partial remission or partial response
PRCA	Pure red cell aplasia
PRD	Prednisone
PRES	Posterior reversible encephalopathy syndrome
PT-CY	Post-HSCT cyclophosphamide
PTLD	Post-transplant lymphoproliferative disorder
PUVA	Psoralen–ultraviolet A irradiation
PV	Polycythemia vera
QLQ	Quality of Life Questionnaire
QOL	Quality of life
qRT-PCR	Quantitative reverse transcription polymerase chain reaction
QW	Once weekly

RA	Refractory anemia
RAEB	Refractory anemia with excess blasts
RAEB-T	Refractory anemia with excess blasts in transformation
RARS	Refractory anemia with ringed sideroblasts
RBC	Red blood cell
RCMD	Refractory cytopenia with multilineage dysplasia
RFS	Relapse-free survival
Rh	Rhesus
RI	Relapse incidence
RIC	Reduced-intensity conditioning
R/R	Relapsing/resistant
RR	Relapse rate/Relative risk
RRT	Regimen-related toxicity
RSV	Respiratory syncytial virus
RT-PCR	Real-time polymerase chain reaction
RTx	Radiotherapy
RTX	Rituximab
SAA	Severe aplastic anemia
SARS	Severe acute respiratory syndrome
SC	Subcutaneous
SCD	Sickle cell disease
SCF	Stem-cell factor
SCID	Severe combined immunodeficiency syndrome
SD	Standard deviation
SE	Standard error
SIR	Sirolimus
SLE	Systemic lupus erythematosus
SNP	Single nucleotide polymorphism
SOP	Standard operating procedure
SOS	Sinusoidal obstruction syndrome
SOT	Solid organ transplantation
SPECT	Single-photon emission computed tomography
SR	Standard risk
SS	Sézary syndrome
SSc	Systemic sclerosis
SSOP	Sequence-specific oligonucleotide probe
t-AML	Therapy-related acute myeloid leukemia
t-MDS	Therapy-related myelodysplastic syndrome
TA-GVHD	Transfusion-associated GVHD
TAC	Tacrolimus
TAI	Thoracoabdominal irradiation
TAM	Transplant-associated microangiopathy
TBI	Total body irradiation
TCD	T-cell depletion
TED	Thromboembolic disease
TGF-β	Transforming growth factor beta
THAL	Thalidomide
TKI	Tyrosine kinase inhibitor

TLC	Total lung capacity
TLI	Total lymphoid irradiation
TLR	Toll-like receptor
TLS	Tumor lysis syndrome
TM	Thalassemia major
TMA	Thrombotic microangiopathy
TMP–SMX	Trimethoprim–sulfamethoxazole
TNC	Total nucleated cell
TNF	Tumor necrosis factor
TNF-α	Tumor necrosis factor α
TPN	Total parenteral nutrition
TRALI	Transfusion-related acute lung injury
TREC	T-cell receptor excision circles
Treg	Regulatory T (cell)
TREO	Treosulfan
TRM	Transplant-related mortality
TRT	Transplant-related toxicity
TT	N-Triethylenethiophosphoramide, thioTEPA
TTP	Thrombotic thrombocytopenic purpura
Tx	Therapy/Treatment
UBC	Umbilical cord
UCB	Umbilical cord blood
UCBT	Umbilical cord blood transplant
URD	Unrelated donor
UV	Ultraviolet
VCR	Vincristine
VEGF	Vascular endothelial growth factor
VGPR	Very good partial remission
VIN	Vinblastine
VIND	Vindesine
VINO	Vinorelbine
VOD	Veno-occlusive disease
VP	Etoposide
VRE	Vancomycin-resistant *Enterococcus*
vWF	von Willebrand factor
VZIg	Varicella zoster immune globulin
VZV	Varicella zoster virus
WBC	White blood cell
WBMT	Worldwide Network for Blood & Marrow Transplantation
WMDA	World Marrow Donor Association
Wt	Wild-type
X-ALD	X-linked adrenoleukodystrophy
ZAP-70	Zeta-associated protein

Part I

Introduction

Topic leaders: Mohamad Mohty and Jane Apperley

1 HSCT: Historical Perspective

Rainer Storb

1.1 Introduction

HSCT has evolved from a field that was declared dead in the 1960s to the amazing clinical results obtained today in the treatment of otherwise fatal blood disorders. This chapter will reflect upon how HSCT has progressed from the laboratory to clinical reality.

1.2 Early Enthusiasm and Disappointment

Research efforts on how to repair radiation effects resulted from observations on radiation damage among survivors of the atomic bomb explosions in Japan (reviewed in van Bekkum and de Vries 1967). In 1949, Jacobson and colleagues discovered protection of mice from TBI by shielding their spleens with lead. Two years later, Lorenz and colleagues reported radiation protection of mice and guinea pigs by infusing marrow cells. Initially many investigators, including Jacobson, thought that the radiation protection was from some humoral factor(s) in spleen or marrow. However, by the mid-1950s, this "humoral hypothesis" was firmly rejected, and several laboratories convincingly demonstrated that the radiation protection was due to seeding of the marrow by donor cells.

This discovery was greeted with enthusiasm because of the implications for cell biology and for therapy of patients with life-threatening blood disorders. The principle of HSCT was simple: high-dose radiation/chemotherapy would both destroy the diseased marrow and suppress the patient's immune cells for a donor graft to be accepted. Within 1 year of the pivotal rodent studies, Thomas and colleagues showed that marrow could safely be infused into leukemia patients and engraft, even though, in the end, the leukemia relapsed. In 1958, Mathé's group attempted the rescue, by marrow transplantation, of six nuclear reactor workers accidentally exposed to TBI. Four of the six survived, although donor cells persisted only transiently. In 1965, Mathé and colleagues treated a leukemia patient with TBI and then marrows from six relatives, absent any knowledge of histocompatibility (Mathe et al. 1965). A brother's marrow engrafted. The patient went into remission but eventually succumbed to a complication, GVHD. Following up on early observations by Barnes and Loutit in mice, Mathé coined the term "graft-vs.-leukemia effect." In 1970, Bortin summarized results of 200 human marrow grafts reported between 1957 and 1967 (Bortin 1970). All 200 patients died of either graft failure, GVHD, infections, or recurrence of leukemia.

R. Storb (✉)
Clinical Research Division,
Fred Hutchinson Cancer Research Center and
University of Washington, School of Medicine,
Seattle, WA, USA
e-mail: rstorb@fredhutch.org

E. Carreras et al. (eds.), *The EBMT Handbook*, https://doi.org/10.1007/978-3-030-02278-5_1

These transplants were performed before a clear understanding of conditioning regimens, histocompatibility matching, and control of GVHD. They were based directly on work in inbred mice, for which histocompatibility matching is not absolutely required. In 1967, van Bekkum and de Vries stated, "These failures have occurred mainly because the clinical applications were undertaken too soon, most of them before even the minimum basic knowledge required to bridge the gap between mouse and patient had been obtained." Clinical HSCT was declared a total failure and prominent immunologists pronounced that the barrier between individuals could never be crossed.

1.3 Back to the Laboratory: Focus on Animal Studies

Most investigators left the field, pronouncing it a dead end. However, a few laboratories continued animal studies aimed at understanding and eventually overcoming the obstacles encountered in human allogeneic HSCT. Van Bekkum's group in Holland used primates, George Santos at Johns Hopkins chose rats, and the Seattle group chose outbred dogs as experimental models. One reason behind using dogs was that, besides humans, only dogs combine unusual genetic diversity with a widespread, well-mixed gene pool. Also, dogs share spontaneous diseases with humans, such as non-Hodgkin lymphoma and X-linked SCID. In addition to determining the best ways to administer TBI, new drugs with myeloablative or immunosuppressive qualities were introduced, including cyclophosphamide, ATG, and BU (Santos 1995). These agents improved engraftment and provided for tumor cell killing similar to TBI. Based on the mouse histocompatibility system defined 10 years earlier, in vitro histocompatibility typing for dogs was developed. Studies from 1968 showed that dogs given grafts from dog leukocyte antigen (DLA)-matched littermates or unrelated donors survived significantly longer than their DLA-mismatched counterparts, even though typing techniques were very primitive and the complexity of the genetic region coding for major antigens was far from understood (Epstein et al. 1968). Serious GVHD was first described in H-2 mismatched mice and in randomly selected monkeys. However, the canine studies first drew attention to fatal GVHD across minor histocompatibility barriers.

These pivotal observations drove the search for Post transplant drug regimens to control GVHD. The most promising drug was the folic acid antagonist, MTX (Storb et al. 1970). Further work in canines showed that transfusion-induced sensitization to minor antigens caused rejection of DLA-identical grafts (reviewed in Georges and Storb 2016). Subsequent canine studies eventually led to ways of understanding, preventing, and overcoming transfusion-induced sensitization. Next, mechanisms of graft-host tolerance were investigated. It turned out that IS could often be discontinued after 3–6 months, and donor-derived T lymphocytes were identified that downregulated immune reactions of other donor T cells against GVHD targets. Immune reconstitution was found to be complete in long-term canine chimeras, enabling them to live in an unprotected environment. Techniques for isolating transplantable stem cells from peripheral blood were refined in dogs and primates. Importantly, studies in pet dogs with non-Hodgkin lymphoma showed cures, in part due to graft-vs.-tumor effects.

1.4 Resuming Clinical Transplantation: 1968–1980s

The second half of the 1960s saw the refinement of high-intensity conditioning regimens, including fractionated TBI and maximally tolerated doses of CY or BU (Santos 1995). Histocompatibility matching was confirmed to be of utmost importance for reducing both graft rejection and GVHD (Thomas et al. 1975). However, even when donor and recipient were well matched, GVHD was a problem unless postgrafting MTX was given, which slowed donor lymphocyte replication. Rapid progress in understanding the molecular nature of the major human histocompatibility complex—HLA—improved matching of donor recipient pairs.

By 1968, the stage was set to resume clinical trials. The first successful transplants were for patients with primary immune deficiency disorders. A 5-month-old boy with "thymic alymphoplasia and agammaglobulinemia" was not perfectly matched with his sister (Gatti et al. 1968). Marrow and peripheral blood cells were infused intraperitoneally without conditioning. After a booster infusion several months later, the patient fully recovered with donor hematopoiesis and is well. A patient with Wiskott-Aldrich syndrome received a first unsuccessful marrow infusion from an HLA-identical sister without conditioning (Bach et al. 1968). A second transplant following CY conditioning resulted in full T- and B-cell recovery, but thrombocytopenia persisted.

During the first 7 or 8 years, most clinical studies were for patients with advanced hematological malignancies and SAA, who were in poor condition and presented tremendous challenges in supportive care (Thomas et al. 1975). They required transfusions and prophylaxis or treatment of bacterial, fungal, and viral infections. Therefore, in addition to discoveries made in marrow transplantation, these early trials stimulated advances in infectious diseases and transfusions (reviewed in Forman et al. 2016). The longest survivors from that era are patients with aplastic anemia who are approaching their 47th anniversary from HSCT with fully recovered donor-derived hematopoiesis and leading normal lives. Chronic GVHD emerged as a new problem among long-term survivors.

The initial studies saw GVHD among approximately half of the patients, despite HLA matching and despite receiving methotrexate. This stimulated further research in the canine system. Major improvements in GVHD control and patient survival were made when combining MTX with CNI inhibitors such as CSA or TAC (Storb et al. 1986). Combinations of drugs have remained a mainstay in GVHD prevention. GVHD treatment with PRD was introduced.

Early results with marrow grafts from HLA-identical siblings after CY for SAA showed 45% long-term survival (reviewed in Georges and Storb 2016). The major cause of failure was graft rejection as expected from canine studies on transfusion-induced sensitization to minor antigens. Canine studies identified dendritic cells in transfusions to be the key element in sensitization. Depleting transfusions of white cells, therefore, reduced the rejection risk. Further canine studies generated a clinical conditioning regimen that alternated CY and ATG, which greatly reduced the rates of both graft rejection and chronic GVHD (Storb et al. 1994). Finally, irradiation of blood products with 2000 cGy in vitro almost completely averted sensitization to minor antigens. Consequently, graft rejection in transplantation for AA has become the exception, and current survivals with HLA-identical sibling and HLA-matched unrelated grafts range from 90% to 100%. First successful grafts for thalassemia (Thomas et al. 1982) and sickle cell disease were reported.

For patients with leukemia and other malignant blood diseases, disease relapse after HSCT has remained a major problem. Attempts to reduce relapse by increasing the intensity of systemic conditioning regimens have met with success, but this benefit was offset by higher non-relapse mortality. Reports by Weiden and the Seattle group in 1979/1981 firmly established the existence of graft-vs.-leukemia (GvL) effects in humans (Weiden et al. 1979). DLI to combat relapse were introduced by Kolb and colleagues in 1990 (Kolb et al. 1990) (see Chap. 59).

Some investigators have removed T cells from the marrow as a means of preventing GVHD (reviewed in Soiffer 2016). Early studies showed high incidences of graft rejection, relapse of underlying malignancies, and infections. More recent studies showed that relapse seemed a lesser problem in patients with acute leukemia. Others have used T-cell depletion with close disease monitoring and treating recurrence with DLI in hopes of initiating GvL responses without causing GVHD. Most recently, younger patients have been given high-intensity conditioning for grafts which were depleted of naïve T cells with a resulting decrease in GVHD (Bleakley et al. 2015).

The late 1980s saw the introduction of G-CSF-mobilized PBSC (reviewed in Schmitz and

Dreger 2016). These were equivalent to marrow as far as engraftment and survival were concerned; however, they seemed to increase the risk of chronic GVHD. For patients with nonmalignant diseases, marrow has therefore remained the preferred source of stem cells in order to keep the rate of chronic GVHD low.

Only approximately 35% of patients have HLA-identical siblings. Therefore, alternative donors have been explored, predominantly HLA-matched unrelated volunteers. The first successful unrelated transplant for leukemia was reported in 1980. In order to expand the donor pool, national registries were established, with currently more than 30 million HLA-typed unrelated volunteers (reviewed in Confer et al. 2016). The likelihood of finding suitable unrelated donors is approximately 80% for Caucasians, although this percentage declines dramatically for patients from minority groups. A second, important alternative stem cell source has been unrelated cord blood (Gluckman et al. 1989), not requiring complete HLA matching and resulting in encouraging outcomes among patients with malignant blood diseases. First attempts with yet another donor source have included TCD megadose CD34+ cell grafts from related HLA-haploidentical donors to treat acute leukemia (Aversa et al. 1998).

1.5 Moving Ahead: The 1990s and Beyond

Conventional HSCT following high-intensity conditioning is risky and requires specialized intensive care wards. The associated toxicities restrict the therapy to younger, medically fit patients. To allow the inclusion of older (highest prevalence of hematological malignancies), medically infirm or very young immunodeficiency patients, less intensive conditioning programs have been developed. In patients with malignancies, these rely less on high-dose chemoradiation therapy and more on graft-vs.-tumor effects. One outpatient transplant strategy combines FLU and 2–3 Gy TBI conditioning with Post transplant IS using an inhibitor of purine synthesis MMF and CSA or TAC. Figure 1.1 illustrates the spectrum of current conditioning regimens (reviewed in Storb and Sandmaier 2016).

A transplant regimen combining fludarabine and 2 Gy TBI conditioning with additional cyclophosphamide before and after HSCT has encouraged widespread use of unmodified HLA-haploidentical grafts (Luznik et al. 2008). It is well tolerated with low incidences of graft rejection and of acute and chronic GVHD, but relapse remains a problem. Strategies addressing relapse have included infusion of donor lymphocytes or NK cells. Retrospective multicenter analyses show comparable outcomes after HLA-matched vs. HLA-haploidentical HSCT.

While reduced-intensity regimens have been well tolerated, relapse and GVHD need improving. Adding targeted radioimmunotherapy against host hematopoietic cells, using anti-CD45 antibody coupled to beta and alpha emitting radionuclides to standard conditioning, has the potential to decrease the pre-transplant tumor burden, thereby lessening the relapse risk (Chen et al. 2012; Pagel et al. 2009). As for GVHD, a recent phase III randomized trial convincingly demonstrated that a triple combination of MMF/cyclosporine/sirolimus significantly reduced both acute GVHD and non-relapse mortality and improved survival (Sandmaier et al. 2016).

Survival of patients with primary immune deficiency diseases given NMA conditioning before HLA-matched and HLA-mismatched grafts between 1998 and 2006 has stabilized at 82% (Moratto et al. 2011).

In the future, better understanding of hematopoietic cell-specific polymorphic minor histocompatibility antigens might result in ways of directing donor immune cells toward hematopoietic targets, thereby controlling relapse without inducing GVHD. Another major research target is containment of chronic GVHD.

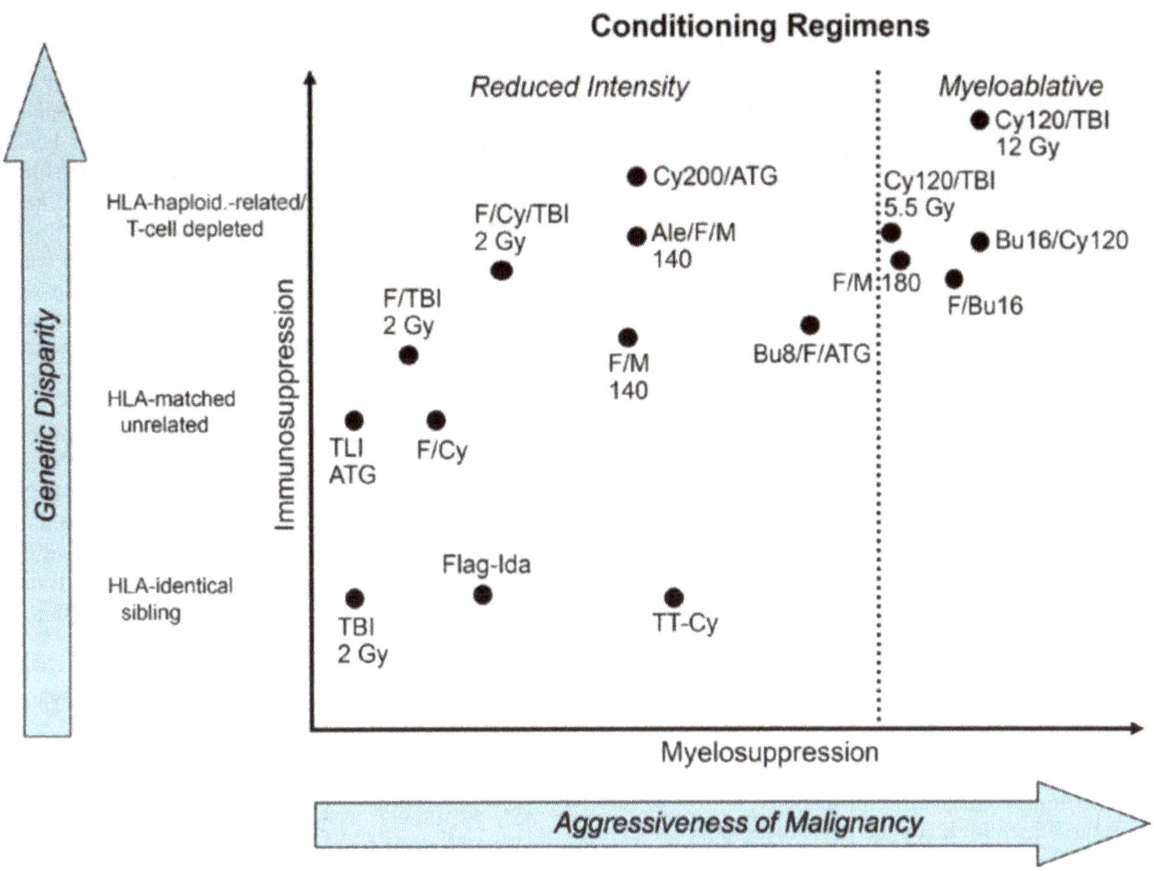

Fig. 1.1 Spectrum of current conditioning regimens. Reproduced with permission from Sandmaier, B.M. and Storb, R. Reduced-intensity allogeneic transplantation regimens (Ch. 21). In Thomas' Hematopoietic Cell Transplantation, fifth edition (ed. by Forman SJ, Negrin RS, Antin JH, & Appelbaum FR) 2016, pp. 232–243. John Wiley & Sons, Ltd., Chichester, UK

Key Points

- Radiation protection of rodents by shielding the spleen or marrow infusion
- First human transplants all failed
- Allogeneic HSCT called a total failure
- HSCT studies in large animals: Histocompatibility matching; MTX for GVHD prevention; CY, ATG, and BU; rejection from transfusion-induced sensitization; PBSC; graft-versus-lymphoma effect
- Fractionated TBI
- HSCT for patients with immunodeficiency diseases, aplastic anemia, leukemia, hemoglobinopathies
- Advances in infection prophylaxis and treatment
- Graft-versus-leukemia effects
- Donor lymphocyte infusions
- ATG conditioning
- Unrelated donors
- Cord blood transplants
- Mega CD34+ HLA-haploidentical grafts
- MTX/CNI GVHD prophylaxis
- Reduced and minimal intensity conditioning
- Outpatient transplantation
- PT-CY GVHD prophylaxis
- Targeted radioimmunotherapy

References

Aversa F, Tabilio A, Velardi A, et al. Treatment of high-risk acute leukemia with T-cell-depleted stem cells from related donors with one fully mismatched HLA haplotype. N Engl J Med. 1998;339:1186–93.

Bach FH, Albertini RJ, Joo P, et al. Bone-marrow transplantation in a patient with the Wiskott-Aldrich syndrome. Lancet. 1968;2:1364–6.

van Bekkum DW, de Vries MJ. Radiation chimaeras. London: Logos Press; 1967.

Bleakley M, Heimfeld S, Loeb KR, et al. Outcomes of acute leukemia patients transplanted with naive T cell-depleted stem cell grafts. J Clin Invest. 2015;125:2677–89.

Bortin MM. A compendium of reported human bone marrow transplants. Transplantation. 1970;9:571–87.

Chen Y, Kornblit B, Hamlin DK, et al. Durable donor engraftment after radioimmunotherapy using alpha-emitter astatine-211-labeled anti-CD45 antibody for conditioning in allogeneic hematopoietic cell transplantation. Blood. 2012;119:1130–8.

Confer DL, Miller JP, Chell JW. Bone marrow and peripheral blood cell donors and donor registries. In: Forman SJ, Negrin RS, Antin JH, Appelbaum FR, editors. Thomas' hematopoietic cell transplantation. 5th ed. Chichester: Wiley; 2016. p. 423–30.

Epstein RB, Storb R, Ragde H, Thomas ED. Cytotoxic typing antisera for marrow grafting in littermate dogs. Transplantation. 1968;6:45–58.

Forman SJ, Negrin RS, Antin JH. F.R.A. complications of hematopoietic cell transplantation. (Ch. Part 7). In: Thomas' hematopoietic cell transplantation. 5th ed. Chichester: Wiley; 2016. p. 944–1306.

Gatti RA, Meuwissen HJ, Allen HD, et al. Immunological reconstitution of sex-linked lymphopenic immunological deficiency. Lancet. 1968;2:1366–9.

Georges GE, Storb R. Hematopoietic cell transplantation for aplastic anemia. In: Forman SJ, Negrin RS, Antin JH, Appelbaum FR, editors. Thomas' hematopoietic cell transplantation. 5th ed. Chichester: Wiley; 2016. p. 517–36.

Gluckman E, Broxmeyer HE, Auerbach AD, et al. Hematopoietic reconstitution in a patient with Fanconi's anemia by means of umbilical-cord blood from an HLA-identical sibling. N Engl J Med. 1989;321:1174–8.

Kolb HJ, Mittermüller J, Clemm C, et al. Donor leukocyte transfusions for treatment of recurrent chronic myelogenous leukemia in marrow transplant patients. Blood. 1990;76:2462–5.

Luznik L, O'Donnell PV, Symons HJ, et al. HLA-haploidentical bone marrow transplantation for hematologic malignancies using nonmyeloablative conditioning and high-dose, post-transplantation cyclophosphamide. Biol Blood Marrow Transplant. 2008;14:641–50.

Mathe G, Amiel JL, Schwarzenberg L, Cattan A, Schneider M. Adoptive immunotherapy of acute leukemia: experimental and clinical results. Cancer Res. 1965;25:1525–31.

Moratto D, Giliani S, Bonfim C, et al. Long-term outcome and lineage-specific chimerism in 194 patients with Wiskott-Aldrich syndrome treated by hematopoietic cell transplantation in the period 1980-2009: an international collaborative study. Blood. 2011;118:1675–84.

Pagel JM, Gooley TA, Rajendran J, et al. Allogeneic hematopoietic cell transplantation after conditioning with 131 I-anti-CD45 antibody plus fludarabine and low-dose total body irradiation for elderly patients with advanced acute myeloid leukemia or high-risk myelodysplastic syndrome. Blood. 2009;114:5444–53.

Sandmaier BM, Maloney DG, Storer BE, et al. Sirolimus combined with mycophenolate mofetil (MMF) and cyclosporine (CSP) significantly improves prevention of acute graft-versus-host-disease (GVHD) after unrelated hematopoietic cell transplantation (HCT): results from a phase III randomized multi-center trial. Blood. 2016;128:#506. (abstract); http://www.bloodjournal.org/content/128/522/506

Santos GW. Preparative regimens: chemotherapy versus chemoradiotherapy. A historical perspective. (review). Ann N Y Acad Sci. 1995;770:1–7.

Schmitz N, Dreger P. Peripheral blood hematopoietic cells for allogeneic transplantation. (Ch. 41). In: Forman SJ, Negrin RS, Antin JH, Appelbaum FR, editors. Thomas' hematopoietic cell transplantation. 5th ed. Chichester: Wiley; 2016. p. 460–8.

Soiffer RJ. T-cell depletion to prevent graft-versus-host disease. (Ch. 82). In: Forman SJ, Negrin RS, Antin JH, Appelbaum FR, editors. Thomas' hematopoietic cell transplantation. 5th ed. Chichester: Wiley; 2016. p. 965–72.

Storb R, Deeg HJ, Whitehead J, et al. Methotrexate and cyclosporine compared with cyclosporine alone for prophylaxis of acute graft versus host disease after marrow transplantation for leukemia. N Engl J Med. 1986;314:729–35.

Storb R, Epstein RB, Graham TC, Thomas ED. Methotrexate regimens for control of graft-versus-host disease in dogs with allogeneic marrow grafts. Transplantation. 1970;9:240–6.

Storb R, Etzioni R, Anasetti C, et al. Cyclophosphamide combined with antithymocyte globulin in preparation for allogeneic marrow transplants in patients with aplastic anemia. Blood. 1994;84:941–9.

Storb R, Sandmaier BM. Nonmyeloablative allogeneic hematopoietic cell transplantation. Haematologica. 2016;101:521–30.

Thomas ED, Buckner CD, Sanders JE, et al. Marrow transplantation for thalassaemia. Lancet. 1982;2:227–9.

Thomas ED, Storb R, Clift RA, et al. Bone-marrow transplantation. N Engl J Med. 1975;292:832–43. 895–902.

Weiden PL, Flournoy N, Thomas ED, et al. Antileukemic effect of graft-versus-host disease in human recipients of allogeneic-marrow grafts. N Engl J Med. 1979;300:1068–73.

2 The EBMT: History, Present, and Future

Alois Gratwohl, Mohamad Mohty, and Jane Apperley

2.1 Introduction

"Only he/she who knows the past has a future" is a proverb attributed to Wilhelm von Humboldt (1767–1835), a great historian, scientist, and philosopher (Spier 2015). It appears as an ideal introduction to a chapter on the history of EBMT. The context by which HSCT evolved in the middle of last century fits with modern views on history. The novel "big history" concept attempts to integrate major events in the past, beginning with the "big bang" up to today's industrial revolution number IV (Spier 2015). According to this model, nothing "just happens." Progress occurs when the conditions fit, at the right time and at the right place. Such circumstances are called "Goldilocks conditions," according to the novel by Robert Southey (https://en.wikipedia.org/wiki/Goldilocks_and_the_Three_Bears. accessed November 6, 2018). They hold true for the formation of galaxies, suns, and planets, for the appearance of life on earth, or for the evolution of mankind. They apply specifically to the latter: as the one and only species, *Homo sapiens* managed to create "Goldilocks conditions" by him or herself. They allowed man to fit religion, art, or beliefs in such ways to master society. In our perspective, big history thinking helps to understand the development of HSCT and EBMT and to view it in a broader framework. It provides as well a caveat for the future.

A. Gratwohl (✉)
Hematology, Medical Faculty, University of Basel, Basel, Switzerland
e-mail: alois.gratwohl@unibas.ch

M. Mohty
Hematology, Hôpital St. Antoine, Sorbonne University, Paris, France

J. Apperley
Centre for Haematology, Hammersmith Hospital, Imperial College London, London, UK

2.2 The Past: Development of HSCT and EBMT

The use of bone marrow (BM) for healing purposes dates back long in history, and BM from hunted animals might have contributed as rich nourishment to the evolution of *Homo sapiens* (McCann 2016). Its recognition as primary hematopoietic organ in adult life with a hematopoietic stem cell as source of the circulating blood cells began in the middle of the nineteenth century (Schinck 1920). It did result in some early recommendations on the potential therapeutic use of bone marrow (JAMA 1997; Osgood et al. 1939), but with no broader application. All changed after the explosions of atomic bombs in Hiroshima and Nagasaki in World War II, when survivors of the immediate exposure died from BM failure (Van Bekkum and De Vries 1967). Research was directed to find ways to treat this lethal complication. It led to the discovery that bone marrow-derived stem cells

E. Carreras et al. (eds.), *The EBMT Handbook*, https://doi.org/10.1007/978-3-030-02278-5_2

from a healthy donor could replace hematopoiesis after total body irradiation (TBI); it provided at the same time, a tool, TBI, to eradicate aberrant hematopoiesis (Van Bekkum and De Vries 1967; Jacobson et al. 1949; Lorenz et al. 1951; Ford et al. 1956). The concept of HSCT was born, and "the conditions were right." It is to no surprise that the first clinical BMT centers in Europe started in hospitals with close links to radiobiology research institutes in the UK, the Netherlands, France, and Germany. Funding of radiobiology fostered basic research and stimulated clinical application. In the first series of patients reported in the NEJM in 1957 by the late Nobel Prize winner ED Thomas, all six patients died but two of them with clear signs of donor chimerism (Thomas et al. 1957). And, BMT "saved" accidentally irradiated workers of a radiation facility in Vinca, a town in former Jugoslawia (Mathé et al. 1959). Hence, the clinical results confirmed the "proof of principle" obtained in mice: TBI could eradicate normal and malignant bone marrow cells, and the infusion of healthy donor bone marrow cells could restore the recipient's depleted hematopoiesis with functioning donor cells. In reality, of more than 200 patients reported by M. Bortin for the IBMTR, all patients with leukemia had died, many of them free of their disease. Three patients survived, all with congenital immune deficiency and transplanted from HLA-identical sibling donors (Bortin 1970). Despite the dismal results, Goldilocks conditions prevailed. Armed forces were convinced of the need for a rescue tool in the event of a nuclear war, physicians viewed BMT as an instrument to treat hitherto incurable blood disorders, and patients envisioned a cure of their lethal disease.

In order to improve outcome, the "believers" joined forces. They met each other, openly reviewed their cases and charts one by one, exchanged views on hurdles and opportunities, spent time together on the slopes in the Alps, and became friendly rivals: EBMT was born. Goldilocks conditions still prevailed. Leukemia could be eradicated. BMT with haploidentical donor bone marrow for SAA after conditioning with ATG yielded spectacular results (Speck et al. 1977). Today, we know that ATG, rather than the cells, was responsible for the outcome. The introduction of intensive induction regimens for AML enabled stable phases of complete first remission (CR1) (Crowther et al. 1970). The discovery of CSA, as the first of its kind of novel IS agents, opened new dimensions in BMT and other organ transplantation (Kay et al. 1980). It became acceptable to transplant patients in early phase of their disease, e.g., CR1 or first chronic phase (CP1) (Thomas et al. 1975). The boom of BMT began (Thomas 2007; Gratwohl et al. 2015a). The first patient in the EBMT database dates back to 1965. In 1973, at the first informal gathering in St. Moritz, the database comprised 13 patients; 4 transplanted in that year. In 1980, a total of 285 HSCT were performed, increasing to 4025 10 years later.

HSCT rapidly diversified in terms of donor type, by including autologous and allogeneic stem cells from related and unrelated donors, and of stem cell source, from bone marrow and peripheral blood to cord blood. Indications expanded from the early congenital immunodeficiency, leukemia, and aplastic anemia to a full variety of severe congenital disorders of the hematopoietic system, to other hematological malignancies such as myeloma and lymphoma, and to non-hematological malignancies, e.g., germ cell tumors. The HSCT technology improved to encompass a variety of in vivo and ex vivo GvHD prevention methods and conditioning regimens of varying intensities with or without TBI. HSCT became open to centers with no links to radiobiology institutes and was no longer bound to "sterile units" and to selected countries (Gratwohl et al. 2015a; Copelan, 2006).

The previously informal gatherings and the database no longer sufficed to share the urgently needed information exchange. EBMT became a formal structure, with elections for presidents and working party chairs. It was listed in PubMed for the first time in 1985 (EBMT 1985). The meetings were no longer confined to ski resorts and became open to all involved in patient care and scientific analyses (Table 2.1). Obviously, organization of the annual meeting is today a major undertaking and only possible with the support of corporate sponsors. Still, the initial spirit remains.

Table 2.1 List of EBMT meetings and presidents

Year	Location annual meeting	Participating groups	EBMT president
1974			Informal gathering
1975	St. Moritz, Switzerland	1st P	
1976	St. Moritz, Switzerland	2nd P	B. Speck[a]
1977	Courchevel, France	3rd P	B. Speck[a]
1978	Courchevel, France	4th P	B. Speck[a]
1979	St. Moritz, Switzerland	5th P	E. Gluckman
1980	Sils-Maria, Switzerland	6th P	E. Gluckman
1981	Courchevel, France	7th P	E. Kubanek
1982	Courmayeur, Italy	8th P	E. Gordon-Smith
1983	Oberstdorf, Germany	9th P	E. Gordon-Smith
1984	Granada, Spain	10th P	J. Barrett
1985	Bad Hofgastein, Austria	11th P, 1st N	J. Barrett
1986	Courmayeur, Italy	12th P, 2nd N	A. Marmont[a]
1987	Interlaken, Switzerland	13th P, 3rd N	A. Marmont[a]
1988	Chamonix, France	14th P, 4th N	G. Gharton
1989	Bad Hofgastein, Austria	15th P, 5th N	G. Gharton
1990	The Hague, Netherlands	16th P, 6th N	J. Goldman[a]
1991	Cortina d'Ampezzo, Italy	17th P, 7th N	J. Goldman[a]
1992	Stockholm, Sweden	18th P, 8th N	J. Goldman[a]
1993	Garmisch-Partenkirchen, Germany	19th P, 9th N	J. Goldman[a]
1994	Harrogate, UK	20th P, 10th N	A. Gratwohl
1995	Davos, Switzerland	21st P, 11th N	A. Gratwohl
1996	Vienna, Austria	22nd P, 12th N	A. Gratwohl
1997	Aix-les-bains, France	23rd P, 13th N	A. Gratwohl
1998	Courmayeur, Italy	24th P, 14th N	A. Bacigalupo
1999	Hamburg, Germany	25th P, 15th N	A. Bacigalupo
2000	Innsbruck, Germany	26th P, 16th N	A. Bacigalupo
2001	Maastricht, Netherlands	27th P, 17th N	A. Bacigalupo
2002	Montreux, Switzerland	28th P, 18th N, 1st DM	J. Apperley
2003	Istanbul, Turkey	29th P, 19th N, 2nd DM	J. Apperley
2004	Barcelona, Spain	30th P, 20th N, 3d DM	J. Apperley
2005	Prague, Czech Republic	31st P, 21st N, 4th DM	J. Apperley
2006	Hamburg, Germany	32nd P, 22nd N, 5th DM	D. Niederwieser
2007	Lyon, France	33rd P, 23d N, 6th DM, 1st P&F	D. Niederwieser
2008	Florence, Italy	34th P, 24th N, 7th DM, 2nd P&F	D. Niederwieser
2009	Goteborg, Sweden	35th P, 25th N, 8th DM, 3rd P&F	D. Niederwieser
2010	Vienna, Austria	36th P, 26th N, 9th DM, 4th P&F	A. Madrigal
2011	Paris, France	37th P, 27th N, 10th DM, 5th P&F	A. Madrigal
2012	Geneva, Switzerland	38th P, 28th N, 11th DM, 6th P&F, 1st QM, 1st Ped	A. Madrigal
2013	London, UK	39th P, 29th N, 12th DM, 7th P&F, 2nd QM, 2nd Ped	A. Madrigal
2014	Milan, Italy	40th P, 30th N, 13th DM, 8th P&F, 3d QM, 3d Ped	A. Madrigal
2015	Istanbul, Turkey	41st P, 31st N, 14th DM, 9th P&F, 4th QM, 4th Ped	M. Mohty
2016	Valencia, Spain	42nd P, 32nd N, 15th DM, 10th P&F, 5th QM, 5thPed, 1stPha	M. Mohty
2017	Marseille, France	43rd P, 33rd N, 16th DM, 11th P&F, 6th QM, 6thPed, 2nd Pha	M. Mohty
2018	Lisbon, Portugal	44th P, 34th N, 17th DM, 12th P&F, 7th QM, 7thPed, 3d Pha	M. Mohty
2019	Frankfurt, Germany	45th P, 35th N, 18th DM, 13th P&F, 8th QM, 8th Ped, 4th Pha	N. Kröger

Participating groups: *P* physicians, *N* nurses, *DM* data manager, *P&F* patient and family day, *QM* quality manager, *Ped* pediatricians, *Pha* pharmacists

[a]deceased

2.3 The Present

Today, EBMT (www.ebmt.org) is a nonprofit organization with a clear mission statement: "To save the lives of patients with blood cancers and other life-threatening diseases by advancing the fields of blood and marrow transplantation and cell therapy worldwide through science, education and advocacy" (https://portal.ebmt.org/Contents/About-EBMT/Mission-Vision/Pages/Mission%2D%2DVision.aspx. Accessed 26 Feb 2018). It is formally a professional society with legal residence in the Netherlands and an administrative office in Barcelona, Spain. EBMT is chaired by the president, who is elected by the members for 2 years and for a maximum of two terms. He/she is supported by the board of association as the executive committee and the board of counselors as external advisors. The scientific council which represents the 11 working parties, the seven committees, and the groups guides the scientific work with the help of the seven offices (Table 2.2). The main task of the organizational body of EBMT is to collect, analyze, and disseminate scientific data; to conduct clinical trials; to improve quality through the close cooperation with JACIE and FACT; to plan the annual meeting, the educational events, and training courses, including the EBMT Handbook; and to provide assistance to patients, donors, physicians, and competent authorities.

Members of the EBMT are mainly centers active in transplantation of hematopoietic stem cells (HSC) or any other organization involved in the care of donors and recipients of HSC. Currently (January 1, 2018), EBMT holds 509 full center members and 55 associate center members, 122 individual, and 35 honorary members, from 65 different countries. EBMT is supported in its activities through the membership fees and the revenue of the annual meetings and by its corporate sponsors (https://www2.ebmt.org/Contents/Members-Sponsors/Sponsors/Listofcorporatesponsors/Pages/List-of-corporate-sponsors.aspx. Accessed 26 Feb 2018). EBMT is part of the global network of organizations involved in HSCT, the Worldwide Network for Blood and Marrow Transplantation (WBMT), and in close link with national and other international professional organizations involved in HSCT, such as AFBMT, APBMT, CIBMTR, EMBMT, LABMT, or WMDA. The EBMT database now holds information on more than 500,000 transplants. Over 35,000 new patients were treated annually over the last 5 years and more than 40,000 HSCT performed (Fig. 2.1). An estimated number of more than 400,000 patients are currently alive after HSCT in Europe; they reflect the EBMT achievements and the challenges ahead.

Table 2.2 EBMT working parties, committees, groups and offices

Working parties	
ADWP	Autoimmune Diseases Working Party
ALWP	Acute Leukemia Working Party
CMWP	Chronic Malignancies Working Party
CTIWP	Cellular Therapy & Immunobiology Working Party
IDWP	Infectious Diseases Working Party
IEWP	Inborn Errors Working Party
LWP	Lymphoma Working Party
PDWP	Paediatric Diseases Working Party
SAAWP	Severe Aplastic Anaemia Working Party
STWP	Solid Tumors Working Party
TCWP	Transplant Complications Working Party
Committees	
	Nuclear Accident Committee
	Donor Outcomes Committee
	Statistical Committee
	Registry Committee
	JACIE Committee
	Global Committee
	Legal & Regulatory Affairs Committee
Groups	
	EBMT nurses' group with its own president
	Data managers' group
	Statisticians' group
EBMT units	
	EBMT Executive Office, Barcelona, Spain
	JACIE Accreditation Office, Barcelona, Spain
	EBMT Central Registry Office, London, UK
	EBMT Data Office, Leiden, The Netherlands
	EBMT Clinical Trials Office, Leiden, The Netherlands
	EBMT Data Office/CEREST-TC, Paris, France
	EBMT Activity Survey Office, Basel, Switzerland

Courtesy: EBMT office Barcelona, Marta Herrero Hoces

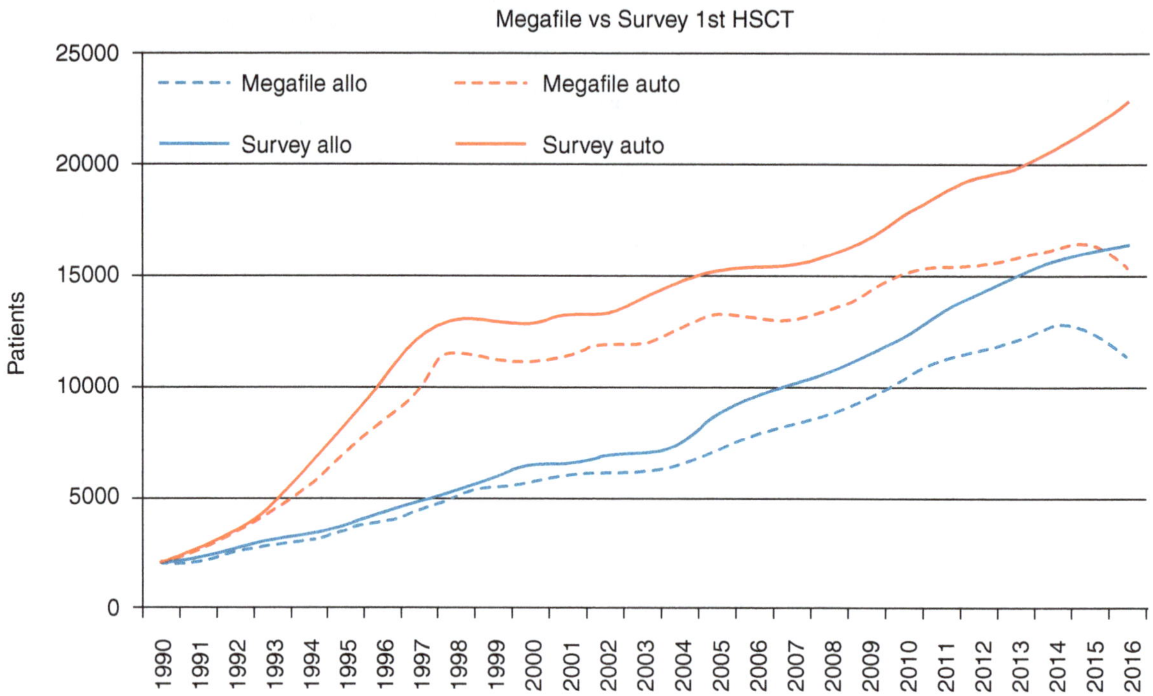

Fig. 2.1 Numbers of patients with a first HSCT by main donor type and year of transplant. The lines reflect the difference in patient numbers with and without information in the database (megafile). Courtesy: Carmen Ruiz de Elvira, EBMT megafile office, London; Helen Baldomero, EBMT activity survey office, Basel

2.4 The Future

Again, according to the Big History concept, predicting the future is a difficult task: "There are no data about the future; from an empirical scientific point of view, it is impossible to say what lies ahead of us." (Spier 2015). But we can project scenarios; we know the past, and we see the today. We live in the rapidly evolving world of the industrial revolution IV, dominated by globalization, digitization, and personalized medicine. Targeted therapies promise cures; gene-modified cells destroy hitherto untreatable cancers; immunomodulation with checkpoint inhibitors has become a reality (Hochhaus et al. 2017; Tran et al. 2017; Le et al. 2015). If HSCT is to remain a valuable treatment, mentalities and methods of the past no longer suffice. The idea of beliefs, hence physicians creating their own Goldilocks conditions, will lead to the end of HSCT. It has to be replaced by a stringent scientific approach. The sad story of HSCT for breast cancer, with more than 40,000 transplants but no clear answer, must not to be repeated (Gratwohl et al. 2010).

Hence, prediction number one: The idea of "a donor for everybody" will be abandoned. HSCT has to provide for the individual patient the best outcome regarding overall survival, quality of life and costs. The outcome after HSCT must be superior, in these three aspects, to any of the modern drugs or treatments, including "watch and wait" strategies or palliation. Assessment of risks needs to integrate risk factors relating to the patient, his or her disease, the donor, the stem cell source, the transplant technology, as well as micro- and macroeconomic risk factors (Gratwohl et al. 2015b; Gratwohl et al. 2017). For some patients, early transplant will be the optimal approach; for others, HSCT may need to be delayed. For others, HSCT will never be the preferred option. Obviously, the transplant physician is no longer in a position to adequately assess risk in comparison to the multiple alternative strategies, as it was possible in the old times of the simple EBMT risk score. Machine-learning algorithms will replace risk assessment; the competent physician will still be needed to discuss the results with his or her patients and their families and to conduct the transplant (Verghese et al. 2018).

Hence, prediction number two: The WHO guiding principles for cell, organ, and tissue transplants, "data collection and data analysis are integral parts of the therapy", need to become a mandatory reality for all transplant teams (WHO 2010). The gap between transplant numbers and reports (Fig. 2.1) has to be closed. Reporting has to become real-time and life-long. The EBMT and transplant centers have to adapt. Data and quality management will become a "condition sine qua non" for all, with close interactions between local, national, and international organizations. Machine learning will end the individualistic center unique transplant techniques. It will no longer be possible to apply hundreds of different GvHD prevention methods and a multitude of conditioning regimens, just by the argument "I have good experience with my method." Standardization will permit correct personalized medicine, as outlined above. Obviously, assessment of outcome can no longer be restricted to transplanted patients; it will need the correct comparison with non-transplant strategies on a routine basis.

Hence, prediction number three: HSCT centers and the EBMT will no longer be isolated in the treatment landscape. HSCT will need to be integrated into the treatment chain, from diagnosis to early treatment, transplant decisions, and secondary treatment, up to life-long follow-up. Not all of these steps have to occur at the transplant center, but they need to be coordinated by the expert team. Data have clearly shown that transplant experience, as measured in patient numbers and years, is associated with outcome (Gratwohl et al. 2015b). No center will have sufficient expertise for all diseases amenable to HSCT or for all transplant techniques, e.g., bone marrow harvest. HSCT centers will have to decide on their priorities, jointly with their referral and their after-care chain, within their city, their country, or with neighboring countries for coordination.

Hence, final prediction: EBMT can take the science-based lead for coordination and standardization, guide in reorganization of networks with non-transplant treatment chains, and prioritize comparative studies, independent of pressure groups. Then, history will tell, whether the proverb from a contemporary of von Humboldt, Georg Wilhelm Friedrich Hegel (1770–1831) "History teaches us that man learns nothing from history." (Spier 2015), can be overcome. The potential is here.

References

11th annual meeting of the EBMT (European Cooperative Group for Bone Marrow Transplantation). Bad Hofgastein (Salzburg). Austria, January 28–30, 1985. Exp Hematol. 1985;13(Suppl 17):1–154.

Bortin MM. A compendium of reported human bone marrow transplants. Transplantation. 1970;9:571–87.

Copelan EA. Hematopoietic stem cell transplantation. N Engl J Med. 2006;354:1813–26.

Crowther D, Bateman CJ, Vartan CP, et al. Combination chemotherapy using L-asparaginase, daunorubicin, and cytosine arabinoside in adults with acute myelogenous leukaemia. Br Med J. 1970;4(5734):513–7.

Ford CE, Hamerton JL, Barnes DW, Loutit JF. Cytological identification of radiation-chimaeras. Nature. 1956;177:452–4.

Gratwohl A, Pasquini MC, Aljurf M, Worldwide Network for Blood and Marrow Transplantation (WBMT), et al. One million haemopoietic stem-cell transplants: a retrospective observational study. Lancet Haematol. 2015a;2:e91–100.

Gratwohl A, Schwendener A, Baldomero H, et al. Changes in the use of hematopoietic stem cell transplantation: a model for diffusion of medical technology. Haematologica. 2010;95:637–43.

Gratwohl A, Sureda A, Baldomero H, Joint Accreditation Committee (JACIE) of the International Society for Cellular Therapy (ISCT), the European Society for Blood and Marrow Transplantation (EBMT), the European Leukemia Net (ELN), et al. Economics and outcome after hematopoietic stem cell transplantation: a retrospective cohort study. EBioMedicine. 2015b;2:2101–9.

Gratwohl A, Sureda A, Cornelissen J, et al. Alloreactivity: the Janus-face of hematopoietic stem cell transplantation. Leukemia. 2017;31:1752–9.

Hochhaus A, Larson RA, Guilhot F, et al. IRIS investigators. Long-term outcomes of Imatinib treatment for chronic myeloid leukemia. N Engl J Med. 2017;376:917–27.

Jacobson LO, Marks EK, Gaston EO, Robson M, Zirkle RE. The role of the spleen in radiation injury. Proc Soc Exp Biol Med. 1949;70:740–2.

Kay HE, Powles RL, Sloane JP, Farthing MG. Cyclosporin A in human bone marrow grafts. Haematol Blood Transfus. 1980;25:255–60.

Le DT, Uram JN, Wang H, et al. PD-1 blockade in tumors with mismatch-repair deficiency. N Engl J Med. 2015;372:2509–20.

Lorenz E, Uphoff D, Reid TR, Shelton E. Modification of irradiation injury in mice and Guinea pigs by bone marrow injections. J Natl Cancer Inst. 1951;12:197–201.

Mathé G, Jammet H, Pendic B, et al. Transfusions and grafts of homologous bone marrow in humans after accidental high dosage irradiation. Rev Fr Etud Clin Biol. 1959;4:226–38.

McCann SR. A history of haematology. From herodotus to HIV. Oxford medical histories. London: Oxford University Press; 2016.

Osgood EE, Riddle MC, Mathews TJ. Aplastic anemia treated with daily transfusions and intravenous marrow; a case report. Ann Intern Med. 1939;13:357–67.

Schinck P. Ernst Neumann als Begründer der Hämatologie. Dissertation Königsberg; 1920.

Speck B, Gluckman E, Haak HL, van Rood JJ. Treatment of aplastic anaemia by antilymphocyte globulin with and without allogeneic bone-marrow infusions. Lancet. 1977;2(8049):1145–8.

Spier F, editor. Big history and the future of humanity. Chichester: Wiley; 2015.

The bone-marrow. JAMA. 1908;LI(23):1997. https://doi.org/10.1001/jama.1908.02540230083025.

Thomas ED. A history of allogeneic hematopoietic cell transplantation. In: Appelbaum FR, Forman SJ, Negrin RS, Blume KG, editors. Thomas' hematopoietic cell transplantation. Chichester: Wiley; 2007. p. 3–7.

Thomas ED, Lochte HL Jr, Lu WC, Ferrebee JW. Intravenous infusion of bone marrow in patients receiving radiation and chemotherapy. N Engl J Med. 1957;257:491–6.

Thomas ED, Storb R, Clift RA, et al. Bone-marrow transplantation (second of two parts). N Engl J Med. 1975;292:895–902.

Tran E, Longo DL, Urba WJ. A milestone for CAR T cells. N Engl J Med. 2017;377:2593–6.

Van Bekkum DW, De Vries MJ. Radiation chimeras. New York: Academic Press; 1967.

Verghese A, Shah NH, Harrington RA. What this computer needs is a physician humanism and artificial intelligence. JAMA. 2018;319:19–20.

World Health Organization. WHO guiding principles on human cell, tissue and organ transplantation. Transplantation. 2010;90:229–33.

3 The Role of Unrelated Donor Registries in HSCT

Irina Evseeva, Lydia Foeken, and Alejandro Madrigal

3.1 Introduction

3.1.1 From Anthony Nolan to 32 Million Volunteer Donors Worldwide

Bone marrow donor registries (hereinafter referred to as registries) have been playing an important role in developing the treatment of HSCT for more than four decades. In 1974, the world's first registry was founded by Shirley Nolan in London. Shirley's son, a 3-year-old, Anthony, had been diagnosed with Wiskott-Aldrich syndrome and needed a transplant. Following the example of Anthony Nolan, a large number of registries have been established around the world, mainly in the late 1980s to early 1990s and have increased over the years. The growing pool of donors has contributed to the development of stem cell transplantation as a treatment method and a field of science (Fig. 3.1).

I. Evseeva
Anthony Nolan, London, UK

L. Foeken
Word Marrow Donor Association (WMDA), Leiden, The Netherlands

A. Madrigal (✉)
Anthony Nolan, London, UK

UCL Cancer Institute, Royal Free Campus, London, UK
e-mail: a.madrigal@ucl.ac.uk

3.1.2 Registry: Structure and Duties

A registry is "an organisation responsible for coordination of the search for haematopoietic progenitor cells from donors (including cord blood) unrelated to the potential recipient" (WMDA International Standards 2017).

Registries play the main role in communication between the physician in the transplant centre and the healthcare professional contacting the donor at national and international level. Search requests for adult unrelated donors (AUDs) and cord blood units (CBUs) are usually sent to the national registry, which facilitates all stages of search and provision of the graft for a patient.

A typical registry performs different interrelated functions, including donor recruitment and management and search and interact with HLA-typing laboratories, apheresis and marrow collection centres, cord blood banks (CBBs), stem cell couriers and transplant centres.

Some registries recruit donors themselves, while others have an agreement with blood banks, donor centres or donor recruitment groups. The donor's or cord blood information is provided by the donor centre or CBB to a registry. The registry is responsible for listing the donors on the global database and handling communication with national and international transplant centres (through their national registries) if a potential match for a patient has been found.

The search for a suitable stem cell source is based on the HLA-type of the patient.

E. Carreras et al. (eds.), *The EBMT Handbook*, https://doi.org/10.1007/978-3-030-02278-5_3

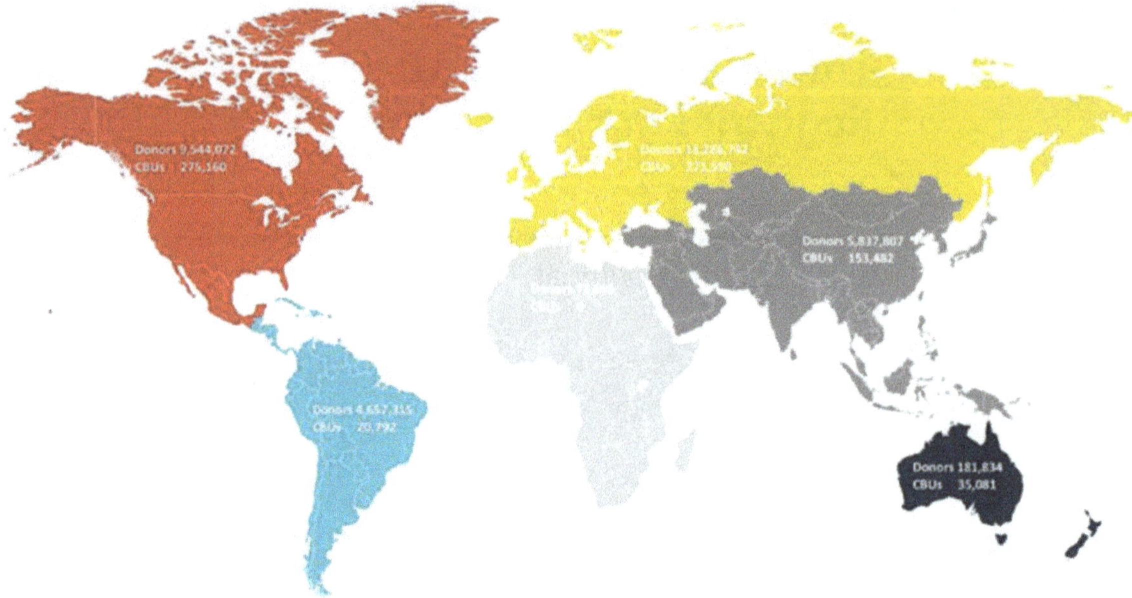

Fig. 3.1 Volunteer donors and cord blood units recruited around the wold (data from WMDA web page)

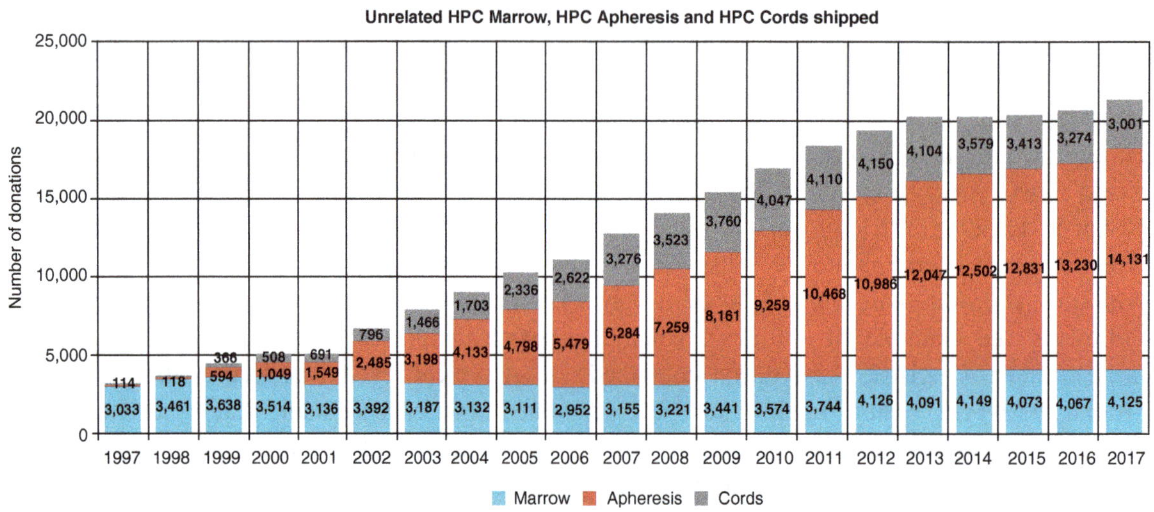

Fig. 3.2 Unrelated HSC from bone marrow, peripheral blood and cord blood shipped annually (data from WMDA)

Transplant centres and search coordinators within donor registries have access to the Search & Match Service of WMDA (https://search.wmda.info/login), where they can register patient data and get a match list to see if there is a potential stem cell source in the global database.

When the transplant centre identifies a potentially matched stem cell source, the national registry will contact the relevant organisation and facilitate the delivery of stem cells for the patient. Annually, more than 20,000 stem cell products of different sources are shipped within and across borders to patients in need of a HSCT (see Fig. 3.2).

3.2 Current Landscape

3.2.1 Ethnic Diversity and Chance to Find a Donor

As of January 2018, more than 32 million potential AUDs and CBUs are listed in the global Search & Match Service of WMDA. Almost 95%

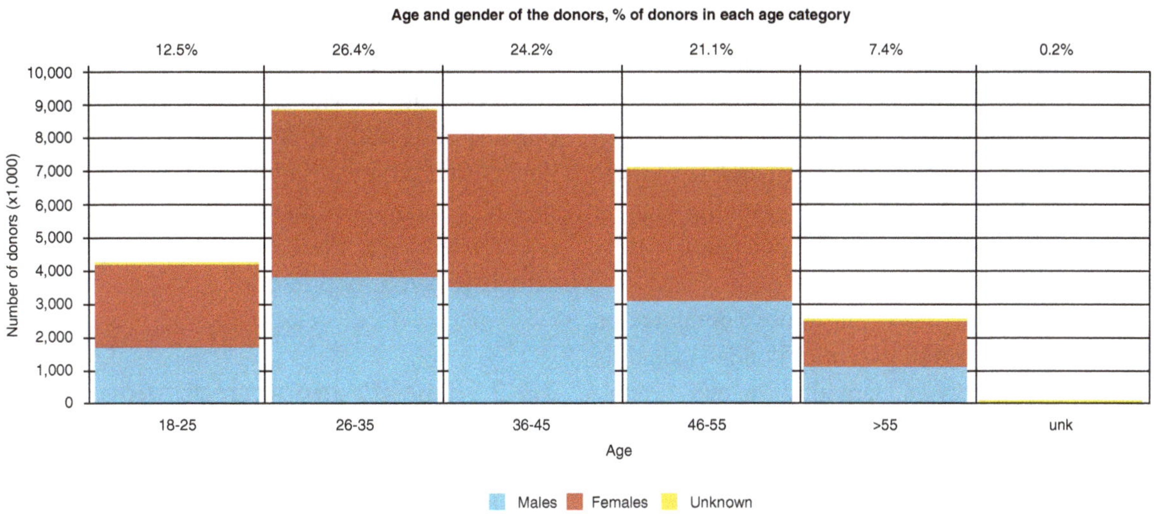

Fig. 3.3 Age and gender of unrelated donors and percentage of donors in each category

of these donors have DNA-based HLA-A, HLA-B and HLA-DRB1 phenotype presented, and more than half are listed with additional information on HLA-C, HLA-DQB1 and HLA-DPB1. Every year, registries across the world add approximately two million new volunteer donors to the worldwide pool, with the vast majority being HLA-typed at high and allelic level resolution.

The chance of finding a well-matched donor varies for patients belonging to different ethnic groups. In 2014, the National Marrow Donor Program (NMDP) study demonstrated that whereas approximately 75% of Caucasian patients are likely to identify an 8/8 HLA-matched AUD, the rate is much lower for ethnic minority and mixed-race patients. This is due to the higher genetic diversity of HLA haplotypes in African and Asian populations compared to Europeans and the lower representation and poorer availability of ethnic minority donors in the worldwide pool (Gragert et al. 2014).

3.2.2 Donor Profile

WMDA defines an unrelated donor as "a person who is the source of cells or tissue for cellular therapy product. Donors are unrelated to the patient seeking a transplant".

Donor centres recruit volunteer donors from 16 to 55 years of age with variations in individual policies. Although donors can remain on the database until they are 60, donor centres try to recruit more young volunteers, as donor age has been proven to be linked to better HSCT outcomes (Kollman et al. 2016). According to the World Marrow Donor Association (WMDA) data, approximately 50% of donors listed globally are younger than 35 (see Fig. 3.3).

Medical suitability for donation, gender diversity, behaviour and psychological risks are constantly changing factors in donor recruitment and management. Donor centres align their policies with national and international standards and recommendations, including donor suitability guidelines produced by the WMDA on https://share.wmda.info/x/FABtEQ and published in 2014 (Lown et al. 2014).

Unrelated donors are acting voluntarily and altruistically and have a right to withdraw from the process at any stage. To avoid such cases, donor centres focus on informing volunteers about all aspects of donation, including risks, at the very early stage of recruitment. When a donor is identified as a potential match for a patient and is asked to provide a blood sample for verification or extended testing, healthcare professionals will have further detailed conversations with the donor addressing any possible questions and concerns. Full informed consent is usually given at the donor's medical, prior to the conditioning of the patient for transplant.

3.2.3 Recruitment, Retention and Data Confidentiality

Recruiting volunteer donors is challenging. Registries and donor centres must ensure they are recruiting the preferred donors (usually younger donors) who are appropriately counselled to fully understand their commitment.

Registries and donor centres use a combination of methods to recruit potential donors including patient-related drives, targeting special groups, e.g. universities, uniformed services, engaging blood donors or online recruitment. The approach depends on the laws of the country and takes traditions, religion and habits into account. The same factors influence donor retention. Considering several options and alternative donors in urgent cases is a recommended practice.

By signing to a donor centre or registry, a potential donor agrees that his/her data are registered in the global database. The donor also provides biological material (blood sample, saliva or buccal swab) for tests, such as HLA typing and infectious disease markers, along with their personal details, in order to be searched as a match for a patient. The registry or donor centre has an obligation to adhere to national and international data protection laws and to keep donor personal and medical information confidentially and use it strictly in line with the donor's informed consent.

While social media helps enormously with donor recruitment and retention, it can present a challenge for confidentiality of both the donor and the recipient. Registries and donor centres in different countries have different policies on donor/patient post-donation contact and on the level of information provided to each other. These should be respected by all sides involved.

3.3 Connections and Worldwide Collaboration

3.3.1 WMDA

In 1988, three pioneers in the field of transplantation, Professors John M. Goldman (United Kingdom), E. Donnell Thomas (United States) and Jon J. van Rood (the Netherlands), informally initiated the WMDA, which became a formal organization in 1994. It is made up of individuals and organizations who promote global collaboration and best practices for the benefit of stem cell donors and patients requiring HSCT. It aims to give all patients worldwide equal access to high-quality stem cells from donors, whose rights and safety are carefully protected.

3.3.2 Quality and Accreditation

In 2017, WMDA took the lead role in the merging of three key organizations: WMDA, BMDW and the NetCord Foundation. This allowed WMDA to streamline resources to provide a global platform for facilitating international search, to support members to develop and grow and to promote safety, quality and global collaboration through accreditation and standardisation. Eighty-four percent of AUDs available for search are provided by WMDA qualified/accredited registries (WMDA Annual Report 2017). WMDA accreditation of the registries along with FACT-NetCord accreditation of the CBBs reassures recipients in the quality of product and services provided. A complete list of the accreditation status of organisations can be found on WMDA Share: https://share.wmda.info/x/4gdcAQ.

3.3.3 Network Formalities

All registries, donor centres and CBBs providing stem cells for HSCT nationally and internationally have legal agreements and contracts with each other within the network. The contracts cover legal, financial and ethical questions of collaboration in respect of obtaining, testing and shipment of stem cells.

3.4 Challenges and Opportunities

3.4.1 Donor Attrition

Time to transplant is reported to be a factor of overall survival (Craddock et al. 2011). Formal search for an unrelated donor on average takes about 2 months. However, more and more urgent search requests are made to the registries, where transplant centres are hoping to get a donor work-up in weeks rather than months.

Not all potential donors listed on the database will be available for donation due to different reasons, including medical or personal circumstances or loss of contact with the registry. It varies in different countries. According to WMDA annual questionnaire, in 2017, the recommended target for donor availability at verification typing stage was 80% and at work-up stage 95%. Registries and donor centres are working hard to keep in contact with their donors to have updated information to help reach the donor without delays. Some donor centres use private healthcare providers to speed-up blood sample collection and increase the number of apheresis centres in order to meet desirable turnaround times.

3.4.2 Ethical Challenges

HSCT is an evolving field of medical science. Volunteer donors can be asked to be a subject of research and clinical trials as part of their stem cell donation for a particular patient or not. In the majority of cases, this is covered by the informed consent given at the recruitment and donor medical stages, but in some cases, additional consent is required. It is the obligation of registries and donor centres to make sure that donors are well informed and free to withdraw.

3.4.3 Donor Pool HLA Diversity

Current trends in HSCT (with high requirements for patient/donor matching, complexity of standard and research protocols and a growing index of indications) present challenges for registries, donor centres and CBBs. Different strategies need to be applied to recruit not only a larger number of potential donors but also increase HLA diversity of the pool. As HLA allele and haplotype frequencies have population-specific patterns, there are limitations to how many different phenotypes can be obtained by adding new donors. In 2016, the WMDA reported no more than 50 different phenotypes per thousand new AUDs and CBUs submitted to the global database. This can be addressed by recruiting among ethnic minority groups or in parts of the world with a wider genetic diversity, e.g. Africa (see Fig. 3.4).

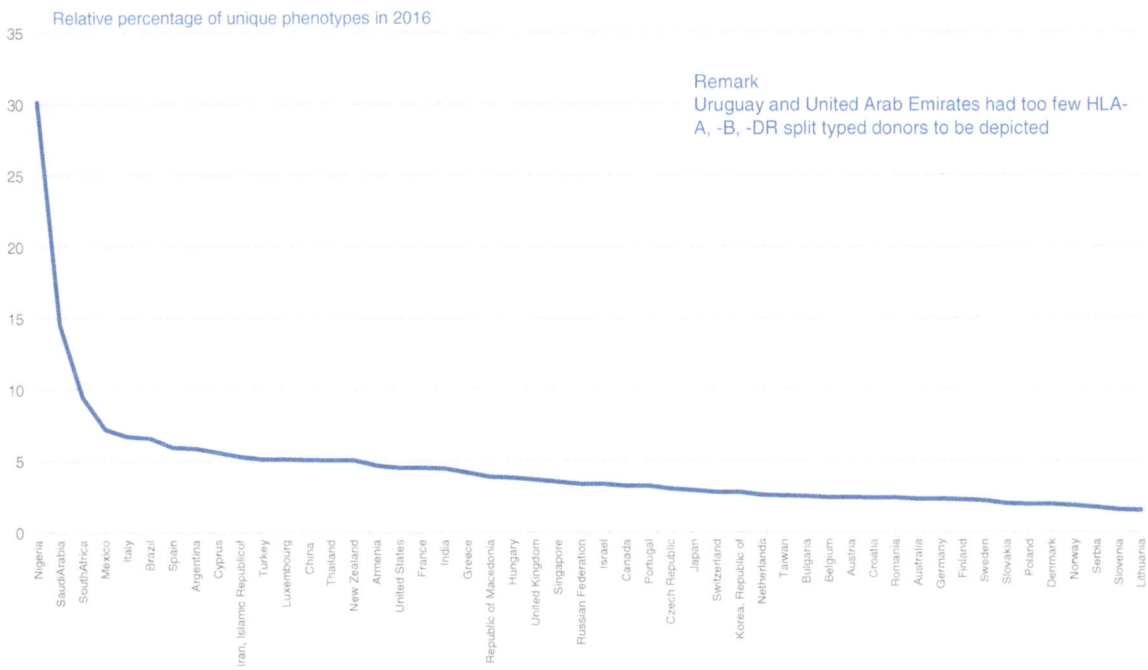

Fig. 3.4 Relative percentage of unique HLA-A, HLA-B and HLA-DR split phenotypes of stem cell donors per country contributed to the entire database of BMDW

Although the majority of stem cell provisions worldwide are currently coming from Northern America and Europe, a few large registries arose in South America and Asia over recent years. WMDA is encouraging and supporting new and growing registries. The WMDA handbook: "A gift for life: the essential WMDA handbook for stem cell donor registries & cord blood banks" (2016) provides all necessary information and advice for starting a registry in your country.

3.5 Future Developments

3.5.1 New Level of HLA Matching

As of January 2018, classic criterion for HLA matching with a patient is 10/10 at HLA-A, HLA-B, HLA-C, HLA-DRB1 and HLA-DQB1 for AUDs and 8/8 on HLA-A, HLA-B, HLA-C and HLA-DRB1 for CBUs, all at high-resolution level, with mismatches associated with inferior patient outcome (Shaw et al. 2017, Eapen et al. 2017). Many transplant centres are now considering HLA-DPB1 allele or epitope matching (Fleischhauer et al. 2012). There are also trends to include other genes like MICA and MICB in donor selection (Fuerst et al. 2016; Carapito et al. 2016; Kitcharoen et al. 2006).

The resolution of HLA matching is important. The advantage of allelic/ultrahigh-resolution HLA matching on OS and NRM compared to high-resolution level was presented by Anthony Nolan at the 2018 BMT Tandem meetings (Mayor et al. 2018). Full/extended gene sequencing results in fully phased phenotypes, thus significantly reduced allelic ambiguity, and can reveal mismatches not otherwise identified by high-resolution typing.

Following these developments, some registries and donor centres have already implemented HLA allelic level typing for their donors and make additional non-HLA genetic information available for transplant centres at the search stage. It is expected that transplant centres will also be able to type patients at this level of resolution to achieve better matching and additional survival advantages.

3.5.2 Related Donors Provision and Follow-Up

Historically, registries have not been closely involved with the provision of related donors. However, in recent years, many registries have begun to support related donors internationally (i.e. where the patient is living in one country and their related donor is living in another) and domestically (e.g. where the patient and donor live far apart or the transplant centre cannot facilitate a collection). Some registries also provide support in following-up related donors post-collection and in providing information and support for related donors.

3.5.3 Advisory Services Provided by Registries

Nowadays, many registries are taking additional advisory roles in supporting transplant centres in stem cell searches as they accumulate knowledge and expertise over an ever-growing number of stem cell provisions. Working closely with clinical teams, national registries may offer advice and consultancy in donor selection, product quality evaluation, education and training.

As part of research and business development strategy, registries are looking at other products and services to further support HSCT. A range of cell therapy products may be provided along with standard stem cell donation or under a separate service agreement.

Key Points

- International collaboration over the last four decades resulted in more than 32 million unrelated donors potentially available to donate stem cells for patients requiring HSCT.
- Donor search and provision are carried out via national registries to ensure quality and legal compliances.
- Unrelated donors act voluntarily and altruistically; their availability varies due to medical and personal reasons.
- Big efforts are made to increase HLA diversity of the donor pool to address the lower chance of finding a well-matched donor for ethnic minority and mixed-race patients.
- Registries continue to develop HSCT by contributing to research, enhancing services and extending the range of cell products provided.

Acknowledgements The authors are grateful to Ms. Ann O'Leary, Ms. Nicola Alderson, Dr. Neema Mayor and Mrs. Pauline Dodi at Anthony Nolan for providing information and advising on the content of this chapter.

References

Carapito R, Jung N, Kwemou M, et al. Matching for the nonconventional MHC-I MICA gene significantly reduces the incidence of acute and chronic GVHD. Blood. 2016;128:1979–86.

Craddock C, Labopin M, Pillai S, et al. Factors predicting outcome after unrelated donor stem cell transplantation in primary refractory acute myeloid leukaemia. Leukemia. 2011;25:808–13.

Eapen M, Wang T, Veys PA, et al. Allele-level HLA matching for umbilical cord blood transplantation for non-malignant diseases in children: a retrospective analysis. Lancet Haematol. 2017;4:325–33.

Fleischhauer K, Shaw BE, Gooley T, et al. Effect of T-cell-epitope matching at HLA-DPB1 in recipients of unrelated-donor haematopoietic-cell transplantation: a retrospective study. Lancet Oncol. 2012;13:366–74.

Fuerst D, Neuchel C, Niederwieser D, et al. Matching for the MICA-129 polymorphism is beneficial in unrelated hematopoietic stem cell transplantation. Blood. 2016;128:3169–76.

Gragert L, Eapen M, Williams E, et al. HLA match likelihoods for hematopoietic stem-cell grafts in the US registry. N Engl J Med. 2014;371:339–48.

Kitcharoen K, Witt C, Romphruk A, et al. MICA, MICB, and MHC beta block matching in bone marrow transplantation: relevance to transplantation outcome. Hum Immunol. 2006;67:238–46.

Kollman C, Spellman SR, Zhang MJ, et al. The effect of donor characteristics on survival after unrelated donor transplantation for hematologic malignancy. Blood. 2016;127:260–7.

Lown RN, Philippe J, Navarro W, et al. Unrelated adult stem cell donor medical suitability: recommendations from the World Marrow Donor Association Clinical Working Group Committee. Bone Marrow Transplant. 2014;49:880–6.

Mayor NP, Hayhurst JD, Turner TR, et al. Better HLA matching as revealed only by next generation sequencing technology results in superior overall survival post-allogeneic haematopoietic cell transplantation with unrelated donors. Biol Blood Marrow Transplant. 2018;24(3):63–4.

Shaw BE, Mayor NP, Szydlo RM, et al. Recipient/donor HLA and CMV matching in recipients of T-cell-depleted unrelated donor haematopoietic cell transplants. Bone Marrow Transplant. 2017;52:717–25.

WMDA Finance and Activities Report. WMDA, 2018. 2017. https://share.wmda.info

WMDA Handbook. A gift for life: the essential handbook for stem cell donor registries and cord blood banks (freely available for WMDA members); 2016.

WMDA International Standards for unrelated haematopoietic stem cell donor registries, January 2017. https://www.wmda.info/professionals/quality-and-accreditation/wmda-standards/.

The HSCT Unit

4

Walid Rasheed, Dietger W. Niederwieser, and Mahmoud Aljurf

4.1 Introduction

HSCT is an advanced therapeutic intervention that is required for a number of malignant and nonmalignant medical conditions, often for critically ill patients. The establishment of an HSCT program requires the efforts of experienced and appropriately trained personnel to lead the program. Clearly, this also requires financial, legal, ethical, and other institutional support. For newly starting programs, it would be essential to identify minimal requirements for establishing an HSCT unit in order to optimize resource utilization as well as maintain safe patient care. While these minimal requirements also apply to well-established units, its structure helps to understand and implement additional steps for larger units which plan to offer additional transplant services and have access to more resources.

Approximately 20 years ago, the EBMT and the ISCT (International Society for Cellular Therapy) formed the Joint Accreditation Committee—ISCT and EBMT (JACIE) based on the FACT (Foundation for the Accreditation of Cellular Therapy) program. Efforts of these bodies have culminated in the establishment of standards related to HSCT and cellular therapies to assure quality and safety in the practice of HSCT. Although program accreditation with JACIE is not mandatory worldwide, these standards are very helpful as guidelines to understand requirements to establish an HSCT unit. Table 4.1 summarizes basic minimal requirements of an HSCT unit, which are discussed in more details in the following sections.

W. Rasheed (✉) · M. Aljurf
King Faisal Specialist Hospital and Research Centre, Riyadh, Saudi Arabia
e-mail: wrasheed@kfshrc.edu.sa

D. W. Niederwieser
University of Leipzig, Leipzig, Germany

4.2 Inpatient Unit

The inpatient HSCT unit should have a minimum number of single-bedded rooms with isolation capability. The number and space of rooms should be adequate for the type and volume of transplant activity performed at the transplant center. These rooms must adhere to the standards of safety and comfort of patients in a tertiary care hospital facility. Every location or room should have a sink and tap for hand washing.

There needs to be a working station or room for nurses involved in patient care. A similar working space for physicians is required. Medical and nursing staff coverage should be available 24 h a day, including public holidays. The ratio of nurses to patient beds depends on the type and intensity of transplants being performed, e.g., autologous versus allogeneic, but generally, a ratio one nurse to three patients is reasonable. Emergency cart with drugs for resuscitation should be available in the inpatient unit.

E. Carreras et al. (eds.), *The EBMT Handbook*, https://doi.org/10.1007/978-3-030-02278-5_4

Table 4.1 HSCT unit minimal requirements

Inpatient unit	– Clean single-bedded rooms with isolation capability
Ancillary medical services	– Intensive care unit – Emergency room service – Gastroenterology and pulmonary service[a]
Outpatient clinic	– Single patient examination rooms
Blood bank	– Twenty-four hour on-site blood bank service: ABO typing and cross match, RBC, and platelets for transfusion – Irradiation and leukocyte depletion of blood products
Laboratory	– Hematology cell count and chemistry lab – Serology for viral screen – Microbiology for basic bacterial and fungal cultures – CMV PCR or antigenemia[a] – Access to CSA/tacrolimus levels[a]
HLA typing lab[a]	– Access to ASHI or similarly accredited HLA typing lab
Stem cell collection	– PBSC apheresis capability – Bone marrow harvesting facility and expertise for matched sibling donor[a]
Stem cell processing facility	– FACS CD34 enumeration – Refrigerator for blood and bone marrow – Controlled cryopreservation capability for freezing of autologous stem cell product – Equipment and expertise to process ABO-mismatched cellular product[a]
Radiology	– Routine x-ray radiology, ultrasound, and CT scanner – Placement of central venous catheters
Pharmacy	– Availability of conditioning chemotherapy drugs – Availability of antimicrobial agents (broad-spectrum antibiotics, antiviral, and antifungal drugs) – Availability of immunosuppressive agents for GVHD prophylaxis and treatment[a]
Human resources	– Medical director: Licensed physician with adequate training and experience in HSCT – Nursing staff with training in chemotherapy administration, infection control, and handling of stem cell products – Clinical laboratory director: Clinical pathology trained. – Appropriately trained lab scientist and technicians – Multidisciplinary medical staff (radiology, pathology, ICU, surgery, gastroenterology[a], pulmonary[a])
Outcome database	– Monitor patient demographics, treatment, and outcomes (level I data reporting)
Quality management	– Written institutional protocols/guidelines – Regular audits of various HSCT procedures and patient treatment outcomes – System to detect errors or adverse events for corrective or preventative actions

[a]Requirements for allogeneic HSCT programs

Infections, including bacterial, viral, or fungal infections, are potential significant complications in transplant recipient and may lead to significant morbidity and mortality. Therefore, HSCT units should have established measures for infection control. Guidelines for infection prevention and prophylaxis in HSCT patients, endorsed by several scientific organizations, are available and highly recommended to follow. HSCT recipients should be placed in single-patient rooms. Furthermore, at a minimum, standard precautions should be followed in all patients including hand hygiene and wearing of appropriate protective equipment (gloves, surgical masks or eye/face protection, gowns) during procedures/activities that are likely to generate splashes or spray of blood, body fluids, or secretions. Hand hygiene is essential, using alcohol-based hand rubs or washing with soap and water. In patients with suspected or proven of having an infection, additional precautions are required accordingly, e.g., airborne, droplet, or contact isolation. HSCT units should be cleaned at least daily with special attention to dust control. During building construction, intensified mold control measures are required, and a multidisciplinary team should be involved.

Other important infection control measures include well-sealed rooms, positive pressure differential between patient rooms and the hallway, self-closing doors, more than 12 air exchanges per hour, and continuous pressure monitoring. HEPA (high efficiency particulate air) filters have shown efficacy in providing protection against acquisition of fungal infections in immune-compromised hematology patients, including HSCT patients, and during hospital construction or renovation works. While HEPA filters are not absolutely required as a minimal requirement in newly established centers with less complicated transplant activities, they are certainly preferred and highly recommended as newly established centers expand their activities to include more complicated (especially allogeneic) transplant activities.

There is no agreed upon minimum number of transplants to be performed in a program. However, to ensure continuing proficiency in a transplant program, the ASBMT recommends for programs performing only one type of HSCT (autologous or allogeneic), at least ten transplants of that type are to be performed per annum; programs performing both allogeneic and autologous transplantations should perform a minimum of ten transplants of each kind per annum.

4.3 Ancillary Medical Services

HSCT patients often require other medical specialties involvement in their complicated care. This includes the risk of developing life-threatening infections or other post transplant complications, hence the importance of having access to emergency room as well as intensive care services at the same tertiary care hospital facility where transplant program is being established. Intensive care units should have the ability of providing inotropic support, respiratory support (including mechanical ventilation) as well as renal replacement (hemodialysis) if required.

Input from infectious disease physicians can be valuable in HSCT patients who are at risk of a multitude of opportunistic and potentially life-threatening infections; this is especially important for programs that perform allogeneic transplants. Availability of gastroenterology specialist with endoscopy services is critical for allogeneic programs, as often diagnostic endoscopy is required to differentiate GVHD from other etiologies of gastrointestinal complications. Similarly, pulmonary medicine service with access to diagnostic bronchoscopies is required for such patients with pulmonary abnormalities.

HSCT programs that perform transplants using radiotherapy as part of conditioning regimen (total body irradiation) should have available radiation oncology service on site. The radiation oncology team, including the radiation oncologist and physicist, should have adequate training in the technique of total body irradiation and appropriate equipment, and procedures must be in place to deliver successful and safe radiation component of these conditioning regimen.

4.4 Outpatient Unit

HSCT patients attend to the outpatient unit, both for pretransplant assessment and work-up and post transplant follow-up and management. Single patient examination rooms are a minimal requirement for the outpatient service of the program. These rooms should be adequately equipped to allow clinical assessment of patients. It is important to implement infection control measures to minimize risk of transmitting infections, including hand hygiene measures and availability of appropriate room to isolate patients who are identified to be potentially infectious to others, e.g., due to herpes zoster infection. A dedicated infusion area would be ideal as transplant recipients often require IV fluid and electrolyte replacement or blood product administration.

4.5 Blood Bank

Availability of blood banking services is a critical component of a successful transplant program. A 24-h on-site blood banking service is required for ABO typing, cross match, and urgent supply of red blood cells and platelets for transfusion. Meeting minimal standard criteria according to recognized international blood bank societies such as the American Association of Blood Banks (AABB) or equivalent is important. Blood bank staff, including blood bank director, scientists, and technicians should be adequately qualified and trained in blood banking procedures.

Transplant recipients are severely immune-compromised and are at risk of transfusion-associated GVHD, caused by unrestricted proliferation of donor lymphocytes in the immune-compromised host. Hence, it is critical that transplant recipients receive irradiated blood products to prevent this complication. The use of leukocyte-depleted blood products is recommended to reduce the risk of HLA alloimmunization in the multiply transfused hematology patients, as well as to reduce the incidence of transfusion reactions. In allogeneic programs, clear documented pathways for transfusion support in cases of ABO mismatch should be available for both blood bank and clinical staff as guidance.

4.6 Laboratory

A 24-h on-site hematology cell count and basic chemistry lab are required. Furthermore, microbiology laboratory service is essential in the clinical management of transplant recipients, including routine bacterial and fungal cultures of various patient specimens. Serology screening for relevant viral and bacterial infections is also required for pretransplant work-up of recipients as well as donor screening. For allogeneic transplant recipients, monitoring for cytomegalovirus (CMV) reactivation is essential, and results must be available in a timely manner to allow therapeutic intervention; both molecular technique by quantitative PCR (preferable) and antigenemia method are acceptable. In the allogeneic setting, monitoring drug levels, e.g., cyclosporine or tacrolimus, is required, and same-day service is recommended to allow interventions aiming at keeping levels of these important drugs within the target therapeutic range.

4.7 HLA Typing Lab

Access to HLA typing laboratory is mandatory for allogeneic programs. Such service can be available on-site or alternatively provided in reference laboratory. JACIE standards state that clinical programs performing allogeneic transplantation shall use HLA testing laboratories that are capable of carrying out DNA-based intermediate and high-resolution HLA typing and are appropriately accredited by the American Society for Histocompatibility and Immunogenetics (ASHI), European Federation for Immunogenetics (EFI), or other accrediting organizations providing histocompatibility services appropriate for hematopoietic cellular therapy transplant patients.

4.8 Stem Cell Collection

Access to peripheral blood stem cell apheresis service on-site is a minimal requirement in each program. This is often part of the blood bank service or alternatively under the administration of the clinical program. Having at least two cell separators would be beneficial, as the second cell separator would be a backup in situations of unexpected machine faults and for routine servicing. Daily operation of apheresis facility requires appropriately trained and experienced nursing staff and a medical director with adequate qualification and experience in clinical and laboratory aspects of the apheresis procedure. Institutional written protocols and policies covering all aspects of apheresis procedure should be available for guidance. JACIE standards require a minimum average of ten cellular therapy products collected by apheresis per year for program accreditation.

A bone marrow stem cell source is sometimes recommended for better patient outcome, e.g., patients with bone marrow failure. Programs performing allogeneic transplants for such indication should have a bone marrow harvest facility on-site. This requires convenient and easy access to surgical operating room with anesthesia service. Appropriate equipment for the bone marrow harvest procedure are required. Physicians with adequate training and experience in bone marrow harvesting are crucial to perform the procedure successfully.

4.9 Stem Cell Processing Facility

The stem cell processing facility requires a designated area, usually within the laboratory. It should be appropriately equipped for the processing of various stem cell products depending on the types of transplants performed and the size of the program. Availability of flow cytometry for the enumeration of CD34 cell count is mandatory. Controlled cryopreservation capability, using liquid nitrogen, for freezing of autologous stem cell product is essential. This may also be used in allogeneic sibling products. Standard quality control measures, including systems to closely monitor and record the temperature in all freezes and refrigerators, are critical. Allogeneic programs should have appropriate equipment and expertise on-site for the timely and safe processing of ABO-mismatched stem cell products as required, including the need to perform red cell or plasma depletion procedures when indicated. The processing facility should be operated by adequately trained staff, including scientist, technicians, and a medical director. Written standard operating procedures explaining all aspects of stem cell processing performed at the facility are required.

4.10 Radiology

Standard routine (X-ray), ultrasound, and computed tomography (CT scan) imaging services are the minimal requirements and should be available on site for the routine diagnostic imaging. Availability of magnetic resonance imaging (MRI) is preferred, as it is often useful in the diagnosis of specific clinical conditions relevant to stem cell transplant recipients, such as iron overload, CNS infections, and posterior reversible encephalopathy syndrome (PRES) related to calcineurin inhibitor toxicity. Placement of central venous catheters in transplant recipients is obviously required in each program. Depending on the institutional setting, this service may be provided by various hospital services; often this is done by the radiology service under ultrasound guidance. Having well trained and experienced interventional radiologist to perform this procedure is crucial for the safety of patients.

4.11 Pharmacy

Pharmacy services are essential in each HSCT program. Availability of conditioning chemotherapy agents is clearly required; specific drugs depend on the type and complexity of transplant procedures performed in each program. Commonly used agents in conditioning regimens include BU, CY, FLU, and MEL. ATG may also be required in the allogeneic setting (e.g., in aplastic anemia) and requires special attention and training by nursing, pharmaceutical, and medical staff in relation to its administration.

Broad-spectrum antibiotics should be available for urgent use as required in transplant recipient. Likewise, access to antiviral and antifungal agents is important for both prophylaxis and treatment. Allogeneic programs should also have access to immunosuppressive drugs used for GVHD prophylaxis such as CSA, MTX, and TAC.

A trained pharmacist is crucial for the HSCT program. The pharmacist should review all conditioning chemotherapy protocols and ensure appropriate dispensing and administration of cytotoxic agents.

4.12 Staffing and Human Resources

Appropriately trained and experienced medical and nursing staffs are crucial for the HSCT program. The clinical medical director of the program should be a licensed physician (specialty certification in hematology, oncology, or immunology) with adequate training at a BMT program. A minimal BMT training duration of 6–12 months is suggested. JAICIE standards indicate that the clinical program director shall have 2 years of experience as an attending physician responsible for the direct clinical management of HSCT patients in the inpatient and outpatient settings. A minimum of one (1) additional attending transplant physician is required in the program.

The success of a transplant program relies heavily on the presence of appropriately trained and experienced nursing staff. This includes training in chemotherapy administration, infection control, management of neutropenic patients, and handling of stem cell products.

Other important staff includes appropriately trained and experienced personnel in the laboratory (including laboratory director, scientist, and technicians), trained pharmacist, as well as medical professionals of ancillary medical services. Continuous education activities are required for all healthcare professionals involved in the management of HSCT patients.

4.13 Institutional Database and Data Manager

Monitoring patient demographics, treatment details, and outcomes is an essential minimal requirement. Each program should keep complete and accurate patient records, and a database containing relevant patient data should be established and regularly maintained. Appropriate patient consent needs to be obtained for such database. An example of the minimal data required to be obtained on each transplant patient is the information required in the CIBMTR or EBMT mid A forms. Having a data manager in a transplant program to initiate and maintain this institutional transplant database is highly recommended. Often data managers have nursing background with experience in stem cell transplantation. Attending training data management courses during international meetings or through links with other experienced and well-established programs would be valuable.

4.14 Quality Control

The JACIE standards require that all essential clinical collection and processing facilities in the transplant center evaluate and report patient outcomes. Regular audits of various HSCT procedures and patient treatment outcomes are required. Essentially, a system is required to be in place to detect errors/adverse events, so that these can be evaluated in order to implement preventative measures to minimize the risk of recurrence of these incidents. Furthermore, each program should have written institutional clinical protocols in relation to the various aspects of the transplant patient care to standardize practice. Likewise, stem cell collection and processing facilities should have standard operating procedures that serve as a guidance for all staff to follow to enhance patient's safety. Access to or relationship with experienced HSCT program is often very helpful and highly recommended via shared protocols/telemedicine and/or web-based conferencing.

4.15 Transplant Coordinator

HSCT is a complex therapeutic intervention, and coordination of the pretransplant, transplant, and post transplant patient care is important. A transplant coordinator can play pivotal role in this context, acting as a facilitator, educator, as well as a point of contact for the patient and their families. Transplant coordinators ensure the smooth and safe running of the HSCT service starting from scheduling and arranging pretransplant work-up of patient and planning the roadmap for the transplant recipient with continued involvement and education of the patients and their families until the time of admission. Furthermore, transplant coordinator would play a significant role in the coordination of post HSCT follow-up and care in clinics. For allo-HSCT, the transplant coordinator would be very valuable in arranging donor search starting from HLA typing of the recipient and his/her family members, in addition to initiating and following a search for unrelated donor in national or international registries.

The transplant coordinator involvement may extend to organizing the logistics of getting the stem cells from the donor from the donor center where the recipient may be in another health facility (national or international). Moreover, transplant coordinators will often lead the HSCT team weekly planning meetings and discussions with the arrangement of the HSCT waiting list. Typically, transplant coordinators have nursing background with significant experience in stem cell transplantation.

Key Points

- The inpatients unit should have single-bedded rooms with isolation capabilities. Single outpatient examination rooms are also required.
- Laboratory, blood bank, and pharmacy services are critical to the success of HSCT programs.
- Stem cell collection and processing capabilities are minimal requirements for any HSCT program; the level of such capabilities depends on the type and complexity of HSCT performed in each center.
- Ancillary medical services are essential components of successful HSCT programs, including intensive care and emergency and radiology services. Additional medical services are required in allogeneic programs.
- Appropriately trained and experienced staff (medical, nursing, laboratory, pharmacy) are crucial for the HSCT program.
- Monitoring patient characteristics and transplant outcomes is essential.
- A local quality control system is required in all aspects involved in the HSCT procedure.
- Having a data manager for the HSCT program, to initiate and maintain institutional minimal transplant data base is highly recommended.
- Transplant coordinators play pivotal role the management of HSCT patients, starting from pre SCT work up, right through post transplant care.

Recommended References

Booth GS, Gehrie EA, Bolan CD, Savani BN. Clinical guide to ABO-incompatible allogeneic stem cell transplantation. Biol Blood Marrow Transplant. 2013;19:1152–8.

Chang CC, Ananda-Rajah M, Belcastro A, et al. Consensus guidelines for implementation of quality processes to prevent invasive fungal disease and enhanced surveillance measures during hospital building works, 2014. Intern Med J. 2014;44:1389–97.

Crysandt M, Yakoub-Agha I, Reiß P, et al. How to build an allogeneic hematopoietic cell transplant unit in 2016: proposal for a practical framework. Curr Res Transl Med. 2017;65:149–54.

Daniele N, Scerpa MC, Rossi C, et al. The processing of stem cell concentrates from the bone marrow in ABO-incompatible transplants: how and when. Blood Transfus. 2014;12:150–8.

FACT/JACIE. FACT-JACIE 7th edition standards; 2018. http://www.jacie.org/.

Hahn T, Cummings KM, Michalek AM, et al. Efficacy of high-efficiency particulate air filtration in preventing aspergillosis in immunocompromised patients with hematologic malignancies. Infect Control Hosp Epidemiol. 2002;23:525–31.

Krüger WH, Zöllner B, Kaulfers PM, Zander AR. Effective protection of allogeneic stem cell recipients against Aspergillosis by HEPA air filtration during a period of construction--a prospective survey. J Hematother Stem Cell Res. 2003;12:301–7.

Leemhuis T, Padley D, Keever-Taylor C, et al. Essential requirements for setting up a stem cell processing laboratory. Bone Marrow Transplant. 2014;49:1098–105.

Napier A, Williamson LM. British Committee for Standards in Haematology, Blood Transfusion Task Force, et al. Guidelines on the clinical use of leucocyte – depleted blood components. Transfusion Med. 1998;81:59–71.

Phillip G, Armitage J, Bearman S. American Society for Blood and Marrow Transplantation guidelines for clinical centers. Biol Blood Marrow Transplant. 1995;1:54–5.

Tomblyn M, Chiller T, Einsele H, et al. Guidelines for preventing infectious complications among hematopoietic cell transplantation recipients: a global perspective. Biol Blood Marrow Transplant. 2009;15:1143–238.

Treleaven J, Gennery A, Marsh J, et al. Guidelines on the use of irradiated blood components prepared by the British committee for standards in haematology blood transfusion task force. Br J Haematol. 2011;152:35–51.

5 JACIE Accreditation of HSCT Programs

Riccardo Saccardi, Eoin McGrath, and John A. Snowden

5.1 Introduction

The complexity of HSCT as a medical technology and the frequent need for close interaction and interdependence between different services, teams, and external providers (donor registries, typing laboratories, etc.) distinguish it from many other medical fields. Approximately 20 years ago, this complexity led to efforts by transplantation professionals to standardize processes based on consensus as a way to better manage inherent risks of this treatment. HSCT was, and continues to be, a pioneer in the area of quality and standards.

R. Saccardi (✉)
Department of Cellular Therapies and Transfusion Medicine, Careggi University Hospital, Florence, Italy
e-mail: riccardo.saccardi@unifi.it

E. McGrath
European Society for Blood and Marrow Transplantation (EBMT), Barcelona, Spain

J. A. Snowden
Department of Haematology, Sheffield Teaching Hospitals NHS Foundation Trust, University of Sheffield, Sheffield, UK

5.2 Background

In 1998, EBMT and the International Society for Cell & Gene Therapy (ISCT) established the Joint Accreditation Committee, ISCT and EBMT (JACIE), aimed to offer an inspection-based accreditation process in HSCT against established international standards. JACIE is a committee of the EBMT, its members are appointed by and are accountable to the EBMT Board, and ISCT is represented through two members of the Committee. JACIE collaborates with the US-based Foundation for the Accreditation of Cellular Therapy (FACT) to develop and maintain global standards for the provision of quality medical and laboratory practice in cellular therapy.

The JACIE and FACT accreditation systems stand out as examples of profession-driven initiatives to improve quality in transplantation and which have subsequently been incorporated by third parties, such as healthcare payers (health insurers, social security) and competent authorities (treatment authorization). The JACIE Accreditation Program was supported in 2004 by the European Commission under the public health program 2003–2008 and was acknowledged as an exemplary project in a 2011 review of spending under the public health program.

E. Carreras et al. (eds.), *The EBMT Handbook*, https://doi.org/10.1007/978-3-030-02278-5_5

5.3 Impact of Accreditation in Clinical Practice

Much literature indicating a better clinical outcome in teaching hospitals and centers of excellence has been available since the 1990s (Hartz et al. 1989; Birkmeyer et al. 2005; Loberiza et al. 2005). Initial evidence of a positive relationship between the implementation of a quality management system and outcome of HSCT in Europe was published in 2011 (Gratwohl et al. 2011). In this paper, patients' outcome was systematically better when the transplantation center was at a more advanced phase of JACIE accreditation, independent of year of transplantation and other risk factors.

Another analysis (Gratwohl et al. 2014) was performed on a large cohort of patients who received either an allogeneic or an autologous transplantation between 1996 and 2006 and reported to the EBMT database. The authors showed that the decrease of overall mortality in allogeneic procedures over the 14-year observation period was significantly faster in JACIE-accredited centers, thus resulting in a higher relapse-free survival and overall survival at 72 months from transplant. Such improvement was not shown in autologous transplantation.

Similar results published by Marmor et al. (2015) in an American study showed that centers accredited by both FACT and Clinical Trial Network (CTN) demonstrated significantly better results for more complex HSCT such as HLA-mismatched transplants.

These data reinforce the concept that clinical improvement is driven by the implementation of a quality management system embedded in external accreditation standards, especially in the context of more complex procedures. This process also results in a wider standardization of procedures across different countries and geographic areas, therefore contributing to providing patients with similar treatment expectations even when accessing different health management systems. A comprehensive review of this was recently published (Snowden et al. 2017).

5.4 JACIE-FACT Accreditation System

JACIE and FACT accreditation systems are based on the development and continuous update of standards covering the entire transplantation process, from selection of the donor/patient to follow-up, including collection, characterization, processing, and storage of the graft. Considering the different competences included in the process, the standards are articulated in four parts:

- Clinical Program,
- Bone Marrow Collection,
- Apheresis Collection and
- Processing Facility.

A quality management (QM) section is embedded in each section, aimed at providing a tool for both the applicants to develop a comprehensive system of quality assessment and for the inspectors to check the compliance of the program to the standard. Stand-alone processing labs can apply; however, the target of the accreditation is the transplantation program, intended as a process in its entirety, thus requiring a full integration of units, laboratories, services, and professionals. Each section focusses on the competence of personnel, listing topics for which the evidence of a specific training is required which also includes the minimum experience requirements for positions of responsibility. Maintaining these competences is also required for all professionals.

The standards are revised on a 3-year basis by a commission formed of experts appointed by JACIE and FACT, including HSCT administration, cell processing and storage, blood apheresis, transplant registries, and QM specialists. The standards are based on published evidence and, when this is not available, on expert consensus. A legal review and comparison with current regulations are carried out for each version. When the developmental phase is finalized, the standards are published for public review and comment and finally approved by JACIE and FACT.

The standards incorporate sound principles of quality medical and laboratory practice in cellular therapy, but do not cover legal requirements of local competent authorities.

The compliance to the standards is ensured through an inspection system, carried out by voluntary inspectors, trained and coordinated by the JACIE office in Barcelona. The JACIE inspection is a multistep procedure: the applicant center is provided with all the application documents and is then required to submit a set of documentation to the JACIE accreditation coordinators. If the first review is positive, the on-site inspection is then planned in agreement with the applicant.

JACIE inspections are carried out in most cases in the language of the applicant. The inspectors' report is then assessed by the JACIE accreditation committee, which may request supplementary information, modifications, or another on-site visit. If all aspects are shown to be compliant, accreditation is awarded. An accreditation cycle is 4 years for JACIE, and facilities must complete an interim desk-based audit after 2 years post-accreditation. Accredited facilities must reapply for reaccreditation and may also be reinspected in response to complaints or information that a facility may be noncompliant with the standards, in response to significant changes in the program and/or facility or as determined by JACIE.

Many tools are made available to prepare the accreditation through the JACIE website, including a quality management guide, the welcome guide, and webinars. JACIE runs training courses throughout the year, and the Barcelona-based staff are available to support the applicants. An accreditation manual provides detailed explanations and examples for each single item of the standards. A special approach is under development for transplant programs in low- and middle-income countries (LMICs), where full accreditation might not be feasible due to resources and/or cultural issues. In this case, a stepped process toward accreditation is being developed, based on the selection of organizational items of the standard which may be fulfilled by the implementation of a QM system, without requiring specific investments in infrastructures and/or equipment. This "stepwise" option will also encourage the programs to connect with an international network of professionals and may also stimulate local authorities to support further progress toward full accreditation in the interests of patients, donors, and the professional community.

The standards cover the use of different sources of hematopoietic stem cells and nucleated cells from any hematopoietic tissue source administered in the context of the transplant process, such as DLI. The term "hematopoietic" in the title is to define the scope of these standards, due to an increasing number of accredited facilities that also support non-hematopoietic cellular therapies. Starting with version 6.1, the standards include new items specifically developed for other cellular therapy products, with special reference to immune effector cells (IECs). This reflects the rapidly evolving field of cellular therapy through mainly, but not exclusively, genetically modified cells, such as CAR-T cells. The standards do not cover the manufacturing of such cells but include the chain of responsibilities where the product is provided by a third party and ensure the competence of the personnel in the management of adverse events related to the infusion.

Another recent development has been the introduction of "benchmarking" standards related to 1-year survival and other patient outcomes. If center performance is below the expected range, then a corrective action plan is mandated. The requirement for a risk-adapted "benchmarking" system is being addressed in the development of the new EBMT MACRO registry, which will enable centers to address these new JACIE standards within their own BMT community and across international boundaries.

JACIE is run on a non-profit basis, resourced almost entirely on application fees. Fees depend on the configuration of the program and its EBMT membership status. At the time of writing in February 2018, the application fee for a transplant program made up of collection, processing, and clinical units is €14,600 for EBMT members and €29,200 for non-EBMT members. Supplementary fees for additional sites and discounts for active inspectors in the team are applied (*see* JACIE website for details).

Overall, over 600 accreditation inspections have been carried out in 25 countries, representing over 40% transplant centers in Europe (Figs. 5.1 and 5.2), many of which have been through more than one accreditation cycle. JACIE accreditation is now mandatory in several European countries, to apply for reimbursement of the procedure and/or to be authorized to perform HSCT. JACIE also represents an opportunity for centers in LMICs to align their organizations with practice in the more advanced HSCT programs.

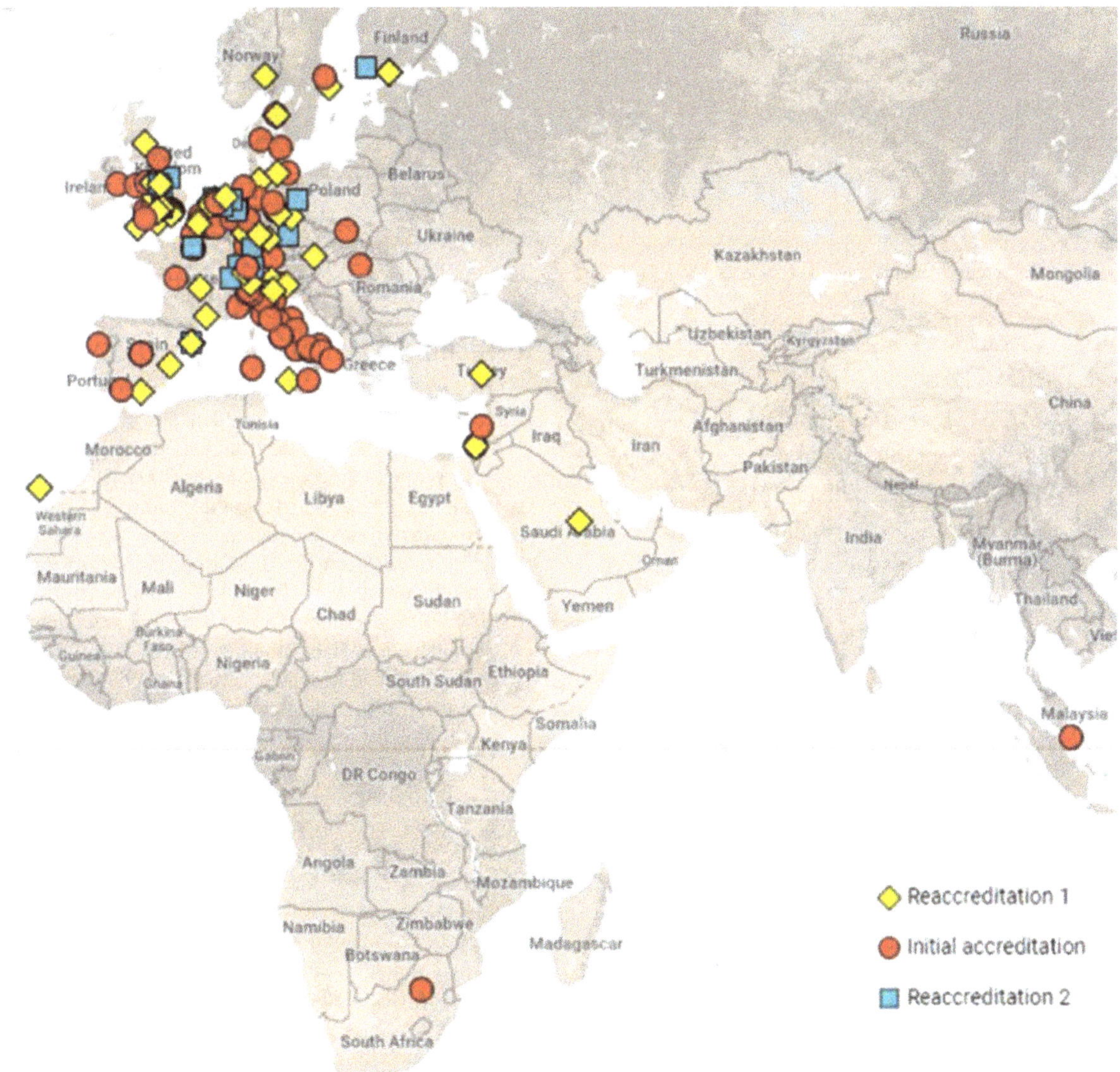

Fig. 5.1 JACIE-accredited programs March 2018

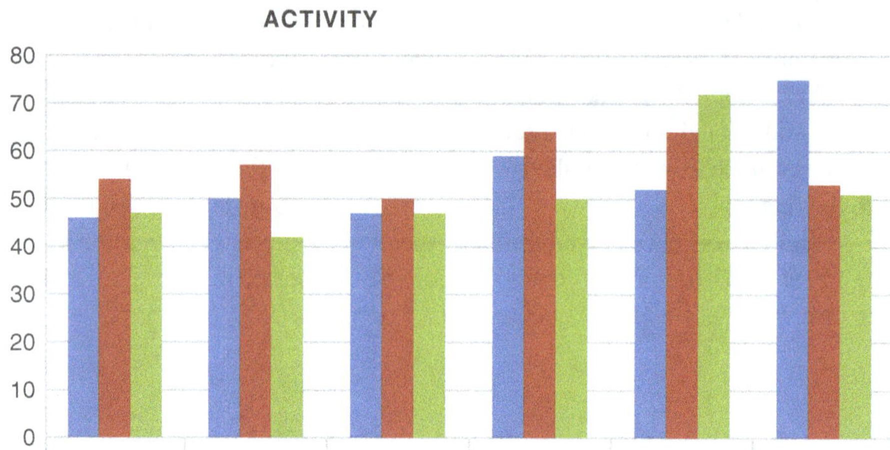

	2012	2013	2014	2015	2016	2017
Applications	46	50	47	59	52	75
Inspections-completed	54	57	50	64	64	53
Accreditations	47	42	47	50	72	51

Fig. 5.2 JACIE activity 2012–2017

Key Points

- JACIE accreditation is based on an internationally agreed quality standard system led and delivered by HSCT and cell therapy professionals.
- The standards are regularly updated, incorporating advances in the evidence base while reflecting the practical view of experienced experts on clinical and laboratory practice of HSCT and cell therapy.
- Published data support a positive improvement in the clinical outcome related to the accreditation process, also promoting a progressive standardization of HSCT practice across different countries.
- Recent developments in the standards include development of standards for CAR-T and other immune effector cells (IEC), "benchmarking" of patient survival and access of centers in LMIC to the "stepwise" accreditation.

References

Birkmeyer NJ, Goodney PP, Stukel TA, et al. Do cancer centers designated by the National Cancer Institute have better surgical outcomes? Cancer. 2005;103:435–41.

Gratwohl A, Brand R, McGrath E, Joint Accreditation Committee of the International Society for Cellular, B. the European Group for, T. Marrow and N. the European Leukemia, et al. Use of the quality management system "JACIE" and outcome after hematopoietic stem cell transplantation. Haematologica. 2014;99:908–15.

Gratwohl A, Brand R, Niederwieser D, et al. Introduction of a quality management system and outcome after hematopoietic stem-cell transplantation. J Clin Oncol. 2011;29:1980–6.

Hartz AJ, Krakauer H, Kuhn EM, et al. Hospital characteristics and mortality rates. N Engl J Med. 1989;321:1720–5.

Loberiza FR, Zhang MJ, Lee SJ, et al. Association of transplant center and physician factors on mortality after hematopoietic stem cell transplantation in the United States. Blood. 2005;105:2979–87.

Marmor S, Begun JW, Abraham J, Virnig BA. The impact of center accreditation on hematopoietic cell transplantation (HCT). Bone Marrow Transplant. 2015;50:87–94.

Snowden JA, McGrath E, Duarte RF, et al. JACIE accreditation for blood and marrow transplantation: past, present and future directions of an international model for healthcare quality improvement. Bone Marrow Transplant. 2017;52:1367–71.

6 Statistical Methods in HSCT and Cellular Therapies

Simona Iacobelli and Liesbeth C. de Wreede

6.1 Introduction

The analysis of data describing the outcomes of patients who have received an HSCT is not only fundamental to assessing the effectiveness of the treatment but can provide invaluable information on the prognostic role of disease and patient factors. Thus, the appropriate analysis and understanding of such data are of paramount importance. This document provides an overview of the main and well-established statistical methods, as well as a brief introduction of more novel techniques. More insight is provided in the *EBMT Statistical Guidelines* (Iacobelli 2013).

6.2 Endpoints

The outcomes most commonly studied in HSCT analyses are the key events occurring at varying times post HSCT, e.g., engraftment, GVHD, relapse/progression, and death. Besides the clinical definition of the event of interest, it is important to define the corresponding statistical endpoint and to use a proper method of measuring the occurrence of the event (Guidelines 2.1).

The main distinction is between events that occur with certainty during a sufficiently long observation period (follow-up), like death, and events which are precluded from occurring once another event occurs, e.g., not all patients will experience a relapse of their disease because some die before. We define death without prior relapse (usually called NRM; see Guidelines 2.1.2) as the "competing event" of relapse. The name "NRM" is preferable to TRM, the proper analysis of which requires individual adjudication of causes of death.

Survival endpoints: In addition to death, other examples of events of the first type are the combinations of (negative) events of interest, which in total have 100% probability of occurrence, for example, PFS which considers as failure of the event "either relapse/progression or death." The components of PFS are the two competing events mentioned above, relapse/progression and NRM.

Competing risks endpoints: In addition to relapse/progression and NRM, other examples are death of a specific cause and all intermediate events during a HSCT history (engraftment, GVHD, achievement of CR, CMV infection) including the long-term (secondary malignancy). Notice that the definition of an endpoint requires specifying which are the competing events. Usually, this will be death without prior event of

S. Iacobelli (✉)
Department of Biology, University of Rome Tor Vergata, Rome, Italy

EBMT, Leiden, The Netherlands
e-mail: simona.iacobelli@ebmt.org

L. C. de Wreede
Department of Biomedical Data Sciences, Leiden University Medical Center, Leiden, The Netherlands

DKMS Clinical Trials Unit, Dresden, Germany

E. Carreras et al. (eds.), *The EBMT Handbook*, https://doi.org/10.1007/978-3-030-02278-5_6

interest, but depending on the disease and the aims of the analysis, other competing events might be included in the analysis, e.g., a second transplantation or other treatment can be considered as competing event for achievement of response.

6.3 Analysis of Time-to-Event Outcomes

Each event of interest may occur at variable times post transplant, so in statistical terms, it has two components—whether it occurs at all and, if it does, when. However, at the end of the follow-up, there can be patients who have not yet had the event of interest but are still at risk for it: their observation times are called "censored." Censoring occurs at different timepoints for different patients. The inclusion of censored data precludes the use of simple statistical methods such as the Chi-Squared or T-test and requires the methods of survival (or competing risks) analysis. The crucial assumption of most methods in survival analysis is that the patients censored at a timepoint are "represented" by those who remain under follow-up beyond that timepoint. In other words, the fact that a patient is censored should not indicate that his/her prognosis is worse or better than the prognosis of a similar patient who remains under observation. This assumption is called "independent and uninformative" censoring.

6.3.1 Kaplan-Meier Curves

The main method to summarize survival endpoints is the Kaplan-Meier curve (Kaplan and Meier 1958), estimating for each point in time t after HSCT the probability S(t) of surviving beyond that time. This curve is decreasing from 100% and will reach 0% with complete follow-up. A long flat tail of the curve (often called "plateau") is often based on a few censored observations at late times, corresponding to very unreliable estimates of the long-term survival. It is useful to report each S(t) with its 95%CI (confidence interval at 95% level, best obtained using the Greenwood formula) or at least the number of patients still at risk at different timepoints. The median survival time is the minimum time when S(t) is equal to 50% (Fig. 6.1).

6.3.2 Cumulative Incidence Curves

The appropriate method to summarize endpoints with competing risks is the cumulative incidence

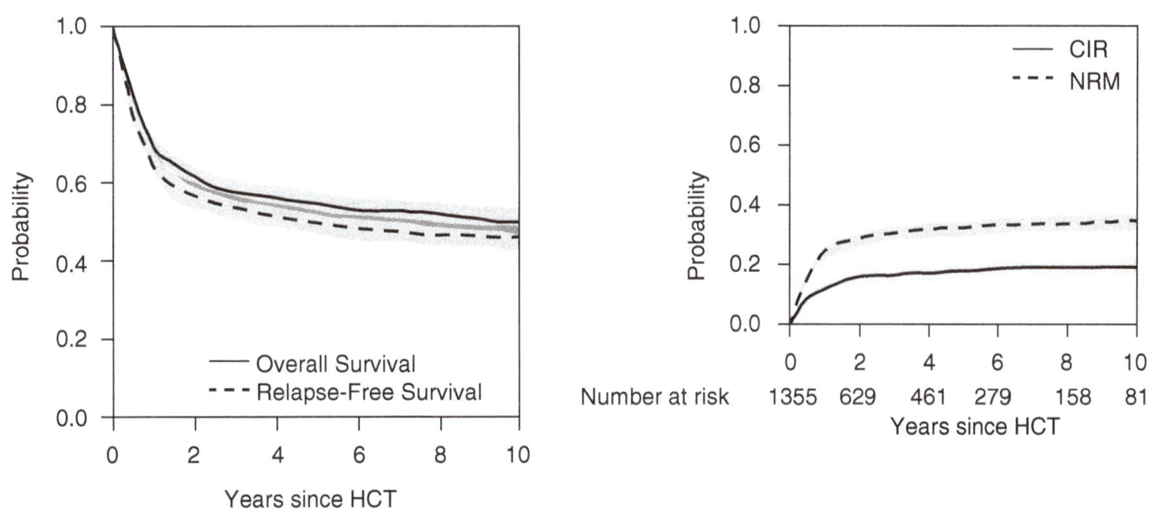

Fig. 6.1 Probability curves of the four main outcomes after HSCT. *CIR* Cumulative Incidence of Relapse. CIR and NRM add up to 1-RFS. Number at risk indicates the number of patients in follow-up who have not experienced an event so far. The grey zones indicate 95% confidence intervals

(CI) curve (Gooley et al. 1999), estimating for each point in time *t* the probability F(t) of having had the event of interest before that time. This curve is increasing from 0% and will not reach 100% even with complete follow-up if the competing event was observed for some patients. It is always useful to interpret CI curves of competing events together, to understand, e.g., when a category of patients has a small risk of relapse, if this means that they have a good prognosis or that they died too early from complications to experience a relapse (shown by a high NRM curve) (Fig. 6.1).

6.3.3 Comparison of Groups

The main method to compare survival curves for two or more independent groups is the Log-Rank test. This test is based on the comparison of the underlying hazard functions, which express the instantaneous probability of the event at a time t among patients currently at risk. It has good properties in the situation of proportional hazards (PH, described in the next section), but it should be avoided (or considered carefully) when the survival curves cross; with converging curve alternatives like the Wilcoxon Signed-Rank test should be preferred.

In the comparison of cumulative incidence curves, the main method is the Gray test. Also the Log-Rank test can be applied to compare groups in the case of competing risks, when the object of interest is not the cumulative probability of occurrence of the event but its instantaneous probability among the cases at risk at each time, which is called "cause-specific hazard." For the interesting difference of the two approaches to the analysis of competing risks endpoints, see Dignam and Kocherginsky (2008).

We refer to Sects. 1.3 and 1.4 of the Guidelines for remarks on statistical testing and about proper settings for comparisons of groups. Importantly, the simple methods described in this chapter can be applied only to groups defined at or before the time origin (e.g., transplantation); assessing differences between groups defined during the follow-up requires other approaches, as those described in Sect. 6.4.1 (Guidelines page 14).

6.3.4 Proportional Hazards Regression Analysis

The above tests do not give a summary measure of the difference in outcomes between groups, nor can they be used when the impact of a continuous risk factor (e.g., age) has to be assessed. Furthermore, any comparison could be affected by confounding. These limitations are typically overcome by applying a (multivariable) regression model. The one most commonly used for survival endpoints is the proportional hazards (PH) Cox model (Cox 1972). Results are provided in terms of hazard ratios (HR), which are assumed to be constant during the whole follow-up (Guidelines 4.3.1). The Cox model in its simplest form is thus not appropriate when a factor has an effect that strongly decreases (or increases) over time, but time-varying effects can be accommodated for in more complex models. Effects of characteristics which change during follow-up can be assessed by including them as time-dependent covariates.

For endpoints with competing risks, two methods can be used, which have a different focus: the Cox model can be used to analyse cause-specific hazards, whereas a regression model for cumulative incidence curves was proposed by Fine and Gray (1999).

The use of these regression models requires a sound statistical knowledge, as there are many potential difficulties with the methods both in application and interpretation of results.

6.4 Advanced Methods

Many more advanced methods than the ones described above exist that help to get more insights from the available data. A good application of these needs expert statistical knowledge. The brief introductions given below are primarily meant to help understanding papers where these methods have been applied. For a more in-depth discussion, see, e.g., Therneau and Grambsch (2000).

6.4.1 Multistate Models

The methodology of multistate models (Putter et al. 2007) has been developed to understand the interplay between different clinical events and interventions after HSCT and their impact on subsequent prognosis. Their primary advantage is that sequences of events, such as HSCT, DLI, GVHD, and death, and competing events, such as relapse and NRM, can be modelled simultaneously (see Fig. 6.2 for an example). This is in contrast to analysing composite survival outcomes such as GVHD-free survival where all failures are combined and resolution of GVHD is not considered. Some studies applying this method that offer new insights into the outcomes after HSCT are Klein et al. (2000) about current leukemia-free survival, Iacobelli et al. (2015) about the role of second HSCT and CR for MM patients, and Eefting et al. (2016) about evalution of a TCD-based strategy incorporating DLI for AML patients.

6.4.2 Random Effect Models

In standard methods, all patients are considered as independent, and each patient only contributes one observation for each endpoint. There are, however, situations when this does not hold, for instance, when patients within the same centre tend to have more similar outcomes than those from another centre or when one patient can experience more than one outcome of the same kind, e.g., infections. In these cases, the outcomes within one "cluster" (a centre or a patient) are more correlated than the outcomes between clusters, which has to be accounted for in the analysis. This is usually done by random effect models, which assume that each cluster shares an unobserved random effect. In survival analysis, these are called frailty models (Therneau and Grambsch 2000, Chap. 9). If the outcome is not an event but a value measured over time, e.g., CD8 counts, the appropriate regression models are called mixed models.

6.4.3 Long-Term Outcomes: Relative Survival/Cure Models

With improved long-term outcomes and increasing numbers of older patients, a substantial number of patients will die from other causes than the disease for which they have been transplanted and the direct and indirect consequences of its treatment. This so-called population mortality can be quantified by methods from relative survival, based on population tables describing mortality of the general population (Pohar Perme et al. 2016).

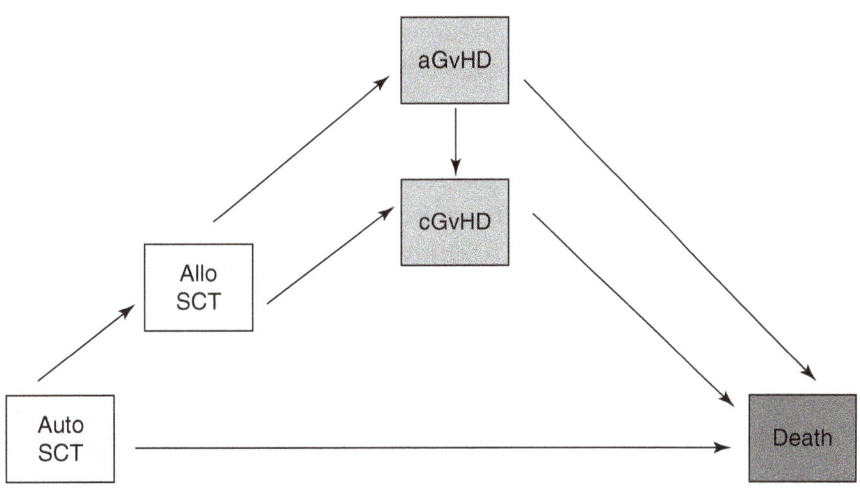

Fig. 6.2 Example of a multistate model. All patients start in state 1 (event-free after HSCT). They can then proceed through the states by different routes. Each arrow indicates a possible transition

Especially for transplanted children, a period with a high risk of mortality can be followed by a very long and stable period where the death risk is (almost) zero. When the focus of an analysis is on the probability of long-term cure, cure models can be used that assess the impact of risk factors on this but only if follow-up is sufficiently long (Sposto 2002).

6.4.4 Propensity Scores

Propensity scores (PS) are useful to compare the outcomes of two treatments in the absence of randomization, to control confounding due to the fact that usually the choice of the treatment depends on patient's characteristics (confounding by indication) (Rosenbaum and Rubin 1983). First, the PS, defined as the probability of receiving one treatment instead of the other, is estimated for each patient. Then PS can be used in various ways (mainly stratification or pair matching), allowing comparison of treatment outcomes among cases with a similar risk profile.

6.4.5 Methods for Missing Values

Missing values in risk predictors are a common problem in clinical studies. The simplest solution is to exclude the patients with missing values from the analysis (complete case analysis). This solution is not optimal, however: firstly, not all information is used (an excluded patient might have other characteristics known), and secondly, this approach can lead to bias if patients with missing values have on average a different outcome from the patients with observed values.

If values can be imputed on the basis of observed values in the dataset, these patients can be retained in the analysis to increase precision of estimates and avoid bias. The method most commonly used is called multiple imputation (White et al. 2011). A major advantage of this method is that it properly takes into account the uncertainty caused by the imputation in the estimates. If data are missing not at random—meaning their values cannot be predicted from the observed variables—multiple imputation can at most decrease the bias but not fully remove it.

Acknowledgements We thank Myriam Labopin, Richard Szydlo and Hein Putter for their contributions to this chapter.

Key Points

- Survival and competing risk endpoints need specific methods.
- Survival analysis methods: Kaplan-Meier, Log-Rank test, Cox model.
- Competing risks methods: Cumulative incidence curve, Gray test, Cox model, and Fine and Gray model.
- Including events/changes of status occurring during follow-up in an analysis requires specific (advanced) methods, like multistate models.

References

Cox DR. Regression models and life tables. J R Stat Soc. 1972;34(Series B):187–220.

Dignam JJ, Kocherginsky MN. Choice and interpretation of statistical tests used when competing risks are present. J Clin Oncol. 2008;26:4027–34.

Eefting M, de Wreede LC, Halkes CJM, et al. Multistate analysis illustrates treatment success after stem cell transplantation for acute myeloid leukemia followed by donor lymphocyte infusion. Haematologica. 2016;101:506–14.

Fine JP, Gray RJ. A proportional hazards models of the subdistribution of a competing risk. J Am Stat Assoc. 1999;94:496–509.

Gooley TA, Leisenring W, Crowley JA, et al. Estimation of failure probabilities in the presence of competing risks: new representations of old estimators. Stat Med. 1999;18:695–706.

Iacobelli S, de Wreede LC, Schönland S, et al. Impact of CR before and after allogeneic and autologous transplantation in multiple myeloma: results from the EBMT NMAM2000 prospective trial. Bone Marrow Transplant. 2015;50:505–10.

Iacobelli S, on behalf of the EBMT Statistical Committee. Suggestions on the use of statistical methodologies in studies of the European Group for Blood and Marrow Transplantation. Bone Marrow Transplant. 2013;48:S1–S37.

Kaplan EL, Meier P. Non-parametric estimation from incomplete observations. J Am Stat Assoc. 1958;53:457–81.

Klein JP, Szydlo RM, Craddock C, et al. Estimation of current leukaemia-free survival following donor lymphocyte infusion therapy for patients with leukaemia who relapse after allografting: application of a multi-state model. Stat Med. 2000;19:3005–16.

Pohar Perme M, Estève J, Rachet B. Analysing population-based cancer survival – settling the controversies. BMC Cancer. 2016;16:933.

Putter H, Fiocco M, Geskus RB. Tutorial in biostatistics: competing risks and multi-state models. Stat Med. 2007;26:2389–430.

Rosenbaum PR, Rubin DB. The central role of the propensity score in observational studies for causal effects. Biometrika. 1983;70:41–55.

Sposto R. Cure model analysis in cancer: an application to data from the Children's Cancer group. Stat Med. 2002;21:293–312.

Therneau TM, Grambsch PM. Modeling survival data: extending the Cox model. New York: Springer; 2000.

White IR, Royston P, Wood AM. Multiple imputation using chained equations: issues and guidance for practice. Stat Med. 2011;30:377–99.

Part II

Biological Aspects

Topic leaders: Chiara Bonini and Jürgen Kuball

7 Biological Properties of HSC: Scientific Basis for HSCT

Alessandro Aiuti, Serena Scala, and Christian Chabannon

7.1 Introduction

Hematopoiesis—from the Greek term for "blood making"—is the adaptive process by which mature and functional blood cells are continuously replaced over the entire lifetime of an individual. Erythrocytes, platelets, and the various subsets of leukocytes all have finite although different life spans. As a consequence, the daily production of red blood cells, platelets, and neutrophils in homeostatic conditions amount to more than 300 billion cells.

In mammals, after the emergence of the first hematopoietic progenitors in extra-embryonic structures such as the yolk sac in mice, cells of hematopoietic nature are first detected in the aorto-gonado-mesonephric (AGM) region of the developing embryo (Costa et al. 2012). The site of hematopoiesis then moves to the fetal liver and next to the BM where it remains established until the death of the individual. Extramedullary hematopoiesis in humans denotes a myeloproliferative syndrome.

The considerable knowledge accumulated over more than a century of experimental hematology led to the early understanding that all hematopoietic lineages are derived from a small subpopulation of undifferentiating and self-renewing stem cells. HSC represent the most accurately explored model of somatic stem cells that are present in most if not all tissues and organs, contributing to tissue homeostasis and repair. Existence of a population of HSC also has practical implications in terms of developing innovative therapies aiming at the definitive replacement or enhancement of a function in cells from one or several hematopoietic lineages, including the possibility to establish durable hematopoietic chimerism in recipients of allogeneic HSCT.

7.2 Self-Renewal

A general property of stem cells is self-renewal, assuming that when these cells divide, at least one of the "daughter cells" fully recapitulate the biological properties of the "mother stem cell." Self-renewal of the HSC population prevents

A. Aiuti
San Raffaele Telethon Institute for Gene Therapy (SR-TIGET)/Pediatric Immunohematology and Bone Marrow Transplantation Unit, IRCCS Ospedale San Raffaele, Vita-Salute San Raffaele University, Milan, Italy

S. Scala
San Raffaele Telethon Institute for Gene Therapy (SR-TIGET), IRCCS Ospedale San Raffaele, Milan, Italy

C. Chabannon (✉)
Institut Paoli-Calmettes, Centre de Lutte Contre le Cancer, Marseille, France

Université d'Aix-Marseille, Marseille, France

Inserm BCT-1409, Centre d'Investigations Cliniques en Biothérapies, Marseille, France
e-mail: chabannonc@ipc.unicancer.fr

E. Carreras et al. (eds.), *The EBMT Handbook*, https://doi.org/10.1007/978-3-030-02278-5_7

exhaustion, while the hematopoietic tissue extensively proliferates and differentiates in steady-state conditions, as well as to repair various damages. Demonstration of self-renewal at the clonal level remains an arduous task, even though high-throughput analytical tools have been adapted. There is a growing body of evidence suggesting aging of the HSC population and decline of stem cell function with age (for a review, see Goodell and Rando 2015; de Haan and Lazare 2018). Appearance of "passenger mutations" in clonal hematopoiesis is one hallmark of aging (Cooper and Young 2017); the significance of such observations remains to be fully elucidated, but obviously raises questions when it comes to solicit elderly individuals to donate HSC for the benefit of a related patient.

7.3 Commitment and Differentiation: New Data Challenge the Historical View of Hematopoietic Hierarchy

The traditional view of HSC differentiation is a hierarchical representation of an inverted tree, where discrete and homogenous populations branch from one another, with successive restrictions in differentiation potentials. This oversimplifying view is increasingly challenged by recent studies reporting on noninvasive genetic experiments and clonal analyses in mice (for a review, see Laurenti and Göttgens 2018; Busch and Rodewald 2016). These studies suggest that hematopoietic differentiation uses different mechanisms under steady-state and stress conditions (Goyal and Zandstra 2015); however, both in steady-state conditions and transplantation models, only a small fraction of HSC contribute to long-term and stable reconstitution without compromising reestablishment of hematopoiesis (Schoedel et al. 2016; Höfer and Rodewald 2016), while most stem cells remain quiescent or proliferate infrequently. Single-cell transcriptional landscapes also suggest that differentiation occurs as a continuous rather than discrete physiological process and that restriction of differentiation is not the result of a "symmetric split" between the myeloid and lymphoid compartments as long thought through the phenotypic identification of "common myeloid progenitors" (CMP) and "common lymphoid progenitors" (CLP).

Commitment to one or several lineages, or conversely restriction in differentiation abilities, results from the expression of a controlled genetic and epigenetic program (Pouzolles et al. 2016; Antoniani et al. 2017; Gottgens, 2015); these mechanisms remain partially understood and thus can only be partially harnessed for in vitro engineering of HSC and their progeny (Rowe et al. 2016). The fate of HSC and their progeny is additionally regulated by extrinsic signals, among which hematopoietic growth factors and cytokines play an important role in survival, proliferation, and amplification (Kaushansky, 2006).

7.4 The Bone Marrow Niches and Maintenance of Stemness (Fig. 7.1)

Recent years have witnessed considerable progress in our understanding of organization and function of the bone marrow microenvironment. HSC establish interactions in the context of microanatomical organizations termed "niches." Progress has been made both in understanding the heterogeneity of niches at and within successive hematopoietic sites and in identifying various categories of cells—either of non-hematopoietic or of hematopoietic origin—that interact with HSC. The various types of bone marrow niches closely associate with the neurovascular network that infiltrates the central bone marrow as well as the endosteal region. The nature of the signaling between these different cell populations is also increasingly deciphered and involves many pathways, some of them unexpected at first (for a review, see Crane et al. 2017; Calvi and Link 2015). Replicating some of these interactions in vitro is key to successful expansion or genetic engineering of isolated HSC. Among the many molecular actors that govern interactions between HSC and the various cells present in niches, the CXCL12 chemokine and its most important

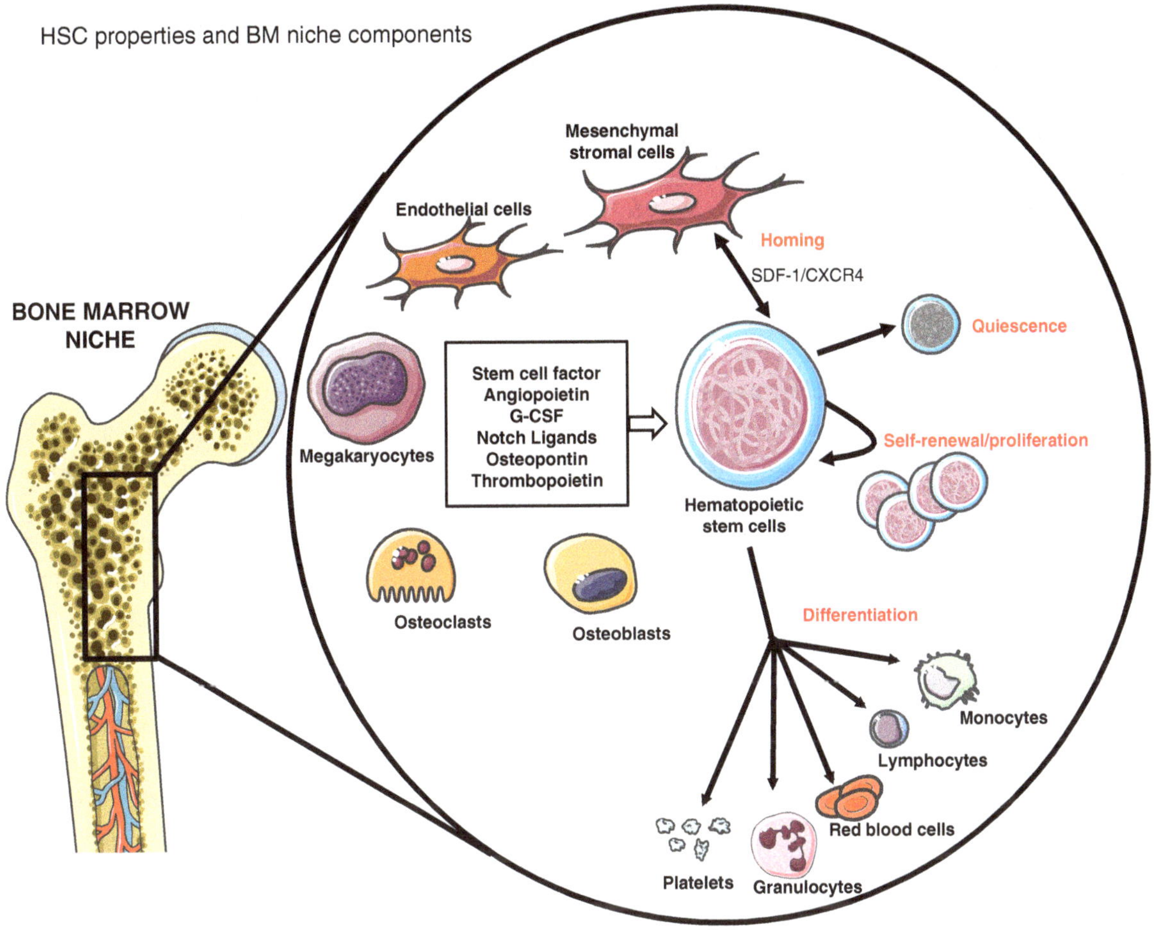

Fig. 7.1 HSC properties and BM niche components

receptor CXCR4 are of particular interest: direct or indirect modulation of this axis is clinically exploited to amplify the compartment of circulating stem cells that exist at low numbers in steady-state conditions.

7.5 Preclinical Models of HSCT

Most of the current knowledge on the biology of HSC and on therapeutic mechanisms of HSCT derives from studies in animal models (Eaves, 2015; Sykes and Scadden 2013). Classical murine transplantation studies showed that single or few engrafting HSC were sufficient and necessary to sustain long-term hematopoiesis in a reconstituted mouse. Human-in-mouse xenografts have become a fundamental tool to study hematopoietic dynamics upon HSCT. The generation of immune-deficient mice bearing a deletion of the interleukin-2 receptor gamma chain on the NOD-SCID background (NSG mice) was instrumental for studying HSC homing, engraftment, lineage differentiation, and serial transplantation capacity. This model has been further modified by introducing human myeloid cytokine genes to increase myeloid differentiation (Doulatov et al. 2012) or loss-of-function mutation in KIT receptor to efficiently support engraftment of human HSC without the need for conditioning therapy (Cosgun et al. 2014). To overcome the lack of human components in the murine BM, humanized-BM niche systems have been recently developed which are based on human stromal cells implanted on specific scaffold or directly injected with extracellular matrix to generate BM micro-ossicles (Di Maggio et al. 2011; Reinisch et al. 2016). These strategies provide novel tools to study the behavior of human HSC in their physiological context and to dissect the role of the niche upon transplantation. However, homing and engraftment parameters in xenografts may be different from the natural setting, and most HSCT models follow recipient mice for few months after transplantations, thus making long-term outcome difficult to assess.

Dogs provide an ideal preclinical modeling system for HSCT studies due to their large body size, life span, and high genetic diversity, which more appropriately recapitulate the human scenario. Preclinical canine modeling has been fundamental for the clinical translation of conditioning regimens and the importance of MHC donor/recipient matching. However, the lack of canine reagents and the logistic difficulties of working with large animal models have precluded widespread availability (Stolfi et al. 2016). Auto-HSCT in nonhuman primates is arguably the experimental model most closely resembling humans; their treatment conditions—including the use of CD34+ cells, mobilization, and conditioning regimens—all parallel those commonly exploited in human transplantation. While the ethical issues and costs have limited their use to selected centers, these animals are able to maintain long-term hematopoiesis up to several years after transplantation allowing the study of HSCT dynamics in a close-to-human fashion (Koelle et al. 2017).

7.6 Gene Transfer/Gene Editing/ Gene Therapy Targeting HSC (Fig. 7.2)

Ex vivo HSC gene therapy (GT) is based on the genetic modification of autologous HSC to correct monogenic disorders or to provide novel features to hematopoietic cells for treating infectious diseases or cancers (Naldini, 2011). It is now well established that HSC can be efficiently gene modified to continuously produce a cell progeny expressing the therapeutic gene while maintaining the ability to engraft long-term, for at least 15 years (Cicalese et al. 2016). Potential advantages of this approach over allogeneic HSCT include the lack of GVHD or rejection and the possibility of engineering HSC in order to achieve supra-physiological level of the corrected protein (Naldini, 2011; Aiuti and Naldini 2016).

Currently, integrating vectors derived from retroviruses represent the most efficient platform for engineering HSC and to provide permanent and heritable gene correction. γ-Retroviral vectors (RV) have been used in many clinical applications including GT of inherited blood disorders and cancer therapy. HSC-GT in primary immunodeficiencies was shown to provide clinical benefit, but the use of γ-RV was associated with risks of insertional mutagenesis due to activation of proto-oncogenes with the exception of ADA deficiency (Cicalese et al. 2016). Self-inactivating (SIN)-lentiviral vectors (LV) are currently the tools of choice for most of the HSC-GT applications given their ability to transduce at higher efficiency non-dividing cells, to carry larger and more complex gene cassettes, and to display a safer insertion site (InS) pattern in human HSC (Naldini, 2011). The recent development of designer endonucleases led to the advent of gene targeting approaches. In contrast to viral vectors, which can mediate only one type of gene modification (gene addition), genome-editing technologies can mediate gene addition, gene disruption, gene correction, and other targeted genome modifications (Dunbar et al. 2018). These strategies have the potential to overcome vector InS genotoxicity and to handle diseases due to dominant negative mutations. Despite the great promises, several challenges need to be addressed. Primitive, slow-cycling human BM-derived HSC are very resistant to ex vivo manipulations required for gene targeting, and the current efficiency of gene editing into repopulating HSC may not be suitable for clinical applications requiring high levels of correction (Dunbar et al. 2018; Kohn, 2017).

Thus, there remains a pressing need to develop methods to expand HSC or gene-corrected HSC while maintaining their repopulating capacity. Various cytokines and growth factors derived from BM niche, such as SCF, TPO, and Flt-3 ligand, are able to regulate HSC stemness and differentiation and are commonly used in HSC transduction protocols. However, even efficiently supporting GT, the balance between self-renewal/differentiation still hangs toward differentiation. High-throughput screening of chemical compounds has resulted in the identification of two promising molecules (StemRegenin1, SR1 (Wagner et al. 2016) and a

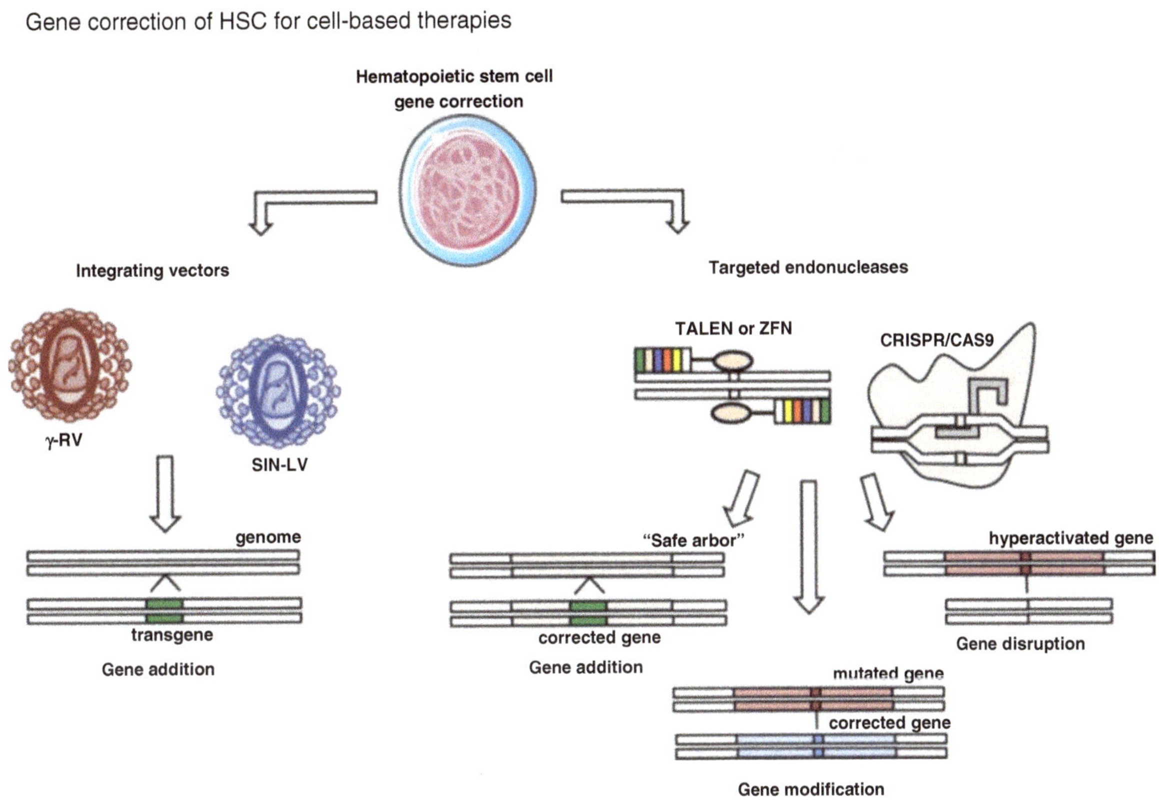

Fig. 7.2 Gene correction of HSC for cell-based therapies

pyrimidole derivative UM171 (Fares et al. 2014)) that are able to achieve great expansion of long-term repopulating HSC. Several small molecules have been identified that may support modest degrees of HSC expansion, but the ideal drug or combination has not yet been reported.

7.7 Studying Dynamics of Hematopoietic Reconstitution upon HSCT (Fig. 7.3)

Upon gene correction, each transduced cell and its progeny become univocally marked by a specific insertion site (InS). The analysis of RV or LV InS has emerged as one of the most effective strategies allowing tracing the activity of genetically engineered hematopoietic cells directly in vivo in animal models as well as in GT-treated patients. Retrieving InS from mature blood cells after HSCT allowed studying the kinetics of blood cell production from individual stem cells within a heterogeneous population (Scala et al. 2016).

In the murine setting, the finding that the vast majority of the InS after transplant were present in either lymphoid or myeloid cells with few InS shared by both lineages led to the concept that murine HSC are heterogeneous and already biased for their fate. The possibility to directly translate these models on human beings is currently under investigation (Lu et al. 2011; Yamamoto et al. 2013).

Clonal tracking studies in nonhuman primates have been pivotal in studying HSCT dynamics in an experimental setting close to humans. The results of these works showed common pattern of hematopoietic reconstitution upon transplantation: clonal fluctuation in the early phases post-HSCT, potentially due to the initial contribution to the hematopoiesis of short-term unilineage progenitors, followed by a recovery of a stable hematopoietic output likely related to the take-over of long-term multipotent HSC contribution. Thus, differently from murine studies, long-term HSC are able to provide multi-lineage engraftment, and there is no evidence of predetermined lineage choice at stem cell level in primates (Koelle et al. 2017; Kim et al. 2014).

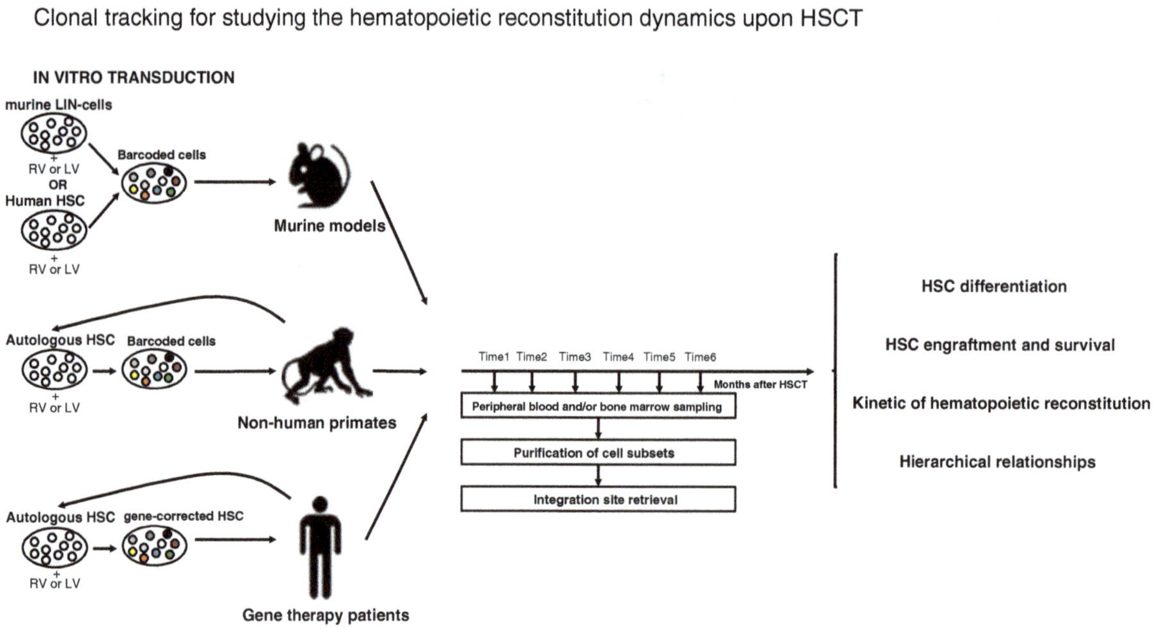

Fig. 7.3 Clonal tracking for studying the hematopoietic reconstitution dynamics upon HSCT

To date, few cutting-edge studies have exploited InS retrieval from GT-treated patients allowing for the first time to study the complexity of hematopoietic system and hematopoietic reconstitution upon HSCT in humans (Biasco et al. 2016; Wang et al. 2010). These studies showed that transplanted gene-repaired HSC are able to engraft and to generate polyclonal multi-lineage output overtime. Longitudinal analyses allowed unveiling that unilineage clones active during the first 6 months after GT tend to be replaced by multilineage long-term clones, indicating HSC-derived activity. Finally, based on the number of InS recaptured overtime, it has been estimated that about 1 in 10^5–10^6 infused gene-corrected cells had the potential to engraft long term. Recently our group unveiled for the first time that primitive HSPC have a distinct role in sustaining human hematopoiesis after transplantation. While MPP are more active in the early phases, long-living HSC are on top of the hematopoietic hierarchy at steady state. Importantly we found that long-term HSC, that were activated in vitro, were capable of homing and resilience upon re-infusion (Scala et al. 2018). These approaches represent a prototypical example of the power of translational studies, providing information relevant on human hematopoietic system complementing and expanding the data derived from animal models.

7.8 From Experimental Hematology to Medical Practices and Hematopoietic Cellular Therapies

As already stressed in this brief review, a considerable amount of knowledge has accumulated over years allowing us to understand part of the mechanisms that control HSC behavior and take advantage of this knowledge; many of these observations cross-fertilized other disciplines. A large gap however persists between the technological sophistication of research tools and the rudimentary nature of clinical grade reagents, devices, and laboratory tests. In clinical transplantation or even in the most modern forms of hematopoietic cellular therapies, stem cells remain identified as "CD34$^+$ cells," which can at best be considered as a gross approach to stemness; functional assays are limited to clonogenic cultures in routine practice; flow cytometry-activated cell sorting barely entered the clinical field, and most cell selection procedures rely on immune selection with magnetic beads. Despite these limitations, and as can be seen from the content of the other chapters in this book, HSCT remains as the only example of a worldwide and widely used cell transplant procedure, with many of its underlying conceptual aspects and techniques being used to design innovative and highly personalized somatic cell therapy or gene therapy medicinal products.

Key Points

HSC characteristics

- Self-renewal: ability of HSC to divide maintaining their biological properties
- Multipotency: ability of HSC to generate all mature hematopoietic cell types
- Quiescence: ability of HSC to remain inactive and unresponsive to external stimuli

Models of hematopoietic hierarchy

- Classical model: HSC differentiate into discrete and homogenous populations with successive restrictions in differentiation potentials
- Functional model: HSC differentiate according to hematopoietic state (stressed vs. unperturbed hematopoiesis)
- Progressive model: HSC differentiate through a continuous rather than discrete physiological process as result of a controlled genetic and epigenetic programs

Preclinical models of HSCT

- Murine models: study of HSC homing, engraftment, lineage differentiation, and serial transplantation capacity
- Canine models: validation of conditioning regimens and assessment of MHC donor/recipient matching significance
- Nonhuman primates: evaluation of mobilization procedures, conditioning regimens, and long-term maintenance of hematopoiesis

Ex vivo *gene therapy*

- Integrating vectors: γ-retroviral vectors (RV) and self-inactivating (SIN)-lentiviral vectors
- Genome editing: zinc-finger nucleases (ZFN), transcription activator-like effector nucleases (TALEN), and clustered, regularly interspaced, short palindromic repeat (CRISPR) nucleases

References

Aiuti A, Naldini L. Safer conditioning for blood stem cell transplants. Nat Biotechnol. 2016;34:721–3.

Antoniani C, Romano O, Miccio A. Concise review: epigenetic regulation of hematopoiesis: biological insights and therapeutic applications. Stem Cells Transl Med. 2017;6:2106–14.

Biasco L, Pellin D, Scala S, et al. In vivo tracking of human hematopoiesis reveals patterns of clonal dynamics during early and steady-state reconstitution phases. Cell Stem Cell. 2016;19:107–19.

Busch K, Rodewald HR. Unperturbed vs. post-transplantation hematopoiesis: both in vivo but different. Curr Opin Hematol. 2016;23:295–303.

Calvi LM, Link DC. The hematopoietic stem cell niche in homeostasis and disease. Blood. 2015;126:2443–52.

Cicalese MP, Ferrua F, Castagnaro L, et al. Update on the safety and efficacy of retroviral gene therapy for immunodeficiency due to adenosine deaminase deficiency. Blood. 2016;128:45–55.

Cooper JN, Young NS. Clonality in context: hematopoietic clones in their marrow environment. Blood. 2017;130:2363–72.

Cosgun KN, Rahmig S, Mende N, et al. Kit regulates HSC engraftment across the human-mouse species barrier. Cell Stem Cell. 2014;15:227–38.

Costa G, Kouskoff V, Lacaud G. Origin of blood cells and HSC production in the embryo. Trends Immunol. 2012;33:215–23.

Crane GM, Jeffery E, Morrison SJ. Adult haematopoietic stem cell niches. Nat Rev Immunol. 2017;17:573–90.

Di Maggio N, Piccinini E, Jaworski M, et al. Toward modeling the bone marrow niche using scaffold-based 3D culture systems. Biomaterials. 2011;32:321–9.

Doulatov S, Notta F, Laurenti E, et al. Hematopoiesis: a human perspective. Cell Stem Cell. 2012;10:120–36.

Dunbar CE, High KA, Joung JK, et al. Gene therapy comes of age. Science. 2018;359:1–10.

Eaves CJ. Hematopoietic stem cells: concepts, definitions, and the new reality. Blood. 2015;125:2605–14.

Fares I, Chagraoui J, Gareau Y, et al. Pyrimidoindole derivatives are agonists of human hematopoietic stem cell self-renewal. Science. 2014;345:1509–12.

Goodell MA, Rando TA. Stem cells and healthy aging. Science. 2015;350:1199–204.

Gottgens B. Regulatory network control of blood stem cells. Blood. 2015;125:2614–21.

Goyal S, Zandstra PW. Stem cells: chasing blood. Nature. 2015;518:488–90.

de Haan G, Lazare S. Aging of hematopoietic stem cells. Blood. 2018;131:479–87.

Höfer T, Rodewald HR. Output without input: the lifelong productivity of hematopoietic stem cells. Curr Opin Cell Biol. 2016;43:69–77.

Kaushansky K. Lineage-specific hematopoietic growth factors. N Engl J Med. 2006;354:2034–45.

Kim S, Kim N, Presson AP, et al. Dynamics of HSPC repopulation in nonhuman primates revealed by a decade-long clonal-tracking study. Cell Stem Cell. 2014;14:473–85.

Koelle SJ, Espinoza DA, Wu C, et al. Quantitative stability of hematopoietic stem and progenitor cell clonal output in transplanted rhesus macaques. Blood. 2017;129:1448–57.

Kohn DB. Historical perspective on the current renaissance for hematopoietic stem cell gene therapy. Hematol Oncol Clin North Am. 2017;31:721–35.

Laurenti E, Göttgens B. Review from haematopoietic stem cells to complex differentiation landscapes. Nature. 2018;553:418–26.

Lu R, Neff NF, Quake SR, et al. Tracking single hematopoietic stem cells in vivo using high-throughput sequencing in conjunction with viral genetic barcoding. Nat Biotechnol. 2011;29:928–33.

Naldini L. Ex vivo gene transfer and correction for cell-based therapies. Nat Rev Genet. 2011;12:301–15.

Pouzolles M, Oburoglu L, Taylor N, et al. Hematopoietic stem cell lineage specification. Curr Opin Hematol. 2016;23:311–7.

Reinisch A, Thomas D, Corces MR, et al. A humanized bone marrow ossicle xenotransplantation model enables improved engraftment of healthy and leukemic human hematopoietic cells. Nat Med. 2016;22:812–21.

Rowe RG, Mandelbaum J, Zon LI, et al. Engineering hematopoietic stem cells: lessons from development. Cell Stem Cell. 2016;18:707–20.

Scala S, Leonardelli L, Biasco L. Current approaches and future perspectives for in vivo clonal tracking of hematopoietic cells. Curr Gene Ther. 2016;16:1–10.

Scala S, Basso-Ricci L, Dionisio F, Pellin D, Giannelli S, Salerio FA, Leonardelli L, Cicalese MP, Ferrua F, Aiuti A, Biasco L. Dynamics of genetically engineered hematopoietic stem and progenitor cells after autologous transplantation in humans. Nat Med. 2018;24(11):1683–90. https://doi.org/10.1038/s41591-018-0195-3.

Schoedel KB, Morcos MNF, Zerjatke T, et al. The bulk of the hematopoietic stem cell population is dispensable for murine steady-state and stress hematopoiesis. Blood. 2016;128:2285–96.

Stolfi JL, Pai C-CS, Murphy WJ. Preclinical modeling of hematopoietic stem cell transplantation—advantages and limitations. FEBS J. 2016;283:1595–606.

Sykes SM, Scadden DT. Modeling human hematopoietic stem cell biology in the mouse. Semin Hematol. 2013;2:1–14.

Wagner JE, Brunstein CG, Boitano AE, et al. Phase I/II trial of stemregenin-1 expanded umbilical cord blood hematopoietic stem cells supports testing as a stand-alone graft. Cell Stem Cell. 2016;18:144–55.

Wang GP, Berry CC, Malani N, et al. Dynamics of gene-modified progenitor cells analyzed by tracking retroviral integration sites in a human SCID-X1 gene therapy trial. Blood. 2010;115:4356–66.

Yamamoto R, Morita Y, Ooehara J, et al. Clonal analysis unveils self-renewing lineage-restricted progenitors generated directly from hematopoietic stem cells. Cell. 2013;154:1112–26.

8 Biological Properties of Cells Other Than HSCs

Attilio Bondanza, Ulrike Koehl, Andrea Hoffmann, and Antoine Toubert

8.1 Introduction

The array of cellular players involved in the biology of HSCT clearly extends beyond HSC themselves and, in the case of transplantation from allogeneic sources, importantly includes cells of the innate and adaptive immune system. Historically, the discovery of the HLA system and the functional characterization of the different immune cell types had a transformational impact on our current understanding of the pathobiological *sequelae* of allo-HSCT (rejection, GVHD, the GVL effect). This body of knowledge coupled to the most recent *exploit* of biotechnology nowadays allows us to design strategies for in vivo stimulation or adoptive transfer of specific immune cell types with the potential to dramatically improve transplantation outcome.

In this chapter, we will review the biological properties of cells other than HSCs that so far have Since apart from vaccination antigen presenting cells and myeloid cells at large have seldom been subject of this type of studies been therapeutically investigated in human allo-HSCT, they will not be discussed here. Conversely, we will briefly touch on mesenchymal stromal cells (MSCs), which, although not classifiable as immune cells *stricto* sensu, have been widely employed in allo-HSCT.

8.2 Conventional or Alpha-Beta T Cells

The majority of mature T cells is characterized by the expression of the αβ TCR, which endows MHC-restricted recognition of peptides derived from non-self-proteins. Mutually exclusive co-expression of CD8 or CD4 further conveys specificity for MHC class I/MHC class II/peptide complexes, respectively. CD8+ T cells recognize intracellular peptides, mainly derived from viruses or mutated genes, mediating cytotoxicity of infected or transformed cells, thence the name cytotoxic T lymphocytes (CTLs). Conversely, CD4+ T cells recognize extracellular pathogen-derived peptides, providing antigen-specific

A. Bondanza (✉)
Innovative Immunotherapies Unit, Division of Immunology, Transplantation and Infectious Diseases, University Vita-Salute San Raffaele and Ospedale San Raffaele Scientific Institute, Milan, Italy
e-mail: Bondanza.Attilio@hsr.it

U. Koehl
University Hospital and Fraunhofer IZI, Leipzig, Germany

Hannover Medical School, Hannover, Germany

A. Hoffmann
Department of Orthopaedic Surgery, Laboratory of Biomechanics and Biomaterials, Hannover Medical School, Hannover, Germany

A. Toubert
University Paris Diderot and Hopital Saint Louis, Paris, France

E. Carreras et al. (eds.), *The EBMT Handbook*, https://doi.org/10.1007/978-3-030-02278-5_8

specific "help" to bystander immune cells, such as B cells in antibody production and phagocytes in killing of engulfed pathogens. Alloreactivity occurs because of αβ TCR-mediated recognition of mismatched HLAs or of non-HLA polymorphic peptides presented in the context of matched HLAs, e.g., those derived from H-Y (male-specific histocompatibility antigen). The latter are known as minor histocompatibility antigens (mHag) and play a major role in GVHD and the GVL effect after HLA-matched transplantation.

The adoptive transfer of CTLs specific for important opportunistic viruses in allo-HSCT (CMV, EBV, ADV) has been one of the first manipulated cellular immunotherapies to be tested in humans (Bollard and Heslop 2016) and in some EU countries is now available as an off-the-shelf therapy from HLA-matched donors. Conversely, it has been proposed that naïve T cells, i.e., cells that have never encountered their cognate antigen, may be more alloreactive than memory T cells, i.e., antigen-experienced cells that have persisted after clearing the infection. This concept is at the basis of protocols for the depletion of naïve T cells from the graft as a way to prevent GVHD while retaining a strong GVL effect (Bleakley et al. 2015). Promising are also attempts at translating this approach against hematological tumor antigens for treating overt leukemia relapse after allo-HSCT (Chapuis et al. 2013). On a different page, given the overall complexity of immune responses, it is not surprising that during evolution, some immune cell types have evolved with the specific task of immune regulation. T regulatory cells (Tregs) are thymus-derived cells characterized by constitutive expression of the transcription factor FoxP3. Tregs are potent suppressors of alloreactivity and are now being investigated for GVHD management after their ex vivo expansion (Brunstein et al. 2016).

8.3 Unconventional T Cells

Unconventional T cells include T cells expressing the γδ TCR, invariant natural killer T cells (iNKT) cells, and mucosal-associated invariant (MAIT) T cells—which will not be treated here—and are an abundant component of the immune system. Although originating from the thymus, they all share lack of MHC-restricted peptide recognition and mainly reside within epithelial tissues. They have a limited TCR repertoire diversity and get activated quickly, bridging innate to adaptive immunity.

1. A subset of γδ T cells (Vγ2Vδ9) are activated by phosphoantigens, non-peptidic metabolites produced by mammalian cells and intracellular pathogens (*M. tuberculosis*, *M. leprae*, *Listeria* species, *Plasmodium* species) after interacting with intracellular butyrophilin 3A1. Gamma-delta T cells can also recognize stress molecules such as MICA, MICB, and ULBPs through the NK receptor NKG2D. The possibility to expand Vγ2Vδ9 effector T cells in vivo by administering the therapeutic bisphosphonate zoledronate has originated many clinical trials in hematological tumors, also in the context of transplantation (Airoldi et al. 2015).
2. Type I invariant NKT is a distinct population of αβ T cells characterized in humans by the expression of α24-Jα18 preferentially paired to Vβ11. They recognize lipids presented in the context of broadly distributed CD1d (monocytes/macrophages, B cells, epithelial cells). Upon activation, iNKT cells produce immune regulatory cytokines and kill tumor targets. Failure to reconstitute iNKT cells after Allo-HSCT (Rubio et al. 2012) or lower iNKT cells in the graft (Chaidos et al. 2012) has been linked to GVHD and relapse. Alpha-galactosyl ceramide is a marine sponge-derived lipid antigen known to expand iNKT cells in vivo and is currently under investigation in Allo-HSCT (Chen et al. 2017).

8.4 NK Cells

Natural killer (NK) cells belong to the innate immune system and provide immediate reactivity against virally infected, as well as tumor targets. NK cytotoxicity is controlled by a balance of several germ-line encoded inhibitory and activating receptors, such as killer immunoglobulin-like receptors (KIRs) and natural cytotoxicity receptors (Vivier et al. 2011). The importance of NK cells in allo-HSCT has surfaced after the demonstration of their pivotal role in preventing leukemia relapse and decreasing GVHD risk after grafting from HLA-haploidentical donors (Ruggeri et al. 2002). Since then, there has been a growing interest in using both autologous and allogeneic NK cells in patients with leukemia or other high-risk hematological tumors, also in the non-transplant setting (Koehl et al. 2016). These trials have uniformly shown safety and potential efficacy of infused NK cells. Nevertheless, they have also documented the emergence of powerful immune escape mechanisms, raising the question on how to improve NK cell-based therapies (Koehl et al. 2018). Various trials are under way in order to investigate ways to achieve better NK cell cytotoxicity and overcome the immunosuppressive tumor microenvironment, including:

1. Combination of novel checkpoint inhibitors with activated NK cells
2. Bi- or tri-specific antibodies for directly binding NK cells to cancer cells
3. Chimeric antigen receptor (CAR)-modified NK cells for direct targeting of cancer cells

The latter strategy is particularly interesting since CAR-NK cells are expected to retain their natural antitumor reactivity, opening for potentially synergistic effects. The first clinical CAR-NK cell studies targeting CD19 and NKG2D ligands have been initiated (ClinGov. No NCT03056339, NCT01974479, NCT00995137, NCT03415100) and will likely be instrumental to demonstrate proof of concept.

8.5 Mesenchymal Stromal Cells

Mesenchymal stroma cells (MSCs) are multipotent cells capable of differentiating into cells and tissues of the mesodermal lineage (bone, cartilage, and adipose cells) (Pittenger et al. 1999). Apart from their regenerative properties, MSCs have been discovered to secrete a variety of soluble factors and exosomes with paracrine actions. Instead of focusing on MSC regenerative properties, most clinical studies have investigated their immunomodulatory (often immunosuppressive) properties, as well as their trophic influence on tissue repair, especially in GVHD (Fibbe et al. 2013). Interestingly, subsequent to hematopoietic stem cells, MSCs are the second most frequently used cell source for therapeutic applications. Notwithstanding their widespread use, MSCs are currently the stem cell population with the least defined identity and properties (Hoffmann et al. 2017).

Important studies have demonstrated that the physiological counterpart of ex vivo-expanded MSCs can be both CD146+ adventitial reticular cells in the subendothelial layer of microvessels (Tormin et al. 2011) and CD146- pericytes surrounding large vessels (Corselli et al. 2013). MSC biological functions are also highly debated and conflicting results were reported in vitro and, more importantly, in clinical trials (Fibbe et al. 2013). Considerable lack of consensus exists within the field as to how MSCs exert their multipronged effects. This is due to several facts: Firstly, MSCs are isolated from many tissues and by different protocols. Secondly, due to the mode of isolation, these cells present heterogeneous cell populations. Thirdly, protocols for in vitro expansion, including the culture conditions (culture vessels, media, additives, passaging), are different. Fourthly, MSCs have often been reported to survive in vivo only for short time (days). A recent comparison of MSC preparations from eight different centers using BM aspirates as starting material for GMP-guided processes revealed considerable variability between the centers (Liu et al. 2017). Cells from six centers were compared in vivo for bone formation and hematopoiesis support. The quantity of deriving bone was highly variable, and only MSCs from three centers supported hematopoiesis. A critical reappraisal of these cell populations and harmonization of the methods for their isolation and expansion, as well as the development of validated potency assays, is therefore necessary for harnessing their full therapeutic potential.

Key Points

- HSCT rather than a solo play is an orchestral concert, where different cellular players contribute to the overall final result of the symphony.
- Besides obviously HSCs, key contributors are cells of the innate and adaptive immune system. Both have evolved for the key task of self/non-self-discrimination, each however focusing on the recognition of different class of molecules, from proteins to glycolipids.
- The tremendous knowledge in immunobiology acquired in the last few decades has enabled to start exploiting the properties of these cells or ameliorating the outcome of HSCT.

References

Airoldi I, Bertaina A, Prigione I, et al. γδ T-cell reconstitution after HLA-haploidentical hematopoietic transplantation depleted of TCR-αβ+/CD19+ lymphocytes. Blood. 2015;125:2349–58.

Bleakley M, Heimfeld S, Loeb KR, et al. Outcomes of acute leukemia patients transplanted with naive T cell-depleted stem cell grafts. J Clin Invest. 2015;125:2677–89.

Bollard CM, Heslop HE. T cells for viral infections after allogeneic hematopoietic stem cell transplant. Blood. 2016;127:3331–40.

Brunstein CG, Miller JS, McKenna DH, et al. Umbilical cord blood-derived T regulatory cells to prevent GVHD: kinetics, toxicity profile, and clinical effect. Blood. 2016;127:1044–51.

Chaidos A, Patterson S, Szydlo R, et al. Graft invariant natural killer T-cell dose predicts risk of acute graft-versus-host disease in allogeneic hematopoietic stem cell transplantation. Blood. 2012;119:5030–6.

Chapuis AG, Ragnarsson GB, Nguyen HN, et al. Transferred WT1-reactive CD8+ T cells can mediate antileukemic activity and persist in post-transplant patients. Sci Transl Med. 2013;5:174ra27.

Chen Y-B, Efebera YA, Johnston L, et al. Increased Foxp3+Helios+ regulatory T cells and decreased acute graft-versus-host disease after allogeneic bone marrowtransplantation in patients receiving sirolimus and RGI-2001, an activator of invariant natural killer T cells. Biol Blood Marrow Transplant. 2017;23:625–34.

Corselli M, Crisan M, Murray IR, et al. Identification of perivascular mesenchymal stromal/stem cells by flow cytometry. Cytom Part J Int Soc Anal Cytol. 2013;83:714–20.

Fibbe WE, Dazzi F, LeBlanc K. MSCs: science and trials. Nat Med. 2013;19:812–3.

Hoffmann A, Floerkemeier T, Melzer C, Hass R. Comparison of in vitro-cultivation of human mesenchymal stroma/stem cells derived from bone marrow and umbilical cord. J Tissue Eng Regen Med. 2017;11:2565–81.

Koehl U, Kalberer C, Spanholtz J, et al. Advances in clinical NK cell studies: donor selection, manufacturing and quality control. Oncoimmunology. 2016;5:e1115178.

Koehl U, Toubert A, Pittari G. Editorial: tailoring NK cell receptor-ligand interactions: an art in evolution. Front Immunol. 2018;9:351.

Liu S, de Castro LF, Jin P, et al. Manufacturing differences affect human bone marrow stromal cell characteristics and function: comparison of production methods and products from multiple centers. Sci Rep. 2017;7:46731.

Pittenger MF, Mackay AM, Beck SC, et al. Multilineage potential of adult human mesenchymal stem cells. Science. 1999;284:143–7.

Rubio M-T, Moreira-Teixeira L, Bachy E, et al. Early posttransplantation donor-derived invariant natural killer T-cell recovery predicts the occurrence of acute graft-versus-host disease and overall survival. Blood. 2012;120:2144–54.

Ruggeri L, Capanni M, Urbani E, et al. Effectiveness of donor natural killer cell alloreactivity in mismatched hematopoietic transplants. Science. 2002;295:2097–100.

Tormin A, Li O, Brune JC, et al. CD146 expression on primary nonhematopoietic bone marrow stem cells is correlated with in situ localization. Blood. 2011;117:5067–77.

Vivier E, Raulet DH, Moretta A, et al. Innate or adaptive immunity? The example of natural killer cells. Science. 2011;331:44–9.

9 Histocompatibility

Eric Spierings and Katharina Fleischhauer

9.1 Introduction

Immune-mediated rejection of tissue allografts was first described in 1945 by the British immunologist Peter Medawar, followed by the discovery of the major histocompatibility complex (MHC) carrying the histocompatibility genes by Peter Gorer and George Snell in 1948, and of the human leukocyte antigen (HLA) molecules by Jean Dausset, Jon van Rood, and Rose Payne a decade later (Thorsby 2009). The importance of these discoveries was recognized by the Nobel Prices in Physiology and Medicine to Medawar, Snell, and Dausset in 1960 and 1980, respectively. Since then, the MHC has emerged as the single most polymorphic gene locus in eukaryotes, with 17,695 HLA alleles reported to date in the IMGT/HLA database, Release 3.31.0, 2018/01/19 (Robinson et al. 2015). While the main barrier to successful tissue grafting remain the HLA incompatibilities, also non-HLA polymorphisms have been recognized as important players, in particular minor histocompatibility antigens (mHAg), killer immunoglobulin-like receptors (KIR), and other polymorphic gene systems (Dickinson and Holler 2008; Gam et al. 2017; Heidenreich and Kröger 2017; Spierings 2014).

9.2 The Biology of Histocompatibility

9.2.1 Major Histocompatibility Antigens

The human MHC is located within ~4 Mbp of DNA on the short arm of chromosome 6 (6p21.3) and contains ~260 genes, many of which with immune-related functions (Trowsdale and Knight 2013). The MHC falls into three main regions, class I, II, and III, containing HLA A, B, and C; HLA DR, DQ, and DP; and complement factor as well as tumor necrosis factor genes, respectively. MHC genes are codominantly expressed and inherited following Mendelian rules, with a resulting 25% probability for two siblings to be genotypically HLA identical, i.e., to have inherited the same MHC from both parents. An additional hallmark of the MHC is linkage disequilibrium (LD), i.e., the nonrandom association of alleles at different HLA loci, and relatively high recombination rates of over 1%, also referred to as "crossing over" (Martin et al. 1995).

E. Spierings
Laboratory for Translational Immunology, University Medical Center, Utrecht, The Netherlands

K. Fleischhauer (✉)
Institute for Experimental Cellular Therapy, University Hospital, Essen, Germany
e-mail: katharina.fleischhauer@uk-essen.de

E. Carreras et al. (eds.), *The EBMT Handbook*, https://doi.org/10.1007/978-3-030-02278-5_9

9.2.2 HLA Class I and II Structure and Function

The classical HLA class I and II molecules are cell surface immunoglobulins (Ig) presenting peptides in their highly polymorphic antigen-binding groove (Madden 1995). HLA class I A, B, and C molecules are heterodimers of a polymorphic α chain of higher molecular weight (MW) than the monomorphic β2 microglobulin (heavy and light chain of 45 kDa and 12 kDa, respectively). The α-chain contains three hypervariable Ig-like domains, two of which form the antigen-binding groove while the third is involved in contacting the CD8 coreceptor on T cells, and the transmembrane region. HLA class I molecules are expressed on all healthy nucleated cells. They present peptides, i.e., protein fragments of mostly intracellular origin generated by proteasomal cleavage and transported to the endoplasmic reticulum via the transporter associated with antigen processing (TAP) (Vyas et al. 2008). Cell surface HLA class I peptide complexes can be recognized by the T cell receptor (TCR) of CD8+ T cells, leading to the activation of cytotoxic and/or cytokine effector functions, or by KIR on natural killer (NK) cells, leading to the inhibition of effector functions. HLA class II DR, DQ, and DP molecules are heterodimers of an α- and a β-chain of similar MW of approximately 30 KDa each, both with a transmembrane part anchored to the cell membrane. Most of the polymorphism is clustered in the β-chain Ig-like domain forming the antigen-binding groove, whose overall structure is similar to that of HLA class I, and the region contacting the CD4 coreceptor on T cells is also located in the β-chain. HLA class II proteins are expressed on professional antigen-presenting cells, as, for example, B cells, macrophages, and dendritic cells. Moreover, HLA class II protein expression on various cell types can be upregulated by proinflammatory cytokines such as IFNγ and TNFα. HLA class II presents peptides generally of extracellular origin generated through degradation of proteins in the phagolysosome (Vyas et al. 2008). Peptide loading onto HLA class II molecules takes place in the dedicated MIIC compartment and is catalyzed by two nonclassical HLA molecules equally encoded in the MHC, HLA DM, and DO. After transport to the cell surface, HLA class II peptide complexes can be recognized by the TCR of CD4+ T cells, leading to the activation of cytokine-mediated helper or regulatory functions. HLA class II receptors on NK cells, analogous to KIR for HLA class I, have not been described to date.

9.2.3 HLA Polymorphism and Tissue Typing

HLA molecules were first detected by serological methods, through the ability of sera from sensitized individuals to agglutinate some but not all leukocytes (hence the term "human leukocyte antigen") (Thorsby 2009). Until the mid-1990s, serological typing was the main method for tissue typing. With the advent of polymerase chain reaction (PCR) techniques, molecular tissue typing took over and unraveled a far greater degree of HLA allelic polymorphism than previously appreciated (Erlich 2012). HLA nucleotide polymorphism is clustered in so-called hypervariable regions (HvR) mainly in exons 2, 3, and 4 of HLA class I and exons 2 and 3 of HLA class II, encoding the functional antigen-binding groove and CD4/CD8 coreceptor-binding regions. Therefore, PCR-based molecular typing focused on these exons, leading to different levels of typing resolution (Table 9.1). With the advent of next-generation sequencing (NGS) for tissue typing purposes (Gabriel et al. 2014), allelic or at least high-resolution typing can be achieved in most cases. Moreover, NGS enables high-throughput sequencing of the entire HLA coding and noncoding regions, unraveling an additional layer of polymorphism with hundreds of new alleles reported to the IMGT/HLA database every month.

9.2.4 T Cell Alloreactivity

The ability of T cells to specifically recognize non-self, allogeneic tissues is called T cell

Table 9.1 HLA typing resolution and appropriate typing methods

HLA typing resolution[a]	Appropriate typing methods[b]
Low (first field)	Serology, SSP, SSOP, others
High (second field)	NGS, SBT
Allelic (all fields)	NGS, SBT
Intermediate	SSP, SSOP, SBT

[a]As defined in (Nunes et al. 2011). *Low:* A serological typing result or DNA-based typing at the first field in the DNA-based nomenclature. *High:* A set of alleles that encode the same protein sequence in the antigen binding site and that exclude alleles not expressed at the cell surface. High resolution thus includes alleles reported with the suffix G (set of alleles with identical nucleotide sequence across the exons encoding the antigen binding site) or the suffix P (set of alleles encoding the same protein sequence at the antigen binding site). *Allelic:* Unique nucleotide sequence for a gene as defined by the use of all of the digits in a current allele name. Intermediate: A level of resolution that falls between high and low resolution, as agreed with the entity requesting the testing. Examples are restriction to common and well-documented (CWD) alleles (Sanchez-Mazas et al. 2017) or reporting by NMDP codes (https://bioinformatics.bethematchclinical.org/hla-resources/allele-codes/allele-code-lists/).
[b]*Serology* complement-dependent cytotoxicity of specific antisera, *SSP* sequence-specific priming, *SSOP* sequence-specific oligonucleotide probing, *Others* additional molecular typing approaches including quantitative PCR and restriction fragment length polymorphism (RFLP), *SBT* sequencing-based typing (Sanger sequencing), *NGS* next-generation sequencing

alloreactivity. It can be either direct or indirect. Direct T cell alloreactivity is targeted to intact mismatched HLA peptide complexes expressed on the cell surface of allogeneic cells and can be mediated by both naïve and memory T cells (Archbold et al. 2008). Indirect T cell alloreactivity refers to the recognition of peptides derived by proteasomal cleavage from mismatched HLA and presented in the antigen-binding groove of self HLA molecules (Gokmen et al. 2008). These peptides are also referred to as Predicted Indirectly ReCognizable HLA Epitopes (PIRCHE, see Sect. 9.3.3) (Geneugelijk and Spierings 2018). A special form of indirect T cell alloreactivity is the recognition of foreign peptides not deriving from mismatched HLA but from any other expressed polymorphic gene and presented by self HLA molecules. These peptides are referred to as minor histocompatibility antigens (mHAg) (Spierings 2014). mHAg are the only targets of T cell alloreactivity in HLA-matched hematopoietic cell transplantation (HSCT) and are mainly recognized by naïve T cells. T cell alloreactivity is the main mediator of both the major benefit and the major toxicity of allogeneic HSCT, represented by immune control of residual malignant disease (graft versus leukemia; GvL) and immune attack of healthy tissues (graft versus host disease; GvHD), respectively.

Key Points

- HLA molecules are encoded by highly polymorphic genes in the human MHC and play a crucial role for peptide antigen recognition by T cells.
- HLA tissue typing can be performed at different levels of resolution, the highest being attainable only by NGS-based methods, which are unraveling an unprecedented degree of polymorphism in the MHC.
- Alloreactive T cells can recognize non-self HLA molecules on healthy and malignant cells after Allo-HSCT, mediating both toxic GvHD and beneficial GvL.

9.3 HLA Matching in Allogeneic HSCT

9.3.1 Donor Types

In HLA identical sibling HSCT, patient and donor have inherited the same parental MHCs, an event occurring with a likelihood of 25% according to Mendelian rules. Genotypic HLA identity should be confirmed by family studies for all six HLA loci (to exclude recombination). Haploidentical donors share only one MHC haplotype while the other haplotype is different. These donors are available for more than 90% of patients and can be found in parents or offsprings (100% likelihood), siblings (50% likelihood), as well as the extended family. Also HLA haploidentity should be confirmed by family studies wherever possible. Unrelated donors (UD) can be found among over 30 million volunteers enrolled in the worldwide registries or from over 700,000 banked cord blood units. The probability to find a volunteer UD matched for 8/8 HLA A, B, C, and DRB1 alleles varies according to the ethnic group of the patient between 30% and over 90% (Gragert et al. 2014). For UD HSCT, HLA identity should be confirmed at the highest resolution level possible (allelic, high, or intermediate resolution, Table 9.1), to be agreed between the transplant center and the tissue typing laboratory.

Table 9.2 Confounding factors of HLA/non-HLA immunogenetics and HSCT outcome

Confounding factor[a]	
Patient related	Age, sex, ABO, CMV serostatus, diagnosis, disease status
Donor related	Age, sex, ABO, CMV serostatus
Transplant related	Conditioning, GvHD prophylaxis, stem cell source, and composition

[a]The impact of HLA matching is additionally confounded by non-HLA immunogenetic factors and vice versa

9.3.2 Clinical Impact of HLA Mismatches

The clinical relevance of histocompatibility for the outcome of HSCT is significantly influenced by different patient-, donor-, and transplant-related factors (Table 9.2). The most striking example for the impact of these confounding factors is the advent of haploidentical HSCT, in which successful transplantation across an entire mismatched haplotype was rendered possible by extensive T cell depletion of the graft and, more recently, by innovative schemes of pharmacological GvHD prophylaxis (Slade et al. 2017). On the other hand, haploidentical HSCT has been associated with a particular form of immune escape relapse characterized by the selective genomic loss of the mismatched HLA haplotype, with important implications for treatment strategies (Vago et al. 2012). In UD HSCT, high-resolution matching for 8/8 HLA A, B, C, and DRB1 alleles has been shown to be associated with the best clinical outcomes, with an approximately 10% decrease in survival probabilities for every (antigenic or allelic) HLA mismatch at these four loci (Lee et al. 2007). On the other hand, the impact of HLA disparity was shown to be significantly reduced by advanced disease status at transplant, again demonstrating the inextricable link between HLA mismatches and confounding factors. The notion that there will be no "one-size-fits-all" solution to the question on the impact of histocompatibility in HSCT has to be taken into account when critically interpreting studies in this complex field.

9.3.3 Models of High-Risk/Nonpermissive HLA Mismatches

HLA mismatches that are clinically less well tolerated than others are referred to as high risk or nonpermissive. This is based on the observation that limited T cell alloreactivity is generally sufficient for the beneficial effect of GvL without inducing clinically uncontrollable GvHD, while intolerable toxicity can be induced by excessive T cell alloreactivity leading to severe treatment refractory GvHD. Therefore, high-risk or nonpermissive HLA mismatches are those associated with excessive T cell alloreactivity compared to their low-risk or permissive counterparts. Different models have been developed over the past years for their identification (Table 9.3). They rely on the presence of shared or nonshared T cell epitope (TCE) groups between mismatched HLA DPB1 alleles (Fleischhauer and Shaw 2017), genetically controlled expression levels of mismatched HLA C or DPB1 alleles in the patient (Petersdorf et al. 2014, 2015), specific high-risk HLA C and DPB1 allele mismatch combinations identified by retrospective statistical association between mismatch status and clinical outcome (Fernandez-Vina et al. 2014; Kawase et al. 2009), and the total number of PIRCHEI (presented by HLA class I) and PIRCHEII (presented by HLA class II) as a measure of the potential level of indirect alloreactivity after transplantation (Geneugelijk and

Table 9.3 Models of high-risk/nonpermissive HLA mismatches

Model	HLA locus, donor type, and clinical association
T cell epitope (TCE) groups[a]	HLA-DPB1; 8/8 UD; mortality and acute GvHD
Expression levels[b]	HLA C and DPB1; 7–8/8 UD; acute GvHD
Mismatch combinations[c]	HLA C and DPB1; 7–8/8 UD; mortality, acute GvHD and relapse
PIRCHE[d]	HLA C and DPB1; 8/8 UD; acute GvHD

[a]*TCE groups:* HLA DPB1 mismatches involving alleles from the same (permissive) or different (nonpermissive) TCE groups (Fleischhauer and Shaw 2017)

[b]*Expression levels:* HLA C or DPB1 mismatches involving a high-expression allele in the patient, as predicted by noncoding single nucleotide expression polymorphisms (Petersdorf et al. 2014, 2015)

[c]*Mismatch combinations*, high-risk allele mismatches defined by statistical associations (Fernandez-Vina et al. 2014; Kawase et al. 2009)

[d]*PIRCHE*, predicted indirectly recognizable HLA epitope numbers as predicted by online tools (Geneugelijk and Spierings 2018)

Spierings 2018). It should be noted that HLA DPB1 mismatches are present in over 80% of 8/8 matched UD HSCT, and models for high-risk or nonpermissive mismatches at this locus are therefore of particular practical relevance. The PIRCHE model is attractive since it is potentially applicable to any HLA-mismatched donor transplantation including <8/8 matched UD and haploidentical HSCT; on the other hand, clinical evidence for its validity in HSCT has so far been obtained only on relatively limited transplant cohorts. As stated above (Sect. 9.3.2), it is crucial that any of these or future models be tested in independent cohorts of sufficient statistical size and that they be continuously revalidated as clinical transplant practice and hence potential confounding factors evolve.

9.3.4 Guidelines for UD Selection by Histocompatibility

Consensus guidelines for donor selection have been established in many countries both in Europe and overseas, through the collaboration between donor registries and national immunogenetic societies. The general recommendation is the selection of an 8/8 HLA A, B, C, and DR (in Europe often 10/10, i.e., including the HLA DQ locus) matched UD if an HLA identical sibling is not available, followed by a 7/8 (or 9/10) UD or a haploidentical donor. Avoidance of high-risk or nonpermissive HLA mismatches according to any of the models outlined in Table 9.3 is usually regarded as optional, with particular emphasis on the avoidance of nonpermissive HLA DPB1 TCE mismatches since the TCE model is the only one to have been validated in different independent clinical studies to date (Fleischhauer and Shaw 2017). Also the inclusion of some of the non-HLA immunogenetic factors outlined in Sect. 9.4 can be considered, in particular with regard to donor KIR typing in haploidentical HSCT (Heidenreich and Kröger 2017).

Key Points

- HSCT donor types (in parenthesis the % probability of their identification for a given patient) include genotypically HLA identical siblings (25%), HLA haploidentical family donors (>90%), UD (30–90%), and cord blood donors (>80%).
- HLA typing strategies including family studies for related donors and typing resolution level for UD should be agreed between the transplant center and the tissue typing laboratory.
- The clinical relevance of HLA matching for the outcome of HSCT is critically dependent on numerous patient-, donor-, and transplant-related factors.
- In UD HSCT, survival probability decreases by 10% with every mismatch at HLA A, B, C, and DRB1, in patients transplanted at early disease stage.
- Models for high-risk nonpermissive HLA mismatches eliciting excessive T cell alloreactivity with intolerable toxicity include structural TCE, expression levels, specific allele

combinations, and PIRCHE. All these and future models need to be tested in independent cohorts of sufficient statistical size and be continuously revalidated as clinical transplant practice evolves.
- Consensus guidelines established at the national level between donor registries and immunogenetic societies aid in the selection of HSCT donors.

9.4 Non-HLA Immunogenetic Factors

9.4.1 Overview

HLA alleles are the most but not the only polymorphic genes in humans. Overall, interindividual gene variability by single nucleotide polymorphism (SNP) or copy-number variation (CNV) affects 0.5% of the 3 × 10^9 bp in the human genome. Although most of these polymorphisms are probably nonfunctional, some of them can give rise to polymorphic proteins that can be mHAg as described in Sect. 9.2.2, affect the expression of different genes including those encoding immunologically active cytokines, or act themselves as immune ligands or receptors relevant to transplantation biology. Among the latter, the KIR gene locus on the long arm of human chromosome 19 displays considerable polymorphism, with 907 alleles reported to the IPD/KIR database, Release 2.7.0, July 2017 (Robinson et al. 2005). Similar to high-risk or nonpermissive HLA mismatches, the role of non-HLA polymorphism in allo-HSCT is still incompletely defined. It is impossible to give a comprehensive overview of all non-HLA factors under study, and the list of factors listed in Table 9.4 and discussed in Sect. 9.4.2 is only a selection based on existing evidence for their clinical impact in certain transplant settings.

Table 9.4 Non-HLA immunogenetic factors and HSCT outcome

Non-HLA factor	Clinical outcome association
mHAg[a]	GvHD and relapse
KIR[b]	Relapse and mortality
MIC[c]	GvHD, relapse, and transplant-related mortality
Others[d]	GvHD and transplant-related mortality

[a]*Minor histocompatibility antigens* (Spierings 2014)
[b]*Killer Ig-like receptors* (Heidenreich and Kröger 2017; Shaffer and Hsu 2016)
[c]*MHC class I-related chain* (Isernhagen et al. 2016)
[d]*Cytokine, chemokine, and immune response gene polymorphisms* including tumor necrosis factor, interleukin (IL)10, the IL1 gene family, IL2, IL6, interferon γ, tumor growth factor β and their receptors, NOD-like receptors (NOD2/CARD15), toll-like receptors, micro-RNAs (Dickinson and Holler 2008; Gam et al. 2017; Chen and Zeiser 2018)

9.4.2 Clinical Impact of Non-HLA Immunogenetic Factors

mHAg are the only targets of T cell alloreactivity in HLA identical HSCT (see Sect. 9.2.2) and as such play an important role for both GvHD and GvL (Spierings 2014). This dual function is related to their different modes of tissue and cell expression, i.e., hematopoietic system restricted or broad. Broadly expressed mHAg can cause both GvHD and GvL, and donor-recipient matching for these mHAg is therefore desirable yet virtually impossible due to their large number, with many of them probably currently undefined. In contrast, mHAg restricted to hematopoietic cells are more prone to induce selective GvL. The latter are being explored as targets for HSCT-based immunotherapy of hematological malignancies, in which mHAg-specific responses are specifically enhanced to promote GvL.

KIR are predominantly expressed by NK cells and recognize certain HLA class I specificities on target cells. KIR have either long inhibitory or short activating cytoplasmic domains and are stochastically coexpressed on NK cells. The eventual outcome of KIR interaction (or lack thereof) with its HLA class I ligand (inhibition or activation) is a complex process that depends on the relative number of inhibitory or activatory KIR and on the state of education of the NK cell. Educated NK cells from individuals expressing the cognate HLA ligand are strongly reactive against cells missing that ligand. This "missing self" reactivity is at the basis for the potent GvL effect attributed to NK cells in the setting of HLA-mismatched transplantation, in particular haploidentical HSCT (Heidenreich and Kröger 2017). Depending on the donor KIR gene asset, a role for NK cell-mediated GvL has also been postulated in the HLA-matched setting (Shaffer and Hsu 2016). Based on all this evidence, KIR typing is increasingly being adopted as an additional criterion for donor selection.

MHC class I chain-related (MIC) A and B are nonclassical MHC class I genes. MICA encodes a ligand for NKG2D, an activating NK receptor. The SNP Val/Met at position 129 of the MICA protein results in isoforms with high (Met) and low affinities (Val) for NKG2D. Consequently, various studies suggest a role for this SNP in SCT outcome, including GvHD, relapse and survival (Isernhagen et al. 2016).

Immune response gene polymorphisms have also been reported to contribute to the risks associated with HSCT (Dickinson and Holler 2008; Gam et al. 2017; Chen and Zeiser 2018). They often comprise SNPs in cytokine or chemokine-coding genes or their regulatory elements such as micro-RNAs (miRNAs). These variations in both the donor and the recipient can have a significant impact on transplant outcome and the development of GvHD; however, their relative role in different transplant settings is not yet fully elucidated.

Key Points

- Non-HLA immunogenetic factors that have been associated with clinical outcome of HSCT include polymorphic mHAg, KIR, MIC, and immune response genes.
- Hematopoietic tissue-specific mHAg are being exploited for specific cellular immunotherapy of hematologic malignancies.
- Polymorphic KIR are responsible for "missing self" recognition by alloreactive NK cells mediating selective GvL after HSCT, and KIR genotyping is therefore increasingly included into donor selection algorithms.

References

Archbold JK, Ely LK, Kjer-Nielsen L, et al. T cell allorecognition and MHC restriction–a case of Jekyll and Hyde? Mol Immunol. 2008;45:583–98.

Chen S, Zeiser R. The role of microRNAs in myeloid cells during graft-versus-host disease. Front Immunol. 2018;9:4.

Dickinson AM, Holler E. Polymorphisms of cytokine and innate immunity genes and GVHD. Best Pract Res Clin Haematol. 2008;21:149–64.

Erlich H. HLA DNA typing: past, present, and future. Tissue Antigens. 2012;80:1–11.

Fernandez-Vina MA, Wang T, Lee SJ, et al. Identification of a permissible HLA mismatch in hematopoietic stem cell transplantation. Blood. 2014;123:1270–8.

Fleischhauer K, Shaw BE. HLA-DP in unrelated hematopoietic cell transplantation revisited: challenges and opportunities. Blood. 2017;130:1089–96.

Gabriel C, Fürst D, Fae I, et al. HLA typing by next-generation sequencing–getting closer to reality. Tissue Antigens. 2014;83:65–75.

Gam R, Shah P, Crossland RE, Norden J, et al. Genetic association of hematopoietic stem cell transplantation outcome beyond histocompatibility genes. Front Immunol. 2017;8:380.

Geneugelijk K, Spierings E. Matching donor and recipient based on predicted indirectly recognizable human leucocyte antigen epitopes. Int J Immunogenet. 2018;45:41–53.

Gokmen MR, Lombardi G, Lechler RI. The importance of the indirect pathway of allorecognition in clinical transplantation. Curr Opin Immunol. 2008;20:568–74.

Gragert L, Eapen M, Williams E, et al. HLA match likelihoods for hematopoietic stem-cell grafts in the U.S. registry. N Engl J Med. 2014;371:339–48.

Heidenreich S, Kröger N. Reduction of relapse after unrelated donor stem cell transplantation by KIR-based graft selection. Front Immunol. 2017;8:41.

Isernhagen A, Malzahn D, Bickeboller H, Dressel R. Impact of the MICA-129Met/Val dimorphism on NKG2D-mediated biological functions and disease risks. Front Immunol. 2016;7:588.

Kawase T, Matsuo K, Kashiwase K, et al. HLA mismatch combinations associated with decreased risk of relapse: implications for the molecular mechanism. Blood. 2009;113:2851–8.

Lee SJ, Klein J, Haagenson M, et al. High-resolution donor-recipient HLA matching contributes to the success of unrelated donor marrow transplantation. Blood. 2007;110:4576–83.

Madden DR. The three-dimensional structure of peptide-MHC complexes. Annu Rev Immunol. 1995;13:587–622.

Martin M, Mann D, Carrington M. Recombination rates across the HLA complex: use of microsatellites as a rapid screen for recombinant chromosomes. Hum Mol Gen. 1995;4:423–8.

Nunes E, Heslop H, Fernandez-Vina MA, et al. Definitions of histocompatibility typing terms. Blood. 2011;118:e180–3.

Petersdorf EW, Gooley TA, Malkki M, et al. HLA-C expression levels define permissible mismatches in hematopoietic cell transplantation. Blood. 2014;124:3996–4003.

Petersdorf EW, Malkki M, O'HUigin C, et al. High HLA-DP expression and graft-versus-host disease. N Engl J Med. 2015;373:599–609.

Robinson J, Halliwell JA, Hayhurst JD, et al. The IPD and IMGT/HLA database: allele variant databases. Nucleic Acids Res. 2015;43:D423–31.

Robinson J, Waller MJ, Stoehr P, Marsh SG. IPD–the immuno polymorphism database. Nucleic Acids Res. 2005;33:D523–6.

Sanchez-Mazas A, Nunes JM, Middleton D, et al. Common and well-documented HLA alleles over all of Europe and within European sub-regions: a catalogue from the European Federation for Immunogenetics. HLA. 2017;89:104–13.

Shaffer BC, Hsu KC. How important is NK alloreactivity and KIR in allogeneic transplantation? Best Pract Res Clin Haematol. 2016;29:351–8.

Slade M, Fakhri B, Savani BN, Romee R. Halfway there: the past, present and future of haploidentical transplantation. Bone Marrow Transplant. 2017;52:1–6.

Spierings E. Minor histocompatibility antigens: past, present, and future. Tissue Antigens. 2014;84:374–60.

Thorsby E. A short history of HLA. Tissue Antigens. 2009;74:101–16.

Trowsdale J, Knight JC. Major histocompatibility complex genomics and human disease. Anuu Rev Genomics Hum Genet. 2013;14:301–23.

Vago L, Toffalori C, Ciceri F, Fleischhauer K. Genomic loss of mismatched human leukocyte antigen and leukemia immune escape from haploidentical graft-versus-leukemia. Semin Oncol. 2012;39:707–15.

Vyas JM, Van der Veen AG, Ploegh HL. The known unknowns of antigen processing and presentation. Nat Rev Immunol. 2008;8:607–18.

10 Clinical and Biological Concepts for Mastering Immune Reconstitution After HSCT: Toward Practical Guidelines and Greater Harmonization

Jürgen Kuball and Jaap Jan Boelens

10.1 Introduction/Background

The main mechanisms of action resulting in a long-term cure, but also in many life-threatening side effects after HSCT, are mediated by the rapidly reconstituting immune repertoire, which depends on the conditioning regimen, cell dose and graft composition, as well as the type of immune suppression. However, knowledge of these mechanisms is limited, due to many variations in clinical programs, including the specific type of transplantation procedure, as well as a lack of standardized immune monitoring after HSCT.

To date, only the process of donor selection has been significantly impacted by new biological insights, but little attention has been given to the design of the cell product in terms of numbers and composition, to avoid variations between different patients. In addition, high variations between patients in the clearance of agents used during the conditioning are rarely investigated. Given the dearth of prospective clinical studies addressing these important concepts, and the fact that such studies will most likely never be performed, due to the lack of interest from pharmaceutical companies, we aim to initiate a consensus discussion. Our goal is to harmonize the intervention HSCT by exploring how individual differences between patients and overall transplantation strategies impact the final effector mechanisms of HSCT, namely, a timely and well-balanced immune reconstitution.

J. Kuball (✉)
Department of Hematology, UMC, Utrecht, The Netherlands

Laboratory of Translational Immunology, UMC, Utrecht, The Netherlands
e-mail: J.H.E.Kuball@umcutrecht.nl

J. J. Boelens
Laboratory of Translational Immunology, UMC, Utrecht, The Netherlands

Memorial Sloan Kettering Cancer Center, New York, NY, USA

10.2 Impact of Conditioning Regimens on Immune Reconstitution and Outcomes: Pharmacokinetics-Pharmacodynamics (PK-PD), Individualized Dosing

Various groups have recently demonstrated that agents administered as part of the conditioning regimen, as well as after HSCT, will influence both short-term and long-term immune reconstitution (Soiffer and Chen 2017; Admiraal et al. 2015). These agents may, therefore, have an unknown effect on also other cell-based therapeutics. In the context of HSCT, "predictable" immune reconstitution is important when studying maintenance therapies with novel drugs, DLI,

E. Carreras et al. (eds.), *The EBMT Handbook*, https://doi.org/10.1007/978-3-030-02278-5_10

and advanced cell therapy interventions. Therefore, it is essential to understand the impact of the agents used on the immune reconstitution. Comprehensive pharmacokinetic (PK) and pharmacodynamic (PD) information can help to illuminate the effects that exposure of agents in the conditioning have on immune reconstitution and subsequent outcomes (e.g., GvHD, relapse and non-relapse mortality).

The recent discovery that the pharmacokinetics of serotherapy (e.g., ATG and ATLG) is highly dependent on receptor load (represented by absolute lymphocyte count; ALC) before the first dosing is one example. In adults, receptor load was the only predictor for ATG clearance, while in pediatric patients (<40 kg), weight also influenced clearance. While prospective validation trials of novel ATG nomograms currently include patients linked to defined transplantation regimens, initial recommendations for dosing serotherapy on lymphocyte count rather than body weight seem to be reasonable, e.g., within the context of T cell-replete reduced conditioning regimens (Admiraal et al. 2015) (Table 10.1). From a post hoc analysis of a recent randomized controlled trial allowing three different types of regimens, we learned that different regimens had the reverse effects of ATLG on the outcomes, resulting in overlapping curves for the primary endpoint, chronic-GvHD-free, leukemia-free survival (Soiffer et al. 2017).

Table 10.1 Suggested novel ATG dosing nomograms based on PK-PD modeling for (non-)myelo-ablative settings in pediatrics and adults[a]

Setting	Dosing on	Target AUC after HSCT (AU*d/mL) and donor source	Starting day
Pediatrics; MAC Admiraal et al. (2015)	Weight ALC Cell source	<20 for cord blood <50 for bone marrow	9
Adults: Non-MAC Admiraal et al. (2017)	ALC	60–90 for peripherally mobilized stem cells	9

ALC absolute lymphocyte count, *AUC* area under the curve

[a]Level C evidence (retrospective studies)

Serotherapy is not the only agent in a conditioning regimen with variable PK that can have a dramatic impact on the chances for survival. In a recent retrospective cohort analysis that included more than 650 pediatric and young adult patients, cumulative exposure to BU was found to influence outcomes (Bartelink et al. 2016). The optimal BU exposure, for the main outcome of EFS, was found to be independent of indication, combination (BU/FLU, BU/CY, or BU/CY/MEL), age, and donor source. BU/FLU within the optimal BU exposure (80–100 mg*h/L) was associated with the highest survival chances and lowest toxicity compared to other combinations. More recently, fludarabine exposure was also found to influence survival (in an ATG-FLU/BU: Boelens et al. 2018). These studies further illustrate that pharmacokinetic variations in individuals can have significant effects on survival. Historically, and still in daily practice, a variety of conditioning regimens are used, which complicates comparisons of HSCT outcomes across different centers and even within trials.

10.3 Graft Composition as an Additional Predictor for Immune Reconstitution and Clinical Outcomes

Although transplant physicians carefully monitor the levels of many drugs, such as CSA or antibiotics, an additional opportunity to further harmonize the transplantation procedure arises from the surprising clinical observation that substantial cell dose variations are currently accepted across patients. The hesitation to monitor cell numbers in the graft or after HSCT, and to act on them, is of course partially driven by the confusing magnitude of immunological subsets, the narrow nature of many immunological programs with a lack of consensus on immune monitoring, and also rather limited immunological education across the majority of transplant physicians. However, currently available retrospective and prospective studies can provide guidance. A retrospective EBMT study indicated that T cell numbers vary frequently between 50 and

885 × 10^6/kg and the highest quartile in CD34+ cells, as well as T cells associate with an inferior clinical outcome (5). As we cannot expect in the future randomized trials addressing the impact of different graft compositions in T cell-replete transplantations on clinical outcomes, avoiding higher numbers of CD34 and T cells within the highest quartile might be reasonable (Czerw et al. 2016). Higher numbers of NKT cells (Malard et al. 2016) and γδT cells (Perko et al. 2015) in the graft have been reported to associate with favorable immune reconstitution, and a positive clinical outcome, most likely due to their impact on controlling GVHD (Du et al. 2017) and acting on CMV, as well as on leukemia (Scheper et al. 2013; de Witte et al. 2018). However, these variables are more difficult to control in daily clinical practice. Direct ex vivo graft engineering provides an elegant solution to further control immune subsets in the graft and the consecutive immune reconstitution. It also allows for the standardization of cell numbers, as well as subsets per patient, e.g., selecting CD34-positive stem cells alone has been reported to associate with less chronic GVHD, while the graft versus leukemia effect is maintained (Pasquini et al. 2012). As the next generation of graft engineering, depletion of αβT cells has been reported to associate with lower frequencies of infection and very low GVHD rates (Locatelli et al. 2017).

10.4 Immune Monitoring

10.4.1 Immune Cell Phenotyping

The most important questions that arise when monitoring immune therapeutic interventions are:

1. How many cells within each leukocyte subset are present in patients at different stages of disease, before immune intervention?
2. What is the immune composition of the graft?
3. Which immune subsets are reconstituting at what points in time?
4. What is the functional response of these cells to additional immunotherapeutic or drug interventions after transplantation (Table 10.1)?

These questions are particularly important in an era when post-HSCT pharmaceutical maintenance interventions and DLI or the administration of other ATMPs (advanced therapy medicinal products) have become daily practice for many different disease categories (Soiffer and Chen 2017).

Flow cytometry is often available for comprehensive immune phenotyping, usually in accredited laboratories within transplant centers. Markers identifying the most common leukocyte subsets are broadly used and can therefore be considered as a "standard" panel: CD45 (lymphocytes), CD3 (T cells), CD19 (B cells), αβTCR, γδTCR, and CD16/CD56 (NK) cells. In some centers/studies, this panel has been extended to identify the differentiation and activation state of subsets of T (T-helper, regulatory T cells), B, and NK(T) cells, as well as cells from the myeloid lineage (monocytes, dendritic cell subsets). This knowledge is important because the success of cell-based immunotherapies, as well as agents modulating the immune system after transplantation, will significantly depend on the presence or absence of different immune subsets. Mastering the diversity might allow for the definition of subpopulations who would benefit from checkpoint-inhibitor treatment after HSCT, as well as characterize patients who would be at high risk for GVHD, while currently this intervention is considered to be very toxic (Davids et al. 2016). Also, other subsets may be suitable as biomarkers to predict clinical efficacy. Given the potential impact of sorafenib on post-HSCT outcomes through the induction of IL15 (Mathew et al. 2018), additional immune subsets associating with improved leukemia control need to be identified. In another study, high baseline frequencies of peripheral blood dendritic cells (DC) correlated with a clinical response to high-dose IL-2 (Finkelstein et al. 2010). These data emphasize the importance of DC in endogenous and therapy-induced antitumor immunity and arguably warrant the incorporation of DC markers in immune-monitoring panels.

Taken together, a variety of specialized subsets may have potential as predictive markers for clinical efficacy, but they require more sophisticated staining protocols, making more cumbersome staining techniques less broadly applicable for harmonized panels across centers or in multicenter clinical trials. Furthermore, it is important to note that trials using whole blood assays may produce different percentages of cell subsets when compared with studies using PBMCs. The same is true when comparing freshly isolated PBMCs with biobanked material, which has been subjected to freeze/thaw procedures that affect expression levels of various markers. Even when the same samples are collected, variations can be introduced by the selection of antibody clones, combination of clones and fluorochromes, and the gating strategies. In sum, minimizing the variability in sample handling and the pre-analysis phase is critical for standardization.

10.4.2 Immune Monitoring: Secretome Analyses

Measuring the production of cytokines, chemokines, and growth factors and their profiles (i.e., the secretome) represents an integral part of immunomonitoring during immunotherapeutic treatments. These biomarkers may distinguish diverse disease/response patterns, identify surrogate markers of efficacy, and provide additional insight into the therapeutic mode of action. Peripheral blood is often the only source for protein analysis, which may lack the sensitivity to reflect local responses in affected tissues. As examples, proteins, such as interleukin-6, granulocyte-macrophage colony-stimulating factor (GM-CSF), hepatocyte growth factor (HGF), ST2 (suppressor of tumorigenicity), and soluble IL-2a, have been suggested as potential biomarkers for GvHD, whereas increased levels of TNF-a and IL-6 are associated with robust immune responses to viral reactivation (de Koning et al. 2016).

The most commonly used methods to identify these markers include antibody-based ELISA or multiplex platforms, such as protein microarrays, liquid chromatography-mass spectrometry (LC-MS), electro-chemiluminescence, and bead-based multiplex immunoassays (MIA). Again, different technologies and reagents (e.g., antibodies and recombinants for standard curves) may lead to different concentrations and dramatic variability in results, depending on how the pre-analytic samples are handled (e.g., differences in processing and storage, including duration of storage). Cytokine levels differ considerably between serum and plasma samples obtained from the same donor, due to release of platelet-associated molecules into serum. Moreover, the type of anticoagulant used in plasma isolation and time- and/or temperature-sensitive changes need to be considered (Keustermans et al. 2013). These phenomena underscore the need for extensive documentation with respect to all biomarker analysis before any conclusions can be made when comparing patient cohorts treated at multiple sites.

10.5 Summary

The failure or success of HSCT is significantly impacted by the patient's immune status. However, only a minority of HSCT programs systematically consider individualized drug monitoring during conditioning, graft design, and immune monitoring as key for patient surveillance, in order to maximally control and capture essential details of the intervention HSCT. Therefore, guidelines are needed to further harmonize the procedure HSCT as well as standardized immune monitoring to allow for distillation of key features for success and failure. First, careful recommendations for individualized drug dosing as well as graft compositions can be made based on available data sets. However, it will be key to register within the new cellular therapy registry of EBMT additional details of drug dosages, graft compositions, as well as immune reconstitution, to capture clinical variations in programs, as well as defined immune reconstitutions. This will enable a retrospective

Table 10.2 Panels under consideration in the panel discussion of the CTIWP (Greco et al. 2018)[a]

	General		Advanced
Graft composition	αβT γδT Treg B NK/NKT	αβTCR, CD45RO/RA, CD3, CD4, CD8, CD27 γδTCR, CD45RO/RA, CD3, CD27 CD45, CD4, CD25, CD127, FoxP3 CD45, CD19, CD38, CD27, IgM/G/D, CD21 CD45, CD3, CD56, TCRα24/β11)	Intracellular cytokines after PMA/ionomycin stimulation Specific TCR by multimer approach
Cell phenotyping pre- and post transplantation	αβT γδT Treg B NK/NKT DC/mono	αβTCR, CD45RO/RA, CD3, CD4, CD8, CD27 γδTCR, CD45RO/RA, CD3, CD27 CD45, CD4, CD25, CD127, FoxP3 CD45, CD19, CD38, CD27, IgM/G/D, CD21 CD45, CD3, CD56, TCRα24/β11) CD11c, HLA-DR, CD14, CD16, CD1c, CD141, CD303	Intracellular cytokines after PMA/ionomycin stimulation Specific TCR by multimer approach αβTCR and γδTCR repertoire
Secretome	–		Multiplex panel (e.g., IL-7, ST2, TNF-a, IL-6, HGF, IL-2R, IL-8, GM-CSF, etc.)
Cell function	–		NK cell lyses T cell proliferation upon antigens and mitogens B cell maturation
PK	BU, FLU, ATG, Campath (if part of conditioning)		Trial drug
MRD	qPCR (targets expressed, flow cytometry)		Next-generation sequencing
Viral load	CMV, EBV, HV6, adenovirus		–

[a]General parameters that could be included in harmonized immune-monitoring protocols across most studies/centers and advanced parameters that may be of great value in specific studies and that can only be performed in specialized immunology labs or analyzed in a central laboratory

increase in insight into daily clinical practice, and its impact on immune reconstitution, as well as clinical outcome. Also, clinical trials should adopt such consensus measurements. Nevertheless, the markers and phenotypes studied in one setting may not be considered relevant in another, supporting the definition of a set of general recommended protocols and a set of add-on trial-specific parameters (Table 10.2). A consensus panel is currently prepared by the cellular therapy and immunobiology working party (CTIWP) of EBMT (Greco et al. 2018). A harmonization procedure to achieve a more balanced immune reconstitution might have a more profound impact on patient survival than any other novel maintenance therapy (Admiraal et al. 2017; Boelens et al. 2018) and allow for a better success rate for novel drugs tested as maintenance therapy.

Key Points

- The failure or success of HCT is significantly impacted by the patient's immune status.
- Harmonizing individualized drug monitoring during conditioning, graft design, and immune monitoring is key for patient surveillance and needs to be registered within the new cellular therapy registry of EBMT.
- A harmonization procedure to achieve a more balanced immune reconstitution might have a more profound impact on patient survival than any other novel maintenance therapy and allow for a better success rate for novel drugs tested as maintenance therapy.

References

Admiraal R, van Kesteren C, Jol-van der Zijde CM, et al. Association between anti-thymocyte globulin exposure and CD4+ immune reconstitution in paediatric haemopoietic cell transplantation: a multicentre, retrospective pharmacodynamic cohort analysis. Lancet Haematol. 2015;2:e194–203.

Admiraal R, Nierkens S, de Witte MA, et al. Association between anti-thymocyte globulin exposure and survival outcomes in adult unrelated haemopoietic cell transplantation: a multicentre, retrospective, pharmacodynamic cohort analysis. Lancet Haematol. 2017;4:e183–91.

Bartelink IH, Lalmohamed A, van Reij EM, et al. Association of busulfan exposure with survival and toxicity after haemopoietic cell transplantation in children and young adults: a multicentre, retrospective cohort analysis. Lancet Haematol. 2016;3:e526–36.

Boelens JJ, Admiraal R, Kuball J, Nierkens S. Fine-tuning antithymocyte globulin dosing and harmonizing clinical trial design. J Clin Oncol. 2018;36:1175–6.

Czerw T, Labopin M, Schmid C, et al. High CD3+ and CD34+ peripheral blood stem cell grafts content is associated with increased risk of graft-versus-host disease without beneficial effect on disease control after reduced-intensity conditioning allogeneic transplantation from matched unrelated donors for acute myeloid leukemia - an analysis from the Acute Leukemia Working Party of the European Society for Blood and Marrow Transplantation. Oncotarget. 2016;7(19):27255–66.

Davids MS, Kim HT, Bachireddy P, et al. Ipilimumab for patients with relapse after allogeneic transplantation. N Engl J Med. 2016;375:143–53.

de Koning C, Plantinga M, Besseling P, et al. Immune reconstitution after allogeneic hematopoietic cell transplantation in children. Biol Blood Marrow Transplant. 2016;22:195–206.

de Witte MA, Sarhan D, Davis Z, et al. Early reconstitution of NK and gammadelta T cells and its implication for the design of post-transplant immunotherapy. Biol Blood Marrow Transplant. 2018;24(6):1152–62.

Du J, Paz K, Thangavelu G, et al. Invariant natural killer T cells ameliorate murine chronic GVHD by expanding donor regulatory T cells. Blood. 2017;129:3121–5.

Finkelstein SE, Carey T, Fricke I, et al. Changes in dendritic cell phenotype after a new high-dose weekly schedule of interleukin-2 therapy for kidney cancer and melanoma. J Immunother. 2010;33:817–27.

Greco R, Ciceri F, Noviello M, et al. Immune monitoring in allogeneic hematopoietic stem cell transplant recipients: a survey from the EBMT-CTIWP. Bone Marrow Transplant. 2018;53:1201–5.

Keustermans GC, Hoeks SB, Meerding JM, et al. Cytokine assays: an assessment of the preparation and treatment of blood and tissue samples. Methods. 2013;61:10–7.

Locatelli F, Merli P, Pagliara D, et al. Outcome of children with acute leukemia given HLA-haploidentical HSCT after alphabeta T-cell and B-cell depletion. Blood. 2017;130:677–85.

Malard F, Labopin M, Chevallier P, et al. Larger number of invariant natural killer T cells in PBSC allografts correlates with improved GVHD-free and progression-free survival. Blood. 2016;127:1828–35.

Mathew NR, Baumgartner F, Braun L, et al. Sorafenib promotes graft-versus-leukemia activity in mice and humans through IL-15 production in FLT3-ITD-mutant leukemia cells. Nat Med. 2018;24:282–91.

Pasquini MC, Devine S, Mendizabal A, et al. Comparative outcomes of donor graft CD34+ selection and immune suppressive therapy as graft-versus-host disease prophylaxis for patients with acute myeloid leukemia in complete remission undergoing HLA-matched sibling allogeneic hematopoietic cell transplantation. J Clin Oncol. 2012;30:3194–201.

Perko R, Kang G, Sunkara A, et al. Gamma delta T cell reconstitution is associated with fewer infections and improved event-free survival after hematopoietic stem cell transplantation for pediatric leukemia. Biol Blood Marrow Transplant. 2015;21:130–6.

Scheper W, van Dorp S, Kersting S, et al. Gammadelta T cells elicited by CMV reactivation after Allo-SCT cross-recognize CMV and leukemia. Leukemia. 2013;27:1328–38.

Soiffer RJ, Chen YB. Pharmacologic agents to prevent and treat relapse after allogeneic hematopoietic cell transplantation. Blood Adv. 2017;1:2473–82.

Soiffer RJ, Kim HT, McGuirk J, et al. Prospective, randomized, double-blind, phase III clinical trial of anti-T-lymphocyte globulin to assess impact on chronic graft-versus-host disease-free survival in patients undergoing HLA-matched unrelated myeloablative hematopoietic cell transplantation. J Clin Oncol. 2017;35:4003–11.

Part III

Methodology and Clinical Aspects

Topic leaders: Arnon Nagler and Nicolaus Kröger

11 Evaluation and Counseling of Candidates

Enric Carreras and Alessandro Rambaldi

11.1 Evaluation of Candidates and Risk Factors for HSCT

Enric Carreras

11.1.1 Introduction

The evaluation of candidates and the analysis of individual risk factors for HSCT permit to establish four fundamental aspects:

1. The HSCT indication
2. To inform the patient properly
3. To choose the best donor, conditioning, and post-HSCT IS
4. To evaluate the results of the transplant in large series

E. Carreras
Spanish Bone Marrow Donor Registry,
Josep Carreras Foundation and Leukemia Research Institute, Barcelona, Catalunya, Spain

Hospital Clinic Barcelona, Barcelona University, Barcelona, Spain

A. Rambaldi(✉)
Department of Hematology-Oncology,
Azienda Socio Sanitaria Territoriale Papa Giovanni XXIII, Bergamo, Università Statale di Milano, Milano, Italy
e-mail: alessandro.rambaldi@unimi.it

11.1.2 Candidates' Evaluation Work Flow

11.1.2.1 First Visit

The most relevant aspects to take into account in this first visit are:

- Medical history (past and present) and physical examination (see Sect. 11.1.2.4).
- Review of diagnostic tests (in referred patients).
- Revaluate HLA typing of patient and potential donors (if allo-HSCT).
- Preliminary information on:
  - Therapeutic options and results
  - HSCT procedure
  - Possible complications and side effects (see specific chapters in Part V)
- Schedule reevaluation of the current status of the disease (see Sect. 11.1.3).
- Schedule visits with radiation therapist (if TBI), dentist, gynecologist, blood bank (list of blood/platelet donors), HSCT unit supervisor nurse, etc.
- Signature of the informed consent for HSCT and for procurement of HSC (if auto-HSCT).

11.1.2.2 Visit Preharvesting (Auto-HSCT)

- Assess the results of complementary explorations.
- Complete information on the procedure.

E. Carreras et al. (eds.), *The EBMT Handbook*, https://doi.org/10.1007/978-3-030-02278-5_11

- If PBSC, assess the status of venous accesses. Program CVC (if necessary) and mobilization schedule.
- If BM: preanesthetic visit.
- Program manipulation of HSCT (if applicable) and/or cryopreservation.

11.1.2.3 Last Visit Before Admission

- Final and complete patient information (see Sect. 11.1.2.5).
- Evaluate reevaluation studies performed (see Sect. 11.1.3).
- Schedule admission and conditioning treatment.
- If necessary, program CVC placement.
- If allo-HSCT: confirm that the donor's evaluation is correct and there are no contraindications for donation (see Chap. 12).
- If auto-HSCT: confirm that the cryopreserved cellularity is correct.
- Submit donor and recipient information to the blood bank (group, CMV serology, previous transfusions, etc.).
- If TBI: confirm that the dosimetry has been carried out and the RT has been programmed.
- Confirm storage of patient and donor samples for serotheque and cellular library.

11.1.2.4 Medical History

Collect information on:

Medical background; childhood illnesses and vaccines; allergies and adverse drug reactions; surgical interventions (previous anesthesia); medications not related to the basic process; previous transfusion history, family tree, and family history valuable; in women, menarche/menopause, pregnancy and childbirth, contraceptive methods, date last rule, and gynecological checkups

Travel to malaria, trypanosomiasis, and HTLV-I/II endemic areas

Previous relevant infections

Data about the current illness:

- Start date and initial symptomatology
- Diagnostic methodology used (staging)
- Chemotherapy and radiotherapy treatments (doses and dates)
- Complications from such treatments
- Result of these treatments
- Recurrences and their treatment
- Transfusions received
- Current state of the disease

Social aspects

- Smoking, alcoholism, and other drug use
- Sexual habits
- Availability of accommodation close to the center and means of transport
- Support family members
- Ethnic, cultural, and intellectual aspects

11.1.2.5 Information to Provide (See Detailed Information in Counseling Section)

Ask the patient (privately) which escorts he or she wishes to have present in this session. For adolescents follow the rules of each country respecting the right of information. Transmit as much information as possible in writing. She/he must be informed about:

- Most frequent early and late complications (see specific chapters in Parts V and VI) including graft failure, GI complications, alopecia, SOS/VOD, acute GVHD, early infections, chronic GVHD, late infections, relapse of the disease, infertility, endocrine complications, neoplasms, and other secondary.
- Treat specifically serious complications (ICU admissions) and possibility of death. Inform about the advance directive registry. Agreeing with the patient on an interlocutor in case at some point they may not be able to make decisions.
- Estimated duration of admission, approximate day of admission.
- Most frequent complications on discharge, outpatient follow-up, likelihood of readmission, and need for caregivers at discharge.

11.1.3 Complementary Explorations

All the following studies must be performed within 30 days prior to the HSCT except the assessment of baseline disease status (7–15 days) and the pregnancy test (7 days):

- CBC and basic coagulation; complete biochemistry (including ferritin); blood type and

Rh/irregular antibodies; dosage of Igs; serology CMV, EBV, VHS, VVZ, toxoplasma, syphilis, HBsAg, HBcAb, and anti-HBsAb (HTLV-I/II, and Chagas disease according to the patient's origin); NAT for HCV, HBV, and HIV; pregnancy test
- Chest x-ray; respiratory function tests (including FEV1 and DLCO); electrocardiogram; echocardiogram or isotopic ventriculography (depending on previous treatment)
- Reevaluation of the disease (MRD) (see specific chapters in part IX)
- Dental evaluation; gynecological evaluation; psychological/psychiatric evaluation
- Nutritional assessment
- HLA typing (recheck) (see Chap. 9)

11.1.4 Risk Assessment

11.1.4.1 Individual Risk Factors

There are a group of variables that have a prognostic value in all predictive models

Variables	High risk
Age	Older. Do not use as a single criterion. Relative importance
General condition	Karnofsky index <80%
Disease	Not in remission. See specific chapters
Type of donor	Others than HLA-identical siblings
HLA compatibility	Any HLA-A, HLA-B, HLA-C, and DRB1 difference
CMV serology	Different serology than the donor
Donor	Age >35–40 years For male recipient, female donor (especially if multiparous)
Interval diagnosis-HSCT	Prolonged (relevant in CML and SAA)
Comorbidities	See HCT-CI model
Iron overload	Present
Experience of the center	Non-JACIE/FACT accredited centers

11.1.4.2 Predictive Models

Disease Risk Index (DRI) (Armand et al. 2012, 2014)

Prognostic index based in the disease and its status at HSCT. It doesn't take into account factors as age or comorbidities. This score index classifies the disease in four prognostic groups and anticipates overall survival, progression-free survival, cumulative incidence of relapse, and cumulative incidence of non-relapse mortality (see Table 11.1).

Table 11.1 Disease risk index (Armand 2012, 2014)

Risk	Disease		
Low	AML with favorable cyt., CLL, CML, indolent B-cell NHL		
Intermediate	AML intermediate cyt., MDS intermediate cyt., myeloproliferative neoplasms, MM, HL, DLBCL/transformed indolent B-NHL, MCL, T-cell lymphoma nodal		
High	AML adverse cyt, MDS adverse cyt, T-cell lymphoma extranodal		
Risk	**Stage**		
Low	CR1, CR≥2, PR1, untreated, CML CP, PR≥2 (if RIC)		
High	PR≥2 (if MAC), induction failure, active relapse, CML AP or BP		
Disease risk	**Stage risk**	**Overall risk**	**OS at 4 years**
Low	Low	Low	64% (56–70%)
Low	High	Intermediate	46%
Intermediate	Low		(42–50%)
Intermediate	High	High	26%
High	Low		(21–31%)
High	High	Very high	6 (0–21%)

Adapted from Armand (2012). *Cyt.* cytogenetics

EBMT Risk Score (Gratwohl et al. 1998, 2009)

This predictive score, validated with 56,505 patients, permits to predict approximately the 5-year probability of OS and the TRM for the main diseases (see Tables 11.2, 11.3, and 11.4).

EBMT risk score is also useful to predict OS and TRM in patients receiving a second HSCT (Rezvani et al. 2012) and in those receiving a TCD HSCT (Lodewyck et al. 2011).

Some authors have introduced modifications in this risk score (including the concept of disease stage) to improve its predictivity (Terwey et al. 2010; Hemmati et al. 2011). Similarly, it has been associated with the HCT-CI (Barba et al. 2014).

This score has been validated by many groups and for many diseases (AML, ALL, PMF, CLL, and CML, among others).

Table 11.2 EBMT risk score (Gratwohl 2009)

Variables	Value of variables	Points
Age	<20 years	0
	20–40 years	1
	>40 years	2
Disease status[a]	Early	0
	Intermediate	1
	Advanced	2
Interval diagnosis-HSCT[b]	<12 months	0
	≥12 months	1
Donor	HLA-identical sibling	0
	Unrelated donor	1
Gender donor – recipient	Female to male	1
	Other combinations	0

Adapted from Gratwohl (2009)

[a]Do not apply in patients with SAA. Early = AL in CR1; MDS in CR1 or untreated; CML in 1st chronic phase; NHL/MM untreated or in CR1. Intermediate = AL in CR2; CML in other status than accelerated phase or blastic phase; MDS in CR2 or in PR; NHL/MM in CR2, PR, or stable dis. Late = AL in other stages; CML in blastic crisis; MDS in all other stages; NHL/MM in all other stages

[b]Do not apply to patients in CR1

Table 11.3 Probability (%) of TRM at 5 years applying the EBMT risk score

Points	0	1	2	3	4	5	6–7
AML	14	20	25	30	36	40	41
ALL	15	23	24	30	40	47	53
CML	15	22	30	38	45	52	55
AA	18	26	40	49	52		
MDS	25	28	30	35	38	46	50
MM			29	35	40	42	52
NHL	15	24	28	30	34	36	38

Extracted from Gratwohl (2009)

Table 11.4 Probability (%) of OS at 5 years applying the EBMT risk score

Points	0	1	2	3	4	5	6–7
AML	68	59	52	38	30	23	18
ALL	66	52	43	38	22	16	14
CML	76	72	60	51	39	26	14
AA	81	72	60	49	45		
MDS	56	52	46	40	35	28	25
MM			48	40	36	22	17
NHL	75	59	50	48	43	40	38

Extracted from Gratwohl (2009)

HCT-Comorbidity Index (HCT-CI) (Sorror et al. 2005)

Developed in Seattle in 2005. It is an adaptation to the HSCT of the classical Charlson Comorbidity Index (CCI). Validated in several cohorts and widely used. The score analyzes 17 comorbidities as well as their degree (see Table 11.5).

Given the impact of age on outcomes, the authors modified the model (Sorror et al. 2014), including a 1-point score for patients aged 40. This modification significantly improved the predictive capacity of the model. Consequently, the patients could be classified in three different risk groups (0 points, low risk; 1–2 points, intermediate risk; 3 or more, high risk) that clearly correlated with 2-year NRM.

Other authors re-stratified the HCT-CI index (flexible HCT-CI) as low risk, 0–3 points; intermediate risk, 4–5 points; and high risk, >5 points, being this classification a better predictor for NRM. In RIC setting, the 100-day and 2-year NRM incidence in these risk categories was 4%, 16%, and 29% and 19%, 33%, and 40%, respectively. They do find this predictive NRM value using neither the original HCT-CI nor the PAM or CCI models. Regarding the 2-year OS, this flexible HCT-CI score was also associated with the highest predictive hazard ratio (Barba et al. 2010).

HCT-CI has also been validated in CD34+ selected HSCT (Barba et al. 2017) and associated with the EBMT risk score that permits a better stratification (Barba et al. 2014).

Pretransplantation Assessment of Mortality (PAM) Score (Parimon et al. 2006; Au et al. 2015)

Developed in Seattle in 2006 but underused and poorly validated. It combines eight variables from patients and HSCT. Only useful for assessing mortality at 2 years.

Variables included age, type of donor, risk of disease, intensity of conditioning, DLCO, FEV1, creatinine, and ALT.

EBMT Machine Learning Algorithm (Shouval et al. 2015)

Based in an alternating decision tree able to detect variables associated with the primary

Table 11.5 HSCT-comorbidity index including age variable (Sorror 2005, 2014)

Comorbidity/definition	Points
Age ≥ 40 years	1
Arrhythmia Atrial fibrillation, flutter, sick sinus node syndrome, or ventricular arrhythmias	1
Cardiac Coronary heart disease, congestive heart failure, IAM, FEVE ≤50%	1
Inflammatory bowel disease Crohn's disease or ulcerative colitis that has required treatment	1
Diabetes Requiring insulin or oral antidiabetic medication in the 4 weeks prior to HSCT	1
Cerebrovascular CVA or TIA or cerebral thrombosis	1
Psychiatric Depression or anxiety or others requiring ongoing treatment (not on demand)	1
Mild liver Chronic hepatitis, elevated bilirubin <1.5 × NV or AST/ALT <2.5 × NV Previous HBV or HCV infection	1
Obesity BMI >35 kg/m^2	1
Previous infection Infection in admission requiring continuation of treatment beyond day 0	1
Moderate lung DLCO and/or FEV1 66–80% or minimal stress dyspnea	2
Rheumatology Systemic lupus, rheumatoid arthritis, polymyositis, polymyalgia rheumatica, connective tissue disease	2
Peptic ulcer Endoscopic or radiological diagnosis (does not score if only reflux or gastritis)	2
Renal Creatinine >176 mcmol/L, dialysis, or previous kidney transplant	2
Previous tumor[a] Neoplasia at some point (excludes non-melanoma skin tumor)	3
Heart valve Diagnosed (except mitral prolapse)	3
Severe pulmonary DLCO and/or FEV1 ≤%, dyspnea at rest or oxygen at home	3
Severe liver disease Bilirubin ≥0.5 for VN or AST or ALT ≥0.5 for VN or cirrhosis	3

[a]A most recent version also includes in this category hematological/tumors of a different lineage to that which motivates the transplant (e.g., lymphoma in an AML patient but not previous MDS in AML patient)

outcome, assigning weights and ignoring redundancies. This score was developed to analyze the NRM at day +100 in patients with acute leukemia but also predict NRM, LFS, and OS at 2 years.

The variables included in the model are age, Karnofsky (≥80; <80), diagnostic (AML; ALL), disease stage (CR1; CR2; all other stages), interval diagnostic-HSCT (<142 days; ≥142 days), donor-recipient CMV status (both (sero +); both (sero -); any other combination), donor type (MSD; MUD), conditioning (MAC; RIC), and annual allo-HSCT performed in the center (<20; ≥21). The total +100 NRM and 2-year NRM, LFS, and OS could be obtained through a web page: http://bioinfo.lnx.biu.ac.il/~bondi/web1.html.

Recently this algorithm has also been validated by an independent set of data from GITMO (Shouval et al. 2017).

11.1.4.3 Predictive Capacity of These Models

Unfortunately, all these models have a relatively low predictive capacity, and none of them stand out more than the rest.

Author	Predictive/s model/s	Predictive capacity
Sorror et al. (2005)	HCT-CI	0.65
Xhaard (2008)	rHCT-CT, PAM	0.49, 0.57
Gratwohl (2009)	EBMT	0.63
Barba et al. (2010)	fHCT-CI, PAM	0.67, 0.63
Barba et al. (2014)	HCT-CI, EBMT	0.60, 0.54
Versluis (2015)	(HCT-CI-EBMT)	0.58, 0.58 (0.64)

Courtesy of P. Barba, MD. rHCT-CI = reduced model, without PFTs; fHSCT = flexible model (modified scale)

11.1.5 Practical Applications of Risk Assessment

Election of the conditioning	In patients with a high risk of NRM following one of the mentioned risk scores, a RIC should be considered
Relative contraindications	Uncontrolled infection, severe or chronic liver disease (excluding cirrhosis), severe disturbances in heart function (FEV <40%), respiratory (DLCO <40%) or renal (creatinine clearance <30 mL/min)
Absolute contraindications	Pregnancy Cirrhosis. Even compensated cirrhosis receiving RIC have a high likelihood of hepatic decompensation (Hogan et al. 2004)

Key Points

- The evaluation of a candidate must be carried out according to a preestablished work plan designed by each institution. The use of standardized procedures reduces the risk of errors or omissions
- Several pretransplant variables (such as age) have a clear impact on the results of the procedure but, when assessed in isolation, are highly insufficient to predict the results
- Predictive models (DRI, EBMT risk score, HCT-CI, PAM) allow a much more realistic approach to the real possibilities of a given candidate and adapt the procedure to their needs

11.2 Counseling of Candidates

Alessandro Rambaldi

11.2.1 Introduction

Allo-HSCT is a potentially curative treatment modality for otherwise incurable diseases. Unfortunately, after transplantation patients may experience not only the persistence or recurrence of their own disease but also some dramatic clinical complications and toxicities, including death. The clinical indications to transplant have been addressed in the section "indications" of this book, but in general, when the allo-HSCT is advised, the strength of the indication (the likelihood to be cured by transplant), the patient fitness, and his/her personal commitment to transplant must be carefully evaluated for each candidate.

Obviously, a first distinction must be done between patients with a neoplastic versus a non-neoplastic disease, and the transplant option should be progressively discussed with the patient during the course of the disease, particularly in the case of hematologic malignancies. Many professionals should concur to illustrate the patients the curative potential of an allo-HSCT and to help understanding the severe complications that can eventually develop. It is clear that different indications remarkably affect the way a patient is advised. However, there is a time when the transplant option must be formally presented and advised. Therefore, evaluation of each transplant candidate must be based on well-predefined formal standard operating procedures to collect exhaustive clinical, instrumental, and laboratory data that may lead to a robust definition of the risks and benefits related to allo-HSCT. All in all, the counseling is to tailor such evaluation to the individual patients (Shouval et al. 2015), according to both objective data and subjective data such as patient propensity and fear of side effects. At the end of this process, the patient should be aware of the rationale, the benefit and the toxicity associated with each step, and component of the transplant procedure. In this chapter, I will hereby summarize the main topics I cover with my patients when they come to my office to discuss the option of the allo-HSCT.

11.2.2 Understanding the Benefit and Risk of Allogeneic Transplant

Patients must be informed that allo-HSCT is a therapeutic option that is always proposed with the intent to achieve a permanent cure of the underlying disease, but despite this premise, disease progression or relapse may eventually happen. The indication to allo-HSCT depends not only on the disease characteristics but also on patient-related factors such as age and comorbidities (Sorror et al. 2007) so that the transplant proposal is the result of an accurate and wise evaluation of both these factors (Sorror et al. 2013; Wang et al. 2014).

The patient should understand the specific risk/benefit balance associated with a conventional versus a transplant-based proposal, and this may be remarkably different if he has been diagnosed with a non-neoplastic disease such as thalassemia or sickle cell anemia, a bone marrow failure syndrome like aplastic anemia, or a blood cancer, such as an acute leukemia. Even when allo-HSCT may in theory represent the most efficacious treatment modality to get a permanent cure of a specific disease, an accurate description of the available alternatives must be presented. This is particularly important when the non-transplant options, albeit not curative, may have the chance to keep the patient alive for a long time (Samuelson Bannow et al. 2018) or, even more importantly, when the conventional treatment may lead to a definitive cure such as in the case of some patients with acute leukemia with intermediate-risk genetic factors or those achieving a deep molecular remission after conventional chemotherapy (Cornelissen and Blaise 2016).

11.2.3 Understanding the Transplant Procedure: The Donor, the Conditioning Regimen, and the Clinical Complications

Once the indication to transplant has been confirmed, patients and their relatives must be informed on how the transplant is performed. Patients should understand that identifying a stem cell donor is an absolute prerequisite to perform a transplant. Accordingly, patients should be informed about the human leukocyte antigen (HLA) genetic system, its specificity for each individual, how it is inherited by parents according to the Mendelian laws, and what is the probability to find a compatible donor in the family group. Understanding the HLA system is crucial to explain why the use of a HLA family-matched sibling donors is considered standard and when such a sibling is not available; an international search has to be performed to identify a HLA-compatible unrelated donor. It is important to underline that more than 30 million of potentially available donors are registered by the World Marrow Donor Association (WMDA), and the probability to find a compatible donor is between 50 and 80% according to the ethnical origin of each patient.

Once such matched unrelated donor is identified, this type of transplant is considered a standard of care, and its clinical outcome is fully comparable to what was observed when using an HLA-identical sibling. In patients for whom a MSD or a MUD is not available, the patient should be informed that two additional options are available, namely, the use of HSC obtained by a family mismatched donor (commonly defined as haploidentical because sharing only one of the patient's HLA haplotypes) or a banked cord blood units. Patients should understand how the HLA diversity between patient and donor has been overcome by specific programs of in vitro or in vivo manipulation of the graft.

Patients should be reassured that the incidence and severity of GvHD, the most important side effect of allo-HSCT, seems not to be higher than observed with MUD. In addition, patients should know that many single-arm studies reported that transplants performed with these alternative stem cell sources proved to be effective and safe even when offered to patients of advanced age and/or with existing accompanying illnesses or when the disease was refractory to conventional treatment. All in all, at the present time, the clinical outcome of these alternative types of transplants compares reasonably well with those achieved with MUD. Therefore, the decision to use this type of stem cell source only when an HLA-matched donor is not available is mostly related to the lack of randomized clinical trials that are planned to be performed in the near future.

The goal of an allo-HSCT is to eradicate the patient's hematopoiesis either neoplastic or normal. This is achieved by the delivery of the conditioning regimen and by the lifelong in vivo effect played by the donor's immune system. Most often, high doses of chemotherapy and/or radiation are included in the preparations although remarkable differences exist depending on the disease needing transplant and patient tolerance. The patient should understand that the intensity of the conditioning regimen may be particularly important in the case of hematologic malignancies when the aim to remove most of the neoplastic cells present in the patient's body is the first goal. However, to avoid at least part of the treatment toxicity, the intensity of the preparative regimen can be down-modulated leading to the definition of this preparative regimen as non-myeloablative or reduced intensity. The depletion of the patient bone marrow stem cells induces a prolonged pancytopenia and the need of donor-derived healthy stem cells to grow and establish a new blood cell production system.

The allogeneic HSC, collected from the donor's BM or PB or a frozen CBU, are infused through the central venous catheter into the bloodstream: HSCT is not a surgical procedure and it is very similar to receiving a blood transfusion. The stem cells find their way into the bone marrow and begin reproducing and growing new, healthy blood cells. It is very important to explain how the donor immune system will develop progressively after transplantation and will either exert a crucial beneficial role against residual neoplastic cells or restore the immune competence against infections, but it could mediate the most harmful GvHD effect against the patient.

After the transplant, supportive care is given to prevent and treat infections, side effects of treatments, and complications. Prolonged anemia, thrombocytopenia, and leukopenia can be dangerous and even life-threatening. A low platelet count can be potentially associated with bleeding in the lungs, GI tract, and brain. Leukopenia, including either a defect of neutrophils and lymphocytes, leads to the development of frequent infections, the most common clinical complications after transplantation. Infections can include not only bacterial, most likely when the patient has a severe bone marrow suppression, but also viral and fungal pathogens. Infections can require an extended hospital stay, prevent or delay engraftment, and/or cause permanent organ damage. On average the time to hematologic engraftment (recovery of the neutrophil and platelet function) is about 2–3 weeks, but a protective recovery of the immune system can take months and sometimes years. High doses of chemotherapy and radiation can cause remarkable toxicities that include but not limited to severe mucositis (inflammation of the mouth and GI tract) that favors bacterial translocation with related infections and GvHD and multi-organ failure mainly the lung, heart, liver, and kidney.

A particular attention should be paid to risk of graft failure that can occur early or late after transplantation. A graft failure is more frequent in some diseases such as myelofibrosis or as the results of infections or when the stem cell content of the graft is insufficient to guarantee a durable engraftment. A graft rejection can also happen after reduced intensity conditioning regimen (when the immune system of the host is not completely eradicated and can actively reject the donor stem cells).

Finally, and most importantly, patients must be aware of what GvHD is, when and how it may develop, and why it represents the most serious complication of a HSCT, being not only life-threatening but also the principal reason of a long-lasting poor quality of life. Transplant candidates should be aware that GvHD is the negative counterpart of the deep interaction of the donor immune system within patient body that at the same time may lead to definitive cure of an otherwise incurable disease. In other words, when transplant is advised, patients must realize that they are accepting the possible onset of a chronic, often invalidating, autoimmune disease. GVHD can appear at any time after transplant. GvHD is conventionally distinguished in an acute form that usually develops within the first 100 days after transplant and the chronic form that occurs later in the transplant course. Patients who develop acute GVHD are more likely to also develop the chronic form of GVHD. Patients must understand the importance of their compliance to all the treatments given post transplant to prevent GvHD and how this is instrumental for a successful transplant. GvHD occurs when the donor's immune system reacts against the recipient's tissue. At variance to what happens after a solid organ transplant where the patient's immune system is driven to reject only the transplanted organ, in GVHD, the donor immune system can react against many different organs of the recipient. This is why the new cells do not recognize the tissues and organs of the recipient's body as self. Over time, thanks to the effect of immune suppressive drugs, a progressive tolerance can develop. The most common sites for GVHD are the GI tract, liver, skin, and lungs.

Key Points

Counseling of patients should be carefully performed to inform candidates that:

- Disease and patient's specific characteristics are equally important to advise transplant
- Allo-HSCT is performed to cure otherwise incurable diseases
- Despite transplant, disease persistence or relapse may occur
- Transplant can severely compromise the quality of life of patients
- Transplant is a form of immunotherapy requiring long-term follow-up care
- Logistics are important to ensure adequate care and assistance

11.2.4 Logistics

After discharge for the transplant ward, patients are followed up in the outpatient clinic two to three times per week until day +100. Patients should be helped to realize how complex is the transplant procedure and that the time spent in the hospital represents only the first part of the treatment program. All allo-HSCT patients should ideally stay within 1 h of the hospital until it is about 3 months from the day of the transplant. Patients and their families should also realize that the overall recovery time varies from person to person and in general this process takes about 1 year to be satisfactory. Allogeneic transplantation is therefore a long-lasting immunotherapy, and the interaction between the donor immune system and the patient requires a careful and prolonged medical assistance, quite often long life.

References

Armand P, Gibson CJ, Cutler C, et al. A disease risk index for patients undergoing allogeneic stem cell transplantation. Blood. 2012;120:905–13.

Armand P, Kim HT, Logan BR, et al. Validation and refinement of the disease risk index for allogeneic stem cell transplantation. Blood. 2014;123:3664–71.

Au BK, Gooley TA, Armand P, et al. Reevaluation of the pretransplant assessment of mortality score after allogeneic hematopoietic transplantation. Biol Blood Marrow Transplant. 2015;21:848–54.

Barba P, Piñana JL, Martino R, et al. Comparison of two pretransplant predictive models and a flexible HCT-CI using different cut off points to determine low-, intermediate-, and high-risk groups: the flexible HCT-CI Is the best predictor of NRM and OS in a population of patients undergoing allo-RIC. Biol Blood Marrow Transplant. 2010;16:413–20.

Barba P, Martino R, Pérez-Simón JA, et al. Combination of the hematopoietic cell transplantation comorbidity index and the European Group for blood and marrow transplantation score allows a better stratification of high-risk patients undergoing reduced-toxicity allogeneic hematopoietic cell transplantation. Biol Blood Marrow Transplant. 2014;20:66–72.

Barba P, Ratan R, Cho C, et al. Hematopoietic cell transplantation comorbidity index predicts outcomes in patients with acute myeloid leukemia and myelodysplastic syndromes receiving CD34(+) selected grafts for allogeneic hematopoietic cell transplantation. Biol Blood Marrow Transplant. 2017;23:67–74.

Cornelissen JJ, Blaise D. Hematopoietic stem cell transplantation for patients with AML in first complete remission. Blood. 2016;127:62–70.

Gratwohl A, Hermans J, Goldman JM, et al. Risk assessment for patients with chronic myeloid leukaemia before allogeneic blood or marrow transplantation. Chronic Leukemia Working Party of the European Group for Blood and Marrow Transplantation. Lancet. 1998;352:1087–92.

Gratwohl A, Stern M, Brand R, et al. Risk score for outcome after allogeneic hematopoietic stem cell transplantation: a retrospective analysis. Cancer. 2009;115:4715–26.

Hemmati PG, Terwey TH, le Coutre P, et al. A modified EBMT risk score predicts the outcome of patients with acute myeloid leukemia receiving allogeneic stem cell transplants. Eur J Haematol. 2011;86:305–16.

Hogan WJ, Maris M, Storer B, et al. Hepatic injury after nonmyeloablative conditioning followed by allogeneic hematopoietic cell transplantation: a study of 193 patients. Blood. 2004;103:78–84.

Lodewyck T, Oudshoorn M, van der Holt B, et al. Predictive impact of allele-matching and EBMT risk score for outcome after T-cell depleted unrelated donor transplantation in poor-risk acute leukemia and myelodysplasia. Leukemia. 2011;25:1548–54.

Parimon T, Au DH, Martin PJ, Chien JW. A risk score for mortality after allogeneic hematopoietic cell transplantation. Ann Intern Med. 2006;144:407–14.

Rezvani K, Kanfer EJ, Marin D, Gabriel I, et al. EBMT risk score predicts outcome of allogeneic hematopoietic stem cell transplantation in patients who have failed a previous transplantation procedure. Biol Blood Marrow Transplant. 2012;18:235–40.

Samuelson Bannow BT, Salit RB, Storer BE, et al. Hematopoietic cell transplantation for myelofibrosis: the dynamic international prognostic scoring system plus risk predicts post-transplant outcomes. Biol Blood Marrow Transplant. 2018;24:386–92.

Shouval R, Labopin M, Bondi O, et al. Prediction of allogeneic hematopoietic stem-cell transplantation mortality 100 days after transplantation using a machine learning algorithm: a European Group for Blood and Marrow Transplantation Acute Leukemia Working Party retrospective data mining study. J Clin Oncol. 2015;33:3144–51.

Shouval R, Bonifazi F, Fein J, et al. Validation of the acute leukemia-EBMT score for prediction of mortality following allogeneic stem cell transplantation in a multi-center GITMO cohort. Am J Hematol. 2017;92:429–34.

Sorror ML. How I assess comorbidities before hematopoietic cell transplantation. Blood. 2013;121:854–63.

Sorror ML, Maris MB, Storb R, et al. Hematopoietic cell transplantation (HCT)-specific comorbidity index: a new tool for risk assessment before allogeneic HCT. Blood. 2005;106:2912–9.

Sorror ML, Giralt S, Sandmaier BM, et al. Hematopoietic cell transplantation specific comorbidity index as an outcome predictor for patients with acute myeloid leukemia in first remission: combined FHCRC and MDACC experiences. Blood. 2007;110:4606–13.

Sorror ML, Storb RF, Sandmaier BM, et al. Comorbidity-age index: a clinical measure of biologic age before allogeneic hematopoietic cell transplantation. J Clin Oncol. 2014;32:3249–56.

Terwey TH, Hemmati PG, Martus P, et al. A modified EBMT risk score and the hematopoietic cell transplantation-specific comorbidity index for pretransplant risk assessment in adult acute lymphoblastic leukemia. Haematologica. 2010;95:810–8.

Versluis J, Labopin M, Niederwieser D, et al. Prediction of non-relapse mortality in recipients of reduced intensity conditioning allogeneic stem cell transplantation with AML in first complete remission. Leukemia. 2015;29:51–7.

Wang HT, Chang YJ, Xu LP, Liu DH, Wang Y, Liu KY, Huang XJ. EBMT risk score can predict the outcome of leukaemia after unmanipulated haploidentical blood and marrow transplantation. Bone Marrow Transplant. 2014;49:927–33.

Xhaard A, Porcher R, Chien JW, et al. Impact of comorbidity indexes on non-relapse mortality. Leukemia. 2008;22:2062–9.

12 Donor Selection for Adults and Pediatrics

Francis Ayuk and Adriana Balduzzi

12.1 Introduction

It is known that multiple factors impact on transplantation outcome; the heaviest ones are disease-related (disease refractoriness, phase, clonal abnormalities, etc. in malignancies and disease type and associated rejection risk in non-malignant diseases) and patient-related (age, comorbidities, infectious diseases/colonization, etc.). Moreover, donor-related issues and stem cell source may influence the extent of disease control and transplant-related mortality.

The availability of a suitable stem cell graft is an absolute prerequisite for the performance of allo-HSCT. Beyond donor-recipient histocompatibility, other factors such as stem cell source, donor age and gender, donor-recipient CMV status, and ABO compatibility may play a role on transplant outcome.

In this chapter we discuss results of studies investigating these factors and conclude with an algorithm for donor selection. Issues which are peculiar to pediatric recipients are also analyzed and discussed.

F. Ayuk
Department of Stem Cell Transplantation, University Medical Center Hamburg-Eppendorf (UKE), Hamburg, Germany

A. Balduzzi (✉)
Outpatient Hematology and Transplant Department, Clinica Pediatrica, Università degli Studi di Milano Bicocca, Ospedale San Gerardo, Monza, Italy
e-mail: abalduzzi@fondazionembbm.it

12.2 Donor HLA Compatibility (See Chap. 9)

The outcome of HSCT depends in part on the matching between the donor and the recipient for the human leukocyte antigens (HLA), encoded by a group of genes on chromosome 6; genes and products are labelled as major histocompatibility complex (MHC). The HLA system is the most polymorphic genetic region known in the human genome. A set of HLA gene alleles, called haplotype, is inherited from each parent; therefore, the probability that a child inherited and shares both parental haplotypes with a full sibling is 25%. Such HLA-identical sibling is still considered an optimal donor.

The most relevant genes for transplantation belong to class I (HLA-A, HLA-B, and HLA-Cw) and class II (HLA-DR, HLA-DQ, and HLA-DP). HLA compatibility with the donor is usually defined by high-resolution typing (four digits) for ten alleles, HLA-A, HLA-B, HLA-C, HLA-DR, and HLA-DQ (Petersdorf 2013), even though there is an increasing evidence supporting the relevance of DPB1 matching (reviewed by Fleischhauer and Shaw 2017).

The concept of "compatibility" for CB donor-recipient pairs is still under debate. Any CB unit which was 6/6 or 5/6 matched was labelled HLA compatible (MD), in the past as defined by low-resolution typing at A and B loci and high-resolution typing at the DRB1 locus; more recently, high resolution for at least A, B,

E. Carreras et al. (eds.), *The EBMT Handbook*, https://doi.org/10.1007/978-3-030-02278-5_12

C, and DRB1 loci is requested, and progressively the same criteria used for volunteer donors are considered to define CB HLA matching (Eapen et al. 2017).

12.3 Donor Selection for Adult Patients

12.3.1 Donor Type (Summarized in Fig. 12.1)

12.3.1.1 Matched Related Siblings and Unrelated Donors

Donor-recipient histocompatibility is one of the key variables in allo-HSCT. An HLA-identical sibling donor is generally considered the best donor for allo-HSCT; however less than a third of patients will have one available. Unrelated donor registries worldwide now include more than about 30 million volunteer donors, most of them in North America and Europe (www.bmdw.org). The probability of finding a fully MUD (8/8 or 10/10) varies on average between 16% and 75% (Gragert et al. 2014; Buck et al. 2016) depending on ethnicity, with lowest and highest probabilities in patients of African and European descent, respectively. Increasing ethnic diversity will with time further limit the chances of finding a fully matched unrelated donor.

Till date no randomized trial has compared outcome of transplants from different donors. However, one prospective (Yakoub-Agha et al. 2006) and several retrospective analyses indicate that outcomes after MSD and fully MUD (8/8 or 10/10) HSCT are comparable (Schetelig et al. 2008; Szydlo et al. 1997; Arora et al. 2009; Ringden 2009; Gupta et al. 2010; Woolfrey et al. 2010; Saber et al. 2012). Increase in donor-recipient HLA disparity in HLA-A, HLA-B, HLA-C, or HLA-DRB1 is associated with poorer outcome after unrelated donor transplantation (Lee et al. 2007; Shaw et al. 2010; Woolfrey et al. 2011; Horan et al. 2012; Fürst et al. 2013; Pidala et al. 2014; Verneris et al. 2015). The overall decrease in survival can be explained by the increase in NRM with no positive effect on relapse. Disparities in HLA-DQB1 as well as C-allele disparities in C*03:03 vs 03:04 have been reported to be permissive with no negative effects on outcome (Lee et al. 2007; Fürst et al. 2013; Morishima et al. 2015; Pidala et al. 2014; Crivello et al. 2016). Disparities in HLA-DPB1 are observed in the majority of HLA-A, HLA-B, HLA-C, and HLA-DQB1

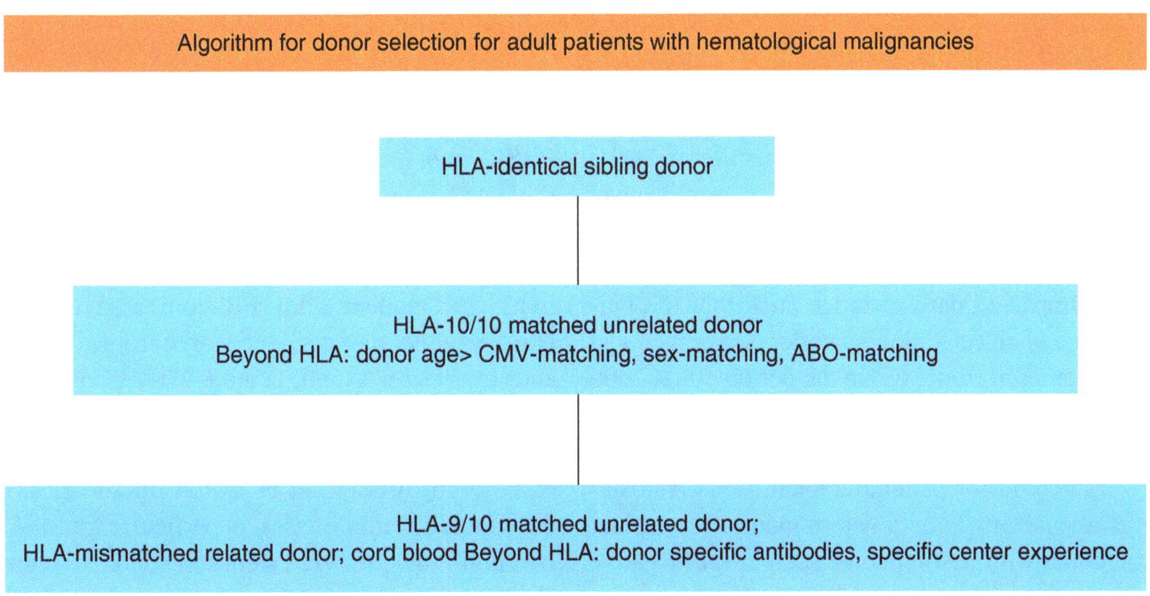

Fig. 12.1 Algorithm for donor selection

(10/10) MUD transplants. Nonpermissive mismatches in DPB1 defined according to T-cell epitope matching (Zino et al. 2004; Crocchiolo et al. 2009; Fleischhauer et al. 2012; Pidala et al. 2014; Oran et al. 2018) or allele cell-surface expression levels (Petersdorf et al. 2015) are associated with poorer outcome compared to full matches or permissive mismatches. Associations of permissive DPB1 mismatches with lower relapse incidence are currently being explored (Fleischhauer and Beelen 2016; Fleischhauer and Shaw 2017).

12.3.1.2 Haploidentical Related Donors

Improvements in transplant technology including pre-transplant ATG (Huang et al. 2006), PT-CY (Luznik et al. 2008), and alpha-beta TCD (Bertaina et al. 2014) have led to improved outcome and rapidly increasing use of haploidentical related donor transplantation (Passweg et al. 2014). Several retrospective comparison studies have reported similar outcome for haploidentical and MUD transplants (summarized by Fuchs 2017). The results of prospective comparative trials are eagerly awaited.

12.3.2 Role of Non-HLA Donor Characteristics

Besides donor-recipient histocompatibility, donor age is now considered one of, if not the most relevant, the non-HLA donor characteristics in unrelated donor HSCT (Kollman et al. 2001, 2016; Wang et al. 2018) with a 2-year survival being 3% better when a donor 10 years younger is selected (Shaw et al. 2018). These findings have impacted daily practice such that the percentage of selected donors under 30 years of age has increased from 36% in the period 1988–2006 to 51% in 1999–2011 up to 69% in 2012–2014 (Kollman et al. 2016).

Matching for patient/recipient CMV serostatus also seems to be a determinant of transplant outcome with best outcome seen in seronegative patients receiving seronegative grafts (Ljungman 2014; Kalra et al. 2016; Shaw et al. 2017).

The impact of sex mismatch on outcome is more controversial, possibly reflecting different definitions of sex mismatch, which has been considered only for male recipients (Gratwohl et al. 2009, 2017; Nakasone et al. 2015) or for both male and female in others (Kollman et al. 2016). Interestingly, all three studies confining sex mismatch to male recipients reported a significant impact for this variable, albeit possibly dependent on conditioning regimen.

The impact of ABO (blood group) compatibility on outcome has been reported to be modest and seems to have further diminished in recent years probably due to changes in transplant practice including less frequent use of bone marrow grafts (Seebach et al. 2005; Kollman et al. 2016; Shaw et al. 2018).

The impact of non-HLA donor characteristics may be less conspicuous in matched and mismatched related donor transplantations using PT-CY. It must however be taken into consideration that the close association of donor age and donor-patient relation on the one hand with patient age on the other hand makes these analyses more complex (McCurdy et al. 2018; Robinson et al. 2018). Larger patient cohorts and prospective studies are required for more definite conclusions.

12.3.3 Donor Choice According to Stem Cell Source

The three graft sources for allo-HSCT are BM, PBSC, and CB. In matched related donor and unrelated donor HSCT, survival outcome has been similar for BM and PBSC. However hematological recovery is more rapid and graft rejection less frequent after PB compared to BM HSCT, while the incidence of chronic GvHD and, to a lesser extent, acute GvHD tends to be higher after PB HSCT (Bensinger et al. 2001; Couban et al. 2002; Schmitz et al. 2002; Couban et al. 2016; Anasetti et al. 2012). In allo-HSCT for nonmalignant diseases, in particular for SAA, BM is still the preferred stem cell source in high-income countries, despite improvements in outcome after PB HSCT (Schrezenmeier et al. 2007;

Chu et al. 2011; Bacigalupo et al. 2012; Kumar et al. 2016).

Traditionally BM has been used as stem cell source for haploidentical HSCT with PT-CY (Luznik et al. 2008), while GCSF-stimulated BM has been used for haploidentical HSCT with ATG (Huang et al. 2006) and PBSC for haploidentical HSCT with alpha-beta T-cell depletion (Bertaina et al. 2014). There are no prospective studies comparing different stem cell sources within these strategies. When PT-CY is used, PBSC seems to be associated with a higher risk of acute and chronic GvHD and lower risk of relapse in patients with leukemia (Bashey et al. 2017).

The use of umbilical CB grafts continues to decrease with the rise in numbers of haploidentical transplants performed (Passweg et al. 2014). Due to the limited number of stem cells per unit, CB grafts have been more frequently used in pediatric HSCT and will be discussed in that section and in the specific CB Chapter.

12.3.4 Anti-HLA Antibodies

The abovementioned improvements in transplant technology have led to an increased use of grafts from HLA-mismatched donors. Detection of donor-specific anti-HLA antibodies in the patients' serum has been associated with increased risk of graft failure and also poorer survival of those patients with graft failure (Ciurea et al. 2015) after haploidentical HSCT. The risk of graft failure and overall mortality may however also depend on the type and intensity of TCD used. The EBMT recently published a consensus guideline on detection and treatment of donor-specific antibodies in haploidentical HSCT (Ciurea et al. 2018).

12.4 Donor Selection for Pediatric Patients

Donor selection criteria may vary between adult and pediatric recipients. According to the "motto" of the Pediatric Disease Working Party, "children are not small adults," besides the size, what makes HSCT in children different is mainly related with indications and the biology of a growing individual.

12.4.1 Pediatric Recipient Size

In terms of size, the recipient weight may vary between few Kg in most patients transplanted for immunodeficiencies and a full adult size in some adolescents. The recommended cell dose in the graft is shown in Table 12.1 (Gluckmann 2012). The lower the recipient weight, the smaller is the amount of the requested absolute count in the graft, which makes the harvest easier, often matching the transplant center requests. An appropriate cell dose in the graft yields a lower risk of rejection, which is actually lowest in pediatrics. On the other hand, the lower amount of cells requested to ensure engraftment in children makes CB a more valuable source than in adults.

12.4.2 Indications

In terms of indications, according to the EBMT, nowadays 46% of the patients younger than 18 years who undergo HSCT are affected with non-malignant diseases (Passweg et al. 2014), which are mainly inherited disorders, namely, immunodeficiencies, hemoglobinopaties, inborn errors of

Table 12.1 Number of cells according to stem cell source

	Volume collected	Med CD34 content	Med CD3 content	Target cell dose
Bone marrow	10–20 mL/kg	$2–3 \times 10^6$/kg[a]	25×10^6/kg	$>2 \times 10^8$ TNC/kg
Peripheral blood	150–400 mL	8×10^6/kg	250×10^6/kg	$5–10 \times 10^6$ CD34+/kg
Umbilical cord blood	80–160 mL	0.2×10^6/kg	2.5×10^6/kg	$>3 \times 10^7$ TNC/kg

[a]Per kg recipient body weight

metabolism, and congenital bone marrow failures. As nonmalignant diseases do not benefit of any alloreactivity, the closest HLA matching (possibly "10 out of 10" HLA alleles) is recommended. On the contrary, a small degree of HLA incompatibility is tolerated in malignancies, as the detrimental effect of HLA disparity, triggering higher risk of GvHD and consequent higher risks of toxicity and mortality, might be counterbalanced by the so-called "graft-versus-leukemia" or "graft-versus-tumor" effect, which is the alloreactivity of immunocompetent donor cells potentially eradicating residual malignant cells in the patient and playing a role in the prevention of malignant disease recurrence.

12.4.3 Donor Type

Due to the decreasing size of modern families in the so-called Western countries, HLA-identical siblings are available in less than 25% of the children in need of a transplant, as shown by the few studies performing a "randomization by genetic chance," based on the availability of an HLA-identical sibling or not (Balduzzi et al. 2005). As a consequence, 75% of the patients may need to run a search for an unrelated donor.

Eligibility criteria for HSCT in malignant diseases varied overtime, resulting from the balance between the outcome of frontline and relapse chemotherapy protocols and the outcome of transplantation, which partially depends on the degree of compatibility within each donor-recipient pair. Similarly, the eligibility for transplantation in nonmalignant diseases increased as the safety profile of the procedure improved. Some patients are considered eligible for transplantation only in case an HLA-identical sibling is available; as the risk profile of the patient worsens, a broader degree of HLA mismatching is considered acceptable.

Within the International BFM Study Group, regardless of their relationship with their recipient, donors are defined as HLA-matched (MD) if the donor-recipient pairs are fully matched (10/10) or have a single allelic or antigenic disparity (9/10) or are defined mismatched donor (MMD) if the donor-recipient pairs have two (8/10) or more allelic or antigenic disparities, up to a different haplotype (Peters et al. 2015). Any donor who is not an HLA-identical sibling or a MD, as defined above, is considered a MMD. Both MD and MMD could be either related or unrelated to their recipient. A related donor who is not an HLA-identical sibling is actually regarded as a MD, and GvHD prophylaxis is planned accordingly (Peters et al. 2015).

Recently, results from a BFM study showed that transplantation from a "10 or 9 out of 10" matched donor, either related or unrelated, was not inferior to transplantation from an HLA-identical sibling in terms of EFS, OS, and CIR in pediatric patients with ALL (Peters et al. 2015). As a consequence eligibility criteria for HSCT might be reviewed and extended to those for MSD HSCT, at least in ALL, and, possibly, considered for other malignant diseases. Therefore, an unrelated donor search activation and transplantation might be recommended in the future virtually for every child for whom an allo-HSCT is indicated. Disparities within donor-recipient pairs are progressively accepted as the risk profile of the patient increases.

Unfortunately some inherited disorders, in particular sickle cell disease (Gluckman et al. 2017) or other recessively inherited disease, which incidence is highly increased by a parental blood relation, have higher incidences in non-Caucasian ethnicities, which are less represented within stem cell donor banks. The consequence is that well-matched donors often lack when a perfect matching is crucial; progresses in haploidentical HSCT broadened its indications and may overcome this issue.

Depending on each transplant center experience, MMD might be preferred, carrying the advantage of prompt donor availability and flexible schedule and bringing higher degree of alloreactivity, potentially associated with lower relapse risk. HSCT from MMD is widely recommended when timing adjustment is crucial, as in advanced disease phase in malignancies and in case of post transplant relapse.

12.4.4 Haploidentical Donors in Pediatrics

Successful haploidentical HSCT mainly evolved in pediatrics over the last two decades from ex vivo T-cell depletion by CD34+-positive selection, to CD34+-negative selection, up to selective CD3 αβ depletion, to allow other cells in the graft, potentially protecting from viral infections (Handgretinger et al. 2001; Klingebiel et al. 2010). In pediatrics, an improved immune recovery after TCR αβ-depleted haploidentical HSCT (Lang et al. 2015), a similar outcome between TCR αβ-depleted and matched sibling and matched unrelated donors HSCT in children with acute leukemia (Locatelli et al. 2017) and in nonmalignant diseases (Bertaina et al. 2014), was recently reported and confirmed by a multicenter phase I/II study (Lang et al. 2017). Moreover, some reports of PT-CY in pediatric show promising results (Jaiswal et al. 2016; Sawada et al. 2014; Wiebking et al. 2017).

One of the parents mostly serves as a donor in haploidentical donors for pediatric recipients. The choice between the mother and the father is still debated. Better survival was shown in patients transplanted from the mother than from the father (51% vs 11%; $P < 0.001$), due to both reduced incidence of relapse and TRM, with a protective effect on the risk of failure (HR 0.42; $P = 0.003$), possibly explained by transplacental leukocyte trafficking during pregnancy, inducing long-term, stable, reciprocal microchimerism in mother and child (Stern et al. 2008).

As donor-derived alloreactive NK cells have been shown to play a key role in the eradication of leukemic cells, favorable NK matching should guide donor selection (Stringaris and Barrett 2017; Mavers and Bertaina 2018). Moreover, anti-HLA antibodies should be checked and accounted for to guide donor selection.

12.4.5 Stem Cell Source

BM is usually recommended as stem cell source. A donor with a body weight allowing for a graft containing at least 3×10^8 nucleated cells/kg recipient body weight and 3×10^6 CD34+ cells/kg body weight should be selected, in order to yield more than 95% neutrophil engraftment chances at a median of 21 days in the setting of hematological malignant diseases (Simonin et al. 2017).

It is rare in pediatrics to require PB just in order to obtain an adequate amount of cells to ensure engraftment, as the absolute cell dose needed rarely overcomes the maximum amount which could be harvested from a donor. As higher numbers of CD3 cells are obtained in PB grafts, it is recommended not to exceed an amount of 10×10^8 CD3+ cells/kg recipient body weight.

The increased risk of chronic GvHD, and possibly acute, after PBSC transplantation, as compared to BM, is commonly reported. In a recent European retrospective study, including 2584 pediatric patients transplanted from 2003 to 2012 for ALL, both TRM and chronic GvHD appeared significantly higher after PBSC, as compared with other SC sources, despite the overall survival was similar for both stem cell sources (Simonin et al. 2017). In the prospective ALL-SCT-BFM 2003 study, the same OS was reported, and no difference could be demonstrated in TRM, acute GvHD, and relapse, whichever the stem cell source in the two cohorts of patients transplanted from HLA-identical siblings and other matched donors. Nevertheless, within patients transplanted from HLA-identical siblings, the cumulative incidence of chronic GvHD was higher in PB compared with BM recipients (Peters et al. 2015).

Reinforced GvHD prophylaxis may be recommended when PBSC are used, mainly when no serotherapy is included as for GvHD prophylaxis, as in most protocols in the HLA-identical sibling setting in malignancies (Simonin et al. 2017).

Nowadays, in the ongoing prospective ALL-I-BFM HSCT trial (FORUM), the algorithm for choosing stem cell source recommends BM as the first choice. To date, there is no demonstration for a better GVL effect after PB HSCT in the pediatric population.

Due to the increased risk of cGvHD after PB transplant, which is almost consistent among investigators, it is definitely recommended to avoid PB in nonmalignant disorders.

From the first CB transplantation performed for a Fanconi anemia patient in 1987, CB appeared as a useful and an efficient stem cell source, due to two major features: high proliferative capacity, allowing engraftment despite 1-log fewer cells, and immune plasticity, allowing a wider HLA disparity within each donor recipient pair (Gluckman et al. 1989).

The possibility to adopt less stringent HLA-matching criteria enlarged the availability of grafts to at least 90% of the pediatric patients in need of an allogeneic transplant (Eapen et al. 2017). According to Eurocord consortium recommendations, unrelated CB with two or less HLA disparities typed in low resolution (i.e., two digit) for class I (A and B loci) and high resolution (i.e., four-digit) for class II (DRB1 locus) and with more than 2.5×10^7 nucleated cell dose/kg or 2×10^5 CD34+ cells/kg are suitable for engraftment (Gratwohl et al. 2009). Recent studies from both Eurocord, NetCord, EBMT, and CIBMTR recommend high-resolution HLA typing for A, B, C, and DRB1 and a maximum of 1 or 2 mismatched loci with a cellularity of 3×10^7 TNC/kg or higher (Eapen et al. 2014).

Two prospective studies could demonstrate no benefit of double CB in pediatric patients transplanted for malignant diseases (Wagner et al. 2014; Michel et al. 2016).

12.4.6 Other Donor-Recipient-Related Factors

Besides HLA compatibility and stem cell source, also donor age, gender, female parity, weight, ABO blood group, and viral serological status should be considered in the decision-making process for donor selection, whenever more than one donor were available, which may not be often the case (Wang et al. 2018).

Most studies report that a young donor is better than an older one. Few studies also report that a male donor is better for a male recipient and better than a multiparous woman for any recipient, even though this finding is not consistent through the literature. The donor gender effect may be mild and need larger series of patients to be demonstrated (Friedrich et al. 2018). Unfavorable weight disparity, with donors weighing less than their recipient, should be avoided, when possible (Styczynski et al. 2012). CMV-IgG, as well as EBV-positive patients, should be grafted from CMV- and EBV-positive donors, respectively (Jeljeli et al. 2014; Bontant et al. 2014). ABO matching is usually preferred, especially instead of a major or even minor incompatibility (Booth et al. 2013). Donor location might also be considered, as oversea deliveries increase the time elapsing between collection and infusion, thus reduce cell viability and potentially jeopardize engraftment. More recently, KIR genotyping would allow to identify alloreactive donors who may contribute to prevent relapse also in the non-haploidentical setting (Mavers and Bertaina 2018).

Even though it is mainly clear which variant should be preferred within each variable, there is no consensus regarding the hierarchical order by which the factors above should be combined. In a recent survey within the Pediatric Diseases Working Party of the EBMT, the features above were listed in the following order of importance, on the average, but evaluations widely differed among responders:

1. HLA compatibility, with 10/10 better than 9/10 or worse matching
2. CMV serological status of positive donors in case of positive recipients
3. BM as stem cell source
4. Donor age, being preferable a younger donor compared with an older one

5. Donor gender, with a male donor preferred, particularly for a male recipient
6. ABO major compatibility
7. Donor center location
8. ABO minor compatibility (unpublished data)

Moreover, the presence of anti-HLA antibodies directed to any mismatched HLA alleles should be ruled out, mainly in heavily transfused nonmalignant diseases, such as hemoglobinopaties or bone marrow failures (Ciurea et al. 2018).

Key Points

- An HLA-identical sibling is considered a donor of first choice.
- For patients with hematological malignancies, transplantation from fully HLA-MUD (8/8 or 10/10) is not inferior to transplantation from HLA-identical siblings in terms of EFS.
- The choice of alternative donors (haploidentical related donors, cord blood, mismatched unrelated donors) depends on center experience, urgency of transplant procedure, and detection of donor-specific anti-HLA antibodies.
- For pediatric patients and patients with nonmalignant disorders, BM is the preferred stem cell source.
- For adult patients with hematological malignancies, survival outcome after HSCT with PBSC and BM is comparable.
- In URD transplantation, donor age is probably the most relevant non-HLA donor factor.

References

Anasetti C, Logan BR, Lee SJ, et al. Peripheral-blood stem cells versus bone marrow from unrelated donors. N Engl J Med. 2012;367:1487–96.

Arora M, Weisdorf DJ, Spellman SR, et al. HLA-identical sibling compared with 8/8 matched and mismatched unrelated donor bone marrow transplant for chronic phase chronic myeloid leukemia. J Clin Oncol. 2009;27:1644–52.

Bacigalupo A, Socie G, Schrezenmeier H, et al. Bone marrow versus peripheral blood as the stem cell source for sibling transplants in acquired aplastic anemia: survival advantage for bone marrow in all age groups. Haematologica. 2012;97:1142–8.

Balduzzi A, Valsecchi MG, Uderzo C, et al. Chemotherapy versus allogeneic transplantation for very-high-risk childhood acute lymphoblastic leukaemia in first complete remission: comparison by genetic randomisation in an international prospective study. Lancet. 2005;366:635–42.

Bashey A, Zhang MJ, McCurdy SR, et al. Mobilized peripheral blood stem cells versus unstimulated bone marrow as a graft source for T-cell-replete haploidentical donor transplantation using post-transplant cyclophosphamide. J Clin Oncol. 2017;35:3002–9.

Bensinger WI, Martin PJ, Storer B, et al. Transplantation of bone marrow as compared with peripheral-blood cells from HLA-identical relatives in patients with hematologic cancers. N Engl J Med. 2001;344:175–81.

Bertaina A, Merli P, Rutella S, et al. HLA-haploidentical stem cell transplantation after removal of αβ+ T and B cells in children with nonmalignant disorders. Blood. 2014;124:822–6.

Bontant T, Sedlaçek P, Balduzzi A, et al. Survey of CMV management in pediatric allogeneic HSCT programs, on behalf of the inborn errors, infectious diseases and pediatric diseases working parties of EBMT. Bone Marrow Transplant. 2014;49:276–9.

Booth GS, Gehrie EA, Bolan CD, Savani BN. Clinical guide to ABO-incompatible allogeneic stem cell transplantation. Biol Blood Marrow Transplant. 2013;19:1152–8.

Buck K, Wadsworth K, Setterholm M, et al. High-Resolution Match Rate of 7/8 and 9/10 or Better for the Be The Match Unrelated Donor Registry. Biol Blood Marrow Transplant. 2016;22:759–63.

Chu R, Brazauskas R, Kan F, et al. Comparison of outcomes after transplantation of G-CSF-stimulated bone marrow grafts versus bone marrow or peripheral blood grafts from HLA-matched sibling donors for patients with severe aplastic anemia. Biol Blood Marrow Transplant. 2011;17:1018–24.

Ciurea SO, Thall PF, Milton DR, et al. Complement-binding donor-specific anti-HLA antibodies and risk of primary graft failure in hematopoietic stem cell transplantation. Biol Blood Marrow Transplant. 2015;21:1392–8.

Ciurea SO, Cao K, Fernadez-Vina M, et al. The European Society for Blood and Marrow Transplantation (EBMT) consensus guidelines for the detection and treatment of donor-specific anti-HLA antibodies (DSA) in haploidentical hematopoietic cell transplantation. Bone Marrow Transplant. 2018;53:521–34.

Couban S, Simpson DR, Barnett MJ, et al. A randomized multicenter comparison of bone marrow and peripheral blood in recipients of matched sibling allogeneic transplants for myeloid malignancies. Blood. 2002;100:1525–31.

Couban S, Aljurf M, Lachance S, et al. Filgrastim-stimulated bone marrow compared with filgrastim-mobilized peripheral blood in myeloablative sibling allografting for patients with hematologic malignancies: a randomized Canadian Blood and Marrow Transplant Group Study. Biol Blood Marrow Transplant. 2016;22:1410–5.

Crivello P, Heinold A, Rebmann V, et al. Functional distance between recipient and donor HLA-DPB1 determines nonpermissive mismatches in unrelated HCT. Blood. 2016;128:120–9.

Crocchiolo R, Zino E, Vago L, et al. Gruppo Italiano Trapianto di Midollo Osseo, Cellule Staminale Ematopoietiche (CSE) e Terapia Cellulare; Italian Bone Marrow Donor Registry. Nonpermissive HLA-DPB1 disparity is a significant independent risk factor for mortality after unrelated hematopoietic stem cell transplantation. Blood. 2009;114:1437–44.

Eapen M, Klein JP, Ruggeri A, et al. Impact of allele-level HLA matching on outcomes after myeloablative single unit umbilical cord blood transplantation for hematologic malignancy. Blood. 2014;123:133–4.

Eapen M, Wang T, Veys PA, et al. Allele-level HLA matching for umbilical cord blood transplantation for non-malignant diseases in children: a retrospective analysis. Lancet Haematol. 2017;4:e325–33.

Fleischhauer K, Beelen DW. HLA mismatching as a strategy to reduce relapse after alternative donor transplantation. Semin Hematol. 2016;53:57–64.

Fleischhauer K, Shaw BE. HLA-DP in unrelated hematopoietic cell transplantation revisited: challenges and opportunities. Blood. 2017;130:1089–96.

Fleischhauer K, Shaw BE, Gooley T, et al. Effect of T-cell-epitope matching at HLA-DPB1 in recipients of unrelated-donor haemopoietic-cell transplantation: a retrospective study International Histocompatibility Working Group in hematopoietic cell transplantation. Lancet Oncol. 2012;13:366–74.

Friedrich P, Guerra-García P, Stetson A, et al. Young female donors do not increase the risk of graft-versus-host disease or impact overall outcomes in pediatric HLA-matched sibling hematopoietic stem cell transplantation. Biol Blood Marrow Transplant. 2018;24:96–102.

Fuchs EJ. Related haploidentical donors are a better choice than matched unrelated donors: point. Blood Adv. 2017;1:397–400.

Fürst D, Müller C, Vucinic V, et al. High-resolution HLA matching in hematopoietic stem cell transplantation: a retrospective collaborative analysis. Blood. 2013;122:3220–9.

Gluckman E, Broxmeyer HA, Auerbach AD, et al. Hematopoietic reconstitution in a patient with Fanconi's anemia by means of umbilical-cord blood from an HLA-identical sibling. N Engl J Med. 1989;321:1174–8.

Gluckman E, Cappelli B, Bernaudin F, et al. Sickle cell disease: an international survey of results of HLA-identical sibling hematopoietic stem cell transplantation. Blood. 2017;129:1548–56.

Gluckmann E (2012) Choice of the donor according to HLA typing and stem cell source. EBMT handbook.

Gragert L, Eapen M, Williams E, et al. HLA Match likelihoods, for hematopoietic stem-cell grafts in the U.S. registry. N Engl J Med. 2014;371:339–48.

Gratwohl A, Stern M, Brand R, et al. European Group for Blood and Marrow Transplantation and the European Leukemia Net. Risk score for outcome after allogeneic hematopoietic stem cell transplantation: a retrospective analysis. Cancer. 2009;115:4715–26.

Gratwohl A, Sureda A, Cornelissen J, et al. Alloreactivity: the Janus-face of hematopoietic stem cell transplantation. Leukemia. 2017;31:1752–9.

Gupta V, Tallman MS, He W, et al. Comparable survival after HLA-well-matched unrelated or matched sibling donor transplantation for acute myeloid leukemia in first remission with unfavorable cytogenetics at diagnosis. Blood. 2010;116:1839–48.

Handgretinger R, Klingebiel T, Lang P, et al. Megadose transplantation of purified peripheral blood CD34(+) progenitor cells from HLA-mismatched parental donors in children. Bone Marrow Transplant. 2001;27:777–83.

Horan J, Wang T, Haagenson M, et al. Evaluation of HLA matching in unrelated hematopoietic stem cell transplantation for nonmalignant disorders. Blood. 2012;120:2918–24.

Huang XJ, Liu DH, Liu KY, et al. Haploidentical hematopoietic stem cell transplantation without in vitro T-cell depletion for the treatment of hematological malignancies. Bone Marrow Transplant. 2006;38:291–7.

Jaiswal SR, Chakrabarti A, Chatterjee S, et al. Haploidentical peripheral blood stem cell transplantation with post-transplantation cyclophosphamide in children with advanced acute leukemia with fludarabine-, busulfan-, and melphalan-based conditioning. Biol Blood Marrow Transplant. 2016;22:499–504.

Jeljeli M, Guérin-El Khourouj V, Porcher R, et al. Relationship between cytomegalovirus (CMV) reactivation, CMV-driven immunity, overall immune recovery and graft-versus-leukaemia effect in children. Br J Haematol. 2014;166:229–39.

Kalra A, Williamson T, Daly A, et al. Impact of donor and recipient cytomegalovirus serostatus on outcomes of antithymocyte globulin-conditioned hematopoietic cell transplantation. Biol Blood Marrow Transplant. 2016;22:1654–63.

Klingebiel T, Cornish J, Labopin M, et al. Results and factors influencing outcome after fully haploidentical hematopoietic stem cell transplantation in children with very high-risk acute lymphoblastic leukemia: impact of center size: an analysis on behalf of the Acute Leukemia and Pediatric Disease Working Parties of the European Blood and Marrow Transplant group. Blood. 2010;115:3437–46.

Kollman C, Howe CW, Anasetti C, et al. Donor characteristics as risk factors in recipients after transplantation of bone marrow from unrelated donors: the effect of donor age. Blood. 2001;98:2043–51.

Kollman C, Spellman SR, Zhang MJ, et al. The effect of donor characteristics on survival after unrelated donor transplantation for hematologic malignancy. Blood. 2016;127:260–7.

Kumar R, Kimura F, Ahn KW, et al. Comparing outcomes with bone marrow or peripheral blood stem cells as graft source for matched sibling transplants in severe aplastic anemia across different economic regions. Biol Blood Marrow Transplant. 2016;22:932–40.

Lang P, Feuchtinger T, Teltschik HM, et al. Improved immune recovery after transplantation of TCRαβ/CD19-depleted allografts from haploidentical donors in pediatric patients. Bone Marrow Transplant. 2015;50(Suppl 2):S6–10.

Lang PL, Schlegel PG, Meisel R, et al. Safety and efficacy of Tcr alpha/beta and CD19 depleted haploidentical stem cell transplantation following reduced intensity conditioning in children: results of a prospective multicenter phase I/II clinical trial. Blood. 2017;130:214.

Lee SJ, Klein J, Haagenson M, et al. High-resolution donor-recipient HLA matching contributes to the success of unrelated donor marrow transplantation. Blood. 2007;110:4576–83.

Ljungman P. The role of cytomegalovirus serostatus on outcome of hematopoietic stem cell transplantation. Curr Opin Hematol. 2014;21:466–9.

Locatelli F, Merli P, Pagliara D, et al. Outcome of children with acute leukemia given HLA-haploidentical HSCT after αβ T-cell and B-cell depletion. Blood. 2017;130:677–85.

Luznik L, O'Donnell PV, Symons HJ, et al. HLA-haploidentical bone marrow transplantation for hematologic malignancies using nonmyeloablative conditioning and high-dose, posttransplantation cyclophosphamide. Biol Blood Marrow Transplant. 2008;14:641–50.

Mavers M, Bertaina A. High-risk leukemia: past, present, and future role of NK cells. J Immunol Res. 2018 Apr;15:2018.

McCurdy SR, Zhang MJ, St Martin A, et al. Effect of donor characteristics on haploidentical transplantation with posttransplantation cyclophosphamide. Blood Adv. 2018;2:299–307.

Michel G, Galambrun C, Sirvent A, et al. Single- vs double-unit cord blood transplantation for children and young adults with acute leukemia or myelodysplastic syndrome. Blood. 2016;127:3450–7.

Morishima Y, Kashiwase K, Matsuo K, et al. Biological significance of HLA locus matching in unrelated donor bone marrow transplantation. Japan Marrow Donor Program. Blood. 2015;125:1189–97.

Nakasone H, Remberger M, Tian L, et al. Risks and benefits of sex-mismatched hematopoietic cell transplantation differ according to conditioning strategy. Haematologica. 2015;100:1477–85.

Oran B, Saliba RM, Carmazzi Y, et al. Effect of nonpermissive HLA-DPB1 mismatches after unrelated allogeneic transplantation with in vivo T-cell depletion. Blood. 2018;131:1248–57.

Passweg JR, Baldomero H, Peters C, et al. European Society for Blood and Marrow Transplantation EBMT. Hematopoietic SCT in Europe: data and trends in 2012 with special consideration of pediatric transplantation. Bone Marrow Transplant. 2014;49:744–50.

Peters C, Schrappe M, von Stackelberg A, et al. Stem-cell transplantation in children with acute lymphoblastic leukemia: a prospective international multicenter trial comparing sibling donors with matched unrelated donors-The ALL-SCT-BFM-2003 trial. J Clin Oncol. 2015;33:1265–74.

Petersdorf EW. The major histocompatibility complex: a model for understanding graft-versus-host disease. Blood. 2013;122:1863–72.

Petersdorf EW, Malkki M, O'hUigin C, et al. High HLA-DP expression and graft-versus host disease. N Engl J Med. 2015;373:599–609.

Pidala J, Lee SJ, Ahn KW, et al. Nonpermissive HLA-DPB1 mismatch increases mortality after myeloablative unrelated allogeneic hematopoietic cell transplantation. Blood. 2014;124:2596–606.

Robinson TM, Fuchs EJ, Zhang MJ, et al. Related donor transplants: has posttransplantation cyclophosphamide nullified the detrimental effect of HLA mismatch? Blood Adv. 2018;2:1180–6.

Saber W, Opie S, Rizzo JD, et al. Outcomes after matched unrelated donor versus identical sibling hematopoietic cell transplantation in adults with acute myelogenous leukemia. Blood. 2012;119:3908–16.

Sawada A, Shimizu M, Isaka K, et al. Feasibility of HLA-haploidentical hematopoietic stem cell transplantation with post-transplantation cyclophosphamide for advanced pediatric malignancies. Pediatr Hematol Oncol. 2014;31:754–64.

Schetelig J, Bornhauser M, Schmid C, et al. Matched unrelated or matched sibling donors result in comparable survival after allogeneic stem-cell transplantation in elderly patients with acute myeloid leukemia: a report from the cooperative German Transplant Study Group. J Clin Oncol. 2008;26:5183–91.

Schmitz N, Beksac M, Hasenclever D, et al. Transplantation of mobilized peripheral blood cells to HLA-identical siblings with standard-risk leukemia. Blood. 2002;100:761–7.

Schrezenmeier H, Passweg JR, Marsh JC, et al. Worse outcome and more chronic GVHD with peripheral blood progenitor cells than bone marrow in HLA-matched sibling donor transplants for young patients with severe acquired aplastic anemia. Blood. 2007;110:1397–400.

Seebach JD, Stussi G, Passweg JR, et al. ABO blood group barrier in allogeneic bone marrow transplantation revisited. Biol Blood Marrow Transplant. 2005;11:1006–13.

Shaw BE, Arguello R, Garcia-Sepulveda CA, Madrigal JA. The impact of HLA genotyping on survival following unrelated donor haematopoietic stem cell transplantation. Br J Haematol. 2010;150:251–8.

Shaw BE, Mayor NP, Szydlo RM, et al. Recipient/donor HLA and CMV matching in recipients of T-cell-

depleted unrelated donor haematopoietic cell transplants. Bone Marrow Transplant. 2017;52:717–25.
Shaw BE, Logan BR, Spellman SR, et al. Development of an unrelated donor selection score predictive of survival after HCT: donor age matters most. Biol Blood Marrow Transplant. 2018;24:1049–56.
Simonin M, Dalissier A, Labopin M, et al. More chronic GvHD and non-relapse mortality after peripheral blood stem cell compared with bone marrow in hematopoietic transplantation for paediatric acute lymphoblastic leukemia: a retrospective study on behalf of the EBMT Paediatric Diseases Working Party. Bone Marrow Transplant. 2017;52:1071–3.
Stern M, Ruggeri L, Mancusi A, et al. Survival after T cell-depleted haploidentical stem cell transplantation is improved using the mother as donor. Blood. 2008;112:2990–5.
Stringaris K, Barrett AJ. The importance of natural killer cell killer immunoglobulin-like receptor-mismatch in transplant outcomes. Curr Opin Hematol. 2017;24:489–95.
Styczynski J, Balduzzi A, Gil L, et al. Risk of complications during hematopoietic stem cell collection in pediatric sibling donors: a prospective European Group for Blood and Marrow Transplantation Pediatric Diseases Working Party study. Blood. 2012;119:2935–42.
Szydlo R, Goldman JM, Klein JP, et al. Results of allogeneic bone marrow transplants for leukemia using donors other than HLA-identical siblings. J Clin Oncol. 1997;15:1767–77.
Verneris MR, Lee SJ, Ahn KW, et al. HLA mismatch is associated with worse outcomes after unrelated donor reduced-intensity conditioning hematopoietic cell transplantation: an analysis from the Center for International Blood and Marrow Transplant Research. Biol Blood Marrow Transplant. 2015;21:1783–9.
Wagner JE, Eapen M, Carter S, et al. One-unit versus two-unit cord-blood transplantation for hematologic cancers. N Engl J Med. 2014;371:1685–94.
Wang Y, Wu DP, Liu QF, et al. Donor and recipient age, gender and ABO incompatibility regardless of donor source: validated criteria for donor selection for haematopoietic transplants. Leukemia. 2018;32:492–8.
Wiebking V, Hütker S, Schmid I, et al. Reduced toxicity, myeloablative HLA-haploidentical hematopoietic stem cell transplantation with post-transplantation cyclophosphamide for sickle cell disease. Ann Hematol. 2017;96:1373–7.
Woolfrey A, Lee SJ, Gooley TA, et al. HLA-allele matched unrelated donors compared to HLA-matched sibling donors: role of cell source and disease risk category. Biol Blood Marrow Transplant. 2010;16:1382–7.
Woolfrey A, Klein JP, Haagenson M, et al. HLA-C antigen mismatch is associated with worse outcome in unrelated donor peripheral blood stem cell transplantation. Biol Blood Marrow Transplant. 2011;17:885–92.
Yakoub-Agha I, Mesnil F, Kuentz M, et al. Allogeneic marrow stem-cell transplantation from human leukocyte antigen-identical siblings versus human leukocyte antigen-allelic-matched unrelated donors (10/10) in patients with standard-risk hematologic malignancy: a prospective study from the French Society of Bone Marrow Transplantation and Cell Therapy. J Clin Oncol. 2006;24:5695–702.
Zino E, Frumento G, Marktel S, et al. A T-cell epitope encoded by a subset of HLA-DPB1 alleles determines nonpermissive mismatches for hematologic stem cell transplantation. Blood. 2004;103:1417–24.

Conditioning

13

Arnon Nagler and Avichai Shimoni

13.1 Overview

HSCT is a therapeutic procedure that can cure and/or prolong life in a broad range of hematologic disorders including malignant and nonmalignant pathologies. Conditioning is the preparative regimen that is administered to the patients undergoing HSCT before the infusion of the stem cell grafts. Historically, the pre-HSCT conditioning had to:

1. Eradicate the hematologic malignancy in case of malignant indication for HSCT.
2. Provide sufficient IS to ensure engraftment and to prevent both rejection and GVHD.
3. Provide stem cell niches in the host BM for the new stem cells.

The third purpose is controversial as it was demonstrated in animal models that with mega doses of HSC and repeated administrations engraftment can be achieved without conditioning.

A. Nagler (✉)
Department of Medicine, Tel Aviv University, Tel-Hashomer, Israel

Hematology Division, BMT and Cord Blood Bank, Chaim Sheba Medical Center, Tel-Hashomer, Israel
e-mail: arnon.nagler@sheba.health.gov.il

A. Shimoni
Bone Marrow Transplantation, Chaim Sheba Medical Center, Tel-Aviv University, Tel Hashomer, Israel

From the theoretic point of view, the conditioning consisted of two components:

1. Myelo-depletion which targets the host stem cells
2. Lymphodepletion which targets the host lymphoid system, respectively

Some of the compounds used in the conditioning are more myeloablative (MA) in nature, for example, MEL or BU, while some are more lymphodepleting like FLU or CY. The pretransplant conditioning may include TBI or in rare and specific instances other types of irradiations like TLI that is applied, for example, in haplo-HSCT, or TAI that was used in the past in Fanconi anemia. Alternatively, the pre-HSCT conditioning can be radiation-free including only chemotherapy. In recent years, serotherapy, specific targeted novel compounds, and MoAb and radiolabeled Ab started to be incorporated into specific disease-oriented conditioning regimens.

Not just the constituents but also the schedule (days) of administration and doses may differ in the various conditioning regimen protocols. The pretransplantation conditioning regimens depend on the type of the HSC donor. For example, in auto-HSCT, the pre-HSCT conditioning consisted of chemotherapy alone, and in some transplant centers, it may include also irradiation, while, in allo-HSCT from unrelated or mismatched donors

E. Carreras et al. (eds.), *The EBMT Handbook*, https://doi.org/10.1007/978-3-030-02278-5_13

as well as in HSCT from alternative donors, the pre-HSCT conditioning usually includes serotherapy with ATG or ALEM (Campath; anti-CDW52 MoAb). Similarly, the intensity of the conditioning is traditionally higher in unrelated and mismatched transplants as well as in transplants from alternative donors in comparison to transplants from HLA MSD. The pre-HSCT conditioning regimen takes into account also the specific disease for which the HSCT is being performed, more so in auto-HSCT than in the allogeneic setting aiming to include an effective anti-disease-specific chemotherapy, for example, MEL for MM or BCNU and CY in lymphoma.

Other factors to be taken into account while choosing the optimal conditioning for a specific patient besides the disease he is afflicted with and the type of donor are age, comorbidities, and organ-specific toxicity risk. The conditioning protocols also differ between pediatrics and adults as in pediatric more emphasis should be given to growth and puberty issues. It also differs between nonmalignant and malignant disorders; the former are not just more frequent in pediatrics, but of major importance is the fact that in nonmalignant indications, there is no need for the GVL, and a main goal is to ensure absolutely no GVHD.

Historically, the conditioning protocols were MA in nature, and the two most popular ones were the CY/TBI (TBI 12Gy followed by IV CY 60 mg/kg × 2 days) and the BU/CY protocol (BU 4 mg/kg × 4 days and CY 60 mg/kg × 2 days). However, MAC is associated with significant organ- and transplant-related toxicity (TRT), limiting allo-HSCT to younger patients in good medical conditioning, typically up to age of 55 and 50 years old in allo-HSCT from sibling and URD, respectively. During the past two decades, non-MA (NMA), RIC, and reduced toxicity conditioning (RTC) regimens have been developed aiming in reducing the organ and TRM while keeping the anti-malignant effect and allowing allo-HSCT in elderly and medically infirm patients. These are relatively nontoxic and tolerable regimens designed not to maximally eradicate the malignancy but rather to provide sufficient IS to achieve engraftment and to allow induction of GVL as the primary treatment. Furthermore, special conditioning protocols have been developed for allo-HSCT from alternative donors including from MMUD, CB donors, and haploidentical family-related donors. These relatively new pre-HSCT conditioning typically includes new drug formulations like IV BU, compounds from the oncology field that are newcomers in HSCT like TREO or TT, new compounds like clofarabine (CLO), or new schedules sequentially administrating novel chemotherapy combination (FLAMSA) to be followed by RIC containing reduced doses of TBI.

13.2 Total Body Irradiation

TBI is a major constituent of MAC regimens. Historically, TBI combined with CY has been the standard regimen used to condition patients with acute leukemia prior to HSCT. TBI is typically given at a dose of 12 Gy (Thomas et al. 1982). Higher doses of TBI up to 14.25 Gy resulted in improved antileukemic effect, but this was counterbalanced by increased toxicity and TRM (Clift et al. 1990). TBI provides both MA and IS ensuring engraftment in combination with optimal antileukemic effect. It provides homogeneous dose distribution in the whole body including sanctuaries for systemic chemotherapy such as the CNS and testicles. Fractionation of 12 Gy TBI in six doses of 2 Gy delivered twice a day over 3 days became the standard over time (Thomas et al. 1982).

The Acute Leukemia Working Party (ALWP) of the EBMT recently showed that 12 Gy fractionated TBI dose delivered either in two fractions or in one fraction per day over 3 or 4 days prior to HSCT resulted in similar outcome, in both ALL and AML patients (Belkacemi et al. 2018). Dose fractionation and dose rate have been shown to be of importance determining both efficacy and toxicity which includes mucositis, interstitial pneumonia, SOS/VOD, hemorrhagic cystitis, and long-term toxicity including growth retardation, endocrine problems, cataracts, and secondary malignancies.

As for mode of TBI administration across Europe, the ALWP of the EBMT performed a questionnaire-based study focusing on technical practices across 56 EBMT centers and 23 countries demonstrating an extremely high heterogeneity of fractionation schedules. The total doses delivered ranged between 8 and 14.4 Gy with dose per fraction varying between 1.65 and 8 Gy. The dose rate at the source ranged between 2.25 and 37.5 Gy/min. This resulted in 40 different reported schedules, to which variations in beam energy, dosimetry, in vivo techniques, and organ shielding disparities had to be added (Giebel et al. 2014). Regarding TBI-mediated antileukemic effect, most studies have shown the equivalence of chemotherapy-based MAC mostly BU/CY and CY/TBI conditioning for AML (Nagler et al. 2013). In contrast, despite the absence of consensus, TBI has remained the first choice in many centers for ALL (Cahu et al. 2016).

13.3 Myeloablative Non-TBI-Containing Conditioning

The MAC are a high-dose chemotherapy mostly alkylating agent-based regimens used in both auto- and allo-HSCT. They cause by definition profound and prolong cytopenia that lasts up to 21 days and necessitates stem cell graft in order to recover (Bacigalupo et al. 2009). Historically, BU/CY is the prototype of chemotherapy-based MAC. It was developed by the Johns Hopkins group as early as 1983 as an alternative to TBI in an effort to reduce the incidence of long-term radiation-induced toxicities and improve the planning of HSCT in institutions lacking easy availability of linear accelerators (Tutschka et al. 1987). A considerable number of studies have shown the equivalence of BU/CY and CY/TBI for allo-HSCT in AML (Nagler et al. 2013) and recently also in ALL (Mohty et al. 2010) although most centers still use TBI-based MAC as the preferred pre-HSCT conditioning for ALL in fit patients with low comorbidities.

The original studies used oral BU that has an erratic and unpredictable absorption with wide inter- and also intra-patient variability with the risk of increased toxicity mainly SOS/VOD in patients with a high area under the curve of BU plasma concentration versus time, while low BU concentrations may be associated with a higher risk of graft rejection and relapse (Hassan 1999). The common solution was monitoring of BU levels and dose adjustments that allowed for better control of the dose administered and reduction of the abovementioned risks (Deeg et al. 2002). The development of the IV BU with more predictable pharmacokinetics, achieving tight control of plasma levels, and less need for plasma level testing and dose adjustments significantly reduced BU-mediated SOS/VOD and TRM (Nagler et al. 2014).

Some other MAC regimens include MEL in combination with BU (Vey et al. 1996), while others incorporated VP (Czyz et al. 2018). Subsequently, in an attempt to further reduce regimen-related toxicity, CY was replaced with FLU, a nucleoside analog with considerable IS properties that also has a synergizing effect with alkylators by inhibiting DNA repair. The combination of BU and FLU used in patients with AML was found to have more favorable toxicity profile with similar efficacy. Recently a well-designed two-arm study compared BU/CY to BU/FLU, demonstrating a significant reduction of TRM in the FLU/BU arm with no difference in RI (Rambaldi et al. 2015). Recently, other alkylators like TT (Eder et al. 2017) and CLO (Chevallier et al. 2012) have been incorporated into MAC protocols for both AML and ALL in an attempt to reduce risk of relapse with equivalent results to TBI-containing conditioning protocols.

13.4 Nonmyeloablative, Reduced Intensity and Reduced Toxicity Conditioning

NMA and RIC have been widely introduced over the past 20 years in an attempt to reduce organ toxicity and TRM allowing HSCT in elderly and medically infirm patients not eligible for standard MAC (Slavin et al. 1998). In addition, RTC based on FLU and MA alkylating agent doses were designed to allow safer administration of dose-intensive therapy. Multiple such protocols have been reported over the years with somewhat overlapping dose intensity and to a certain extent unclear categorization among NMA versus RIC and RTC.

A group of experts had an attempt to define and dissect the conditioning regimen intensity based on the expected duration and reversibility of cytopenia after HSCT (Bacigalupo et al. 2009). MAC was defined as a conditioning regimen that results in irreversible cytopenia in most patients, and stem cell support after HSCT is required. Truly NMA regimens cause minimal cytopenia and can theoretically be given without stem cell support. RIC regimens cause profound cytopenia and should be given with stem cells, but cytopenia may not be irreversible. The original NMA conditioning protocols were the TBI 2 Gy in combination with MMF and CSA (the so-called Seattle protocol that subsequently incorporated FLU 90 mg because of high non-engraftment in the original protocol) (McSweeney et al. 2001) and the FLAG conditioning protocol (FLU, Ara-C, idarubicin, and G-CSF) pioneered in MD Anderson (Giralt et al. 1997).

Additional very popular protocol is the FLU/BU conditioning regimen we pioneered in Jerusalem initially with oral but subsequently with the IV formulation of BU that is given 2–4 days determining the intensity of the conditioning being NMA, RIC/RTC, and MAC, respectively (Kharfan-Dabaja et al. 2014). Overall multiple studies indicated that the conditioning dose intensity is highly correlated with outcome after HSCT. Increased dose intensity is associated with reduced RI but also with higher NRM (Aoudjhane et al. 2005). For example, few studies compared the FLU/BU RIC to another frequently used RIC regimen, namely, the FLU/MEL protocol demonstrating lower RI but higher toxicity with the FLU/MEL protocol which is more intense (Shimoni et al. 2007). Subsequently TREO (L-threitol-1,4-bis-methanesulfonate, dihydroxybusulfan) with activity against both on committed and noncommitted stem cells as well as potent IS properties (Danylesko et al. 2012) was combined with FLU as an effective conditioning regimen pre-HSCT for both myeloid and lymphatic malignancies with a favorable toxicity profile with little extramedullary toxicity (Nagler et al. 2017).

Overall outcome comparing these low-intensity conditioning protocols versus MAC was determined by the net effect of the opposing effects, i.e., reduction in TRM, while higher RI, leading to similar LFS and OS with patient age, comorbidities, and disease status at transplantation being significant prognostic factors. Retrospective comparative trials showed that while outcome may be similar with the various regimens in patients given HSCT in remission, NMA/RIC are inferior when HSCT is given in advanced disease, due to high RI. These observations were confirmed in some of the long-term studies but not in others (Shimoni et al. 2016). Interestingly, no disadvantage was observed for the low-intensity protocols in comparison to MAC even in high-risk disease like AML with monosomal karyotype or secondary leukemia (Poiré et al. 2015). RTC regimens are typically with more intensive antileukemic activity but limited toxicity and thus better tolerated by patients not eligible for myeloablative conditioning (Shimoni et al. 2018).

New novel conditioning protocols that may be categorized in this family of conditioning although no consensus was established are the regimens that incorporate CLO and TT and especially the TBF regimen (TT, BU, FLU) (Saraceni et al. 2017). Another worth mentioning conditioning that was developed for high-risk leukemia with encouraging results is the FLAMSA conditioning which comprised sequential chemotherapy including FLU, Ara-C, and amsacrine followed by RIC pre-allo-HSCT (Malard et al. 2017). Only few randomized studies compared head-to-head MAC to RIC or RTC regimens mostly confirming the above findings. A French well-designed two-arm study compared BU/FLU to TBI (low dose)/FLU demonstrating less RI with the BU/FLU regimen but higher TRM resulting in similar LFS and OS (Blaise et al. 2013). Similarly, a German randomized study compared RIC regimen of four doses of 2 Gy of TBI and 150 mg/m^2 FLU versus MAC of six doses of 2 Gy of TBI and 120 mg/kg CY demonstrating reduced toxicity in the RIC arm but similar RI, TRM, LFS, and OS between both study arms (Bornhäuser et al. 2012). These results were recently confirmed with longer follow-up.

Finally, a recent CTN phase III randomized trial compared MAC (BU/CY, FLU/BU, or CY/TBI) with RIC (FLU/BU or FLU/MEL) in patients with AML and MDS (Scott et al. 2017). RIC resulted in lower TRM but higher RI compared with MAC, with a statistically significant advantage in RFS and a trend to an advantage in OS with MAC. Another randomized study comparing RIC and MAC in patients with MDS demonstrated similar 2-year RFS and OS with no difference between the two conditioning regimens (Kröger et al. 2017). As for the issue of higher risk of RI post RIC, novel immunological and pharmacologic approaches are being currently explored (as will be discussed in Chap. 69). Treatment options include second HSCT or DLI with similar results (Kharfan-Dabaja et al. 2018).

13.5 Conditioning Regimens for Allo-HSCT from Alternative Donors: MMUD, CB, and Haploidentical

Historically, these types of allo-HSCT were the most challenging ones with relatively high incidence of non-engraftment and high TRM. Notably, recent development in the field of transplantation including novel conditioning regimens resulted in major improvement in the results of allo-HSCT from alternative donors with the haplo-HSCT being of the most interest (Lee et al. 2017). A key component of the conditioning regimen for MMUD and haplo-HSCT is ATG, recently reviewed for the ALWP of the EBMT (Baron et al. 2017). In previous well-designed randomized clinical trials in allo-HSCT from URD and in a single study also from MSD, ATG was demonstrated to reduce GVHD and TRM without jeopardizing the GVL effect, and thus there is no increase in RI (Baron et al. 2017). In contrast and somewhat still puzzling in CBT, ATG is a negative factor associated with decreased OS and EFS rates and a high incidence of NRM (Pascal et al. 2015).

In an analysis performed by Eurocord, the MAC regimen for CBT included TBI 12 Gy—or BU—with or without FLU, TBI 12 Gy + CY, and more recently TBF (TT, BU, FLU) (Ruggeri et al. 2014). Comparing these regimens in single (s) (with >2.5 × 10^7 cells/kg) and double (d) CBT resulted in similar outcomes, NRM and RI incidence, which were not statistically different among the groups. LFS was 30% for sUCBT using TBI- or BU-based MAC compared with 48% for sUCBT TBF and 48% for dUCBT ($P = 0.02$ and $P = 0.03$, respectively), and it was not statistically different between sUCBT with TBF and dUCBT. They concluded that the choice of TBF conditioning regimen for sUCBT may improve results, and whether this regimen may be effective in dUCBT should be further analyzed (Ruggeri et al. 2014). In the haploidentical setting, the field moved from T-depleted to T-repleted haplo-HSCT and in recent years from ATG-based anti-GVHD prophylaxis to PT-CY pioneered by the Baltimore group (reviewed in Lee et al. 2017). Initial conditioning protocols in the Baltimore approach were RIC with BM grafts, but subsequently MAC regimens and PB grafts were introduced. In recent years, the TBF condoning is increasingly used for haplo-HSCT in Europe. Similarly, the PT-CY strategy for GVHD prophylaxis is being adopted to allo-HSCT from MUD, MMUD, and sibling donors (Ruggeri et al. 2018). In general comparing RIC to MAC for MMUD, CBT, and haplo-HSCT demonstrated in large similar transplantation global outcome for RIC versus MAC with some differences in the various alternative donors (Baron et al. 2016). For example, in the allo-HSCT from MMUD in patients >50 years, RIC resulted in reduced TRM and better LFS and OS in comparison to MAC, while in those <50 years, no difference was observed (Savani et al. 2016). In CBT, RIC resulted in a higher RI and a lower NRM, translating to comparable LFS, GVHD and relapse-free survival (GRFS), and OS (Baron et al. 2016). In the haplo-setting, no significant difference was observed (Rubio et al. 2016).

13.6 Preparative Conditioning for Autologous HSCT

Auto-HSCT are performed mainly for malignant lymphoma and MM. The most popular conditioning protocol for auto-HSCT in lymphoma is BEAM (BCNU, VP, Ara-C, and MEL) (Mills et al. 1995) or BEAC (with CY instead of MEL), while some centers substitute the BCNU with TT (the so-called TEAM or TECAM protocol), especially in patients with pulmonary problems in order to prevent the BCNU-mediated lung toxicity. Others tried to replace the BCNU by bendamustine (the so-called BeEAM protocol). Adding anti-CD20 radiolabeled MoAb like yttrium-90-ibritumomab tiuxetan (Zevalin) to the condition improved results in some studies, but a large randomized multicenter study with 131I-tositumomab (Bexxar) was negative (Vose et al. 2013).

As for auto-HSCT in MM, high-dose MEL has been shown to be superior to TBI/MEL. Recently some centers incorporated IV BU into the auto-HSCT in MM, while others included BOR. The numbers of auto-HSCT in acute leukemia went down in the last two decades in parallel to the increase in the numbers of allo-HSCT with RIC and from alternative donors (Gorin et al. 2015). The most popular preparative regimen for AML is BU/CY. Recently on behalf of the ALWP of the EBMT, we demonstrated that BU/MEL is a better preparative regimen as compared to BU/CY with lower RI, better LFS and OS, and no difference in TRM. Similar results were obtained in the subgroup of patients with high-risk AML. Patients with negative MRD before auto-HSCT did better (Gorin et al. 2017).

Key Points

- Conditioning regimens are integral and important part of HSCT enabling engraftment and provide an antitumor effect.
- The conditioning regimen pretransplantation should take into consideration patient and disease characteristics including age, comorbidities, disease status, and most probably measurable residual disease.
- Conditioning regimens may include irradiation, chemotherapy, serotherapy, monoclonal antibodies, and targeted therapy which varied in different malignancies and types of donors.
- The dose intensity of the pre-HSCT conditioning varied between MAC, RTC, RIC, and NMA in decreasing intensity order.
- The NMA and RIC significantly reduced transplant-related organ toxicity and mortality enabling transplant in elderly and medically infirm patients.
- The conditioning regimens for allo-HSCT from cord blood and haploidentical donors are somewhat specific.

References

Aoudjhane M, Labopin M, Gorin NC, et al. Comparative outcome of reduced intensity and myeloablative conditioning regimen in HLA identical sibling allogeneic haematopoietic stem cell transplantation for patients older than 50 years of age with acute myeloblastic leukaemia: a retrospective survey from the Acute Leukemia Working Party (ALWP) of the European Group for Blood and Marrow Transplantation (EBMT). Leukemia. 2005;19:2304–12.

Bacigalupo A, Ballen K, Rizzo D, et al. Defining the intensity of conditioning regimens: working definitions. Biol Blood Marrow Transplant. 2009;15:1628–33.

Baron F, Ruggeri A, Beohou E, et al. RIC versus MAC UCBT in adults with AML: a report from Eurocord, the ALWP and the CTIWP of the EBMT. Oncotarget. 2016;7:43027–38.

Baron F, Mohty M, Blaise D, et al. Anti-thymocyte globulin as graft-versus-host disease prevention in the setting of allogeneic peripheral blood stem cell transplantation: a review from the Acute Leukemia Working Party of the European Society for Blood and Marrow Transplantation. Haematologica. 2017;102:224–34.

Belkacemi Y, Labopin M, Giebel S, et al. Single dose daily fractionated is not Inferior to twice a day fractionated total body irradiation prior to allogeneic stem cell transplantation for acute leukemia: a useful practice simplification resulting from the Sarasin Study. Int J Radiat Oncol Biol Phys. 2018;102:515–26.

Blaise D, Tabrizi R, Boher JM, et al. Randomized study of 2 reduced-intensity conditioning strategies for human leukocyte antigen-matched, related allogeneic peripheral blood stem cell transplantation: prospective clinical and socioeconomic evaluation. Cancer. 2013;119:602–11.

Bornhäuser M, Kienast J, Trenschel R, et al. Reduced-intensity conditioning versus standard conditioning before allogeneic haemopoietic cell transplantation in patients with acute myeloid leukaemia in first complete remission: a prospective, open-label randomised phase 3 trial. Lancet Oncol. 2012;13:1035–44.

Cahu X, Labopin M, Giebel S, et al. Impact of conditioning with TBI in adult patients with T-cell ALL who receive a myeloablative allogeneic stem cell transplantation: a report from the acute leukemia working party of EBMT. Bone Marrow Transplant. 2016;51:351–7.

Chevallier P, Labopin M, Buchholz S, et al. Clofarabine-containing conditioning regimen for allo-SCT in AML/ALL patients: a survey from the Acute Leukemia Working Party of EBMT. Eur J Haematol. 2012;89:214–9.

Clift RA, Buckner CD, Appelbaum FR, et al. Allogeneic marrow transplantation in patients with acute myeloid leukemia in first remission: a randomized trial of two irradiation regimens. Blood. 1990;76:1867–71.

Czyz A, Labopin M, Giebel S, et al. Cyclophosphamide versus etoposide in combination with total body irradiation as conditioning regimen for adult patients with Ph-negative acute lymphoblastic leukemia undergoing allogeneic stem cell transplant: on behalf of the ALWP of the European Society for Blood and Marrow Transplantation. Am J Hematol. 2018;93:778–85.

Danylesko I, Shimoni A, Nagler A. Treosulfan-based conditioning before hematopoietic SCT: more than a BU look-alike. Bone Marrow Transplant. 2012;47:5–14.

Deeg HJ, Storer B, Slattery JT, et al. Conditioning with targeted busulfan and cyclophosphamide for hemopoietic stem cell transplantation from related and unrelated donors in patients with myelodysplastic syndrome. Blood. 2002;100:1201–7.

Eder S, Canaani J, Beohou E, et al. Thiotepa-based conditioning versus total body irradiation as myeloablative conditioning prior to allogeneic stem cell transplantation for acute lymphoblastic leukemia: a matched-pair analysis from the Acute Leukemia Working Party of the European Society for Blood and Marrow Transplantation. Am J Hematol. 2017;92:997–1003.

Giebel S, Miszczyk L, Slosarek K, et al. Extreme heterogeneity of myeloablative total body irradiation techniques in clinical practice: a survey of the Acute Leukemia Working Party of the European Group for Blood and Marrow Transplantation. Cancer. 2014;120:2760–5.

Giralt S, Estey E, Albitar M, et al. Engraftment of allogeneic hematopoietic progenitor cells with purine analog-containing chemotherapy: harnessing graft-versus-leukemia without myeloablative therapy. Blood. 1997;89:4531–6.

Gorin NC, Giebel S, Labopin M, et al. Autologous stem cell transplantation for adult acute leukemia in 2015: time to rethink? Present status and future prospects. Bone Marrow Transplant. 2015;50:1495–502.

Gorin NC, Labopin M, Czerw T, et al. Autologous stem cell transplantation for adult acute myelocytic leukemia in first remission-Better outcomes after busulfan and melphalan compared with busulfan and cyclophosphamide: a retrospective study from the Acute Leukemia Working Party of the European Society for Blood and Marrow Transplantation (EBMT). Cancer. 2017;123:824–31.

Hassan M. The role of busulfan in bone marrow transplantation. Med Oncol. 1999;16:166–76.

Kharfan-Dabaja MA, Labopin M, Bazarbachi A, et al. Comparing i.v. BU dose intensity between two regimens (FB2 vs FB4) for allogeneic HCT for AML in CR1: a report from the Acute Leukemia Working Party of EBMT. Bone Marrow Transplant. 2014;49:1170–5.

Kharfan-Dabaja MA, Labopin M, Polge E, et al. Association of second allogeneic hematopoietic cell transplant vs donor lymphocyte infusion with overall survival in patients with acute myeloid leukemia relapse. JAMA Oncol. 2018. https://doi.org/10.1001/jamaoncol.2018.2091.

Kröger N, Iacobelli S, Franke GN, et al. Dose-reduced versus standard conditioning followed by allogeneic stem-cell transplantation for patients with myelodysplastic syndrome: a prospective randomized phase III study of the EBMT (RICMAC trial). J Clin Oncol. 2017;35:2157–64.

Lee CJ, Savani BN, Mohty M, et al. Haploidentical hematopoietic cell transplantation for adult acute myeloid leukemia: a position statement from the Acute Leukemia Working Party of the European Society for Blood and Marrow Transplantation. Haematologica. 2017;102:1810–22.

Malard F, Labopin M, Stuhler G, et al. Sequential intensified conditioning regimen allogeneic hematopoietic stem cell transplantation in adult patients with intermediate- or high-risk acute myeloid leukemia in complete remission: a study from the Acute Leukemia Working Party of the European Group for Blood and Marrow Transplantation. Biol Blood Marrow Transplant. 2017;23:278–84.

McSweeney PA, Niederwieser D, Shizuru JA, et al. Hematopoietic cell transplantation in older patients with hematologic malignancies: replacing high-dose cytotoxic therapy with graft-versus-tumor effects. Blood. 2001;97:3390–400.

Mills W, Chopra R, McMillan A, et al. BEAM chemotherapy and autologous bone marrow transplantation for patients with relapsed or refractory non-Hodgkin's lymphoma. J Clin Oncol. 1995;13:588–95.

Mohty M, Labopin M, Volin L, et al. Reduced-intensity versus conventional myeloablative conditioning allogeneic stem cell transplantation for patients with acute lymphoblastic leukemia: a retrospective study from the European Group for Blood and Marrow Transplantation. Blood. 2010;116:4439–43.

Nagler A, Rocha V, Labopin M, et al. Allogeneic hematopoietic stem-cell transplantation for acute myeloid leukemia in remission: comparison of intravenous busulfan plus cyclophosphamide (Cy) versus total-body irradiation plus Cy as conditioning regimen—a report from the acute leukemia working party of the European group for blood and marrow transplantation. J Clin Oncol. 2013;31:3549–56.

Nagler A, Labopin M, Berger R, et al. Allogeneic hematopoietic SCT for adults AML using i.v. BU in the conditioning regimen: outcomes and risk factors for the occurrence of hepatic sinusoidal obstructive syndrome. Bone Marrow Transplant. 2014;49:628–33.

Nagler A, Labopin M, Beelen D, et al. Long-term outcome after a treosulfan-based conditioning regimen for patients with acute myeloid leukemia: a report from the Acute Leukemia Working Party of the European Society for Blood and Marrow Transplantation. Cancer. 2017;123:2671–9.

Pascal L, Mohty M, Ruggeri A, et al. Impact of rabbit ATG-containing myeloablative conditioning regimens on the outcome of patients undergoing unrelated single-unit cord blood transplantation for hematological malignancies. Bone Marrow Transplant. 2015;50:45–50.

Poiré X, Labopin M, Cornelissen JJ, et al. Outcome of conditioning intensity in acute myeloid leukemia with monosomal karyotype in patients over 45 year-old: a study from the acute leukemia working party (ALWP) of the European Group of Blood and Marrow Transplantation (EBMT). Am J Hematol. 2015;90:719–24.

Rambaldi A, Grassi A, Masciulli A, et al. Busulfan plus cyclophosphamide versus busulfan plus fludarabine as a preparative regimen for allogeneic haemopoietic stem-cell transplantation in patients with acute myeloid leukaemia: an open-label, multicentre, randomised, phase 3 trial. Lancet Oncol. 2015;16:1525–36.

Rubio MT, Savani BN, Labopin M, et al. Impact of conditioning intensity in T-replete haplo-identical stem cell transplantation for acute leukemia: a report from the acute leukemia working party of the EBMT. J Hematol Oncol. 2016;9:25.

Ruggeri A, Sanz G, Bittencourt H, et al. Comparison of outcomes after single or double cord blood transplantation in adults with acute leukemia using different types of myeloablative conditioning regimen, a retrospective study on behalf of Eurocord and the Acute Leukemia Working Party of EBMT. Leukemia. 2014;28:779–86.

Ruggeri A, Labopin M, Bacigalupo A, et al. Post-transplant cyclophosphamide for graft-versus-host disease prophylaxis in HLA matched sibling or matched unrelated donor transplant for patients with acute leukemia, on behalf of ALWP-EBMT. J Hematol Oncol. 2018;11:40.

Saraceni F, Labopin M, Hamladji RM, et al. Thiotepa-busulfan-fludarabine compared to busulfan-fludarabine for sibling and unrelated donor transplant in acute myeloid leukemia in first remission. Oncotarget. 2017;9:3379–93.

Savani BN, Labopin M, Kröger N, et al. Expanding transplant options to patients over 50 years. Improved outcome after reduced intensity conditioning mismatched-unrelated donor transplantation for patients with acute myeloid leukemia: a report from the Acute Leukemia Working Party of the EBMT. Haematologica. 2016;101:773–80.

Scott BL, Pasquini MC, Logan BR, et al. Myeloablative versus reduced-intensity hematopoietic cell transplantation for acute myeloid leukemia and myelodysplastic syndromes. J Clin Oncol. 2017;35:1154–61.

Shimoni A, Hardan I, Shem-Tov N, et al. Comparison between two fludarabine-based reduced-intensity conditioning regimens before allogeneic hematopoietic stem-cell transplantation: fludarabine/melphalan is associated with higher incidence of acute graft-versus-host disease and non-relapse mortality and lower incidence of relapse than fludarabine/busulfan. Leukemia. 2007;21:2109–16.

Shimoni A, Labopin M, Savani B, et al. Long-term survival and late events after allogeneic stem cell transplantation from HLA-matched siblings for acute myeloid leukemia with myeloablative compared to reduced-intensity conditioning: a report on behalf of the acute leukemia working party of European group for blood and marrow transplantation. J Hematol Oncol. 2016;9:118.

Shimoni A, Labopin M, Savani B, et al. Intravenous busulfan compared with treosulfan-based conditioning for allogeneic stem cell transplantation in acute myeloid leukemia: a study on behalf of the Acute Leukemia Working Party of European Society for Blood and Marrow Transplantation. Biol Blood Marrow Transplant. 2018;24:751–7.

Slavin S, Nagler A, Naparstek E, et al. Nonmyeloablative stem cell transplantation and cell therapy as an alternative to conventional bone marrow transplantation with lethal cytoreduction for the treatment of malignant and nonmalignant hematologic diseases. Blood. 1998;91:756–63.

Thomas ED, Clift RA, Hersman J, et al. Marrow transplantation for acute nonlymphoblastic leukemic in first remission using fractionated or single-dose irradiation. Int J Radiat Oncol Biol Phys. 1982;8:817–21.

Tutschka PJ, Copelan EA, Klein JP. Bone marrow transplantation for leukemia following a new busulfan and cyclophosphamide regimen. Blood. 1987;70:1382–8.

Vey N, De Prijck B, Faucher C, et al. A pilot study of busulfan and melphalan as preparatory regimen prior to allogeneic bone marrow transplantation in refractory or relapsed hematological malignancies. Bone Marrow Transplant. 1996;18:495–9.

Vose JM, Carter S, Burns LJ, et al. Phase III randomized study of rituximab/carmustine, etoposide, cytarabine, and melphalan (BEAM) compared with iodine-131 tositumomab/BEAM with autologous hematopoietic cell transplantation for relapsed diffuse large B-cell lymphoma: results from the BMT CTN 0401 trial. J Clin Oncol. 2013;31:1662–8.

14 Bone Marrow Harvesting for HSCT

Norbert Claude Gorin

14.1 Introduction

Historically, the bone marrow (BM) has been the first source of stem cells considered since the early 1960s for HSCT (Santos 1990; Thomas et al. 1979; Mathe 1964; Gorin et al. 1990). Parallel attempts at using fetal liver cells at that time have remained unsuccessful. In 1986 the first success of an unrelated cord blood (UCB) transplantation in a child promoted UCB (Gluckman et al. 1997) as an alternative source in certain settings.

Since 1994 and the initial demonstration that PBSC mobilized by cytokines (G-CSF first and more recently when needed plerixafor) could be used as well as BM, the proportion of PB transplants has considerably increased to reach about 70–95% of all stem cell transplants (Passweg et al. 2012, 2016), so that nowadays BM transplantation accounts for a minority of transplants.

There remain however several situations where and when a marrow harvest can still be of interest or even is highly recommended.

This chapter indicates the principal indications of BM transplantation, compares schematically the advantages of BM versus PB, and details the technique of BM harvesting.

N. C. Gorin MD, PhD (✉)
Department of Hematology and Cell Therapy, EBMT Paris Office, Hôpital Saint Antoine APHP, Paris, France

Paris Sorbonne University, Paris, France
e-mail: norbert-claude.gorin@aphp.fr

14.2 Indications for Considering and Possibly Selecting BM as a Preferred Source of HSC

It is not the purpose of this chapter to review the benefit/risk ratio of BM versus peripheral mobilized blood as sources of HSC. Several studies, including prospective randomized studies, have shown in general with BM when compared to PB slower engraftment but lower incidence and lower severity of acute and chronic GVHD with in the end similar disease free and overall survivals (Schmitz et al. 2005). However, some retrospective studies for both auto- and allo-HSCT have shown better survival with rich BM collections (Gorin et al. 2003) or BM versus PB (Gorin et al. 2009, 2010). Also, the quality of life has not been carefully analyzed (Sun et al. 2010), and further studies may be in favor of BM (Ruggeri et al. 2018; Lee et al. 2016).

Time and cost constraints have however in general favored leukaphereses and PB transplants which represent about 95% of all auto-HSCT and 70% of allo-HSCT (Passweg et al. 2016). Table 14.1 lists the situations when nowadays marrow may appear as a better choice.

For allo-HSCT, BM is preferred/mandatory whenever the wish to reduce toxicity, NRM, and most of all GVHD (particularly extensive chronic)

E. Carreras et al. (eds.), *The EBMT Handbook*, https://doi.org/10.1007/978-3-030-02278-5_14

Table 14.1 Preferences for BM as source of stem cells in ALLO-HSCT

Allo-HSCT	Rationale	Justification 1	Justification 2	Reference
Children donors and/or recipients	Administration of GCSF to and leukapheresis of the donor more difficult to set	More cGVHD and NRM after PB compared with BM	In some countries, the use of GCSF (and plerixafor) is not allowed in children	Simonin et al. (2017)
Aplastic anemia	BM mandatory, associated with better results	Higher risk of GVHD with PB	Included in EBMT and CIBMTR guidelines	Bhella et al. (2018), Schrezenmeier et al. (2007), Bacigalupo et al. (2012), Eapen et al. (2011), and Barone et al. (2015)
MAC with a MUD and no ATG	BM associated with better results and less cGVH	Randomized trial with no ATG showing less cGVH and better QOL with BM	If a suitable BM donor is available. Otherwise PB with ATG	Anasetti et al. (2012), Lee et al. (2016), Eapen et al. (2007), and Walker et al. (2016)
Haploidentical transplantation	BM or combination of PB and BM favored by some teams	Team choice or clinical trial	High-dose CY for GVH prevention	Kasamon et al. (2017) and Luznik et al. (2010)

is considered as priority, such as for children with aplastic anemia and for some teams for haploidentical transplantation (see Table 14.1). The outcome considered to favor this choice is the GRFS (GVHD and relapse-free survival) as defined by EBMT (Ruggeri et al. 2016).

Conversely, PB can be a first choice in patients with hematological malignancies at high or very high risk of progression/relapse, such as AML FLT3ITD positive, lymphomas in progression after relapse from auto-HSCT, etc. for whom the risk of relapse is considered as first priority despite the risk of increasing NRM. Usually, this choice is made in parallel to the decision whether the conditioning regimen should be MAC or RIC (Gilleece et al. 2018).

For autologous HSCT (Table 14.2) the two major reasons for using BM are autologous transplantation for AML in remission and attempts at increasing the stem cell dose infused following poor marrow collections.

14.3 Mobilized or Primed Marrow

Following the discovery of cytokines, G-CSF in particular, the use of BM collected after 2–4 days of GCSF administration has been investigated in the year 2000–2005. G-CSF-primed marrow harvesting results in a graft with more mononuclear cells collected and higher CD34(+) stem and progenitor cell doses s (Grupp et al. 2006). The clinical significance of different HSC sources (primed marrow, mobilized blood, and steady-state marrow) in auto- and allo-HSCT was reviewed in 2004 (Elfenbein and Sackstein 2004). Mobilized marrow speeds up engraftment for both auto- and allo-HSCT, with a possible (unproven) reduction of GVHD rate and severity. Its use nowadays is rare, but it is for some teams the preferred stem cell source or part of a combination of primed marrow + PB as stem cell source for haploidentical donor transplantation (Huang et al. 2009; Ly et al. 2015).

14.4 Technique of BM Collection and Impact of the Dose of Nucleated Cells Infused

Marrow is collected from the posterior superior iliac crests, usually under general anesthesia, although few teams have used sedation or locoregional anesthesia (Fig. 14.1).

Marrow is aspirated with bone needles with multiple holes all around, which makes collection easier and the procedure more rapid. However, to avoid large dilution with blood, it is recommended to limit each aspiration to a volume of less than 5 mL, before transferring the

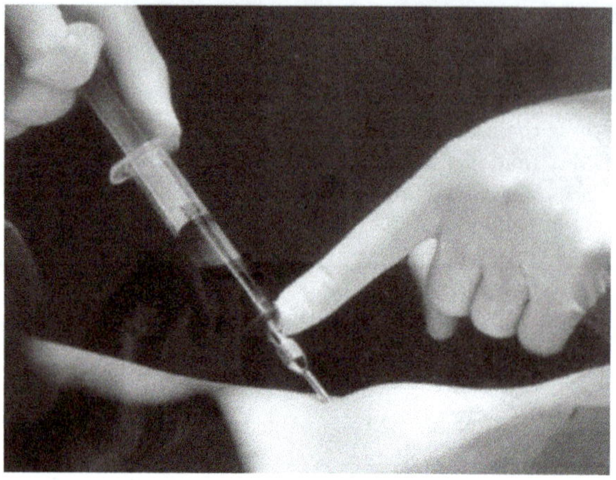

Fig. 14.1 Bone marrow harvest

aspirate through a three-way tap to the collection bag. The collection bag contains ACD anticoagulant solution and the syringes are rinsed with heparin (5.000 U/mL).

The goal is nowadays to obtain typically at least 3 × 10^8 nucleated cells/kg, although 2 × 10^8 nucleated cells/kg has long been in the past the usual target and remains acceptable. However, it should be kept in mind that old studies in the early development of BMT have indicated better results both in terms of engraftment but also decrease in NRM and RI and better outcome, with higher marrow doses (Gorin et al. 1999, 2003; Sierra et al. 1997):

- For Allo-HSCT with identical siblings, an early EBMT retrospective study evaluated the impact of the marrow cell dose infused: The median BM cell dose was 2.7 × 10^8/kg (0.17–29 × 10^8/kg). In multivariate analyses, high-dose BM compared to PB was associated with lower NRM, better LFS, and better OS (RR = 0.64; 95% CI, 0.44–0.92; $P = 0.016$). Results in patients with AML receiving allografts in CR1 indicated a better outcome with BM as compared to PB, when the dose of BM infused was above the median value.
- For Allo-HSCT fully with matched unrelated donors (Sierra et al. 1997), transplantation of a marrow cell dose above the median value of 3.65 × 10^8/kg was associated with faster neutrophil and platelet engraftment and decreased incidence of severe acute GVHD. Transplant in remission of acute leukemia with a high dose of marrow cells was associated with the best outcome in both children and adults.

If the targeted goal cannot be achieved, additional collection can be made from the anterior iliac crests, although it is time consuming and potentially more harmful for the patient or the donor, who must be turned over with all sterile fields to be reinstalled.

All things considered the maximum accepted volume collected should not go over 20 mL/kg donor body weight. Depending on the volume collected, three attitudes regarding transfusion during marrow collection may be followed: no transfusion and liquid replacement is the first option for many teams. Autotransfusion (to prepare beforehand in the 3 weeks preceding marrow collection, which adds some constraint) is the other recommended transfusional option. In rare circumstances allo-transfusion remains possible; usually two packs of concentrated red cells are enough.

Another option to consider to increase the stem cell dose to infuse when marrow collection has been insufficiently productive is the addition of PBSC. This however can be a complex decision which should take into account the disease and disease status, whether it concerns an autograft or an allograft or in this last situation whether a possible increase in the incidence and severity of GVHD associated with GVL/tumor is potentially beneficial or harmful. Two examples of this dilemma are summarized below:

1. In the context of auto-HSCT for leukemias or lymphomas, when analyzing patients receiving combinations of BM and PBSC (either because PBSC were collected to supplement poor BM or the reverse), outcomes are poor. One likely explanation is the existence of a bias since in most of these patients, poor collections (either BM or PBSC or both) are surrogate markers of multiple previous lines of chemotherapy for resistant/progressing diseases.
2. In contrast, for some teams, the combination of BM and PBSC has become the standard stem cell source for HSCT (see Table 14.1).

Table 14.2 Preferences for BM as source of stem cells in AUTO-HSCT

Auto-HSCT	Rationale	Justification	Comments
Poor PB collection	Increase the dose of HSC in the autograft	Ensure safer engraftment	However, poor mobilizers are likely to also produce poor marrow collection*
AML	Outcome better when compared to PB		Several EBMT retrospective studies

*Although there are biases, data from the EBMT registry indicate that poor mobilizers (often previously heavily treated with chemotherapy) have a poor outcome Shouval et al. (2018)

14.5 Complications of Bone Marrow Collections

One cannot ignore that on theoretical grounds two major hazards of marrow collection although very rare are death secondary to general anesthesia (<1/200,000) and major organ damage by mechanical mismanipulation of the bone needles that may sideslip if sufficient expertise and caution are not present.

The NMDP analyzed in 1993, 493 volunteers who donated unrelated marrow from October 1991 in 42 centers (Stroncek et al. 1993). The median volume of marrow collected was 1050 mL (range 180–2983 mL). Autologous red blood cells were transfused to 90% of donors, but only three donors received allogeneic blood. Apnea during anesthesia occurred in one donor. Other acute complications related to the collection procedure occurred in 6% of donors. Following marrow collection 75% experienced tiredness, 68% experienced pain at the marrow collection site, and 52% of the donors experienced low back pain. Mean recovery time was 16 days, but 42 donors felt that it took them at least 30 days to recover fully. The duration of the marrow collection procedure and duration of anesthesia both positively correlated with donor pain and/or fatigue following the collection. The recommendation of this study was the duration of the collection procedure and probably the duration of anesthesia, and therefore the volume of marrow collected should be kept to a minimum, but this conclusion is to be weighed against the wish to collect stem cell doses as high as possible to ensure fast engraftment and improve outcome.

14.6 Bone Marrow Cryopreservation

In the context of auto-HSCT, BM and PBSC are almost always cryopreserved and stored either in liquid nitrogen (−196 °C) or the gas phase of liquid nitrogen (−140 °C). The technique of freezing at −1 °C/min with dimethyl sulfoxide (DMSO) and the technique of rapid thawing are well established (Gorin 1986). Harmless long duration of storage has been reported up to 11 years (Aird et al. 1992). Recently some attempts at avoiding cryopreservation to replace it by storage at 4 °C in the refrigerator have produced interesting results, but using refrigerator storage is not presently validated and cannot be recommended by EBMT (Sarmiento et al. 2018).

Cryopreservation and storage of a marrow in view of an allo-HSCT is possible. However, it should be kept in mind that any cryopreservation procedure, would it seem perfect, results in some measurable (CFU-GM, BFU-E) and many less measurable (immune functions, etc.) damages. Therefore, it should be reserved to special situations when, for instance, the donor cannot be available at the very time of the transplantation procedure. As a rule, fresh marrow is preferable to frozen marrow.

14.7 Quality Control for BM Harvesting and Cryopreservation

The major indicator for successful BM collection is the dose collected, as discussed above, i.e., the number of nucleated cells expressed per kg of body weight for the recipient. It is very usual to have a blood count done at the mid time of the collection to ensure proper richness. With a goal of a minimum of 3×10^8 nucleated cells/kg, any richness above this value can be seen as a bonus. Harvest below this level, around 2×10^8 or even lower, however has been associated with correct engraftment.

CD34+ evaluation is not routinely performed for BM, while it is the rule for PB.

For cryopreserved marrow, some teams routinely cryopreserve small samples in minibags or ampoules, enabling viability testing before thawing the graft (usually an autograft). However, and importantly, a technical bias has been observed with ampoules since differences in cooling rates prevent ampoules from being a reliable index of HSC cryopreservation in large volumes (Douay et al. 1986a).

More pertinent testing consists in the evaluation of CFU-GM which represents in this setting the most reliable functional viability indicator (Douay et al. 1986b). Although there is no guideline, experience has shown that the results in CFUGM/kg are about 1–1.5 log below the expected or calculated results in CD34+ cells /kg (therefore expressed in 10^5/kg). CFU-GM evaluation is not a consensual prerequisite since it is an additional time-consuming effort, but it may bring important information in some cases, for instance, when dealing with marrow collections below 2×10^8/kg.

14.8 Conclusions

PB collections and transplantation nowadays represent 70–90% of all stem cell sources for transplants.

However, BM transplantation has not disappeared and is likely to persist in some limited situations and indications.

Further studies may revisit and increase the choice of marrow as stem cell source.

The Five Key Points of Marrow Collection

- Harvest with small (2–5 mL) aspirate volumes to avoid dilution with blood.
- The goal should be at least 3×10^8 nucleated cells per kg, but the more the better. The maximum volume collected should not go over 20 mL/kg donor body weight. Decision for no transfusion with liquid replacement (recommended) or autotransfusion (second best option) or in rare cases Allotransfusion during collection relies on the judgment of the local medical team.
- Cryopreservation is the rule for auto-BMT, while it should be avoided and used only in rare specific conditions for allogeneic transplantation.
- BM is mandatory in children and patients with aplastic anemias. It is presently favored by some teams in the context of haploidentical transplantation.
- BM when compared with PBSC results in less NRM, less GVHD (in particular less chronic extensive GVHD), but less GVL/lymphoma/tumor effect.

References

Aird W, Labopin M, Gorin NC, Antin JH. Long-term cryopreservation of human stem cells. Bone Marrow Transplant. 1992;9:487–90.

Anasetti C, Logan BR, Lee SJ, et al. Peripheral-blood stem cells versus bone marrow from unrelated donors. N Engl J Med. 2012;367:1487–96.

Bacigalupo A, Socie G, Schrezenmeier H, et al. Bone marrow versus peripheral blood as the stem cell source for sibling transplants in acquired aplastic anemia: survival advantage for bone marrow in all age groups. Haematologica. 2012;97:1142–8.

Barone A, Lucarelli A, Onofrillo D, et al. Diagnosis and management of acquired aplastic anemia in childhood. Guidelines from the marrow failure study group of the pediatric haemato-oncology Italian association (AIEOP). Blood Cells Mol Dis. 2015;55:40–7.

Bhella S, Navneet S, Majhail NS, Betcher J, et al. Choosing wisely BMT: American society for blood and marrow transplantation and Canadian blood and marrow transplant group's list of 5 tests and treatments to question in blood and marrow transplantation. Biol Blood Marrow Transplant. 2018;24:909–13.

Douay L, Lopez M, Gorin NC. A technical bias: differences in cooling rates prevent ampoules from being a reliable index of stem cell cryopreservation in large volumes. Cryobiology. 1986a;23:296–301.

Douay L, Gorin NC, Mary JY, et al. Recovery of CFUGM from cryopreserved marrow and in vivo evaluation after autologous bone marrow transplantation are predictive of engraftment. Exp Hematol. 1986b;14:358–65.

Eapen M, Logan BR, Confer DL, et al. Peripheral blood grafts from unrelated donors are associated with increased acute and chronic graft-versus-host disease without improved survival. Biol Blood Marrow Transplant. 2007;13:1461–8.

Eapen M, Le Rademacher J, Antin JH, et al. Effect of stem cell source on outcomes after unrelated donor transplantation in severe aplastic anemia. Blood. 2011;118:2618–21.

Elfenbein GJ, Sackstein R. Primed marrow for autologous and allogeneic transplantation: a review comparing primed marrow to mobilized blood and steady-state marrow. Exp Hematol. 2004;32:327–39.

Gilleece M, Labopin M, Yakoub-Agha I, et al. Measurable residual disease, conditioning regimen intensity and age predict outcome of allogeneic hematopoietic cell transplantation for acute myeloid leukaemia in first remission: a registry analysis of 2292 patients by the acute leukemia working party European society of blood and marrow transplantation. Am J Hematol. 2018;93:1142–52.

Gluckman E, Rocha V, Boyer-Chammard A, et al. Outcome of cord-blood transplantation from related and unrelated donors. Eurocord transplant group and the European blood and marrow transplantation group. N Engl J Med. 1997;337:373–81.

Gorin NC. Collection, manipulation and freezing of haemopoietic stem cells. Clin Haematol. 1986;15:19–48.

Gorin NC, Aegerter P, Auvert B, et al. Autologous bone marrow transplantation for acute myelocytic leukemia in first remission: a European survey of the role of marrow purging. Blood. 1990;75:1606–14.

Gorin NC, Labopin M, Laporte JP, et al. Importance of marrow dose on posttransplant outcome in acute leukemia: models derived from patients autografted with mafosfamide-purged marrow at a single institution. Exp Hematol. 1999;27:1822–30.

Gorin NC, Labopin M, Rocha V, et al. Marrow versus peripheral blood for geno-identical allogeneic stem cell transplantation in acute myelocytic leukemia: influence of dose and stem cell source shows better outcome with rich marrow. Blood. 2003;102:3043–51.

Gorin NC, Labopin M, Blaise D, et al. Higher incidence of relapse with peripheral blood rather than marrow as a source of stem cells in adults with acute myelocytic leukemia autografted during the first remission. J Clin Oncol. 2009;27:3987–93.

Gorin NC, Labopin M, Reiffers J, et al. Higher incidence of relapse in patients with acute myelocytic leukemia infused with higher doses of CD34+ cells from leukapheresis products autografted during the first remission. Blood. 2010;116:3157–62.

Grupp SA, Frangoul H, Wall D, et al. Use of G-CSF in matched sibling donor pediatric allogeneic transplantation: a consensus statement from the Children's Oncology Group (COG) Transplant Discipline Committee and Pediatric Blood and Marrow Transplant Consortium (PBMTC) Executive Committee. Ped Blood Cancer. 2006;46:414–21.

Huang XJ, Liu DH, Liu KY, et al. Treatment of acute leukemia with unmanipulated HLA-mismatched/haploidentical blood and bone marrow transplantation. Biol Blood Marrow Transplant. 2009;15:257–65.

Kasamon YL, Ambinder RF, Fuchs EJ, et al. Prospective study of nonmyeloablative, HLA-mismatched unrelated BMT with high-dose posttransplantation cyclophosphamide. Blood Adv. 2017;1:288–92.

Lee SJ, Logan B, Westervelt P, et al. Comparison of patient-reported outcomes in 5-year survivors who received bone marrow vs peripheral blood unrelated donor transplantation: long-term follow-up of a randomized clinical trial. JAMA Oncol. 2016;2:1583–9.

Luznik L, Bolanos-Meade J, Zahurak M, et al. High-dose cyclophosphamide as single-agent, short-course prophylaxis of graft-versus-host disease. Blood. 2010;115:3224–30.

Ly M, Zhao XS, Hu Y, et al. Monocytic and promyelocytic myeloid-derived suppressor cells may contribute to G-CSF-induced immune tolerance in haplo-identical allogeneic hematopoietic stem cell transplantation. Am J Hematol. 2015;90:E9–E16.

Mathe G. Treatment of leukemia with allogenic bone marrow transplantation. Brux Med. 1964;44:559–62.

Passweg JR, Baldomero H, Gratwohl A, Bregni M, Cesaro S, Dreger P, et al. The EBMT activity survey: 1990–2010. Bone Marrow Transplant. 2012;47:906–23.

Passweg JR, Baldomero H, Bader P, et al. Hematopoietic stem cell transplantation in Europe 2014: more than 40 000 transplants annually. Bone Marrow Transplant. 2016;51:786–92.

Ruggeri A, Labopin M, Ciceri F, et al. Definition of GvHD-free, relapse-free survival for registry-based studies: an ALWP-EBMT analysis on patients with AML in remission. Bone Marrow Transplant. 2016;51:610–1.

Ruggeri A, Labopin M, Bacigalupo A, et al. Bone marrow versus mobilized peripheral blood stem cells in haploidentical transplants using posttransplantation cyclophosphamide. Cancer. 2018;124:1428–37.

Santos GW. Bone marrow transplantation in hematologic malignancies. Current status. Cancer. 1990;65(3 Suppl):786–91.

Sarmiento M, Ramirez P, Parody R, et al. Advantages of non-cryopreserved autologous hematopoietic stem cell transplantation against a cryopreserved strategy. Bone Marrow Transplant. 2018;53:960–6. https://doi.org/10.1038/s41409-018-0117-5.

Schmitz N, Beksac M, Bacigalupo A, et al. Filgrastim-mobilized peripheral blood progenitor cells versus bone marrow transplantation for treating leukemia: 3-year results from the EBMT randomized trial. Haematologica. 2005;90:643–8.

Schrezenmeier H, Passweg JR, Marsh JC, et al. Worse outcome and more chronic GVHD with peripheral blood progenitor cells than bone marrow in HLA-matched sibling donor transplants for young patients with severe acquired aplastic anemia. Blood. 2007;110:1397–400.

Shouval R, Labopin M, Bomze D, et al. Prediction of leukemia free survival following autologous stem cell transplantation in AML. A risk score developed by the ALWP of the EBMT. EHA 23rd annual meeting, Stockholm, 2018. Abstract.

Sierra J, Storer B, Hansen JA, et al. Transplantation of marrow cells from unrelated donors for treatment of high-risk acute leukemia: the effect of leukemic burden, donor HLA matching and marrow cell dose. Blood. 1997;89:4226–35.

Simonin M, Dalissier A, Labopin M, et al. More chronic GvHD and non-relapse mortality after peripheral blood stem cell compared with bone marrow in hematopoietic transplantation for paediatric acute lymphoblastic leukemia: a retrospective study on behalf of the EBMT Paediatric Diseases Working Party. Bone Marrow Transplant. 2017;52:1071–3.

Stroncek DF, Holland PV, Bartch G, et al. Experiences of the first 493 unrelated marrow donors in the National Marrow Donor Program. Blood. 1993;81:1940–6.

Sun CLFL, Kawashima T, Leisenring W, et al. Prevalence and predictors of chronic health conditions after hematopoietic cell transplantation: a report from the bone marrow transplant survivor study. Blood. 2010;116:3129–39.

Thomas ED, Buckner CD, Clift RA, et al. Marrow transplantation for acute non lymphoblastic leukemia in first remission. N Engl J Med. 1979;301:597–9.

Walker I, Panzarella T, Couban S, et al. Pretreatment with anti-thymocyte globulin versus no anti-thymocyte globulin in patients with haematological malignancies undergoing haemopoietic cell transplantation from unrelated donors: a randomised, controlled, open-label, phase 3, multicentre trial. Lancet Oncol. 2016;17:164–73.

15 Mobilization and Collection of HSC

Kai Hübel

15.1 Introduction

The intravenous infusion of patient's own HSC to restore BM damage is the basic principle of high-dose chemotherapy, since otherwise the patient would expect long-lasting aplasia with life-threatening infections. Therefore, a sufficient collection of HSC before application of high-dose therapy is mandatory. Since HSC expresses CD34 on their surface, the number of CD34+ cells in the transplant material is considered as an indicator of the HSC content.

In principle, there are two ways how to collect stem cell: by repeated aspiration of BM from the pelvic crest or by leukapheresis after mobilization of HSC into the PB. The latter one is favored and considered as standard because it is less stressful for the patient and leads to faster engraftment and hematologic reconstitution which may improve patient outcomes (Gertz 2010).

Usually, HSC circulates in a very small number in the PB. Therefore, mobilization of HSC from the BM to the PB is an essential part of auto-HSCT programs. Following sufficient mobilization, patient will need leukapheresis which is often performed by central lines to facilitate the procedure. Finally, HSC will be cryopreserved using dimethyl sulfoxide (DMSO) until transfusion.

15.2 Strategies of Mobilization

There are two different strategies to mobilize HSC from the BM to the PB: the so-called "steady-state" mobilization and the mobilization by chemotherapy.

15.2.1 Mobilization Without Chemotherapy ("Steady State")

Using this approach, HSC will be mobilized by the use of cytokines only. The only recommended cytokine for mobilization is G-CSF, since GM-CSF is no longer available in many countries after commercial failure and withdrawal. G-CSF induces myeloid hyperplasia and the release of CD34+ cells into the circulation through proteolytic cleavage of adhesion molecules (Lapidot and Petit 2002). Currently, the G-CSF cytokines filgrastim and lenograstim have market approval for mobilization of HSC in Europe.

The recommended doses are filgrastim 10 μg/kg/day SC for 5–7 consecutive days and lenograstim 10 μg/kg/day SC for 4–6 consecutive days. The use of biosimilar G-CSF has equivalent efficacy (Schmitt et al. 2016).

K. Hübel (✉)
University of Cologne, Department of Internal Medicine, Cologne, Germany
e-mail: kai.huebel@uni-koeln.de

E. Carreras et al. (eds.), *The EBMT Handbook*, https://doi.org/10.1007/978-3-030-02278-5_15

Leukapheresis usually is performed on day 5 independent whether filgrastim or lenograstim was used for mobilization. The measurement of CD34+ cells in the PB before leukapheresis is not mandatory but could help to estimate the expected collection yield and the duration of leukapheresis. If the number of cells collected is inadequate, mobilization with G-CSF may be continued for 1–2 days. However, if the collection goal is not reached after the third leukapheresis, a successful mobilization is unlikely.

The major advantages of steady-state mobilization are the relatively low toxicity, the predictable time of leukapheresis, the outpatient administration, and the reduced costs compared to chemo-mobilization. The major disadvantages are variable mobilization failure rates and the lower CD34+ cell yields compared to chemo-mobilization. Mobilization with G-CSF only may be used in patients without further need of chemotherapy, e.g., in patients with a stable remission of the underlying disease.

15.2.2 Mobilization with Chemotherapy

The use of chemotherapy in combination with G-CSF is the preferred way of mobilization for all patients who will need further decrease of tumor burden and/or who have to collect a high number of HSC.

CY in a dose of 2–4 g/m^2 is widely used for HSC mobilization. It is also possible to mobilize HSC not by a separate chemotherapy but as part of the disease-specific chemotherapy, e.g., to mobilize HSC following salvage treatment with R-DHAP or R-ICE in lymphoma patients. The choice of a specific chemo-mobilization approach is based on patient's disease characteristics and local clinical practice guidelines.

Approved doses of G-CSF for HSC mobilization after myelosuppressive therapy are filgrastim 5 μg/kg/day SC and lenograstim 150 μg/m^2/day SC. There are reports of the use of higher doses of G-CSF (Romeo et al. 2010), but there are no randomized trials and additional side effects are possible. Mobilization with G-CSF should start after completion of chemotherapy at the earliest and at the leukocyte nadir at the latest and should continue until the last leukapheresis. Most protocols recommend the initiation of G-CSF within 1–5 days after the end of chemotherapy.

The major advantage of adding chemotherapy to cytokines, besides the effect on the tumor, is the expected improvement of the collection yield with fewer apheresis sessions (Sung et al. 2013). The major disadvantages of chemo-mobilization are the therapy-related toxicity, the requirement of in-hospital treatment in most cases, the bone marrow damage by the chemotherapy which may impair future mobilizations, and higher mobilization costs. Furthermore, an exact prognosis of the CD34+ cell peak in the PB and the optimal start of leukapheresis are difficult and require daily monitoring of CD34+ cells in the PB. Table 15.1 summarizes a recommendation of timing of G-CSF following most used chemotherapy regimens and start of monitoring of CD34+ cells in the PB.

In several clinical trials, it was documented that relapse rate after auto-HSCT following mobilization with and without chemotherapy is comparable (Tuchman et al. 2015).

Table 15.1 Recommended start of G-CSF and start of CD34+ monitoring for most used mobilization chemotherapy regimens

Chemotherapy	Start G-CSF	Start CD34+ monitoring
CY 2 g/m^2	Day 5	Day 10
CAD	Day 9	Day 13
(R)CHOP/CHOEP	Day 6	Day 11
(R)DHAP	Day 9	Day 14
(R)ICE	Day 6	Day 12
(R)AraC/TT	Day 5	Day 10

Day 1: first day of chemotherapy application (without rituximab). Adapted from (Kriegsmann et al. 2018)

15.3 CD34+ Cell Count and Timing of Leukapheresis

Up to date, CD34+ cell count in mobilized peripheral blood product is the most important parameter of graft quality, as it is the only recognized predictor of stable hematopoietic engraftment after auto-HSCT (Saraceni et al. 2015). Monitoring of CD34+ cells in the PB is optional in steady-state mobilization but an essential part of chemo-mobilization. Following chemotherapy, the daily measurement of leukocytes and thrombocytes is recommended. If not otherwise specified by the protocol, CD34 monitoring should be initiated at the latest if leukocytes increase up to 1000/μL during recovering from aplasia. This increase of leukocytes is mostly accompanied with an increase of thrombocytes. A prompt start of leukapheresis is required of CD34+ cell count of ≥20/μL (Mohty et al. 2014); for more details, please see Sect. 15.6.

15.4 Target HSC Collection Count

The target quantity of HSC to be collected is dependent on the underlying disease. Most patients with NHL or HL (expect for rare case of patients with HL who require double auto-HSCT) will need one autograft. The generally accepted minimum CD34+ cell yield to proceed to transplantation is 2×10^6 cells/kg (Mohty et al. 2014); however, higher yields of $4–5 \times 10^6$ CD34+ cells/kg are aimed for at many centers since they have been associated with faster neutrophil and platelet recovery, reduced hospitalization, blood transfusions, and antibiotic therapy (Stiff et al. 2011; Giralt et al. 2014). Patients mobilizing >8–10 × 10^6 cells/kg are called "super mobilizer"; however, the reported positive effect after infusion of such a high number of HSC on the outcome and prognosis of the patient is highly speculative. For patients with a chance of two or even more transplantations (mainly patients with MM), it is essential to collect the required number of HSC before the first high-dose therapy since mobilization after high-dose therapy has an increased risk of failure. For tandem transplantation, the required cell dose for one transplantation is also at least 2×10^6 CD34+ cells/kg.

15.5 Leukapheresis

Collection of peripheral HSC for auto-HSCT is a well-established process. The duration of one leukapheresis session should not exceed 5 h, and the total number of leukapheresis session should not exceed four procedures since more sessions are useless in most cases and will stress the patient. CD34+ cell collection has been shown to be more effective with larger apheresis volume (4.0–5.3 times the patient's total blood volume), and no difference in CD34+ cell viability was observed compared with normal-volume apheresis (2.7–3.5 times the patient's total blood volume) (Abrahamsen et al. 2005). Enhanced volumes are especially recommended for patients with a high risk of mobilization failure or for patients with a high individual CD34+ cell collection goal. However, not all patients are eligible for enhanced volume strategies. Larger transfusion volumes and related higher DMSO contents have been associated with increased risk of cardiac side effects (Donmez et al. 2007).

15.6 Poor Mobilizer

Despite widespread and established practice, current mobilization strategies vary between centers and differ in terms of feasibility and outcome. Although the majority of patients are able to mobilize sufficient CD34+ cells for at least a single auto-HSCT, approximately 15% fail to do so (Wuchter et al. 2010).

Poor mobilizers are usually defined as patients with less than 2×10^6 CD34+ cells/kg collected or patients mobilizing less than 10–20 CD34+ cells/µl into the PB. In general, there are two groups of poor mobilizers: predicted poor mobilizers and proven poor mobilizers (Olivieri et al. 2012). Proven poor mobilizers have low CD34+ peripheral counts circulating or do not achieve adequate HSC on day 1 of apheresis. Based on CD34+ cells, it is possible to identify the following subgroups: "borderline poor mobilizer" (11–19 CD34+ cells/µL), "relative poor mobilizer" (6–10 CD34+ cells/µL), and "absolute poor mobilizer" (0–5 CD34+ cells/µL) (Wuchter et al. 2010). If a patient has ≥20 CD34+ cells/µL at time of apheresis, the collection process should start. Between 15 and 20 CD34+ cells/µL, collection might be sufficient if not more than two transplantations are planned and the patient has no risk factors for poor mobilization (see below).

Otherwise, the use of plerixafor (recommended dose 0.24 mg/kg/day SC) should be considered. If a patient has 10–15 CD34+ cells/µL, plerixafor application should be discussed. Below 10 CD34+ cells/µl, the use of plerixafor is clearly indicated to avoid mobilization failure. That means that there is a "gray area" between 10 and 20 CD34+ cells/µL, and the decision to use plerixafor in this situation is based on disease characteristics and treatment history (Fig. 15.1). Furthermore, if it is not possible to collect at least one third of the collection goal with the first apheresis, plerixafor should be applied because of high risk of mobilization failure (Mohty et al. 2014; Cheng et al. 2015).

Predicted poor mobilizers are defined by baseline patient or disease characteristics which are

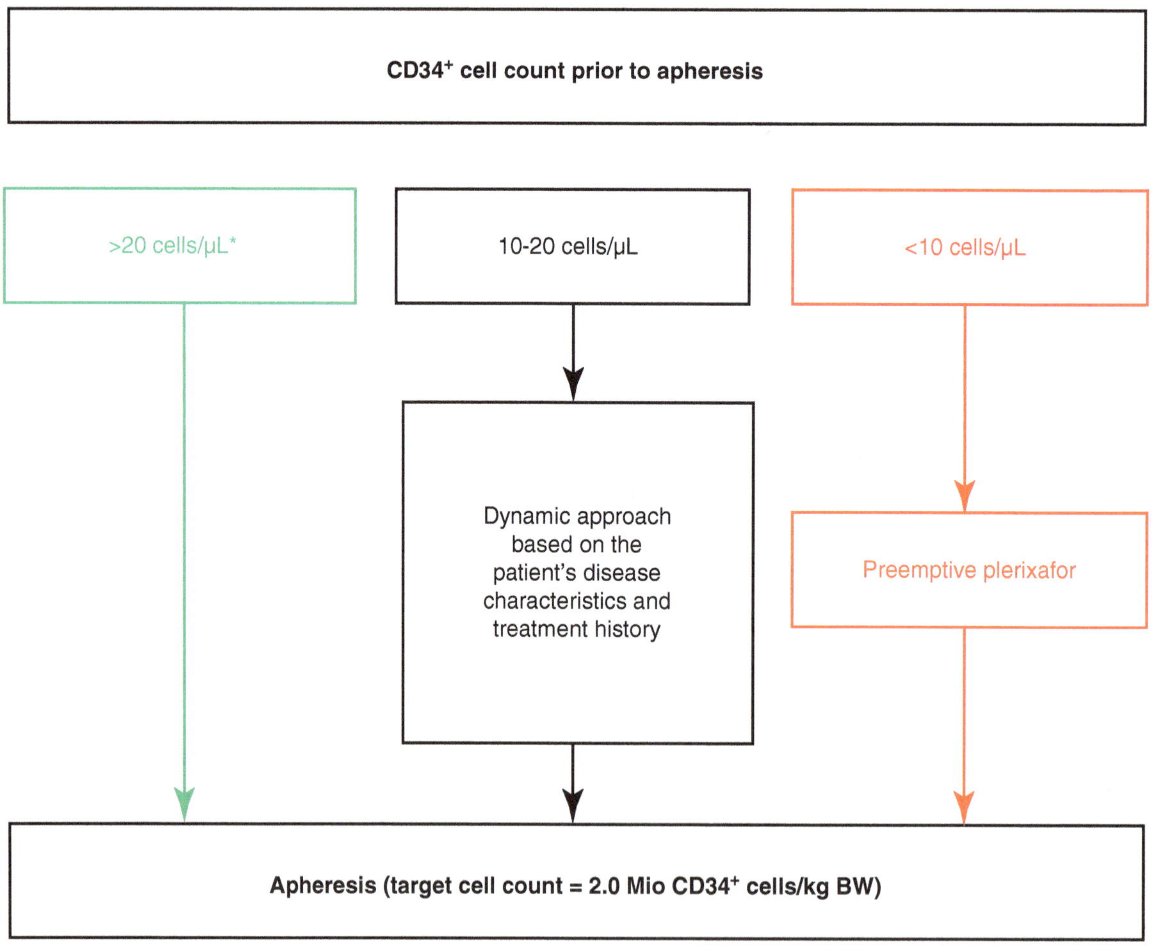

Fig. 15.1 Proactive intervention to rescue mobilization failure (Adapted from Mohty et al. 2014). *No active intervention required

Table 15.2 Factors described as predictive of poor mobilization or mobilization failure

Risk factors for poor mobilization
Age >60 years
Advanced stage of underlying disease
High number of prior treatment lines
Therapy with fludarabine, melphalan, and lenalidomide *(controversial)*
Low CD34+ cell count before apheresis
Low platelet count before mobilization *(controversial)*

Adapted from (Mohty et al. 2014)

associated with poor mobilization. These factors are listed in Table 15.2. In patients with one or more of these risk factors, the preemptive use of plerixafor should be considered. It is generally accepted that the most robust predictive factor for poor mobilization is the CD34+ cell count in PB before apheresis.

The use of plerixafor is not only valuable to avoid a failed mobilization in the described risk groups, bit it has also a documented effect on the resources of the centers. With the use of plerixafor, patients spend less time on apheresis with less blood volume processed and collect more CD34+ cells with the first apheresis, leading to a decreased number of apheresis sessions needed (Mohty et al. 2018). This has a direct effect on reducing mobilization costs. In case of a failed first mobilization attempt, the use of plerixafor for remobilization is clearly indicated (Hubel et al. 2011).

15.7 Future Directions

At this time, the number of CD34+ cells in the graft is the major and most important indicator for graft quality. A sufficient number of CD34+ cells are essential to overcome the toxicity of high-dose chemotherapy and to facilitate hematopoietic recovery. However, there is an increasing understanding that other graft subsets, e.g., CD34+ subpopulations or immune cell subsets (B cells, T cells, NK cells, dendritic cells), influence immune recovery. There are also reports that the mobilization regimen has a major impact on graft immune composition and patient's outcome (Saraceni et al. 2015). Therefore, stem cell mobilization could not only be an important part of high-dose therapies but could also be part of an effective immunotherapy. The delineation of this approach has just been started.

Key Points

- Mobilization with chemotherapy plus G-CSF is the preferred method for patients who will need decrease of tumor burden or who have to collect a high number of HSC.
- Up to date, CD34+ cell count in the PB is the most important parameter of graft quality.
- The required HSC dose for one transplantation is at least 2 × 10^6 CD34+ cells/kg.
- The indication for the use of plerixafor depends on the CD34+ cell count in the PB, the collection goal, the collection yield with the first apheresis, and/or the presence of risk factors.

References

Abrahamsen JF, Stamnesfet S, Liseth K, et al. Large-volume leukapheresis yields more viable CD34+ cells and colony-forming units than normal-volume leukapheresis, especially in patients who mobilize low numbers of CD34+ cells. Transfusion. 2005;45:248–53.

Cheng J, Schmitt M, Wuchter P, et al. Plerixafor is effective given either preemptively or as a rescue strategy in poor stem cell mobilizing patients with multiple myeloma. Transfusion. 2015;55:275–83.

Donmez A, Tombuloglu M, Gungor A, et al. Clinical side effects during peripheral blood progenitor cell infusion. Transfus Apher Sci. 2007;36:95–101.

Gertz MA. Current status of stem cell mobilization. Br J Haematol. 2010;150:647–62.

Giralt S, Costa L, Schriber J, et al. Optimizing autologous stem cell mobilization strategies to improve patient outcomes: consensus guidelines and recommendations. Biol Blood Marrow Transplant. 2014;20:295–308.

Hubel K, Fresen MM, Salwender H, et al. Plerixafor with and without chemotherapy in poor mobilizers: results from the German compassionate use program. Bone Marrow Transplant. 2011;46:1045–52.

Kriegsmann K, Schmitt A, Kriegsmann M, et al. Orchestration of chemomobilization and G-CSF administration for successful hematopoietic stem cell collection. Biol Blood Marrow Transplant. 2018;24:1281–8.

Lapidot T, Petit I. Current understanding of stem cell mobilization: the roles of chemokines, proteolytic enzymes, adhesion molecules, cytokines, and stromal cells. Exp Hematol. 2002;30:973–81.

Mohty M, Azar N, Chabannon C, et al. Plerixafor in poor mobilizers with non-Hodgkin's lymphoma: a multicenter time-motion analysis. Bone Marrow Transplant. 2018;53:246–54.

Mohty M, Hubel K, Kroger N, et al. Autologous haematopoietic stem cell mobilisation in multiple myeloma and lymphoma patients: a position statement from the European group for blood and marrow transplantation. Bone Marrow Transplant. 2014;49:865–72.

Olivieri A, Marchetti M, Lemoli R, et al. Proposed definition of 'poor mobilizer' in lymphoma and multiple myeloma: an analytic hierarchy process by ad hoc working group Gruppo Italiano Trapianto di Midollo Osseo. Bone Marrow Transplant. 2012;47:342–51.

Romeo A, Chierichini A, Spagnoli A, et al. Standard- versus high-dose lenograstim in adults with hematologic malignancies for peripheral blood progenitor cell mobilization. Transfusion. 2010;50:2432–46.

Saraceni F, Shem-Tov N, Olivieri A, Nagler A. Mobilized peripheral blood grafts include more than hematopoietic stem cells: the immunological perspective. Bone Marrow Transplant. 2015;50:886–91.

Schmitt M, Hoffmann JM, Lorenz K, et al. Mobilization of autologous and allogeneic peripheral blood stem cells for transplantation in haematological malignancies using biosimilar G-CSF. Vox Sang. 2016;111:178–86.

Stiff PJ, Micallef I, Nademanee AP, et al. Transplanted CD34(+) cell dose is associated with long-term platelet count recovery following autologous peripheral blood stem cell transplant in patients with non-Hodgkin lymphoma or multiple myeloma. Biol Blood Marrow Transplant. 2011;17:1146–53.

Sung AD, Grima DT, Bernard LM, et al. Outcomes and costs of autologous stem cell mobilization with chemotherapy plus G-CSF vs G-CSF alone. Bone Marrow Transplant. 2013;48:1444–9.

Tuchman SA, Bacon WA, Huang LW, et al. Cyclophosphamide-based hematopoietic stem cell mobilization before autologous stem cell transplantation in newly diagnosed multiple myeloma. J Clin Apher. 2015;30:176–82.

Wuchter P, Ran D, Bruckner T, et al. Poor mobilization of hematopoietic stem cells-definitions, incidence, risk factors, and impact on outcome of autologous transplantation. Biol Blood Marrow Transplant. 2010;16:490–9.

16 Collection of HSC in Children

Volker Witt and Christina Peters

16.1 Introduction

Collecting or harvesting HSCs from children is a challenge, not only because children have different physiological and therefore anatomical situations but also because psychological, legal and ethical concerns in minors are sometimes more difficult compared to adult donors. In addition, parents and/or legal guardians have to be addressed in all issues. This chapter will focus on the technical, physiological, and ethical problems in the field of HSC collection from children rather than indications.

The main difference to the adult setting is the small bodyweight; the difficulties in accessing venous access, especially in the leukapheresis setting; and the need for blood cell substitution in case of BM harvest. In children the indications for autologous HSC harvesting is well-established (Passweg et al. 2014). Using children in the allogeneic setting as donors is a complete different issue (Bitan et al. 2016). Children should not donate HSCs if a comparable compatible adult volunteer HSC donor is available, if the indication for the stem cell therapy is not first line, or if the therapy is experimental (Sheldon 2004; Zinner 2004).

The main resources to harvest HSCs are BM and PBSCs. The basic techniques are quite similar to the techniques used in adults. For BM collection punctures of the iliac crests or in very small children, the tibia is used. For harvesting HSCs from the PB, leukapheresis is used with the same apheresis systems as in adults.

To perform these procedures in children, physicians and nursing practitioners must have working knowledge about the normal age-dependent physiological parameters, like vital signs, growth, and psychological and motorical development, and should be trained in the communication with children, parents, and/or their legal guardians (Anthias et al. 2016).

16.2 Bone Marrow Harvest (See Chap. 14)

The collection of HSCs from the BM is the historical oldest technique. Multiple punctures of the iliac crest are performed in general anesthesia by experienced physicians and practitioners. The bone marrow is harvested by aspirations through adequately dimensioned needles. In very small children and if the iliac crest is anatomically not suitable for punctures, the aspirations could also be performed by punctures of the proximal tibia.

V. Witt
Department of Pediatric Hematology and Oncology, St. Anna Kinderspital, Medical University Vienna, Vienna, Austria

C. Peters (✉)
Stem Cell Transplantation Unit, St. Anna Children's Hospital, Vienna, Austria
e-mail: christina.peters@stanna.at

E. Carreras et al. (eds.), *The EBMT Handbook*, https://doi.org/10.1007/978-3-030-02278-5_16

For successful HSCT, it is necessary to obtain enough progenitor cells during the BM harvesting procedure. Most centers are using multiple aspirations of maximum 2 mL BM, while other centers are using few larger amount aspirations for BM harvesting (20–100–250 mL). It could be shown that the latter methods result in comparable grafts for transplantation (Witt et al. 2016). For some young donors with anatomically tiny situations or in diseases where a suitable donor should be used for more than one recipient a minimal harming procedure is warranted for the bone marrow harvest (Biral et al. 2008; Furey et al. 2018).

More recently, adult donors have received G-CSF because stimulated BM is richer in HSCs and therefore results in quicker engraftment (Ji et al. 2002). Experience with G-CSF-mobilized BM in pediatrics is limited. Recent data showed that a dose of 3–5 × 10^6 CD34+ HPC/kg of recipient bodyweight is the optimal CD34+ cell dose infused to attain GVHD relapse-free survival in children with an HLA-matched sibling donor. A higher CD34+ cell dose did not impact clinical outcome. G-CSF-primed BM harvest might have a better impact on smaller amount of BM harvest volume needed for a sufficient stem cell graft, but the study was underpowered to give an answer on this urgent question (Frangoul et al. 2007; Furey et al. 2018).

16.3 Peripheral Blood Stem Cell Harvest

PBSCs are harvested by leukapheresis in very small children even below 6 kg bodyweight and are described since the 1990s of the last century (Kanold et al. 1994; Klingebiel et al. 1995; Diaz et al. 1996; Moon et al. 2013). Special experience and techniques are required to perform safe leukapheresis procedures in pediatric patients using apheresis systems who are constructed for the use in adults. Due to the large extracorporeal volume of the apheresis systems available on the market (ca. 160–220 mL), there is a need to calculate the expected blood loss in the set during procedure (Witt et al. 2007). This has to be done in each procedure to decide whether a priming of the set is needed with blood (Moon et al. 2013). In most of the newest versions of the apheresis systems, an algorithm guides the user through this pediatric priming procedure. For priming only irradiated and leukodepleted packed RBCs should be used. In order to gain enough flow for the apheresis systems in very small children, a central venous catheter is needed, but also alternative line management with arterial lines is possible (Goldstein 2012; Even-Or et al. 2013; Hunt et al. 2013). It is important to know that in reports from registries, up to 50% of vascular access lines were peripheral venous access lines only in pediatric patients (Witt et al. 2008). For anticoagulation, citrate is used even in very small children. To avoid side effect, a calcium substitution is recommended (Kreuzer et al. 2011; Maitta et al. 2014).

For mobilization of the HPC into the PB, the longest experience exists with G-CSF in combination with chemotherapy in the autologous setting, but also plerixafor is reported in case series as suitable and safe in the use in children (Chambon et al. 2013). As in adults, a leukapheresis should be performed if a meaningful number of CD34+ HPCs are mobilized in the peripheral blood, to achieve the harvest of 2–5 × 10^6/kg recipient with a minimum number of procedures (Fritsch et al. 2010).

16.4 Risk Analysis BM Versus PBMNC

A study from the EBMT Pediatric Diseases Working Party describes which factors influenced the safety of HSC collection. In this prospective evaluation, 453 pediatric donors were included. The children donated either BM or PBSCs according to center policy. A large variability in approach to donor issues was observed between the participating centers. Significant differences were observed between BM and PBSC donors regarding pain, need for blood allotransfusion, duration of hospital stay, and iron supplementation; however, differences between the groups undergoing BM vs PBSC donation preclude direct risk comparisons between the two procedures. The most common adverse event was pain, reported mainly by older children after BM harvest but also observed after CVC placement for PBSC collection. With regard to severe adverse events, one patient developed a pneumothorax with hydrothorax after CVC placement for PBSC collection. The risk of allo-transfusion after BM harvest was associated with a donor age of <4 years and a BM harvest volume of >20 mL/kg. Children <4 years were at higher risk than older children for allo-transfusion after BM harvest, and there was a higher risk of complications from CVC placement before apheresis. It was concluded that PBSC and BM collection are both safe procedures in children (Styczynski et al. 2012).

16.5 Pediatrics as Allogeneic Donors

Pediatric-aged donors vary widely in their ability to assent or consent to the risks of a donation procedure. There are key regulations and ethical imperatives, which must be addressed in deciding which donation procedure is appropriate for minors (van Walraven et al. 2013). In order to have general guidance, the American Academy of Pediatrics published in 2010 a recommendation on this issue. The authors strongly recommend the inclusion of the potential child donor in all decision-making process to the extent that they are capable. A minor's advocate should be an independent person who will help to prevent the delay of the donation procedure (Chan and Tipoe 2013).

The decision to take a minor family donor especially in inherited diseases is complicated to the fact that phenotypically healthy or minor symptomatic siblings with mild carrier status might be eligible for the severely ill recipient. One simple example is a sibling with thalassemia minor for a recipient with a thalassemia major (Biral et al. 2008). There are many other major diseases, including primary immunodeficiencies, chronic granulomatous disease, or sickle cell disease, where carriers are used as HSC donors. Potential family sibling donors with medical or psychological reasons not to donate should not be HLA typed (Bitan et al. 2016).

Key Points

- Pediatric donors can safely donate HSCs if an experienced team is performing the harvest procedure.
- Donors below 4 years of age have a higher risk for harvest-associated complications: With BM harvest, they have a higher need for Allo-transfusions, and there is a higher risk of complications from CVC placement before apheresis.
- Minors should only be recruited as HSC donors if no medically equivalent histocompatible adult person is available for donation and if there is a reasonable likelihood that the recipient will benefit.
- An informed consent (child assent) for the HSC donation has to be obtained by the legal guardians and from the pediatric donor. A donor advocate with expertise in pediatric development should be appointed for all individuals who have not reached the age of majority and who are considered as potential HSC donor.
- Long-term follow-up data should be collected to help determine the actual medical and psychological benefits and risks of child donors.

References

Anthias C, O'Donnell PV, Kiefer DM, et al. European group for blood and marrow transplantation centers with FACT-JACIE accreditation have significantly better compliance with related donor care standards. Biol Blood Marrow Transplant. 2016;22:514–9.

Biral E, Chiesa R, Cappelli B, et al. Multiple BM harvests in pediatric donors for thalassemic siblings: safety, efficacy and ethical issues. Bone Marrow Transplant. 2008;42:379–84.

Bitan M, van Walraven SM, Worel N, et al. Determination of eligibility in related pediatric hematopoietic cell donors: ethical and clinical considerations. Recommendations from a working group of the Worldwide Network for Blood and Marrow Transplantation Association. Biol Blood Marrow Transplant. 2016;22:96–103.

Chambon F, Merlin E, Rochette E, et al. Mobilization of hematopoietic stem cells by plerixafor alone in children: a sequential Bayesian trial. Transfus Apher Sci. 2013;49:453–8.

Chan TK, Tipoe GL. The policy statement of the American Academy of Pediatrics–children as hematopoietic stem cell donors–a proposal of modifications for application in the UK. BMC Med Ethics. 2013;14:43.

Diaz MA, Villa M, Alegre A, et al. Collection and transplantation of peripheral blood progenitor cells mobilized by G-CSF alone in children with malignancies. Br J Haematol. 1996;94:148–54.

Even-Or E, Grunspan A, Swerdlow Y, et al. Peripheral blood stem-cell harvest using percutaneous arterial lines in children. Pediatr Blood Cancer. 2013;60:946–8.

Frangoul H, Nemecek ER, Billheimer D, et al. A prospective study of G-CSF primed bone marrow as a stem-cell source for allogeneic bone marrow transplantation in children: a Pediatric Blood and Marrow Transplant Consortium (PBMTC) study. Blood. 2007;110:4584–7.

Fritsch P, Schwinger W, Schwantzer G, et al. Peripheral blood stem cell mobilization with pegfilgrastim compared to filgrastim in children and young adults with malignancies. Pediatr Blood Cancer. 2010;54:134–7.

Furey A, Rastogi S, Prince R, et al. Bone marrow harvest in pediatric sibling donors: role of granulocyte colony-stimulating factor priming and CD34(+) cell dose. Biol Blood Marrow Transplant. 2018;24:324–9.

Goldstein SL. Therapeutic apheresis in children: special considerations. Semin Dial. 2012;25:165–70.

Hunt EA, Jain NG, Somers MJ. Apheresis therapy in children: an overview of key technical aspects and a review of experience in pediatric renal disease. J Clin Apher. 2013;28:36–47.

Ji SQ, Chen HR, Wang HX, et al. Comparison of outcome of allogeneic bone marrow transplantation with and without granulocyte colony-stimulating factor (lenograstim) donor-marrow priming in patients with chronic myelogenous leukemia. Biol Blood Marrow Transplant. 2002;8:261–7.

Kanold J, Rapatel C, Berger M, et al. Use of G-CSF alone to mobilize peripheral blood stem cells for collection from children. Br J Haematol. 1994;88:633–5.

Klingebiel T, Handgretinger R, Herter M, et al. Autologous transplantation with peripheral blood stem cells in children and young adults after myeloablative treatment: nonrandomized comparison between GM-CSF and G-CSF for mobilization. J Hematother. 1995;4:307–14.

Kreuzer M, Ahlenstiel T, Kanzelmeyer N, et al. Regional citrate anticoagulation—a safe and effective procedure in pediatric apheresis therapy. Pediatr Nephrol. 2011;26:127–32.

Maitta RW, Vasovic LV, Mohandas K, et al. A safe therapeutic apheresis protocol in paediatric patients weighing 11 to 25 kg. Vox Sang. 2014;107:375–80.

Moon JH, Kim MJ, Song SY. Safety and efficacy of G-CSF mobilization and collection of autologous peripheral blood stem cells in children with cerebral palsy. Transfus Apher Sci. 2013;49:516–21.

Passweg JR, Baldomero H, Peters C. Hematopoietic SCT in Europe: data and trends in 2012 with special consideration of pediatric transplantation. Bone Marrow Transplant. 2014;49:744–50.

Sheldon M. Children as organ donors: a persistent ethical issue. Camb Q Healthc Ethics. 2004;13:119–22.

Styczynski J, Balduzzi A, Gil L, et al. Risk of complications during hematopoietic stem cell collection in pediatric sibling donors: a prospective European Group for Blood and Marrow Transplantation Pediatric Diseases Working Party study. Blood. 2012;119:2935–42.

van Walraven SM, Straathof LM, Switzer GE, et al. Immediate and long-term somatic effects, and health-related quality of life of BM donation during early childhood. A single-center report in 210 pediatric donors. Bone Marrow Transplant. 2013;48:40–5.

Witt V, Beiglbock E, Ritter R, et al. Performance of a new separator system for routine autologous hematopoietic progenitor cell collection in small children. J Clin Apher. 2007;22:306–13.

Witt V, Pichler H, Fritsch G, Peters C. Multiple small versus few large amount aspirations for bone marrow harvesting in autologous and allogeneic bone marrow transplantation. Transfus Apher Sci. 2016;55:221–4.

Witt V, Stegmayr B, Ptak J, et al. World apheresis registry data from 2003 to 2007, the pediatric and adolescent side of the registry. Transfus Apher Sci. 2008;39:255–60.

Zinner S. Cognitive development and pediatric consent to organ donation. Camb Q Healthc Ethics. 2004;13:125–32.

17 Processing, Cryopreserving and Controlling the Quality of HSCs

Patrick Wuchter

17.1 Assessment of HSCs by Measuring CD34 and the Presence of Other Cell Subsets

The efficiency of an autologous, as well as an allogeneic, HSCs graft is mainly determined by the number of $CD34^+$ cells present. The dose of transplanted $CD34^+$ cells per kg body weight (BW) determines the kinetics of the neutrophil and platelet engraftment after auto-HSCT (Weaver et al. 1995). The measurement of $CD34^+$ cells by flow cytometry is, therefore, an important method to assess the graft quantity.

The minimal number of $CD34^+$ cells for an autologous transplant is $\geq 2.0 \times 10^6$ $CD34^+$ cells/kg BW. Transplants below this threshold should only be used in cases where no additional stem cell collection is feasible and there is a vital indication for the autologous stem cell transplantation. Most transplant centres regard a cell dose of $2.5–6 \times 10^6$ $CD34^+$ cells/kg BW as optimal, based on published clinical data (Duong et al. 2014; Perez-Simon et al. 1999; Giralt et al. 2014; Lisenko et al. 2017b; Mohty et al. 2014). For an allo-HSCT, a cell dose of $\geq 4.0 \times 10^6$ $CD34^+$ cells/kg BW is regarded as adequate.

P. Wuchter (✉)
Institute of Transfusion Medicine and Immunology, German Red Cross Blood Service Baden-Württemberg – Hessen, Medical Faculty Mannheim, Heidelberg University, Mannheim, Germany
e-mail: Patrick.Wuchter@medma.uni-heidelberg.de

In the autologous setting, it has been speculated that the quality of $CD34^+$ cells from poor mobilizers may be inferior. However, studies have found that the proportions of primitive and quiescent $CD34^+$ subsets were comparable across mobilization groups (Jiang et al. 2012), and leukocyte and platelet recovery after transplantation was not different (Wuchter et al. 2010).

The application of plerixafor in order to overcome insufficient HSCs mobilization not only increases the number of $CD34^+$ cells but also the proportion of more primitive HSCs subsets, the absolute lymphocyte count and the numbers of lymphocytes in various subsets ($CD19^+$ cells, $CD3^+$ cells, T-cells and NK-cells) in the autograft (Fruehauf et al. 2009; Taubert et al. 2011; Varmavuo et al. 2013). However, these variances do not translate into relevant clinical differences regarding haematopoietic recovery. Taken together, the graft quality from poor mobilizers can be regarded equivalent compared to that from good mobilizers, regardless of the use of plerixafor.

It was further speculated that the composition of cellular subsets in the transplant may have an influence on the haematopoietic reconstitution. However, based on the currently published data, no final conclusion can be drawn, and further investigations are warranted to determine the potential effects of autograft cell subsets on the patients' clinical outcomes. As delineated in an EBMT position statement from 2014, determination of cell subsets other than $CD34^+$ cells is not routinely performed in clinical practice but only

E. Carreras et al. (eds.), *The EBMT Handbook*, https://doi.org/10.1007/978-3-030-02278-5_17

in clinical trials (Mohty et al. 2014). Accordingly, assessment of tumour cell contamination is usually not part of the clinical routine but can be of interest in clinical trials.

17.2 HSCs Cryopreservation

HSCs should be processed and stored in accordance with the respective Medical Council, responsible local and overarching authorities as well as scientific society's guidelines (e.g. EU: Guideline 2004/23/EG and 2006/17/EG, EU-GMP-Guideline).

If necessary, collected cells can be stored for a maximum of up to 72 h at 2–6 °C before cryopreservation. However, cryopreservation within 48 h or less is recommended to maintain an optimal viability of the cells. In the case of storage for >24 h prior to cryopreservation, the maximum nucleated cell (NC) concentration should not exceed 2×10^8/mL.

For cryopreservation, a number of different protocols are used worldwide. Usually, the maximum accepted NC concentration is $\leq 4 \times 10^8$/mL. If necessary, PBSC products can be diluted with autologous plasma or commercial resuspension medium. Increasing the cell concentration by volume depletion minimizes the number of cryostored bags needed, but the upper limit of the NC concentration needs to be considered. The final product includes 5–10% dimethyl sulfoxide (DMSO) as a cryoprotectant and 0.05–0.25 mL of ACD-A stabilizer solution per ml of transplant. Freezing at a controlled rate of 1–2 °C per minute is recommended. Cells need to be stored in vapour phase nitrogen at a temperature of ≤ -140 °C. Cross-contamination while preparing and storing the cells must be prevented by taking appropriate measures.

At the time of auto-HSCT, cryopreserved bags must be thawed at the site of transplantation, and PBSCs should be reinfused within a maximum time span of 10–20 min of thawing using standard transfusion filters in order to minimize the detrimental effect of DMSO upon HSCs. Previous washing for purposes of DMSO depletion is not routinely performed, as the loss and damage of HSCs are regarded as too high.

Several studies demonstrated that under these storage conditions, $CD34^+$ HSCs remained viable for up to 19 years (Fernyhough et al. 2013; McCullough et al. 2010; Spurr et al. 2002). In addition, a recent study demonstrated that the duration of cryostorage of the transplant had no impact on the haematologic reconstitution after transplantation (Lisenko et al. 2017a).

17.3 HSCs Quality Assessment

HSCs product quality assessment needs to be performed at several time points during cell processing and storage. Volume measurement, enumeration of NC and red blood cells and flow cytometry-based $CD34^+$ cell quantification should be performed directly after PBSC collection in accordance with the Stem Cell Enumeration Committee Guidelines of the International Society of Hematotherapy and Graft Engineering (ISHAGE) (Sutherland et al. 1996). A validated protocol and external quality control (e.g. the round robin test) is strongly recommended (Whitby et al. 2012).

Shortly before freezing, microbiological culture samples must be obtained. NC enumeration and NC viability measurement (e.g. by staining with trypan blue, 7-aminoactinomycin D [7-AAD] or propidium iodide) should be performed from aliquots of the final cell product after freezing and thawing. This viability testing is only valid for a defined and limited time span, often 2–5 years based on local guidelines, before it needs to be repeated prior to transplantation. As a result, a sufficient number of reference samples should be prepared for each HSCs product (the recommended minimum number is 3).

Target values need to be defined for the final product, mostly in accordance with local authorities. In most transplant centres in Europe, the following criteria are mandatory (together with additional criteria) for the release of an autologous transplant: NC concentration $\leq 4 \times 10^8$/mL, $CD34^+$ cell number $\geq 2 \times 10^6$/kg BW, red blood concentration ≤ 0.1 mL per mL of transplant, no microbial growth and minimum NC viability of >50% after freezing and thawing.

17.4 Collection of Reference (Retention) Samples for Quality Control

Reference samples for quality control must be taken and stored from the cell product. These samples allow the proof of quality and potency of the transplant in terms of sterility, purity and viability of the cells. In the case of an allo-HSCT, reference samples may also need to be collected from the donor, depending on the respective local legal situation, to allow for a retrospective analysis in terms of serological testing.

Reference samples are prepared in parallel with the cell product and stored under the same cryoconditions until they are analysed. As a release criterion for an autologous stem cell transplant, a reference sample should be cryopreserved for >24 h under the identical conditions as the cell product before the viability of $CD34^+$/$CD45^+$ cells is analysed. Performing a clonogenic assay (e.g. colony-forming assay) from the reference samples can assess the haematopoietic potency of the cells. However, this is not regarded as a release criterion but should be performed for process validation or in the case of prolonged cryostorage of a transplant (>2–5 years).

The final cell product must be labelled in accordance with respective legal requirements. In order to transport cryopreserved HSCs products, a validated shipping container is required, preferably with continuous temperature monitoring. The treating physician is responsible for application of the HSCs transplant after evaluating its integrity and the accompanying documents.

Key Points

- Minimal number of $CD34^+$ cells is $\geq 2.0 \times 10^6$/kg BW for an auto-HSCT and $\geq 4.0 \times 10^6$/kg BW for an Allo-HSCT.
- Determination of cell subsets other than $CD34^+$ is not routinely required.
- Cryopreservation needs to be performed within 72 h, preferably <48 h.
- The maximum NC concentration in the cryostored transplant should be $\leq 4 \times 10^8$/mL.
- The final product includes 5–10% DMSO as a cryoprotectant and 0.05–0.25 mL of ACD-A stabilizer solution per ml of transplant.
- Freezing at a controlled rate of 1–2 °C per minute is recommended, and cells need to be stored in vapour phase nitrogen at a temperature of ≤−140 °C.
- NC viability should be >50% after freezing and thawing.
- At the time of ABSCT, cryopreserved bags must be thawed and reinfused within a maximum of 10–20 min of thawing.
- Reference samples for quality control must be prepared and cryostored in parallel and under identical conditions as the cell product.

References

Duong HK, Savani BN, Copelan E, et al. Peripheral blood progenitor cell mobilization for autologous and allogeneic hematopoietic cell transplantation: guidelines from the American Society for Blood and Marrow Transplantation. Biol Blood Marrow Transplant. 2014;20:1262–73.

Fernyhough LJ, Buchan VA, McArthur LT, Hock BD. Relative recovery of haematopoietic stem cell products after cryogenic storage of up to 19 years. Bone Marrow Transplant. 2013;48:32–5.

Fruehauf S, Veldwijk MR, Seeger T, et al. A combination of granulocyte-colony-stimulating factor (G-CSF) and plerixafor mobilizes more primitive peripheral blood progenitor cells than G-CSF alone: results of a European phase II study. Cytotherapy. 2009;11:992–1001.

Giralt S, Costa L, Schriber J, et al. Optimizing autologous stem cell mobilization strategies to improve patient outcomes: consensus guidelines and recommendations. Biol Blood Marrow Transplant. 2014;20:295–308.

Guidelines 2004/23/EG des Europäischen Parlaments und des Rates vom 31. März 2004 zur Festlegung von Qualitäts- und Sicherheitsstandards für die Spende, Beschaffung, Testung, Verarbeitung, Konservierung, Lagerung und Verteilung von menschlichen Geweben und Zellen. Amtsblatt der Europäischen Union.

Guidelines 2006/17/EG der Kommission vom 8. Februar 2006 zur Durchführung der Richtlinie 2004/23/EG des Europäischen Parlaments und des Rates hinsichtlich technischer Vorschriften für die Spende, Beschaffung und Testung von menschlichen Geweben und Zellen. Amtsblatt der Europäischen Union.

Guidelines EU-Leitfaden der Guten Herstellungspraxis – Humanarzneimittel und Tierarzneimittel (EU-GMP). Europäische Kommission: EudraLex;4.

Jiang L, Malik S, Litzow M, et al. Hematopoietic stem cells from poor and good mobilizers are qualitatively equivalent. Transfusion. 2012;52:542–8.

Lisenko K, Pavel P, Kriegsmann M, et al. Storage duration of autologous stem cell preparations has no impact on hematopoietic recovery after transplantation. Biol Blood Marrow Transplant. 2017a;23:684–90.

Lisenko K, Wuchter P, Hansberg M, et al. Comparison of different stem cell mobilization regimen in AL amyloidosis patients. Biol Blood Marrow Transplant. 2017b;23:1870–8.

McCullough J, Haley R, Clay M, et al. Long-term storage of peripheral blood stem cells frozen and stored with a conventional liquid nitrogen technique compared with cells frozen and stored in a mechanical freezer. Transfusion. 2010;50:808–19.

Mohty M, Hubel K, Kroger N, et al. Autologous haematopoietic stem cell mobilisation in multiple myeloma and lymphoma patients: a position statement from the European Group for Blood and Marrow Transplantation. Bone Marrow Transplant. 2014;49:865–72.

Perez-Simon JA, Martin A, Caballero D, et al. Clinical significance of CD34+ cell dose in long-term engraftment following autologous peripheral blood stem cell transplantation. Bone Marrow Transplant. 1999;24:1279–83.

Spurr EE, Wiggins NE, Marsden KA, et al. Cryopreserved human haematopoietic stem cells retain engraftment potential after extended (5–14 years) cryostorage. Cryobiology. 2002;44:210–7.

Sutherland DR, Anderson L, Keeney M, Nayar R, Chin-Yee I. The ISHAGE guidelines for CD34+ cell determination by flow cytometry. International Society of Hematotherapy and Graft Engineering. J Hematother. 1996;5:213–26.

Taubert I, Saffrich R, Zepeda-Moreno A, et al. Characterization of hematopoietic stem cell subsets from patients with multiple myeloma after mobilization with plerixafor. Cytotherapy. 2011;13:459–66.

Varmavuo V, Mantymaa P, Silvennoinen R, et al. CD34+ cell subclasses and lymphocyte subsets in blood grafts collected after various mobilization methods in myeloma patients. Transfusion. 2013;53:1024–32.

Weaver CH, Hazelton B, Birch R, et al. An analysis of engraftment kinetics as a function of the CD34 content of peripheral blood progenitor cell collections in 692 patients after the administration of myeloablative chemotherapy. Blood. 1995;86:3961–9.

Whitby A, Whitby L, Fletcher M, et al. ISHAGE protocol: are we doing it correctly? Cytometry B Clin Cytom. 2012;82:9–17.

Wuchter P, Ran D, Bruckner T, et al. Poor mobilization of hematopoietic stem cells-definitions, incidence, risk factors, and impact on outcome of autologous transplantation. Biol Blood Marrow Transplant. 2010;16:490–9.

18 Procurement and Management of Cord Blood

Sergio Querol and Vanderson Rocha

18.1 Introduction

Umbilical cord blood (UCB) cells for allogeneic use are collected and frozen in more than 130 public CB banks worldwide. More than seven hundred and fifty thousands CB units (CBU) are available for transplantation. In this chapter we will describe some procedures for cord blood collection, processing, banking and recommendations on how to choose a single or double UCB unit for transplantation (Garcia 2010).

18.2 Collection

Donor recruitment usually starts during the antenatal period, with objective information given by woman's health-care provider. After consent, trained personnel need to determine donor eligibility to ensure that donation is safe for future patients. To assess donor eligibility, a donor medical history interview shall be conducted identifying risk factors for transmissible and genetic disease. In addition, infectious disease markers (IDM) performed to maternal blood samples will be obtained within 7 days before or after the collection of the UCB unit. These samples will be tested for evidence of infection of HIV-1, HIV-2, hepatitis B, hepatitis C, HTLV-I, HTLV-II, syphilis and any additional markers according to local regulations.

Collection must not interfere with normal delivery attention. A successful collection should have a high collection volume and a high total nucleated cell count, be non-contaminated and have the proper documentation. A UCB collection typically involves cord clamping (delayed clamping up to 1–2 min is still compatible with public donations) (Frändberg et al. 2016), disinfection, venipuncturing of umbilical vein and draining by gravity avoiding clotting. Collection bag should be appropriately labelled.

There are two main techniques to collect UCB from the cord vein: before the placenta is delivered (in utero) or after the placenta is delivered (ex utero). Both collection techniques have their own unique advantages and disadvantages, but both techniques require that the individuals performing the collections be adequately trained.

After collection, typically health-care provider will complete a report describing labour and completing variables that could be useful to release the unit like the presence of fever, complications, type of delivery, etc. In case of unexpected adverse reactions during collection they need to be communicated to the competent authority. After collection, it may be required a follow-up of the donor including health questionnaires. Additionally, if

S. Querol (✉)
Banc Sang i Teixits, Barcelona, Spain
e-mail: squerol@bst.cat

V. Rocha
University of São Paulo, São Paulo, Brazil

University of Oxford, Oxford, UK

E. Carreras et al. (eds.), *The EBMT Handbook*, https://doi.org/10.1007/978-3-030-02278-5_18

any abnormal result is detected during testing, a counseling process should be in place.

UCB units shall be transported to the processing facility, and sometimes, these facilities could be far away from the collection sites. A validated procedure for transportation between these two facilities is needed to demonstrate a reliable method. Standard procedures shall be in place to describe time and temperature of storage and transportation methods. All transportation records shall allow tracking back from the collection site to the UCB bank, and any deviation should be recorded.

18.3 Processing and Banking

18.3.1 UCB Cell Processing

Unrelated UCB unit must arrive at the processing laboratory in time to allow initiation of cryopreservation within 48 h of collection (this time is extended to 72 h for related or directed UCB donations). The decision as to whether a collected UCB unit will be acceptable for processing and banking will be made based on the acceptance criteria specified by the UCB bank. Many banks have further refined their acceptance criteria based on economics and the desire to build an international inventory of UCB units with very high TNC or percentage of ethnic minorities. Many UCB banks are now committed to processing and storing only those UCB units with high TNC (e.g. >20 × 10^7 TNC or higher), based on the greater likelihood of these units being used (Saccardi et al. 2016).

Volume reduction of UCB is considered essential to the provision of a high-quality product and cost-effective UCB banking. Reducing the volume of the final product allows for storage efficiency in terms of space and cost and, most importantly, reduces the risk of ABO incompatibility and DMSO toxicity to the potential recipient. Despite some loss of cells, volume reduction has additional practical and clinical benefits; the process yields RBC and plasma components as waste products that can be used for immediate or future testing, thereby minimizing the loss of the actual stem cell product for testing purposes. Different methods for volume reduction are available (Hough et al. 2016).

The selection of a suitable protocol for cryopreservation of UCB for use in transplantation is critical to optimize the recovery of functionally viable progenitor cells, most of which lie within the $CD34^+$ compartment. Some important considerations that are potential sources of cell damage include the type and concentration of cryoprotectant, the cell concentration and the cooling and warming rates. UCB units must be stored in freezing bags designed and approved for the cryopreservation of human cells and placed into metal canisters to afford protection during freezing, storage, transportation and shipping. It is important that after filling, each freezing bag is visually examined for possible leaking and breakage of seals.

UCB units should be cryopreserved using a controlled rate freezer with a validated freezing programme. Liquid nitrogen-based controlled rate freezers have been used to ensure long-term maintenance. Minimizing transient-warming events is very important for that. Stability programmes should be designed in order to establish the expiration time of the UCB stored.

18.3.2 Testing and Quality Assessment

Table 18.1 shows release specification for UCB units. Quality assessment is written below:

Safety It is essential that UCB is screened for those infectious diseases which can be transmitted via blood (as described above). In addition, product should be free of microbial contamination (or with an appropriate antibiogram for related uses). Prior to release for administration, each UCB unit must have undergone hemoglobinopathy screening.

Identity At least, HLA-A, HLA-B, HLA-C and DRB1 loci must be determined using DNA-based methods and result included when listing a UCB unit on the search registries. It is recommended that HLA typing is performed in an accredited laboratory. ABO blood group and Rh type must be reported prior to listing a UCB

Table 18.1 Lists the specification requirements for CBU stored for clinical application, according to the sixth edition NetCord-FACT International Standards for Cord Blood Collection, Banking, and Release for Administration (www.factwebsite.org)

Specification requirements for cord blood units stored for clinical administration				
	Unrelated specification		Related specification	
Test	Fresh post-processing sample	Post-thaw attached segment or representative sample prior to release	Fresh post-processing sample	Post-thaw attached segment or representative sample prior to release
Total nucleated cell count	$\geq 5.0 \times 10^8$		Enumerated	
Total nucleated cell recovery	Should be ≥60%		Should be ≥60%	
Total viability	≥85%		≥70%	
Viable CD34 count	$\geq 1.25 \times 10^6$			
Viability of CD34 cells	≥85%	≥70%	≥85%	≥70%
Viability of CD45 cells		≥40%		≥40%
CFU (or other validated potency assay)[a]		Growth (or positive result for potency)		Growth (or positive result for potency)
Sterility	Negative for aerobes, anaerobes, fungus		Negative for aerobic and anaerobic bacteria and fungi—OR—identify and provide results of antibiotic sensitivities	
Donor screening and testing	Acceptable as defined by Applicable Law and NetCord-FACT standards		Acceptable as defined by Applicable Law and NetCord-FACT standards	
Identity		Verified		Verified

[a]There should be evidence of potency by CFU or other validated potency assay on a fresh post-processing sample

unit for search. Prior to release of a UCB unit for administration, it is imperative that HLA identity is confirmed. Ideally, confirmatory typing will be performed on a sample taken from a contiguous segment. HLA typing on maternal blood may also be performed prior to release of a UCB unit. Haplotype matching between maternal donor and infant donor confirms linkage between the two and serves as a secondary confirmation of identity.

Purity UCB unit specifications report total nucleated cells, total nucleated RBC count and $CD34^+$ cells, and a cell blood count with differential should be performed, with parameters for neutrophils, lymphocytes, monocytes and platelets defined.

Potency Potency testing to determine the growth potential and viability of progenitor cells in a UCB unit should be performed post-processing (prior to cryopreservation), in addition to being performed on a representative thawed sample prior to release for administration.

18.4 Selecting CBU for Transplantation

The success of the UCB transplantation (UCBT) will depend on the characteristics of the CBU. Tables 18.2 and 18.3 list the recommendation of choosing single and double cord blood units, respectively, for transplantation.

Table 18.2 Recommendations for unrelated CBU selection and transplantation[a]

Initial selection of single CBU should be based upon	
(a) HLA matching of the recipient and CBU	
(b) CBU collected cell dose (TNC ± $CD34^+$)	
(c) Patient's diagnosis (malignant versus non-malignant)	
(d) Avoiding CBU containing Ag that match the specificity of any pre-transplant donor-specific anti-HLA Ab in the recipient	
HLA matching	
• *Malignant disorders* (Eapen et al. 2014)	
HLA matching should be based upon allelic typing for HLA-A, HLA-B, HLA-C and HLA-DRB1 for single CBT	
1. Select an HLA-matched (8/8) CBU. TNC dose should be >3 × 10^7/kg	
2. If an HLA-matched (8/8) CBU is unavailable, select a CBU matched at 7/8 HLA loci. HLA-A or HLA-B mismatches are preferable to HLA-DRB1 mismatches. TNC dose should be >5 × 10^7/kg for 5–7/8 matched units	
3. If a CBU matched at 8/8 or 7/8 HLA loci is unavailable, consider a CBU matched at 5 or 6/8 HLA loci. Avoid mismatches in HLA-DRB1	
4. If CBU 4/8 matched, CBU may rarely be considered as a single CB graft if no other option is available. TNC dose should be >5 × 10^7/kg for 4/8 matched units	
5. CBU 3/8 HLA-matched CBU are not recommended	
• *Non-malignant disorders* (Eapen et al. 2017)	
1. CBU with HLA 8/8 or 7/8 give same survival results	
2. CBU with HLA 6/8 and 5/8 give inferior survival rates and are alternative options	
3. We do not recommend selecting cord blood units with more HLA disparities	
TNC and $CD34^+$ cell dose	
• *Malignant disorders*	
Nucleated cell dose[b]	At freezing, minimum TNC dose 3.0 × 10^7/kg, or After thawing, minimum TNC of 2.0–2.5 × 10^7/kg
$CD34^+$ cell dose[c]	At freezing, 1.0–1.7 × 10^5/kg, or After thawing, around 1.0–1.2 × 10^5/kg
• *Non-malignant disorders*[d]	
Nucleated cell dose	At freezing, minimum cell dose 3.5 × 10^7/kg, or After thawing, minimum cell dose 3.0 × 10^7/kg
$CD34^+$ cell dose	At freezing or after thawing, >1.7 × 10^5/kg
Colony-forming unit assay: This assay is important to evaluate the functional capacity of HPCs after thawing an aliquot or after thawing the product; however it is difficult to establish a generalized CFU-GM dose due to variations of colony setup and counting between centres	
Other considerations when selecting single CB units	
If many CBU meeting the criteria above are available, the following factors should also be considered	
• *Use accredited cord blood banks.* For safety, only accredited banks recognized by national and international organizations should be used	
• *ABO compatibility:* ABO compatibility may be associated with improved outcomes, although the data are conflicting	
• *NIMA*: If the cord banks have the mother's HLA typing, the potential effect of NIMA should be noted in context of clinical trials	
• *KIR ligand:* Due to conflicting data, KIR ligand matching should not be used in the selection of CBUs	
• *Sex matching:* Sex matching between CBUs and patients in single or double UCBT is not necessary	

[a]Based on Eurocord and British Society of Blood and Marrow Transplantation recommendations (Hough et al. 2016, modified)

[b]If the infused TNC dose is 1.0–2.0 × 10^7/kg, the number of $CD34^+$ cells or CFU-GM should be taken into consideration to predict the probability of neutrophil recovery and to discuss the possibility of a second transplant. If both cell doses are lower than recommended, a BM aspirate and chimerism analysis should be performed between days +20–28. The absence of engraftment indicates the need for a second transplant; preliminary data shows that haploidentical or double CBT should be considered

[c]Due to variation in counting $CD34^+$ cells, this recommendation should be taken with caution. However, if colonies are not growing, the transplant physicians should consider a second transplant after day +30

[d]For patients with BMF syndromes (aplastic anaemia or congenital bone marrow failure states) or haemoglobinopathies, the number of TNC at freezing should be greater than 5 × 10^7/kg

Table 18.3 Additional criteria for double CBU selection

– When a single CBU unit contains insufficient cells (as specified above), double UCBT is recommended for the treatment of malignant disorders	
– There are currently insufficient data to make recommendations for double UCBT in the treatment of non-malignant disorders	
HLA matching	
• The historical stringency of HLA matching for CBUs with the recipient for double UCBTs should be used, i.e. the minimum acceptable HLA matching between either CBU and the recipient is 4/6 using low/intermediate typing (antigen) for HLA-A and HLA-B and high- resolution typing (allelic) for HLA-DRB1	
• There is no requirement for inter-cord HLA matching	
• The role of high-resolution (allele) typing is not yet defined for double CBT	
Cell dose	
Nucleated cell dose	At freezing, the sum of both CBUs >3.5 × 10^7/kg
	The minimum cell dose of each unit should be >1.5 × 10^7/kg
$CD34^+$ cell dose	At freezing or after thawing, the sum of both CBUs >1.8 × 10^5/kg
ABO matching	
Recently, a retrospective study of Eurocord of almost 1000 double UCBT recipients has shown an important association between ABO compatibility of 2 units with the patient on acute GVHD, NRM and OS. Thus, ABO compatibility between units and patients should be preferred over minor or major compatibility of one of the units between CB and patient (V Rocha on behalf of Eurocord, personal recommendation)	

Key Points

- Cord blood donation comprises the following steps: informative and consent process, revision of eligibility criteria, cord blood collection and finally fresh storage before a standardized transportation to the processing cell lab.
- Cell processing labs require coordination of production and quality control labs to transform the altruistically donated raw material in a medicinal product with predefined specifications that ensure its safety, identity, purity and potency.
- A public cord blood bank is a stem cell registry that provides ready-to-use banked medicinal products for any patient in need through international networking of stem cell donor organizations.
- Cord blood selection is based on sorting CB units using primary criteria (cell content and HLA matching) followed by ranking based in secondary criteria depending on disease status, conditioning, age and recipient's weight.

References

Eapen M, Klein JP, Ruggeri A, Spellman S, Lee SJ, Anasetti C, Arcese W, Barker JN, Baxter-Lowe LA, Brown M, Fernandez-Vina MA, Freeman J, He W, Iori AP, Horowitz MM, Locatelli F, Marino S, Maiers M, Michel G, Sanz GF, Gluckman E, Rocha V, Center for International Blood and Marrow Transplant Research, Netcord, Eurocord, and the European Group for Blood and Marrow Transplantation. Impact of allele-level HLA matching on outcomes after myeloablative single unit umbilical cord blood transplantation for hematologic malignancy. Blood. 2014;123:133–40.

Eapen M, Wang T, Veys PA, Boelens JJ, St Martin A, Spellman S, Bonfim CS, Brady C, Cant AJ, Dalle JH, Davies SM, Freeman J, Hsu KC, Fleischhauer K, Kenzey C, Kurtzberg J, Michel G, Orchard PJ, Paviglianiti A, Rocha V, Veneris MR, Volt F, Wynn R, Lee SJ, Horowitz MM, Gluckman E, Ruggeri A. Allele-level HLA matching for umbilical cord blood transplantation for non-malignant diseases in children: a retrospective analysis. Lancet Haematol. 2017;4:e325–33.

Frändberg S, Waldner B, Konar J, Rydberg L, Fasth A, Holgersson J. High quality cord blood banking is feasible with delayed clamping practices. The eight-year experience and current status of the national Swedish Cord Blood Bank. Cell Tissue Bank. 2016;17(3):439–48.

Garcia J. Allogeneic unrelated cord blood banking worldwide: an update. Swedish bank reference delay clamping. Transfus Apher Sci. 2010;42:257–63.

Hough R, Danby R, Russell N, Marks D, Veys P, Shaw B, Wynn R, Vora A, Mackinnon S, Peggs KS, Crawley C, Craddock C, Pagliuca A, Cook G, Snowden JA, Clark A, Marsh J, Querol S, Parkes G, Braund H, Rocha V. Recommendations for a standard UK approach to incorporating umbilical cord blood into clinical transplantation practice: an update on cord blood unit selection, donor selection algorithms and conditioning protocols. Br J Haematol. 2016;172:360–70.

Saccardi R, Tucunduva L, Ruggeri A, Ionescu I, Koegler G, Querol S, Grazzini G, Lecchi L, Nanni Costa A, Navarrete C, Pouthiers F, Larghero J, Regan D, Freeman T, Bittencourt H, Kenzey C, Labopin M, Baudoux E, Rocha V, Gluckman E. Impact of cord blood banking technologies on clinical outcome: a Eurocord/Cord Blood Committee (CTIWP), European Society for Blood and Marrow Transplantation and NetCord retrospective analysis. Transfusion. 2016;56:2021–9.

19 Graft Manipulation

Michael Schumm, Peter Lang, and Rupert Handgretinger

19.1 Introduction

Graft manipulation is performed to define and to optimize the volume and cellular composition of stem cell sources like apheresis products, bone marrow, or umbilical cord blood.

Basic manipulations comprise centrifugation procedures for depletion of erythrocytes and volume reduction and are required to cryopreserve grafts in the presence of cryoprotectants like DMSO (Dimethylsulfoxide) (Rowley 1992). These are standard procedures for BM and CB, while apheresis products usually can be cryopreserved without further manipulation.

More complex manipulations are used to optimize the cellular composition and to meet requirements of the individual transplant regimen. Selection of CD34+ or AC133+ progenitors from apheresis or BM has been used to produce concentrated stem cell grafts. In recent years, the selective depletion of unwanted cells like CD3+ T cells, TcRαβ+ T cells, and others provides a custom-tailored graft. For both enrichment and depletion, immunomagnetic cell sorting using monoclonal antibodies and paramagnetic microbeads in combination with semi- or fully automated devices has become the standard technique in most laboratories.

M. Schumm · P. Lang · R. Handgretinger (✉)
Department of Hematology/Oncology and General Pediatrics, Children's University Hospital, University of Tuebingen, Tuebingen, Germany
e-mail: rupert.handgretinger@med.uni-tuebingen.de

19.2 Graft Manipulation

19.2.1 Physical Manipulations

19.2.1.1 Volume Reduction

Volume reduction might be necessary in small children and is done by a simple centrifugation process and removal of the supernatant.

19.2.1.2 Washing to Reduce Plasma Antibodies or Anticoagulants

Washing might be necessary in case of unwanted isoagglutinins or to lower the heparin concentration and is also done by centrifugation in a bag or dedicated devices and by exchange of plasma with a suitable solution like 0.9% NaCl. Addition of anticoagulant is not necessary as coagulating agents are washed out by the treatment.

19.2.1.3 Depletion of Erythrocytes

Depletion of erythrocytes is necessary in case of blood group incompatibilities and usually confined to bone marrow. Several procedures

E. Carreras et al. (eds.), *The EBMT Handbook*, https://doi.org/10.1007/978-3-030-02278-5_19

are employed including centrifugation with an apheresis device or centrifugation in bags or tubes and subsequent harvest of the buffy coat. In special cases, a separation using density gradient centrifugation (e.g., Ficoll) might be useful with an even stronger depletion of erythrocytes.

19.2.2 Immunomagnetic Procedures

19.2.2.1 CD34 Enrichment

Enrichment of CD34+ stem cells was the first method which provided grafts with a very low number of T cells and therefore allowed to avoid GvHD highly effective even in haploidentical HSCT (Ringhoffer et al. 2004; Handgretinger et al. 2001).

The method has also been successfully used in MSD and MUD HSCT to minimize the rate of GvHD (Pasquini et al. 2012; Lang et al. 2003) and showed a clear advantage regarding combined cGVHD-free and relapse-free survival compared to unmanipulated grafts in myeloid diseases (Tamari et al. 2018).

Moreover, CD34 selection is used as a graft backbone to which other cell types (unmanipulated DLI, CD45RA depleted DLI, and others) can be added.

Enrichment can be performed with the Miltenyi Biotec CD34 reagent system which uses a mAb for the CD34 class 2 epitope and therefore has to be detected by an Ab to a different epitope (normally class 3). Stem cells after separation normally show a high purity with extremely low amounts of other contaminating cell types. In some cases various amounts of monocytes are found without detrimental effect on the graft. Due to the small size of the graft, absolute numbers of contaminating T cells remain low even if a significant percentage persists. B cells are passively depleted as well, whereas CD34+CD19+ B-cell precursors are retained: 1–3% in PB, up to 30% in BM preparations.

Recovery of CD34+ cells is in the range of 50–90% (Schumm et al. 1999).

19.2.2.2 CD133 Enrichment

CD133 detects a slightly smaller subpopulation of CD34+ cells and can also be used for enrichment of stem cells with similar results (Koehl et al. 2002; Lang et al. 2004).

19.2.2.3 T-Cell Depletion

Immunomagnetic TCD is technically more demanding than CD34+ enrichment as the processed grafts contain a much higher overall number of cells and even extremely low percentages of contaminating T cells can endanger the success of the manipulation. Moreover, the correct enumeration of T cells in a depleted graft is challenging and needs special protocols.

CD3 Depletion

Depletion of CD3+ T cells provides almost untouched grafts with potential antileukemic effectors (e.g., NK cells) enabling fast engraftment and reliable prevention of GvHD. Prospective phase I/II trials showed low TRM rates after haplo-HSCT in combination with toxicity- and intensity-reduced conditioning regimens in children and adults (Lang et al. 2014; Federmann et al. 2012).

Depletion can be done using the CliniMACS LS tubing set or the DTS tubing set. In both cases the depletion efficacy can be 0.5 log lower than in CD34+ selection. Since in haplo-HSCT residual T cells should not exceed 50×10^3/kg, it might be occasionally necessary to perform a CD34+ selection with parts of the apheresis to remain below the requested thresholds and to guarantee a sufficient number of progenitor cells (Lang et al. 2014; Federmann et al. 2012; Huenecke et al. 2016).

It should be ensured that during the incubation process, all cells come into contact with the CD3 reagent to avoid unstained T cells which can impair the result of the depletion significantly. This may happen when transferring stained cells into a second bag system leaving unstained cells in the tubing ends and crinkles of the bag behind. Even smallest amounts of 20–50 μL can contain more T cells than the whole graft should have.

Analysis of CD3 depleted grafts needs special protocols and has to take into account the rare number of T cells among the huge overall number of cells. Therefore, a multigating strategy should be implemented and validated, and T cells should be determined using several parameters. Exclusion of myeloid cells by CD33 could be helpful as well as the use of CD3 in a bright fluorochrome like APC. Gating can be facilitated by using a "spiked" probe with cells of the negative fraction and a small percentage of cells from the positive fraction added to set the gate for subsequent analysis of the negative fraction. For statistical reasons, a minimum of 1×10^6 events should be acquired. To prevent takeover of cells from a previous tube, special care should be taken like flushing the cannula with water before the actual acquisition or to clean the cannula on the outside (Schumm et al. 2013).

TcRαβ Depletion

This procedure removes αβ + T lymphocytes via a biotinylated anti-TcRαβ Ab followed by an anti-biotin Ab conjugated to magnetic microbeads while retaining both γδ + T lymphocytes and natural killer cells in the graft.

Depletion with the TcRab reagent has been shown to be associated with a high depletion efficacy (4.7 log), better than after CD3 depletion (4.0 log) and similar to CD34+ enrichment (4.6 log). Moreover, the results differ less than those after CD3 depletion, resulting in $<50 \times 10^3$/kg infused residual TCRαβ+ T cells, even in small children (Schumm et al. 2013).

Compared to CD34 selected grafts, a faster expansion was seen for CD3+ and for CD56+ in the early phase after haplo-HSCT, probably caused by expansion of co-transfused γδ T cells and NK cells (Lang et al. 2015). Moreover, clinical trials in children and adults demonstrated a very low incidence of acute and chronic GvHD as well as favorable engraftment and TRM rates (Locatelli et al. 2017; Kaynar et al. 2017). The method was successfully used to avoid GvHD also in MUD HSCT (Maschan et al. 2016).

Detection of TcRαβ+ T cells should be done with the same precaution used for CD3 depleted cells, with a minimum of 1×10^6 events and several parameters for the identification of the TcRαβ+ cells. Pregating on CD3-PE vs 7-AAD has been shown to be very helpful as well as gating on TcRαβ and TcRγδ cells in the consecutive dot plot (Schumm et al. 2013).

CD19 Depletion

Depletion of CD19+ B cells can be done together with CD3 or TcRαβ depletion and prevents effectively the occurrence of EBV-associated PTLD. Although the threshold dose of contaminating B cells is still not defined, no cases of PTLD were observed in two multicenter trials with 104 children and adults after infusion of median numbers of 28 and 7×10^3 CD20+ cells/kg BW, respectively (Lang et al. 2014; Federmann et al. 2012).

Alternatively, B-cell depletion can be done in vivo by infusion of therapeutic anti-CD20 mAbs (Locatelli et al. 2017).

Detection of CD19+ B cells needs special attention as the binding of fluorescence-labeled antibody is impaired when cells were preincubated with the CD19 reagent. Therefore, the detection has to be done with an antibody for CD20 which is co-expressed on B cells (Schumm et al. 2006).

Stem Cell Boosts

Poor graft function after HSCT is a relevant complication and is defined as at least bilinear severe cytopenia and/or transfusion requirement, which occurs in a situation of full donor chimerism.

Administration of stem cell boosts from the original donor offers a therapeutic option (Remberger et al. 1998).

To reduce the risk of GvHD, ex vivo TCD procedures as mentioned above are recommended (Olsson et al. 2013). Most experience exists with CD34 selected boosts. Response rates of 80% and a low risk of de novo GvHD between 6% and 22% were observed, even in the case of mismatched donors (Askaa et al. 2014; Mainardi et al. 2018).

19.2.3 DLI and T Cells

T cells may be added to a graft or administered post transplant to provide T cell immunity in various situations. The tolerable dose of T cells varies strongly depending on the HLA disparity, the T cell chimerism in the patient, and the time after transplantation. In MUD HSCT or in haploidentical HSCT, it can be helpful to cryopreserve a number of vials with a defined number of T cells (i.e., 100×10^3 CD3+/kg and 25×10^3 CD3+/kg, respectively) for easy access in case of increasing recipient chimerism.

19.2.3.1 CD45RA Depletion

DLI with CD45RA+-depleted T cells takes advantage of the CD45R0+ T cells which obviously exert little graft-versus-host reaction but can provide antileukemic and antiviral activity. Depletion can be done using the same equipment and reagents for depletion. Depletion is highly effective, and contaminating CD45RA+ cells cannot be found at all (Teschner et al. 2014).

19.2.3.2 DLI in Relapse

DLI has been first used in CML patients after relapse and was given as unmanipulated non-mobilized apheresis in the HLA-matched setting.

19.2.3.3 DLI in Mixed Chimerism

Repetitive DLI can be used to revert a mixed T cell chimerism. Depending on the type of the donor, various cell numbers are employed. In MSD or MUD HSCT, doses between 1×10^5 and 1×10^6/kg are usual, whereas after mismatched or haploidentical HSCT, starting doses of 25×10^3 CD3/kg are recommended (Haines et al. 2015) (and own experience).

19.2.3.4 Virus-Specific T Cells

Virus-specific T cells can be enriched from peripheral blood or an unstimulated apheresis of the original (seropositive) stem cell donor or—if not possible—alternatively from a partially matched third-party donor.

Donor-derived-specific T cells against ADV-, CMV-, or EBV-associated antigens have been already used in many patients suffering from life-threatening infections post transplant, and clinical or virological response rates between 70% and 86% were observed (Icheva et al. 2013; Feucht et al. 2015; Feuchtinger et al. 2010).

The most common technique in the field of graft manipulation is the cytokine capture system which employs the secretion of IFNg after stimulation with appropriate Ag or peptide mixtures for immunomagnetic selection of specific T cells. Simultaneous stimulation with several Ag is possible and generates multispecific T cells.

The selection procedure can be done with a CliniMACS Prodigy® from a maximum of 1×10^9 cells from a non-mobilized or a mobilized apheresis and yields 6–7 ml of cells, with $0.1–2 \times 10^6$ CD3+IFNg+ target cells.

Accompanying debris and dead cells require an accurate analysis. Moreover, the small amount of target cells limits the sample size available for analysis, and therefore a single platform procedure including cell count and viability in one measurement is recommended. The first step should be done without washing and includes a cell gate to exclude debris. CD45 and 7-AAD can be used for proper determination of cell viability. A second sample can be analyzed after washing for CD3+, CD4+, and CD8+ numbers and the percentage of IFNg+ cells in these subsets. Bystander cells like B cells, monocytes, and granulocytes can be found in low numbers (Feuchtinger et al. 2006).

19.3 Regulatory Issues

Graft manipulation is regarded as drug manufacturing in most countries and has to follow the requirements of the EU GMP guidelines, the European Pharmacopoeia, and several EU directives. Therefore clean room areas are required for the manufacturing and a manufacturing license, and a marketing authorization is mandatory for distribution of the product. A quality assurance system has to be implemented, and specifications have to be in place for both raw material and drug product. In most cases, volume, cell number, cell dose, viability, and composition are minimum parameters. Sterility in the form of microbiological examination of cell-based preparations according to Pharm. Eu. 2.6.27 has to be shown either before release of the product or, in the case of limited stability, after release.

Peripheral blood stem cells from both blood and bone marrow for hematopoietic reconstitution are regarded as non-ATMP.

Key Points

- CD34 enrichment yields stem cell preparations with low contaminating T and B cells
- CD3/CD19 depletion preserves large numbers of NK cells in the grafts
- TcR αβ/CD19 depletion provides large numbers of NK cells and γδ T cells with very low amounts of TcRαβ T cells
- DLI with CD45RA-depleted T cells might reduce the risk of GvHD
- Virus antigen-specific donor- or third-party-derived T cells can be utilized post transplant in patients with therapy-refractory viral infections

References

Askaa B, Fischer-Nielsen A, et al. Treatment of poor graft function after allogeneic hematopoietic cell transplantation with a booster of CD34-selected cells infused without conditioning. Bone Marrow Transplant. 2014;49:720–1.

Federmann B, Bornhauser M, Meisner C, et al. Haploidentical allogeneic hematopoietic cell transplantation in adults using CD3/CD19 depletion and reduced intensity conditioning: a phase II study. Haematologica. 2012;97:1523–31.

Feucht J, Opherk K, Lang P, et al. Adoptive T-cell therapy with hexon-specific Th1 cells as a treatment of refractory adenovirus infection after HSCT. Blood. 2015;125:1986–94.

Feuchtinger T, Matthes-Martin S, Richard C, et al. Safe adoptive transfer of virus-specific T-cell immunity for the treatment of systemic adenovirus infection after allogeneic stem cell transplantation. Br J Haematol. 2006;134:64–76.

Feuchtinger T, Opherk K, Bethge WA, et al. Adoptive transfer of pp65-specific T cells for the treatment of chemorefractory cytomegalovirus disease or reactivation after haploidentical and matched unrelated stem cell transplantation. Blood. 2010;116:4360–7.

Haines HL, Bleesing JJ, Davies SM, et al. Outcomes of donor lymphocyte infusion for treatment of mixed donor chimerism after a reduced-intensity preparative regimen for pediatric patients with nonmalignant diseases. Biol Blood Marrow Transplant. 2015;21:288–92.

Handgretinger R, Klingebiel T, Lang P, et al. Megadose transplantation of purified peripheral blood CD34(+) progenitor cells from HLA-mismatched parental donors in children. Bone Marrow Transplant. 2001;27:777–83.

Huenecke S, Bremm M, Cappel C, et al. Optimization of individualized graft composition: CD3/CD19 depletion combined with CD34 selection for haploidentical transplantation. Transfusion. 2016;56:2336–45.

Icheva V, Kayser S, Wolff D, et al. Adoptive transfer of Epstein-Barr virus (EBV) nuclear antigen 1-specific t cells as treatment for EBV reactivation and lymphoproliferative disorders after allogeneic stem-cell transplantation. J Clin Oncol. 2013;31:39–48.

Kaynar L, Demir K, Turak EE, et al. TcRalphabeta-depleted haploidentical transplantation results in adult acute leukemia patients. Hematology. 2017;22:136–44.

Koehl U, Zimmermann S, Esser R, et al. Autologous transplantation of CD133 selected hematopoietic progenitor cells in a pediatric patient with relapsed leukemia. Bone Marrow Transplant. 2002;29:927–30.

Lang P, Bader P, Schumm M, et al. Transplantation of a combination of CD133+ and CD34+ selected progenitor cells from alternative donors. Br J Haematol. 2004;124:72–9.

Lang P, Feuchtinger T, Teltschik HM, et al. Improved immune recovery after transplantation of TCRalphabeta/CD19-depleted allografts from haploidentical donors in pediatric patients. Bone Marrow Transplant. 2015;50(Suppl 2):S6–10.

Lang P, Handgretinger R, Niethammer D, et al. Transplantation of highly purified CD34+ progenitor cells from unrelated donors in pediatric leukemia. Blood. 2003;101:1630–6.

Lang P, Teltschik HM, Feuchtinger T, et al. Transplantation of CD3/CD19 depleted allografts from haploidentical family donors in paediatric leukaemia. Br J Haematol. 2014;165:688–98.

Locatelli F, Merli P, Pagliara D, et al. Outcome of children with acute leukemia given HLA-haploidentical HSCT after alphabeta T-cell and B-cell depletion. Blood. 2017;130:677–85.

Mainardi C, Ebinger M, Enkel S, et al. CD34(+) selected stem cell boosts can improve poor graft function after paediatric allogeneic stem cell transplantation. Br J Haematol. 2018;180:90–9.

Maschan M, Shelikhova L, Ilushina M, et al. TCR-alpha/beta and CD19 depletion and treosulfan-based conditioning regimen in unrelated and haploidentical transplantation in children with acute myeloid leukemia. Bone Marrow Transplant. 2016;51:668–74.

Olsson R, Remberger M, Schaffer M, et al. Graft failure in the modern era of allogeneic hematopoietic SCT. Bone Marrow Transplant. 2013;48:537–43.

Pasquini MC, Devine S, Mendizabal A, et al. Comparative outcomes of donor graft CD34+ selection and immune suppressive therapy as graft-versus-host disease prophylaxis for patients with acute myeloid leukemia in complete remission undergoing HLA-matched sibling allogeneic hematopoietic cell transplantation. J Clin Oncol. 2012;30:3194–201.

Remberger M, Ringden O, Ljungman P, et al. Booster marrow or blood cells for graft failure after allogeneic bone marrow transplantation. Bone Marrow Transplant. 1998;22:73–8.

Ringhoffer M, Wiesneth M, Harsdorf S, et al. CD34 cell selection of peripheral blood progenitor cells using the CliniMACS device for allogeneic transplantation: clinical results in 102 patients. Br J Haematol. 2004;126:527–35.

Rowley SD. Hematopoietic stem cell cryopreservation: a review of current techniques. J Hematother. 1992;1:233–50.

Schumm M, Handgretinger R, Pfeiffer M, et al. Determination of residual T- and B-cell content after immunomagnetic depletion: proposal for flow cytometric analysis and results from 103 separations. Cytotherapy. 2006;8:465–72.

Schumm M, Lang P, Bethge W, et al. Depletion of T-cell receptor alpha/beta and CD19 positive cells from apheresis products with the CliniMACS device. Cytotherapy. 2013;15:1253–8.

Schumm M, Lang P, Taylor G, et al. Isolation of highly purified autologous and allogeneic peripheral CD34+ cells using the CliniMACS device. J Hematother. 1999;8:209–18.

Tamari R, Oran B, Hilden P, et al. Allogeneic stem cell transplantation for advanced myelodysplastic syndrome: comparison of outcomes between CD34(+) selected and unmodified hematopoietic stem cell transplantation. Biol Blood Marrow Transplant. 2018;24:1079–87.

Teschner D, Distler E, Wehler D, et al. Depletion of naive T cells using clinical grade magnetic CD45RA beads: a new approach for GVHD prophylaxis. Bone Marrow Transplant. 2014;49:138–44.

20 Documentation of Engraftment and Chimerism After HSCT

Peter Bader

20.1 Introduction

It is of central interest to document that the newly developing hematopoiesis post-transplant is of donor or recipient origin. The investigations of the genotype origin of post-transplant hematopoiesis are called chimerism analysis. The term "chimerism" was first introduced into medicine in 1951. Andresen wrote that an organism with cells from two or more distinct zygote lineages is a "chimera." Since 1956 this term was used in field of transplantation (Ford et al. 1956). Chimera refers itself to the Greek mythology where Homer described a fire-spitting monster with the head of a lion, a tail of a serpent, and the body of a goat terrorizing Lycia, a region in Minor Asia.

For a long time, it was believed that complete donor hematopoiesis is necessary to maintain engraftment after allo-HSCT. A few decades ago, it became apparent that donor and recipient hematopoiesis may coexist. This state of coexistence of hematopoietic cells is called mixed chimerism (MC). If all cells are of donor origin, the patient is referred to as "complete chimera," and he shows a "complete chimerism."

P. Bader (✉)
Division for Stem Cell Transplantation and Immunology, University Hospital for Children and Adolescents, Goethe University Frankfurt am Main, Frankfurt, Germany
e-mail: peter.bader@kgu.de

It is important to note that the state of hematopoietic chimerism may underlay a certain dynamic. Patients with a complete chimerism may develop a "mixed chimerism" at a later time point or vice versa. In the later patients, the amount of autologous cells may "increase" or "decrease." The patients then develop an "increasing mixed chimerism" or a decreasing mixed chimerism. To avoid misunderstandings as to whether donor or recipient hematopoiesis changes, it is recommended to report "increasing mixed donor chimerism" or "increasing mixed recipient chimerism."

Nowadays, it has become possible to analyze hematopoietic chimerism also in single cell subpopulations. If a patient's hematopoiesis is mixed only in different cell lines, these patients are referred to have a "split chimerism." Finally the applied method for chimerism analysis has also an impact on the degree of chimerism. A patient could be complete chimera with a method detecting about 1% autologous cells, whereas recipient cells could have been detected with a more sensitive technique (Bader et al. 2005).

20.2 Methods for Chimerism Analysis

Different methods have been developed for the assessment of hematopoietic chimerism. All these methods followed the same principle using

E. Carreras et al. (eds.), *The EBMT Handbook*, https://doi.org/10.1007/978-3-030-02278-5_20

differences in polymorphic genetic markers and their products. Historically restriction fragment length polymorphism (RFLP), cytogenetics, red cell phenotyping, and fluorescence in situ hybridization techniques were used for the assessment of hematopoietic chimerism. All of these techniques have been very time-consuming and did not always offer the possibility to be used in every patient-donor constellation.

Widespread and timely clinical applicability has become possible after polymerase-chain-reaction (PCR) techniques were developed. During the 1990s, these analyses were mainly performed by amplification of variable number of tandem repeats (VNTR). Later in the decade short tandem repeats (STR) were used. Fluorescent labeling of the primers and resolution of PCR products with capillary electrophoresis allowed immediate and accurate quantification of the degree of chimerism. Semiautomated PCR analysis using the appropriate hardware allowed moreover high sample throughput. This made it possible to study chimerism in all patients and in short time intervals already early after transplantation. Accurate monitoring of engraftment as well as surveillance of impending graft rejection in patients transplanted for nonmalignant disease has become possible (McCann and Lawler 1993; Alizadeh et al. 2002; Thiede et al. 2001).

Recently, real-time PCR (rPCR) approaches using single nucleotide polymorphism (SNP) have also become available for the detection of chimerism. SNPs are biallelic variants that differ from each other only at a single nucleotide and occur on average every 1.3 kb in the human genome. This rPCR has an even higher sensitivity compared to STR-PCR assays, but their quantitative accuracy with a variation coefficient of only 30–50% is lower compared to 1–5% of the STR systems.

The latest developments for the detection of chimerism are the analysis using digital PCR (dPCR) procedures. This technology allows accurate and absolute quantification of DNA. This dPCR system is based on deletion/insertion polymorphism (DIP/INDEL) analysis. Clinical studies using this technique, however, are not yet performed (Jacque et al. 2015; Clark et al. 2015).

Based on these issues, the STR-PCR with fluorescent-labeled primers and resolution of the fragments with capillary electrophoresis is currently still considered to be the gold standard for the assessment of post-transplant chimerism. It is important to stress that whatever method is employed to study chimerism, it is important that the procedure is standardized and the chimerism laboratory is accredited and is participating in quality control rounds (Lion et al. 2012).

20.3 Chimerism Investigation in the Clinical Setting

20.3.1 Chimerism in Nonmalignant Diseases

Allo-HSCT is the only curative treatment option for many patients with inherited or acquired nonmalignant diseases such as immunodeficiency, storage diseases, osteopetrosis, thalassemia, sickle cell disease, severe aplastic anemia, bone marrow failure syndromes, and many others.

The aim of the transplant procedure in these diseases is to achieve stable and durable engraftment to (1) improve the hematopoietic function, to (2) correct the immune competence, and/or to (3) increase or normalize the respective enzyme shortage. As a consequence, it is not always necessary to replace the recipient hematopoiesis completely. For many diseases, it is sufficient to implement a state of mixed hematopoietic chimerism to improve the patients' well-being. To minimize toxic side effects intensity of conditioning regimens in these diseases is often reduced and therefore less myeloablative. MC is more likely, and graft rejection or non-engraftment remained the major causes of treatment failures in these patients (Bader et al. 2005; Thiede et al. 2001).

It could be shown that rapid donor cell presence and maintenance of early complete donor chimerism in NK and T cells may play an important role in achieving sustained engraftment especially in patients who were treated with reduced intensity conditioning regimens. Analysis of chimerism in disease characterizing cell subpopulations in patients with nonmalignant disease, e.g., in patients with severe combined immune deficiencies (SCID) or in patients with storages disease, enables the documentation of success of the transplant procedures (Preuner et al. 2016).

20.3.1.1 Intervention to Influence the Evolution of Chimerism: Transfusion of DLI

In patients with nonmalignant diseases, MC occurs frequently. The question whether individual patients with MC are at risk to reject their graft depends on the diagnosis and on the conditioning regimens. Studies have clearly shown that MC can be influenced by DLI. MC can be stabilized or even converted to complete donor chimerism by DLI. However, in treating patients with MC and DLI, physicians have to bear in mind the potential risk to induce GVHD which should be avoided in patients with nonmalignant disease with all efforts.

Hemoglobinopathies

In *thalassemia patients*, large studies have been published already from the Pesaro group of Guido Lucarelli, evaluating the influence of MC and disease recurrence. In general it was found that patients whose recipient MC increased to >30% autologous cells were by far more likely to ultimately reject and be transfusion dependent. However, there are patients with persisting high level MC who remained transfusion independent. Retrospective studies have been performed evaluating the possibility of influencing MC by DLI. It could be shown that a state of MC may be sufficient to remain transfusion independent. It was also shown that DLI is capable to convert MC to CC. However, no general recommendation could be given at the time being (Fitzhugh et al. 2014; Karasu et al. 2012; Abraham et al. 2017).

In *sickle cell disease (SCD)*, the impact of MC has been studied intensively as more and more patients with SCD were transplanted from matched but also from mismatched donors. In the late 1990s, first studies concluded that 10% of donor cell engraftment and persistence were needed for effective treatment of SCD in patients who were treated with a homozygous healthy donor; however, if the patient was grafted with the stem cells of a heterozygous HbAS donor, 30–40% donor cells are required. The presence of MC in patients transplanted for sickle cell disease does not warrant DLI per se. In patients with less than 30% of donor chimerism, DLI might be considered. In a most recent study, Fitzhugh and colleagues developed a mathematical model by which they could show that a donor chimerism in the myeloid compartment of 20% is necessary to reverse the sickle cell phenotype and to prevent patients from disease recurrence (Fitzhugh et al. 2017).

20.3.2 Chimerism in Malignant Diseases

Chimerism detected by molecular methods allows the assessment of persisting or reappearing recipient cells after allo-HSCT. These cells might be a reflection of either survival of malignant cells or of survival or recurrence of recipient hematopoietic cells or a combination of both. It could be shown by prospective studies already in the early 1990s that a MC frequently occurs in the mononuclear cell fraction, weakens thereby the GvL effect, and facilitates recurrence of the underlying leukemia.

Chimerism analysis does provide information about the alloreactivity and/tolerance induction of the graft and thereby serves more likely a "prognostic factor" than as an indirect marker for MRD. It has become evident that the development of post-transplant chimerism is a dynamic process. Hence, if chimerism analyses are performed in the intention to detect impending relapse, investigations need to be performed in short time intervals (Bader et al. 2004b; Thiede et al. 2001; Kröger et al. 2010a, b).

Initially, many pediatric studies using serial analysis of chimerism could clearly demonstrate that patients who develop a MC Post transplant have an increased risk for future relapse of their leukemia. This could later also be confirmed by studies in adult patients.

Moreover these and subsequent studies undoubtedly showed that by immunotherapeutic interventions, e.g., withdrawal of IS or transfusion of DLI, MC could be converted to complete chimerism, GvL effect restored, and many patients prevented from developing overt hematological relapse (Platzbecker et al. 2012; Bader et al. 2004a).

Based on its limited sensitivity to detect minor cell population of about 1%, chimerism analysis in the whole blood is not suitable to serve as a MRD marker. For the assessment of MRD, other techniques should be used, if possible. In patients and diseases lacking a disease-specific marker, for example, regularly in patients with MDS and often in patients with AML, chimerism analysis could be performed in cell subpopulations. Thiede et al. could clearly demonstrate that by the characterization of chimerism in the CD34-positive cell fraction, leukemia relapse could be anticipated in advance in many patients with AML and MDS. In ALL patients, several studies have been performed investigating the impact of MC after enrichment of entity specific subpopulation, e.g., CD 10, CD19, and CD 34 for precursor B ALL and CD3, CD4, CD5, and CD8 for T-lineages. Remarkable correlation between MRD and chimerism in different subsets could be proven (Platzbecker et al. 2012; Bornhäuser et al. 2009; Rettinger et al. 2011).

Serial and quantitative analysis of chimerism allows the identification of patients at highest risk for relapse. Not all patients can be identified, and time interval between the onset of MS and relapse is often short. It is essential to perform the analysis frequently and ideally: chimerism should be combined with MRD analysis to optimize the predictive value. These investigations can form the basis for individual preemptive immunotherapy strategies to prevent recurrence of the underlying disease.

Key Points

- Documentation of engraftment is the important step on the way to successful HSCT
- Post-transplant patients are carrying two different genetic profiles and are called chimera
- Analysis of hematopoietic chimerism offers the possibility to realize impending graft rejection and may also serve as an indicator for the recurrence of the underlying disease
- Since several years, these investigations have become the basis for intervention strategies to:
  - Avoid graft rejection
  - Maintain engraftment
  - To treat imminent relapse by preemptive immunotherapy

References

Abraham A, Hsieh M, Eapen M, et al. Relationship between mixed donor-recipient chimerism and disease recurrence after hematopoietic cell transplantation for sickle cell disease. Biol Blood Marrow Transplant. 2017;23:2178–83.

Alizadeh M, Bernard M, Danic B, et al. Quantitative assessment of hematopoietic chimerism after bone marrow transplantation by real-time quantitative polymerase chain reaction. Blood. 2002;99:4618–25.

Bader P, Kreyenberg H, Hoelle W, et al. Increasing mixed chimerism is an important prognostic factor for unfavorable outcome in children with acute lymphoblastic leukemia after allogeneic stem-cell transplantation: possible role for immuno-therapy. J Clin Oncol. 2004a;22:1696–705.

Bader P, Kreyenberg H, Hoelle W, et al. Increasing mixed chimerism defines a high-risk group of childhood acute myelogenous leukemia patients after allogeneic stem cell transplantation where pre-emptive immunotherapy may be effective. Bone Marrow Transplant. 2004b;33:815–21.

Bader P, Niethammer D, Willasch A, et al. How and when should we monitor chimerism after allogeneic stem cell transplantation? Bone Marrow Transplant. 2005;35:107–19.

Bornhäuser M, Oelschlaegel U, Platzbecker U, et al. Monitoring of donor chimerism in sorted CD34+ peripheral blood cells allows the sensitive detection of imminent relapse after allogeneic stem cell transplantation. Haematologica. 2009;94:1613–7.

Clark JR, Scott SD, Jack AL, et al. Monitoring of chimerism following allogeneic haematopoietic stem cell transplantation (HSCT). Br J Haematol. 2015;168:26–37.

Fitzhugh CD, Abraham A, Hsieh MM. Alternative donor/unrelated donor transplants for the β-thalassemia and sickle cell disease. Adv Exp Med Biol. 2017;1013:123–53.

Fitzhugh CD, Abraham AA, Tisdale JF, et al. Hematopoietic stem cell transplantation for patients with sickle cell disease. Hematol Oncol Clin North Am. 2014;28:1171–85.

Ford CE, Hamerton JL, Barnes DW, et al. Cytological identification of radiation-chimaeras. Nature. 1956;177:452–4.

Jacque N, Nguyen S, Golmard J-L, et al. Chimerism analysis in peripheral blood using indel quantitative real-time PCR is a useful tool to predict post-transplant relapse in acute leukemia. Bone Marrow Transplant. 2015;50:259–65.

Karasu GT, Yesilipek MA, Karauzum SB, et al. The value of donor lymphocyte infusions in thalassemia patients at imminent risk of graft rejection following stem cell transplantation. Pediatr Blood Cancer. 2012;58:453–8.

Kröger N, Bacher U, Bader P, et al. NCI first international workshop on the biology, prevention, and treatment of relapse after allogeneic hematopoietic stem cell transplantation. Biol Blood Marrow Transplant. 2010a;16:1325–46.

Kröger N, Bacher U, Bader P, et al. NCI first international workshop on the biology, prevention, and treatment of relapse after allogeneic hematopoietic stem cell transplantation. Biol Blood Marrow Transplant. 2010b;16:1187–211.

Lion T, Watzinger F, Preuner S, et al. The EuroChimerism concept for a standardized approach to chimerism analysis after allogeneic stem cell transplantation. Leukemia. 2012;26:1821–8.

McCann SR, Lawler M. Mixed chimaerism; detection and significance following BMT. Bone Marrow Transplant. 1993;11:91–4.

Platzbecker U, Wermke M, Radke J, et al. Azacitidine for treatment of imminent relapse in MDS or AML patients after allogeneic HSCT. Leukemia. 2012;26:381–9.

Preuner S, Peters C, Pötschger U, et al. Risk assessment of relapse by lineage-specific monitoring of chimerism in children undergoing allogeneic stem cell transplantation for acute lymphoblastic leukemia. Haematologica. 2016;101:741–6.

Rettinger E, Willasch AM, Kreyenberg H, et al. Preemptive immunotherapy in childhood acute myeloid leukemia for patients showing evidence of mixed chimerism after allogeneic stem cell transplantation. Blood. 2011;118:5681–8.

Thiede C, Bornhäuser M, Oelschlägel U, et al. Sequential monitoring of chimerism and detection of minimal residual disease after allogeneic blood stem cell transplantation (BSCT) using multiplex PCR amplification of short tandem repeat-markers. Leukemia. 2001;15:293–302.

21 Short- and Long-Term Controls After HSCT

Montserrat Rovira and Maria Suárez-Lledó

21.1 Introduction

Patients undergoing HSCT (mainly allo-HSCT) have a risk of developing complications related to pre-, peri-, and post-HSCT. The resulting morbidity of the HSCT process makes it necessary for patients to adopt a healthy lifestyle that promotes health and contemplate preventive measures for the detection and treatment of possible complications.

The short- and long-term controls allow for regular and systematic screening and at the same time are an opportunity to give advice on healthy lifestyle habits. Monitoring should be multidisciplinary with involvement of hematology, other medical specialties, physicians of primary care, nursing, and mental health professionals.

Early and late complications, as well as psychological problems, are discussed in Parts IV, V and VI of the Handbook.

After discharge, it is important that the patient has a summary of the treatment received and a long-term follow-up plan appropriate to the exposure and individual risk factors.

The recommendations related to screening and prevention post-HSCT can be consulted in several web pages (see references).

M. Rovira (✉) · M. Suárez-Lledó
HSCT Unit, Hematology Department, Hospital Clínic de Barcelona, University of Barcelona, Barcelona, Catalunya, Spain
e-mail: mrovira@clinic.cat

E. Carreras et al. (eds.), *The EBMT Handbook*, https://doi.org/10.1007/978-3-030-02278-5_21

21.2 Monitoring Depending on the Type of HSCT

21.2.1 Autologous HSCT

Timing	Monitoring
From discharge to day +100	Until full hematologic recovery, it is recommended to live near the hospital Recommended controls[a]: – Clinical evaluation and transfusions when necessary – Basic hematological and biochemical tests – Specific markers for different diseases
At +3 months	Evaluate the status of the primary disease Recommended controls[a]: – Hematological and biochemical tests, specific tumoral markers – MRD evaluation: Immunophenotype and molecular specific adapted to each disease – BM biopsy in case of NHL, HL, MPS, and solid neoplasms with previous marrow affectation, in the remaining disease BM smears (see specific chapters) – Imaging tests depending on primary disease
Long term	Visits every 6 months up to 2 years and then annually Recommended controls[a]: – Analytical and complementary explorations: See Table 21.1 – Baseline disease: Control of possible progression or relapse during at least 5 years – In patients treated with chemotherapy + radiotherapy, assess the risk of second malignancies or MDS after HSCT

[a]Variable frequency depending on the patient's condition

21.2.2 Allogeneic HSCT

Timing	Monitoring
From discharge to day +100	It is recommended that the patient resides near the transplant center during the first 3–6 months after HSCT Recommended controls[a]: – Weekly clinical evaluation, during the first month, every other week until 2 m, and then monthly up to 6–12 m, unless problems arise. It must include complete physical examination, with special emphasis on data of acute GvHD, infections, and pulmonary complications – Blood samples: Complete blood count, liver and kidney function, Mg, levels of IS agents, quantify CMV by PCR (and EBV if ATG); chimerism evaluation at 1 month – BM aspirate (or biopsy) in diseases with previous marrow affectation (usually within 1 month of HSCT)
At 3 months	Usually, this moment marks the turning point so that, if the patient does not have major problems, he/she can be monitored by the referring doctor. However, the patient should be periodically reevaluated at the transplant center (every 3–4 months during the first year, every 4–6 months during the second year, and annually after the third year) Recommended controls[a]: – Visit and complete physical exploration with special emphasis on the signs of acute and chronic GvHD (assessment by organs as indicated in Chaps. 43 and 44 and paragraph 21.3) – Blood test: Complete blood count, kidney function, liver function, clearance creatinine, IS levels; chimerism and sample for MRD follow-up. In patients aged <17 years, weight and height every 3 months
Long term	It depends on the complications that arise during follow-up. If there are no complications, it is recommended that a patient visits to the center every 6 months up to 3 years and annually thereafter Recommended controls: – Visit and complete physical examination including gynecological evaluation and endocrinological, if appropriate – Analytical and complementary explorations: See Sect. 21.3 – Specific controls: Specific MRD studies on diseases with markers (see corresponding chapters) – In patients treated with chemotherapy + radiotherapy, the risk of secondary neoplasms

[a]Variable frequency depending on the patient's condition

21.3 Organ-Specific Long-Term Monitoring

Table 21.1 analyzes organ by organ the long-term follow-up recommendations.

Table 21.1 Organ-specific monitoring[a]

Recommended screening[b]	6 months	1 year	An.	Comments
Ocular (see Chap. 48)				
– Clinical symptom evaluation	1	1	1	– Immediate exam if visual symptoms
– Visual acuity and fundus exam	+	1	+	– Special attention to *sicca* syndrome
Oral (Chap. 50)				
– Preventive oral health and dental maintenance	1	1	1	– Avoid smoking, sugar beverages, or oral piercing
– Clinical assessment	1	1	1	– If oral cGvHD, high-risk squamous cell cancer; evaluation every 6 months
– Dental assessment (+children)	+	1	1	
Respiratory (Chap. 52)				
– Clinical pulmonary assessment	1	1	1	* Active or passive
– Smoking tobacco avoidance*	1	1	1	– If cGVHD, spirometry test in each control (recommended for many authors)
– PFT (+chest Rx if symptoms)	+	+	+	
Cardiac and vascular[c] (Chap. 55)				
– CV risk factor assessment	+	1	1	– Counseling on heart healthy lifestyle – Active treatment of risk factors
Liver (Chaps. 38 and 49)				
– Liver function testing	1	1	1	– Monitor viral load by PCR if HCV or HBV
– Serum ferritin testing		1	+	– Additional testing if high ferritin levels (MRI/ FerriScan®)
Kidney (Chap. 51)				
– Blood pressure screening	1	1	1	– Hypertension should be investigated and treated appropriately
– Urine protein screening	1	1	1	
– BUN/creatinine testing	1	1	1	– Avoid nephrotoxins
Muscle and connective (Chap. 54)				
– Physical activity counseling	1	1	1	– If risk of cGvHD, test joint mobility and touch skin to detect sclerotic changes
– Evaluation muscle weakness	2	2	2	– Treat cramps symptomatically
Skeletal (Chap. 54)				
– Bone density testing[d]		1	+	– Prevent bone loss and fractures with exercise, vitamin D, and calcium
Nervous system (Chap. 53)				
– Neurologic clinical evaluation	+	1	1	* Special attention of cognitive development in pediatric patients
– Cognitive development*		1	1	
Endocrine (Chap. 56)				
– Thyroid function testing		1	1	– Annual gynecological evaluation in women
– Growth speed in children		1	1	– Hormonal replacement if necessary
– Gonadal function assessment[e]	1	1	1	
– Gonadal function assessment[f]		1	+	
– Gonadal function assessment[g]		+	+	

Table 21.1 (continued)

Recommended screening[b]	6 months	1 year	An.	Comments
Mucocutaneous (Chap. 54)				
– Skin self-exam, sun counseling	1	1	1	– Avoid sunlight without adequate protection
– Gynecological exam in women		1	1	
Immunity				
– Encapsulated Microorg. Prophylaxis*	2	2	2	* If chronic GvHD and IS therapy, consider endocarditis prophylaxis in high-risk patients
– PJP prophylaxis (see Chap. 39)	1	2	2	
– Immunizations (see Chap. 29)	1	1	1	
Secondary neoplasia (Chap. 47)				
– Counseling and autoexamination		1	1	– Reduce UV skin exposure
– Same population screening		1	1	– Special attention to high-risk organs – If TBI, increase frequency mammography
Psychosocial and sexual				
– Psychosocial assessment (see Chap. 30)	1	1	1	– Add spousal/caregiver psychological adjustment and family functioning
– QOL assessment (see Chap. 34)	1	1	1	
– Evaluation of Sexual function	1	1	1	

An. annually, *1* recommended for all transplant recipients, *2* recommended for patients with ongoing chronic GvHD or IS, + reassessment recommended for abnormal testing in a previous time period or for new signs/symptoms
[a]Adapted from Majhail et al. (2012). Similar recommendations but focused in children have been elaborated by the Children's Oncology Group http://www.survivorshipguidelines.org
[b]In patients with chronic GVHD, these controls should be tightened, and their frequency increased
[c]Follow the American Heart Association for endocarditis prophylaxis in high-risk HSCT recipients
[d]Adult women, all allo-HSCT, and patients at high risk for bone loss
[e]Prepubertal men and women
[f]Postpubertal women
[g]Postpubertal men

21.4 Fertility (See Chap. 56)

21.5 Quality of Life (See Chap. 34)

- Monitoring should be multidisciplinary with involvement of hematology, other medical specialties, physicians of primary care, nursing, and mental health professionals

Key Points

- Patients auto- and mainly allo-HSCT have a risk of developing complications related to pre-, peri-, and post-HSCT
- The resulting morbidity of the HSCT process makes it necessary for patients to adopt a healthy lifestyle that promotes health and contemplate preventive measures for the detection and treatment of possible complications
- The short- and long-term controls allow for regular and systematic screening and at the same time are an opportunity to give advice on healthy lifestyle habits

Recommended References

DeFilipp Z, Duarte RF, Snowden JA, et al. Metabolic syndrome and cardiovascular disease after hematopoietic cell transplantation: screening and preventive practice recommendations from the CIBMTR and EBMT. Biol Blood Marrow Transplant. 2016;22:1493–503.

Dietz AC, Mehta PA, Vlachos A, et al. Current knowledge and priorities for future research in late effects after hematopoietic cell transplantation for inherited bone marrow failure syndromes: consensus statement from the Second Pediatric Blood and Marrow Transplant Consortium International Conference on Late Effects after Pediatric Hematopoietic Cell Transplantation. Biol Blood Marrow Transplant. 2017;23:726–35.

Dyer G, Gilroy N, Bradford J, et al. A survey of fertility and sexual health following allogeneic haematopoietic stem cell transplantation in New South Wales, Australia. Br J Haematol. 2016;172:592–601.

Elad S, Raber-Durlacher JE, Brennan MT, et al. Basic oral care for hematology-oncology patients and hematopoietic stem cell transplantation recipients: a position paper from the joint task force of the Multinational Association of Supportive Care in Cancer/International Society of Oral Oncology (MASCC/ISOO) and the EBMT. Support Care Cancer. 2015;23:223–36.

Fred Hutchinson Cancer Research Center/Seattle Cancer Care Alliance Version June 03, 2015. Long-Term Follow-Up After Hematopoietic Stem Cell Transplant General Guidelines For Referring Physicians.

Heimall J, Buckley RH, Puck J, et al. Recommendations for screening and management of late effects in patients with severe combined immunodeficiency after allogenic hematopoietic cell transplantation: a consensus statement from the Second Pediatric Blood and Marrow Transplant Consortium International Conference on Late Effects after Pediatric HCT. Biol Blood Marrow Transplant. 2017;23:1229–40.

Inamoto Y, Shah NN, Savani BN, et al. Secondary solid cancer screening following hematopoietic cell transplantation. Bone Marrow Transplant. 2015;50:1013–23.

Majhail NS, Rizzo JD, Lee SJ, et al. Recommended screening and preventive practices for long-term survivors after hematopoietic cell transplantation. Biol Blood Marrow Transplant. 2012;18:348–71.

National Marrow Donor Program Guidelines.: www.BeTheMatch.org/md-guidelines. For patients: www.BeTheMatch.org/Patient; For Pediatric patients: www.survivorshipguidelines.org.

Parsons SK, Tighiouart H, Terrin N. Assessment of health-related quality of life in pediatric hematopoietic stem cell transplant recipients: progress, challenges and future directions. Expert Rev Pharmacoecon Outcomes Res. 2013;13:217–25.

Persoon S, Kersten MJ, van der Weiden K, et al. Effects of exercise in patients treated with stem cell transplantation for a hematologic malignancy: a systematic review and meta-analysis. Cancer Treat Rev. 2013;39:682–90.

Shenoy S, Gaziev J, Angelucci E, et al. Late effects screening guidelines after Hematopoietic Cell Transplantation (HCT) for hemoglobinopathy: consensus statement from the Second Pediatric Blood and Marrow Transplant Consortium International Conference on Late Effects after Pediatric HCT. Biol Blood Marrow Transplant. 2018;24(7):1313–21.

Tichelli A, Rovó A. Survivorship after allogeneic transplantation-management recommendations for the primary care provider. Curr Hematol Malig Rep. 2015;10:35–44.

Part IV

General Management of the Patient

Topic leaders: Carlo Dufour, Silvia Montoto and John Murray

22 Vascular Access

Simone Cesaro and Federica Minniti

22.1 Introduction

The central venous catheter (CVC) is a key tool for patients undergoing a HSCT, and its introduction in the oncology setting has represented a clear improvement in the quality of patient health care. The use of a CVC requires correct maintenance to prevent malfunctioning due to partial or complete occlusion, dislodgement, kinking, rupture, thrombosis, or life-threatening complications such as catheter-related bloodstream infections (CRBSI).

CVCs are being designated by:

- Duration (e.g., temporary or short-term versus permanent or long-term)
- Site of insertion (e.g., subclavian vein, femoral vein, jugular vein, basilic vein)
- Number of lumens (single, double, or triple lumen)
- Characteristic of tip (open tip or closed tip)
- Materials to reduce complications (e.g., impregnation with heparin, antibiotics, or silver)

Table 22.1 shows the main maintenance actions for CVC (Cesaro et al. 2016).

Table 22.1 CVC maintenance: suggested main rules

1. Assessment of line functionality and dressing site daily for inpatients or every 2–3 days for outpatients
2. CVC care and maintenance as dictated by local policy or standard operating procedure[a]
3. Vigorous mechanical scrub for manual disinfection prior to each CVC access and allow it to dry. Acceptable disinfecting agents include 70% isopropyl alcohol, iodophors (i.e., povidone-iodine), or >0.5% chlorhexidine in alcohol solution
4. Change gauze dressing every 7 days or before in case of soiled, dampened, and loosened
5. Change the transfusion administration set and filter after the completion of each unit or every 4 h. If more than 1 unit can be infused in 4 h, the transfusion set can be used for a 4-h period
6. Change intermittent administration sets every 24 h
7. Replace administration sets for parenteral nutrition solutions at least every 24 h
8. Replace administration sets used for intravenous fat emulsions infused separately every 12 h
9. Change caps every 72 h (or 7 days if pressure-positive device is used)

[a]There may be a variability among EBMT centers regarding the practice of CVC care and maintenance such as the use of sterile gloves and mask by provider/assistant, the adoption of aseptic technique for all catheter entries, the use of prepackaged dressing change kit, the frequency of flushing, and the type of solution used for flushing CVC

S. Cesaro (✉)
Pediatric Hematology Oncology, Azienda Ospedaliera Universitaria Integrata, Verona, Italy
e-mail: simone.cesaro@aovr.veneto.it

F. Minniti
Mother and Child Department, Ospedale della Donna e del Bambino, University of Verona, Verona, Italy

E. Carreras et al. (eds.), *The EBMT Handbook*, https://doi.org/10.1007/978-3-030-02278-5_22

22.2 Type of CVC Materials

Catheter materials should be biocompatible, kink resistant, inherently chemically resistant and neutral, biostable, soft, and deformable and should have a high tensile strength (Lim et al. 2018; Frasca et al. 2010). The most commonly used materials are polyurethane, polyethylene and polytetrafluoroethylene (Teflon), polyvinylchloride (PVC), silicone, and Vialon (Borretta et al. 2018). Silicone catheters are flexible, chemically stable, and well tolerated. Polyurethane catheters are preferred to those made of polyethylene or PVC because of their lower rate of CRBSI and their lower friability (Frasca et al. 2010). Polytetrafluoroethylene catheters are rigid and lose X-ray transparency when injected with opaque solutions. Polyurethane has a superior tensile strength.

Non-tunneled, semirigid catheters are usually made of polyurethane, while tunneled catheters are usually made of both silicone and polyurethane (Lim et al. 2018). The superiority of polyurethane catheters compared with silicone is debated. The two catheter types have no difference in surface degradation; however, silicone catheters are more prone to material failure as a result of the development of surface irregularities due to loss of barium sulfate molecules and thrombotic occlusion. Conversely, polyurethane catheters have a higher susceptibility for catheter-induced venous thrombosis and CRBSI (Blanco-Guzman 2018; Wildgruber et al. 2016).

22.3 Type of CVC

CVCs are classified in two main categories: *tunneled and non-tunneled*, according to whether or not they follow a subcutaneous route before accessing the central vein. Non-tunneled catheters are directly inserted into a peripheral or large central vein. Both tunneled and non-tunneled CVCs may have a single or multiple lumen. Tunnelization of CVCs was introduced to reduce the risk of infectious and mechanical (dislodgement) complications, and this type of CVC is ideal for long-term care (Cesaro et al. 2009). Non-tunneled CVCs are usually inserted for a short to medium period (from 2–4 weeks to 1–3 months) (Lee and Ramaswamy 2018; Padmanabhan 2018). Tunneled CVCs are in turn classifiable in two subgroups: partially implanted and totally implanted. Partially implanted CVCs are characterized by an external part outside the patient's body whose extremity (hub) is used to draw blood sampling or to connect the infusion lines, a tunneled subcutaneous part with a Dacron cuff at a few centimeters from the skin entry point, and a final intravenous part with the tip positioned at the border between the superior vena cava and the right atrium (Padmanabhan 2018; Blanco-Guzman 2018). The Dacron cuff stimulates a fibrotic reaction of the subcutaneous tissues over 2–4 weeks ensuring stability and CVC securement. Both cuff and subcutaneous course are fundamental to prevent the CVC from becoming infected due to the migration of external microbes along the CVC. Broviac, Hickman, and Groshong CVCs belong to this group. Broviac-Hickman CVCs have an open tip and require the clamping of the external part of the CVC when they are not in use to avoid the backflow of the blood from the tip with breath or body movements. Groshong CVCs have a closed tip with lateral valves on their terminal part that open as fluid is withdrawn or infused, while they remain closed when the CVC is not in use. The CVC has to be clamped only if the catheter does not have a needle-free connector. The ideal situation to avoid backflow of blood is a neutral pressure needle-free connector with an open clamp (Padmanabhan 2018).

Totally implanted catheters (porth) consist of a reservoir (port) placed in a pocket in the subcutaneous tissue anteriorly on the chest wall, below the clavicle, that is connected to the catheter (Padmanabhan 2018; Blanco-Guzman 2018). This type of CVC has no part outside of the body, thus preserving the patient's body image and ensuring almost no limitations on sports activities, and body hygiene. The main drawback of this type of CVC is that its accessing needs a skin puncture with a special "non-coring" needle (Huber needle or gripper system). In case of frequently repeated port accesses, the procedure can be painful or discomforting for the patient, requiring the application of topical skin anesthetics for its prevention. Moreover, the needle does not permit the infusion or the extraction of high volumes making it less suitable for patients requiring high infusion or blood extraction rates. The recent introduction of port models with a modified reservoir chamber (vortex, tidal, power port) has allowed to obtain a higher flow rate suitable for leukapheresis, red blood cell exchange, extracorporeal photopheresis, and therapeutic plasma exchange (Blanco-Guzman 2018; Lim et al. 2018).

The *peripherally inserted central catheter (PICC)* is a CVC inserted into a vein of the arm, usually the basilic or cephalic veins; its tip is advanced through the axillary and subclavian veins up to the cavoatrial junction (Hashimoto et al. 2017; Cornillon et al. 2017). For more information on PICCs, see Chap. 32.

22.4 Venous Access

Central lines are usually inserted through the subclavian, the jugular, or, less frequently, the femoral vein. This last venous access is associated with a higher risk of infectious complications (O'Leary 2016), and it is more commonly used in critically ill patients admitted to intensive care units who require a non-tunneled CVC. Using the subclavian or jugular access, the tip of the catheter has to lie in the superior vena cava, just before the entrance of the right atrium, about 29–55 mm below the level of trachea carina (in adults). The incidence of pneumothorax after CVC insertion is about 1.5–3.1%, and it is higher with subclavian vein catheterization, whereas the risk of hemorrhage and bruise is slightly more common with the jugular venous line access.

In the positioning of a PICC, the incannulation of the basilic vein is preferred to that of the cephalic vein as it has low risk of complications. To minimize the risk of complications due to venous catheterizations, the routine use of ultrasound guidance to cannulate the vein is recommended instead of the classical (blind) technique (Cornillon et al. 2017; Crocoli et al. 2015).

A chest X-ray must be performed at the end of the CVC insertion procedure to confirm that the line is positioned inside the superior vena cava and, for the cannulation of subclavian or jugular veins, no pneumothorax was inadvertently caused. Recently, the use of intracavitary ECG (electrocardiographic method) has also been approved for clinical use to evaluate the correct position of the catheter tip (Borretta et al. 2018).

22.5 CVC Complications

Catheter-related complications may be classified into *infectious* (local or systemic) and *mechanical* (occlusion, rupture, dislodgement, accidental self-removal, and thrombosis) (Cesaro et al. 2009). As the catheter is itself a risk for developing complications, when there is no further need for a catheter, it should be removed. Removal of the catheter must also be considered in the event of catheter dysfunction; CRBSI by *Candida* spp., *Pseudomonas* spp., *Klebsiella* spp., and *Staphylococcus aureus*; persistent bacteria colonization or recurrent CRBSI; or contraindications against anticoagulant therapy.

22.5.1 Special Measures to Prevent Catheter-Related Infections

The key rules to prevent infections are proper handwashing by the performing provider, the use of aseptic technique over the patient at insertion time, thorough cleaning of the insertion site, and periodic review of the CVC exit site (Cesaro et al. 2016). Impregnation of the CVC with heparin may reduce the incidence of infectious and thrombotic complications. To prevent CRBSI and tunnel or exit-site infection, medication-impregnated dressings with different antimicrobial materials were developed to decrease the production of the biofilm by microorganisms and decrease the adhesion of them to the catheter walls. The most commonly used impregnating medications are chlorhexidine gluconate, silver sulfadiazine, rifampin, and minocycline (Frasca et al. 2010). Chlorhexidine gluconate impregnates the whole dressing or is applied using an impregnated sponge (e.g., Biopatch®) and covered by a transparent polyurethane semipermeable transparent dressing (Ullman 2015).

22.6 Catheters for Leukapheresis

The procedure of stem cell collection by apheresis is performed both for auto- and allo-HSCT to obtain PBSC (O'Leary 2016). As the procedure requires sustained high blood flow rates (50–100 mL/min), an adequate venous access is needed (O'Leary 2016). Peripheral access placed in the basilic, cephalic, brachial, median cubital and radial veins is recommended (Padmanabhan 2018; Lim et al. 2018; Hölig et al. 2012). Considering that the placement of a central CVC is associated with potentially life-threatening complications such as pneumothorax, bleeding, and embolism (Hölig et al. 2012), its use is not recommended for PBSC collection of a healthy volunteer donor. Conversely, in the case of auto-PBSC, if the patient has no adequate peripheral or central venous access, a temporary non-tunneled CVC may be placed in the internal jugular, subclavian, or femoral veins (Padmanabhan 2018; Lim et al. 2018; Vacca et al. 2014; Hölig et al. 2012; Cooling 2017a). Catheter removal is performed on donor laboratory values (PLT >50 × 10^9/L) or after the assessment of an adequate CD34+ dose and successful cryopreservation of the HPC product (O'Leary 2016; Vacca et al. 2014).

Partially implanted silicone CVCs are often used by pediatric oncologists-hematologists because they are most suitable for long-term complex treatment (Wildgruber et al. 2016). In the case of leukapheresis procedure, silicone CVCs are not ideal because they are more prone to collapse during automatic apheresis (Ridyard et al. 2017). On the other hand, the harvesting procedure of PBSC, which requires high blood flow rates and a large needle, may be difficult in children below 10 kg using a temporary peripheral venous access due to the small size of veins (Padmanabhan 2018; Cesaro et al. 2016). In this case, the placement of a short-term CVC made of polyurethane may be needed (Cooling 2017a, b). However, in younger children, the rigidity of such material and the narrower lumens of the veins may represent a potential risk for thrombosis and infection (Ridyard et al. 2017; Cooling 2017b; Vacca et al. 2014).

Key Points

CVC indications and insertion		
1. Type of CVC	Tunneled CVCs/Port/PICCs	Long-term therapy (months, years) Port for intermittent use, tunneled CVC for continuous use Suitable for inpatient and outpatient
	Non-tunneled CVCs	Short-term therapy (2–4 weeks, 1–3 months) Suitable for inpatient
2. Number of lumens	Single lumen vs Double lumen	Double lumen in patients undergoing HSCT, critically ill patients, intensive intravenous therapy
3. Insertion	Percutaneous/minimally invasive	Ultrasound guidance recommended Adequate training required
	Cutdown approach	Very limited indication (premature infants) Experienced operator
4. Material	Silicone	Tunneled CVC
	Polyurethane	Tunneled and non-tunneled CVC

References

Blanco-Guzman MO. Implanted vascular access device options: a focus review on safety and outcomes. Transfusion. 2018;58:558–68.

Borretta L, MacDonald T, Digout C, et al. Peripherally inserted central catheters in pediatric oncology patients: a 15-year population-based review from Maritimes, Canada. J Pediatr Hematol Oncol. 2018;40:e55–60.

Cesaro S, Cavaliere M, Pegoraro A, et al. A comprehensive approach to the prevention of central venous catheter complications: results of 10-year prospective surveillance in pediatric hematology-oncology patients. Ann Hematol. 2016;95:817–25.

Cesaro S, Tridello G, Cavaliere M, et al. Prospective, randomized trial of two different modalities of flushing central venous catheters in pediatric patients with cancer. J Clin Oncol. 2009;27:2059–65.

Cooling L. Performance and safety of femoral central venous catheters in pediatric autologous peripheral blood stem cell collection. J Clin Apher. 2017a;32:501–16.

Cooling L. Procedure-related complications and adverse events associated with pediatric autologous peripheral blood stem cell collection. J Clin Apher. 2017b;32:35–48.

Cornillon J, Martignoles JA, Tavernier-Tardy E, et al. Prospective evaluation of systematic use of peripherally inserted central catheters (PICC lines) for the home care after allogenic hematopoietic stem cells transplantation. Support Care Cancer. 2017;25:2843–7.

Crocoli A, Tornesello A, Pittiruti M,. et al. Central venous access devices in pediatric malignancies: a position paper of Italian Association of Pediatric Hematology and Oncology. J Vasc Access. 2015;16(2):130–6.

Frasca D, Dahyot-Fizelier C, Mimoz O. Prevention of central venous catheter-related infection in the intensive care unit. Crit Care. 2010;14:212.

Hashimoto Y, Fukuta T, Maruyama J, et al. Experience of peripherally inserted central venous catheter in patients with hematologic disease. Intern Med. 2017;56:389–93.

Hölig K, Blechschmidt M, Kramer M, et al. Peripheral blood stem cell collection in allogeneic donors: impact of venous access. Transfusion. 2012;52(12):2600–5.

Lee K, Ramaswamy RS. Intravascular access devices from an interventional radiology perspective: indications, implantation techniques, and optimizing patency. Transfusion. 2018;58(Suppl 1):549–57.

Lim HS, Kim SM, Kang DW. Implantable vascular access devices–past, present and future. Transfusion. 2018;58:545–8.

O'Leary MF. Venous access for hematopoietic progenitor cell collection: an international survey by the ASFA HPC donor subcommittee. J Clin Apher. 2016;31(6):529–34.

Padmanabhan A. Cellular collection by apheresis. Transfusion. 2018;58:598–604.

Ridyard CH, Plumpton CO, Gilbert RE, Hughes DA. Cost-effectiveness of pediatric central venous catheters in the UK: a secondary publication from the CATCH clinical trial. Front Pharmacol. 2017;8:644.

Ullman AJ, Cooke ML, Mitchell M, et al., Dressings and securement devices for central venous catheters (CVC). Cochrane Database Syst Rev. 2015;(9):CD010367.

Vacca M, Perseghin P, Accorsi P, et al. Central venous catheter insertion in peripheral blood hematopoietic stem cell sibling donors: the SIdEM (Italian Society of Hemapheresis and Cell Manipulation) point of view. Transfus Apher Sci. 2014;50:200–6.

Wildgruber M, Lueg C, Borgmeyer S, et al. Polyurethane versus silicone catheters for central venous port devices implanted at the forearm. Eur J Cancer. 2016;59:113–24.

23 Transfusion Support

Hubert Schrezenmeier, Sixten Körper, Britta Höchsmann, and Christof Weinstock

23.1 General Aspects

Transfusions are an essential part of supportive care in the context of HSCT. RBC and platelet concentrates (PCs) are the main blood products transfused in the peri-transplant period. Many recommendations in this chapter are based on evidence from studies including a broad variety of diseases. Only a few studies addressed transfusion strategy specifically in patients undergoing HSCT (see review Christou et al. 2016). Many recommendations are derived from patients with cytopenia in non-transplant settings. There are both need and opportunity to address issues regarding transfusion of HSCT patients in clinical trials. So far, there is a paucity of studies on the impact of transfusion on HSCT-specific outcomes.

RBC, PC, and FFP for patients who are candidates for HSCT should be leukocyte-reduced, i.e., should contain <1 × 10^6 leukocytes/unit. Leukocyte reduction reduces febrile non-hemolytic transfusion reactions and decreases the incidence of alloimmunization to leukocyte antigens and the risk of CMV transmission. Also all cellular blood components (RBC, PC, granulocyte transfusions) must be irradiated (see below).

H. Schrezenmeier (✉) · S. Körper · B. Höchsmann
C. Weinstock
Institute of Clinical Transfusion Medicine and Immunogenetics Ulm, German Red Cross Blood Transfusion Service Baden-Württemberg-Hessen and University Hospital Ulm, Ulm, Germany

Institute of Transfusion Medicine, University of Ulm, Ulm, Germany
e-mail: h.schrezenmeier@blutspende.de

23.2 Irradiation for Prevention of Transfusion-Associated GvHD (ta-GvHD)

Ta-GvHD is a rare complication of transfusion wherein viable donor T lymphocytes in cellular blood products mount an immune response against the recipient (Kopolovic et al. 2015). Some of the clinical presentations of ta-GvHD resemble that of GvHD (fever, cutaneous eruption, diarrhea, liver function abnormalities). Also many patients develop pancytopenia. Since mortality is high (>90%), prevention of ta-GvHD is critical (Kopolovic et al. 2015). HSCT recipients are at risk of ta-GvHD and should receive irradiated cellular blood products (Kopolovic et al. 2015). It is recommended that no part of the component receives a dose <25 Gy and >50 Gy (European Committee (Partial Agreement) on Blood Transfusion (CD-P-TS) 2017). Some pathogen-reduction technologies have been shown to inactivate lymphocytes, and additional gamma-irradiation is not required (Cid 2017).

There is no consensus on the duration of the use of irradiated blood products in HSCT recipients. Standard practice is (1) auto-HSCT, at

E. Carreras et al. (eds.), *The EBMT Handbook*, https://doi.org/10.1007/978-3-030-02278-5_23

least 2 weeks prior to stem cell collection until at least 3 months after HSCT, and (2) allo-HSCT, at the latest starting with conditioning until at least 6 months after HSCT or until immune reconstitution. However, some centers recommend lifetime use of irradiated products since it is difficult to confirm complete and sustained immunological reconstitution.

23.3 Prevention of CMV Transmission

The highest risk of transfusion-transmitted CMV (TT-CMV) remains in CMV-seronegative recipients of matched CMV-negative HSCT (Ljungman 2014). Risk of TT-CMV can be reduced by transfusion of leukocyte-reduced blood products (i.e., <1 to 5 × 10^6 residual leukocytes per unit) or by transfusion of blood components from CMV-seronegative donors (Ziemann and Thiele 2017). However, it is unclear whether the "belt and suspender approach," i.e., the use of both leukocyte-reduced and seronegative products, further reduces the risk of TT-CMV. Donations from newly CMV-IgG-positive donors bear the highest risk for transmitting CMV infections (Ziemann and Thiele 2017). Currently no international consensus on risk mitigation for CMV transmission exists. A recent snapshot of current practice revealed that about half of the countries use either leukocyte-reduced or seronegative products and the other half use the combination of both (Lieberman et al. 2014). Also, there is no consensus how long CMV-seronegative products should be given to transplant recipients: the current practice ranges from 100 days after transplant till lifelong (or until CMV seroconversion) (Lieberman et al. 2014).

23.4 Red Blood Cell Concentrates (RBCs)

A restrictive RBC transfusion threshold of 7–8 g/dL hemoglobin is recommended for adult patients who are hemodynamically stable. A restrictive RBC transfusion threshold of 8 g/dL is recommended for patients with existing cardiovascular disease (Carson et al. 2016). These cutoffs are derived from studies on a broad range of indications. Only one randomized clinical trial is available specifically for patients undergoing HSCT (TRIST trial, NCT01237639). It compared a liberal strategy (Hb threshold <90 g/L) with a restrictive strategy (Hb threshold <70 g/L). Health-related quality of life was similar between groups, and no appreciable differences in HSCT-associated outcomes were reported (Tay et al. 2016). The median number of RBC units transfused was lower in the restrictive strategy compared to the liberal strategy group, but this did not reach statistical significance (Tay et al. 2016).

In adult recipients, one unit of RBC increases the hemoglobin concentration by about 1 g/dl. In children, the dose should be calculated by the formula:

Volume (mL RBC): Target Hb after transfusion (g/dL) − pretransfusion Hb (g/dL) × 4 × weight (kg)

In recent years, several randomized trials showed no evidence that transfusion of fresh RBC reduced morbidity or mortality compared to standard issue RBCs. Thus, the AABB recommends that patients should receive RBC selected at any point within their licensed dating period (Carson et al. 2016).

Chronic RBC transfusions result in iron overload. Hyperferritinemia and iron overload before HSCT are associated with reduced overall survival and incidence of non-relapse mortality after allo-HSCT. However, a meta-analysis (Armand et al. 2014) and a prospective cohort study suggest that iron overload, as assessed by liver iron content, is not a strong prognostic factor for overall survival in a general adult HSCT population. Thus, ferritin alone is an inadequate surrogate for iron overload in HSCT.

23.5 Platelet Concentrates (PCs)

PC should be transfused prophylactically to nonbleeding, nonfebrile patients when platelet counts are ≤10 × 10^9/L (Schiffer et al. 2018). Prophylactic platelet transfusions may be administered at higher counts based on clinical judgment (Schiffer et al. 2018). Patients with active bleeding, febrile conditions, or active infections should receive prophylactic PC transfusions at a threshold of 20×10^9/L. Also, in case of specific transplant-related toxicity which might increase the risk of bleeding (acute GvHD, mucositis, hemorrhagic cystitis, or diffuse alveolar hemorrhage), a threshold of 20×10^9/L or even higher, based on careful clinical observation, might be justified.

Two prospective randomized control trials comparing prophylactic versus therapeutic PC transfusion in adult patients (≥16 years) suggest that a therapeutic transfusion strategy might be feasible in patients after auto-PBSCT but cannot be easily transferred to other indications (AML, allo-HSCT) for whom special attention to the increased risk of bleeding, in particular, CNS bleeding, is needed (Stanworth et al. 2013; Wandt et al. 2012). The results may not be generalizable to children since a subset analysis of the PLADO trial demonstrated that bleeding rates were significantly increased among children, particularly among those undergoing autologous HSCT (Josephson et al. 2012).

The randomized PLADO trial compared different doses of PC transfusions ("low dose," "medium dose," and "high dose" defined as 1.1×10^{11}, 2.2×10^{11}, and 4.4×10^{11} platelets per m^2 BSA) (Slichter et al. 2010). While a strategy of "low-dose" transfusion significantly reduces the overall quantity of platelets transfused, patients required more frequent PC transfusion events (Slichter et al. 2010). At doses between 1.1×10^{11} and 4.4×10^{11} platelets/m^2, the number of platelets in the prophylactic transfusions had no effect on the incidence of bleeding.

Both apheresis PC and pooled PC from whole blood donations are safe and effective. Available data suggest equivalence of the products in non-allosensitized recipients (Schrezenmeier and Seifried 2010). A clear advantage of apheresis PCs can only be demonstrated in allosensitized patients with HLA- and/or HPA-antibodies who receive antigen-compatible apheresis PCs.

Some patients experience inadequate increment after PC transfusions, i.e., a corrected count increment (CCI) below 5000/μL at 1 h after transfusion of fresh, ABO-identical PCs on at least two subsequent transfusions. Refractoriness can be caused by non-immunological factors (>80%) or immunological factors (<20%) (Fig. 23.1). If platelet refractoriness is suspected and no apparent nonimmune causes can be identified, screening for the presence of HLA-Ab is recommended. If HLA-Ab are present, the patient should receive apheresis PCs from matched donors (Juskewitch et al. 2017; Stanworth et al. 2015): ideally all four antigens (HLA-A, HLA-B) of donor and

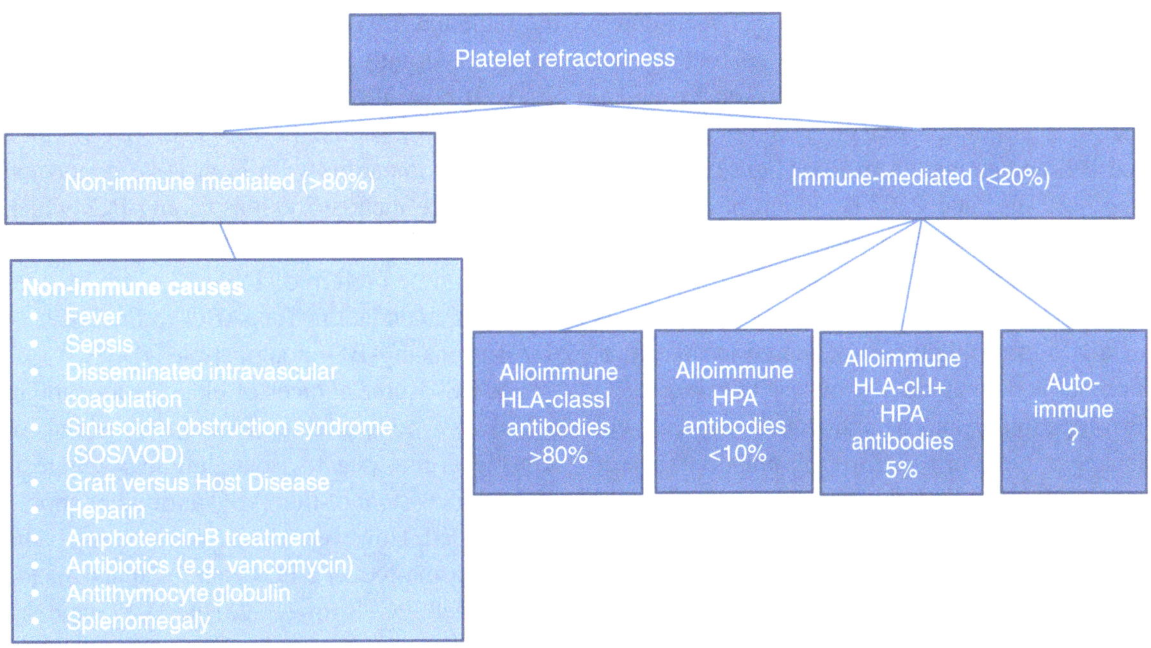

Fig. 23.1 Etiology of platelet transfusion refractoriness (modified according to Pavenski et al. 2012)

recipient are identical. Also PCs from donors expressing only antigens which are present in the recipient can be used. If PCs from such donors are not available, donors with "permissive" mismatches in HLA-A or HLA-B shall be selected (e.g., based on cross-reactive groups or computer algorithms that determine HLA compatibility at the epitope level). If no better-matched donor is available, antigen-negative platelets, i.e., not expressing the target antigen(s) of the recipients' HLA allo-Ab, can be transfused. Screening for antibodies against human platelet antigens (HPA) should be performed if refractoriness persists also after transfusion of HLA-matched PCs and nonimmune causes are unlikely. Approaches for patients without compatible platelet donors are autologous cryopreserved platelets (e.g., collected in remission prior to allogeneic HSCT), IS (e.g., rituximab), and high-dose IVIg and plasmapheresis.

23.6 Immunohematological Consequences of ABO-Mismatched Transplantation

About 40–50% of allo-HSCT are ABO mismatched. While transplantation across the ABO barrier is possible, immunohematological problems have to be taken into account. There is a risk that ABO incompatibility between donor and recipient causes hemolytic transfusion reactions. In case of major ABO mismatch and a recipient anti-donor isoagglutinin titer ≥1:32, the red cell contamination in PBSC graft should be kept <20 mL, and RBC depletion of BM grafts must be performed. If recipient anti-donor isoagglutinin titers are low (≤1:16), no manipulation of the PBSC graft is required, and RBC depletion of a BM graft might be considered in this situation but is not mandatory. In case of minor ABO incompatibility and a high donor anti-recipient isoagglutinin titer (≥1:256), plasma depletion of both PBSC and BM grafts should be performed. If the donor anti-recipient isoagglutinin titer is low (≤1:128), no manipulation of the PBSC graft is required, and plasma depletion of a BM graft might be considered but is not mandatory. In case of bidirectional ABO incompatibility and high titers of anti-recipient isoagglutinins, both RBC and plasma depletion is required.

Delayed hemolysis can occur in minor ABO-mismatched HSCT, in particular after RIC, due to hemolysis of remaining recipient red cells by isoagglutinins produced by donor B lymphocytes.

Major or bidirectional ABO-incompatible HSCT can cause pure red cell aplasia (PRCA), delayed engraftment, and increased RBC transfusion requirement. The risk is higher if a group O recipient with high-titer anti-A isoagglutinins receives a group A graft. If no spontaneous remission of PRCA occurs and anti-donor isoagglutinins persist, various treatments to remove isoagglutinins, to reduce their production, or to stimulate erythropoiesis can be used (see review Worel 2016).

23.7 Transfusion in ABO- or RhD-Incompatible HSCT

The change of blood group and the persistence of recipient isoagglutinins require a special approach for transfusion support in ABO-incompatible HSCT considering several aspects: isoagglutinins might target engrafting progenitors and transfused platelets to which variable amounts of ABO antigens can be bound. ABO blood group antigens are expressed in many non-hematopoietic tissues which continue to express the recipients' ABO antigens also after engraftment. ABO antigens can be secreted into body fluids. If possible, exposure of HSC recipients to isoagglutinins should be avoided. RBCs which are ABO compatible with both HSC donor and recipient are mandatory. Plasma and PCs which are compatible with both the donor and the recipient should be preferred. Table 23.1 summarizes the recommendation for ABO preference of transfusions in ABO-incompatible HSCT.

For PCs, some choices of blood groups might not always be available. To reduce the risk of adverse events due to isoagglutinins, apheresis PC donors with high-titer ABO antibodies should be excluded. However, a preferred strategy is the use of plasma-reduced PC (both for apheresis PC and pooled PC from whole blood donations). These are suspended in platelet additive solution with only about 30% plasma volume remaining.

Table 23.1 RBC, platelet, and plasma transfusion support for patients undergoing ABO-incompatible HSCT

			Phase I[c]	Phase II and phase III[c]				
				RBC	Platelets		Plasma	
ABO incompatibility	Recipient	Donor	All products	Choice[a]	First choice	Second choice[a]	First choice	Second choice
Major	O	A	Recipient	O	A	AB, B, O	A	AB
	O	B	Recipient	O	B	AB, A, O	B	AB
	O	AB	Recipient	O	AB	A, B, O	AB	–
	A	AB	Recipient	A, O	AB	A, B, O	AB	–
	B	AB	Recipient	B, O	AB	B, A, O	AB	–
Minor	A	O	Recipient	O	A[b]	AB, B, O	A	AB
	B	O	Recipient	O	B[b]	AB, A, O	B	AB
	AB	O	Recipient	O	AB[b]	A, B, O	AB	–
	AB	A	Recipient	A, O	AB[b]	A, B, O	AB	–
	AB	B	Recipient	B, O	AB[b]	B, A, O	AB	–
Bidirectional	A	B	Recipient	O	AB	B, A, O	AB	–
	B	A	Recipient	O	AB	A, B, O	AB	–

– not applicable
[a]Choices are listed in the order of preference
[b]For practical reasons, the use of donor type platelets might be defined as first choice, in phase III, i.e., after complete engraftment
[c]Phase I until preparative regimen, phase II until complete engraftment, phase III after complete engraftment.

HSC recipients should receive RhD-negative RBC and also RhD-negative PC except when both HSC donor and recipient are RhD-positive. If the HSC donor is RhD-positive and the recipient is RhD-negative, platelet transfusion can be switched to RhD-positive products after erythroid engraftment, i.e., appearance of RhD-positive red cells.

Whenever possible, RBC should be compatible both with HSCT donor and recipient for CcEe antigens. If Rh antigens of HSCT donor and recipient differ in a way that compatibility with both is not possible (e.g., recipient CCD.ee, donor ccD.EE), then RBC compatible with the recipient shall be chosen in the period until engraftment. After the appearance of donor-derived red cells, RBC supply should switch to compatibility with the graft. Patients should receive K-negative RBC except when both recipient and donor are K positive.

23.8 Granulocyte Concentrates

In life-threatening non-viral infections during neutropenia, the use of irradiated granulocyte transfusions should be considered. Response and survival after granulocyte transfusion correlate strongly with hematopoietic recovery. Thus, granulocyte transfusions may mainly bridge the gap between specific treatment and neutrophil recovery. Granulocyte transfusions can help to control active fungal infections in a very high-risk population of patients who otherwise are denied by transplant program. A retrospective study suggested that granulocyte transfusion might maintain the mucosal integrity and thus reduces bacterial translocation and triggers for GvHD. In the randomized RING trial, success rates for granulocyte and control arms did not differ within any infection type. The overall success rates for the control and granulocyte transfusion group were 41% and 49% (n.s.) (Price 2015). However, patients who received high dose ($\geq 0.6 \times 10^9$ granulocytes/kg per transfusion) fared better than patients who received lower doses. The collection center should ensure to provide a high-dose concentrate by appropriate donor selection, pre-collection stimulation, and apheresis techniques. The optimal number of granulocyte transfusions is unclear. Adverse events of granulocyte infusions are fever, chills, pulmonary reactions, and alloimmunization. Studies demonstrated that overall risk of alloimmunizations was low and there was no effect of alloimmunization on the primary outcome (survival, microbial response), the occurrence of transfusion reactions, or post transfusion neutrophil increments. Alloimmunization remains a problem because of its negative impact on increments after platelet transfusion and potential increase of graft failure after HSCT. Donor-specific HLA-Ab might be implicated in early graft failure (Spellman et al. 2010). If granulocyte transfusions are used prior to a planned unrelated HSCT, recipients should be monitored for the development of HLA-Ab, and the search algorithm for the UD should take into account donor-specific antibodies. All granulocyte concentrates must be gamma-irradiated and should be obtained from CMV-seronegative donors, ideally also confirmed by CMV-PCR to avoid donations in the serological window period.

Key Points

- Patients undergoing HSCT must be transfused with irradiated blood products (at least 2 weeks prior to stem cell collection in auto- and starting with the conditioning in allo-HSCT)
- A restrictive RBC transfusion threshold of 7–8 g/dL hemoglobin is recommended for adult patients who are hemodynamically stable
- RBC must be compatible with both the HSC donor and the recipients
- Platelet concentrates should be transfused to non-bleeding, nonfebrile patients when platelet counts are $\leq 10 \times 10^9$/L
- Prophylactic platelet transfusion remains the standard of care for thrombocytopenic patients undergoing allogeneic HSCT
- RBC must be compatible with both the HSC donor and the recipient

References

Armand P, Kim HT, Virtanen JM, et al. Iron overload in allogeneic hematopoietic cell transplantation outcome: a meta-analysis. Biol Blood Marrow Transplant. 2014;20:1248–51.

Carson JL, Guyatt G, Heddle NM, et al. Clinical practice guidelines from the AABB: red blood cell transfusion thresholds and storage. JAMA. 2016;316: 2025–35.

Christou G, Iyengar A, Shorr R, et al. Optimal transfusion practices after allogeneic hematopoietic cell transplantation: a systematic scoping review of evidence from randomized controlled trials. Transfusion. 2016;56:2607–14.

Cid J. Prevention of transfusion-associated graft-versus-host disease with pathogen-reduced platelets with amotosalen and ultraviolet A light: a review. Vox Sang. 2017;112:607–13.

European Committee (Partial Agreement) on Blood Transfusion (CD-P-TS). Guide to the preparation, use and quality assurance of blood components. 19th. 2017. EDQM.

Josephson CD, Granger S, Assmann SF, et al. Bleeding risks are higher in children versus adults given prophylactic platelet transfusions for treatment-induced hypoproliferative thrombocytopenia. Blood. 2012;120:748–60.

Juskewitch JE, Norgan AP, De Goey SR, et al. How do I … manage the platelet transfusion-refractory patient? Transfusion. 2017;57:2828–35.

Kopolovic I, Ostro J, Tsubota H, et al. A systematic review of transfusion-associated graft-versus-host disease. Blood. 2015;126:406–14.

Lieberman L, Devine DV, Reesink HW, et al. Prevention of transfusion-transmitted cytomegalovirus (CMV) infection: standards of care. Vox Sang. 2014;107:276–311.

Ljungman P. The role of cytomegalovirus serostatus on outcome of hematopoietic stem cell transplantation. Curr Opin Hematol. 2014;21:466–9.

Pavenski K, Freedman J, Semple JW. HLA alloimmunization against platelet transfusions: pathophysiology, significance, prevention and management. Tissue Antigens. 2012;79:237–45.

Price TH, Boeckh M, Harrison RW, et al. Efficacy of transfusion with granulocytes from G-CSF/dexamethasone-treated donors in neutropenic patients with infection. Blood. 2015;126:2153–61.

Schiffer CA, Bohlke K, Delaney M, et al. Platelet transfusion for patients with cancer: American Society of Clinical Oncology clinical practice guideline update. J Clin Oncol. 2018;36:283–99.

Schrezenmeier H, Seifried E. Buffy-coat-derived pooled platelet concentrates and apheresis platelet concentrates: which product type should be preferred? Vox Sang. 2010;99:1–15.

Slichter SJ, Kaufman RM, Assmann SF, et al. Dose of prophylactic platelet transfusions and prevention of hemorrhage. N Engl J Med. 2010;362:600–13.

Spellman S, Bray R, Rosen-Bronson S, et al. The detection of donor-directed, HLA-specific alloantibodies in recipients of unrelated hematopoietic cell transplantation is predictive of graft failure. Blood. 2010;115:2704–8.

Stanworth SJ, Estcourt LJ, Powter G, et al. A no-prophylaxis platelet-transfusion strategy for hematologic cancers. N Engl J Med. 2013;368:1771–80.

Stanworth SJ, Navarrete C, Estcourt L, Marsh J. Platelet refractoriness–practical approaches and ongoing dilemmas in patient management. Br J Haematol. 2015;171:297–305.

Tay J, Allan DS, Chatelein E, et al. Transfusion of red cells in hematopoietic stem cell transplantation (TRIST study): a randomized controlled trial evaluating 2 red cell transfusion thresholds. Blood. 2016;128:1032.

Wandt H, Schaefer-Eckart K, Wendelin K, et al. Therapeutic platelet transfusion versus routine prophylactic transfusion in patients with haematological malignancies: an open-label, multicentre, randomised study. Lancet. 2012;380:1309–16.

Worel N. ABO-mismatched allogeneic hematopoietic stem cell transplantation. Transfus Med Hemother. 2016;43:3–12.

Ziemann M, Thiele T. Transfusion-transmitted CMV infection–current knowledge and future perspectives. Transfus Med. 2017;27:238–48.

24 Nutritional Support

Annic Baumgartner and Philipp Schuetz

24.1 Introduction

Patients undergoing HSCT, particularly allo-HSCT, are at risk for malnutrition (Fuji et al. 2012). Malnutrition is associated with poor clinical outcome, decreased OS, higher risk of infectious and immunologic complications, delayed neutrophil engraftment and prolonged hospital stay (Baumgartner et al. 2016, 2017). Importantly, most patients are well-nourished or even overweight upon admission to HSCT but experience rapid deterioration of nutritional status during treatment (Fuji et al. 2014). Weight loss results from a complex interplay of toxic, inflammatory and immunological mechanisms leading to caloric deficits by anorexia as well as a catabolism of the metabolism.

Nutritional support is meant to reduce caloric deficit and reduce the risks for negative metabolic effects. However, there is a lack of large-scale trials proving benefit of nutritional interventions in this setting (Baumgartner et al. 2017). The current nutritional approach is thus based on physiological considerations and results of observational and some smaller interventional trials and needs to be adapted to an individual patient's situation.

24.2 Screening for Malnutrition

Pre-existing malnutrition is an important additional risk factor in patients undergoing HSCT. International guidelines such as the European Society of Enteral and Parenteral Nutrition (ESPEN) recommend screening for malnutrition at admission for transplantation (Bozzetti et al. 2009). There is no international consensus on how to assess malnutrition in this patient population. For reasons of practicability, the use of the NRS 2002 is generally recommended (Bozzetti et al. 2009). In the acute setting, weight assessment may be inaccurate because of inflammatory fluid retention.

Based on "Supportive Care" in EBMT Handbook, 2009, by Tamás Masszi and Arno Mank.

A. Baumgartner (✉)
Internal Medicine and Endcrinology/Diabetology/Clinical Nutrition and Metabolism, Medical University Clinic of Kantonsspital Aarau, University of Basel, Aarau, Switzerland
e-mail: annic.baumgartner@ksa.ch

P. Schuetz
Department of Endocrinology, Diabetes and Metabolism and Internal Medicine, Kantonsspital Aarau, University of Basel, Aarau, Switzerland

E. Carreras et al. (eds.), *The EBMT Handbook*, https://doi.org/10.1007/978-3-030-02278-5_24

24.3 Nutritional Recommendations (See General Recommendations in Table 24.1 and Fig. 24.1; Monitoring in Table 24.2 and Nutritional Strategies in Fig. 24.1)

24.3.1 Nutrition in Allo-HSCT

24.3.1.1 Route of Administration

Due to its positive effects on GI integrity and microbiome, enteral nutritional (EN) support is generally preferred over parenteral nutrition (PN) in case of a functioning GI tract.

During allo-HSCT, patients often experience GI failure so PN is used instead. Yet, higher risk of central line infections as well as hyperglycaemia associated with PN demand restricted use (Seguy et al. 2012).

Small, prospective, non-randomized trials on EN found satisfying results on feasibility and safety with lower infection rates as well as beneficial effects such as earlier neutrophil engraftment and lower rates of severe GI GvHD (Seguy et al. 2012; Guièze et al. 2014). Some studies even report higher OS (Seguy et al. 2012). Results of a large prospective trial are expected (Lemal et al. 2015).

We encourage the use of EN as a first-line measure. Indication for PN should be limited to

Table 24.1 Summary of general recommendations for nutritional support

Screening for malnutrition	
Indication	All patients to estimate risk for pre-existing malnutrition
Tools	NRS 2002
Nutritional support	
General management	1. Early involvement of dietitians 2. Consider placement of nasogastric tube on day +1 3. Standardized monitoring of nutritional intake 4. Nutritional reassessment every 3 days using the NRS 2002
Indication of intervention	1. Oral intake <60% for 3 days consecutively 2. Consider nutritional support in all patients with preexisting malnutrition and/or BMI < 18
Discontinuation	Oral intake >50% for 3 days consecutively
Estimation of caloric needs	According to Harris Benedict formula (ideal body weight) OR BASA-ROT table/(25–30 kcal/kg ideal body weight)
Route of nutritional support	1. Intensification of oral nutrition 2. Enteral nutrition 3. Parenteral nutrition
Forms of nutritional support	
Intensified oral nutrition	*Indication*: Malnutrition or underweight (BMI < 18 kg/m^2) and preserved oral intake *Options*: Additional snacks rich in proteins and energy, protein or calorie enrichment of main courses, additional protein and energy drinks (ONS) *Standardized supplementation*: None
Enteral nutrition	*Indication*: If nutritional goals cannot be reached by oral support alone *Standardized supplementation:* Vitamin K once weekly
Parenteral nutrition	*Indication*: If nutritional goals cannot be reached in patients with gastrointestinal failure and/or intolerance for NGT *Standardized supplementation:* Lipid-soluble vitamins (ADEK) Water-soluble vitamins Trace elements
Vitamin and trace elements	Multivitamin generally recommended Vitamin D: Supplementation recommended (Bolus of 40000E at admission, maintenance therapy with 1500E orally per day Other vitamins or trace elements if overt deficiency
Immunonutrition	Generally not recommended

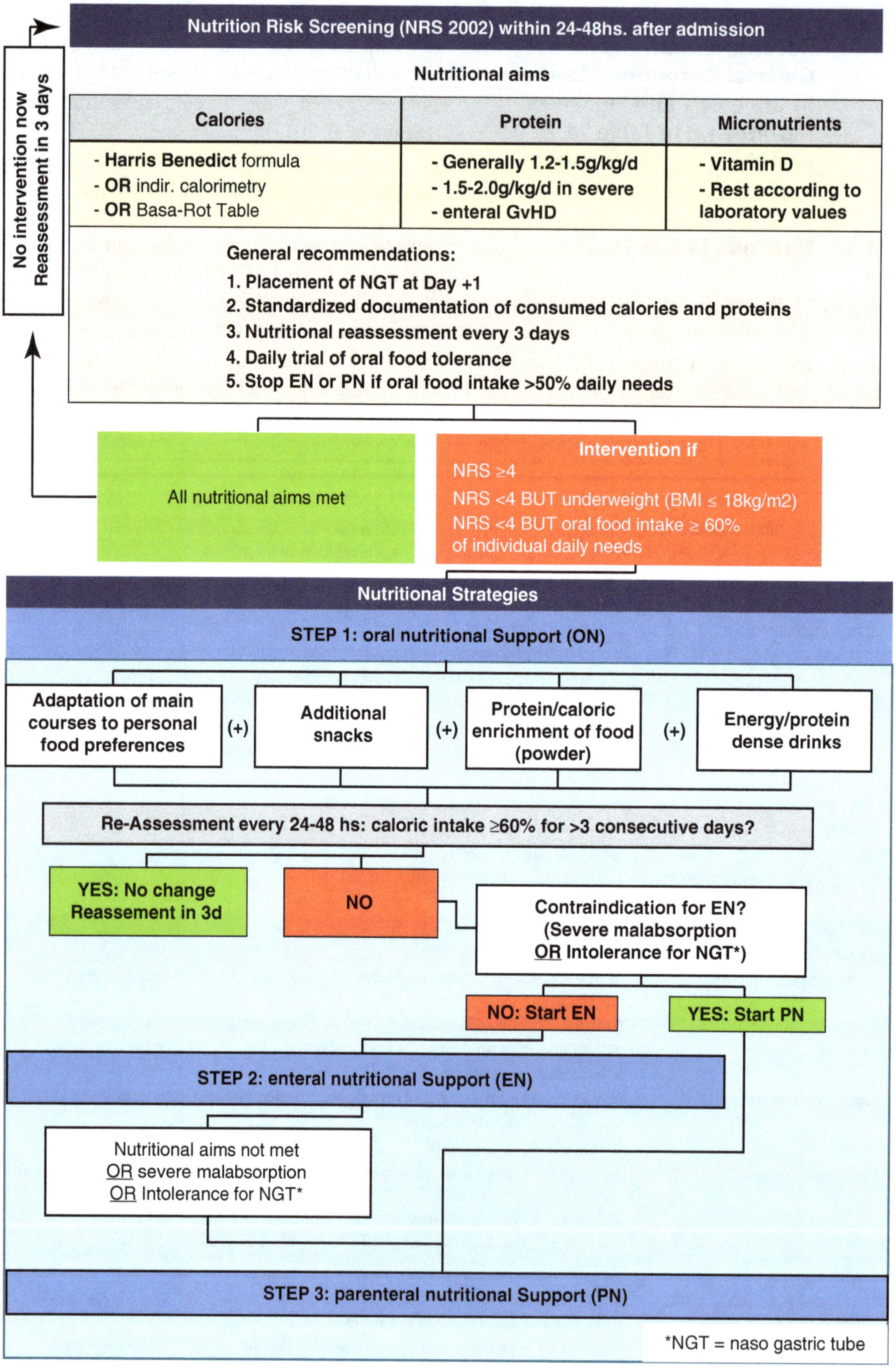

Fig. 24.1 Algorithm for guided nutritional support

intolerance for nasogastric tube and GI failure including severe malabsorption or limited gastroenteral passage.

24.3.1.2 Indications and Timing

There are few study data regarding optimal timing of nutrition. The ESPEN guidelines recommend implementation of nutritional support if oral caloric intake falls below 60–70% of basic requirements for 3 days consecutively (Bozzetti et al. 2009).

Discontinuation of EN or PN should be considered, if >50% of daily requirements are met by oral intake (Bozzetti et al. 2009). To enhance early return to oral food intake patients should be encouraged to maintain minimal oral intake throughout therapy.

24.3.1.3 Estimation of Caloric Needs

Most studies investigating energy expenditure by indirect calorimetry have been performed in small paediatric populations. Validity of the data for adults therefore is limited, and results are controversial (Sharma et al. 2012; Duro et al. 2008).

Determination of energy requirements based on calculations, e.g., by the BASA-ROT table or Harris-Benedict Formula, does not differ significantly from results by indirect calorimetry (Sharma et al. 2012; Valentini 2012; Harris 1918). Therefore, we recommend estimation of energy requirements according to an adjusted Harris-Benedict formula.

24.3.2 Nutrition in Auto-HSCT

In general, effects of auto-HSCT on nutritional status are less pronounced. Nutritional support is not generally recommended and has to be evaluated individually in patients experiencing severe complications or in patients with pre-existing malnutrition.

Table 24.2 Monitoring of nutritional parameters

Parameter	Frequency of assessment	Significance and implications
Anthropometry		
Weight	Daily	Correlation with fluid balance Evaluation of diuretics and Albumin supplementation
Bioimpedance assessment	Individually	Uncontrolled, unexplained weight loss Severe, prolonged inflammation
Nutritional assessment		
Oral food consumption	3× daily	Evaluation of nutritional support
Laboratory parameter		
Albumine	Weekly	Evaluation of supplementation in anasarca
Sodium, Potassium	Daily	Adaptation of potassium supplementation
Calcium, Magnesium, Phosphate	Twice weekly	Adaptation of supplementation CAVEAT refeeding, gastrointestinal loss
INR, Quick	Twice weekly	Evaluation of supplementation CAVEAT low content in certain products for EN/PN
Glucose	3–6× daily if PN or preexisting diabetes mellitus otherwise twice weekly	Adaptation of insulin dose
Creatinine	Daily	Correction of fluid balance CAVEAT toxic damage
Liver function tests	Twice weekly	Evaluation of toxic damage, infection, hepatic GvHD, VOD or relapse
Triglycerides	Twice weekly if PN	Adaptation of PN
Vitamin D	At admission	Begin routine supplementation
Vitamin B12	At admission	Supplementation pretransplantational individually

24.3.3 Nutrition in Acute Gastrointestinal GvHD

GvHD of the digestive tract leads to excessive diarrhoea, abdominal pain, nausea, vomiting, gastrointestinal bleeding, dysphagia and malabsorption. Patients experience malnutrition to a higher extent and show significantly more additional complications (van der Meij et al. 2013).

Caloric demands are mainly driven by energy loss through diarrhoea. Enteral solutions should be low in fibre and fat and not contain lactose. Maintaining a minimal amount of oral or enteral nutrition facilitates early dietary recovery (Imataki et al. 2006; Andermann et al. 2016). Complete bowel rest and total PN are indicated in severe GvHD grade IV and stool volume >1500 ml in 24 h (Bozzetti et al. 2009; Imataki et al. 2006).

Protein requirements are elevated. Recommendations range from 1.2 to 2.5 g/kg/day. We recommend aiming for 1.5–2 g/kg/day in the absence of severe renal impairment (Bozzetti et al. 2009; Muscaritoli et al. 2002).

Vitamin and trace elements are often deficient and need to be measured regularly to evaluate need of supplementation.

24.3.4 Low Bacterial Diet/Low Microbial Diet/Neutropenic Diet

A low microbial diet has been installed in the 1980s to prevent potential threat of food-borne infections from organisms colonizing the gastrointestinal tract.

There is no standardized protocol, and variations amongst centres, contradictions even, are high. Yet, there is no proof of efficacy in preventing infections or death.

In line with most current publications, we recommend safe food handling and strict hand hygiene as proposed by the FDA or the EC over a neutropenic diet.

24.4 Immunonutrition

A meta-analysis on glutamine found reduced severity and duration of mucositis and GvHD (Kota and Chamberlain 2017). To date, no randomized controlled trial showed a benefit on overall survival or reduction of infection rates (Crowther et al. 2009).

Pre- and probiotics may enhance diversity of the GI microbiome. So far, no study has evaluated their effects compared to placebo. Again, there might be a benefit on severity of GvHD (Ladas et al. 2016). Safety has been evaluated in a pilot study in children and adolescents and proved satisfying.

There are no randomized controlled trials assessing the benefits of omega-3 fatty acids or trace elements. Except for vitamin D, there is no proven benefit of a routine supplementation (Hall and Juckett 2013). Based on this data, we do not recommend routine use of immunonutrients.

24.5 Long-Term Follow-Up

Follow-up should include regular nutritional screening and documentation of weight, BMI, appetite and functional status based on patients' history. A balanced, Mediterranean diet can be recommended along with regular physical training to regain muscle mass. An increase in weight should be addressed early to avoid full development of a metabolic syndrome because of high baseline cardiovascular risk in transplanted patients.

Persisting malnutrition, especially in chronic GvHD, should be handled by an interdisciplinary team. Caloric needs seem to be elevated and often require in- and out-hospital nutritional support.

Key Points

- There is high risk for malnutrition upon HSCT treatment
- Malnutrition is an independent risk factor in these patients
- The potential benefit of all nutritional interventions remains largely unproven
- All dietary recommendations are based on physiological considerations and results of mainly observational trials
- Adherence to a systematic approach to nutritional support improves transparency, comparability and generally reduces use of unnecessary PN

- Oral and enteral nutritional support is recommended over parenteral support in case of functioning gastrointestinal tract
- A minimal oral or enteral food intake is beneficial for recovery of mucosa and microbiome
- Immunonutrients did not show significant beneficial effects and therefore are not recommended for routine use
- Neutropenic diets did not show a benefit over safe food handling approaches

References

Andermann TM, Rezvani A, Bhatt AS. Microbiota manipulation with prebiotics and probiotics in patients undergoing stem cell transplantation. Curr Hematol Malig Rep. 2016;11:19 28.

Baumgartner A, Bargetzi A, Zueger N, et al. Revisiting nutritional support for allogeneic hematologic stem cell transplantation—a systematic review. Bone Marrow Transplant. 2017;52:506–13.

Baumgartner A, Zueger N, Bargetzi A. Association of nutritional parameters with clinical outcomes in patients with acute myeloid leukemia undergoing hematopoietic stem cell transplantion. Ann Nutr Metab. 2016;69:89–98.

Bozzetti F, Arends J, Lundholm K, Micklewright A, Zurcher G, Muscaritoli M. ESPEN guidelines on parenteral nutrition: non-surgical oncology. Clin Nutr. 2009;28:445–54.

Crowther M, Avenell A, Culligan D. Systematic review and meta-analyses of studies of glutamine supplementation in haematopoietic stem cell transplantation. Bone Marrow Transplant. 2009;44:413–25.

Duro D, Bechard LJ, Feldman HA, et al. Weekly measurements accurately represent trends in resting energy expenditure in children undergoing hematopoietic stem cell transplantation. J Parenter Enter Nutr. 2008;32:427–32.

Fuji S, Mori T, Khattry N, et al. Severe weight loss in 3 months after allogeneic hematopoietic SCT was associated with an increased risk of subsequent non-relapse mortality. Bone Marrow Transplant. 2014;50:100–5.

Fuji S, Mori T, Lee V, et al. A multi-center international survey related to the nutritional support after hematopoietic stem cell transplantation endorsed by the ASIA Pacific Blood and Marrow Transplantation (APBMT). Food Nutr Sci. 2012;3:417–21.

Guièze R, Lemal R, Cabrespine A, et al. Enteral versus parenteral nutritional support in allogeneic haematopoietic stem-cell transplantation. Clin Nutr. 2014;33:533–8.

Hall AC, Juckett MB. The role of vitamin D in hematologic disease and stem cell transplantation. Nutrients. 2013;5:2206–21.

Harris JA, Benedict FG. A biometric study of human basal metabolism. Proc Natl Acad Sci U S A. 1918;4:370–3.

Imataki O, Nakatani S, Hasegawa T, et al. Nutritional support for patients suffering from intestinal graft-versus-host disease after allogeneic hematopoietic stem cell transplantation. Am J Hematol. 2006;81:747–52.

Kota H, Chamberlain RS. Immunonutrition is associated with a decreased incidence of graft-versus-host disease in bone marrow transplant recipients: a meta-analysis. JPEN J Parenter Enteral Nutr. 2017;41:1286–92.

Ladas EJ, Bhatia M, Chen L, et al. The safety and feasibility of probiotics in children and adolescents undergoing hematopoietic cell transplantation. Bone Marrow Transplant. 2016;51:262–6.

Lemal R, Cabrespine A, Pereira B, et al. Could enteral nutrition improve the outcome of patients with haematological malignancies undergoing allogeneic haematopoietic stem cell transplantation? A study protocol for a randomized controlled trial (the NEPHA study). Trials. 2015;16:136.

Muscaritoli M, Grieco G, Capria S, Iori AP, Rossi Fanelli F. Nutritional and metabolic support in patients undergoing bone marrow transplantation. Am J Clin Nutr. 2002;75:183–90.

Seguy D, Duhamel A, Rejeb MB, et al. Better outcome of patients undergoing enteral tube feeding after myeloablative conditioning for allogeneic stem cell transplantation. Transplantation. 2012;94:287–94.

Sharma TS, Bechard LJ, Feldman HA, et al. Effect of titrated parenteral nutrition on body composition after allogeneic hematopoietic stem cell transplantation in children: a double-blind, randomized, multicenter trial. Am J Clin Nutr. 2012;95:342–51.

Valentini L. The BASA-ROT table: an arithmetic-hypothetical concept for easy BMI-, age-, and sex-adjusted bedside estimation of energy expenditure. Nutrition. 2012;28:773–8.

van der Meij BS, de Graaf P, Wierdsma NJ, et al. Nutritional support in patients with GVHD of the digestive tract: state of the art. Bone Marrow Transplant. 2013;48:474–82.

25 GVHD Prophylaxis (Immunosuppression)

David Michonneau and Gérard Socié

25.1 Introduction

The most life-threatening complication of allo-HSCT is the graft-versus-host disease (GVHD) which occurs when T cells from the recipient recognize the host as foreign. Despite 50 years of history and nearly half a million of procedures performed worldwide, GVHD remains the most challenging issue physicians are facing on a daily basis.

Overall, 30–50% of the patients will develop acute GVHD, and around 15% will have severe GVHD (grades III–IV). The main risk factor for developing chronic GVHD is the previous development of the acute form of the disease.

The pathophysiology, diagnosis, and management of both acute and chronic GVHD will be covered by other chapters in this Handbook (Chaps. 43 and 44). This chapter will summarize the use of IS to prevent the development of acute GVHD since attempt to prevent chronic GVHD basically rely on the ability to prevent the acute disease. Readers with interest on a more detailed overview of the acute GVHD biological process, prevention, and therapy can refer to an excellent recent review (Zeiser and Blazar 2017).

25.2 GVHD Prophylaxis After MAC; The "Gold" Standard; CNI in Combination with MTX

Back in the mid-1980s, Storb and colleagues reported that the combination of CSA/MTX (Table 25.1) was superior to CSA in a series of prospective randomized phase 3 trials (Storb et al. 1986). This gold standard regimen remains the most widely used in Europe today as prophylaxis regimen especially after MAC.

In the late 1990s, another CNI-based prophylactic regimen using tacrolimus (TAC) in conjunction with MTX was developed, and two randomized phase 3 trials were published after MAC in HLA-identical and URD, respectively (Ratanatharathorn et al. 1998; Nash et al. 2000). Although both reported a significant decreased in the incidence of grade II–IV acute GVHD, none of the two could demonstrate an improved survival rate with TAC/MTX as compared to CSA/MTX. The reasons for this lack of improvement are twofold: (1) in the trial performed from HLA-identical sibling D, there was an imbalanced of disease risk among the two groups with higher risk patients with leukemia among patients receiving TAC/MTX, and (2) for the trial in URD, the HLA-typing methodology at

D. Michonneau · G. Socié (✉)
Hematology/Transplantation, AP/HP Hospital St Louis, Paris, France

University Paris VII, Denis Diderot, Paris, France

INSERM UMR 1160, Paris, France
e-mail: gerard.socie@aphp.fr

E. Carreras et al. (eds.), *The EBMT Handbook*, https://doi.org/10.1007/978-3-030-02278-5_25

Table 25.1 CSA/MTX for GVHD prophylaxis

	Cyclosporine	Methotrexate
Drug posology	3 mg/kg/day IV till engraftment then orally	15 mg/m² day +1 10 mg/m² day +3, +6, +11
Adjusting dose	Target dose to 150–200 ng/mL; adjust to renal function	Day 11 may be omitted if grade III/IV mucositis
Interaction	Numerous; ++ with azoles	
Secondary effects	Numerous Renal insufficiency, CNS, and endothelial toxicities	Mucositis

that time was serologically based and thus included a very high proportion of patients with almost certainly high degree of mismatching. Nevertheless it should be stressed that the TAC/MTX regimen is currently considered as the American gold standard, while it never reached popularity in Europe.

CSA and TAC inhibit GVHD by preventing the activation of the nuclear factor of activated T-cell (NFAT) family of transcription factors, thereby reducing the transcription of interleukin-2 and the activation of effector T cells, albeit with a concurrent reduction in levels of interleukin-2-dependent anti-inflammatory Tregs.

25.3 GVHD Prophylaxis After RIC; Is CNI Plus MMF Standard?

From the early development of the RIC, two regimens have been used in the setting of RIC, CSA (or TAC) alone or in combination with MMF (reviewed in; Zeiser and Blazar 2017). Somewhat surprisingly the association of CSA/MMF while largely used worldwide has never been tested stringently in the setting of a large randomized prospective randomized trial. CNI in this setting are usually used at the same dose (and share the same toxicity profile) as after MAC. MMF's toxicity mainly relies on sometimes unpredictable hematological toxicity. Attention must be paid to the use of ganciclovir (for CMV reactivation) in addition to MMF because of the risk of severe pancytopenia. MMF is usually delivered at the dose of 30 mg/kg/day split into two to three doses. Anecdotal evidence suggests depending on the transplant situation (i.e., HLA-identical vs. URD) that MMF should be delivered (till day + 80?) in recipients from URD.

25.4 Can PT-CY Be Considered as Standard GVHD Prophylaxis in Transplantation from Haploidentical Donors and Beyond?

There is a recent bloom in the use of haploidentical donor during the past few years worldwide. While initial attempt was to use megadose of CD34+ selected HSC, the advent of PT-CY has really revolutionized this procedure. The PT-CY designed by Baltimore's group includes CY 50 mg/kg on day +3 and +4 followed by TAC/MMF. Toxicities include those associated with CNI and MMF. Specific toxicity associated with CY includes hemorrhagic cystitis and the rare but potentially serious early cardiologic dysfunction. Although the incidence of acute GVHD remains significant (in around 1/3 of the patients), there is now some evidence that PT-CY might be associated with low rate of chronic GVHD (reviewed in; Fuchs 2017).

Furthermore, beyond the setting of haploidentical transplant, PT-CY has gained popularity in other setting including transplantation from URD and HLA-identical sibling. Although it seems unlikely today that any formal randomized trial (vs. ATG) will be launched after haplo-HSCT, it would be of major scientific interest to prospectively compare within a phase 3 trial ATG vs. PT-CY.

Finally, whether PT-CY is equally effective after RIC and MAC regimen is currently unknown as it is unknown if other combination like sirolimus (SIR) + MMF can be as effective as (or less effective as) CNI/MMF in addition to PT-CY in the haploidentical situation or even if PT-CY can safely be used as a single agent after HLA-identical sibling transplants, as recently reported (Mielcarek et al. 2016).

CY administered in two doses scheduled soon after transplantation depletes highly proliferating alloreactive conventional T cells while helping to preserve Tregs.

25.5 ATG or Alemtuzumab for GVHD Prophylaxis in HSCT

Since almost two decades, both ATG and alemtuzumab (ALEM) have been used to prevent GVHD especially after transplantation from URD. ALEM although efficacious in preventing acute GVHD has never been tested prospectively in a randomized phase 3 trial and has almost exclusively been developed in the UK. ATG however has been tested in four prospective randomized phase 3 trials. Three out of these four used anti-T-lymphocyte globulin (ATLG) and one rabbit ATG (rATG). However, the design, the time period, patients' selection, donor type, and primary end point of these four randomized trials differ (see Table 25.2 for references). From the perspective of GVHD prophylaxis efficacy, all four trials demonstrated a significant decrease in chronic GVHD rate and in three out of the four a statistical significant decrease in the rate of acute GVHD. Other end points varied among the four trials. In particular the American trial by Soiffer et al. was the only one in which patients who received ATLG experienced an increased rate of relapse mainly in patients with AML who received TBI as part of a MAC pre-transplant.

25.6 New Immunosuppressive Regimens for GVHD Prophylaxis

With current treatment strategies summarized above, the rate of moderate to severe acute GVHD remains of concern in the range of 20–50%. As reviewed elsewhere in the Handbook, the treatment of acute and of chronic GVHD with high-dose steroids remains unsatisfactory with 30–50% of the patients being steroid resistant or dependent. There is thus an unmet clinical need in GVHD prophylaxis. After years of lack of new agent in this setting, the better knowledge of basic T-cell immunology, of the pathophysiology of the disease, and new drug development by the industry, new agents have been tested mostly in phase 2 trials which appeared to be promising. This section summarized the drugs with most advanced development that reported an acute GVHD incidence in the 20% range (i.e., a range that may warrant development of subsequent phase 3 trials). Readers with interest on a more detailed portfolio of current drug development and new targets could refer to a recent review (Zeiser and Blazar 2017).

In contrast to CNI, SIR, an mTOR inhibitor, is a more potent suppressor of the expansion of conventional T cells than Tregs, owing to the greater dependence of conventional T cells on the mTOR-protein kinase B pathway. This was the basis of the development by the Dana-Farber Cancer Institute (DFCI) group of a regimen that leads to an estimated cumulative incidence of acute GVHD grades II–IV of 20.5% and of less than 5%

Table 25.2 Four randomized trials using ATG as a GVHD prophylaxis

	Finke et al. (2009)	Kroger et al. (2016)	Soiffer et al. (2017)	Walker et al. (2016)
N	202	168	254	203
Product	ATLG	ATLG	ATLG	rATG
Primary end point	GVHD	cGVHD	cGVHD-free survival	Freedom from all IST
Conditioning	MAC	MAC	MAC	MAC+RIC
Donor	URD	Id. Sibling	URD	URD
GvHD prophylaxis	CSA +MTX	CSA +MTX	TAC +MTX	CSA or TAC+MTX or MMF
Acute GVHD	33 vs. 51% (grade II–IV)	11 vs. 18% (grade II–IV)	23 vs. 40% (grade II–IV)	50 vs. 65% (any grade)
Chronic GVHD	Decreased	Decreased	Decreased	Decreased

grades III–IV. This prompted a large trial of the BMTCTN comparing TAC/SIR to TAC/MTX. The primary end point of the trial was to compare grade II–IV acute GVHD-free survival using an intention-to-treat analysis of 304 randomized subjects. There was no difference in the probability of day 114 grade II–IV acute GVHD-free survival (67% vs. 62%, $P = 0.38$). Grade II–IV GVHD was similar in the TAC/SIR and TAC/MTX arms (26% vs. 34%, $P = 0.48$) (Cutler et al. 2014). A smaller randomized single-center phase 2 study found however less cumulative incidence with 43% grade II–IV after TAC/SIR (as compared to an unexpected high rate of 89% after TAC/MTX) (Pidala et al. 2012).

Encouraging rates have also been reported by two other compounds: Bortezomib (BOR) (Koreth et al. 2012) and Maraviroc in 2012 (Reshef et al. 2012) delivered in addition to TAC/MTX. These two drugs as well as CY have been then tested in randomized phase 2 trials in the setting of HSCT (BMTCTN 1203 trial) after RIC in a pick-the-winner-designed trial (i.e., aimed to test in a multicenter setting the three drugs) and compared to prospective contemporary cohort of patients who received TAC/MTX. The final results of this trial closed for recruitment will be available in 2018. Finally, in an open-label three-arm phase 2 randomized controlled trial, investigator at the DFCI compared grade II–IV acute GVHD between conventional TAC/MTX (A) vs. BOR/TAC/MTX (B) and vs. BOR/SIR/TAC (C), in RIC-HSCT recipients from URD in 138 patients. Day +180 grade II–IV acute GVHD rates were similar (A 32.6%, B 31.1%, C 21%) as was the 2-year NRM. Overall, the BOR-based regimens evaluated did not seem to improve outcomes compared with TAC/MTX therapy (Koreth et al. 2018).

Finally, based on preclinical works in mice models, two drugs Vorinostat and Tocilizumab provided exciting results and were supported by ancillary biological data in humans.

- Vorinostat, a histone deacetylase inhibitor, at low concentration has anti-inflammatory and immunoregulatory effects. Pavan Reddy's group in Michigan provided compelling evidences that in preclinical models Vorinostat reduced GVHD rate, suppressed pro-inflammatory cytokines, regulated APCs, and enhanced Treg functions. In two separate trials (Choi et al. 2014, 2017), authors translated their findings in the clinical setting. In one trial where Vorinostat was added to standard prophylaxis after RIC in HLA-identical siblings, acute GVHD grade II–IV rate was 22% and that of grades III–IV of 6%. In another trial after MAC in URD, the acute GVHD rates were similar.
- The addition of Tocilizumab to CNI+ MTX standard prophylaxis has been tested by two different groups (Kenedy et al. 2014; Dorobyski et al. 2018). Tocilizumab is a humanized anti-IL-6 receptor monoclonal antibody. IL-6 levels are increased early during GVHD and are present in all target tissues. Blockade of the IL-6 signaling pathway has been shown to reduce the severity of GVHD and to prolong survival in experimental models. Investigators in Milwaukee and in Brisbane conducted two separate phase 2 trials using Tocilizumab, and both found very low rate of grade II–IV acute GVHD (less than 15%).

Other new agents are currently either tested in preclinical models or are in the early stage of development in clinical trials (reviewed in Zeiser and Blazar 2017). New strategies that have shown efficacy in preclinical models of GVHD include the inhibition of Janus kinase (JAK) and rho-associated protein kinase 1 (ROCK-1). The blockade of phosphatidylinositol 3-kinase (PI3K), mitogen-activated protein kinase (MEK) proteins 1 and 2, aurora A kinase, and cyclin-dependent kinase 2 (CDK2) have been shown to reduce acute GVHD in murine models.

25.7 Conclusion and Perspective

Despite decades of experience with transplantation, GVHD still occurs in over 40% of the patients. When acute GVHD develops, the main treatment is high-dose steroids. However around one third of the patients will be steroid resistant.

Steroid resistance remains associated with a dismal prognosis (30–40% 1-year survival). These data urge for developing new strategies to prevent GVHD. Fortunately enough, based on preclinical findings and improved knowledge on the immune biology of HSCT, recent drug combination opens the gate for future development.

Key Points

- Current GVHD prophylaxis relies on CNI + short-term MTX after MAC and of CSA ± MMF after RIC
- ATG has been demonstrated to decrease acute GVHD after URD transplant and of chronic GVHD
- Despite the above two points, new prophylactic regimens are clearly warranted since severe GVHD rates still lie on the 25% range

References

Choi SW, Braun T, Chang L, et al. Vorinostat plus tacrolimus and mycophenolate to prevent graft-versus-host disease after related-donor reduced intensity conditioning allogeneic haematopoietic stem-cell transplantation. Lancet Oncol. 2014;15:87–95.

Choi SW, Braun T, Henig I, et al. Vorinostat plus tacrolimus/methotrexate to prevent GVHD after myeloablative conditioning, unrelated donor HSCT. Blood. 2017;130:1760–7.

Cutler C, Logan B, Nakamura R, et al. Tacrolimus/sirolimus vs tacrolimus/methotrexate as GVHD prophylaxis after matched, related donor allogeneic HCT. Blood. 2014;124:1372–7.

Dorobyski WR, Szabo A, Zhu F, et al. Tocilizumab, tacrolimus and methotrexate for prevention of acute graft-versus-host disease: low incidence of lower gastrointestinal tract disease. Haematologica. 2018;103:717–27.

Finke J, Bethge WA, Schmoor C, et al. Standard graft-versus-host disease prophylaxis with or without anti-T-cell globulin in haematopoietic cell transplantation from matched unrelated donors: a randomised, open-label, multicentre phase 3 trial. Lancet Oncol. 2009;10:855–64.

Fuchs EJ. Related haploidentical donors are better choice than matched unrelated donors: point. Blood Adv. 2017;1:397–400.

Kenedy GA, Varelias A, Vuckovic S, et al. Addition of interleukin-6 inhibition with tocilizumab to standard graft-versus-host disease prophylaxis after allogeneic stem-cell transplantation: a phase 1/2 trial. Lancet Oncol. 2014;15:1451–9.

Koreth J, Kim HT, Lange PB, et al. Bortezomib-based immunosuppression after reduced-intensity conditioning hematopoietic stem cell transplantation: randomized phase II results. Haematologica. 2018;103:522–30.

Koreth J, Stevenson KE, Kim HT, et al. Bortezomib-based graft-versus-host disease prophylaxis in HLA-mismatched unrelated donor transplantation. J Clin Oncol. 2012;30:3202–8.

Kroger N, Solano C, Wolschke C, et al. Antilymphocyte globulin for prevention of chronic graft-versus-host disease. N Engl J Med. 2016;374:43–53.

Mielcarek M, Furlong T, O'Donnell PV, et al. Post-transplant cyclophosphamide for prevention of graft-versus-host disease after HLA-matched mobilized blood cell transplantation. Blood. 2016;127:1502–8.

Nash RA, Antin JH, Karanes C, Fay JW, et al. Phase 3 study comparing methotrexate and tacrolimus with methotrexate and cyclosporine for prophylaxis of acute graft-versus-host disease after marrow transplantation from unrelated donors. Blood. 2000;96:2062–8.

Pidala J, Kim J, Jim H, et al. A randomized phase II study to evaluate tacrolimus in combination with sirolimus or methotrexate after allogeneic hematopoietic cell transplantation. Haematologica. 2012;97:1882–9.

Ratanatharathorn V, Nash RA, Przepiorka D, et al. Phase III study comparing methotrexate and tacrolimus (prograf, FK506) with methotrexate and cyclosporine for graft-versus-host disease prophylaxis after HLA-identical sibling bone marrow transplantation. Blood. 1998;92:2303–14.

Reshef R, Luger SM, Hexner EO, et al. Blockade of lymphocyte chemotaxis in visceral graft-versus-host disease. N Engl J Med. 2012;367:135–45.

Soiffer RJ, Kim HT, McGuirk J, et al. Prospective, randomized, double-blind, phase III clinical trial of anti–T-lymphocyte globulin to assess impact on chronic graft-versus-host disease–free survival in patients undergoing HLA-matched unrelated myeloablative hematopoietic cell transplantation. J Clin Oncol. 2017;35:4003–11.

Storb R, Deeg HJ, Whitehead J, et al. Methotrexate and cyclosporine compared with cyclosporine alone for prophylaxis of acute graft versus host disease after marrow transplantation for leukemia. N Engl J Med. 1986;314:729–35.

Walker I, Panzarella T, Couban S, et al. Pre-treatment with anti-thymocyte globulin versus no anti-thymocyte globulin in patients with haematological malignancies undergoing haemopoietic cell transplantation from unrelated donors: a randomised, controlled, open-label, phase 3, multicentre trial. Lancet Oncol. 2016;17:164–73.

Zeiser R, Blazar BR. Acute graft-versus-host disease; biologic process, prevention and therapy. N Engl J Med. 2017;377:2167–79.

26 Management ATG (SIRS)

Francesca Bonifazi

26.1 Introduction

Currently horse and rabbit anti-lymphoglobulins (ATLG) or antithymocyte globulin (ATG) is available; the main, although not exclusive, use is for the treatment of aplastic anemia (horse) and for GVHD prophylaxis (rabbit). They differ in the manufacturing process (i.e., used animal, pulsed antigens, antibody specificities, and cellular targets): for this reason, dose, timing, and setting cannot be interchangeable, and also clinical results are different. As they are polyclonal serum-derived products from nonhuman organisms, they can cause serum sickness and infusion reactions.

26.2 ATLG/ATG Infusion Protocol (See Table 26.1)

ATLG/ATG infusion should be performed in trained centers. Standard hygienic handling of the injection site, careful evaluation of the infusion speed, and appropriate choice of the venous access are crucial. Medical personnel should carefully watch over patients for adverse events not only during but also after infusion.

During administration, the patient needs to be monitored for symptoms related to infusion reactions or anaphylaxis. The first dose should be administered at a reduced speed for the first 30 min. If no symptoms of intolerance occur, infusion rate may be increased. In case of anaphylactic or anaphylactoid reactions, physicians must be prepared to promptly manage this event, and appropriate medical treatment has to be implemented.

A central venous catheter is preferred, although a peripheral large high-flow access may be acceptable, if a central line is not available. Thrombophlebitis is the major risk when a peripheral vein is used. The availability of a high-flow access is important in case of treatment of infusion reactions.

Premedication is mandatory in order to improve systemic and local tolerance (see later). Stability, compatibility, and dilution are different for each product, and specific manufacturer recommendations should be followed carefully.

Preinfusion intraepidermal tests are not yet validated for rabbit ATG but, according to manufacturer indications, are recommended for horse ATLG.

—Although standard infusion time is between 4 and 12 h, a longer administration time correlates with milder side effects, thus making infusions of 12 h highly advised.

F. Bonifazi (✉)
Institute of Hematology "Seràgnoli", University Hospital S. Orsola-Malpighi, Bologna University, Bologna, Italy
e-mail: francesca.bonifazi@unibo.it

E. Carreras et al. (eds.), *The EBMT Handbook*, https://doi.org/10.1007/978-3-030-02278-5_26

Table 26.1 Infusion of ATLG/ATG

Factors	Comments
Infusion site	– Central line is highly preferred – Risk of thrombophlebitis and drug precipitation are higher in peripheral veins
Dilution	Avoid to inject undiluted preparation; follow the manufacturer instructions for each ATLG/ATG type
Compatibility	– rATLG-Grafalon: avoid to mix concentrate solution with glucose, blood, blood derivatives, sodium heparin, and lipid-containing solutions – rATG-Thymoglobulin: avoid dilutions with other than saline and dextrose – Horse ATGAM: avoid dextrose injection or acidic solution because of precipitation or instability
Stability	Diluted solutions up to 24 h (infusion time included) stored in refrigerator
Duration of infusion	4–12 h – Slower infusion results in a lower incidence and severity of infusion reactions; therefore ≥12 h infusion is recommended Start first administration at low infusion rate (at least for the first 30–60 min)
Drug interactions	Not reported
Premedication	Mandatory; steroids, acetaminophen, antihistamines
Preinfusion test	– Not advised for rabbit sera – Recommended for ATGAM – Skin and conjunctival tests not extensively validated
Criteria for permanent discontinuation	Anaphylaxis: severe anaphylaxis, always. De-sensitization protocols: not validated
What does D/C stand for?	SIRS: depending on grading and clinical evaluation of pros and cons. In case of rechallenge, more stringent monitoring is required

26.3 ATLG/ATG Dose

Dose and timing of ATLG/ATG administration vary substantially among transplant centers (Bacigalupo et al. 2001; Finke et al. 2009; Walker et al. 2016; Kröger et al. 2016; Soiffer et al. 2017).

The currently used doses of ATLG/ATG are calculated and validated in clinical trials, according to body weight. A strong rationale and some preliminary data (Admiraal et al. 2017) suggest that calculating the ATG/ATLG dose according to the cellular target, i.e., the number of total lymphocyte before infusion of the first dose, can provide the optimal drug exposure and therefore maximize the benefit (GVHD decrease) over the potential risks (increase of relapses and infections). Since ATLG and ATG are different preparations arising from different manufacturing processes and different pulsed antigens, no dose equivalence can be established.

26.4 Infusion Reactions

ATLG/ATG administration can be complicated by several infusion reactions including fever, chills, erythema, dyspnea, oxygen desaturation, nausea/vomiting, diarrhea, abdominal pain, hyperkalemia, tachycardia, hypo- or hypertension, malaise, rash, urticaria, headache, arthralgia, myalgia (serum sickness, after 5–15 days from infusion), hepatic cytolysis, and even systemic anaphylaxis.

Even if the NCI Terminology Criteria for Adverse Events (CTCAE) use different scales for grading reactions to infusion of chemotherapy and allergic/anaphylaxis reactions, there are no specific symptoms enabling to distinguish "standard" infusion reaction from an allergic one that can evolve to anaphylaxis.

Anaphylaxis and acute allergic reactions are based on IgE effect and histamine release by mastocytes, but the vast majority of symptoms can be attributed to the cytokine release syndrome (CRS) and are generally reversible. CRS is a form of systemic inflammatory response syndrome (SIRS) (Matsuda and Hattori 2006; Balk 2014). CRS can follow not only ATG/ATLG infusion but also chemotherapy, MoAb (Remberger et al. 1999; Feng et al. 2014), bispecific antibodies, or CAR-T cell therapies (Lee et al. 2014). All these (both allergic and nonallergic, such as CRS) are infusion reactions. Serum sickness is a hypersensitivity phenomenon that can develop after 5–15 days after the infusion, and it is well responsive to steroid treatment.

26.5 SIRS

SIRS is a clinical syndrome due to dysregulated inflammation. SIRS may occur in several conditions, such as infection, autoimmune disorders, vasculitis, thromboembolism, chemotherapy infusion, surgery, and burns. The denomination originates from changes of some parameters (temperature, heart and respiratory rates, and white blood cell count) occurring after infection/sepsis according to Bone (Bone et al. 1992). A pediatric version tailored on patient age is also available (Goldstein 2005). More recently, some authors (Lee et al. 2014) revised the classification of the cytokine release syndrome according to the treatment required (oxygen, vasopressors, organ toxicity).

26.5.1 Risk Factors for SIRS

SIRS after ATLG/ATG infusion cannot be predicted and the risk factors are not well known.

The binding of ATLG/ATG to the surface of target cells (lymphocytes, monocytes, dendritic cells) elicits cytokine production and systemic inflammation (Bone et al. 1992).

Thus, that the higher the number of lymphocytes at the moment of the (first) infusion, the more likely is the risk of systemic activation of inflammation and then SIRS.

Accordingly, RIC regimens are reported to be associated with greater cytokine release syndrome (Remberger and Sundberg 2004) because of the likely higher number of residual lymphocytes in RIC in comparison with MAC regimens.

26.5.2 Management of SIRS

26.5.2.1 Prophylaxis

ATLG/ATG infusion reactions can be reduced in frequency and severity by two factors: premedication and speed of infusion. Premedication is performed with steroids, antihistamine, and acetaminophen. The optimal schedule of premedication is not yet well established. Doses of prednisolone of 250 mg (higher than 1 mg/kg), given before the first infusion and followed by an additional dose in the same day, reduce the incidence of infusion reactions and cytokine release as reported (Pihusch et al. 2002).

The rate of infusion is one of the most important factors to reduce the incidence and severity of infusion reactions since lower infusion rates are associated with a lower incidence and the severity of reactions. Administration time ≥12 h is the preferred schedule to yield high compliance to ATLG/ATG infusion.

26.5.2.2 Treatment

If symptoms of SIRS appear, the drug should be discontinued, at least temporarily.

Treatment is symptomatic and depends upon the clinical manifestations. Intensive care for respiratory and hemodynamic support should be given according to international guidelines for critical patients, and the intervention of an intensive specialist may be requested. SIRS after ATLG/ATG is different from sepsis-induced SIRS where steroids failed to achieve a significant benefit (Cronin et al. 1995). Symptoms due to ATLG/ATG-related SIRS are more pronounced on day +1 and then tend to decrease. Steroids, widely used preemptively, provide high response rates also as a treatment measure.

Permanent Discontinuation/Rechallenge

Rechallenge after anaphylaxis and after standard infusion reactions >3 is strongly discouraged.

Non-controlled life-threatening infections are contraindications to transplant and should not modify ATLG/ATG administration per se.

Desensitization protocols are not yet clearly validated.

Key Points

- SIRS is a systemic reaction related to cytokine release after ATLG/ATG infusion.
- The infusion reactions can be reduced by premedication (steroids, antihistamines, and acetaminophen) and by a low infusion rate (12 h or longer).

References

Admiraal R, Nierkens S, de Witte MA, et al. Association between anti-thymocyte globulin exposure and survival outcomes in adult unrelated haemopoietic cell transplantation: a multicentre, retrospective, pharmacodynamic cohort analysis. Lancet Haematol. 2017;4:e183–91.

Bacigalupo A, Lamparelli T, Bruzzi P, et al. Antithymocyte globulin for graft-versus-host disease prophylaxis in transplants from unrelated donors: 2 randomized studies from Gruppo Italiano Trapianti Midollo Osseo (GITMO). Blood. 2001;98:2942–7.

Balk RA. Systemic inflammatory response syndrome (SIRS): where did it come from and is it still relevant today? Virulence. 2014;5:20–6.

Bone RC, Balk RA, Cerra FB, et al. American College of Chest Physicians/Society of Critical Care Medicine Consensus Conference: definitions for sepsis and organ failure and guidelines for the use of innovative therapies in sepsis. Crit Care Med. 1992;20:864–74.

Cronin L, Cook DJ, Carlet J, et al. Corticosteroid treatment for sepsis: a critical appraisal and meta-analysis of the literature. Crit Care Med. 1995;23:1430–9.

Feng X, Scheinberg P, Biancotto A, et al. In vivo effects of horse and rabbit antithymocyte globulin in patients with severe aplastic anemia. Haematologica. 2014;99:1433–40.

Finke J, Bethge WA, Schmoor C, et al. Standard graft-versus-host disease prophylaxis with or without anti-T-cell globulin in haematopoietic cell transplantation from matched unrelated donors: a randomised, open-label, multicentre phase 3 trial. Lancet Oncol. 2009;10:855–64.

Goldstein B, Giroir B, Randolph A, International Consensus Conference on Pediatric Sepsis. International pediatric sepsis consensus conference: definitions for sepsis and organ dysfunction in pediatrics. Pediatr Crit Care Med. 2005;6:2–8.

Kröger N, Solano C, Wolschke C, et al. Antilymphocyte globulin for prevention of chronic graft-versus-host disease. N Engl J Med. 2016;374:43–53.

Lee DW, Gardner R, Porter DL, et al. Current concepts in the diagnosis and management of cytokine release syndrome. Blood. 2014;124:188–95.

Matsuda N, Hattori Y. Systemic inflammatory response syndrome (SIRS): molecular pathophysiology and gene therapy. J Pharmacol Sci. 2006;101:189–98.

Pihusch R, Holler E, Mühlbayer D, et al. The impact of antithymocyte globulin on short-term toxicity after allogeneic stem cell transplantation. Bone Marrow Transplant. 2002;30:347–54.

Remberger M, Sundberg B. Cytokine production during myeloablative and reduced intensity therapy before allogeneic stem cell transplantation. Haematologica. 2004;89:710–6.

Remberger M, Svahn BM, Hentschke P, et al. Effect on cytokine release and graft-versus-host disease of different anti-T cell antibodies during conditioning for unrelated haematopoietic stem cell transplantation. Bone Marrow Transplant. 1999;24:823–30.

Soiffer RJ, Kim HT, McGuirk J, et al. Prospective, randomized, double-blind, phase III clinical trial of anti-t-lymphocyte globulin to assess impact on chronic graft-versus-host disease-free survival in patients undergoing HLA-matched unrelated myeloablative hematopoietic cell transplantation. J Clin Oncol. 2017;35:4003–11.

Walker I, Panzarella T, Couban S, et al. Pretreatment with anti-thymocyte globulin versus no anti-thymocyte globulin in patients with haematological malignancies undergoing haemopoietic cell transplantation from unrelated donors: a randomised, controlled, open-label, phase 3, multicentre trial. Lancet Oncol. 2016;17:164–73.

27 Infection Control and Isolation Procedures

Malgorzata Mikulska

27.1 Introduction

Infection control is defined as a set of measures aimed at preventing or stopping the spread of infections in healthcare settings. All HSCT recipients should follow general guidelines (e.g. CDC) for preventing healthcare-associated infections through hand hygiene, disinfection and sterilization, environmental infection control, isolation precautions and prevention of intravascular catheter-related infection (Sehulster et al. 2004; Guidelines for Hand Hygiene in Healthcare Settings (2002), Guideline for Isolation Precautions: Preventing Transmission of Infectious Agents in Healthcare Settings (2007), Guidelines for Environmental Infection Control in Health-Care Facilities (2003), all available at https://www.cdc.gov/infectioncontrol/guidelines/index.html; Freifeld et al. 2011).

Dedicated and detailed international recommendations for HSCT recipients on preventing infectious complications have been published in 2009 (Tomblyn et al. 2009; Yokoe et al. 2009). As there were no well-executed randomized or controlled trials and little evidence to hand from cohort case-controlled or multiple time-series studies or uncontrolled experiments, reliance had to be placed on descriptive studies, reports of expert committees or on the opinions of respected authorities. Hence, most of these recommendations on infection control could only be graded as level III.

Isolation procedures in HSCT recipient comprise precautions universal for all healthcare settings (Standard Precautions and Transmission-Based Precautions) and those specific for HSCT and employed to prevent transmission of spores of filamentous fungi, mainly *Aspergillus*, with unfiltered air.

There is no consensus on specific *protective environment*, called also reverse isolation, for neutropenic patients. HSCT recipients should be placed in single-patient room, with adequate ventilation system (see below), if possible. However, no clear benefit of routine footwear exchange, or use of disposable gloves and gowns on the rate of infections have been demonstrated, and procedures vary significantly between institutions, with routine use of masks and disposable gloves and gowns in some but not others. On the contrary, the negative effect of strict protective isolation on patient's quality of life and well-being should be acknowledged and weighted against the evidence of benefits of single protective measures (Abad et al. 2010).

M. Mikulska (✉)
Division of Infectious Diseases, Department of Health Sciences (DISSAL), IRCCS Ospedale Policlinico San Martino, University of Genova, Genova, Italy
e-mail: m.mikulska@unige.it

E. Carreras et al. (eds.), *The EBMT Handbook*, https://doi.org/10.1007/978-3-030-02278-5_27

27.2 Standard Precautions

Should be used universally for all patients and they include:

1. Proper hand hygiene
2. Use of standard personal protective equipment (PPE)
3. Appropriate cleaning and disinfection protocols (including those for shared equipment or toys and play areas in paediatric units)
4. Safe injection practices
5. Infection control practices for special procedures (e.g. surgical masks for lumbar puncture)

27.2.1 Hand Hygiene

It is by far the most effective means of prevention of pathogen transmission (Freifeld et al. 2011; Tomblyn et al. 2009). The preferred method of hand decontamination is with an alcohol-based hand rub, due to its superior convenience and reduced drying of the skin. Handwashing with soap and water is recommended if hands are visibly soiled, for example, with blood or body fluids, or after potential contact with spores of *Clostridium difficile* or with *Norovirus*. Of note, 15–30 s is the minimum necessary handwashing time.

PPE used routinely by healthcare workers during patient care and procedures are gloves, gowns (used if direct contact with patient's fluids is expected) and mouth, nose and eye protection (used during procedures which are likely to generate splashes or sprays of blood, body fluids, secretions and excretions). Routine donning of gowns upon entrance into a high-risk unit, including HSCT unit, is not indicated.

27.3 Transmission-Based Precautions

These are the measures used in addition to standard precautions for patients with documented or suspected infection or colonization with highly transmissible or epidemiologically important pathogens for which additional precautions are necessary to prevent transmission. The main types of transmission-based precautions are *contact* precautions, *airborne* precautions and *droplet* precautions. The specific PPE and the examples of pathogens which require each type of transmission-based precautions are outlined in Table 27.1.

Contact precaution should be also applied in a *pre-emptive* way, e.g. in case of patients transferred from high-risk facilities, pending the results of surveillance cultures. Clear criteria should be provided for appropriate discontinuation of contact precautions (usually when three different swabs from a known multidrug-resistant (MDR) positive site, taken 1–7 days apart, are negative). In case of contact precautions, and particularly if a patient is still colonized with a resistant pathogen, this information should be clearly stated on the discharge information form for the centres which will care for this patient subsequently. In case of MDR Gram-negative pathogens, full antibiotic susceptibility results should be provided to allow appropriate empirical therapy in case of severe subsequent infection.

Cough etiquette should be promoted. Additionally, transplant recipients, particularly those with respiratory symptoms, should use surgical masks and maintain special separation from others in common waiting areas, ideally a distance of at least 1 m.

Upon entering HSCT unit, *visitors* should be screened for the presence of symptoms of easily transmissible diseases such as *viral respiratory tract infections*, gastroenteritis, etc. and, if present, advised to postpone their visit until no longer symptomatic. Also, healthcare workers with respiratory symptoms should refrain from direct patient care until the symptoms resolve. Sero negative persons who were exposed to communicable diseases such as measles or chickenpox should refrain from contact with HSCT recipients or transplant candidates until the incubation period passes without developing the disease. Instructional materials for patients and visitors on recommended hand hygiene, respiratory hygiene/cough etiquette practices and the application of transmission-based precautions should be provided. Vaccination of healthcare workers

Table 27.1 Transmission-based precautions, to be applied in addition to standard precautions

Type of precaution	Patients placement and PPE to be used by patients	PPE for healthcare personnel	Example of pathogens and comments
Contact	– Single room; if not available, cohorting of those colonized/infected by the same pathogen – During transport, cover patient's colonized/infected areas	– Disposable gloves and gowns – Use patient-dedicated or disposable equipment; if not feasible, clean and disinfect thoroughly	– Infection with *Clostridium difficile* – Colonization or infection with MDR pathogens – Infectious diarrhoea due to pathogens such as *Salmonella*, *Norovirus*, *Rotavirus*, etc All the units or other hospitals involved in patient's care should be notified about all the isolated pathogens requiring contact precautions
Droplet	– Single room; if not available, cohorting of those infected by the same pathogen – Surgical mask – Follow CDC's respiratory hygiene/cough etiquette in healthcare setting	– Mask (surgical) – Disposable gloves and gowns	– Pathogens transmitted by respiratory droplets (i.e. large-particle droplets >5 μ in size) that are generated by a patient who is coughing, sneezing or talking, e.g. influenza or other respiratory viruses In case of transplant recipients, the duration of precautions should be extended due to the possibility of prolonged shedding caused by immunodeficiency
Airborne	– Rooms with at least 6 (existing facility) or 12 (new construction/renovation) air changes per hour and direct exhaust of air to the outside (if not possible, the air may be returned to the air-handling system or adjacent spaces if all air is directed through HEPA filters) – Surgical mask – Follow CDC's respiratory hygiene/cough etiquette in healthcare setting	– N95 or higher-level respirator for respiratory protection	– *Mycobacterium tuberculosis* (patients with respiratory tuberculosis and sputum with direct evidence of mycobacteria) – Measles, chickenpox and disseminated herpes zoster

HEPA high-efficiency particulate air, *MDR* multidrug resistant, *PPE* personal protective equipment

and household contacts is paramount and discussed in the dedicated chapter.

27.4 Management of the Threat of MDR Bacteria

In the era of increasing bacterial resistance, an important part of infection control deals with *prevention of colonization and infection with MDR bacteria* (Siegel et al. 2007). Active surveillance, for example, with rectal swabs for detecting colonization with vancomycin-resistant enterococci (VRE) or carbapenem-resistant *Enterobacteriaceae* or nasal swabs for methicillin-resistant *Staphylococcus aureus*, should be performed in institutions where these pathogens are regularly encountered or in patients coming from such institutions.

The need for screening for different pathogens may vary according to local epidemiology. For instance, Italian statement on the management of carbapenem-resistant *Klebsiella pneumoniae* (CR-*Kp*) infections in HSCT was published (Girmenia et al. 2015). Briefly, they recommended active detection of CR-*Kp* carriers before and after HSCT, since the carriers have approximately 30% risk of developing CR-*Kp* bloodstream infection; staff education and monitoring of adherence to contact precautions; a cautious approach to declare a patient no longer colonized and a need for coordinated effort to intra- or inter-hospital transmission. HSCT is not contraindicated in MDR carriers, but establishing upfront the appropriate empirical therapy to be administered in case of fever during neutropenia is mandatory, and careful evaluation of the possibility of decolonization in selected cases through oral administration of non-absorbable molecules or faecal microbiota transplantation is warranted (Girmenia et al. 2015; Bilinski et al. 2017).

In order to counteract the threat of MDR pathogens and the shortage of agents active against Gram-negative MDR bacteria, *antimicrobial stewardship program* should be implemented in every centre (Gyssens et al. 2013). Additionally, national systems for surveillance, with obligation for notification and recommendations for containment and infection control measures, should be put in place (Tacconelli et al. 2014).

The aim of *antimicrobial stewardship* is to limit the negative impact of MDR pathogens on patients' outcome, and its *main elements* are detailed in Table 27.2.

Successful implementation of antimicrobial stewardship is based on a multidisciplinary approach and close collaboration between the treating haematologists, microbiology laboratory and infectious diseases consultation service, including infection control unit, hospital pharmacy and hospital authorities who should recognize that this is an important step in high-quality management of infectious complications after HSCT.

Surveillance of effectiveness of infection control practices should be put in place, with regular monitoring of adherence. In case of contact-transmission pathogens, such as *Clostridium difficile* or MDR bacteria, laboratory data should be regularly analysed to detect any trends indicating possible increase in transmission.

Table 27.2 Main elements of antimicrobial stewardship program

1. Regularly updated (e.g. every 6–12 months) surveillance of local epidemiology of infections in HSCT recipients, through reports on:
   (a) Resistance rates to main antibiotics in top 10 most frequent pathogens
   (b) Data on antibiotic consumption
   (c) Data on patient outcomes in case of most frequent/difficult infections
2. Implementation of updated diagnostic methods and prompt reporting of microbiologic results by the laboratory in order to provide clinicians with
   (a) Correct and timely diagnosis (e.g. of viral or fungal infections or *Clostridium difficile*, which may allow to avoid unnecessary antibiotic therapy)
   (b) Rapid results of antimicrobial susceptibility testing to allow choosing the best targeted antibiotic therapy
3. Promoting appropriate antibiotic use, for example
   (a) Implementing timely de-escalation or discontinuation of antibiotic treatment, particularly during neutropenia
   (b) Appropriate dosing for different indications
   (c) Optimized infusion strategies for time- and dose-dependent molecules, e.g. use of extended or continuous infusion of time-dependent molecules such as beta-lactams
4. Establishing and regularly updating protocols for prevention and treatment of infections, e.g. identifying antibiotic and antifungal regimens for empirical therapy in accordance with local epidemiology (e.g. prevalence of extended spectrum beta-lactamase (ESBL) producing Enterobacteriaceae, methicillin-resistant staphylococci, azole-resistant aspergilli, etc.)

27.5 HSCT Environment

Flowers, fountains, water leaks and water-retaining bath toys carry the risk of *water-associated infections* with Gram-negative bacilli such as *Pseudomonas aeruginosa* or *Legionella* and thus should be avoided in the areas where severely immunocompromised patients are being cared for (Yokoe et al. 2009). In addition, there are issues specific for HSCT recipients, such as room ventilation, intensified protective measures applied during hospital construction and renovations, avoidance of contact with soil (including potted plants) and avoidance of dust both permanently (e.g. non-carpeting and no porous surfaces) and while cleaning, all aimed at decreasing the risk of invasive aspergillosis (Yokoe et al. 2009).

CIBMTR/ASBMT/EBMT global recommendations on protective environment concerning hospital *room design and ventilation* are available (Yokoe et al. 2009). Briefly, allo-HSCT recipients should ideally be placed in protective environment rooms that incorporate several features including central or point-of-use HEPA (high-efficiency particulate air) filters with 99.97% efficiency for removing particles ≤0.3 μm in diameter and ≥12 air exchanges/hours, with directed airflow and consistent positive air pressure differential between the patient's room and the hallway ≥2.5 Pa. All these measures remove airborne fungal spores and are aimed at preventing airborne infections with filamentous fungi such as aspergilli. The efficacy of protective isolation measures in case of auto-HSCT recipients is less well established.

Currently *HEPA-filtered rooms* are probably available in almost all centres, while few centresfulfilled all the CIBMTR/ASBMT/EBMT requirements. However, the knowledge on the details and maintenance of protective environments in the HSCT setting was recently found inadequate, requiring education efforts and cooperation with hospital infection control and the hospital maintenance services (Styczynski et al. 2018).

During *construction and renovations*, due to high density of fungal spores, protective environmental measures are particularly important, and mould-control measures should be intensified and filtration efficiency should be monitored frequently to best determine appropriate time for replacement. Specific recommendations are available and should be followed (Sehulster et al. 2004). For example, construction and renovation areas should have negative air pressure relative to HSCT patient care areas to ensure that air flows from patient care areas toward construction areas, and a portable, industrial-grade HEPA filter should be used between a construction zone and the HSCT unit if a large area is under construction and negative pressure differential cannot be guaranteed. In addition, HSCT recipients may benefit from wearing N95 respirators outside HEPA-filtered areas, particularly during ongoing constructions, since unlike surgical masks, higher efficiency ones offer protection against *Aspergillus* spores. Active monitoring of cases of invasive mould infections should be performed in order to detect any possible outbreak.

27.6 Food Safety in Transplant Recipients

Drinking *water* should be safe; thus boiled or bottled water is to be preferred. Tap water in highly populated areas is usually regarded as safe from bacterial contamination because regularly tested for it. However, it may still contain *Cryptosporidiums*. Water from private wells should be avoided.

The use of *low-microbial diet*, which prohibits fresh fruits and vegetables and unprocessed food, did not result in a decreased incidence of infections in neutropenic patients (Sonbol et al. 2015; van Dalen et al. 2016). Standard food safety practices that emphasize safe handling and washing or thoroughly cooking food were found to be just as safe and produced no increase in infection rates or incidence of neutropenic fever. Similarly, to other immunocompromised patients, HSCT recipients should avoid foods possibly contaminated by *Listeria monocytogenes*, *Campylobacter jejuni*, *Salmonella enteritidis*, *Toxoplasma gondii*, etc. *Main high-risk foods* to avoid include:

- Raw or undercooked meat, poultry, fish or shellfish
- Refrigerated smoked fish
- Unpasteurized milk
- Foods with raw or undercooked eggs
- Unwashed fruits and vegetables
- Raw sprouts
- Soft cheeses made from unpasteurized milk like brie, camembert and blue-veined and fresh cheese (can be eaten if cooked)
- Hot dogs, deli meats and luncheon meats that have not been reheated to steaming hot or to 75 °C
- Unsafe water and ice made of it

Food safety practices for food handling should be followed, and specific information for cancer patients is available online (https://www.fda.gov/downloads/Food/FoodborneIllnessContaminants/

UCM312793.pdf). Too restrictive diet recommendations, in the absence of the clear benefit of avoiding foods other than abovementioned, may have negative impact on patient's nutritional status and/or quality of life.

Key Points

- General guidelines for preventing healthcare-associated infections should be followed, and hand hygiene is the single most effective measure.
- Mandatory isolation procedures comprise Standard Precautions and Transmission-Based Precautions if appropriate: airborne, contact or droplets.
- Specific recommendations on ventilation, room design and protective environment during construction/renovation are provided to protect HSCT from transmission of spores of filamentous fungi, mainly *Aspergillus*.
- Protocols for prevention of colonization and infection with multidrug-resistant bacteria should be put in place, particularly in centres where these bacteria are already present.
- Antimicrobial stewardship program should be implemented in every centre to promote optimal use of antibiotics.
- Standard food safety practices should be applied, and only selected foods should be avoided (e.g. raw/undercook/underheated meat, fish or eggs, unpasteurized milk, unwashed fruits and vegetables, unsafe water).

References

Abad C, Fearday A, Safdar N. Adverse effects of isolation in hospitalised patients: a systematic review. J Hosp Infect. 2010;76:97–102.

Bilinski J, Grzesiowski P, Sorensen N, et al. Fecal microbiota transplantation in patients with blood disorders inhibits gut colonization with antibiotic-resistant bacteria: results of a prospective, single-center study. Clin Infect Dis. 2017;65:364–70.

Centers for Disease Control and Prevention. Guideline for hand hygiene in health-care settings: recommendations of the Healthcare Infection Control Practices Advisory Committee and the HICPAC/SHEA/APIC/IDSA Hand Hygiene Task Force. MMWR Recomm Rep. 2002;51(RR16):1.

Freifeld AG, Bow EJ, Sepkowitz KA, et al. Clinical practice guideline for the use of antimicrobial agents in neutropenic patients with cancer: 2010 update by the Infectious Diseases Society of America. Clin Infect Dis. 2011;52:427–31.

Girmenia C, Viscoli C, Piciocchi A, et al. Management of carbapenem resistant Klebsiella pneumoniae infections in stem cell transplant recipients: an Italian multidisciplinary consensus statement. Haematologica. 2015;100:e375.

Gyssens IC, Kern WV, Livermore DM, ECIL-4, a joint venture of EBMT, EORTC, ICHS and ESGICH of ESCMID. The role of antibiotic stewardship in limiting antibacterial resistance among hematology patients. Haematologica. 2013;98:1821–5.

Sehulster LM, Chinn RYW, Arduino MJ, et al. Guidelines for environmental infection control in health-care facilities. Recommendations from CDC and the Healthcare Infection Control Practices Advisory Committee (HICPAC). Chicago: American Society for Healthcare Engineering/American Hospital Association; 2004.

Siegel JD, Rhinehart E, Jackson M, Chiarello L, Healthcare Infection Control Practices Advisory Committee. Guideline for isolation precautions: preventing transmission of infectious agents in healthcare settings. 2007. http://www.cdc.gov/ncidod/dhqp/pdf/isolation2007.pdf.

Sonbol MG, Firwana B, Diab M, et al. The effect of a neutropenic diet on infection and mortality rates in cancer patients: a meta-analysis. Nutr Cancer. 2015;67:1230–8.

Styczynski J, Tridello G, Donnelly P, et al. Protective environment for hematopoietic cell transplant (HSCT) recipients: the Infectious Diseases Working Party EBMT analysis of global recommendations on health-care facilities. Bone Marrow Transplant. 2018;53:1131. https://doi.org/10.1038/s41409-018-0141-5.

Tacconelli E, Cataldo MA, Dancer SJ, et al. ESCMID guidelines for the management of the infection control measures to reduce transmission of multidrug-resistant Gram-negative bacteria in hospitalized patients. Clin Microbiol Infect. 2014;20(Suppl 1):1–55.

Tomblyn M, Chiller T, Einsele H, et al. Guidelines for preventing infectious complications among hematopoietic cell transplantation recipients: a global perspective. Biol Blood Marrow Transplant. 2009;15:1143–38.

van Dalen EC, Mank A, Leclercq E, et al. Low bacterial diet versus control diet to prevent infection in cancer patients treated with chemotherapy causing episodes of neutropenia. Cochrane Database Syst Rev. 2016;4:CD006247.

Yokoe D, Casper C, Dubberke E, et al. Infection prevention and control in health-care facilities in which hematopoietic cell transplant recipients are treated. Bone Marrow Transplant. 2009;44:495–7.

28 General Management of the Patient: Specific Aspects of Children

Francesca Riccardi and Elio Castagnola

28.1 Introduction

Many of the conditions requiring allo-HSCT and related complications are similar in adults and children and are covered in other chapters of this handbook.

However, since pediatric age is a continuum between newborns and adults, there are at least two aspects, psychological and infectious disease issues, that may require a dedicated approach for the following reason:

1. *Psychological aspects*. Childhood encompasses different ages and consequently different cognitive, decisional, and emotional capacities that make psychological intervention far more faceted than in adults. In addition, psychological intervention should also take in charge at higher extent the needs and the expectations of the patient's family.
2. *Infectious diseases*. Data on epidemiology and management of infections in children are far less numerous and consistent than in adults. In addition most of the available data are derived from studies in adults, and they cannot always simply be transposed to children for an effective application.

In the following paragraphs, we will analyze the specific approaches related to these aspects in children undergoing HSCT.

28.2 Psychological Aspects (Table 28.1)

Children who undergo HSCT experience several *numerous psychological reactions*: anxiety, depression, behavioral and social problems, and post-traumatic stress symptoms. In the stages before HSCT, anxiety increases, and the emotional distress continues to rise until 1 week after transplant, whereas depression is heightened by hospitalization and physical isolation. Age (<7 years) and severity of the illness influence the level of emotional reactions. Especially, children <5 years are more likely to withdraw and to be deprived of their self-help skills and even of their mobility and speech skills. The level of pre-HSCT emotional disturbance is strongly predictive of post-HSCT emotional functioning; therefore early intervention appears of critical importance (Packman et al. 2010).

The most studied psychological treatments for children with cancer are *cognitive behavioral therapies* (CBT) that are considered to improve emotional adjustment, compliance with medical

F. Riccardi
Consultant Hematology Unit, Hemato-Oncology and SCT Pole, Istituto Giannina Gaslini, Genoa, Italy

E. Castagnola (✉)
Infectious Diseases Unit, Department of Pediatrics, Istituto Giannina Gaslini, Genoa, Italy
e-mail: eliocastagnola@gaslini.org

E. Carreras et al. (eds.), *The EBMT Handbook*, https://doi.org/10.1007/978-3-030-02278-5_28

Table 28.1 Main psychological problems in HSCT in pediatric age

	Problems	Suggested intervention
Patients	*Emotional disturbance*: anxiety, depression, behavioral and social problems, post traumatic stess symptoms *HRQOL*: compromission is evident before and soon after HSCT. Start to improve between 4 and 6 months after HSCT *Neurocognitive area*: impairment is associated with younger age at diagnosis and treatment. Adaptive skills and social competence are affected in the first year after HSCT	– Individual therapies to improve emotional adjustment, compliance with medical treatment and behavioral problems associated with HSCT – Guided imagery, distraction, rhythmic breathing, relaxation to decrease the distress due to medical procedures – Clinical assessment is recommended: before the recovery period 1 year after HSCT annually thereafter
Siblings	Post-traumatic stress reactions, anxiety, low self-esteem, feelings of guilt and school problems	Open communication Facilitate the access of sibling to the hospital
Parents	Parental distress, anxiety, depression, post traumatic stress symptoms. Take care of additional burden due to medical complications	Familial intervention Crisis intervention approach Stress and coping models

treatment, and behavioral problems associated with HSCT. Effective interventions are clearly largely dependent on social skills and emotional well-being. Techniques such as guided imagery, distraction, rhythmic breathing, and relaxation are commonly used to decrease the acute psychological distress due to medical procedures including HSCT (Packman et al. 2010). Psychiatric assessment and pharmacological approach should be advisable when other approaches are not sufficient for children with preexisting psychiatric diagnoses who are vulnerable to worsening of the psychiatric disorders (Steele et al. 2015).

Health-related quality of life (HRQOL) compromission is usually evident prior to and soon after transplant and starts to improve between 4 and 6 months after HSCT. Child psychosocial problems, caregiver stress, and social support emerged as significant predictors of physical and emotional outcome after discharging. Indeed, high level of stress of caregivers and/or low perceived social support was associated with higher risk of psychologically complicated outcome. On the contrary emotional and behavioral problems of the child at discharge were not associated to substantially slower improvements in overall HRQOL that usually occurred between 3 and 9 months after discharge. This is because reestablishment of usual activities that were precluded during HSCT outbalances emotional problems due to the return to "normal" life (Loiselle et al. 2016).

As for neurocognitive functions, long-term studies are not fully concordant, but some findings (Kelly et al. 2018) seem to suggest that *children's intelligence quotient* (IQ) scores post HSCT are inferior to those before HSCT. In particular adaptive skills and social competence domains are affected in the first year after HSCT and so do self-esteem and emotional well-being. Impairment in neurocognitive area is associated with younger age at diagnosis and treatment and may occur even if school performance remains in normal ranges. Children may also experience decrements in executive functioning skills, like deficits in fine motor abilities usually seen in patients who received cranial irradiation at younger age. Clinical assessment is recommended before the recovery period, at 1 year after HSCT and annually thereafter, or, at least, at the beginning of each stage of education. In the post-HSCT assessment, clinicians should also consider the impact of factors such as isolation, missed schooling, and impaired socialization with peers. Encouraging results in cognitive rehabilitation come from intensive therapist-delivered training since the systematic use of computer-based training appeared to improve working memory and processing speed (Kelly et al. 2018).

Siblings, either donors or non-donors, are at risk of developing emotional disturbances such as post-traumatic stress reactions, anxiety, low self-esteem, feelings of guilt, and school problems. Indeed, researches are needed to identify the most useful intervention to cope with negative effects of HSCT on siblings (Packman et al. 2010; Gerhardt et al. 2015). Currently adopted strategies include open communication about the patient's medical situation and transplant process, favoring the idea of accepting help from friends and family members, and facilitating the access of sibling to the hospital arranging visits in a way that they look like a special event or assigning a sibling a special role (Gerhardt et al. 2015; White et al. 2017).

Parental distress, anxiety, and depression levels are often increased as a result of their child undergoing HSCT. The distress and anxiety may be even greater for parents whose healthy child also becomes part of the HSCT process through donating his/her marrow (Packman et al. 2010). Significant determinants of parental distress include prior parent and patient experience of distress associated with the child's illness, the child's tendency of internalizing or externalizing behavior problems, the family's attitude to provide support, and a parental proneness toward avoidant coping behaviors (Phipps et al. 2005). Parents mostly experience post-traumatic stress symptoms that manifest in cognitive and behavioral efforts to avoid reminders of the HSCT and intrusive thoughts about it (Virtue et al. 2014).

Early and late HSCT medical complications significantly increase the psychological involvement of the caregiver. HSCT healthcare professionals should also take care of the additional burden that complications generate on the parents and should proactively link parents to resources aimed to help them coping with this extra load (Heinze et al. 2015). Despite the recognized needs, very few caregivers seek out psychological service. The most frequent barriers are that clinicians prioritize medical patient's needs and cover tasks usually deemed to social support, lack of adequate locations, and embarrassment about seeking psychological counseling (Devine et al. 2016).

Familial interventions aimed to enhance protective factors, improve communication, and decrease parental anxiety and depression are crucial. In this respect, cancer-specific psychological interventions may serve as a template to delivering HSCT-tailored interventions (Packman et al. 2010). Traditional individual therapy is very useful even if in adapted forms. Usually it includes crisis intervention approach and stress and coping models to reduce HSCT-related stress. CBT can encompass different strategies such as the expression of emotional feelings, identification of distorted automatic thoughts, the use of problem-focused coping skills, discussion of psychosocial impact on the family, and training in assertiveness and communication skills (Steele et al. 2015).

28.3 Infectious Diseases

Infections represent one of the most frequently occurring and feared complications of HSCT.

Antibacterial prophylaxis for febrile neutropenia is frequently administered in pediatric HSCT but never specifically analyzed in a randomized clinical trial. Its use can be associated with selection of resistant strains.

In the pre-engraftment phases, *empirical antibiotic therapy* for febrile neutropenia could be represented by monotherapy with an anti-*Pseudomonas* beta-lactam, but it is mandatory its adaptation to local epidemiological data (Lehrnbecher et al. 2017). Moreover, empirical antibiotic therapy should be considered also after engraftment because of the important risk of morbidity and mortality. Antibiotic-resistant pathogens represent a new challenge because of the high mortality rates (>50%) observed in pediatric HSCT (Girmenia et al. 2015; Caselli et al. 2016).

Clostridium difficile may represent a cause of severe, and sometimes recurrent, disease, but it must be kept in mind that children aged below 2 years may harbor this pathogen in their intestinal tract (Lees et al. 2016;

Enoch et al. 2011) and that other pathogens (e.g., viruses or *Cryptosporidium*) could be the cause of gastroenteritis (Castagnola et al. 2016). Table 28.2 summarizes antibacterial drugs for prophylaxis and treatment of invasive diseases.

Invasive fungal disease (IFD) is associated with high mortality in pediatric HSCT (Cesaro et al. 2017; Castagnola et al. 2018b). Increasing age has been identified as a risk factor for the development of IFD (Fisher et al. 2017), but recent multivariable analyses showed that age is no longer significant in the presence of severe acute or chronic extensive GvHD or in cases of primary graft failure or rejection (Castagnola et al. 2014, 2018a).

Primary prophylaxis should be implemented in the highest-risk groups like patients with primary graft failure or rejection, or with severe acute or chronic extensive GvHD, or in centers with high incidence of IFD (Groll et al. 2014).

Table 28.2 Prophylaxis and therapy of invasive bacterial infections in children undergoing allogeneic HSCT

	Prophylaxis for febrile neutropenia
Ciprofloxacin	Oral or IV until neutrophil recovery or start of empirical therapy for febrile neutropenia *Notes*: Never analyzed in a randomized clinical trial in HSCT. Risk of selection of resistant strains
Amoxicillin-clavulanate	Oral or IV until neutrophil recovery or start of empirical therapy for febrile neutropenia *Notes*: Never analyzed in a randomized clinical trial in HSCT. Risk of selection of resistant strains
	Empirical therapy for febrile neutropenia, or fever after engraftment, especially in presence of GvHD
Pipera-tazo	100 mg/kg (max 4000 mg) of piperacillin q6h
Cefepime	33 mg/kg (max 2000 mg) q8h
Ceftazidime	33 mg/kg (max 2000 mg)
Meropenem	20 mg/kg (max 1000 mg) q8h *Notes*: Risk of selection of resistant Gram-negatives or *C. difficile* associated disease. Higher doses could be necessary for treatment of carbapenem resistant pathogen when MIC is ≤16 mg/L. For higher MIC values carbapenems are not indicated
Combination therapy	Aminoglycoside [e.g. amikacin 20 mg/kg (max 1500 mg) q24h] + beta-lactam *Notes*: According to local susceptibility, and proportions of resistance to beta-lactams indicated for monotherapy
	Documented infections: according with localizations and antibiotic susceptibility tests
Antibiotics for resistant pathogens, combinations could be needed	*Gram-positives*: vancomycin, teicoplanin daptomycin, linezolid, tigecycline, fosfomycin *Gram-negatives*: ciprofloxacin, colistin, tigecycline (not active against P. aeruginosas), fosfomycin, ceftazidime-avibactam (not active against metallo beta-lactamases), ceftolozane-tazobactam (not active against carbapenemases) *Notes*: – According to ATB susceptibility tests in documented infections – Beta-lactams should be preferred to glycopeptides in case of infections due to oxacillin-susceptible staphylococci – Do not use empirical glycopeptides for persistent fever without signs of localizations attributable to Gram-positives or high suspicion or risk by patient's history or local epidemiology of oxacillin-resistant staphylococci or ampicillin-resistant enterococci – For vancomycin resistant staphylococci or enterococci daptomycin, linezolid or tigecycline could represent therapeutic options – No PK data for ceftazidime-avibactam or ceftolozane-tazobactam available in children
	Clostridium difficile associated disease
Vancomycin, metronidazole, fidaxomicin	Oral therapy, vancomycin 10 mg/kg (max 125 mg) q6h as 1st choice Fidaxomicin is not registered for <18 years *Notes*: No data are available for fecal transplantation in immunocompromised children. Different dosages proposed for recurrent disease

MIC minimally inhibitory concentration, *GvHD* graft vs. host disease, *Pipera-tazo* Piperacillin-Tazobactam

Diagnosis of IFD is based on isolation of fungal pathogens from cultures of sterile sites or tissue invasion demonstrated by histology or by the presence of fungal antigens in blood or cerebrospinal fluid or bronchoalveolar lavage, associated with suggestive imaging (Castagnola et al. 2016; Tomà et al. 2016) in children with a compatible clinical picture. Detection of galactomannan and 1-3-beta-D-glucan is widely used for the diagnosis of (probable) IFD also in children. However, a recent meta-analysis (Lehrnbecher et al. 2016) and new clinical data (Calitri et al. 2017) showed highly variable and generally poor sensitivity, specificity, and predictive values of these tests, especially when used for screening. PCR should still be considered as an investigative test (Lehrnbecher et al. 2016). Also, for the use of antifungal drugs, there are caveats.

Treatment: Voriconazole frequently needs to be administered at higher dosages in the youngest patients (<5 years) to achieve and maintain effective plasma concentrations (Xu et al. 2016; Soler-Palacın et al. 2012; Neely et al. 2015; Castagnola and Mesini 2018). Inflammation, steroid administration, or obesity can further modify its concentrations (Castagnola and Mesini 2018; Natale et al. 2017) and so do genetic factors (Teusink et al. 2016). Finally, severe cutaneous adverse events can be observed also in children when voriconazole is administered for prolonged periods, especially in concomitance with sun exposure (Goyal et al. 2014; Bernhard et al. 2012). Posaconazole oral suspension has variable absorption implying the risk of sub-therapeutic concentrations (Jancel et al. 2017), especially in the presence of intestinal acute GvHD (Heinz et al. 2016). This can be at least partially avoided by fatty meal and/or other "bundle" measures or using doses based on body surface area (Castagnola and Mesini 2018). Posaconazole tablets have no absorption problems, and pediatric pharmacological data show that their use determines effective concentrations also in children (Castagnola and Mesini 2018). However, tablets are slightly less than 2 cm long and should be swallowed whole with water and should not be crushed, chewed, or broken (EMA 2018) thus limiting their use in youngest patients, but alternate day administration could represent an effective strategy (Mesini et al. 2018). Triazoles have also many drug interactions that must be kept in mind during their use. For all these reasons, therapeutic drug monitoring is mandatory both for prophylactic and therapeutic uses (Groll et al. 2014).

Pneumocystis jirovecii pneumonia is a severe, life-threatening fungal infection in allo-HSCT recipients. Primary prophylaxis is highly recommended in children undergoing allo-HSCT at least in the post-engraftment. Prophylaxis is highly effective, and in case of documented failure, especially in adolescents, compliance must be checked (Castagnola and Mesini 2018). Table 28.3 summarizes dosages of drugs for prevention or treatment of IFD in children.

Viral Infections No major differences between children and adults are expected. However, primary viral infections are more frequent in pediatrics, and in this setting, it must be stressed that healthy household contacts and healthcare workers may represent important sources, with possible hospital spreading.

Screening and Isolation Application of bundle procedures for patients as well as correct hand hygiene, correct vascular access manipulation, correct isolation procedures according to the via of pathogen spreading, and the use of HEPA filters can be all of great utility in the prevention of difficult to treat infections in HSCT.

Vaccines represent also an important tool for prevention of viral and bacterial (*S. pneumoniae*) infections in the post transplant setting.

Table 28.3 Prophylaxis and therapy of IFI in children undergoing allogeneic HSCT

Voriconazole

Spectrum of activity: molds, yeasts

Prophylaxis: No evidence to support this indication in children. Dosage in children aged 2 to <12 years or 12–14 years with weight <50 kg: 9 mg/kg q12h; In children aged ≥15 years or 12–14 years and with weight ≥50 kg: 4 mg/kg q12h (1st day, 6 mg/kg). Target concentration >1 and <6 mg/L at steady state

Therapy: Dosage in children aged 2 to <12 years or 12–14 years with weight <50 kg: 9 mg/kg q12h; In children aged ≥15 years or 12–14 years with weight ≥50 kg: 4 mg/kg q12h (1st day, 6 mg/kg). Target concentration >1 and <6 mg/L at steady state.

Notes: Measure serum concentrations (mandatory) before the 5th dose (2 days of treatment); before the 5th dose following any dose adjustment; routinely every 1–2 weeks after achievement of steady-state; when interacting drugs start or stop in case of potential clinical or laboratory manifestations of toxicity

Posaconazole

Spectrum of activity: molds, yeasts

Prophylaxis: Oral suspension: 120 mg/m^2 q8h for children who can not swallow tablets. Tablets: loading dose of 300 mg q12h (1st day) then maintenance 300 q24h, independently from meal. According with BW:

Body weight	*Load (1st day)*	*Maintenance*
15–21 kg	150 mg q12h	100 mg q24h
22–30 kg	150 mg q12h	150 mg q24h
31–35 kg	200 mg q12h	200 mg q24h
35–40 kg	250 mg q12h	250 mg q24h
>40 kg or 13 years	300 mg q12h	300 mg q24h

Target concentration for prophylaxis 0.7 mg/L at steady state. Not registered for use <18 years

Therapy: Oral suspension: 120 mg/m^2 q8h for children who cannot swallow tablets. Tablets: loading dose of 300 mg q12h (1st day) then maintenance 300 q24h, independently from meal. According with BW:

Body weight	*Load (1st day)*	*Maintenance*
15–21 kg	150 mg q12h	100 mg q24h
22–30 kg	150 mg q12h	150 mg q24h
31–35 kg	200 mg q12h	200 mg q24h
35–40 kg	250 mg q12h	250 mg q24h
>40 kg or 13 years	300 mg q12h	300 mg q24h

Target concentration for therapy ≥1 mg/L at steady state. Not registered for use <18 years

Notes: When using oral suspension remove acid suppression if possible and use "posaconazole bundle":

- ascorbic acid 500 mg per os with each dose of posaconazole
- 120–180 mL of carbonated soda beverage (i.e.: cola or ginger ale) or acidic fruit juice (e.g.: cranberry or orange juice) with each dose of posaconazole
- heavy snack or food with each dose, preferably high-fat, including
- use a more fractionated schedule (q 6-8h)

With any formulation measure serum concentrations (mandatory): 7 days after initiation of therapy or following dose adjustment or when interacting drugs start or stop or in case of concerns about GI absorption, especially for prolonged periods of time or in case of potential clinical or laboratory manifestations of toxicity

Itraconazole

Spectrum of activity: molds, yeasts

Prophylaxis: Moderate evidence to support a recommendation in children. Oral solution 2.5 mg/kg per day orally (in children aged ≥2 years) q12h, with empty stomach. Target concentration for prophylaxis 0.5 mg/L at steady state

Notes: Measure serum concentrations. For oral administration use oral solution. Administer with empty stomach

Fluconazole

Spectrum of activity: yeast

Prophylaxis: Not highly recommendable because of the narrow spectrum (yeasts only). 6 mg/kg/ day (maximum 400 mg/ day) intravenously or orally q24h

Therapy: 10–20 mg/kg/day, maximum 800 mg/day) intravenously or orally q24h

Liposomal amphotericin B

Spectrum of activity: molds, yeasts

Prophylaxis: Moderate evidence to support intravenous, no evidence for nebulized administration Intravenous: 1 mg/kg q24h every other day or 2.5 mg/kg q24h twice weekly; Nebulized: 25 mg q12h on 2 consecutive days per week associated with fluconazole

Therapy: Intravenous: 3–5 mg/kg according to etiology. Doses up to 10 mg/kg have been proposed for mucormycosis

Table 28.3 (continued)

Micafungin
Spectrum of activity: yeast (not *Cryptococcus*) (molds?) *Prophylaxis*: Not highly recommendable because of the narrow spectrum (yeasts only) 1 mg/kg (in children weighing ≥50 kg, 50 mg) q24h *Therapy*: 2–4 mg/kg (max 100 mg/kg) q24h
Isavuconazole
Spectrum of action: molds, yeasts *Prophylaxis*: No evidence for this indication. No data for pediatric use and dosage. Not registered <18 years *Therapy*: No data for pediatric use and dosage. Not registered <18 years
Corimoxazole, dapsone, atovaquone, pentamidine
Spectrum of action: *P. Jirovecii* *Prophylaxis*: Cotrimoxazole 1st choice: 2.5 mg/kg of trimethoprim (max 180 mg) q12h, 1–3 days/week *Therapy*: Cotrimoxazole 1st choice: 5 mg/kg of trimethoprim q8h *Notes*: In case op pneumonia add prednisone at 2 mg/kg/day. Nebulized pentamidine requires special tools for administration

IFI invasive fungal infection

Key Points

Many of the conditions requiring allo-HSCT and related complications are similar in adults and children and are covered in other chapters of this handbook.

However, since pediatric age is a continuum between newborns and adults, there are at least two aspects:

- Psychological aspects. Childhood encompasses different ages and consequently different cognitive, decisional, and emotional capacities that make psychological intervention far more faceted than in adults.
- Infectious diseases. Data on epidemiology and management of infections in children are far less numerous and consistent than in adults. Despite that there are many differential aspects in its management.

References

Bernhard S, Kernland Lang K, et al. Voriconazole-induced phototoxicity in children. Pediatr Infect Dis J. 2012;31:769–71.

Calitri C, Caviglia I, Cangemi G, et al. Performance of 1,3-β-D-glucan for diagnosing invasive fungal diseases in children. Mycoses. 2017;60:789–95.

Caselli D, Cesaro S, Fagioli F, et al. Incidence of colonization and bloodstream infection with carbapenem-resistant Enterobacteriaceae in children receiving antineoplastic chemotherapy in Italy. Infect Dis (Lond). 2016;48:152–5.

Castagnola E, Bagnasco F, Amoroso L, et al. Role of management strategies in reducing mortality from invasive fungal disease in children with cancer or receiving hemopoietic stem cell transplant: a single center 30-year experience. Pediatr Infect Dis J. 2014;33:233–7.

Castagnola E, Bagnasco F, Menoni S, et al. Risk factors associated with development and mortality by invasive fungal diseases in pediatric allogeneic stem cell transplantation. A pediatric subgroup analysis of data from a prospective study of the Gruppo Italiano Trapianto di Midollo Osseo (GITMO). Bone Marrow Transplat. 2018;53:1193. https://doi.org/10.1038/s41409-018-0160-2.

Castagnola E, Mesini A. Antifungal prophylaxis in children receiving antineoplastic chemotherapy. Curr Fungal Infect Rep. 2018;12:78. https://doi.org/10.1007/s12281-018-0311-3.

Castagnola E, Ruberto E, Guarino A. Gastrointestinal and liver infections in children undergoing antineoplastic chemotherapy in the years 2000. World J Gastroenterol. 2016;22:5853–66.

Cesaro S, Tridello G, Castagnola E, et al. Retrospective study on the incidence and outcome of proven and probable invasive fungal infections in high-risk pediatric onco-hematological patients. Eur J Haematol. 2017;99:240–8.

Devine KA, Manne SL, Mee L, et al. Barriers to psychological care among primary caregivers of children undergoing hematopoietic stem cell transplantation. Support Care Cancer. 2016;24:2235–42.

Enoch DA, Butler MJ, Pai S, et al. Clostridium difficile in children: colonisation and disease. J Infect. 2011;63:105–13.

European Medicine Agency. Posaconazole summary of product characteristics. www.ema.europa.eu. Last check 15 Mar 2018.

Fisher BT, Robinson PD, Lehrnbecher T, et al. Risk factors for invasive fungal disease in pediatric cancer and hematopoietic stem cell transplantation: a systematic review. J Pediatr Infect Dis Soc. 2017. https://doi.org/10.1093/jpids/pix030. [Epub ahead of print].

Gerhardt CA, Lehmann V, Long KA, Alderfer MA. Supporting siblings as a standard of care in pediatric oncology. Pediatr Blood Cancer. 2015;62(Suppl 5):S750–804.

Girmenia C, Rossolini GM, Piciocchi A, et al. Infections by carbapenem-resistant Klebsiella pneumoniae in SCT recipients: a nationwide retrospective survey from Italy. Bone Marrow Transplant. 2015;50:282–8.

Goyal RK, Gehris RP, Howrie D. Phototoxic dermatoses in pediatric BMT patients receiving voriconazole. Pediatr Blood Cancer. 2014;61:1325–8.

Groll AH, Castagnola E, Cesaro S, et al. Fourth European Conference on Infections in Leukaemia (ECIL-4): guidelines for diagnosis, prevention, and treatment of invasive fungal diseases in paediatric patients with cancer or allogeneic haemopoietic stem-cell transplantation. Lancet Oncol. 2014;15(8):e327–40.

Heinz WJ, Cabanillas Stanchi KM, Klinker H, et al. Posaconazole plasma concentration in pediatric patients receiving antifungal prophylaxis after allogeneic hematopoietic stem cell transplantation. Med Mycol. 2016;54:128–37.

Heinze KE, Rodday AM, Nolan MT, et al. The impact of pediatric blood and marrow transplant on parents: introduction of the parent impact scale. Health Qual Life Outcomes. 2015;13:46.

Jancel T, Shaw PA, Hallahan CW, et al. Therapeutic drug monitoring of posaconazole oral suspension in paediatric patients younger than 13 years of age: a retrospective analysis and literature review. J Clin Pharm Ther. 2017;42:75–9.

Kelly DL, Buchbinder D, Duarte RF, et al. Neurocognitive dysfunction in hematopoietic cell transplant recipients: expert review from the late effects and Quality of Life Working Committee of the Center for International Blood and Marrow Transplant Research and complications and Quality of Life Working Party of the European Society for Blood and Marrow Transplantation. Biol Blood Marrow Transplant. 2018;24:228–41.

Lees EA, Miyajima F, Pirmohamed M, Carroll ED. The role of Clostridium difficile in the paediatric and neonatal gut—a narrative review. Eur J Clin Microbiol Infect Dis. 2016;35:1047–57.

Lehrnbecher T, Robinson PD, Fisher BT, et al. Galactomannan, β-D-glucan, and polymerase chain reaction–based assays for the diagnosis of invasive fungal disease in pediatric cancer and hematopoietic stem cell transplantation: a systematic review and meta-analysis. Clin Infect Dis. 2016;63:1340–8.

Lehrnbecher T, Robinson P, Fisher B, et al. Guideline for the management of fever and neutropenia in children with cancer and hematopoietic stem-cell transplantation recipients: 2017 update. J Clin Oncol. 2017;35:2082–94.

Loiselle KA, Rausch JR, Bidwell S, et al. Predictors of health-related quality of life over time among pediatric hematopoietic stem cell transplant recipients. Pediatr Blood Cancer. 2016;63:1834–9.

Mesini A, Faraci M, Giardino S, et al.. Alternate day dosing of posaconazole tablets in children leads to efficient plasma levels. Eur J Haematol. 2018 Mar 15. https://doi.org/10.1111/ejh.13063. [Epub ahead of print].

Natale S, Bradley J, Huy Nguyen W, et al. Pediatric obesity: pharmacokinetic alterations and effects on antimicrobial dosing. Pharmacotherapy. 2017;37:361–78.

Neely M, Margol A, Fu X, et al. Achieving target voriconazole concentrations more accurately in children and adolescents. Antimicrob Agents Chemother. 2015;59:3090–7.

Packman W, Weber S, Wallace J, Bugescu N. Psychological effects of hematopoietic SCT on pediatric patients, siblings and parents: a review. Bone Marrow Transplant. 2010;45:1134–46.

Phipps S, Dunavant M, Lensing S, Rai SN. Psychosocial predictors of distress in parents of children undergoing stem cell or bone marrow transplantation. J Pediatr Psychol. 2005;30:139–53.

Soler-Palacın P, Frick MA, Martın-Nalda A, et al. Voriconazole drug monitoring in the management of invasive fungal infection in immunocompromised children: a prospective study. J Antimicrob Chemother. 2012;67:700–6.

Steele AC, Mullins LL, Mullins AJ, Muriel AC. Psychosocial interventions and therapeutic support as a standard of care in pediatric oncology. Pediatr Blood Cancer. 2015;62(Suppl 5):S585–618.

Teusink A, Vinks A, Zhang K, et al. Genotype-directed dosing leads to optimized voriconazole levels in pediatric patients receiving hematopoietic stem cell transplantation. Biol Blood Marrow Transplant. 2016;22(3):482–6. e-pub ahead of print 2015/12/01. https://doi.org/10.1016/j.bbmt.2015.11.011.

Tomà P, Bertaina A, Castagnola E, et al. Fungal infections of the lung in children. Pediatr Radiol. 2016;46:1856–65.

Virtue SM, Manne SL, Mee L, et al. Psychological distress and psychiatric diagnoses among primary caregivers of children undergoing hematopoietic stem cell transplant: an examination of prevalence, correlates, and racial/ethnic differences. Gen Hosp Psychiatry. 2014;36:620–6.

White TE, Hendershot KA, Dixon MD, et al. Family strategies to support siblings of pediatric hematopoietic stem cell transplant patients. Pediatrics. 2017;139(2):e20161057. e-pub ahead of print 2017/01/26. https://doi.org/10.1542/peds.2016-1057.

Xu G, Zhu L, Ge T, Liao S, Qi F. Pharmacokinetic/pharmacodynamic analysis of voriconazole against Candida spp. and Aspergillus spp. in children, adolescents and adults by Monte Carlo simulation. Int J Antimicrob Agents. 2016;47:439–45.

29 Vaccinations

Rafael de la Cámara

29.1 General Concepts

Vaccination should be considered a *routine practice for all HSCT receptors*, either autologous or allogeneic, adults or children. It should be implemented in all HSCT programs. Adult cover is particularly important as they represent 90% of HSCTs. To obtain this objective, the following are necessary:

- To have in place a standardized program specific for HSCT patients.
- The collaboration of the Preventive Department of the hospital and primary care physicians.
- The program must be simple, with a clear chronology, and convenient for the patient and physician (no increase in the number of visits).
- FACT-JACIE Standards (version 7.0, March 2018) require that policies/SOP are in place for post transplant vaccination schedules and indications.

The vaccination program should include not only the patient but also those who live with the patient and the healthcare workers (HCWs).

R. de la Cámara (✉)
Department of Hematology, Hospital de la Princesa, Madrid, Spain
e-mail: jrcamara@telefonica.net

There is no a unique vaccine schedule for all HSCT patients. Each center should discuss and adapt a specific vaccine program.

- The practical application of the immunization programs shows important variations across centers (Miller et al. 2017).
- Auto-HSCT is generally vaccinated with the schedule used for allogeneic patients with small differences (see Tables 29.1 and 29.2).

Reasons for universal vaccination of HSCT patients:

- *General interest*: as a general healthcare principle, all the population should be correctly vaccinated, including adults and of course HSCT patients. If an increasing collective of patients, like HSCT, is not well vaccinated, that can generate holes of immunity that can be a risk for the health of the general population.
- *Individual interest for each HSCT patient*: vaccination protects the patient against infections that can cause important morbi-mortality. There are frequent infections in HSCT that have safe vaccines (pneumococcus, influenza, HBV) and other rare infections associated with high mortality that have an unsatisfactory prevention/treatment but can be prevented by immunization (tetanus, diphtheria, measles, polio).

E. Carreras et al. (eds.), *The EBMT Handbook*, https://doi.org/10.1007/978-3-030-02278-5_29

Table 29.1 International consensus recommendations (Ljungman et al. 2009)

Vaccine	No. of doses	Time post-HSCT to initiate vaccine	Grading
Influenza (inactivated)	1 2 for children <9 years, or if <6 m from HSCT (C III)	4–6 months, yearly, lifelong seasonal vaccination	AII
Measles[a]	1 (2 in children)	24 months	AII children BII seronegative adults
Mumps[a]			CIII
Rubella[a] (in adults for sero(-) females with pregnancy potential)			BIII
Hepatitis B virus (HBV) (follow country recommendations for general population)[b]	3	6–12 months	BII
Human papillomavirus	Follow recommendations for general population in each country		CIII
Inactivated polio	3	6–12 months	BII
Pneumococcal conjugate (PCV)	3	3–6 months	BI
– polysaccharide pneumococcal vaccine (PPS)	1	6 months after last PCV	BII
– in case of GVHD, use PCV instead of PPS for this 4th dose	1		CIII
Meningococcal conjugate (follow country recommend for general population)	1	6–12 months	BII
Haemophilus influenzae conjugate	3	6–12 months	BII
Diphtheria-tetanus (DT preferred over Td)	3	6–12 months	BII
Pertussis (acellular) (DTaP preferred over Tdap)	3	6–12 months	CIII

[a]MMR. These vaccines are contraindicated (EIII) before 24 months post-HSCT or in case of active GVHD or IS. These vaccines are usually given together as a combination vaccine

[b]VHB. Vaccination is recommended for HBV surface Ag-negative or HBV core Ab-positive patients, as vaccination can reduce the risk of reverse seroconversion (BII). For HBV surface Ag-negative or HBV core Ab-negative HSCT patients, recommendations for the general population in their country of residence should be followed

29.2 General Principles of Vaccination in HSCT Patients

29.2.1 The Pretransplant Vaccination

The pretransplant vaccination is not effective to maintain a prolonged post transplant immunity. In other to protect the HSCT patient, a complete series of post transplant vaccinations is required. This is different from what is recommended for solid organ transplant (SOT) recipients for whom pretransplant vaccination is an essential part of the vaccination program. Post-HSCT patients should be viewed as "never vaccinated" regardless of the pre-HSCT vaccination history of the patient or the donor (Rubin et al. 2014).

29.2.2 The Pre-HSCT Immunity

The pre-HSCT immunity for a specific pathogen is not a reason to withhold vaccination after transplant. The majority of patients will lose their immunity after HSCT.

As general rule, *live vaccines should be considered contraindicated* (there are exceptions, see later). The inactivated, subunit, or protein/polysaccharide vaccines can be safely administered.

There are few randomized trials in HSCT patients, and many of the studies have been done in patients transplanted with BM/PB, using

Table 29.2 ECIL recommendations for allo-HSCT recipients (Cordonnier et al. 2017)

Vaccine	No. of doses[a]	Time post-HSCT to initiate vaccine	Grading
Influenza (inactivated)	1 (or 2, special cases)[b]	>6 months	AIIr
		As long as patient is judged to be IS	BIIr
		Yearly, lifelong from 3 months in case of a community outbreak	BIIr
Measles–mumps–rubella			
• Measles In sero(-) patients, with no GVHD, no IS, no REL of underlying disease, and no IGIV at least 8 months	1 (2 in children) MMR	≥24 months	BIIu
		≥12 months in case of measles outbreak in patients with low grade IS	CIII
• Rubella In sero(-) women and of childbearing potential, with same precautions as for measles vaccine	1 MMR	≥24 months	CIIu
Virus hepatitis B[c]			
• Sero(-) patients before HSCT and patients vaccinated pre-HSCT but lost their immunity at 6 months)	3[d]	6–12 months	BIIt
• Previously infected and anti-HBs <10 IU/L		6–12 months	BIII
• Sero(-) patients with a donor with positive anti HBc		Vaccine before transplant	BIII
Human papilloma virus (HPV) Follow recommendations for general population in each country	According to official label	From 6–12 months	BIIu
Inactivated polio	3[e]	6–12 months	BIIu
Live-attenuated varicella vaccine	1	Can be considered in sero(-) patients, with ALL the following: >24 m from HSCT, no GVHD, no IS, no REL of the underlying disease, and no IGIV in the last 8 months	BIIr
	2	The addition of a second dose in adults may be considered in patients who were sero(-) before HSCT or had no history of VZ infect	
Live-attenuated zoster vaccine	Not recommended		DIII
Pneumococcal conjugate (PCV)	3	3 months	AI
Polysaccharidic vaccine In case of GVHD, use PCV instead of PPS for this 4th dose (BIIr)	1	12 months (no earlier than 8 weeks after last PCV)	BI
Meningococcal conjugate (in accordance with country recommendations and local prevalence)	2	From 6 months	
		For men-C or tetravalent vaccine	BIIu
		For men-B vaccine	BIII
Haemophilus influenzae conjugate	3	3 months or 6 months	BIIr
Diphtheria-tetanus (DT is preferred to Td)	3[e]	From 6 months	BIu
Pertussis (acellular) (DTaP is preferred over Tdap)	3	From 6–12 months	CIII

[a]If not specified otherwise, the interval between dose is 1 month

[b]Influenza: A second dose of influenza vaccine, after 3–4 weeks from the first, may have a marginal benefit and should preferably be considered in patients with severe GVHD or low lymphocyte count (B II r) and also for the patients vaccinated early (from 3 months after transplant) (B II r). Children ≥6 months through 8 years, receiving influenza for the first time after transplant, should receive a second dose at least 4 weeks after the first dose

[c]HBV. After post transplant vaccination, if anti-HBs is <10 mIU/ml, an additional three doses should be considered, but the benefit of this second series of vaccination is uncertain. IDSA guidelines (Rubin et al. 2014) give the same recommendations (strong, low). For adolescents and adults, a high dose of vaccine (40 μg) is recommended for these booster doses (strong, low)

[d]Three doses: interval 0, 1, and 6 months

[e]At 1–2 months interval

Note for auto-HSCT: same recommendations but grading changes for some vaccines: influenza BIIr (instead AII); PCV BIII (instead AI)

MAC. The experience with other sources (CBU), conditioning regimens (RIC), and donors (haplo) is scarce.

Many vaccines are administered by *intramuscular route*, which can be a problem for severe thrombocytopenic patients (less than 50 × 10^9 platelets/L). For severe thrombocytopenic patients, some vaccines can be safely administered SC (inactivated poliomyelitis, conjugate pneumococcal vaccine) or even intradermic route (for influenza vaccine). Clinical experience suggests that intramuscular injections are safe if the platelet count is ≥30 to 50 × 10^9/L, a ≤23-gauge needle is used, and constant pressure is maintained at the injection site for 2 min (Rubin et al. 2014).

29.2.3 The Dose of Vaccine

The dose of vaccine used is the same for general population, with some exceptions (see Table 29.2). A uniform specific interval between doses cannot be recommended, as various intervals have been used in studies. As a general guideline, a minimum of 1 month between doses may be reasonable.

29.2.4 Several Patient and Vaccine Characteristics Impact on the Vaccine Response

Time from Transplantation As a general rule, the later time a vaccine is administered, the better response is obtained (there are exceptions; see pneumococcal vaccine section). Usually >12 months from transplant is associated with better responses.

Type of Vaccine T-cell-dependent vaccine obtains better response than T-cell-independent vaccines, because it triggers memory response that leads to a longer protection compared with T-cell-independent vaccine.

The presence of GVHD or ongoing IS treatment has been associated with a decrease in vaccine response, particularly for polysaccharide-based vaccines.

- Some vaccine responses seem to be not impaired by the presence of GVHD/IS treatment. This is the case of conjugated *Haemophilus* vaccine, conjugated pneumococcal vaccine, conjugated meningococcal vaccine, inactivated polio vaccine, and diphtheria-tetanus vaccine.
- International guidelines recommend different attitudes in patients with GVHD for the moment of vaccine administration.
- The international consensus guidelines (Ljungman et al. 2009) recommend to not postpone vaccinations with non-live vaccines in patients with ongoing active or resolved cGVHD of any severity grade.
- However, the International Consensus Conference on Clinical Practice in chronic GVHD (Hilgendorf et al. 2011) recommends postponing vaccination in patients with GVHD: if patients receive prednisone >0.5 mg/kg bodyweight as part of a combination therapy or a three-agent IS treatment is given, vaccination may be postponed until IS is reduced to a double combination or prednisone <0.5 mg/kg bodyweight in order to achieve better vaccine response. In any case, IS therapy should not lead to postponing vaccination for more than 3 months, and this applies for patients with ongoing active or resolved cGVHD of any severity grade.
- In practices, the majority of centers seems to delay vaccinations if GVHD is present (Miller et al. 2017).

The use of rituximab decreases serological vaccine response at least to tetanus and influenza.

- ECIL 2017 guidelines (Cordonnier et al. 2017): patients who have received rituximab from transplant should have their vaccine

program delayed at least more than 6 months after the last dose.
- As the antibody response is uncertain, specific antibody assessment after vaccination can be helpful.

29.2.5 Types of Vaccines in HSCT Patients

Generally recommended for all HSCT (auto and allogeneic)

- Influenza (inactivated/subunit), poliomyelitis (inactivated), human papillomavirus, pneumococcus, *Haemophilus influenzae*, hepatitis B, meningococcus, tetanus, diphtheria, pertussis, and measles–mumps–rubella (special conditions, see Sects. 29.4 and 29.5).

Optional/special situations, to cover situations such as after disease exposure or before travel to areas endemic for infections:

- Hepatitis A, tick-borne encephalitis, Japanese B encephalitis, rabies, yellow fever (live), varicella (Varivax®, live).

Contraindicated: As general rule, *all live vaccines*:

- Oral polio vaccine, bacillus Calmette-Guérin, oral typhoid, zoster vaccine (Zostavax®), intranasal influenza vaccine, oral rotavirus vaccine.
- The exceptions for this rule are live vaccines for measles–mumps–rubella that are recommended following strict safety rules (see Sect. 29.4), yellow fever (live) (see specific section), and varicella (Varivax®, live); all these vaccines are contraindicated (EIII) before 24 m post-HSCT or in case of active GVHD or IS.

Use of IVIG and Vaccines For inactivated vaccines, Ig do not inhibit immune responses. For live virus vaccines, vaccination should be delayed 8 months after the last dose of Ig administration.

29.3 Benefits and Risks of Vaccination in HSCT Patients

29.3.1 Benefits

Direct Benefits The prevention of the specific infectious disease, as shown by influenza and varicella vaccination. Nonetheless, the majority of the efficacy studies in HSCT patients are based on surrogate markers (serology response) and not on the demonstration of a reduced risk of the infectious disease.

Indirect Benefits The benefits of vaccination can go beyond the prevention of a particular infection, as shown by influenza vaccine. Influenza immunization with inactivated vaccine is recommended by cardiologists as part of comprehensive secondary prevention with the same enthusiasm as the control of cholesterol, blood pressure, and other modifiable risk factors (Davis et al. 2006). It reduces cardiovascular mortality (risk ratio (RR) 0.45) (Clar et al. 2015), all-cause mortality (odds ratio (OR) 0.61), myocardial infarction (OR 0.73), and major adverse cardiovascular events (OR 0.47) (Loomba et al. 2012). Although all these studies were performed in general population, it is logical to assume a similar trend in HSCT patients.

29.3.2 Risks

Limited evidence indicates that *inactivated vaccines* have the same safety profile in immunocompromised patients as in immunocompetent individuals (Beck et al. 2012; Rubin et al. 2014; Cordonnier et al. 2017), and there is no evidence that they induce or aggravate GVHD (Cordonnier et al. 2017).

Live vaccines represent a real risk for HSCT and should not be used except in special situations with strict requirements (see section of varicella vaccine and ECIL vaccination guidelines table). Fatal disseminated VZV infections due to vaccine strain have been reported in HSCT patients after varicella vaccine and zoster vaccine, even when vaccine was administered several years after transplant (Cordonnier et al. 2017).

29.4 Vaccination Recommendations

There are several international recommendations focused on HSCT patients. The best known are those by the Infectious Disease Working Party (IDWP) of the EBMT, ECIL, CDC, and Infectious Diseases Society of America (IDSA).

The IDWP of the EBMT was one of the first cooperative groups that published recommendations specific for HSCT patients. The first ones were published in 1995, with updates in 1999 and 2005. In 2017 guidelines were reviewed and updated under the umbrella of the ECIL group, available online (Cordonnier et al. 2017) (Table 29.2).

In 2009 an international consensus guideline was published cosponsored by the main groups involved in HSCT and immunocompromised hosts (Ljungman et al. 2009) and probably is the most widely used in practice (Table 29.1).

The IDSA published their last recommendations in 2014 (Rubin et al. 2014).

There are other more specific guidelines focused on one pathogen (Engelhard et al. 2013) or on patients with GVHD (Hilgendorf et al. 2011).

29.5 Specific Vaccines

29.5.1 Influenza

29.5.1.1 Clinical Manifestations (Ljungman et al. 2011; Engelhard et al. 2013)

Twenty percent of HSCT with confirmed influenza are afebrile.

It is a serious disease in HSCT: One third develop pneumonia, 10% require mechanical ventilation, and 6% died (Ljungman et al. 2011) (i.e., 100–300 times higher the mortality of influenza in general population). Other complications include encephalitis that can be lethal and myocarditis.

29.5.1.2 Influenza and Cardiovascular Disease (CVD)

The majority of influenza deaths are related to lung complications. Nonetheless, in general population up to a third of deaths related to influenza are CV deaths (Loomba et al. 2012).

The risk of acute myocardial infarction is significantly increased after laboratory-confirmed influenza infection (Kwong et al. 2018).

HSCT patients are at high risk of developing CVD. At 10 years, 8% will develop CVD (Armenian et al. 2012).

29.5.1.3 Vaccine

Evidence of Vaccine Efficacy

- A retrospective study showed a protection rate of 80% in the rates of virologically confirmed influenza (Machado et al. 2005).
- A systematic review and meta-analysis showed significantly lower odds of influenza-like illness after vaccination in transplant recipients (HSCT and SOT) compared with patients receiving placebo or no vaccination (Beck et al. 2012). Seroconversion and seroprotection were lower in transplant recipients compared with immunocompetent controls.
- Given the suboptimal immunogenicity in HSCT patients, family members and healthcare professionals involved in the care of these populations should be vaccinated.

Vaccine Response (Engelhard et al. 2013; Cordonnier et al. 2017)

- Longer interval from transplant is associated with better serology response. Vaccination within the first 6 months after transplant produces poor serology responses. Nonetheless, seasonal vaccination against

influenza can boost the cellular immune response in HSCT patients as early as 3 months after HSCT, but the protective effect is lower compared with healthy controls (Engelhard et al. 2013).
- Conflicting data exist on the benefit of a second dose of vaccine, and marginal benefit was seen with the use of GM-CSF.
- In HSCT the superiority of high-dose influenza vaccine has not been demonstrated (Halasa et al. 2016).
- Rituximab administration during the year before vaccination was associated with a lack of seroprotective titer.
- Active GVHD and low lymphocyte counts at vaccination are associated with poor immune response.

Live, attenuated influenza vaccine is contraindicated in HSCT patients (Rubin et al. 2014).

There is a difference in *the duration of influenza vaccine recommendation* in the European (Cordonnier et al. 2017) and US guidelines (Rubin et al. 2014):

- ECIL recommends vaccination as long as patient is judged to be immunosuppressed (A II r) although considered, with a lower strength, the use of yearly, lifelong (B II r) (Cordonnier et al. 2017).
- IDSA recommends lifelong immunization (Rubin et al. 2014).
- There are no trials to support one or other recommendations, but a lifelong immunization seems logical as fatal influenza illness can occur several years after HSCT, without clear risk factors in some patients, particularly in auto-HSCT (Ljungman et al. 2011), and the proved safety of influenza vaccine in this population. Moreover, for general population, the CDC recommends routine annual influenza vaccination for all persons aged ≥6 months (Grohskopf et al. 2017).

For severe thrombocytopenic patients, the intradermic influenza vaccine can be safely administered although it has not yet been evaluated in transplant recipients.

29.5.2 Measles, Mumps, and Rubella

The clinical impact and the reasons for immunization in HSCT patients differ among these viruses:

- *Measles*: Severe and also fatal measles infections (pneumonia, encephalitis) have been reported in SCT recipients. The aim of vaccination is to protect the patient of severe consequences of infection.
- *Rubella*: There are no reports of severe rubella disease occurring in HSCT recipients. The main indication for rubella vaccination is prevention of congenital rubella in fertile women.
- *Mumps*: There are no reports of severe mumps occurring in HSCT recipients. The indication for mumps vaccination is therefore weak. There is no indication for routine mumps vaccination after HSCT. However, mumps is included in combination vaccines with measles and rubella.

Vaccines Only live-attenuated vaccines are available. Presentations: measles alone, combined measles–mumps–rubella, combined measles–mumps–rubella–varicella (live).

29.5.3 Hepatitis B Virus (HBV)

Prevention of infection and reverse seroconversion:

- Approximately 40–70% of HSCT patients obtain a titer of anti-HBs of >10 mIU/mL after post-HSCT vaccination, a rather low response compared with healthy controls. Even those who fail to obtain a response may benefit from vaccination as it can prevent reverse seroconversion.
- Patients that have evidence of a previously resolved hepatitis B infection prior to the transplant (i.e., HBsAg negative but anti-HBs and/or anti-HBc) are at risk or reverse seroconversion.

- Immunization for HBV can prevent HBV reverse seroconversion even in non-responders to hepatitis B vaccine after allo-HSCT (Takahata et al. 2014). Probably, antigen-specific memory T cells and cytotoxic T cells induced by hepatitis B vaccine are largely responsible for prevention of reverse seroconversion in non-responders to the vaccine. This reinforces the need of HBV vaccination.

29.5.4 Human Papilloma Virus (HPV)

In HSCT women nearly 40% will have genital HPV infection in long-term follow-up (Shanis et al. 2018). HPV is associated with cervical, vulvar, and vaginal cancer in females, penile cancer in males, and anal cancer and oropharyngeal cancer in both females and males.

In long-term survivors, second neoplasias are a significant complication after allo-HSCT. Cervix cancer is one of the most frequent. Squamous cell cancers, the commonest post transplant solid tumors, are associated with HPV infection. Genital HPV disease is a significant late complication of allo-HSCT, occurring in one third of women. Prolonged systemic IS treatment for cGVHD is associated with a higher risk of developing HPV-related squamous intraepithelial lesions.

Regular gynecologic examination, cervical cytology, and HPV testing after HSCT is recommended for all women (Majhail et al. 2012) as preventing measure for HPV-related cancer and as a tool for early diagnose and treatment of genital GVHD.

29.5.4.1 Vaccine

- HPV vaccine is a noninfectious, virus-like particle (VLP) vaccine. There are three formulations of HPV vaccines that differ in the number of HPV covered: a 9-valent HPV vaccine (6, 11, 16, 18, 31, 33, 45, 52, and 58 VLPs) (Gardasil 9®), quadrivalent HPV vaccine (6, 11, 16, and 18 VLPs) (Gardasil®), and bivalent vaccine (16, 18 VLPs) (Cervarix®).
- The experience with HPV vaccine in HSCT is limited, 20 children (MacIntyre et al. 2016) and 64 adults (Stratton et al. 2018), but shows a good immune response, similar to health women, with no specific safety issue.
- HPV vaccine is recommended in all guidelines (Ljungman et al. 2009; Hilgendorf et al. 2011; Rubin et al. 2014; Cordonnier et al. 2017) but with a low grade of recommendation (B II u to C III) due to the limited experience in HSCT patients. The recommended number of doses is three (Hilgendorf et al. 2011; Rubin et al. 2014).

29.5.5 Poliovirus

The WHO European Region was declared polio-free in 2002. Imported wild-type and vaccine-type polioviruses still remain a threat to unvaccinated people in the EU/EEA. Maintaining high vaccination coverage in all population groups remain an essential tool for keeping Europe polio-free.

Only inactivated poliovirus vaccines are used in all EU/EEA countries.

Oral polio vaccine (OPV) is contraindicated for HSCT patients due to the risk of paralytic poliomyelitis. This complication has occurred after vaccination of patients with severe combined immune deficiency but has not been described in HSCT patients.

29.5.6 Varicella Zoster Virus (VZV)

Prevention of VZV After HSCT Antiviral prophylaxis (acyclovir/valacyclovir) is the primary mode of prevention. It should be given for at least 1 year after allo-HSCT and for 3–6 months after auto-HSCT (Cordonnier et al. 2017).

Types of Vaccines There are three types of available vaccines and one not commercially available. None is licensed for use in IS patients.

- Live-attenuated varicella vaccine, a low-titer VZV vaccine (Varivax®, Varilix®). It is also available in combination in the same vaccine with measles, mumps, and rubella.

 - Varicella vaccine can be used in HSCT following strict requirements (see ECIL and IDSA vaccination guidelines) (Cordonnier et al. 2017; Rubin et al. 2014). Although vaccination with varicella-attenuated vaccine is indicated/considered in guidelines, in practice it is rarely used due to concerns of safety, particularly in adults (Miller et al. 2017). The commercial availability of the VZ subunit vaccine and maybe in the future the inactivated vaccine will make the use of the attenuated vaccines even lower.
- Live-attenuated zoster vaccine, a high-titer vaccine (Zostavax®). It contains more than 14 times more virus than varicella vaccine. In all guidelines, this vaccine is contraindicated in HSCT patients.
- New phase III studies with new VZL vaccines in auto-HSCT.
  - *Adjuvanted VZV subunit vaccine* (Shingrix®) (de la Serna et al. 2018; Sullivan et al. 2018) consists of recombinant VZV gE antigen mixed with AS01B adjuvant. It was recently approved by the FDA (October 2017) and EMA (March 2018) for prevention of herpes zoster (HZ) and post-herpetic neuralgia, in adults 50 years of age or older. It is administered IM in two doses separated by 60 days.
  - *Inactivated VZV-vaccine (V212), in auto-HSCT* (Winston et al. 2018), is not yet commercially available. It is administered in four doses by SC injection, beginning ~5 days prior to chemotherapy or ~30 days prior to auto-HSCT and the remaining doses being administered at 30, 60, and 90 days later.
  - Both vaccines showed a high vaccine efficacy for preventing zoster which was 68–64%, post-herpetic neuralgia 89–84%, VZV-related hospitalizations 85%, and for other VZV complications 78–75%. The positive results of these studies probably are going to change the prevention of VZV complications after auto-HSCT.

29.5.7 Pneumococcus

Pneumococcus is a frequent and *serious complication in HSCT*. The incidence of invasive pneumococcal disease (IPD) in HSCT is 50 times higher compared to the general population (Shigayeva et al. 2016). In spite of this high incidence of IPD, less than one in five HSCT patients with IPD had received pneumococcal vaccine.

29.5.7.1 Types of Vaccine

- Polysaccharidic (PS) vaccine
  - 23-valent polysaccharidic (PS) vaccine (Pneumo 23®, Pneumovax23®): poor immunogenic, T-cell-independent response, no boost benefit
  - Poor responses, particularly in patients with GVHD
  - PS after PCV vaccine increases and expands the response obtained with PCV. Some non-responders to PCV will achieve a response with PS vaccine.
- Conjugate vaccine (PCV): highly immunogenic, T-cell-dependent response, with boost benefit
  - 13-valent in the majority of countries (Prevenar 13r®) (that replace the previous 7-valent vaccine) or 10-valent available in some countries (Synflorix®).
  - Five trials have shown a good response to PCV after three doses (range 54–98%). Four trials used 7-valent conjugated vaccine and one the 13-valent vaccine (Cordonnier et al. 2017). These responses are much better compared with what is obtained with PS vaccine.
  - Early vaccination at 3 months is not inferior to late vaccination (9 months) after allo-HSCT.
  - PCV should always be administered before PS vaccine.

29.5.8 Diphtheria-Tetanus-Pertussis

The exposure to *tetanus* in the environment is a real risk for HSCT patients, so the aim of vaccination after transplant is to protect the patient.

Diphtheria has essentially been eradicated but ongoing vaccination is critical for immunity. Diphtheria cases are still happening in Europe with an increase of 280% from 2009 to 2014. The reappearance of diphtheria cases in countries like Spain diphtheria-free for more than 30 years (Jane et al. 2018) is alarming and another reason to vaccine all our HSCT patients.

There are very limited published data of *pertussis* in HSCT and no reported case of severe or fatal pertussis infection after SCT in adults. Therefore, the objective of vaccination in these patients is avoiding pertussis transmission by HSCT patients.

29.6 Vaccinations Before Travel to Areas Endemic for Infections (See Table 29.3) (Ljungman et al. 2009)

29.7 Serological Testing

For the majority of vaccines, no pre- or postvaccination serology is recommended. Nonetheless, there are exceptions for this rule (Ljungman et al. 2009).

29.7.1 Pre-Vaccination

Testing for Abs to measles is recommended in adults, with vaccination performed only if the patient is seronegative (CIII).

If vaccination against varicella is contemplated, testing of immunity should be carried out and vaccination should be administered to seronegative patients only (CIII).

29.7.2 Postvaccination

Pneumococcal vaccine: Testing to assess the response to vaccination is recommended at

Table 29.3 Vaccinations before travel to areas endemic for infections (Ljungman et al. 2009)

If contraindications for the vaccine exist, the patient should be advised not to travel to endemic areas (CIII) Vaccination is one of the precautions that the HSCT patients should observe. There are other equal important measures that should be followed: chemoprophylaxis against malaria; mosquito-oriented precautions; food safety to prevent traveler's diarrhea; avoiding sun exposure, particularly for those under treatments associated with photosensitivity (like voriconazole)	
Tick-borne and Japanese B encephalitis	• According to local policy in endemic areas (CIII)No data exist regarding the time after HCT when vaccination can be expected to induce an immune response
Rabies	• Rabies vaccine is made from killed virus and cannot cause rabies. Nonetheless, there are no data regarding safety, immunogenicity, or efficacy among HCT recipients • Preexposure rabies vaccination should probably be delayed until 12–24 months after HCT • Postexposure administration of rabies vaccine with human rabies Ig can be administered any time after HCT, as indicated
Yellow fever (live)	• Limited data regarding safety and efficacy (C III). Yellow fever vaccine has been safely administered to a limited number of post-HSCT patients (Rubin et al. 2014) • The risk–benefit balance may favor the use of the vaccine in patients residing in or traveling to endemic areas
Hepatitis A	• Follow recommendations for general population in each country (CIII) • Ig should be administered to hepatitis A-susceptible HCT recipients who anticipate hepatitis A exposure (for example, during travel to endemic areas) and for postexposure prophylaxis
Typhoid (IM), inactivated vaccine	• No data were found regarding safety, immunogenicity, or efficacy among HCT recipients. DIII. Remember that typhoid oral vaccine is live attenuated and is contraindicated in HSCT patients (EIII)
Cholera	• No data were found regarding safety and immunogenicity among HCT recipients. Vaccine is not recommended (DIII)

1 month or later after the third or fourth dose of pneumococcal vaccine (BIII). As a widely accepted definition of adequate response to pneumococcal vaccine is lacking, guidelines for revaccination of non-responders are not given. Testing for immunity to pneumococcus might reasonably be repeated every 2 years for the first 4 years (BIII).

Hepatitis B: Testing should be carried out 1 month or later after the third vaccine dose (BIII). A second three-dose vaccination schedule is recommended in non-responders (CIII)

Testing should be conducted approximately every 4–5 years to assess for immunity to HBV, measles, tetanus, diphtheria, and polio (BIII).

29.8 Vaccinations for Donors, Close Contacts/Family, and HCWs of HSCT Recipients (See Table 29.4) (Ljungman et al. 2009; Cordonnier et al. 2017; Rubin et al. 2014)

Table 29.4 Vaccinations for donors, close contacts/family, and HCWs of HCT recipients

General comments		
Inactivated vaccines can be safely given for donors, close contacts, and HCWs of HSCT patients For live vaccines a careful evaluation should be done (see below). Some have no safety issues for HSCT recipients but other can cause severe damage		
Donors		
Guidelines do not recommend donor vaccination for the benefit of the recipient[a,b] • Only vaccines that are indicated and recommended based on the donor's age, vaccination history, and exposure history should be administered • Nonetheless, vaccination of the donor has been shown to improve the post transplant immunity of the patient in the case of tetanus, diphtheria, 7-valent pneumococcal conjugate vaccine (PCV), and *Haemophilus influenzae* type b-conjugate vaccines. Donation is an opportunity to update the donor vaccination calendar. If the donor has to receive any of these vaccines in his/her own interest, the administration of at least one dose pre-collection of stem cells could benefit also the receptor Administration of MMR, MMRV, varicella, and zoster vaccines should be avoided within 4 weeks of stem cell harvest[b]. By extension, all live vaccines should be avoided before stem cell collection due to the risk of transmission of the pathogen with the graft[c]		
Vaccines recommended for close contacts and HCWs of HSCT recipients		
Who?	*Vaccine*	*Dose/notes*
All	Influenza, inactivated	•Annually, as long as there is contact with an IS recipient[a]: Close contacts: AII[a]-AIII[c]; HCWs: AI[a]-AIIt[c]
All sero(-) VZ	Varicella: AIII[a]	• 2 doses, separated by at least 28 days
HCWs Sero(-)	Measles	• AIII[a]; recommended, not graded[b,c]
Live vaccines given for *close contacts or HCWs* of HCST patients: precautions		
Intranasal influenza vaccine		• If live influenza vaccine is administered to a close contact/HCWs, contact between the IS patient and household member should be avoided for 7 days (weak, very low)[b]
Measles-mumps-rubella		• No risk for the HSCT patient
Varicella		• The vaccination dose or doses should be completed >4 weeks before the conditioning regimen begins or >6 weeks (42 days) before contact with the HCT recipient is planned (BIII)[a] • If a varicella vaccinee develops a postvaccination rash within 42 days of vaccination, the vaccinee should avoid contact with HCT recipients until all rash lesions are crusted or the rash has resolved[a]

(continued)

Table 29.4 (continued)

Oral polio vaccine (OPV)	• Oral polio vaccine (OPV) should not be administered to individuals who live in a household with IS patients (strong, moderate)[b]. These vaccinated contacts shed the live-attenuated poliovirus strains of the vaccine in the stools that can induce paralytic poliomyelitis in immunocompromised patients like HSCT • If live-attenuated oral polio vaccine, that is still available in some non-US/non-European countries, is given to a household contact, a 4- to 6-week furlough is advised
Rotavirus	• Rotavirus vaccine is included in the children vaccine calendar of many countries, so it will be frequent that a HSCT patient has a child candidate for the vaccine • Virus is shed in stools for 2–4 weeks after vaccination. Transmission from vaccinated to IS person has been confirmed, but there are no reported cases of symptomatic infection in contacts • Highly IS patients should avoid handling diapers of infants who have been vaccinated with rotavirus vaccine for 4 weeks after vaccination (strong, very low) • HSCT recipients should have no contact with the stools or diapers of vaccinated children for 4 weeks following vaccination[c]
Vaccines for travel: yellow fever vaccine; oral typhoid vaccine	• Can safely be administered[b]

HCWs healthcare workers
[a]Ljungman et al. (2009)
[b]Rubin et al. (2014)
[c]Cordonnier et al. (2017)

Key Points

- Vaccination should be considered a routine practice for all HSCT receptors, either autologous or allogeneic, adults or children. It should be implemented in all HSCT programs.
- There is no a unique vaccine schedule for all HSCT patients. Each center should discuss and adapt a specific vaccine program.
- To obtain this objective, it is necessary to have in place a standardized program specific for HSCT patients with a simple and clear chronology and the collaboration of the Preventive Department of the hospital and primary care physicians.
- The vaccination program should include not only the patient but also those who live with the patient and the healthcare workers (HCWs).
- There are two main reasons for universal vaccination of HSCT patients: (a) the general interest as all the population should be correctly vaccinated to avoid holes of immunity that can be a risk for the health of the general population and (b) individual interest for each HSCT patient.

References

Armenian SH, Sun CL, Vase T, et al. Cardiovascular risk factors in hematopoietic cell transplantation (HCT) survivors: role in development of subsequent cardiovascular disease. Blood. 2012;120:4505–12.

Beck CR, McKenzie BC, Hashim AB, et al. Influenza vaccination for immunocompromised patients: systematic review and meta-analysis by aetiology. J Infect Dis. 2012;206:1250–9.

Clar C, Oseni Z, Flowers N, et al. Influenza vaccines for preventing cardiovascular disease. Cochrane Database Syst Rev. 2015;5:CD005050.

Cordonnier C, Cesaro S, De Lavallade H, et al. Guidelines for vaccination of patients with hematological malignancies and HSCT recipient. ECIL 2017. 2017; Published online 4-10-2017. www.ecil-leukaemia.com.

Davis MM, Taubert K, Benin AL, et al. Influenza vaccination as secondary prevention for cardiovascular disease: a science advisory from the American Heart Association/American College of Cardiology. J Am Coll Cardiol. 2006;48:1498–502.

Engelhard D, Mohty B, de la Camara R, et al. European guidelines for prevention and management of influenza in hematopoietic stem cell transplantation and leukemia patients: summary of ECIL-4 (2011), on behalf of ECIL, a joint venture of EBMT, EORTC, ICHS, and ELN. Transpl Infect Dis. 2013;15:219–32.

Grohskopf LA, Sokolow LZ, Broder KR, Walter EB, Bresee JS, Fry AM, et al. Prevention and control of seasonal influenza with vaccines: recommendations of the Advisory Committee on Immunization Practices - United States, 2017-18 influenza season. MMWR Recomm Rep. 2017;66:1–20.

Halasa NB, Savani BN, Asokan I, et al. Randomized double-blind study of the safety and immunogenicity of standard-dose trivalent inactivated influenza vaccine versus high-dose trivalent inactivated influenza vaccine in adult hematopoietic stem cell transplantation patients. Biol Blood Marrow Transplant. 2016;22:528–35.

Hilgendorf I, Freund M, Jilg W, et al. Vaccination of allogeneic haematopoietic stem cell transplant recipients: report from the international consensus conference on clinical practice in chronic GVHD. Vaccine. 2011;29:2825–33.

Jane M, Vidal MJ, Camps N, et al. A case of respiratory toxigenic diphtheria: contact tracing results and considerations following a 30-year disease-free interval, Catalonia, Spain, 2015. Euro Surveill. 2018;23. https://doi.org/10.2807/1560-7917.

Kwong JC, Schwartz KL, Campitelli MA, et al. Acute myocardial infarction after laboratory-confirmed influenza infection. N Engl J Med. 2018;378:345–53.

de la Serna J, Campora L, Chandrasekar P, et al. Efficacy and safety of an adjuvanted herpes zoster subunit vaccine in autologous hematopoietic stem cell transplant recipients 18 years of age or older: first results of the phase 3 randomized, placebo-controlled ZOEHSCT clinical trial. 2018. Late break abstract. BMT TANDEM meeting 2018, Salt Lake City.

Ljungman P, Cordonnier C, Einsele H, et al. Vaccination of hematopoietic cell transplant recipients. Bone Marrow Transplant. 2009;44:521–6.

Ljungman P, de la Camara R, Perez-Bercoff L, et al. Outcome of pandemic H1N1 infections in hematopoietic stem cell transplant recipients. Haematologica. 2011;96:1231–5.

Loomba RS, Aggarwal S, Shah PH, Arora RR. Influenza vaccination and cardiovascular morbidity and mortality. J Cardiovasc Pharmacol Ther. 2012;17:277–83.

Machado CM, Cardoso MR, da Rocha IF, et al. The benefit of influenza vaccination after bone marrow transplantation. Bone Marrow Transplant. 2005;36:897–900.

MacIntyre CR, Shaw P, Mackie FE, et al. Immunogenicity and persistence of immunity of a quadrivalent Human Papillomavirus (HPV) vaccine in immunocompromised children. Vaccine. 2016;34:4343–50.

Majhail NS, Rizzo JD, Lee SJ, et al. Recommended screening and preventive practices for long-term survivors after hematopoietic cell transplantation. Bone Marrow Transplant. 2012;47:337–41.

Miller PDE, de Silva TI, Skinner R, et al. Routine vaccination practice after adult and paediatric allogeneic haematopoietic stem cell transplant: a survey of UK NHS programmes. Bone Marrow Transplant. 2017;52:775–7.

Rubin LG, Levin MJ, Ljungman P, et al. 2013 IDSA clinical practice guideline for vaccination of the immunocompromised host. Clin Infect Dis. 2014;58: e44–100.

Shanis D, Anandi P, Grant C, et al. Risks factors and timing of genital human papillomavirus (HPV) infection in female stem cell transplant survivors: a longitudinal study. Bone Marrow Transplant. 2018;53:78–83.

Shigayeva A, Rudnick W, Green K, et al. Invasive pneumococcal disease among immunocompromised persons: implications for vaccination programs. Clin Infect Dis. 2016;62:139–47.

Stratton P, Battiwalla M, Abdelazim S, et al. Immunogenicity of HPV quadrivalent vaccine in women after allogeneic HCT is comparable to healthy volunteers. BMT TANDEM meeting 2018, Salt Lake City. Biol Blood Marrow Transplant. 2018;24: S85–6.

Sullivan K, Abhyankar A, Campora L, et al. Immunogenicity and safety of an adjuvanted herpes zoster subunit vaccine in adult autologous hematopoietic stem cell transplant recipients: phase 3, randomized, placebo-controlled, ZOE-HSCT clinical trial. 44th annual meeting of the European Society for Blood and Marrow Transplantation 18-21 March, Lisbon, Portugal; 2018.

Takahata M, Hashino S, Onozawa M, et al. Hepatitis B virus (HBV) reverse seroconversion (RS) can be prevented even in non-responders to hepatitis B vaccine after allogeneic stem cell transplantation: long-term analysis of intervention in RS with vaccine for patients with previous HBV infection. Transpl Infect Dis. 2014;16:797–801.

Winston DJ, Mullane KM, Cornely OA, Boeckh MJ, Brown JW, Pergam SA, et al. Inactivated varicella zoster vaccine in autologous haemopoietic stem-cell transplant recipients: an international, multicentre, randomised, double-blind, placebo-controlled trial. Lancet. 2018;391:2116–27.

30 Psychological Morbidity and Support

Alice Polomeni, Enrique Moreno, and Frank Schulz-Kindermann

30.1 Introduction

Allo-HSCT is associated with significant physical and psychological morbidity that may have a negative impact on patients' and on their relatives' health-related quality of life (HRQoL) (Majhail and Rizzo 2013). Patients suffer a broad range of acute and chronic impairments of health-related quality of life (HRQoL), concerning physical, emotional, cognitive and social constraints. Psychosocial difficulties have been identified throughout the HSCT process, from pre-transplant to recovery phase and even for long-term survivors. Insofar, psychological support of HSCT recipients and caregivers is based on a—where ever possible—preventive, concrete and sustainable approach, comprising a broad range of aspects of HRQoL. Psychooncological interventions are planned and conducted regularly in an interdisciplinary approach, taking into consideration medical, social and nursing issues.

A. Polomeni (✉)
Service d'Hématologie clinique et thérapie cellulaire, Hôpital Saint Antoine - Assistance Publique-Hôpitaux de Paris, Paris, France
e-mail: alice.polomeni@aphp.fr

E. Moreno
Department of Psychology, Asleuval (Valencian Association of Leukemia), Valencia, Spain

F. Schulz-Kindermann
Pychooncological Outpatient Department, Institute of Medical Psychology, University Cancer Center Hamburg, University of Hamburg, Hamburg, Germany

30.2 The Period Preceding HSCT

Since HSCT often appears to be the only therapeutic cure, this can cause high expectations in patients and their families, who may overestimate HSCT's benefits and underestimate the procedure's morbidity and mortality risks. Several authors are adamant about the importance of pragmatic information, specifically regarding prognosis, post transplant effects and the impact of HSCT on QOL. This information not only could guide patients in their decision to undergo the treatment (or not) but could also help them and their close relatives to face the persistent side effects post-HSCT (Jim et al. 2014). Studies show that specific pre-transplant distress predicts psychosocial problems during and after HSCT (Schulz-Kindermann et al. 2002). This suggests a thorough medical as well as psychosocial preparation about risks and challenges with concomitant illustration of possible coping resources. Understanding of the information about the prognosis can be associated with depression and a worsening QOL over time (Applebaum et al. 2016).

Frequently described are anxious-depressive symptoms and sleep disruption pre-HSCT, linked to the burden of uncertainty about treatment outcomes. Baseline anxiety and depression predict

E. Carreras et al. (eds.), *The EBMT Handbook*, https://doi.org/10.1007/978-3-030-02278-5_30

worsening HRQoL during hospitalisation and post-treatment adjustment, even identifying these symptoms as risk factors for survival (Artherholt et al. 2014). This suggests a thorough survey of the psychosocial anamnesis and a brief screening in the course of treatment and survivorship. To avoid evitable strain, short instruments to measure distress, anxiety, depression and HRQoL—like the Distress Thermometer, Patient Health Questionnaire, Cancer Treatment-Related Distress Scale and EORTC QLQ-C30—should be implemented. Attention should always involve caregivers as well as minor children of patients. Finally, HSCT teams should screen patients' and families' met and unmet needs, including psychosocial support. Regarding preparation for HSCT, patients who are in a fairly stable physical state should take advantage of psychological support before admission to inpatient treatment. Psychological interventions cover different approaches like psychodynamic interviews, introduction in relaxation techniques, communication skills (regarding problem-focused communication with staff and with caregivers) and coping with side effects (pain, nausea, fatigue, restlessness, sleep disorder; see Syrjala et al. 2012).

30.3 Hospitalisation for HSCT

During hospitalisation, patients grapple with considerable changes, including a loss of physical abilities and autonomy. HSCT hospitalisation constraints, combined with poor physical condition, may increase patients' feelings of isolation and dependence, negatively affecting psychological well-being (Tecchio et al. 2013). Symptoms of depression, anxiety, sleep disruption and adjustment disorders are frequently reported (El Jawahri 2015). Unlike anxiety, which does not change over time, depression levels increase more than twofold after 2 weeks of isolation (Tecchio et al. 2013).

These symptoms can go unrecognised and have been known to interfere with HSCT medical treatment. Depression during hospitalisation is associated with longer hospital stay, increased risk of mortality (Prieto et al. 2005), post transplant anxio-depressive symptoms and post traumatic stress syndrome (PTSS) (El-Jawahri et al. 2016).

Depressive symptoms are risk factors for a poorer outcome after HSCT. It is noteworthy to follow a precise diagnostic process, differentiating depression and demoralisation. The latter focuses on an attitude of senselessness and hopelessness, while depression has a pronounced somatic level, overlapping with fatigue. Recent research has explored psychoneuroendocrinology and psychoneuroimmunology to identify pathways that may mediate between psychosocial factors and disease outcomes (Costanzo et al. 2013). These authors have recommended the treatment of sleep and circadian disturbances, as well as the option of psychotropic medications and cognitive behavioural interventions in the HSCT setting.

A significantly positive correlation between the presence of a family caregiver (FC) during hospitalisation and HSCT survival has been established (Foster et al. 2013). The support provided by the HSCT team can also help patients to better cope with hospitalisation and facilitate psychological adjustment after discharge, reducing difficulties in the transition towards outpatient care.

Psychooncological interventions concerning depressive and anxious symptomatology rely on psychoeducational, psychodynamic and biobehavioural approaches, incorporating adequate coping potential. Specific techniques to ameliorate anxiety but also side effects like pain, sleeplessness, nausea or restlessness comprise relaxation, imagery and hypnotherapeutic approaches. Particularly in cases of fear and panic, pharmacological approaches with benzodiazepines and certain antidepressants should be taken into account.

Precise and repeated pain diagnostics are paramount, deriving multidisciplinary pain management, including medication, ongoing information about pain management and psychological interventions. There is some evidence for effectiveness of relaxation, imagery, hypnosis and cognitive-behavioral therapy (Syrjala 2014).

30.4 Post-HSCT

Data show that patients in remission for 2–5 years post-HSCT have a high probability of long-term survival. Nevertheless, HSCT-related morbidity is substantial, negatively affecting psychological functioning and social integration. HSCT's late effects on physical and psychic well-being have been well described, notably for chronic graft versus host disease, the severity of which is significantly related to impaired psychosocial functioning and diminished QOL (Majhail and Rizzo 2013).

Regarding psychopathology post-HSCT, several studies reported high rates of anxiety and depression, even several years after transplantation. Notwithstanding, research on psychological issues after HSCT has shown inconsistent results due to varying outcome measures, participation biases and cohort size and composition (Sun et al. 2011).

Although some studies have shown that depression and anxiety rates do not differ significantly from those of siblings or population norms, others reveal rates of psychological distress of 14% to 90% in survivors of HSCT (Sun et al. 2011). Even though some results demonstrate that physical morbidity tends to decrease by 1-year post-HSCT and psychosocial condition improves gradually over 1–5 years (Sun et al. 2013), other research reports depressive symptoms as long as 5 or even 10 years after HSCT (Jim et al. 2016). An unsettling fact is that depression post-HSCT has been associated with higher mortality and increased risk of suicide (Tichelli et al. 2013).

Depressive symptoms and sleep disorders are related to cognitive dysfunctions. Sleep disruption remains an issue for 43% of HSCT patients after transplant (Jim et al. 2016). These rates of disruption are substantially higher than those of the general population. Incidence of cognitive dysfunction in the first 5 years after HSCT is up to 60% (Scherwath et al. 2013). Poor neurocognitive functioning and psychosocial outcomes lead to lax medication management and adherence to recommended monitoring guidelines, which in turn may increase post-treatment morbi-mortality risks (Mayo et al. 2016).

Psychological interventions for depressive symptoms focus on dysfunctional, exaggerated cognitions and on an increase of activities. Psychopharmacological treatment is often recommended additionally, offering a broad range of substances, which can and should be adapted to respective indications and to the broad range of further medication. In the case of severe demoralisation, existential and meaning-centred approaches are advisable and show some evidence.

Concerning lasting traumatic experiences, in cross-sectional studies between 5 and 19% fulfilled a diagnosis of post-traumatic stress disorder (PTSD). In one of the rare prospective studies, PTSD symptomatology was observable at all time points (Esser et al. 2017a). Therefore, psychological support should not only be offered in the acute phase but already before HSCT and in the long term. Impairment by pain and pain intensity were risk factors for elevated levels of PTSD symptomatology. This highlights the importance of informing patients early enough that pain might occur and to introduce techniques for dealing with it. Since medical complications predicted severity of PTSD symptomatology 1 year after HSCT, medical professionals should be aware of psychological strain among patients suffering from long-term medical complications.

Psychosocial issues have also been explored in QOL research. Some studies in this domain stated that even if medical problems remain, the patients' emotional well-being seems to improve throughout the rehabilitation period. Nonetheless, fatigue, sleep disorders, neurocognitive impairment, neurobehavioural problems and sexual dysfunction persist. Esser et al. (2017b) identified in a prospective study three stable symptom complexes: exhausted (incl. fatigue), affective (incl. irritability and depressive symptoms) and gastrointestinal (incl. nausea). Fatigue was most persistent and also most severe and predictive for HRQoL. Fear of relapse, feelings of disability and barriers to social rehabilitation are frequent concerns, even several years after the procedure, with only a minority of disease-free transplant survivors consider themselves having 'returned to normal' (Syrjala et al. 2012).

These psychosocial difficulties are not systematically approached in current HSCT follow-up: despite their incidence, anxious-depressive symptoms are not often reported which should be treated by HSCT physicians. Barriers to approaching psychosocial issues are, on one hand, patients' fear of being stigmatised and, on the other hand, doctors who tend to prioritise strictly medical aspects. Health professionals often poorly evaluate psychological symptoms: anxiety is overrated, depression is underestimated, and consistency between the patients and the medical team's evaluations seems insufficient. Most patients receive prescriptions for these lingering symptoms, even over long periods, yet half of them benefit of follow-up by specialised professionals due to organisational and emotional obstacles (Mosher et al. 2010).

Anxieties after HSCT may be treated in a cognitive-behavioural approach, relying on working directly with fear-related contents and applying this to the broad range of oversimplified anxieties. For progression anxiety, manualised psychooncological therapies are well-tried, combining psychoeducational elements with group-format psychological therapy. Cognitive-behavioural therapy has demonstrated effectiveness in the treatment of PTSD with cancer patients in a significant number of studies, including patients with HSCT (DuHamel et al. 2010). Concerning fatigue, there are several promising approaches combining psychosocial counselling with physical training.

30.5 Close Relatives

Family caregivers (FC) can contribute to patients' recovery and to better survival following HSCT (Ehrlich et al. 2016). That said, the HSCT impact on FC has not been sufficiently explored, with most studies suffering from limitations due to small and heterogeneous samples.

Current research shows that FC experience a significant burden across the treatment trajectory. At the time of transplant, FC report high levels of fatigue, sleep disorders, depression and anxiety (El Jawahri 2015). FC may have more emotional difficulties than patients, and their well-being can be impaired well past post transplant. FC face negative effects in their own family and professional and social lives and express marital dissatisfaction after HSCT (Langer et al. 2017).

Qualitative data indicate that the main FC difficulties are related to long-term HSCT consequences and the unpredictable, uncertain character of their evolution. Assuming not only daily tasks but also the patients' psychological support, FC may feel overwhelmed by the complex demands of the caregiving role and the social impact of a lengthy rehabilitation (Applebaum et al. 2016).

In spite of the obstacles met during this post transplant period, FC rarely benefit from regular psychosocial support. Attention should also involve patients' minor children. The current trend has been to outsource part of the patient care. Research should better explore FC's real-life experience in order to propose targeted interventions during HSCT's various stages.

30.6 Related Donors

Related donors (RDs) deserve particular attention. Although positive effects of related donation have been demonstrated—such as deep personal satisfaction and a higher degree of self-esteem—there is also a negative impact. The incidence of pain and depressive symptoms is higher in RDs than in unrelated donors. Unexplained chronic pain could be associated with psychological distress related to the recipient's medical condition and HSCT outcomes. Data suggest that psychological support and follow-up should also be offered to RD (Garcia et al. 2013).

Like for patients, sufficient information, preparation and guidance should be available for FC and RD. That is, not only the tremendous task should be emphasised but also probable problems and risks, as well as available resources of care. Several interventions were developed to support FC, like problem-solving skills, cognitive-behavioural interventions and expressive talking (Applebaum et al. 2016).

30.7 Adolescents and Young Adults (AYA)

The adolescent and young adult group (AYA) represents a particular group that significantly varies from non-AYA patients, especially in psychosocial aspects (Pulewka et al. 2017). Research reveals that a quarter of AYA patients who experienced HSCT reported depression and anxiety symptoms, with nearly half meeting the criteria for post-traumatic stress (Syrjala et al. 2012).

HSCT appears to be a risk factor for poor health-related quality of life (HRQoL) and social functioning in AYA cancer survivors (Tremolada et al. 2016). Qualitative studies show that this population encounters difficulties in physical (sexuality and fatigue), psychological (depression, adherence and dependency issues, fear of the future, uncertainty) and social domains (changes in roles and relationships, educations and financial issues, family problems). Evidence-based psychosocial interventions in this population are sparse and should include specific problems, such as family relationships and social integration (school and work). Recent approaches use group formats enhancing self-help resources of peers, activity coaching and motivational interviewing.

30.8 Paediatric Patients

In their review of the literature, Packman et al. (2010) shows that HSCT paediatric patients experience acute psychological symptoms such as anxiety and depression before and during hospitalisation, as well as significant peer isolation, behavioural problems and post-traumatic stress symptoms after HSCT. Declines in cognitive abilities, social functioning and self-esteem have also been observed.

It is noteworthy that the accord between parent and child is better regarding physical conditions than it is with psychological issues. This discrepancy between the child's and the parents' evaluations also holds true regarding HRQoL post-HSCT (Chang et al. 2012).

HSCT may lead to disruptions in family life: parents and siblings (notably, donors) also report high levels of anxiety, depression and post-traumatic stress symptoms (Packman et al. 2010).

Paediatric HSCT survivors report psychosocial difficulties and decreased QOL with a high risk for anxiety, depression and behavioural problems. Childhood survivors' specific issues are related to sexual dysfunction, impoverished self-image and social adjustment. As follow-up of childhood HSCT patients is fundamental, special attention should be paid to the risk of withdrawal as they journey towards adulthood (Cupit et al. 2016).

Key Points

- The previously discussed rates of psychological morbidity in HSCT patients emphasise the need for clinical assessment throughout the procedure and at regular intervals.
- Given their vital role in the patients' recovery process, HSCT teams should also assess FC for psychological adjustment and family functioning.
- Particular attention should be given to RDs, who do not benefit systematically from a medical and psychological follow-up.
- Regardless of the overwhelming evidence of psychological morbidity in HSCT patients and in FC, barriers still exist in discussing psychosocial issues in routine care.
- Systematic screening may contribute to stimulate discussion of psychological symptoms, but quality psychosocial

care requires team training and an effective multidisciplinary approach.
- Psychological support should be installed low threshold and as far as possible attached to the transplant centre.
- Effectiveness of psychooncological interventions is proven widely and should be adapted to patients and FCs all along the course of HSCT.

References

Applebaum AJ, Bevans M, Son T, et al. A scoping review of caregiver burden during allogeneic HSCT: lessons learned and future directions. Bone Marrow Transplant. 2016;51:1416–22.

Artherholt SB, Hong F, Berry DL, Fann JR. Risk factors for depression in patients undergoing hematopoietic cell transplantation. Biol Blood Marrow Transplant. 2014;20:946–50.

Chang G, Ratichek SJ, Recklitis C, et al. Children's psychological distress during pediatric HSCT: parent and child perspectives. Pediatr Blood Cancer. 2012;58:289–96.

Costanzo ES, Juckett MB, Coe CL, et al. Biobehavioral influences on recovery following hematopoietic stem cell transplantation. Brain Behav Immun. 2013;30(Suppl):S68–74.

Cupit MC, Duncan C, Savani BN, et al. Childhood to adult transition and long-term follow-up after blood and marrow transplantation. Bone Marrow Transplant. 2016;51:176–81.

DuHamel KN, Mosher CE, Winkel G, et al. Randomized clinical trial of telephone-administered cognitive-behavioral therapy to reduce posttraumatic stress disorder and distress symptoms after hematopoietic stem-cell transplantation. J Clin Oncol. 2010;28:3754–61.

Ehrlich KB, Miller GE, Scheide T, et al. Pre-transplant emotional support is associated with longer survival after allogeneic hematopoietic stem cell transplantation. Bone Marrow Transplant. 2016;51:1594–8.

El-Jawahri AR, Traeger LN, Kuzmuk K, et al. Quality of life and mood of patients and family caregivers during hospitalization for hematopoietic stem cell transplantation. Cancer, 2015. 121(6): p. 951–9.

El-Jawahri AR, Vandusen HB, Traeger LN, et al. Quality of life and mood predict posttraumatic stress disorder after hematopoietic stem cell transplantation. Cancer. 2016;122:806–12.

Esser P, Kuba K, Scherwath A, et al. Posttraumatic stress disorder symptomatology in the course of allogeneic HSCT: a prospective study. J Cancer Surviv. 2017a;11:203–10.

Esser P, Kuba K, Scherwath A, et al. Stability and priority of symptoms and symptom clusters among allogeneic HSCT patients within a 5-year longitudinal study. J Pain Symptom Manag. 2017b;54:493–500.

Foster LW, McLellan L, Rybicki L, et al. Validating the positive impact of in-hospital lay care-partner support on patient survival in allogeneic BMT: a prospective study. Bone Marrow Transplant. 2013;48:671–7.

Garcia MC, Chapman JR, Shaw PJ, et al. Motivations, experiences, and perspectives of bone marrow and peripheral blood stem cell donors: thematic synthesis of qualitative studies. Biol Blood Marrow Transplant. 2013;19:1046–58.

Jim HS, Quinn GP, Gwede CK, et al. Patient education in allogeneic hematopoietic cell transplant: what patients wish they had known about quality of life. Bone Marrow Transplant. 2014;49:299–303.

Jim HSL, Sutton SK, Jacobsen PB, et al. Risk factors for depression and fatigue among survivors of hematopoietic cell transplantation. Cancer. 2016;122:1290–7.

Langer S, Lehane C, Yi J. Patient and caregiver adjustment to hematopoietic stem cell transplantation: a systematic review of dyad-based studies. Curr Hematol Malig Rep. 2017;12:324–34.

Majhail NS, Rizzo D. Surviving the cure: long term follow up of hematopoietic cell transplant recipients. Bone Marrow Transplant. 2013;48:1145–51.

Mayo S, Messner HA, Rourke SB, et al. Relationship between neurocognitive functioning and medication management ability over the first 6 months following allogeneic stem cell transplantation. Bone Marrow Transplant. 2016;51:841–7.

Mosher CE, KN DuHamel KN, Rini CM, et al. Barriers to mental health service use among hematopoietic SCT survivors. Bone Marrow Transplant. 2010;45:570–9.

Packman W, Weber S, Wallace J, et al. Psychological effects of hematopoietic SCT on pediatric patients, siblings and parents: a review. Bone Marrow Transplant. 2010;45:1134–46.

Prieto JM, Atala J, Blanch J, et al. Role of depression as a predictor of mortality among cancer patients after stem-cell transplantation. J Clin Oncol. 2005;23:6063–71.

Pulewka K, Wolff D, Herzberg PY, et al. Physical and psychosocial aspects of adolescent and young adults after allogeneic hematopoietic stem-cell transplantation: results from a prospective multicenter trial. J Cancer Res Clin Oncol. 2017;143:1613–9.

Scherwath A, Schirmer L, Kruse M, et al. Cognitive functioning in allogeneic hematopoietic stem cell transplantation recipients and its medical correlates: a prospective multicenter study. Psychooncology. 2013;22:1509–16.

Schulz-Kindermann F, Hennings U, Ramm G, et al. The role of biomedical and psychosocial factors for the prediction of pain and distress in patients undergoing high-dose therapy and BMT/PBSCT. Bone Marrow Transplant. 2002;29:341–51.

Sun CL, Francisco L, Baker KS, et al. Adverse psychological outcomes in long-term survivors of hematopoietic cell transplantation: a report from the Bone

Marrow Transplant Survivor Study (BMTSS). Blood. 2011;118:4723–31.

Sun CL, Kersey JH, Francisco L, et al. Burden of morbidity in 10+ year survivors of hematopoietic cell transplantation: report from the bone marrow transplantation survivor study. Biol Blood Marrow Transplant. 2013;19:1073–80.

Syrjala K, Martin PJ, Lee SJ. Delivering care to long-term adult survivors of hematopoietic cell transplantation. J Clin Oncol. 2012;30:3746–51.

Syrjala KL, Jensen MP, Mendoza ME, Yi JC et al. Psychological and behavioral approaches to cancer pain management. J Clin Oncol. 2014; 32 (16): 1703–11.

Tecchio C, Bonetto C, Bertani M, et al. Predictors of anxiety and depression in hematopoietic stem cell transplant patients during protective isolation. Psychooncology. 2013;22:1790–7.

Tichelli A, Labopin M, Rovó A, et al. Increase of suicide and accidental death after hematopoietic stem cell transplantation: a cohort study on behalf of the Late Effects Working Party of the European Group for Blood and Marrow Transplantation (EBMT). Cancer. 2013;119:2012–21.

Tremolada M, Bonichini S, Basso G, et al. Perceived social support and health-related quality of life in AYA cancer survivors and controls. Psychooncology. 2016;25:1408–17.

31 Clinically Relevant Drug Interactions in HSCT

Tiene Bauters

31.1 Introduction

Patients undergoing HSCT often receive polymedication which carries the potential to result in drug interactions. To avoid unexpected outcomes, attention to drug interactions is crucial especially when drugs with a narrow therapeutic index or inherent toxicity profile are involved (Leather 2004; Glotzbecker et al. 2012; Gholaminezhad et al. 2014).

Drug interactions can be defined as changes in a drug's effect due to recent or concurrent use of another drug, food, or environmental agent. The net effect of the combination can result in enhanced activity of the affected drug, possibly leading to toxicity, or reduced activity leading to therapeutic failure (Thanacoody 2012).

In general, drug interactions can be categorized as being pharmacodynamic, pharmacokinetic, or pharmaceutical in nature.

31.1.1 Pharmacodynamic Interactions

Pharmacodynamic interactions occur when the effect of one drug is changed by the presence of another drug at its site of action. They compete for specific receptor sites or interfere indirectly with physiological systems.

The effect can be additive/synergistic or antagonistic. An example of an additive interaction is the concurrent use of QT-prolongating drugs (e.g., ciprofloxacin and fluconazole) which substantially increases the risk of torsades de pointes or other ventricular tachyarrhythmias.

Specific antagonists can be used to reverse the effect of another drug at the receptor site (e.g., naloxone, an opioid receptor antagonist which reverses signs of opioid intoxication) (Lexicomp Drug® Interactions 2018).

31.1.2 Pharmacokinetic Interactions

Pharmacokinetic interactions (PK) occur when one drug alters the rate or extent of absorption, distribution, metabolism, or elimination of another drug resulting in diminished effects or drug potentiation (Palleria et al. 2013). The most frequent and significant drug interactions relate to drug metabolism. These will be further discussed here.

31.1.2.1 Cytochrome P450 Enzyme System

Several enzyme families are involved in drug metabolism, cytochrome P450 (CYP450) being the most important one. CYP450 consists of a unique group of isoenzymes grouped into families (1–3) and divided into subfamilies (A–E).

T. Bauters (✉)
Pharmacy, Pediatric Hemato-Oncology and Stem Cell Transplantation, Ghent University Hospital, Ghent, Belgium
e-mail: Tiene.bauters@uzgent.be

E. Carreras et al. (eds.), *The EBMT Handbook*, https://doi.org/10.1007/978-3-030-02278-5_31

They are primarily found in the liver and are genetically encoded (Ingelman-Sundberg and Rodriguez-Antona 2005; Lynch and Price 2007).

The effect of a CYP450 isoenzyme on a particular substrate can be altered by interaction with other drugs. Drugs can be substrates for a CYP450 isoenzyme and/or may inhibit or induce the isoenzyme (Larson 2018; Glotzbecker et al. 2012; Leather 2004):

Inhibition: Leads to reduced metabolism of the substrate with an increase in the steady-state concentration. It potentiates the effect and might lead to enhanced or toxic effects, especially in drugs with a narrow therapeutic index like cyclosporine and tacrolimus. Its onset occurs within 1–3 days for drugs with a short half-life, while the maximal effect may be delayed for drugs with a long half-life.

Induction: Increases the activity of CYP450 enzymes and usually results in decreased concentration/effect of the affected drug with the risk of therapeutic failure. Since the process of enzyme induction requires new protein synthesis, the effect usually occurs over days to weeks after starting an inducer.

Prodrugs rely on CYP450 enzymes for conversion to their active form(s). The combination of a prodrug (e.g., CFM) with a CYP450 inhibitor may result in therapeutic failure because of little or no production of the active drug. Conversely, an exaggerated therapeutic effect or adverse effect can be expected when a CYP450 inducer is added (Lynch and Price 2007).

In general, any drug metabolized by one of the CYP450 enzymes has the potential for PK- interaction, and concurrent use should be done with caution. As CYP3A4 is responsible for the metabolism of more than 50% of clinically administered drugs (Ingelman-Sundberg and Rodriguez-Antona 2005; Larson 2018), examples of CYP3A4 substrates, inhibitors, and inducers used in HSCT are presented in Table 31.1.

Mutations in CYP genes give rise to four major phenotypes: poor metabolizers, intermediate metabolizers, extensive metabolizers, and ultrarapid metabolizers (Ingelman-Sundberg and Rodriguez-Antona 2005; Ahmed et al. 2016). Polymorphisms in CYP450 are of concern in the study of interindividual altered drug metabolisms and/or adverse drug reactions.

31.1.2.2 Drug Transportation

P-glycoprotein (PgP) is a plasma membrane transporter involved in the excretion of drugs.

Table 31.1 CYP3A4 substrates, inhibitors and inducers commonly used in HSCT (non-limitative list) (Flockhart 2018; Medicines Complete 2018)

Substrates	Inhibitors	Inducers
Benzodiazepines[a]	Amiodarone	**Barbiturates (phenobarbital)**
Budesonide	Aprepitant	**Carbamazepine**
Calcium Channel Blockers[b]	Cimetidine	Corticosteroids
Carbamazepine	Ciprofloxacin	**Phenytoin**
Corticosteroids	**Clarithromycin**	**Rifampicin**
Etoposide	Diltiazem	St John's wort
Immunosuppressives[c]	Erythromycin	
Macrolide antibiotics[d]	Fluconazole	
Statins[e]	Grapefruit juice	
Steroids[f]	**Itraconazole**	
Miscellaneous[g]	**Ketoconazole**	
	Posaconazole	
	Voriconazole	
	Verapamil	

Bold font indicates strong inhibitors/inducers
[a]Alprazolam, diazepam, midazolam
[b]Amlodipine, diltiazem, verapamil
[c]Cyclosporine, tacrolimus, sirolimus
[d]Clarithromycin, erythromycin, NOT azithromycin
[e]Atorvastatin, NOT pravastatin, simvastatin
[f]Estradiol, progesterone, testosterone
[g]Aprepitant, fentanyl, ondansetron, thiotepa, zolpidem

Table 31.2 Drug interactions with busulfan (BU) (non-limitative list)[a]

Interacting drug	Proposed mechanism	Effect	Recommended action
Paracetamol	Competition for glutathione	Increased BU levels	– Avoid paracetamol within 72 h prior to or concurrently with BU – Monitor for increased BU concentrations/toxicity when used concurrently
Metronidazole	CYP3A4 inhibition Competition for glutathione		– Monitor for increased BU concentrations/toxicity when used concurrently
Itraconazole voriconazole	Unclear (probably CYP3A4 inhibition)		
Phenytoin	CYP3A4/glutathione-S-transferase induction	Decreased BU levels	– Use alternative antiepileptic (levetiracetam)

[a]Lexicomp® Drug interactions (2018) and Glotzbecker et al. (2012)

Its activity can be inhibited or induced by other drugs, resulting in increased or decreased bioavailability/clearance of PgP substrates (Ingelman-Sundberg and Rodriguez-Antona 2005; Thanacoody 2012).

Monoclonal Antibodies

Metabolism of monoclonal antibodies (MABs) does not involve CYP450 enzymes or drug transporters; therefore, PK interactions between MABs and conventional drugs are very limited. However, current information in this area is not abundant and more research is needed (Ferri et al. 2016).

31.1.3 Pharmaceutical Interactions

Pharmaceutical interactions manifest when two or more drugs and their diluents are mixed in the same infusion bag/syringe or when infusion lines meet at a Y-site junction. They are the result of incompatibilities as physicochemical reactions (changes in color, turbidimetry, and precipitation). Amphotericin B, for example, should not be diluted or mixed with physiological saline as microprecipitation will occur immediately.

31.2 Drug Interactions in HSCT Practice

Drug interactions can occur as early as during the conditioning regimen. Drugs as etoposide and thiotepa rely on CYP450 enzymes for metabolism, while cyclophosphamide needs to be converted to become functional. A non-limitative list of PK interactions with busulfan and recommendations for management are summarized in Table 31.2.

Many clinically relevant interactions have been reported with calcineurin inhibitors (cyclosporine and tacrolimus) and sirolimus. A non-limitative overview of PK interactions with these drugs is presented in Table 31.3.

31.3 Interactions with Herbal Drugs and Food

31.3.1 Herbal Drugs

The use of herbal drugs is growing worldwide, and a number of serious interactions with conventional drugs have been reported (Enioutina et al. 2017). Patients often do not perceive herbal supplements as drugs and prescribers are not always aware that patients are taking these products. A thorough drug history anamnesis is important and should be performed by asking very specific questions about herbal drug use.

An example of an herbal drug frequently involved in major drug interactions is St John's wort (SJW) (*Hypericum perforatum*). SJW is an over-the-counter product commonly used in HSCT patients for the treatment of mild depression. SJW can reduce the serum concentration of CYP3A4 substrates as cyclosporine and tacrolimus by induction of CYP3A4 or by increasing PgP expression, resulting in lack of response. Concomitant use of SJW with drugs metabolized by CYP3A4 should be avoided or monitored if no

Table 31.3 Pharmacokinetic interactions with cyclosporine (C), tacrolimus (T) and sirolimus (S) (non-limitative list)[a]

Interacting drug	Proposed mechanism	Effect	Recommended action
Anti-epileptics			
Carbamazepine Phenobarbital Phenytoin	CYP3A4 induction	– ▼ C/T/S level	• Monitor C/T/S levels • Increased C/T/S doses will likely be needed • Consider therapy modification (levetiracetam)
Antifungals			
Caspofungin	Unknown	– C: ▲ adverse/toxic effect of caspofungin – ▼ T/S levels	• Monitor liver function/hepatotoxicity in combination with C • Monitor T/S levels and adjust as necessary
Fluconazole Itraconazole Posaconazole Voriconazole	CYP3A4 and/or PgP inhibition	– ▲ C/T/S levels	• Monitor clinical response of C/T/S closely • Monitor C/T/S levels closely • Decreased C/T/S doses will likely be needed • Itraconazole: consider therapy modification (C/T/S) • Posaconazole/voriconazole: consider therapy modification (C/T), avoid combination (S)
Calcium channel blockers			
Diltiazem Verapamil	CYP3A4 inhibition	– ▲ C/T/S levels	• Monitor C/T/S levels • Decreased doses of C/T/S might be needed • Monitor for decreases in blood pressure (C) • Consider therapy modification (C)
Calcineurin inhibitors			
Cyclosporine	CYP3A4 competition	– T: ▲ levels/nephrotoxicity of C/T – S: ▲levels of S (of specific concern with modified C)	• Discontinue C/T therapy at least 24 h prior to initiating therapy with the other agent • C/T: avoid combination • Monitor for toxic effects of S • S: ▲ risk of C-induced HUS/TTP/TMA • Administer oral doses of S 4 h after doses of C • C/S: consider therapy modification
Tacrolimus		– C: ▲ levels/nephrotoxicity of C/T – S: ▲ adverse/toxic effect of T/S, ▼ level of T	• Avoid combination with C/S (enhanced toxicity of C/T/S)
Corticosteroids	CYP3A4/PgP induction CYP3A4 substrate	– ▲/▼ C/T levels – ▲ corticosteroid levels	• Monitor for changes in C/T levels (likely initial increase, possibly decrease thereafter) and toxic effects of corticosteroids and/or C/T if used concomitantly
Macrolide antibiotics (not azithromycin)			
Clarithromycin Erythromycin	CYP3A4/PgP inhibition	– ▲ C/T/S levels – S: ▲ level of erythromycin	• Monitor C/T/S levels and adjust dose accordingly • Avoid concurrent use
Proton pump inhibitors (PPI, not pantoprazole)			
Omeprazole Lansoprazole	C: unclear T: CYP3A4/CYP2C19 inhibition	– ▲ C/T level	• Monitor C/T levels closely when starting or stopping therapy with PPI and adjust dosage if necessary (T) • Inconsistent data (omeprazole), rabeprazole or pantoprazole: less likely to significantly interact

Table 31.3 (continued)

Interacting drug	Proposed mechanism	Effect	Recommended action
Statins			
Atorvastatin Simvastatin	CYP3A4 inhibition and inhibition of OATP1B1-mediated hepatic uptake	– C: ▲ level of atorvastatin/simvastatin – T: limited effect	• Monitor for increased risk for statin-related toxicities (myopathy and rhabdomyolysis) • C: Avoid concurrent use atorvastatin / simvastatin • Consider changing to pravastatin or fluvastatin (less sensitive to this interaction) or alternative therapy • Warn patients to report any unexplained muscle pains or weakness • T: No action needed
Miscellaneous			
Grapefruit juice	CYP3A4 inhibition (intestinal)	– ▲ C/T/S levels (C/T: primarily limited to orally administered C/T)	• Monitor C/T/S levels • Avoid combination with C/S/T
Metronidazole	CYP3A4 inhibition	– ▲ C/T/S levels	• Monitor C/T/S levels
Mycophenolate mofetil (MMF)	Decreased enterohepatic recirculation	– C: ▲ glucuronide metabolite concentrations (associated with mycophenolate adverse effects) – MMF: ▼ C exposure in children – T: does not affect PK of mycophenolic acid (one study suggests ▲ T exposure)	• Monitor MMF dosing and response to therapy particularly closely when adjusting concurrent C (starting, stopping, or changing dose) or if changing from C to T/S
Rifampicin	CYP3A4/PgP induction	– ▼ C/T/S levels	• Monitor levels, increase dose C/T/S accordingly • Avoid combination if possible
St John's wort (SJW)	CYP3A4/PgP induction	– ▼ C/T/S levels	• Consider alternatives to SJW • If it cannot be avoided, monitor C/T/S levels

▼ = decreased; ▲ = increased

[a]Lexicomp® Drug Interactions (2018) and Glotzbecker et al. (2012)

alternative for SJW is available (Enioutina et al. 2017; Lexicomp® Drug Interactions 2018).

31.3.2 Food

Drug interactions with food and drinks are known to occur. Grapefruit juice is a potent inhibitor of intestinal CYP3A4, and many clinically relevant interactions have been reported (e.g., with simvastatin and calcineurin inhibitors). Cruciferous vegetables (Brussels sprouts, cabbage, and broccoli) contain substances that are inducers of CYP1A2 but do not appear to cause clinically important drug interactions (Thanacoody 2012).

31.4 Resources for Drug Interactions

Drug interactions in HSCT can be numerous. Whenever a potential clinically relevant drug interaction is recognized, a management plan should be recommended (modification in drug therapy or closer monitoring of efficacy and adverse reactions) (Tannenbaum and Sheehan 2014). A number of resources are available to help identifying and managing drug interactions (e.g., Lexicomp® Drug Interactions 2018; Clinical Pharmacology® 2018; Medicines Complete® 2018). Interpretation of interactions must be performed carefully to avoid the risk of over-alerting. The patient's clinical status, comorbidities, and severity of the drug interactions presented should always be taken into account.

31.5 Conclusion

Drug interactions can occur at all levels during HSCT. Attention to and management of interactions is crucial to prevent severe clinical consequences. Due to the complexity of the therapy and the risk of drug interactions, an active collaboration in a HSCT multidisciplinary team, including physicians, pharmacists, and nurses, is of paramount importance.

Key Points

- Drug interactions in HSCT are common and can occur at all levels
- Knowledge of mechanisms involved in drug metabolism might help in anticipating interactions
- A multidisciplinary approach is important to reduce the risk of drug interactions

References

Ahmed S, Zhou Z, Zhou J, Chen SQ. Pharmacogenomics of drug metabolizing enzymes and transporters: relevance to precision medicine. Genomics Proteomics Bioinformatics. 2016;14:298–313.

Clinical Pharmacology powered by ClinicalKey. Tampa: Elsevier. http://www.clinicalkey.com. Accessed 16 Jan 2018.

Enioutina EY, Salis ER, Job KM, Gubarev MI, Krepkova LV, Sherwin CM. Herbal Medicines: challenges in the modern world. Part 5. Status and current directions of complementary and alternative herbal medicine worldwide. Expert Rev Clin Pharmacol. 2017;10:327–38.

Ferri N, Bellosta S, Baldessin L, Boccia D, Racagni G, Corsini A. Pharmacokinetics interactions of monoclonal antibodies. Pharmacol Res. 2016;111:592–9.

Flockhart Table P450 Drug Interactions. Indiana University. http://medicine.iupui.edu/clinpharm/ddis/main-table/. Accessed 16 Jan 2018.

Gholaminezhad S, Hadjibabaie M, Gholami K, et al. Pattern and associated factors of potential drug-drug interactions in both pre- and early post-hematopoietic stem cell transplantation stages at a referral center in the Middle East. Ann Hematol. 2014;93:1913–22.

Glotzbecker B, Duncan C, Alyea E, Campbell B, Soiffer R. Important drug interactions in hematopoietic stem cell transplantation: what every physician should know. Biol Blood Marrow Transplant. 2012;18:989–1006.

Ingelman-Sundberg M, Rodriguez-Antona C. Pharmacogenetics of drug-metabolizing enzymes: implications for a safer and more effective drug therapy. Philos Trans R Soc Lond B Biol Sci. 2005;360:1563–70.

Larson AM. Drugs and the liver: metabolism and mechanisms of injury. UpToDate, Post TW (Ed), UpToDate, Waltham, MA. Accessed 16 Jan 2018.

Leather HL. Drug interactions in the hematopoietic stem cell transplant (HSCT) recipient: what every transplanter needs to know. Bone Marrow Transplant. 2004;33:137–52.

Lexicomp Drug Interactions. UpToDate, Post TW (Ed), UpToDate, Waltham, MA. Accessed 16 Jan 2018.

Lynch T, Price A. The effect of cytochrome P450 metabolism on drug response, interactions, and adverse effects. Am Fam Physician. 2007;76:391–6.

MedicinesComplete [online]. London: Pharmaceutical Press. http://www.medicinescomplete.com/. Accessed 16 Jan 2018.

Palleria C, Di Paolo A, Giofrè C, et al. Pharmacokinetic drug-drug interaction and their implication in clinical management. J Res Med Sci. 2013;18:601–10.

Tannenbaum C, Sheehan NL. Understanding and preventing drug-drug and drug-gene interactions. Expert Rev Clin Pharmacol. 2014;7:533–44.

Thanacoody HKR. Drug interactions. In: Walker R, Whittlesea C, editors. Clinical pharmacy and therapeutics. 5th ed. London: Elsevier; 2012.

32 Role of Nursing in HSCT

Aleksandra Babic and John Murray

32.1 Introduction: HSCT Nursing

With the progress of HSCT in the early 1960s, it became clear that nurses play a crucial role within the multidisciplinary team (MDT) caring for patients and their families undergoing this intense treatment. The distress during the time prior to undergoing HSCT, during isolation, in the recovery phase and the time after (long-term recovery) is not to be underestimated.

The best compliment towards nursing was made by Prof. Edward Donnall Thomas, the 1990 Nobel Prize winner in Medicine who stated that 'nurses and nursing are my secret weapon without whom I could not have achieved my goals' (Appelbaum 2013).

Continuity of care is vital to patient's right from their initial attendance in hospital. Nurses are an advocate throughout the transplant and often act as a motivating force, supporting and advising as well as supplying physical, psychological and emotional care whilst patient's transition from acute care to long-term follow-up clinics. Experienced nurses with high levels of technical competencies offer patients and families excellent care and support in this challenging area.

Patient preparation for HSCT involves the use of chemotherapy and/or radiotherapy to eradicate the underlying disease of the patient. Throughout the transplant procedure, the patient needs special care to overcome the complications associated with treatment. Nurses must be aware of the possible complications in order to play a role in prevention or early detection of alarming signs, such as sepsis, fluid overload and organ dysfunction, taking appropriate measures to minimize adverse effects and restore the clinical balance of the patient. This care is very complex and requires a high level of skill (Wallhut and Quinn 2017).

The field of nursing research in HSCT has evolved from reflecting on symptom management and service development to quality of life and long-term survival topics. The FACT-JACIE International Standards Accreditation requires that the clinical programme has access to personnel who are formally trained, experienced and competent in the management of patients receiving cellular therapy (JACIE 7th edition n.d.). Thus, it is important that training and competency programmes are structured and ongoing, with documented evidence of training topics and dates (Babic 2015).

A. Babic (✉)
IOSI-Istituto Oncologico della Svizzera Italiana, OSG, Bellinzona, Switzerland
e-mail: Aleksandra.Babic@eoc.ch

J. Murray
Haematology and Transplant Unit, The Christie NHS Foundation Trust, Manchester, UK

E. Carreras et al. (eds.), *The EBMT Handbook*, https://doi.org/10.1007/978-3-030-02278-5_32

32.2 Role of Nursing Throughout HSCT Patient Pathway

HSCT is a standard therapy in a number of malignant and non-malignant conditions.

Pre-transplant assessments must be undertaken, and the results of these along with suitable donor medical clearance and cell availability are essential to ascertain that transplant is a valid option and can proceed safely.

Nurses are pivotal in implementing practices to prevent and manage infections and other serious effects following HSCT (Sureda et al. 2015; Kenyon and Babic 2018) as:

- Bleeding risk caused by thrombocytopenia
- Tiredness and fatigue caused by the decreased haemoglobin levels and lasting effects of chemo-/radiotherapy and associated medications
- Pain due to mucositis
- Sepsis
- Reduced nutrition
- Psychosocial distress
- Isolation

32.2.1 The Role of the Transplant Coordinator (TC)

Many transplant coordinators are nurse specialists who focus their role on the individual needs of the patient and families; however, some centres have medical staff that organize transplants. TC is the person who should:

- Ensure that timely events occur for each patient and their families undergoing HSCT and that the patients are physically and psychologically prepared for the treatment.
- Provide a high level of care and management, inform and educate the patient, have holistic knowledge of the patient, participate in specific or advanced nursing practices (bone marrow sampling, HLA typing, transplant recipient care) and coordinate all the transplant logistics.
- Ensure that a suitable source of cells is available following the high-dose chemotherapy or immunosuppressive treatment that the patient will receive. Make requests to donor search panels, and order cells once the ideal match has been identified by the transplant physician.
- Support the patient with verbal and written information, and educate them about the whole process from typing to transplant. The TC will coordinate all of the care and embodies a clinical nursing function where emphasis is placed on specialization in a clearly defined area of care.
- Actively participate in the JACIE process of accreditation of transplant centres by writing and evaluating SOPs and being a valued member of the MDT and ward team offering teaching and advice.

32.3 Specific Aspects with a Prominent Role for Nurses

32.3.1 Venous Access Device (VAD)

Education and training should not be limited to the care and maintenance after insertion of the VAD but should be focused on well-being and patient safety. An algorithm for choosing the right VAD for the right patient should start with the diagnosis and treatment plan. The best VAD should be chosen based on the pH and osmolarity of the drugs used during the whole treatment period and the vein condition and should include the option for (partial) home infusion treatment.

Within the range of CVAD (central VAD), a peripherally inserted central catheter (PICC) is seen frequently in haematology patients, often as an alternative for a tunnelled CICC (centrally inserted central catheter) such as a Hickman catheter (see Chap. 22).

Nurses are responsible for the safe administration of drugs such as chemotherapy, IS immunosuppressive drugs and blood products as well as parenteral nutrition and symptom control drugs. The accurate handling and taking care of the central venous catheter and infusion pump systems are vital in the process because the catheter is related to the highest risk of infections. The use of an Aseptic Non Touch Technique (ANTT) (Pratt et al. 2007) and its ten principles of care have led to a decrease in catheter-related infections.

GAVeCeLT (*Gli Accessi Venosi Centrali a Lungo Termine*) (Pittiruti and Scoppettuolo 2017) has developed an algorithm for the choice of the most appropriate VAD, based on the best evidence available in the international guidelines, the bundle for the safe implantation of PICCs (see Table 32.1).

Table 32.1 The bundle for the safe implantation of PICCs[a]

The *goals* of the bundle are to minimize
1. Complications related to venipuncture: failure, repeated punctures, nerve injury, arterial injury
2. Malposition
3. Venous thrombosis
4. Dislocation
5. Infection
In order to reach the goal, *the SIP protocol* was developed and needs to be followed
1. Bilateral US scan of all veins at the arm and neck
2. Handwashing, aseptic technique and maximal barrier protection
3. Choice of the appropriate vein at the midarm (vein mm = or >cath Fr)
4. Clear identification of median nerve and brachial artery
5. Ultrasound-guided venipuncture
6. US tip navigation during introduction of the PICC
7. Electrocardiography method for assessing tip position
8. Securing the PICC with cyanoacrylate glue, sutureless devise and transparent dressing
Infections in PICCs to be close to zero if a bundle of *preventive measures* are taken[b]
• Site selection
• Skin disinfection with 2% chlorhexidine in 70% gluconate
• Hand hygiene
• Maximum barrier precautions
• Daily control on indication and on complications

[a]Pittiruti and Scoppettuolo (2017)
[b]Harnage (2012)

32.3.2 Early and Acute Complications

They occur following transplantation when the patient has reduced tolerance due to neutropenia and/or increased intestinal permeability. In neutropenia, the number of white blood cells decreases significantly, resulting in aplasia with an increased risk of infection. An increased permeability of the intestinal wall is caused by intensive chemotherapy damaging the gastrointestinal mucosa. As a result, pathogenic bacteria (bodily bacteria or bacteria from the diet) can enter the bloodstream and cause sepsis.

Early complications generally occur within 100 days post HSCT. In the early phase of HSCT, the main risk factors for infections are neutropenia-barrier breakdown due to mucositis, indwelling catheters, depressed T-cell and B-cell function and aGvHD.

Two of the most common early complications are oral mucositis and sepsis. Some other relatively rare complications are HC, ES, IPS and DAH. TAM and SOS/VOD are analysed in Chaps. 42, 49 and 50. For all complications there are locally agreed recommendations for prevention and principles for nursing care, with monitoring and prompt intervention that may have an influence on patients' morbidity and mortality.

32.3.2.1 Oral Mucositis (OM)

Oral mucositis (OM) has been defined (Rubenstein et al. 2004) as the inflammation of the mucosal membrane, characterized by ulceration, which may result in pain, swallowing difficulties and impairment of the ability to talk. The mucosal injury caused by OM provides an opportunity for infection to flourish and in particular putting the severely immunocompromised patient in the HSCT setting at risk of sepsis and septicaemia.

OM and oral problems in the HSCT setting can be expected to occur in as many as 68% of patients undergoing autologous HSCT and 98% of patients undergoing allogeneic HSCT (EORTC Guidelines). With the increasing use of targeted drug therapies and approaches in the cancer and haematology setting, problems in the oral cavity will increase and become even more of a challenge (Quinn et al. 2015).

All treatment strategies aimed at improving mouth care are dependent on four key principles: accurate assessment of the oral cavity, individualized plan of care, initiating timely preventative measures and correct treatment (Quinn et al. 2008). The assessment process should begin prior to HSCT by identifying all the patient risks most likely to increase oral damage.

The choice of prevention regimens should be guided by evidence based on expert opinion interventions, working with the patient to reduce their potential risk of oral mucositis occurring.

All treatment plans should be based upon the grading of oral damage and patient reports, and these may include the use of topical analgesics and the use of opiates (Elad et al. 2015).

32.3.2.2 Sepsis

Sepsis is a life-threatening condition caused by aberrant and dysregulated host response to infection (Elad et al. 2015). The most important action to prevent infections acquired by exogenous organisms is good hand hygiene performed correctly (Hand Hygiene Guidelines). Appropriate clean work clothes, with short sleeves, no jewellery and no neck tie are the responsibility of all staff. Protective isolation during the neutropenic phase is recommended, and the patient should not be in contact with any staff or visitors with symptoms of infection. For prevention of endogenous infections, oral hygiene and skin care to maintain the mucosal and skin barrier and use of prophylactic antibiotics are the most important actions. Correct handling of any indwelling catheters is also a key nursing responsibility in infection control.

Other areas where infections can be prevented are air and water quality, food hygiene and environmental cleaning. Environmental cleaning includes medical equipment as well.

Early recognition and treatment are vital for a successful outcome of sepsis. Temperature, pulse, blood pressure, respirations and saturation (vital signs) should be frequently monitored. Signs of infection are not always obvious, but if the patient has a temperature ≥38.0 °C, cultures should be taken, IV antibiotics and IV fluids started or increased and oxygen therapy initiated.

The goal is always to *start antibiotic treatment within 1 h* from detection of fever and is the most critical period in the patient's survival from sepsis. Early recognition and intervention are achieved by frequent monitoring of the patient's vital signs and general condition and paying attention to subtle changes that should be promptly reported, such as mental state alteration or mottled skin.

Alert for immediate action are when a previously well patient only responds to pain or becomes unresponsive, becomes confused and has a systolic blood pressure of <90 mmHg or a fall of >40 mmHg from baseline; an elevated heart rate >130 bpm; a respiratory rate of >25 per min, requiring oxygen to maintain saturations >92%; a non-blanching rash or mottled, ashen or cyanotic skin, not passed urine in the last 18 h; an output of <0.5 ml/kg/h; a lactate of >2 mmol/l; or received recent chemotherapy.

Immediate action is required at the first indication of sepsis. The concept of *the sepsis six and the severe sepsis resuscitation bundle* (Daniels et al. 2011) has been developed as a guide to prioritize interventions in patients where sepsis is suspected:

1. Oxygen therapy aims to keep saturations >94% (88–92% if at risk of CO_2 retention, e.g. COPD).
2. Blood cultures, at least a peripheral set, consider CSF, urine, sputum, chest X-ray and urinalysis.
3. IV antibiotics, according to hospital policy, consider allergies prior to administration.
4. Fluid resuscitation, if hypotensive or lactate >2 mmol/l, 500 ml bolus stat, may be repeated if clinically indicated. Do not exceed 30 ml/kg.
5. Serial serum lactates corroborate high VBG lactate with arterial sample. If lactate >4 mmol/l, call critical care for support. Recheck after each 10 ml/kg challenge.

6. Assess urine output which may require catheterization, and ensure fluid balance chart commenced and completed hourly.

When treatment has been initiated, the patient must be continually monitored to determine the effect of treatment or worsening of the condition. This includes vital signs, fluid balance including weight and assessment of identified and/or potential infection sites (mouth, skin, all indwelling catheters, urine, stools, etc.), mental status, signs of bleeding, pain and general appearance and well-being.

Antibiotics should be delivered with strict adherence to the prescribed time schedule. Antipyretic agents should be avoided since they may mask fever but may under certain circumstances be used to alleviate patient discomfort and pain.

32.3.2.3 Pain

Pain in the HSCT setting is most commonly experienced as a result of mucositis, but patients will also report other pain such as bone pain associated with G-CSF, abdominal pain due to diarrhoea or general discomfort with fluid accumulation. A comprehensive evaluation of the pain, location, characteristics, onset, duration, frequency and severity, exacerbating and relieving factors, should be included. This assessment should be supported by the patient's non-verbal reactions such as facial expression, pallor, tempo of speech, body position, etc. as well as their vital signs.

32.3.2.4 GvHD

GvHD remains a leading cause of non-relapse mortality and is associated with a high morbidity that increasingly affects quality of life (Lee et al. 2003; Dignan 2012). Nursing care of patients with GvHD is highly complex and extremely stressful especially in the acute setting in patients with grades 3–4 skin and GI involvement (Table 32.2). Supportive nursing care to complement medical interventions aims to offer symptomatic comfort and relief.

There are many manifestations of GvHD, and nurses are able to advise patients with respect to many of these including eye, mouth and genital care. Further readings: GvHD chapter in the EBMT Textbook for nurses 2018 (Kenyon and Babic 2018).

Table 32.2 Nursing care of patients with skin and gastrointestinal GvHD

Skin care
1. Maintain integrity of the skin; regular application of cream, ointment or gel; patient choice of vehicle
2. Emollient application, high or low water content to be considered, QV, hydromol or diprobase
3. At least 30-min gap between emollient and steroid cream applications
4. Topical steroids, strength decided by site and length of treatment
5. Menthol cream for painful and pruritic skin, cooling effect
6. Use high-factor sunscreen SPF 50+
7. Always apply creams to make the skin appear shiny; adult body will require 500 g per week
8. Apply in one direction, direction of hair growth, do not scrub on
9. Medical grade silk clothing
10. Good fluid intake and nutrition
11. Organic coconut oil or other natural lipids
12. Aloe vera gels; do not use alone as they will dry the skin
Gastrointestinal
1. Ensure stool samples are taken to exclude infection
2. Adequate oral intake with strict fluid balance
3. Small and frequent high-calorie food and drinks
4. Antiemetics
5. Loperamide, codeine and octreotide may be used to stem diarrhoea
6. Rest bowel and use parenteral feeding
7. Consider the use of radiologically inserted gastrostomy (RIG) feeding
8. Flexi-seal faecal collection device

32.3.3 Long-Term Complications and Side Effects Post Allo-HCST

Long-term side effects after allo-HSCT include non-malignant organ or tissue dysfunction, changes in quality of life, infections related to abnormal immune reconstitution and secondary cancers. Many of these can be attributed to effects of chronic graft-versus-host disease (Dignan 2012; Bhatia 2011; Mohty and Mohty 2011). With advances achieved in terms of supportive care, it is reasonable to expect outcomes to improve steadily, and consequently increasing numbers of transplant survivors will be facing life after the initial transplant experience. For some survivors the burden of long-term morbidity is substantial, and long-term follow-up of patients who received allo-HSCT is now widely recommended.

Key Points

- Specific technical care activities require nursing knowledge and specific skills in the field of HSCT such as instrument manipulation, knowledge of technologies and the use of special protocols to effectively intervene in complex situations and deal with acute and chronic HSCT complications.
- As patients become more complex, so does the care that they require.
- It is essential that nursing adapts to these challenges and improves in both the quality and expertise that is vital to improve patient survival and overall experience of this life-changing treatment.
- The predominant role for nurses is focused to vascular access device, oral mucositis and other early complications as HC, ES, IPS and DAH. TAM and SOS/VOD, sepsis, pain, GVHD and several late complications.

References

Appelbaum FR. 2013. http://www.hematology.org/Thehematologist/Profiles/1088.aspx.

Babic A. Transplant unit personnel competency maintenance: online testing by sharepoint application. EBMT 2015. Oral presentation N003.

Bhatia S. Long-term health impacts of hematopoietic stem cell transplantation inform recommendations for follow-up. 2011. https://www.ncbi.nlm.nih.gov/pmc/articles/PMC3163085/.

Daniels R, Nutbeam T, McNamara G, Galvin C. The sepsis six and the severe sepsis resuscitation bundle: a prospective observational cohort study. Emerg Med J. 2011;28:507–12.

Dignan FL, Amrolia P, Clark A, Haemato-oncology Task Force of British Committee for Standards in Haematology, British Society for Blood and Marrow Transplantation, et al. Diagnosis and management of chronic graft-versus-host disease. Br J Haematol. 2012;158:46–61.

Elad S, Raber-Durlacher JE, Brennan MT, et al. Basic oral care for hematology-oncology patients and hematopoietic stem cell transplantation recipients: a position paper from the joint task force of the Multinational Association of Supportive Care in Cancer/International Society of Oral Oncology (MASCC/ISOO) and the European Society for Blood and Marrow Transplantation (EBMT). Support Care Cancer. 2015;23:223–36.

Harnage S. Seven years of zero central-line-associated bloodstream infections. Br J Nurs. 2012;21:S6, S8, S10-2.

JACIE 7th Edition Standards. www.Jacie.org.

Kenyon M, Babic A. European blood and marrow transplantation textbook for nurses. Cham: Springer; 2018. isbn:978-3-319-50025-6.

Lee SJ, Vogelsang G, Flowers MED. Chronic graft-versus-host disease. Biol Blood Marrow Transplant. 2003;9:215–33.

Mohty B, Mohty M. Long-term complications and side effects after allogeneic hematopoietic stem cell transplantation: an update. Blood Cancer J. 2011;1:e16.

Pittiruti M, Scoppettuolo G. The GAVeVeLT manual of PICC and midline, indications, insertion, management. St. Paul: Edra; 2017.

Pratt RJ, Pellowe CM, Wilson JA, et al. National evidence-based guidelines for preventing healthcare-associated infections in NHS hospitals in England. J Hosp Infect. 2007;65(Suppl 1):S1–64.

Quinn B, Potting C, Stone R, et al. Guidelines for the assessment of oral mucositis in adult chemotherapy, radiotherapy and haematopoietic stem cell transplant patients. Eur J Cancer. 2008;44:61–72.

Quinn B, Thompson M, Treleaven J, et al. United Kingdom oral care in cancer guidance. 2nd ed. 2015. www.ukomic.co.uk. Accessed 03 Sep 2016.

Rubenstein EB, Peterson DE, Schubert M, Mucositis Study Section of the Multinational Association for Supportive Care in Cancer, International Society for Oral Oncology, et al. Clinical practice guidelines for the prevention and treatment of cancer therapy-induced oral and gastrointestinal mucositis. Cancer. 2004;100(Suppl 9):2026–46.

Sureda A, Bader P, Cesaro S, et al. Indications for allo- and auto-SCT for haematological diseases, solid tumours and immune disorders: current practice in Europe, 2015. Bone Marrow Transplant. 2015;50:1037–56.

Wallhut E, Quinn B. Early and acute complications and the principles of HSCT nursing care. In: Wallhult E, Quinn B, Kenyon M, Babic A, editors. The European blood and marrow transplantation textbook for nurses. 2017. https://doi.org/10.1007/978-3-319-50026-3_9.

33 Ethical Issues in HSCT

Khaled El-Ghariani and Jean-Hugues Dalle

33.1 Introduction

Ethics is a branch of philosophy, and, like mathematics, moral philosophy does not give ready-made answers to questions but teaches how one could systematically analyse and resolve a problem. Philosophy's main tool, to achieve this, is logic, where accurate premises are linked together to support a conclusion within a sound and valid ethical argument (West 2009). This chapter aims to explain this process using examples from blood and marrow transplantation practices.

Ethical discourse requires a theory of ethics (Thompson 2005). One requires a landmark to understand their ethical position. One needs to know on what basis one can decide if an action is wrong or right, bad or good; a theory of ethics should help this. It will also allow better understanding of common threats to ethics such as appealing to religion, using relativism to justify accepting different truths to different situations or explaining that ethical stands are unreasonably demanding (Blackburn 2001).

The most known ethical theories are Kant's deontological theory and Bentham and Mill's utilitarianism (Vardy and Grosch 1999). Kant argued for our duty to pursue a set of intrinsically ethical rules that can be universally applied. Ethics is the search for such rules. On the other hand, utilitarianism argues that an action or a rule is moral if their outcomes bring the greatest pleasure and happiness to the greatest numbers of people. No doubt, these theories would ignite an interesting discussion on transplant ethics but may not provide clear enough guidance to healthcare practitioners to help tackle the dilemmas that they regularly encounter.

During the last four decades, Beauchamp and Childress (2013) defended, and significantly developed, the four principles ethical theory for healthcare profession. These principles include:

1. Respect for autonomy: respecting the decision-making capacity of autonomous persons
2. Non-maleficence: avoiding the causation of harm
3. Beneficence: providing benefits as well as balancing such benefits against risks and cost
4. Justice: distributing benefits, risks and costs fairly.

According to Beauchamp and Childress (2013)

K. El-Ghariani (✉)
Department of Hematology, Sheffield Teaching Hospitals Trust and NHSBT, The University of Sheffield, Sheffield, UK
e-mail: Khaled.el-ghariani@nhsbt.nhs.uk

J.-H. Dalle
Department of Pediatric Hematology-Immunology, Hospital Robert-Debré, Assistance Publique-Hôpitaux de Paris, Paris Diderot University, Paris, France

E. Carreras et al. (eds.), *The EBMT Handbook*, https://doi.org/10.1007/978-3-030-02278-5_33

Beneficence is the primary goal of medicine and healthcare, whereas respect for autonomy, along with non-maleficence and justice, sets the moral limits on the professional's actions in pursuit of this goal.

Ethical obligations towards patients (and sometimes their relatives) are well known to healthcare professionals. In the field of transplantation, management of donors adds another dimension to the ethical complexity. Two more areas of work are morally challenging, and although less well argued for, they are critical and have wide implications: firstly, the moral obligations of professionals to engage with fund holders, commissioners and insurers to ensure fair funding of service and, secondly, the ethical role of experts in the management, reporting and publishing of data and information to ensure accurate practice evidence to inform decision-making. Ethical practice requires one to apply the above four principles to all field of work, every time an ethical issue is raised. Transplantation practice is full with issues that can raise serious and sometimes disturbing ethical concerns. The following is a discussion of some aspects of the ethical implications of high-risk treatment, lack of enough funding for healthcare and issues with donor care.

33.2 Ethical Challenges of High-Risk Treatment

Blood and marrow transplantation is mostly used to treat life-threatening illnesses, but also it carries serious complications that are themselves life threatening. Resistance disease or a recipient with significant comorbidities can make transplant risks too high and brings risks of futility to the equation. Although guidelines and outcomes data are available in the literature, the application of such evidence may require the support of colleagues or other experts within a multidisciplinary team. This should help in striking the desirable balance between expected benefits and possible harm (the beneficence and the non-maleficence principles). Although risks may be too high, one ought to ask 'is it the best option available for that particular patient with that particular disease?' (Snyder 2016). Moreover, the implications of undertaking a transplant procedure with limited benefits on resources and other patients ought to be considered. The limitation of transplant rooms, for example, may explain how a decision to transplant a particular patient could affect another.

A transplant procedure that carries only 10–20% chance of success can be a source of worry to staff as it brings the beneficence/non-maleficence balance to a critical point. However, the other two ethical principles may help. What the patient wants to do? And will such a transplant jeopardise other patients care or face funding rejection? Obviously for a keen patient and supportive healthcare payers, the decision is less problematic. The balance of forces may be different in another situation with the same clinical ground. This brings uncomfortable variations into practice which can only be minimised by the development of constructive ethical discourse.

An unbiased list of options ought to be discussed with the patient (and possibly with their relatives and even healthcare payers). To obtain an autonomous consent, staff have to ensure that the patient has fully understood all options and has made a choice that is not influenced by any coercive factors. Obtaining such a valid consent requires arrangements and it will take some time and effort. This, however, not only meets our moral obligations but also has practical benefits, as a well-consented patient is likely to cooperate with the demand of treatment and work with staff to fight complications. Respect of autonomy dictates that patients are well informed about decisions that they make, and it also dictates that staff accept such decisions even if decisions sound counterintuitive. A self-funding patient who refuses life-saving transplant to save the money for their young children may pose difficult and very uncomfortable challenges to staff. This patient can be helped through exploring charitable funds for their treatment, but ignoring their autonomous decisions is not an ethical option.

33.3 Engagement with Funding Issues as a Professional Moral Obligation

Establishing funding rules for transplantation treatment has been, on many occasions, considered the job of healthcare payers or insurers. Medical staff are involved in setting up guidelines, publishing data on outcomes and advising in some complex cases. However, an ethical assessment of the issue will put medical staff in the centre of decision-making. After all, healthcare payers and insurers will base all their decisions not only on medical information but also on the interpretation of such information as provided by medical staff. It is prudent to think that it is unethical that medical staff do not engage actively in this process. The same ethical desire that drives staff to treat illness and complications ought to drive their engagement in mending funding practices that do not meet patients' needs, as both issues are detrimental to patients' outcomes.

The respect to autonomy principle dictates involvement of patients' representatives in funding decisions. Most healthcare services have such an arrangement, and the job of the medical staff is to educate representatives to be able to make valid and informed decisions. The principle of beneficent, in this setting, can be applied by gathering, analysing and publishing good data to support funding decisions. Whilst publishing papers may have been considered as an option for academic progression, it seems that it has become an ethical obligation. Non-maleficence means that delays in introducing new development in the field must be avoided. Transplant field is rapidly changing (for the better), and such delays could devote patients from a helpful treatment modality that could make a difference to them. The principle of justice is in the heart of healthcare funding. However, this ought to not mean 'sticking to the rule'. Most rules have legitimate exceptions and the job of the transplant physician to fight the corner of the patients in this regard. Some healthcare services support cord transplant but not the use of double cord, because of cost implications. This would disadvantage many adult patients with body weight that is too high for a cord blood unit to support. The desire to establish an ethical process of funding may have led the English National Healthcare Service to establish Clinical Reference Groups, including one for transplantation. This group is composed of a medical chair, eight other transplant physicians and three members to represent patient and public voice (NHS England 2018). Medical ethics is mainly seen as a direct issue between a professional and a patient. This discussion showed the ethical obligations of professionals outside the clinic and the hospital ward. This is obviously demanding but also more helpful to patients.

33.4 The Ethical Issues in Donor Management

Transplant donation is a fertile subject for ethical debate as all types of donation carry some moral concerns. These are mainly around respect of donor autonomy, risk of exploitation or possible harm to donor. Unrelated donors are supported by professionals other than staff who look after the recipient, and this is according to national and international guidance. Unrelated donations have some financial and reputational benefits to the donor registries. However, given existing professionalism and code of practice, this has rarely raised concerns. On the other hand, family donors receive less structured protection. The recent success in haploidentical transplantation means that more family donors will be involved, and so ethical grounds of such process needs to be established.

Whilst the balance of risks and benefits of most types of treatment offered to a particular patient can be established, a major dilemma in donor ethics is the fact that assessing harm and inconvenience to one person (the donor) in relation to expected benefits to another (the recipient) is highly problematic. Staff occasionally make the decision themselves and argue that some temporary aches and pains and minimal risks of ruptured spleen (G-CSF side effects) are acceptable risks to justify a life-saving donation, particularly to a family member. Staff position makes 'some sense', but it does not respect donor autonomy, and so it cannot be accepted as a universal rule that could be practiced widely, i.e. it lacks ethical grounds.

Child donors, pregnancies conceived for HCT and donation from a family member who lack capacity have been debated. Minor sibling donors require particular consideration as their autonomy is harder to prove. There is evidence that a child donor is subjected to both physical and psychological implications. This prompted (the) American Academy of Pediatrics Committee on Bioethics to recommend that five conditions are met to ensure morally justified donations from children (AAP 2010). These include lack of suitable adult donor, the expected benefit to recipient is reasonably high, strong relationship between donor and recipient, potential physical and psychological harms to donor must be minimised and, finally, obtaining parents' consent and child assent. Child assent and agreement are hard to confirm, and the availability of independent committee or assessor to look after such donors has been recommended.

Moreover, a family donation from an adult with full capacity can be morally challenging for two reasons. Firstly, not all family members want to donate. Some of them find the process too demanding, and if they were 'given the choice', they will rather not. The story of one such donor was in the news. A newspaper (the Daily Mail, UK) reported the situation using the following headline: 'Sentenced to die by my sister, leukemia victim refused her only chance of transplant' (Oldfield 1997). The sister refused to donate bone marrow because of the phobia of hospitals. The subsequent media debate led the donor to reconsider her position. This is a moral position that is hard to defend. Secondly, the health risks to family donors are not minimum or negligible. They are more likely to encounter significant complications than unrelated donors (Halter et al. 2009). Documented experience from unrelated donations cannot be used to advise family donors, and the comparison between harm to donor and benefit to recipient is even harder in the family donor situation. Many authors (van Walraven et al. 2010; Brand et al. 2011) attempted to raise awareness of these issues, and many argued that a system that is separate to and not influenced by patient care ought to be in place to manage family donors.

Transplantation, like other healthcare practices, requires an accurate balance between expected benefits and possible harm as well as valid patient consent. Given limited resources, the implication of one transplant on another ought to be considered. Given the life-saving and life-threatening nature of this modality of treatment, ethical issues with transplantation are likely to be challenging. Staff are expected to let patients decided for themselves. Moreover, staff ought to escalate complex issues to the legal system or more commonly to the ethics committee within their institution. In the European Union, Directive 2001/20/EC established ethics committees as an independent body to agree complex ethical challenges.

Key Points

- Clinical ethics teaches skills to tackle moral dilemmas but does not provide ready-made answers.
- Clinical ethics now extends, beyond patient clinician relationship, to donor care as well as engagement with fund holders and insurers.
- The four principles ethical theory (autonomy, beneficent, non-maleficence and justices) provides reasonable basis for moral assessment of ethical issues in most fields of practice.
- The donation process requires ethical vigilance. Family donors have high health risks and, given the potential social pressure, are not always autonomous.

References

American Academy of Pediatrics. Policy statement, children as hematopoietic stem cell donors. 2010. http://pediatrics.aappublications.org/content/pediatrics/125/2/392.full.pdf.

Beauchamp TL, Childress JF. Principles of biomedical ethics. 7th ed. Oxford: Oxford University Press; 2013.

Blackburn S. Being good a short introduction to ethics. Oxford: Oxford University Press; 2001.

Brand A, et al. Uniform examination of stem cell donors. ISBT Sci Ser. 2011;6:160–4.

Halter J, Kodera Y, Ispizua AU, et al. Severe events in donors after allogeneic hematopoietic stem cell donation. Haematologica. 2009;94:94–101.

NHS England. NHS commissioning, Specialised, F01. Blood and Marrow Transplantation. 2018. https://www.england.nhs.uk/commissioning/spec-services/npc-crg/blood-and-infection-group-f/f01/.

Oldfield S. Sentenced to die by my sister. Daily Mail. 1997;1:5.

Snyder DS. Ethical issues in haematopoietic cell transplantation. In: Forman SJ, et al., editors. Thomas' hematopoietic cell transplantation. Chichester: Wiley Blackwell; 2016.

Thompson M. Ethical theory. 2nd ed. Coventry: Hodder Murray; 2005.

Vardy P, Grosch P. The puzzle of ethics. London: Fount; 1999.

van Walraven SM, Nicoloso-de Faveri G, Axdorph-Hygell UAI, et al. Family donor care management: principles and recommendations. Bone Marrow Transplant. 2010;45:1269–73.

West AA. Rulebook for arguments. 4th ed. Indianapolis: Hackett Publishing; 2009.

34 Quality of Life Assessment After HSCT for Pediatric and Adults

Anna Barata and Heather Jim

34.1 Introduction

Methodological advances in the HCT field have increased the population of survivors worldwide. However, HCT is associated with significant morbidity that impairs survivors' recovery and adversely affects their QoL. A significant body of literature has addressed QoL after HCT and highlights significant deficiencies in physical, psychological, social, and role functioning both in adult and pediatric survivors (Pidala et al. 2010). These data are clinically relevant as they help to understand the impact of HCT on patient's lives. Clinically, assessment of QoL can inform patient education and be used to evaluate the benefit of supportive care interventions.

34.2 QoL Assessment

QoL can be considered a patient-reported outcome (PRO). PROs are defined by the US Food and Drug Administration (FDA) as the "measurement of any aspect of a patient's health status that comes directly from the patient, without the interpretation of the patient's response by a clinician or anyone else" (US Food and Drug Administration 2009). Thus, PROs specifically describe the impact that HCT has on patients' lives and provide information unavailable from other sources (Kurosawa et al. 2017; Russell et al. 2006). PROs are also used in pediatric populations, although parents or other proxies might be used as source of information when children are unable to report their own QoL. However, the use of patients' own reports is clearly recommended because significant discrepancies are found when comparing patients' self-reported QoL to reports of physicians, parents, or other proxies (Kurosawa et al. 2017; Russell et al. 2006). In general, measures to assess patient- and proxy-reported QoL are questionnaires.

These instruments can be broadly categorized as general or disease- or procedure-specific. General measures assess QoL of the general population and can also be administered to specific populations, such as HCT recipients. These questionnaires allow comparisons of QoL across populations, such as between HCT survivors and individuals without cancer. In contrast, disease- and procedure-specific instruments examine specific aspects of the health conditions assessed. These measures capture specific PROs that are likely to be important to patients.

A. Barata (✉)
Department of Hematology, Hospital de la Santa Creu i Sant Pau, Universitat Autònoma de Barcelona, Barcelona, Spain

José Carreras Leukemia Research Institute, Barcelona, Spain
e-mail: ABarata@santpau.cat

H. Jim
Department of Health Outcomes and Behavior, Moffitt Cancer Center, Tampa, FL, USA

E. Carreras et al. (eds.), *The EBMT Handbook*, https://doi.org/10.1007/978-3-030-02278-5_34

34.3 Measures to Assess QoL in Adults and Pediatric Patients Undergoing HCT

There are numerous measures assessing QoL on adults and pediatric HCT recipients. Measures used have been both general and disease-specific. The following sections list some of the most common used questionnaires in the field of HCT.

34.3.1 Adults

Interest in assessing QoL in adult HCT recipients is reflected in the variety of measures used to assess this outcome. However, there is a need for the scientific community to reach consensus about which questionnaires to use in order to facilitate comparison across studies (Shaw et al. 2016). Table 34.1 summarizes alphabetically some of the most common questionnaires to assess QoL in adults.

Table 34.1 QoL questionnaires assessing QoL in adult HCT survivors

(a) General	
European Quality of Life- 5 Dimensions (EQ-5D-5L) (van Reenen and Jansen 2015)	
Aim	Health status
Items	6
Domains/subscales	Mobility, self-care, usual activities, pain, anxiety, depression
Results	Profile of each of the domains assessed, and an index of the health status. Higher scores indicate better health status
Translations	Available in more than 130 languages
Medical Outcomes Study-Short Form (MOS SF-36) (Ware et al. 1994)	
Aim	QoL
Items	36; shorter versions feature 12 items (SF-12) or 8 items (SF-8)
Domains/subscales	General health, physical, role, emotional and social functioning, mental health, pain, vitality
Results	Physical Component Score; Mental Component Score and Global Score. Higher scores indicate better QoL
Translations	Available in more than 170 languages
Patient-Reported Outcomes Measurement Information System (PROMIS) (Cella et al. 2010)	
Aim	Mental, physical, and social health and QoL in healthy populations as well as those with chronic conditions
Items	Multi-item measures varying in length and complexity; for example, PROMIS-29 has 29 items, PROMIS-43 has 43 items, PROMIS-57 has 57 items
Domains/subscales	Each subscale measures a single domain; PROMIS Profile measures assess multiple domain
Results	Higher scores indicate more of the concept being measured. Measures use standardized T-score metric against normative data for the US population
Translations	Available in Spanish and several other languages
(b) Cancer and HCT specific	
European Organization for Research and Treatment of Cancer QoL Questionnaire Core 30 (EORTC QLQ-C30) version 3.0 (Aaronson et al. 1993)	
Aim	QoL in cancer
Items	30 items
Domains/subscales	Functional scales, symptom scale and a QoL scale
Results	Higher scores in functional and QoL scales indicate better wellbeing. Higher scores in the symptom scale indicate worse symptomatology
Translations	Available in more than 100 languages

Table 34.1 (continued)

Functional Assessment of Cancer Therapy—Bone Marrow Transplant (FACT-BMT) (McQuellon et al. 1997)	
Aim	QoL in HCT
Items	47
Domains/subscales	Consists of the FACT-G (Cella et al. 1993) and the BMT concerns subscale
Results	Higher scores indicate better QoL
Translations	Available in more than 38 languages
Functional Assessment of Cancer Therapy—General Scale (FACT-G) (Cella et al. 1993)	
Aim	QoL in cancer
Items	33
Domains/subscales	Physical, functional, social and emotional well-being
Results	Higher scores indicate better wellbeing and global QoL
Translations	Available in more than 60 languages

34.3.2 Pediatrics

There is less research on QoL on pediatric patients than adult patients. Initial pediatric studies focused on a single aspect of functioning, such as psychosocial and physical limitations. It was not until the early 1990s that pediatric QoL began to be addressed as a multidimensional construct. Most of the measures used in pediatric studies were originally developed to be used in the general population or in children with specific illnesses. Table 34.2 lists alphabetically the most common measures used to assess QoL in pediatric population.

34.4 Challenges when implementing QoL assessment

Improvement in patients' QoL is included among the strategic goals of major cancer organizations such as the American Society of Clinical Oncology and regulatory agencies such as the FDA and the European Medicines Agency. Recognition of the importance of the patient experience is reflected in the increasing incorporation of patient-reported QoL measures in observational research and clinical trials. However, some aspects should be considered when implementing patient-reported QoL measures.

Historically, studies and clinical trials performed in the USA have often used the FACT instruments, whereas studies performed in Europe have chosen the EORTC. This divergence makes results difficult to compare (Shaw et al. 2016), although efforts are underway to map common QoL measures such as the EORTC QLQ-C30 and FACT-G to one another (Young et al. 2015). Second, the mode of administration should also be considered. PRO measures have traditionally been administered by paper and pencil, but new technologies offer the potential to use electronic measures. Electronic measures administered before or during a clinic visit allow results to be available at the time of consultation and may facilitate symptom monitoring to guide supportive treatment. One example is the PROMIS instrument, which is available using computer adaptive testing or through REDCap software. Computer adaptive testing selects questions based on the previous responses that patients have provided to approximate the construct being measured in the fewest number of questions. The implementation of routine assessment of patients' QoL on clinical care and clinical trials has the potential to improve patients' well-being.

Table 34.2 QoL questionnaires assessing QoL in pediatric HCT survivors

(a) General	
Child Health Questionnaire (CHQ) (Landgraf et al. 1996)	
Aim	QoL
Versions	Parent-reported versions feature 50 items (CHQ-PF50) or 28 items (CHQ-PF28) and are intended for parents of children aged 5–18 years. The child-report version (CHQ-87) has 87 items and is appropriate for children aged 10–18
Domains/subscales	Global health, physical functioning, role/social-physical functioning, bodily pain/discomfort, role/social-emotional functioning, role/social -behavior, parental impact -time, parental impact -emotional, self-esteem, mental health, global behavior, family activities, family cohesion, and changes in health
Results	Higher scores indicate higher physical and psychosocial wellbeing
Translations	The CHQ-PF50 and CHQ-PF28 are available in more than 80 languages, and the CHQ-87 to 34
Patient-Reported Outcomes Measurement Information System (PROMIS) (Hinds et al. 2013)	
Aim	Health and QoL in healthy populations as well as those with chronic conditions
Versions	Multi-item measures varying in length and complexity: PROMIS-25 has 25 items, PROMIS-37 37 items, and PROMIS-49 49 items. PROMIS measures are child- and parent-reported. Child-report measures are intended for children aged 8–17, and parent-report for children 5–17
Domains/subscales	Physical, mental and social health, and a global QoL score
Results	Higher scores indicate more of the concept being measured. PROMIS use standardized T-score metric against normative data for the US population
Translations	Children and proxy measures are available in Spanish and in several other languages
Pediatric Quality of Life Inventory (PedsQL™) 4.0 Generic Score Scales (Varni et al. 2001)	
Aim	QoL in healthy children or those diagnosed with an acute or chronic disease
Versions	Parent-report form for children aged 2–4 has 21 items, and child and parent reports for children aged 5–18 have 23 items
Domains/subscales	Physical, emotional, social, and school functioning
Results	Physical health summary score; Psychosocial health summary score; Total score. Higher scores indicate better QoL
Translations	Available in more than 70 languages
(b) Cancer and HCT specific	
Child Health Rating Inventories (CHRIs)-and Disease-Specific Impairment Inventory-Hematopoietic Stem Cell Transplantation (DSII-HCT) (Parsons 2005)	
Aim	The disease specific (DSII-HCT) module assesses QoL of childhood HCT survivors
Versions	10-item module intended to child-report (aged 5–12), adolescent-report (13–18) and parents-report (5–18)
Domains/subscales	Items are grouped in three domains reported by parents and patients to be most salient to the HCT experience: worry, hassless, and body image
Results	Higher scores indicate better QoL
Translations	The questionnaire is available in English
Peds Quality of Life Cancer Module 3.0 (PedsQL CM™) (Varni et al. 2002)	
Aim	QoL in children with cancer
Versions	Parent-report form for children aged 2–4 has 25 items, child and parent reports for children aged 5–7 has 26 items, and child and parents reports for children more than 8 years has 27 items
Domains/subscales	Pain and hurt, nausea, procedural anxiety, treatment anxiety, worry, cognitive problems, perceived physical appearance and communication
Results	Higher scores indicate better QoL
Translations	Available in more than 100 languages
The Behavioral, Affective and Somatic Experiences Scales (BASES) (Phipps et al. 1994)	
Aim	QoL during the acute phase of HCT
Versions	There are separate versions to be completed by nurses (BASES-N), parents (BASES-P) and children (BASES-C). The BASES-N and BASES-P have 38 items and the BASES-C has 14 items. The questionnaire is intended to be used in child aged 5–17
Domains/subscales	Somatic distress, mood disturbance, compliance, quality of interactions and activities
Results	Higher scores indicate more distress/impairment
Translations	Available in English

Key Points

- Assessing HCT survivors' QoL is essential in order to know the impact that the HCT, its morbidity, its treatments, and related interventions have on survivors' well-being.
- Enhanced efforts should be made to in order to include QoL assessment in routine clinical practice. Engaging clinicians in using QoL assessments, potentially by means of electronic administration, as well as broadening the interpretation of their scores into the clinical field, might facilitate incorporation.
- Further efforts should elucidate to what extent QoL results are incorporated into management decisions, treatment recommendations, and patients' education.
- Additional efforts should also be made to include QoL outcomes in clinical trials.
- The incorporation of QoL assessment into clinical and research practice has the potential to improve HCT outcomes.

References

Aaronson NK, Ahmedzai S, Bergman B, et al. The European Organization for Research and Treatment of Cancer QLQ-C30: a quality-of-life instrument for use in international clinical trials in oncology. J Natl Cancer Inst. 1993;85:365–76.

Cella D, Riley W, Stone A, et al. The Patient-Reported Outcomes Measurement Information System (PROMIS) developed and tested its first wave of adult self-reported health outcome item banks: 2005-2006. J Clin Epidemiol. 2010;63:1179–94.

Cella DF, Tulsky DS, Gray G, et al. The Functional Assessment of Cancer Therapy scale: development and validation of the general measure. J Clin Oncol. 1993;11:570–9.

Hinds PS, Nuss SL, Ruccione KS, et al. PROMIS pediatric measures in pediatric oncology: valid and clinically feasible indicators of patient-reported outcomes. Pediatr Blood Cancer. 2013;60:402–8.

Kurosawa S, Oshima K, Yamaguchi T, et al. Quality of life after allogeneic hematopoietic cell transplantation according to affected organ and severity of chronic graft-versus-host disease. Biol Blood Marrow Transplant. 2017;23:1749–58.

Landgraf JM, Abetz L, Ware JE. Child health questionnaire (CHQ): a user's manual. Boston: Health Institute, New England Medical Center; 1996.

McQuellon RP, Russell GB, Cella DF, et al. Quality of life measurement in bone marrow transplantation: development of the Functional Assessment of Cancer Therapy-Bone Marrow Transplant (FACT-BMT) scale. Bone Marrow Transplant. 1997;19:357–68.

Parsons SK, Shih MC, Mayer DK, Barlow SE, Supran SE, Levy SL, Greenield S, Kaplan SH. Preliminary psychometric evaluation of the Child Health Ratings Inventory (CHRIs) and Disease-Specific Impairment Inventory-Hematopoietic Stem Cell Transplantation (DSII-HSCT) in parents and children. Qual Life Res. 2005;14(86):1613–25.

Phipps S, Hinds PS, Channell S, et al. Measurement of behavioral, affective, and somatic responses to pediatric bone marrow transplantation: development of the BASES scale. J Pediat Oncol Nurs. 1994;11:109–17; discussion 118-119.

Pidala J, Anasetti C, Jim H. Health-related quality of life following haematopoietic cell transplantation: patient education, evaluation and intervention. Br J Haematol. 2010;148:373–85.

van Reenen M, Jansen B. EQ-5D-5L user guide. Basic information on how to use the EQ-5D-5L instrument [Internet]. 2015 [cited 2018 Jan 24]. https://euroqol.org/wp-content/uploads/2016/09/EQ-5D-5L_UserGuide_2015.pdf. Accessed 12 Feb 2018.

Russell KMW, Hudson M, Long A, et al. Assessment of health-related quality of life in children with cancer: consistency and agreement between parent and child reports. Cancer. 2006;106:2267–74.

Shaw BE, Lee SJ, Horowitz MM, et al. Can we agree on patient-reported outcome measures for assessing hematopoietic cell transplantation patients? A study from the CIBMTR and BMT CTN. Bone Marrow Transplant. 2016;51:1173–9.

US Food and Drug Administration. Guidance for industry: patient-reported outcome measures: use in medical product development to support labeling claims. US Department of Health and Human Services. Food and Drug Administration. 2009. https://www.fda.gov/downloads/drugs/guidances/ucm193282.pdf. Accessed 12 Feb 2018.

Varni JW, Burwinkle TM, Katz ER, et al. The PedsQL in pediatric cancer: reliability and validity of the Pediatric Quality of Life Inventory generic core scales, multidimensional fatigue scale, and cancer module. Cancer. 2002;94:2090–106.

Varni JW, Seid M, Kurtin PS. PedsQL 4.0: reliability and validity of the Pediatric Quality of Life Inventory version 4.0 generic core scales in healthy and patient populations. Med Care. 2001;39:800–12.

Ware JE, Kosinski M, Keller S. SF-36 physical and mental health summary scales: a user's manual. Boston: Health Institute; 1994.

Young TA, Mukuria C, Rowen D, et al. Mapping functions in health-related quality of life: mapping from two cancer-specific health-related quality-of-life instruments to EQ-5D-3L. Med Decis Mak. 2015;35:912–26.

Part V

HSCT Complications and Management

Topic leaders: Jan Styczynski, Enric Carreras and Per Ljungman

35 Neutropenic Fever

Malgorzata Mikulska

35.1 Introduction

Fever during neutropenia is almost universal after a HSCT. In neutropenic HSCT recipients, clinicians are faced with a unique combination of two issues: (1) high incidence of bacterial bloodstream infections and (2) high mortality in case of infections due to Gram-negative bacteria unless effective antibiotic treatment is provided promptly.

Additionally, in the absence of neutrophils which are responsible for most of clinical signs or symptoms during a localized bacterial infection (abscess formation, prominent lung infiltrates, pyuria, etc.), fever is frequently the only symptom present also in these cases. On the other hand, fever is a highly unspecific sign, and there are numerous causes of fever during neutropenia other than bacterial infections, including (a) viral infections, (b) fungal infections, (c) drug reactions (e.g. ATG), (d) transfusion reactions, (e) mucositis, (f) underlying disease, (g) engraftment syndrome, (h) GvHD, (i) cytokine release syndrome, (j) rejection and (k) haemophagocytosis.

However, since infection due to Gram-negative bacteria, including *Pseudomonas aeruginosa*, can result in rapid deterioration of clinical conditions and death, this possibility should be always considered and appropriate empirical antibiotic therapy started while awaiting the results pointing to the actual cause of fever. The issue of prevention of fever and infections during neutropenia through antibiotic prophylaxis with fluoroquinolones has been seriously challanged by a worldwide increase in antibiotic resistance (Mikulska et al. 2018).

35.2 Initial Management of Fever During Neutropenia

Initial management of fever during neutropenia should include all the following (Freifeld et al. 2011; Averbuch 2013; Lehrnbecher et al. 2017).

35.2.1 Diagnostic Procedures

(a). Two sets (1 set = 1 aerobic and 1 anaerobic bottle) of *blood cultures*
   1. Including at least one set from the central venous catheter (CVC), if present
   2. Using an aseptic methodology to reduce the risk of contamination
   3. Providing adequate blood volume (20 ml in each bottle), since the volume of blood is essential to ensure optimal detection of bacteraemia or candidaemia

(b) *Clinical exam* with particular attention to subtle signs of a localized infection
   4. Signs of infection of exit/entry of CVC

M. Mikulska (✉)
Division of Infectious Diseases, Department of Health Sciences (DISSAL), IRCCS Ospedale Policlinico San Martino, University of Genova, Genova, Italy
e-mail: m.mikulska@unige.it

E. Carreras et al. (eds.), *The EBMT Handbook*, https://doi.org/10.1007/978-3-030-02278-5_35

5. Perineal pain suggestive of an abscess
6. Skin or nail lesions suggestive of fungal infection
7. Abdominal defence or diarrhoea
8. Upper respiratory tract symptoms such as rhinorrhoea suggestive of viral respiratory infection
9. Mucosal lesions
10. CNS sings or symptoms (focal lesions, e.g. with fungal infection or bacteria abscess vs. being confused in severe systemic infection or viral encephalitis)

(c). Any *other microbiological exams* based on the clinical presentation (e.g. sputum culture, pharyngonasal swab for respiratory viruses, urinary antigen for *Legionella*, CMV DNA, *Clostridium difficile* toxin, etc)

(d). *Radiological exams* based on the clinical presentation (for suspected lung involvement, lung CT should be used since chest X-ray has too low sensitivity for detecting pneumonia in neutropenic patients)

35.2.2 Evaluation of the Risk of Clinically Severe Infection

Such an evaluation, based on comorbidities, current clinical presentation, etc. leads to the decision on hospital admission and the need for close monitoring for sings of further clinical deterioration.

35.2.3 Evaluation of the Risk of Infection Due to Resistant Bacteria

This risk is considered high in case of:

(a) Colonization with a resistant bacterial strain
(b) Previous infection caused by resistant bacterial strain
(c) Local epidemiology with high incidence of infections caused by resistant pathogens

35.2.4 Choice of the Appropriate Empirical Antibiotic Therapy

It comprised the choice between escalationa and de-escalation strategy (see Table 35.1) and the subsequent choice of antibiotic agent(s).

35.2.5 In High-Risk Patient's Assessment of the Need for Antifungal Therapy

(a) Assessing the risk of candidaemia in patients not receiving antifungal prophylaxis and presenting with septic shock
(b) Assessing the risk of invasive aspergillosis (IA) based on the incidence of IA (taking into account risk factors, mould-active prophylaxis, etc.) and the results of galactomannan (GM) screening or targeted testing.

Empirical antifungal therapy (adding antifungal agent in patients persistently febrile despite broad-spectrum antibiotics) could be replaced by diagnostic-driven strategy based on the use of diagnostic tools, such as a chest computed tomography scan, fungal serum markers (mainly GM, possibly also β-D-glucan or PCR) and targeted treatment following diagnosis (see Chap. 37).

35.3 Main Changes in the Last Decade and Empirical Therapy Modalities

The main change in the management of febrile neutropenia is due to an increasing rate of *multidrug-resistant (MDR) bacteria* in certain countries or centres, in particular Gram-negative rods resistant to almost all antibiotics available (e.g. *Enterobacteriaceae* resistant to third-generation cephalosporins ± piperacillin-tazobactam, i.e. producers of extended-spectrum β-lactamases [ESBLs]; *Enterobacteriaceae* or *Pseudomonas aeruginosa* or *Acinetobacter baumannii* resistant to carbapenems).

35.3.1 De-escalation Strategy

Thus, it might be no longer possible to imagine a single empirical antibiotic regimen which would be appropriate for all the patients and to use a traditional escalation approach, which means changing empirical antibiotic regimen in case of

Table 35.1 The main characteristics of escalation and de-escalation strategy

Strategy	Escalation	De-escalation
Definition	Empirical treatment active against susceptible *Enterobacteriaceae* and *P. aeruginosa*	Starting upfront an empirical coverage of *MDR* bacteria, particularly Gram-negatives, which is later *(72–96 h) reduced (de-escalated)* if a MDR pathogen is *not* isolated: • Susceptible strain isolated • No microbiological results
Antibiotics usually used	Monotherapy with anti-pseudomonal cephalosporin (cefepime, ceftazidime) or piperacillin-tazobactam	• Carbapenem or potentially a new β-lactam such as ceftolozane/tazobactam or ceftazidime/avibactam (although none of them studied in neutropenic patients yet), to cover ESBL-producers and some resistant *P. aeruginosa* *Combinations*, examples • β-lactam + aminoglycoside • β-lactam + coverage of resistant Gram-positives • Colistin-based combinations
Main advantages	Less induction or selection of resistant strains (carbapenem sparing). Less toxicity	Appropriate therapy before culture results are available > *lower mortality*
Main limitations	In case of infection due to a resistant Gram-negatives, prognosis is significantly worsened	*Overuse of broad-spectrum antibiotics/combinations > high antibiotic pressure, particularly in case of failure to de-escalate*
Who	All patients, unless criteria for de-escalation approach are present	Patients at risk for infections due to *resistant bacteria, such as*: • *Colonization with a resistant pathogen* • *Previous infection with a resistant pathogen* • *Centres in which resistant pathogens are frequently isolated* *Particularly* if presenting in *severe clinical conditions*

MDR multidrug resistant

persistent (48–72 h) fever. Indeed, patients who are at high risk of infections due to resistant bacteria, particularly if presenting in severe clinical conditions, should immediately receive agents targeting these strains since any delay in starting effective antimicrobial therapy has been associated with an increased mortality (Tumbarello et al. 2008). Therefore, a de-escalation strategy, typically used in critically ill patients in intensive care units, has been proposed also for neutropenic haematology patients (Averbuch et al. 2013).

Traditional *escalation empirical therapy* is defined as starting with piperacillin-tazobactam or ceftazidime or cefepime and then changing/adding antibiotics if necessary. This approach is still appropriate in most of cases, especially in countries or centres when resistance rates are low among pathogens commonly causing infections in neutropenia. With this approach, carbapenems are used as second-line therapy in patients either failing the initial therapy or in case of a documented infection, and adding an aminoglycoside to a β-lactam, which has been shown in numerous studies as associated with more toxicity and no clinical advantage, is avoided (Averbuch et al. 2013; Drgona et al. 2007). The empirical use of an antibiotic active against resistant Gram-positive bacteria (such as vancomycin) is not recommended neither as initial therapy nor in persistently febrile patients, unless the patient has signs or symptoms suggesting a Gram-positive aetiology (e.g. skin or CVC involvement or pneumonia) or a documented Gram-positive infection (Freifeld et al. 2011; Beyar-Katz et al. 2017).

De-escalation strategy consists of starting with a very broad initial empirical regimen, chosen due to on the severity of the patient's clinical presentation and the risk of infection due to resistant (mainly Gram-negative) bacteria based on individual factors for harbouring MDR bacteria and the local bacterial epidemiology.

The key issues of de-escalation approach are (1) providing immediately effective treatment of a potentially life-threatening MDR pathogen and (2) reducing as much as possible the unnecessary use of precious broad-spectrum drugs, such as carbapenems, colistin, novel beta-lactams or anti-MRSA agents. Data from neutropenic cancer patients in ICU, and more recently from neutropenic haematopoietic stem cell transplant recipients, showed that de-escalation approach is safe and feasible (Mokart et al. 2014; Snyder et al. 2017; Gustinetti et al. 2018). Main characteristics of escalation and de-escalation approach are reported in Table 35.1.

35.3.2 Antibiotic Discontinuation

Another issue of management of febrile neutropenia is the *length of antibiotic therapy*, particularly in the absence of clinically or microbiologically documented infection. Traditionally, antibiotic treatment was continued until neutrophil recovery, with the aim of avoiding infection relapse. In the last decade, this issue has been challenged by IDSA and ECIL guidelines, with the latter stating that antibiotics can be safely discontinued after ≥72 h of IV therapy in patients that are and have been haemodynamically stable since the onset of fever and are without fever for ≥48 h, irrespective of the granulocyte count and the expected duration of neutropenia. The rational for this recommendation was the fact that alteration of patient's microbiota leads to an increased risk of colonization/selection of resistant pathogens, which might subsequently cause life-threatening infections.

The safety of *discontinuation of empirical antibiotic* therapy after few days of treatment, provided the antibiotic treatment is restarted immediately if case of fever reappearance, has been reported and demonstrated in several studies (Orasch et al. 2015). Recently, the first randomized multicentre, open-label superiority trial was performed in 157 high-risk haematology patients with febrile neutropenia without etiological diagnosis. It showed that antimicrobial therapy can be safely discontinued after 72 h of apyrexia and clinical recovery, irrespective of the neutrophils count, and it saves exposure to antimicrobials (mean difference of 4.5 days of antibiotics in the per-protocol analyses). Of note, there were no differences in the number of total days of fever and the crude mortality, and the incidence of recurrent fever during neutropenia and secondary infections was also similar in both groups (Aguilar-Guisado et al. 2017).

35.4 Fever Persistent Despite Empirical Antibiotic Therapy

Fever persistent despite empirical antibiotic therapy is not an infrequent event. Patient's general clinical conditions are the most important factor to consider.

If no signs or symptoms of clinical deterioration (e.g. septic shock, confusion, worsening respiratory function) are present, slow response to antibiotic treatment should be considered, particularly if accompanied by improvement in inflammatory markers such as C-reactive protein, or procalcitonin (particularly for Gram-negative bloodstream infections). In alternative, nonbacterial infections (e.g. viral) or non-infectious causes, such as mucositis, should be considered. Usually, changes in antibiotic regimen are not necessary if clinical conditions are stable. Routine addition of antibiotics against resistant Gram-positives (glycopeptides) has not been shown effective (Beyar-Katz et al. 2017).

Results of GM or other non-invasive fungal tests, performed either in screening or at the onset of fever, should be available by day 2–3 of fever and should guide antifungal treatment. In selected patients at high risk of IA, lung CT scan may be performed to exclude pulmonary fungal disease. *Empirical antifungal treatment* has been introduced when non-invasive diagnostic tests were not available and CT scan availability was extremely limited. When these diagnostic measures became available, *pre-emptive approach* has been shown able to provide earlier treatment than empirical approach (Maertens et al. 2005) (see Chap. 37). Empirical antifungals might be provided while awaiting the results of diagnostic tests or, in case of mould-active prophylaxis, the confirmation of adequate blood levels, but every effort should be made to confirm or exclude the presence of invasive fungal disease. Two meta-analyses in which empirical treatment was compared with no treatment or pre-emptive therapy confirmed that empirical antifungal treatment was associated with a lower rate of (diagnosed) invasive fungal diseases and higher exposure to antifungals but gave no significant advantage in terms of overall mortality (Goldberg et al. 2008; Fung et al. 2015). Similar results were provided by a randomized trial comparing empirical vs. pre-emptive antifungal treatment in which 30% of patient received autologous SCT (Cordonnier et al. 2009).

If clinical conditions deteriorate, usual management steps are:

1. *Aggressive diagnostic workup* (repeated blood cultures, CT scan, BAL lavage in case of pneumonia, lumbar puncture in case of CNS symptoms, etc.)
2. *Escalation* of antibacterial treatment
3. Starting an *antifungal therapy*

There is no universal scheme for antibiotic escalation therapy, but it usually covers resistant Gram-negatives (including those producing extended-spectrum beta-lactamases, ESBLs, e.g. with a carbapenem or an addition of aminoglycoside) and methicillin-resistant staphylococci or ampicillin-resistant enterococci (e.g. with a vancomycin or novel agents). Coverage of other resistant bacteria should be based on the local epidemiology, the epidemiology of a centre where the patient was cared for before transplant and on patient's past history of infections and colonization. Less frequent agents, such as legionella, mycobacteria, *Nocardia* and nonbacterial infections (viral, fungal and parasitic) should be considered in differential diagnosis and tested for, based on clinical presentation and patient's past exposure. Empirical antifungal treatment in this setting might be warranted while awaiting the results of all diagnostic workup.

Key Points

- Numerous causes of fever during neutropenia exist, but usually it should be managed as suspected bloodstream infection unless proven otherwise.
- The initial management includes diagnostics (mandatory blood cultures) and the assessment of the risk of (1) clinically severe infection and (2) infection due to resistant bacteria.
- In patients with severe presentation and the risk of resistant bacteria, de-escalation approach should be used in order to cover the most probable resistant strain(s).
- In other cases, escalation approach is appropriate, and the choice of the first-line empirical antibiotic therapy should be based on antibiotic susceptibility of Gram-negative bacteria most frequently isolated in a given centre.
- Empirical antifungal therapy could be replaced in most cases by diagnostic-driven (pre-emptive) strategy.
- In the absence of clinically or microbiologically documented infection, empirical antibiotic can be safely discontinued after 72 h of apyrexia and clinical recovery, irrespective of the neutrophils count, and it saves exposure to antimicrobials.
- In case of clinical worsening and persistence of fever, extensive diagnostic workup is mandatory.

References

Aguilar-Guisado M, Espigado I, Martín-Peña A, et al. Optimisation of empirical antimicrobial therapy in patients with haematological malignancies and febrile neutropenia (How Long study): an open-label, randomised, controlled phase 4 trial. Lancet Haematol. 2017;4:e573–83.

Averbuch D, Orasch C, Cordonnier C, ECIL4, a joint venture of EBMT, EORTC, ICHS, ESGICH/ESCMID and ELN, et al. European guidelines for empirical antibacterial therapy for febrile neutropenic patients in the era of growing resistance: summary of the 2011

4th European Conference on Infections in Leukemia. Haematologica. 2013;98:1826–35.

Beyar-Katz O, Dickstein Y, Borok S, et al. Empirical antibiotics targeting gram-positive bacteria for the treatment of febrile neutropenic patients with cancer. Cochrane Database Syst Rev. 2017;6:CD003914.

Cordonnier C, Pautas C, Maury S, et al. Empirical versus preemptive antifungal therapy for high-risk, febrile, neutropenic patients: a randomized, controlled trial. Clin Infect Dis. 2009;48:1042–51.

Drgona L, Paul M, Bucaneve G, et al. The need for aminoglycosides in combination with β-lactams for high-risk, febrile neutropaenic patients with leukaemia. Eur J Cancer Suppl. 2007;5:13–22.

Freifeld AG, Bow EJ, Sepkowitz KA, et al. Clinical practice guideline for the use of antimicrobial agents in neutropenic patients with cancer: 2010 update by the Infectious Diseases Society of America. Clin Infect Dis. 2011;52:427–31.

Fung M, Kim J, Marty FM, et al. Meta-analysis and cost comparison of empirical versus pre-emptive antifungal strategies in hematologic malignancy patients with high-risk febrile neutropenia. PLoS One. 2015;10:e0140930.

Goldberg E, Gafter-Gvili A, Robenshtok E, et al. Empirical antifungal therapy for patients with neutropenia and persistent fever: systematic review and meta-analysis. Eur J Cancer. 2008;44:2192–203.

Gustinetti G, Raiola A, Varaldo R, et al. De-escalation and discontinuation of empirical antibiotic treatment in a cohort of allogeneic hematopoietic stem cell transplantation recipients during the pre-engraftment period. Biol Blood Marrow Transplant. 2018;24:1721.

Lehrnbecher T, Robinson P, Fisher B, et al. Guideline for the management of fever and neutropenia in children with cancer and hematopoietic stem-cell transplantation recipients: 2017 update. J Clin Oncol. 2017;35:2082–94.

Maertens J, Theunissen K, Verhoef G, et al. Galactomannan and computed tomography-based preemptive antifungal therapy in neutropenic patients at high risk for invasive fungal infection: a prospective feasibility study. Clin Infect Dis. 2005;41:1242–50.

Mikulska M, Averbuch D, Tissot F, et al. Fluoroquinolone prophylaxis in haematological cancer patients with neutropenia: ECIL critical appraisal of previous guidelines. J Infect. 2018;76:20–37.

Mokart D, Slehofer G, Lambert J, et al. De-escalation of antimicrobial treatment in neutropenic patients with severe sepsis: results from an observational study. Intensive Care Med. 2014;40:41–9.

Orasch C, Averbuch D, Mikulska M, 4th European Conference on Infections in Leukemia (ECIL-4), et al. Discontinuation of empirical antibiotic therapy in neutropenic leukaemia patients with fever of unknown origin is ethical. Clin Microbiol Infect. 2015;21:e25–7.

Snyder M, Pasikhova Y, Baluch A. Early antimicrobial de-escalation and stewardship in adult hematopoietic stem cell transplantation recipients: retrospective review. Open Forum Infect Dis. 2017;4:ofx226.

Tumbarello M, Sali M, Trecarichi EM, et al. Bloodstream infections caused by extended-spectrum-beta-lactamase- producing Escherichia coli: risk factors for inadequate initial antimicrobial therapy. Antimicrob Agents Chemother. 2008;52:3244–52.

36 Bacterial Infections

Diana Averbuch

36.1 Introduction

Bloodstream infections (BSI) are the most frequent bacterial infections in HSCT patients; they occur in 5–10% of auto-HSCT and 20–50% of allo-HSCT patients, with higher rates before engraftment, and are associated with increased morbidity and mortality (Tomblyn et al. 2009; Girmenia et al. 2017; Weisser et al. 2017; Mikulska et al. 2018a). Microbiological documentation of skin and soft tissue infection, pneumonia, and typhlitis is frequently missing.

Patient-related risk factors for bacterial infections include older age, comorbidities, low functional capacity, and high-risk hematological disease (active malignancy, aplastic anemia).

Transplant-related risk factors are specific to the post-HSCT period. During the early pre-engraftment phase, neutropenia and disruption of anatomical barriers (mucosal damage and vascular devices) predispose to infections resulting from Gram-positive cocci (GPC) and Gram-negative bacilli (GNB)—mainly bacteremia/sepsis, pneumonia, sinusitis, proctitis, and cellulitis. In regimens with minimal myelosuppression and mucosal toxicity, as with some non-myeloablative protocols, the risk of infection in the immediate post transplant period is reduced. Conversely, CBT is associated with slower engraftment delayed immune reconstitution, and higher infection risks. During the intermediate phase, starting at engraftment (days +30 to +100), the main risk factors are CVC, GVHD-related organ damage and its treatment, and lack of immune reconstitution. Later, incompetent humoral and cellular immunity (resulting from GVHD, among other factors) predisposes to encapsulated pathogen-associated infections (*Streptococcus pneumoniae* and *Haemophilus influenzae*).

36.2 Epidemiology of Bacteremia

GNB has become an increasingly common cause of bacteremia. They almost equal GPC in a review of studies and ECIL-4 survey (2011) on bacteremia surveillance in European centers. A remarkable variation between centers was shown, from 85%/15% to 26%/74% GPC to GNB ratio (Mikulska et al. 2014). Attribute mortality and TRM are usually higher in patients with GNB-BSI compared with GPC-BSI (Girmenia et al. 2017; Mikulska et al. 2018a).

Emergence of antibacterial resistance complicates treatment of infections. An increase in infections caused by multidrug-resistant (MDR) bacteria (non-susceptible to ≥1 agent in ≥3 therapeutically relevant antimicrobial categories) has been observed in some centers.

D. Averbuch (✉)
Pediatric Infectious Diseases, Hadassah Medical Center, Hebrew University, Jerusalem, Israel
e-mail: adiana@hadassah.org.il

E. Carreras et al. (eds.), *The EBMT Handbook*, https://doi.org/10.1007/978-3-030-02278-5_36

Extensively, drug-resistant bacteria (susceptible to ≤2 antimicrobial categories) have also been reported (Averbuch et al. 2017). Prevalence of resistance is influenced by local antibiotic use policies in prophylaxis and treatment, infection control measures, as well as local resistance patterns throughout the specific hospital and countrywide.

In this session, we address infections caused by the most frequent GPC and GNB.

36.3 Gram-Positive Infections

Coagulase-negative Staphylococcus (CoNS) is the most frequent etiology of BSI (Mikulska et al. 2014). True CoNS BSI, defined as at least two consecutive positive blood cultures, is usually CVC-related. Methicillin resistance is frequent (>50%), prompting treatment with glycopeptides. The prognosis is usually good.

Staphylococcus aureus is rare, reported in a median 6% of HSCT patients, and its attribute mortality is high (12–40%). Cefazolin and oxacillin are the therapeutic mainstays against methicillin-susceptible *Staphylococci*. Methicillin-resistant *Staphylococcus aureus* (MRSA) is frequent; these bacteria are usually susceptible to glycopeptides (vancomycin and teicoplanin). Reduced vancomycin susceptibility has, however, been reported (VISA). Other active agents include daptomycin, linezolid, and tigecycline. The main disadvantages of these agents include:

(a) Linezolid: myelosuppression.
(b) Daptomycin: inactivation by surfactant, it should not be used to treat pneumonia; reduced susceptibility among VISA.
(c) Tigecycline: monotherapy for BSI is not recommended due to low blood levels. Increased mortality has been reported, in comparison with other agents for treating severe infections; a better outcome has been, however, reported with loading and increased daily dosages.

Some newer antibiotics are active against MRSA: ceftaroline, ceftobiprole, dalbavancin, oritavancin, telavancin, and tedizolid.

Enterococci cause a median 5–8% of BSI in HSCT patients, usually occurring later after HSCT, near the time of neutrophil recovery; *E. faecium* is more common than *E. faecalis* (Satlin and Walsh 2017). VRE is an increasing threat in some centers. Previous colonization, mucositis, and broad-spectrum antimicrobial exposure predispose to VRE BSI, which typically occurs in patients in poor clinical condition, perhaps explaining high associated mortality. Main treatment options include linezolid and daptomycin, with VRE sometimes susceptible to quinupristin–dalfopristin (*E. faecium* only), tigecycline, fosfomycin, tedizolid, oritavancin, dalbavancin, and telavancin. Reduced daptomycin susceptibility was reported among VRE; thus, increased dosage (>8 mg/kg/day) is recommended.

Streptococcus viridans (VS) (Freifeld et al. 2011) causes median 5–13% of BSI, usually occurring soon after HSCT (median 4 days); ARDS and septic shock accompany 7–39% of episodes. Mucositis, especially following cytarabine, exposure to fluoroquinolone or ceftazidime, antiacids, MAC, and haploidentical HSCT predispose to VS infections. VS is usually susceptible to most β-lactams used in empirical therapy for febrile neutropenia, with the exception of ceftazidime. The possibility of β-lactam-resistant VS infections, mainly observed after exposure to β-lactams or in nosocomial BSI, justifies addition of vancomycin in neutropenic patients with septic shock.

HSCT patients are at risk for *invasive pneumococcal disease* (IPD), mainly bacteremia and pneumonia, late (median 17 months, range 4 months to 10 years) after HSCT (Engelhard et al. 2002), with a mortality rate of 13–20%. Predisposing factors include allo- versus auto-HSCT, BM versus PBSCT, hypogammaglobulinemia, specific antipneumococcal antibody, and IgG2 deficiency; memory cell defects, as in cGVHD, may also affect the response to vaccines.

36.4 Gram-Negative Infections (Averbuch et al. 2013a, b, 2017; Mikulska et al. 2014, 2018a; Trecarichi et al. 2015; Girmenia et al. 2017)

GNB infecting HSCT patients include *Enterobacteriaceae* (~70%) and non-fermentative GNB (NFGNB, ~24%); others are rare. GNB infections may present with bacteremia, sepsis, enterocolitis, soft tissue infections, such as ecthyma gangrenosum (typically associated with *Pseudomonas aeruginosa*), and septic shock; death may occur within hours in the absence of appropriate supportive and antibiotic treatment.

Several studies report an increase in MDR-GNB infections in HSCT patients, leading to inadequate empirical therapy and increased mortality. In the multinational prospective EBMT study, half of GNB were resistant to non-carbapenem β-lactams, the first-line treatment for febrile neutropenia; 18.5% (40% in some south-western regions) were carbapenem-resistant (CR); and 35% were MDR (Averbuch et al. 2017). Higher rates of resistance were reported in allo- versus auto-HSCT patients and in the south-eastern Europe, as compared with the northwest. The main risk factors for CRGNB are previous colonization, breakthrough on carbapenems, and hospitalization in an ICU. The main Gram-negatives and their resistance pattern are:

36.4.1 Broad-Spectrum β-Lactamase-Producing *Enterobacteriaceae*

The main resistance mechanism to empirical therapy in *Enterobacteriaceae* is broad-spectrum β-lactamase production. This includes (a) extended-spectrum β-lactamase (ESBL), reported in 2–44% of *Enterobacteriaceae* in HSCT patients, and (b) AmpC enzymes, typically produced by *Serratia*, *Providencia*, *Proteus*, *Citrobacter*, and *Enterobacter* spp. These can be induced by non-carbapenem β-lactam treatment. ESBL- or AmpC-producing organisms may appear susceptible in vitro to third-generation cephalosporins (e.g., ceftazidime) or inhibited by β-lactam/β-lactamase inhibitors (BLBLI: sulbactam, clavulanate, tazobactam) yet still be functionally resistant to these agents (Satlin and Walsh 2017). They are frequently fluoroquinolone-resistant. Carbapenems should be the preferred option for treating severely ill patients with broad-spectrum β-lactamase-producing organisms. High-dose prolonged BLBLI infusion can be used under close clinical monitoring in certain stable patients infected with ESBL+ bacteria, susceptible in vitro to BLBLI (Perez et al. 2014; Gudiol et al. 2017).

36.4.2 Carbapenemase-Producing *Enterobacteriaceae* (CPE) (Averbuch et al. 2013a, 2017; Satlin and Walsh 2017; Bassetti et al. 2018)

The main carbapenem resistance mechanism in *Enterobacteriaceae* is production of carbapenemases, including *Klebsiella pneumoniae* carbapenemase (KPC), New Delhi metallo-β-lactamase (NDM), and OXA-type enzymes. Among *Enterobacteriaceae*, carbapenem resistance is more frequent in *Klebsiella pneumoniae*. Delay in appropriate therapy can explain high mortality (~60%) in CPE infections in the allo-HSCT setting. CPE are frequently resistant to "last resource" antibiotics, e.g., fluoroquinolones (in 80%), amikacin or gentamicin (~40%), tigecycline (30%), and colistin (18%). Colistin/polymyxin B is active against a majority of GNB but not *Proteus*, *Serratia*, and *Providencia* spp. Increased mortality has been demonstrated in some retrospective studies, in comparison with other appropriate regimens. Its main side effects include nephrotoxicity and neurotoxicity. Adequate dosing is important (9 million IU loading dose; 4.5 million IU BID maintenance dose). Emergence of plasmid-associated colistin resistance challenges its utility.

Fosfomycin is in vitro active against some resistant GNB. Intravenous formulation is, however, unavailable in some countries; resistance can develop on treatment.

Two or more active agent combinations, including aminoglycosides, polymyxins, tigecycline, fosfomycin, and high-dose (2 g TID), prolonged infusion meropenem (if MIC is ≤8 mg/L), should be preferred in severely ill patients with CPE infections (Gutierrez-Gutierrez et al. 2017). Other treatment modalities include:

- For KPC-CPE infections:
  - TDM-guided meropenem treatment for more resistant bacteria (MIC >8 mg/L)
  - Double carbapenem therapy (ertapenem + meropenem/doripenem)
  - Ceftazidime/avibactam (also active against some OXA-producing GNB); resistance can, however, develop during treatment
  - Meropenem-vaborbactam
- For NDM-producing GNB: aztreonam + ceftazidime/avibactam

36.4.3 *Pseudomonas aeruginosa* (PA) (Mikulska et al. 2014; Averbuch et al. 2017; Satlin and Walsh 2017)

PA Causes 5–15% of BSI, carrying 39–79% mortality, especially in ICU-acquired and resistant PA infections. In a multicenter Italian study, <40% of patients with MDR PA BSI survived longer than 4 months following HSCT (Girmenia et al. 2017). PA in HSCT patients is frequently resistant to fluoroquinolones, aminoglycosides, and β-lactams; 25–71% are MDR. As prognosis is poor, combination therapy, using β-lactam with aminoglycoside or fluoroquinolone, is frequently used in treating severe PA infections, at least initially until the patient is stabilized. Nephrotoxicity is, however, a concern, and no survival benefit of combination therapy has been demonstrated by meta-analysis (Vardakas et al. 2013). A high-dose extended β-lactam infusion regimen was associated with better survival. Ceftolozane-tazobactam was successfully used in severely ill patients with carbapenem-resistant PA.

36.4.4 Other NFGNB

Other NFGNR rarely cause infections in HSCT patients. *Stenotrophomonas maltophilia* is intrinsically resistant to carbapenems and frequently resistant to aminoglycosides and β-lactams. While TMP/SMX should be considered as the primary therapeutic agent, resistance has been reported, and the sulfonamide can be poorly tolerated. Experience with alternative agents, such as ticarcillin-clavulanate, ceftazidime, fluoroquinolones, and minocycline, is limited. Combination of TMP/SMX with either ticarcillin/clavulanate or ceftazidime can be considered in severely ill patients.

MDR *Acinetobacter* infections have been associated with 49–95% mortality rate in HSCT patients. These bacteria can be susceptible to ampicillin/sulbactam, colistin, and tigecycline. Combination therapy was not associated with decreased mortality.

36.5 Bacterial Infection Syndromes

36.5.1 Central Line-Associated BSI (CLABSI)

CVC infections should be suspected when blood cultures are persistently positive, at the presence of exit site or tunnel infection and when fever and chills develop during CVC flushing. This can be proved by a differential time to positivity of >120 min in blood cultures simultaneously drawn from the CVC and a vein. Catheter removal, in addition to systemic antimicrobial therapy, is recommended for tunnel or port pocket site infection, septic thrombosis, endocarditis, hemodynamic instability, persistently positive (>72 h) blood cultures under appropriate antibiotics, and CLABSI caused by *S. aureus*, *P. aeruginosa*, fungi, or mycobacteria (Freifeld et al. 2011). CVC salvage can be attempted by antimicrobial lock.

36.5.2 Pneumonia

Bacterial pneumonia during the neutropenic phase is due to GNB (including PA) and GPC typical to this stage. Specific entities include *Stenotrophomonas maltophilia* hemorrhagic pneumonia, *VS*-associated ARDS, and nosocomial legionellosis. In the late post-engraftment phase, IPD and *Haemophilus influenzae* should be considered. Symptoms and signs can be atypical and scarce, rapid progression can nonetheless occur. Hypoxemia can be the sole finding and should prompt chest CT; diagnostic bronchoscopy, if feasible; and immediate antibiotic therapy. Empirical therapy should reflect the history of colonization with resistant bacteria.

36.5.3 Diarrhea

Clostridium difficile-associated infection (CDI) is a typical bacterial toxin cause of diarrhea, occurring in 5–30% of HSCT patients following exposure to broad-spectrum antibiotics and chemotherapy. Clinical manifestation may paradoxically be mild. Severe complications, such as toxic megacolon and perforation, can, however, occur. Treatment choice is determined by the severity of CDI, patient's ability to take oral treatment, and recurrence (Debast et al. 2014).

Bacterial diarrhea due to *Shigella*, *Salmonella*, *Yersinia*, *Campylobacter* spp., and enterohemorrhagic *E. coli* is rare and usually occurs in a community-acquired setting. Routine stool culture is, thus, recommended for patients with diarrhea only within 3 days of admission.

36.5.4 CNS Infections

Bacteria rarely cause brain abscess (*Streptococcus epidermidis*, *Staphylococcus aureus*, *Klebsiella pneumonia*) or meningoencephalitis (*Listeria*, IPD). Clinical manifestations include fever, headache, altered mental state, and focal neurological signs and seizures. MRI is more sensitive than CT in identifying brain lesions.

36.6 Improving Management of Bacterial Infection (Averbuch et al. 2013a, b; Satlin and Walsh 2017)

Empirical therapy for febrile neutropenia should be individualized using escalation/de-escalation approach based on local epidemiology and patients' risk factors for infection with resistant bacteria and for complicated course. Early initiation of appropriate therapy improves prognosis and can be achieved by:

(a) Monitoring local department bacterial resistance patterns.
(b) Monitoring colonization with resistant bacteria and empirical administration of active antibiotics in colonized or previously infected febrile neutropenic patients, such as carbapenems in patients colonized with ESBL-GNB. Therapy streamlining, de-escalation, and discontinuation of unnecessary antibiotics should follow culture and susceptibility results.
(c) Novel laboratory techniques (e.g., matrix-assisted laser desorption/ionization–time of flight, MALDI-TOF) that reduce the time for pathogen identification and antibiotic susceptibility testing.

Antibiotic therapy should be optimized in line with pharmacokinetic/pharmacodynamic principles:

1. A loading dose, followed by prolonged or continuous infusion of time-dependent antibiotics, such as β-lactams, has been associated with lower mortality than short-term infusion.
2. Once-daily infusion for concentration-dependent drugs, such as aminoglycosides or daptomycin.

3. A loading dose, when appropriate (tigecycline and colistin).

36.7 Prevention of Bacterial Infection (Tomblyn et al. 2009; Tacconelli et al. 2014; Cordonnier et al. 2015; ECIL-meeting 2017)

General measures to prevent infection include patient's personal hygiene, safe diet, bathing with chlorhexidine-impregnated washcloths, and use of single-patient rooms. Important infection control measures include standard precautions, especially hand hygiene, use of gloves and gowns when soiling is likely, and environmental cleaning. Multifaceted interventions should be practiced to prevent MDR bacteria spread, including patient's screening for colonization in the epidemic setting, using contact precautions, isolation, and cohorting of colonized and/or infected patients and staff (this last, for CPE-colonized patients). Routine CPE-targeted decolonization with nonabsorbable oral antibiotics is not supported; it can select for resistance to the last treatment options.

Antimicrobial stewardship should aim to limit unnecessary antibiotic exposure and to optimize antimicrobial therapy, e.g., using escalation empirical approach (non-carbapenem monotherapy) for stable febrile patients without previous MDR bacteria colonization/infection.

CLABSI prevention includes sterile insertion by a specialized team, avoiding femoral sites, chlorhexidine cleaning during use, and removal of unnecessary catheters.

Fluoroquinolone prophylaxis is recommended in high-risk neutropenic patients with expected neutropenia ≥7 days (Freifeld et al. 2011). Meta-analysis of studies published prior to 2010 demonstrated significantly reduced all-cause mortality, fewer febrile episodes, and reduced GNB-BSI in patients receiving prophylaxis (Gafter-Gvili et al. 2012). Currently, prophylaxis benefit may be less, as fluoroquinolone resistance rates among GNB are high (Averbuch et al. 2017). Meta-analysis of studies published during 2006–2014 does not demonstrate reduction in mortality on fluoroquinolone prophylaxis. The possible benefits of prophylaxis should be weighed against its potential harm, including CDI risk, side effects, and association with colonization or infection with fluoroquinolone- or multidrug-resistant strains (Mikulska et al. 2018b).

Table 36.1 Vaccination schedule (against bacterial infections)

Vaccine	Start after HSCT (months)	Interval between doses (months)	Doses
Pneumococcal conjugate vaccine, PCV13	3	1	3–4[a]
Pneumococcal polysaccharide vaccine, PPV23[b]	12	6 months after last PCV13	1
Haemophilus influenzae B[c]	3–6	1	3
DTP vaccines	6–12	1–2	3
MenC or MCV4[d]	6–12	2	≥2
Men-B[d]	6–12	1–6	2

[a]A fourth dose (6 months after the third dose) if there is GVHD
[b]If no GVHD
[c]Can use combination vaccines
[d]According to country recommendations

Late infection prevention (>100 days post-HCT), targeting mainly encapsulated bacteria, includes:

1. Oral prophylaxis with penicillin (or other agents, according to local antibiotic resistance patterns) in patients with cGVHD or hypogammaglobulinemia
2. IVIg in patients with severe hypogammaglobulinemia (serum IgG level <400 mg/dL)
3. Vaccinations (Table 36.1; also see Chap. 29)

Key Points

- GNB increasingly cause infections in HSCT patients; prognosis is frequently poor.
- Resistant bacteria, such as broad-spectrum β-lactamase-producing (mainly ESBL) *Enterobacteriaceae*, carbapenemase-producing *Enterobacteriaceae* (CPE), MDR *Pseudomonas aeruginosa*, and VRE, are causing an increased number of infections, leading to delay in appropriate therapy and increased mortality.
- Targeted therapy against the main resistant bacteria includes:
  - Linezolid and daptomycin against VRE
  - Carbapenem preferred against severe ESBL+ infections
  - Combination therapy (colistin, aminoglycoside, and carbapenem if low-level resistance) preferred against severe CPE infections
  - β-Lactam with aminoglycoside or fluoroquinolone combination preferred for initial treatment of severe *Pseudomonas aeruginosa* infections
- Antimicrobial stewardship is aimed to individualize empirical approach (escalation vs. de-escalation) to patients with suspected infection, limit unnecessary antibiotic use, and optimize treatment based on pharmacokinetic/pharmacodynamic principles.
- Infection control is crucial to limit the spread of MDR pathogens.
- Fluoroquinolone prophylaxis is recommended for high-risk neutropenic patients; its efficacy, however, can be reduced.
- Encapsulated bacteria (*Streptococcus pneumoniae* and *Haemophilus influenzae*) cause infections during late post-engraftment period; preventive measures include oral prophylaxis, IVIg, and vaccinations.

References

Averbuch D, Cordonnier C, Livermore DM, et al. Targeted therapy against multi-resistant bacteria in leukemic and hematopoietic stem cell transplant recipients: guidelines of the 4th European Conference on Infections in Leukemia (ECIL-4, 2011). Haematologica. 2013a;98:1836–47.

Averbuch D, Orasch C, Cordonnier C, et al. European guidelines for empirical antibacterial therapy for febrile neutropenic patients in the era of growing resistance: summary of the 2011 4th European Conference on Infections in Leukemia. Haematologica. 2013b;98:1826–35.

Averbuch D, Tridello G, Hoek J, et al. Antimicrobial resistance in gram-negative rods causing bacteremia in hematopoietic stem cell transplant recipients: intercontinental prospective study of the infectious diseases working party of the European bone marrow transplantation group. Clin Infect Dis. 2017;65:1819–28.

Bassetti M, Giacobbe DR, Giamarellou H, et al. Management of KPC-producing Klebsiella pneumoniae infections. Clin Microbiol Infect. 2018;24:133–44.

Cordonnier C, Ljungman P, Juergens C, et al. Immunogenicity, safety, and tolerability of 13-valent pneumococcal conjugate vaccine followed by 23-valent pneumococcal polysaccharide vaccine in recipients of allogeneic hematopoietic stem cell transplant aged ≥2 years: an open-label study. Clin Infect Dis. 2015;61:313–23.

Debast SB, Bauer MP, Kuijper EJ, et al. European Society of Clinical Microbiology and Infectious Diseases: update of the treatment guidance document for Clostridium difficile infection. Clin Microbiol Infect. 2014;20(Suppl 2):1–26.

ECIL-meeting. Vaccines in stem cell transplant patients. 2017. http://www.ecil-leukaemia.com/telechargements/ECIL%207%20Vaccine%20Part%20I%20and%20II%20Final.pdf. Retrieved 31 Mar 18, 2018.

Engelhard D, Cordonnier C, Shaw PJ, et al. Early and late invasive pneumococcal infection following stem cell transplantation: a European Bone Marrow Transplantation survey. Br J Haematol. 2002;117:444–50.

Freifeld AG, Bow EJ, Sepkowitz KA, et al. Clinical practice guideline for the use of antimicrobial agents in neutropenic patients with cancer: 2010 update by the infectious diseases society of america. Clin Infect Dis. 2011;52:e56–93.

Gafter-Gvili A, Fraser A, Paul M, et al. Antibiotic prophylaxis for bacterial infections in afebrile neutropenic patients following chemotherapy. Cochrane Database Syst Rev. 2012;1:CD004386.

Girmenia C, Bertaina A, Piciocchi A, et al. Incidence, risk factors and outcome of pre-engraftment gram-negative bacteremia after allogeneic and autologous hematopoietic stem cell transplantation: an Italian prospective multicenter survey. Clin Infect Dis. 2017;65:1884–96.

Gudiol C, Royo-Cebrecos C, Abdala E, et al. Efficacy of beta-lactam/beta-lactamase inhibitor combinations for the treatment of bloodstream infection due to extended-spectrum-beta-lactamase-producing Enterobacteriaceae in hematological patients with neutropenia. Antimicrob Agents Chemother. 2017;61:e00164–17.

Gutierrez-Gutierrez B, Salamanca E, de Cueto M, et al. Effect of appropriate combination therapy on mortality of patients with bloodstream infections due to carbapenemase-producing Enterobacteriaceae (INCREMENT): a retrospective cohort study. Lancet Infect Dis. 2017;17:726–34.

Mikulska M, Raiola AM, Galaverna F, et al. Pre-engraftment bloodstream infections after allogeneic hematopoietic cell transplantation: impact of T cell-replete transplantation from a haploidentical donor. Biol Blood Marrow Transplant. 2018a;24:109–18.

Mikulska M, Averbuch D, Tissot F, et al. Fluoroquinolone prophylaxis in haematological cancer patients with neutropenia: ECIL critical appraisal of previous guidelines. J Infect. 2018b;76:20–37.

Mikulska M, Viscoli C, Orasch C, et al. Aetiology and resistance in bacteraemias among adult and paediatric haematology and cancer patients. J infect. 2014;68:321–31.

Perez F, Adachi J, Bonomo RA. Antibiotic-resistant gram-negative bacterial infections in patients with cancer. Clin Infect Dis. 2014;59(Suppl 5):S335–9.

Satlin MJ, Walsh TJ. Multidrug-resistant Enterobacteriaceae, Pseudomonas aeruginosa, and vancomycin-resistant Enterococcus: three major threats to hematopoietic stem cell transplant recipients. Transpl Infect Dis. 2017;19:e12762. https://doi.org/10.1111/tid.12762. Epub 2017 Oct 25.

Tacconelli E, Cataldo MA, Dancer SJ, et al. ESCMID guidelines for the management of the infection control measures to reduce transmission of multidrug-resistant Gram-negative bacteria in hospitalized patients. Clin Microbiol Infect. 2014;20(Suppl 1):1–55.

Tomblyn M, Chiller T, Einsele H, et al. Guidelines for preventing infectious complications among hematopoietic cell transplant recipients: a global perspective. Preface. Bone Marrow Transplant. 2009;44: 453–5.

Trecarichi EM, Pagano L, Candoni A, et al. Current epidemiology and antimicrobial resistance data for bacterial bloodstream infections in patients with hematologic malignancies: an Italian multicentre prospective survey. Clin Microbiol Infect. 2015;21:337–43.

Vardakas KZ, Tansarli GS, Bliziotis IA, et al. Beta-lactam plus aminoglycoside or fluoroquinolone combination versus beta-lactam monotherapy for Pseudomonas aeruginosa infections: a meta-analysis. Int J Antimicrob Agents. 2013;41:301–10.

Weisser M, Theilacker C, Tschudin Sutter S, et al. Secular trends of bloodstream infections during neutropenia in 15 181 haematopoietic stem cell transplants: 13-year results from a European multicentre surveillance study (ONKO-KISS). Clin Microbiol Infect. 2017;23: 854–9.

37 Invasive Fungal Infections

Johan A. Maertens

37.1 Epidemiology

Invasive fungal diseases (IFD) are frequent infectious complications of HSCT. The 12 m cumulative incidence approaches 8–10% in URD or mismatched allo-HSCT, 6% in MRD allo-HSCT, and less than 2% following auto-HSCT (Kontoyiannis et al. 2010). However, higher incidences (up to 17%) have been reported in haplo-identical HSCT and CBT.

Classical risk periods for IFD include (a) the pre-engraftment period when neutropenia and mucosal damage are most profound, (b) the early post-engraftment period (days +40 to +100) when patients are at highest risk for acute GvHD and viral reactivations due to defective T-cell immunity, and (c) the late post-engraftment period (beyond day +100) complicated by chronic GvHD, delayed immune reconstitution, and occasionally secondary neutropenia. The Gruppo Italiano Trapianto Midollo Osseo (GITMO) has identified period-specific risk factors for proven and probable IFD (Girmenia et al. 2014). The presence of a proven or probable IFD is an independent and strong negative predictor of overall mortality at 1 year after allogeneic HSCT.

Before the introduction of antifungal prophylaxis, *Candida* infections were prevalent in as many as 18–20% of HSCT recipients. However, the widespread use of fluconazole prophylaxis since the late 1990s has significantly reduced the incidence of systemic *Candida* infections and has decreased the transplant-related mortality secondary to *Candida* infections and to gut GvHD. But, this successful approach has also resulted in an epidemiological shift from fluconazole-susceptible *Candida albicans* infections to predominantly fluconazole-resistant non-*albicans Candida* infections (including *Candida glabrata* and *Candida krusei*). Based on a recent EBMT study, the incidence of candidemia by day +100 has now dropped to 1.2% but remains associated with increased NRM and lower short- and long-term OS (with candidemia being an independent risk factor for NRM and OS) (Cesaro et al. 2018).

Over the past two decades, respiratory mould infections caused by *Aspergillus* species (and to a much lesser extent non-*Aspergillus* moulds such as *Mucorales*, *Fusarium* species, and some rare other pathogens) have become much more prevalent. Unlike yeasts, which are acquired through indwelling lines or via intestinal translocation, mould infections are usually acquired by inhalation of airborne spores. In HSCT recipients, the primary lines of defence, including phagocytosing alveolar macrophages and neutrophils, are often nonfunctional in the presence of IS drugs and/or corticosteroids. Hence, *Aspergillus* spores

J. A. Maertens (✉)
Department of Haematology, University Hospital Gasthuisberg, Leuven, Belgium
e-mail: johan.maertens@uzleuven.be

E. Carreras et al. (eds.), *The EBMT Handbook*, https://doi.org/10.1007/978-3-030-02278-5_37

may germinate and produce hyphae, which then invade blood vessels, followed by vascular occlusion and infarction and dissemination to distant organs. The crude mortality rate of invasive mould disease in HSCT recipients can be as high as 60%.

37.2 Diagnosis of Fungal Disease

37.2.1 Mould Infections

Despite a high index of clinical suspicion, diagnosing invasive mould disease remains challenging. The clinical presentation in HSCT patients is often nonspecific and difficult to distinguish from non-fungal infections and even noninfectious complications. A diagnosis of mould disease is based on histopathological examination of infected tissue, imaging (in particular chest CT scan) and microbiological tests, both culture based and non-culture based.

Although *histopathology* remains the gold standard for making a definite diagnosis, many clinicians are reluctant to ask for invasive procedures with biopsy in these vulnerable patients with underlying coagulation problems. As a result, the majority of invasive mould diseases are categorised as probable or even possible.

Culture and direct microscopic examination of sputum, BAL and other body fluids, and skin samples, using staining techniques that allow diagnosis on the same day (e.g. optical brighteners such as calcofluor white), have been the cornerstones for making a microbiological diagnosis of invasive mould disease. Culture has the additional advantage of allowing fungal species identification and determining antifungal susceptibility. Unfortunately, culture is time-consuming and requires considerable expertise. In addition, blood cultures are notoriously negative for moulds, even in disseminated disease, and culture from any respiratory specimen has only low to moderate sensitivity and predictive value.

The (ongoing) development of serological tests has been a major advance in the field (Maertens et al. 2016a, b). *Galactomannan* (GM), a fungal cell wall molecule that is released during fungal growth, can be detected by a commercial enzyme immunoassay (Bio-Rad Platelia™ Aspergillus EIA). Earlier studies used an index of ≥1.5 to define positivity. The ECIL guidelines now support the use of a single serum or plasma value of ≥0.7 or multiple (consecutive) values of ≥0.5 to define positivity. This lower cutoff permits detection of fungal infection before the clinico-radiological manifestations appear. However, improved sensitivity with the use of lower cutoffs comes with a loss of specificity. In addition, false-positive results as well as false-negative results are not uncommon (Table 37.1) and cross-reactivity with non-*Aspergillus* moulds (including but not limited to *Fusarium* spp., *Penicillium* spp., *Acremonium* spp., *Alternaria* spp., and *Histoplasma capsulatum*) may occur, although the assay does not detect *Mucorales*. GM testing can also be applied to other types of specimens, including BAL fluid. Cutoff values of 1.0 have been recommended although it is likely that higher thresholds are needed. Recently, an index cutoff of 1.0 has also been suggested for analysing cerebrospinal fluid samples from patients with (suspected) cerebral aspergillosis.

Unlike GM, *β-d-glucan* (BDG) is a component of the cell wall of many pathogenic fungi including *Candida* spp., *Fusarium* spp., and *Pneumocystis* (Maertens et al. 2016a, b). The main exceptions are *Mucorales* and some *Cryptococcus* species. The Fungitell® assay (Associates of Cape Cod) has been approved by the US FDA and carries the European CE label for the presumptive diagnosis of invasive fungal infection. Most studies report good sensitivity, but specificity and positive predictive value are poor due to a high rate of false-positive results (Table 37.1), regardless of the specimen. However, the negative predictive value is around 80–90%.

PCR-based methods have also been developed. Lack of standardisation has for a long time hampered the acceptance of these diagnostic assays. Fortunately, over the past decade, the

Table 37.1 Limitations of antigen assays in the diagnosis of invasive fungal disease

	Galactomannan	β-D-glucan
Reactivity with fungal species	*Aspergillus* spp., *Fusarium* spp., *Paecilomyces* spp., *Acremonium* spp., *Penicillium* spp., *Alternaria* spp., *Histoplasma capsulatum*, *Blastomyces dermatitidis*, *Cryptococcus neoformans*, *Emmonsia* spp., *Wangiella dermatitidis*, *Prototheca*, *Myceliophthora*, *Geotrichum capitatum*, *Chaetomium globosum*	*Pneumocystis jirovecii*, *Aspergillus* spp., *Fusarium* spp., *Histoplasma capsulatum*, *Candida* spp., *Acremonium* spp., *Trichosporon* sp., *Sporothrix schenckii*, *Saccharomyces cerevisiae*, *Coccidioides immitis*, *Prototheca*
False-positive test results	– Semi-synthetic β-lactam ATB[a] – Multiple myeloma – Blood products collected using Fresenius Kabi bags – Gluconate-containing plasma expanders – Flavoured ice pops/frozen desserts containing sodium gluconate – *Bifidobacterium* spp. (gut) – Severe mucositis or GI GvHD – Enteral nutritional supplements	– Semi-synthetic β-lactam antibiotics – Human blood products, including IVIg, albumin, plasma, coagulation factor infusions, filtered through cellulose membranes – Cellulose haemodialysis/haemofiltration membranes – Exposure to (surgical) gauze – Bacterial bloodstream infections (e.g. *P. aeruginosa)*
False-negative test results	– Concomitant use of mould-active antifungal agents – Mucolytic agents	– Concomitant use of antifungal agents

[a]Including ampicillin, amoxicillin clavulanate, and piperacillin/tazobactam (although this problem seems largely abated compared with previous experience)

European Aspergillus PCR Initiative (EAPCRI) has made tremendous progress in standardising protocols for efficient DNA extraction and amplification (White et al. 2015). Recently a lateral-flow device (LFD) was developed for the point-of-care diagnosis of invasive aspergillosis (Hoenigl et al. 2018); clinical validation studies are currently ongoing.

The sensitivity and specificity of conventional *radiology* are too low to diagnose or to exclude a fungal infection. Thin-section multislice CT scan nowadays is the preferred imaging technique; more recently, computed tomography pulmonary angiography is rapidly gaining popularity as an alternative diagnostic technique (Stanzani et al. 2015). Nodules, with or without a halo sign, are suggestive of invasive mould disease; this 'halo sign' appears early in the course of the infection; thereafter the lesions become more nonspecific. Following neutrophil recovery, an air crescent sign may develop, usually associated with a good outcome. An inversed halo sign has been described as more suggestive of invasive mucormycosis. The added value of PET scan is currently being investigated.

37.2.2 Yeast Infections

Cryptococcal Ag assays have become very sensitive and should be used where cryptococcal meningitis is suspected.

Microbiologic cultures, the gold standard diagnostic method for invasive *Candida* infections and candidemia, have low sensitivity (especially for chronic disseminated candidiasis) and take up to 2–5 days to grow (from blood samples). The T2Candida panel is a novel, fully automated qualitative diagnostic platform for diagnosis of candidemia in whole blood specimens with a mean time to species identification of less than 5 h. The negative predictive value is almost 100% in a population with 5–10% prevalence of candidemia (Mylonakis et al. 2015). Unfortunately, the assay detects only five different *Candida* species.

37.2.3 *Pneumocystis jirovecii* Pneumonia (PJP)

Immunofluorescence assays remain recommended as the most sensitive microscopic method. Real-time PCR on BAL fluid can be used to rule out the diagnosis of PJP. However, a positive PCR test does not necessarily mean that the patient has PJP, since low fungal loads will be picked up in colonised patients. BDG positivity in serum can further contribute to the diagnosis, although a positive test result may also indicate other fungal infections (Alanio et al. 2016).

37.3 Prevention and Prophylaxis

37.3.1 Protective Environment Measures

Protective environment measures (such as the use of HEPA-filtered isolation rooms or the use of portable HEPA filters) are useful to prevent in-hospital acquisition of airborne fungal pathogens. However, many patients develop IFD during the outpatient follow-up period, when these isolation measures are not applicable.

37.3.2 Pharmacological Antifungal Prophylaxis

Pharmacological antifungal prophylaxis; updated ECIL recommendations are phase-specific (ECIL-5 2013).

37.3.2.1 During the (Neutropenic) Pre-engraftment Phase

Fluconazole (400 mg/day) is still recommended for centres with a low incidence of mould infections [i.e. below 5%] but only when combined with a mould-directed diagnostic approach (biomarker and/or CT scan based) or a mould-directed therapeutic approach (empirical antifungal therapy). Centres with a higher incidence of mould infections are advised to adopt an alternative approach.

Voriconazole (400 mg/day following loading) failed to show a difference in fungal-free survival, overall survival, incidence of IFD, invasive aspergillosis, empirical use of antifungals, and toxicity compared with fluconazole. When tested against itraconazole oral solution, voriconazole was superior for the composite endpoint, but the difference was driven by a lower use of systemic antifungals with voriconazole, which could be given for a longer duration than itraconazole, not by better efficacy. Itraconazole (200 mg IV q24h, followed by oral solution 200 mg q12) provided better protection against invasive mould infections than fluconazole. However, drug toxicities and tolerability limited its usefulness as prophylactic agent. Therefore, voriconazole and itraconazole were both given a B-I recommendation.

Data for the echinocandins are limited to micafungin (50 mg IV q24h). The study comparing micafungin versus fluconazole had significant shortcomings, including the overrepresentation of a low-risk population and the lack of a predefined workup for diagnosing IFD. Hence, prophylaxis with micafungin received a B-I recommendation for centres with a low incidence of mould infections and C-I for those with a high incidence.

The addition of aerosolised liposomal amphotericin B (AmB) to fluconazole is not recommended for centres with a low incidence of mould infections, although there is some evidence to do so in higher-risk centres (B-II). IV liposomal AmB for prophylaxis was given a C-II recommendation.

Although there are no specific studies of posaconazole prophylaxis during the pre-engraftment phase, the drug (oral solution 200 mg q8h or gastro-resistant tablet/IV formulation 300 mg q24h following a loading dose of 300 mg q12h on the first day) was given a B-II recommendation based on results inferred from data during the neutropenic phase in AML/MDS patients.

37.3.2.2 During the (GvHD) Post-engraftment Phase

Given the significantly increased risk of invasive mould infection during GvHD (and its associated high mortality), ECIL strongly recommends against the use of fluconazole for prophylaxis in patients with high-risk GvHD. Based on the results of a large, double-blind study, posaconazole (oral solution or gastro-resistant tablet/IV formulation) is the drug of choice for antifungal prophylaxis (AI), although no difference was observed in patients with chronic GvHD.

37.3.2.3 PJP Prophylaxis

Oral TMP/SMX given 2–3 times weekly is the drug of choice for the primary prophylaxis of PJP and should be given during the entire period at risk (from engraftment to ≥6 months and as long as IS is ongoing). All other drugs, including aerosolised or IV pentamidine, atovaquone, and dapsone, are considered second-line alternatives when TMP/SMX is poorly tolerated or contraindicated (Maertens et al. 2016a).

37.4 Treatment of Fungal Disease

Over the last few decades, three basic strategies (apart from prophylaxis) have been developed and investigated in clinical studies to deal with IFD (Mercier and Maertens 2017). For a long time, profound and prolonged neutropenia accompanied by persistent or relapsing fever after 5–7 days of adequate antibacterial coverage has been regarded as a sufficient trigger for starting broad-spectrum antifungals, a strategy referred to as *empirical* antifungal therapy. This practice has never been supported by robust scientific evidence and has important drawbacks, including drug-related toxicity and increased cost due to overtreatment. In spite of this, the empirical use of antifungals became standard of care in many centres. It was also endorsed by consensus guidelines and is relied on by centres that have limited or no access to radiological and mycological diagnostic tools. If relying on this approach, ECIL guidelines recommend the use of caspofungin (50 mg/day following 70 mg on day 1) or liposomal amphotericin B at 3 mg/kg (both have an AI recommendation).

A *diagnostic-driven* approach (also called *pre-emptive*) has been advocated by some centres and guidelines following recent improvements in diagnostic techniques. The aim is to start antifungal therapy in at-risk patients only when they present with an early marker of fungal infections, such as a positive GM, BDG, or PCR screening assay, or a suggestive lesion on imaging. Unfortunately, such a strategy is restricted to centres that perform non-culture-based testing twice weekly and readily have access to chest CT scan and other imaging modalities.

Directed antifungal treatment is used for patients with documented fungal disease, either proven or probable (Table 37.2).

- Voriconazole and isavuconazole are recommended as the first-line treatment for invasive aspergillosis, including cerebral aspergillosis (Tissot et al. 2017). In a randomised clinical trial, voriconazole and isavuconazole had the same efficacy (all-cause mortality at day 42 around 20%), although isavuconazole has a better toxicity profile (including hepatotoxicity) and somewhat fewer drug-drug interactions compared to voriconazole (Maertens et al. 2016c). The upfront combination of antifungals with different mechanisms of action (e.g. an azole plus an echinocandin) is not recommended because superiority over monotherapy could not be demonstrated in a recent trial (Marr et al. 2015). Liposomal AMB at 3 mg/kg is the recommended alternative for primary therapy if these azoles cannot be used due to intolerance, drug interactions, prior exposure to broad-spectrum azoles (e.g. prophylaxis), or documented azole resistance (Resendiz Sharpe et al. 2018), an emerging problem in some European centres. For salvage therapy, the global response is around 40%, irrespective of the antifungal used. Treatment duration is typically between 6 and 12 weeks, followed by secondary prophylaxis in patients with ongoing IS therapy. During the first week of treatment, pulmonary lesions can grow on imaging; this is in line with the normal kinetics of the disease and does not correlate with a poor outcome. When elevated at baseline, reduction in serum GM correlates with treatment response.
- Treatment of mucormycosis includes control of the underlying condition, surgical debridement (often destructive), and antifungal therapy. At present, lipid-based formulations of AmB (at doses of 5–10 mg/kg) are the first-line therapy of choice (Tissot et al. 2017; Cornely et al.

Table 37.2 ECIL-6 guidelines for the *first-line antifungal treatment* of IA and mucormycosis in HSCT patients

	Grade	Comments
Invasive aspergillosis		
Voriconazole	AI	Daily adult dose 2 × 6 mg/kg on day 1 followed by 2 × 4 mg/kg (initiation oral therapy: CIII) Need for therapeutic drug monitoring Check for drug-drug interactions
Isavuconazole	AI	Adult dose 200 mg t.i.d. for 2 days, thereafter 200 mg daily As effective as voriconazole but better tolerated
Liposomal amphotericin B	BI	Daily adult dose, 3 mg/kg
Amphotericin B lipid complex	BII	Daily adult dose, 5 mg/kg
Amphotericin B colloidal dispersion	CI	Not more effective than AmB deoxycholate but less nephrotoxic
Caspofungin	CII	
Itraconazole	CIII	
Combination anidulafungin + voriconazole	CI	
Other combinations	CIII	
Recommendation against the use of amphotericin B deoxycholate	AI	Less effective and more toxic
Invasive mucormycosis[a]		
Amphotericin B deoxycholate	CII	
Liposomal amphotericin B	BII	Daily adult dose, 5 mg/kg. Liposomal AmB should be preferred in CNS infection and/or renal failure
Amphotericin B lipid complex	BII	
Amphotericin B colloidal dispersion	CII	
Posaconazole	CIII	No data to support its use as first-line treatment
Combination therapy	CIII	

[a]Management of mucormycosis includes antifungal therapy, surgery, and control of the underlying condition

2014). Both posaconazole and isavuconazole can be used for oral outpatient therapy following initial stabilisation of the disease.

- Hyalohyphomycosis constitutes a heterogeneous group of fungi, including (but not limited to) *Fusarium*, *Scedosporium*, *Acremonium*, and *Scopulariopsis* species. Clinical manifestations range from colonisation to localised infections to acute invasive and/or disseminated disease. First-line therapy of fusariosis should include voriconazole and surgical debridement where possible; posaconazole can be used as salvage treatment. Voriconazole is also the recommended the first-line treatment of *Scedosporium* infections (except for *Lomentospora prolificans*, previously named *S. prolificans*, for which there is no standard treatment available). The optimal antifungal treatment has not been established for *Acremonium* spp., *Scopulariopsis* spp., and other hyalohyphomycosis (Tortorano et al. 2014).
- Echinocandins are the drugs of choice for the first-line therapy of invasive candidiasis/candidemia, followed by a step-down approach in clinically stable patients upon receipt of the species identification and antifungal susceptibility testing results (Andes et al. 2012). Catheter removal is strongly recommended in patients with candidemia or with *C. parapsilosis* bloodstream infection. Treatment duration typically is 14 days after the last positive blood culture. Of note, echinocandin resistance is on the rise (particularly for *C. glabrata*), and recent outbreaks of multiresistant *C. auris* infections have been reported (Lamoth and Kontoyiannis 2018).
- High-dose trimethoprim/sulfamethoxazole is the treatment of choice for patients with documented PJP; the combination of primaquine plus clindamycin is the preferred alternative. Treatment duration typically is 3 weeks, and secondary anti-PJP prophylaxis

is indicated thereafter. The administration of glucocorticoids must be decided on a case-by-case basis (Maschmeyer et al. 2016).

- Of note, uncertainty about exposure and drug interactions is common when using azole antifungals. Therapeutic drug monitoring for voriconazole (plasma target 1–6 mg/L for prophylaxis and treatment) and posaconazole (plasma target >0.7 mg/L for prophylaxis; >1 mg/L for treatment) is therefore recommended (ECIL-6 guidelines).

Key Points

- *Aspergillus*, *Candida*, and *Pneumocystis jirovecii* are the cause of almost 90% of the invasive fungal diseases following HSCT. Most infections are diagnosed post-engraftment during episodes of acute and/or chronic GvHD.
- Chest and sinus CT scan and non-invasive mycological tools (serology, PCR) are crucial for making an early diagnosis.
- Antifungal prophylaxis, targeting yeast and/or mould infections depending on the post transplant risk period, is highly recommended. TMP/SMX remains the drug of choice for preventing PJP.
- Echinocandins are the preferred first-line therapy for invasive *Candida* infections and candidemia. Voriconazole or isavuconazole is the recommended first-line options for invasive aspergillosis, whereas lipid-based formulations of AmB are the recommended first-line option for mucormycosis.

References

Alanio A, Hauser PM, Lagrou K, et al. ECIL guidelines for the diagnosis of Pneumocystis jirovecii pneumonia in patients with haematological malignancies and stem cell transplant recipients. J Antimicrob Chemother. 2016;71:2386–96.

Andes DR, Safdar N, Baddley JW, et al. Impact of treatment strategy on outcomes in patients with candidemia and other forms of invasive candidiasis: a patient-level quantitative review of randomized trials. Clin Infect Dis. 2012;54:1110–22.

Cesaro S, Tridello G, Blijlevens NS, et al. Incidence, risk factors and long-term outcome of acute leukemia patients with early candidemia after allogeneic stem cell transplantation. A study by the acute leukemia and infectious diseases working parties of EBMT. Clin Infect Dis. 2018;67(4):564–72.

Cornely OA, Arikan-Akdagli S, Dannaoui E, et al. ESCMID and ECMM joint clinical guidelines for the diagnosis and management of mucormycosis 2013. Clin Microbiol Infect. 2014;20(Suppl 3):5–26.

ECIL-5. 2013. http://www.ecil-leukaemia.com.

Girmenia C, Raiola AM, Piciocchi A, et al. Incidence and outcome of invasive fungal diseases after allogeneic stem cell transplantation: a prospective study of the Gruppo Italiano Trapianto Midollo Osseo (GITMO). Biol Blood Marrow Transplant. 2014;20:872–80.

Hoenigl M, Eigl S, Heldt SS, et al. Clinical evaluation of the newly formatted lateral-flow device for invasive pulmonary aspergillosis. Mycoses. 2018;61:40–3.

Kontoyiannis DP, Marr KA, Park BJ, et al. Prospective surveillance for invasive fungal infections in hematopoietic stem cell transplant recipients, 2001-2006: overview of the Transplant-Associated Infection Surveillance Network (TRANSNET) Databasc. Clin Infect Dis. 2010;50:1091–100.

Lamoth F, Kontoyiannis DP. The candida auris alert: facts and perspectives. J Infect Dis. 2018;217:516–20.

Maertens J, Cesaro S, Maschmeyer G, et al. ECIL guidelines for preventing Pneumocystis jirovecii pneumonia in patients with haematological malignancies and stem cell transplant recipients. J Antimicrob Chemother. 2016a;71:2397–404.

Maertens JA, Blennow O, Duarte RFS, et al. The current management landscape: aspergillosis. J Antimicrob Chemother. 2016b;71(Suppl 2):ii23–9.

Maertens JA, Raad II, Marr KA, et al. Isavuconazole versus voriconazole for primary treatment of invasive mould disease caused by Aspergillus and other filamentous fungi (SECURE): a phase 3, randomised-controlled, non-inferiority trial. Lancet. 2016c;387:760–9.

Marr KA, Schlamm HT, Herbrecht R, et al. Combination antifungal therapy for invasive aspergillosis: a randomized trial. Ann Intern Med. 2015;162:81–9.

Maschmeyer G, Helweg-Larsen J, Pagano L, et al. ECIL guidelines for treatment of Pneumocystis jirovecii pneumonia in non-HIV-infected haematology patients. J Antimicrob Chemother. 2016;71:2405–13.

Mercier T, Maertens J. Clinical considerations in the early treatment of invasive mould infections and disease. J Antimicrob Chemother. 2017;72(suppl_1):i29–38.

Mylonakis E, Clancy CJ, Ostrosky-Zeichner L, et al. T2 magnetic resonance assay for the rapid diagnosis of candidemia in whole blood: a clinical trial. Clin Infect Dis. 2015;60:892–9.

Resendiz Sharpe A, Lagrou K, Meis JF, et al. Triazole resistance surveillance in Aspergillus fumigatus. Med Mycol. 2018;56(suppl 1):83–92.

Stanzani M, Sassi C, Lewis RE, et al. High resolution computed tomography angiography improves the radiographic diagnosis of invasive mold disease in patients with hematological malignancies. Clin Infect Dis. 2015;60:1603–10.

Tissot F, Agrawal S, Pagano L, et al. ECIL-6 guidelines for the treatment of invasive candidiasis, aspergillosis and mucormycosis in leukemia and hematopoietic stem cell transplant patients. Haematologica. 2017;102:433–44.

Tortorano AM, Richardson M, Roilides E, et al. ESCMID and ECMM joint guidelines on diagnosis and management of hyalohyphomycosis. Clin Microbiol Infect. 2014;20(Suppl 3):27–46.

White PL, Barnes RA, Springer JS, et al. Clinical performance of aspergillus PCR for testing serum and plasma: a study by the European aspergillus PCR initiative. J Clin Microbiol. 2015;53:2832–7.

38 Viral Infections

Per Ljungman, Jan Styczynski, and Hermann Einsele

38.1 Herpes Viruses

38.1.1 Cytomegalovirus (CMV)

38.1.1.1 Clinical Symptoms

CMV can cause symptoms from almost any organ as well as unspecific symptoms such as fever, malaise, and bone marrow suppression in stem cell transplant patients. However, the most important clinical entities in allo-HSCT patients are pneumonia, gastroenteritis, and retinitis.

The likelihood for symptomatic infection is much higher after allo-HSCT compared to auto-HSCT. Being CMV seropositive (CMV (+)) is also associated with decreased OS after allo-HSCT as is the use of a CMV (+) donor to a CMV-seronegative (CMV (−)) patient.

P. Ljungman (✉)
Department of Cellular Therapy and Allogeneic Stem Cell Transplantation, Karolinska University Hospital, Stockholm, Sweden

Division of Hematology, Department of Medicine Huddinge, Karolinska Institutet, Stockholm, Sweden
e-mail: per.ljungman@ki.se

J. Styczynski
Department of Pediatric Hematology and Oncology, Collegium Medicum, Nicolaus Copernicus University, Bydgoszcz, Poland

H. Einsele
Department of Internal Medicine II, Julius Maximilian University of Würzburg, Würzburg, Germany

In patients undergoing MAC allo-HSCT, the use of a CMV (−) donor to a CMV (+) patient has been associated with an increased risk for NRM and decreased OS. In addition, proof of CMV replication is associated with increased NRM, while the effect on the risk for leukemia relapse is controversial.

38.1.1.2 Diagnostics

CMV antibody status should be determined pretransplant in all patients undergoing HSCT and in allogeneic stem cell donors.

Allo-HSCT patients should be monitored weekly for CMV replication with a sensitive diagnostic technique at least the first 3 months after HSCT. Patients with GVHD and those with documented CMV replication should be monitored longer. There is no need to routinely monitor patients after autologous HSCT.

The most commonly used technique is qPCR, but also the so-called pp65 antigenemia assay and other tests detecting CMV nucleic acids can be used. Recently tests detecting CMV-specific T-cells have become available, but further evaluation of these tests' usefulness in routine care is necessary.

To diagnose CMV disease, it is important to combine symptoms and signs with documentation of the presence of CMV in affected tissue. An exception is CMV retinitis where ophthalmologic findings are characteristic although to detect CMV in vitreous fluid can be helpful. Established techniques for detection of CMV in tissue are

E. Carreras et al. (eds.), *The EBMT Handbook*, https://doi.org/10.1007/978-3-030-02278-5_38

histopathology, immunohistochemistry, and DNA hybridization. High levels of CMV DNA in BAL are associated with CMV pneumonia, while its absence almost excludes CMV pneumonia. PCR in CSF supports the diagnosis of CMV encephalitis. For other end-organ diseases, qPCR needs additional study.

38.1.1.3 Prophylaxis

Letermovir has been shown in a placebo-controlled randomized trial to decrease the risk for clinically significant CMV infection (need for preemptive antiviral therapy and/or CMV disease) and also decrease all-cause mortality in CMV (+) patients.

Ganciclovir can reduce the risk for CMV disease but is associated with significant toxicity.

High-dose acyclovir/valaciclovir can reduce the risk for CMV replication.

The data regarding prophylactic Ig is conflicting and its use is currently not recommended.

38.1.1.4 Treatment

Ganciclovir, valganciclovir, and foscarnet have all been shown to be effective to prevent development of CMV disease in allo-HSCT recipients when used for so-called preemptive therapy based on detection of CMV in blood. Their efficacy is similar, so the choice should be based on the risk for side effects and practical aspects.

It is not possible to give a recommendation on what CMV DNA level preemptive therapy should be initiated since this depends on patient factors, the material used for monitoring (plasma/whole blood), and the performance of the assay used.

Therapy is usually given for at least 2 weeks, but longer therapy courses might be needed. Second episodes of CMV replication are common, and second-line therapy can be given with either the same or other antiviral drugs mentioned above.

Ganciclovir (valganciclovir) and foscarnet are the most used drugs for CMV disease. The addition of high-dose Ig for treatment of CMV pneumonia has been commonly used, but the data supporting this combination is limited. There is no data supporting the addition of Ig to antiviral treatment for other types of CMV disease. Cidofovir can be considered as failure therapy. The duration of therapy has to be decided on a case-by-case basis, but normally longer therapy is needed compared to preemptive therapy (6–8 weeks).

Cidofovir is also a possibility for second- or third-line antiviral therapy. New antiviral drugs are in development but have not been proven efficacious on this indication. Leflunomide and artesunate have been tested, but data supporting their use is very limited.

38.1.1.5 Cellular Immunotherapy

Several groups have tried to prevent or treat CMV infection and disease following allo-HSCT by the transfer of CMV-specific T-cells. The T-cell lines and clones specific for CMV were mostly derived from the HSC donor but in some studies also from a third-party donor or even patient-derived CMV-specific T-cells obtained from the patient prior to conditioning therapy.

New strategies were applied to select CMV-specific T-cell without long-term in vitro culture. Thus, techniques like the cytokine capture assay combined with the Miltenyi CliniMACS system or tetramers, pentamers, or streptamers were applied to generate CMV-specific T-cells for prophylactic or therapeutic transfer. The transfer of these cells was shown to reconstitute virus-specific T-cell immunity. When given therapeutically to patients with chemotherapy-refractory CMV infection, a drop in the viral load after an increase in the number of CMV-specific T-cells could be documented. In patients with chemotherapy-refractory CMV infection post-HSCT, adoptive T-cell therapy is a valid therapeutic option.

The efficacy in patients receiving high-dose ($\geq$2 mg/kg) corticosteroids is likely to be low.

38.1.2 HHV-6

38.1.2.1 Clinical Symptoms

HHV-6A primary infection has so far not been associated with specific symptoms.

HHV-6B primary infection is the main cause of *exanthema subitum* in young children. It has also been associated with febrile seizures. Almost all children are infected by the age of 2 years.

HHV-6B is the main cause of viral encephalitis after allo-HSCT, but HHV-6A has also been documented. Patients undergoing CBT are at an increased risk. Other symptoms suggested to be associated with HHV-6 are bone marrow suppression, pneumonia, and acute GVHD.

38.1.2.2 Diagnostics

Serology is not helpful. HHV-6 DNA can be analyzed in blood by qPCR. The usefulness of monitoring is not established. HHV-6 can be integrated in germline, and these individuals are strongly positive in qPCR, and this is not a proof of viral replication.

MRI is recommended for diagnosis of HHV-6 encephalitis. The typical finding is of limbic encephalitis, but other patterns are also seen. HHV-6 DNA is usually positive in the CSF in patients with encephalitis.

38.1.2.3 Prophylaxis

Foscarnet has been used but its usefulness is not established.

38.1.2.4 Treatment

Either ganciclovir or foscarnet can be used for treatment of HHV-6 encephalitis. There is no established treatment for HHV-6 infection or patients with other suspected HHV-6-associated complications. Cellular immunotherapy was only performed in a few patients.

38.1.3 HHV-7

38.1.3.1 Clinical Symptoms

HHV-7 primary infection in young children occasionally causes *exanthema subitum (roseola)* and rarely status epilepticus with fever. Nearly all children are infected with HHV-7 by the age of 5 years.

HHV-7 detection after HSCT is relatively infrequent, with rare cases in which HHV-7 has been associated with CNS disease (encephalitis, myelitis).

The risk of infection in HSCT patients: allo > auto, TBI-based > chemo-based, children > adults.

Reactivation of HHV-7 occurs in about 10% of patients after allo-HSCT.

38.1.3.2 Diagnostics

HHV-7 DNA by qPCR. HHV-7 might be a cofactor of CMV reactivation.

38.1.3.3 Prophylaxis

Not used.

38.1.3.4 Treatment

Infection by HHV-7 does not require specific treatment.

38.1.4 HHV-8

38.1.4.1 Clinical Symptoms

HHV-8 (KSHV, Kaposi's sarcoma-associated herpesvirus) is the cause of Kaposi's sarcoma (KS), primary effusion lymphoma, or multicentric Castleman's disease.

The prevalence of KSHV infection is high in Africa and parts of the Amazon basin. KS is very rare after HSCT (only 14 cases are described).

Fever and marrow aplasia with plasmacytosis after HSCT can occur. Skin involvement is the dominant clinical presentation in adults, while pediatric cases have visceral involvement.

38.1.4.2 Diagnostics

Detection of HHV-8 DNA by qPCR. KS can be clinically defined on the basis of characteristic skin lesions or histopathologically defined in a malignant tumor.

38.1.4.3 Prophylaxis

Not recommended.

38.1.4.4 Treatment

In disease limited to the skin only, surgical excision or electrochemotherapy is the most preferable approach.

For visceral or disseminated disease, possible options include the use of interferon alpha or chemotherapy. The use of antiviral treatment is considered without benefit. Imatinib showed promising results in HIV-related KS patients.

38.1.5 EBV

38.1.5.1 Clinical Symptoms

Syndromes caused by primary EBV infection include infectious mononucleosis, chronic active EBV infection, and X-linked lymphoproliferative syndrome.

In HCT patients EBV can cause life-threatening complication: post transplant lymphoproliferative disorder (PTLD) or end-organ diseases such as encephalitis/myelitis, pneumonia, or hepatitis. Details on EBV-PTLD are presented in Chap. 45.

Donor EBV seropositivity contributes also to the risk of cGVHD in patients with acute leukemia.

38.1.5.2 Diagnostics

All allo-HCT patients and donors should be tested for EBV Ab before HCT.

38.1.5.3 Prophylaxis

Since EBV sero-mismatch is a risk factor for PTLD, the selection of an EBV-matched donor, if possible, might be beneficial.

As EBV-PTLD after HCT is usually of donor origin and EBV might be transmitted with the graft, the risk of EBV-PTLD is higher when the donor is seropositive.

38.1.5.4 Treatment

Most EBV reactivations are subclinical and require no therapy. Details on treatment of EBV-PTLD are presented in Chap. 45.

38.1.6 Herpes Simplex Virus (HSV)

38.1.6.1 Clinical Symptoms

HSV reactivation can be caused by either type 1 or 2 and is usually associated with localized mucocutaneous disease in the orofacial region (85–90%) and less frequently in the esophageal and genital area. Uncommon manifestations are pneumonia, hepatitis, meningitis (HSV-2), and encephalitis (HSV-1).

38.1.6.2 Diagnostics

All patients should be tested for HSV antibodies before HSCT. The diagnosis of mucocutaneous HSV disease is suspected on clinical grounds, and the diagnosis is usually verified by PCR. PCR in CSF is the technique of choice for the diagnosis of HSV meningitis and encephalitis.

38.1.6.3 Prophylaxis

Primary HSV infection in HSCT patients is unusual, and antiviral drug prophylaxis is thus not recommended in HSV-seronegative patients after HSCT (but might be needed against VZV; see below).

HSV-seropositive patients undergoing allo-HSCT should receive antiviral drug prophylaxis. IV acyclovir 250 mg/m^2 or 5 mg/kg q12h, oral acyclovir 3 × 200 to 2 × 800 mg/day, oral valaciclovir 2 × 500 mg/day, or famciclovir 2 × 500 mg/day can be used.

The duration depends on if also prophylaxis against VZV (see below) is indicated but should be given for at least 4 weeks after HSCT in VZV-seronegative patients.

38.1.6.4 Treatment

IV acyclovir 250 mg/m^2 or 5 mg/kg q8h for 7–10 days is the therapy of choice for severe mucocutaneous or visceral HSV disease.

Oral acyclovir, from 5 × 200 to 5 × 400 mg/day, valaciclovir 2 × 500 mg/day, or famciclovir 2 × 500 mg/day for 10 days are considered as alternatives for less serious manifestations of HSV disease.

For HSV pneumonia or HSV meningitis and encephalitis, IV acyclovir 500 mg/m^2 or 10 mg/kg q8h for at least 14–21 days is recommended.

HSV resistance occurs in approximately 5–15% of patients and is mediated through mutation in the HSV thymidine kinase. Foscarnet or cidofovir are second-line therapy.

38.1.7 Varicella-Zoster Virus (VZV)

38.1.7.1 Clinical Symptoms

Primary infection (varicella) occurs rarely after HSCT, but it might have severe clinical course.

Reactivation as herpes zoster is frequently complicated by prolonged neuralgia and is common unless long-term antiviral prophylaxis is given.

Clinically, severe symptoms include disseminated infection similar to varicella, visceral disease presenting as severe abdominal pain or acute hepatitis, and rarely encephalitis, retinal necrosis, or pneumonitis.

38.1.7.2 Diagnostics

Patients should be tested for VZV antibodies before HSCT. The rash in clinical varicella or zoster is usually characteristic. However, in some cases disseminated HSV can have a similar appearance. PCR on vesicular material for VZV and HSV can differentiate.

Visceral VZV disease can occur without rash and then PCR on blood is diagnostic.

38.1.7.3 Prophylaxis

VZV-seropositive patients should be given antiviral prophylaxis for at least 12 months or up to the end of IS therapy.

Prophylaxis can be given with acyclovir (2 × 800 mg; in children 2 × 20 mg/kg) or valacyclovir (2 × 500 mg).

In seronegative patients exposed to VZV, post-exposure prophylaxis with acyclovir or valacyclovir is recommended.

Prophylaxis should be started as soon as possible and continued until 21 days after exposition.

38.1.7.4 Treatment

First-line therapy for varicella, disseminated zoster, and visceral disease is acyclovir 3 × 500 mg/m^2/d IV.

For localized or limited infections, oral valaciclovir (3 × 1000 mg), acyclovir (5 × 800 mg; in children 4 × 20 mg/kg), or famciclovir (3 × 500 mg) can be given until the lesion crusts over (usually 7–10 days).

In case of resistance to acyclovir, second-line therapies are foscarnet (60 mg/kg q12h) or cidofovir (5 mg/kg weekly, together with probenecid and hydration).

VZIg is not recommended. Only case reports exist on cellular therapy for VZV infection.

38.2 Adenovirus (ADV)

38.2.1 Clinical Symptoms

ADV is transmitted mainly from person to person; however it can persist in epithelial cells and lymphoid tissue and reactivate during IS. Children are more frequently affected than adults.

The spectrum of ADV-associated disease in HSCT patients ranges from mild gastroenteric or respiratory symptoms to severe hemorrhagic enteritis, hemorrhagic cystitis, nephritis, hepatitis, pneumonia, encephalitis, myocarditis, and multiple organ involvement.

Risk factors for ADV infection/disease include haploidentical or URD graft, CBT, TCD, GVHD III–IV, severe lymphopenia, and treatment with alemtuzumab.

38.2.2 Diagnostics

ADV-DNA by qPCR. Monitoring with qPCR of ADV viremia in PB is recommended on at least weekly basis for patients with at least one risk factor. qPCR is also recommended in case of clinical suspicion of ADV infection/disease.

38.2.3 Prophylaxis

Non-pharmacological prophylaxis is mandatory: strict isolation and hygienic measures in patients shedding the virus are absolutely necessary to prevent horizontal transmission and nosocomial outbreaks.

Prophylactic antiviral therapy with available antiviral drugs is not recommended.

38.2.4 Treatment

Patients especially children, with increasing viral load and at least one risk factor, should receive preemptive antiviral treatment with cidofovir 3–5 mg/kg/week for 2–3 weeks and, thereafter, every other week.

Patients with probable or proven ADV disease should be treated with IV cidofovir (5 mg/kg weekly for at least three doses; thereafter, every other week), together with hyperhydration and oral probenecid.

Ribavirin is not recommended for ADV. Donor-derived ADV-specific CTLs are an option for clinically non-responding patients. Oral brincidofovir 2 mg/kg twice weekly might be obtained for compassionate use.

38.3 Respiratory Viruses

38.3.1 Influenza

38.3.1.1 Clinical Symptoms

Influenza is a yearly occurring respiratory viral infection with outbreaks of different sizes depending on the circulating strain.

Influenza can be a very severe infection in HSCT recipients. The risk for lower tract disease (LTD) has been reported to be as high as 33%, and mortality has varied in different reports between 0 and 15%.

The risk for LTD is higher when occurring just prior to or during conditioning, very early after HSCT, with viruses resistant to neuraminidase inhibitors and with new viral strains such as the recent H1N1 ("swine flu").

Symptoms are similar as in the immune-competent individual. Respiratory symptoms vary from very mild to life-threatening symptoms. GI symptoms and CNS symptoms can also occur. Secondary bacterial infections are not uncommon.

38.3.1.2 Diagnostics

Several commercial tests detecting either nucleic acid or influenza antigens are available. Since the symptoms frequently are uncharacteristic, multiplex tests detecting different respiratory viruses are frequently used.

38.3.1.3 Prophylaxis

The most important prophylactic measure is vaccination, which is recommended yearly to all HSCT recipients. The efficacy of the vaccine varies from season to season depending on the fitness of the strains used in preparing the vaccine to the circulating strains.

The immune response to vaccination is better when given at least 6 months after HSCT although vaccination can be considered from 3 months after HSCT in outbreak situations. A second dose of vaccine can be considered.

Antiviral prophylaxis is not generally recommended but can be considered in patients exposed to an infected individual.

38.3.1.4 Treatment

Standard therapy is with neuraminidase inhibitors mainly oseltamivir or zanamivir although no study has shown efficacy specifically in HSCT recipients.

It should be recognized that the normally recommended duration of 5 days often is too short since viral excretion might continue for a long time. Resistance to oseltamivir is not rare although variable with the strain circulating in that particular season.

38.3.2 Other Community-Acquired Respiratory Viruses (CARVs)

38.3.2.1 Clinical Symptoms

Infections with CARVs including respiratory syncytial virus (RSV), parainfluenza viruses (PIV), metapneumovirus, rhinoviruses, and coronaviruses are very common in HSCT recipients.

Most infections are mild causing only upper respiratory symptoms but LTD occurs. Importantly CARV infections occurring before start of conditioning have been associated with severe symptoms and increased NRM, and therefore deferring the start of conditioning shall be considered at least in symptomatic patients.

38.3.2.2 Diagnostics

Multiplex PCR testing of different CARVs is today the most used technique.

38.3.2.3 Prophylaxis

The only available measure is to avoid nosocomial spread of these infections.

38.3.2.4 Treatment

No therapy of a CARV has been proven efficacious in controlled trials.

Ribavirin either given as inhalation or systemically has been suggested to reduce the risk for progression of upper respiratory tract RSV infection to LTD and possibly to reduce mortality in RSV pneumonia. No licensed therapy is available for any other CARV.

38.4 Polyomaviruses

38.4.1 Polyoma JCV

38.4.1.1 Clinical Symptoms

Reactivation of the ubiquitous, neurotropic John Cunningham polyomavirus (JCV) may cause PML, a rare, opportunistic, and severe disease of the CNS.

PML awareness increased following the introduction of new immunomodulatory or IS treatments with natalizumab, rituximab, efalizumab, infliximab, brentuximab, fingolimod, dimethyl fumarate, azathioprine, tacrolimus, and MMF.

38.4.1.2 Diagnostics

JCV-DNA by PCR, especially in CSF (also multiplex PCR).

The new option is high-resolution melting analysis (PCR-HRM) for diagnosis of JCV in patients with PML.

Profound suppression in cellular immunity T-lymphopenia may constitute a primary PML risk factor.

38.4.1.3 Prophylaxis

Not used.

38.4.1.4 Treatment

No specific treatment is currently available.

The application of G-CSF may facilitate immune reconstitution and JCV clearance in the CSF. BKV-specific CTLs might demonstrate anti-JCV activity due to virus homology.

38.4.2 BKV

BKV (See Chap. 51: Hemorrhagic Cystitis and Renal Dysfunction)

38.5 Hepatotropic Viruses

38.5.1 Hepatitis A Virus (HAV)

38.5.1.1 Clinical Symptoms

Enteric transmission via person-to-person contact is the predominant way of spreading.

Infection with HAV in HSCT recipients can increase the risk of SOS/VOD, and HAV has been associated with aplastic anemia.

Due to the scarcity of chronic HAV infection, blood products and HSCT donors are not routinely tested for HAV.

38.5.1.2 Diagnostics

PCR is the preferred method in HSCT setting.

Liver function tests (LFT) should be performed in donors before HSC harvesting. Donors with abnormal LFT should be tested for anti-HAV-IgM. If HAV is detected, donation should be delayed until HAV-RNA is no longer detectable in the donor.

38.5.1.3 Prophylaxis

HSCT is not recommended if the donor or the recipient is viremic for HAV because of an increased risk of SOS/VOD.

Vaccination should be considered in HAV-IgG-negative patients at risk.

38.5.1.4 Treatment

Symptomatic.

38.5.2 Hepatitis B Virus (HBV)

38.5.2.1 Clinical Symptoms

After primary infection, even in case of HBsAg seroconversion, HBV probably persists lifelong in the nucleus of hepatocytes.

HBV can reactivate after treatment-induced loss of immune control.

Hepatitis, including cases of fulminant hepatic failure, typically occurs after immune system reconstitution, de novo recognition, and destruction of HBV-infected hepatocytes.

Fibrosing cholestatic hepatitis can be a consequence of HBV reactivation. The case-fatality rate of HBV reactivation is high in patients with hematological malignancy.

38.5.2.2 Diagnostics

All donors and recipients must be screened for anti-HBsAg, anti-HBc, and anti-HBs and HBV-DNA if anti-HBc is detected.

38.5.2.3 Prophylaxis

Antiviral prophylaxis should be given to anti-HBc-positive patients and those receiving grafts from HBV-infected donors. Tenofovir or entecavir are the drugs of choice.

Vaccination of anti-HBc-negative and anti-HBs-negative patients before and after HSCT is recommended. Double vaccine doses may be required to achieve an anti-HBs response in immunocompromised patients (0–1–2–6 months).

Vaccination of anti-HBc-negative and anti-HBs-negative stem cell donors before HSCT harvesting should be considered; an accelerated single-dose 3-week (0–10–21 days) schedule may be an alternative to the conventional 6-month protocols.

38.5.2.4 Treatment

Indication for treatment includes all HBsAg-positive patients. Vaccination and the addition of hepatitis B immune globulin can be considered in this setting.

Antiviral treatment should be started with the beginning of IST. Tenofovir or entecavir are the drugs of choice. The treatment should be continued 1 year after withdrawal of IST, longer in recipients with cGVHD and patients exposed to depleting Ab.

38.5.3 Hepatitis C Virus (HCV)

38.5.3.1 Clinical Symptoms

Assessment of liver fibrosis in HCV-RNA-positive recipients is recommended, as close monitoring is essential in patients with known underlying fibrosis. Liver fibrosis is a risk factor for SOS/VOD and drug toxicity.

The risk of acute flare-ups is higher in patients on rituximab-containing treatment regimens.

Cirrhosis and a worse outcome have been clearly documented after HSCT.

38.5.3.2 Diagnostics

Close monitoring of LFT and HCV-RNA is recommended in infected patients.

38.5.3.3 Prophylaxis

A HCV-RNA-positive donor could be considered, if other donor options are considered inferior. In this case, the donor should be rapidly evaluated by a hepatologist, and treatment with directly acting antivirals should be considered.

The presence of HCV-RNA positive in the recipient does not constitute a contraindication for HSCT, but antiviral therapy should be considered if it is possible to postpone the HSCT to allow completion of a treatment course.

38.5.3.4 Treatment

Antiviral treatment should be considered for all HCV-RNA-positive hematological patients, once the hematological disease has been brought under control. This should be done in consultation with an expert hepatologist.

38.5.4 Hepatitis E Virus (HEV)

38.5.4.1 Clinical Symptoms

HEV exists in at least four different subtypes that can spread either through water, undercooked food, or blood transfusions. The main source of spread varies between different parts of the world with infected water being the most common route in resource-poor areas. In other areas the most common route of spread is via undercooked food produced from infected animals.

HEV infection in HSCT recipients is usually mildly symptomatic although acute hepatitis with jaundice has been reported and also fatal infections in pregnant women.

The probably more important clinical picture in HSCT recipients is chronic hepatitis since rapid progression to cirrhosis has been reported in IS patients.

38.5.4.2 Diagnostics

Serology to detect previously infected patients or PCR to detect acute or chronic infections.

38.5.4.3 Prophylaxis

None available.

38.5.4.4 Treatment

Ribavirin has been suggested as a treatment for chronic infection based on case reports and small case series. However, no controlled data exists.

38.6 Norovirus

38.6.1 Clinical Symptoms

Noroviruses are the most common cause of foodborne disease and acute nonbacterial gastroenteritis worldwide.

Its prevalence was 2% in adults and up to 22% among pediatric transplant recipients with diarrhea, requiring hospitalization in 55% and ICU admission in 27%. Recurrence rate 29%.

Risk factors: second HSCT, intestinal GVHD, children.

Norovirus can cause severe, prolonged disease complicated by enteritis, fever, recurrent hospitalizations for dehydration, chronic diarrhea, acute renal failure, weight loss, malnutrition, pneumatosis intestinalis, peritonitis, secondary bacteremia, and death.

38.6.2 Diagnostics

Viral RNA by RT-PCT in the stool.

38.6.3 Prophylaxis

Non-pharmacological prophylaxis is mandatory: strict isolation and hygiene measures in patients shedding the virus are absolutely necessary to prevent horizontal transmission and nosocomial outbreaks.

38.6.4 Treatment

Symptomatic. Some reports indicate oral human immunoglobulin therapy. Specific therapies are not available.

38.7 Zika Virus (ZIKV)

38.7.1 Clinical Symptoms

ZIKV infection is transmitted mainly by *Aedes aegypti* mosquitoes, sexual contact, or blood transfusion. It is typically a mild, asymptomatic disease in the general population.

The disease is a self-limiting febrile illness lasting 4–7 days. Infection can be followed by neurological consequences including Guillain-Barre syndromes and microcephaly or other congenital neurological syndromes after vertical transmission from an infected mother to her fetus during pregnancy.

38.7.2 Diagnostics

Direct detection of ZIKV-RNA or specific viral antigens.

38.7.3 Prophylaxis

Blood, tissues, and cells should not be imported from areas of ZIKV transmission or should be tested negative for the presence of ZIKV.

Donor diagnosed with ZIKV infection or who has just returned from an affected area should be deferred for at least 28 days after cessation of symptoms. The deferral should be at least 3 months after sexual contact with person at risk.

38.7.4 Treatment

No specific prophylaxis or therapy is available.

Key Points

- Epidemiology: Latent (especially CMV), endemic (especially CARV), and hepatotropic viruses are the main problem in patients after HSCT
- Diagnosis: Viral diagnostics after HSCT require qPCR or multiplex PCR
- Prophylaxis and treatment: Prophylaxis (pharmacological or environmental) or preemptive treatment is necessary. All patients after HSCT should undergo vaccinations according to current recommendations
- Outcome: Viral infections contribute to non-relapse mortality after HSCT

Recommended References

Engelhard D, Mohty B, de la Camara R, et al. European guidelines for prevention and management of influenza in hematopoietic stem cell transplantation and leukemia patients: summary of ECIL-4 (2011), on behalf of ECIL, a joint venture of EBMT, EORTC, ICHS, and ELN. Transpl Infect Dis. 2013;15:219–32.

Hirsch HH, Martino R, Ward KN, Boeckh M, Einsele H, Ljungman P. Fourth European Conference on Infections in Leukaemia (ECIL-4): guidelines for diagnosis and treatment of human respiratory syncytial virus, parainfluenza virus, metapneumovirus, rhinovirus, and coronavirus. Clin Infect Dis. 2013;56:258–66.

Ljungman P, de la Camara R, Crocchiolo R, et al. CMV and HHV6 update. ECIL-7. 2017. http://www.ecil-leukaemia.com/program2017.htm.

Mallet V, van Bömmel F, Doerig C, et al. Management of viral hepatitis in patients with haematological malignancy and in patients undergoing haemopoietic stem cell transplantation: recommendations of the 5th European Conference on Infections in Leukaemia (ECIL-5). Lancet Infect Dis. 2016;16:606–17.

Matthes-Martin S, Feuchtinger T, Shaw PJ, et al. European guidelines for diagnosis and treatment of adenovirus infection in leukemia and stem cell transplantation: summary of ECIL-4. Transpl Infect Dis. 2012;14:555–63.

Styczynski J, Reusser P, Einsele H, et al. Management of HSV, VZV and EBV infections in patients with hematological malignancies and after SCT: guidelines from the Second European Conference on Infections in Leukemia. Bone Marrow Transplant. 2009;43:757–70.

Styczynski J, Hoek J, Knelange N, et al. No report on Zika virus infection in EBMT registry: Infectious Diseases Working Party statement. Bone Marrow Transplant. 2017;52:1345–6.

Zaia J, Baden L, Boeckh MJ, et al. Viral disease prevention after hematopoietic cell transplantation. Bone Marrow Transplant. 2009;44:471–82.

39 Other Life-Threatening Infections

Rodrigo Martino

39.1 Toxoplasmosis

39.1.1 General Concepts

Toxoplasma gondii is a protozoan that commonly infects animals and birds. Primary *T. gondii* infection in humans and other mammals is usually asymptomatic but leads to lifelong latent infection. Transmission to humans occurs by ingesting tissue cysts from undercooked meat or oocysts (released in the feces of cats). Latent cysts can give rise during immunosuppression to a severe localized reactivation producing, for example, toxoplasma encephalitis or chorioretinitis, with dissemination being common. (Martino et al. 2000; Martino et al. 2005; Tomblyn et al. 2009; Martino 2016).

Although toxoplasmosis is the most common systemic parasitic infection in EBMT centers, it is a relatively rare opportunistic infection following HSCT. Currently we are aware that the patients' seroprevalence explains the wide range of incidences published. Table 39.1 summarizes selected case series of toxoplasmosis in HSCT published to date.

R. Martino (✉)
Hospital de la Santa Creu I Sant Pau, Autonomous University of Barcelona, ES, Barcelona, Spain
e-mail: rmartino@santpau.cat

39.1.2 Risk Factors and Incidence in HSCT

The seroprevalence for *T. gondii* varies greatly between and even within countries, ranging from <15% in Japan and in pediatric wards, 30% in urban adults in North America and the UK, and to 40–80% of adult HSCT recipients in countries with high endemicity such as France or Turkey. This varying seroprevalence is the main reason for the great variability in the incidence of toxoplasmosis after HSCT, which has been estimated to average 0.8%, with <0.4% in areas of low endemicity to 2–3% in those with high-antibody prevalence.

Toxoplasmosis occurs mainly in allo-HSCT recipients, although cases after auto-HSCT have been published. Reactivation of latent tissue cysts in previously infected individuals is the usual mechanism implicated. Thus, it is important to determine the patients' serostatus prior to transplant. However, the disease may also develop if primary (or re-)infection after transplant may occur.

Ninety-five percent of the cases occur within the first 6 months after the procedure, and acute GVHD and its treatment are the main risk factors. Late cases may occur, again usually in patients with chronic GVHD requiring IST. In addition, seropositive patients without GVHD but with severe cellular IS due to in vivo or ex vivo TCD are also at risk.

E. Carreras et al. (eds.), *The EBMT Handbook*, https://doi.org/10.1007/978-3-030-02278-5_39

Table 39.1 Selected case series of toxoplasmosis after HSCT (Martino 2017)

Author (year)[a]	Cases	Number of HSCT (% frequency)	% of sero (+) pre-HSCT	Median (range) day onset
Derouin et al. (1992)	7	296 allo (2.4)	65	74 (55–180)
Slavin et al. (1994)	12	3.803 allo (0.31) 509 auto (0)	15	59 (35–97)
Bretagne et al. (1995)	2	550 allo (0.3)	70	NS
Maschke et al. (1999)	20[b]	655 (3.1)	NS	73 (14–689)
Martino et al. (2003)	41	4.391 allo (0.93) 7.097 auto (0)	Variable (multinational study)	64 (4–516)
Small et al. (2000)	10	463 allo (2.2)	23	78 (36–155)
Aoun et al. (2006)	7	121 allo (5) 204 auto (0.4)	69	45 (13–140)
de Medeiros et al. (2001)	9	789 allo-HSCT (1.14)	NS	69 (13–265)
Mulanovich et al. (2011)	9	3.626 Allo (0.25) – U.S. pt 0.15% – Non-U.S. pt 1.6%	18% U.S. pt >50% non-U.S. pt	56 (12–122)
Bautista et al. (2012) and Martino et al. (2015)	9	148 adult CBT (4%)	45	39 (7–98)
Sumi et al. (2013)	6	279 allo (1.8%) 87 auto (1.1%)	10	NS
Hakko et al. (2017)	5	170 allo (2.9%)	70	42 (26–119)

[a]Not all in references

[b]4 definite and 16 possible cases of toxoplasmosis

39.1.3 Most Common Clinical Presentations

The CNS is the main site of disease, but pneumonitis and myocarditis are also frequent findings.

Toxoplasma encephalitis typically presents with focal neurologic abnormalities of subacute onset, frequently accompanied by non-focal signs and symptoms such as headache, altered mental status, and fever. Meningeal signs are very rare. CT brain scans often show multiple bilateral cerebral lesions, although MRI is more sensitive than CT in the early diagnosis of this infection. Toxoplasma pneumonitis may develop in the absence of extrapulmonary disease. Toxoplasma chorioretinitis is rare compared to AIDS patients.

39.1.4 Diagnosis

In HSCT recipients, the utility of serology is mainly to identify those at risk for developing toxoplasmosis post transplant.

PCR techniques are currently the standard method for its diagnosis. These techniques are applicable in blood, CSF, and BAL, the usual samples that are available in HSCT recipients with this infection. Most centers use qPCR with a level of detection as low as 20 parasites/mL, with parasite loads of >600/mL reported in most patients with toxoplasmosis.

Since histologically proven toxoplasmosis is a very difficult-to-obtain diagnosis, various levels of diagnostic certainty have been proposed. Histologically defined cases are considered as definite cases of toxoplasma disease, PCR-defined cases as probable, and CNS imaging-defined cases as possible ones.

39.1.5 Treatment and Prognosis

Table 39.2 details the recommended treatment and prophylaxis of toxoplasmosis in HSCT recipients. Most patients respond to one or another of these regimens, and neurologic improvement of toxoplasma brain involvement usually occurs within 7 days. If appropriately treated, up to 60% of patients may show clinical–radiologic improvement or even a complete response to therapy. This highlights the importance for a high index of suspicion for toxoplasmosis in immunocompromised patients.

39.1.6 Specific Screening and/or Prophylactic Strategies Available

Current data suggest that infection may precede disease in most cases of toxoplasmosis. Thus, monitoring sero(+) patients with weekly qPCR of blood samples has been advocated, especially when prophylaxis is not being used, in an effort of using a preemptive-type therapeutic approach, as used for CMV infection. Although an optimal qPCR technique has not been standardized, several studies support the usefulness of this approach. Patients on TMP/SMX prophylaxis should not be monitored.

TMP/SMX is useful in minimizing the risk of reactivation of toxoplasmosis, although there are well-reported cases of toxoplasmosis breaking through this prophylaxis in HSCT recipients. Suboptimal dosing may have contributed to some of these "breakthrough" infections, since these cases occur when TMP/SMX is taken less than 3 days per week. Thus, using either one standard-dose tablet (80/400 mg) daily or a double-strength tablet (160/800 mg) 4 days per week is the recommended dosing, as shown in Table 39.2.

Avoiding primary or reinfection after HSCT is always important, avoiding the most common sources of infection: uncooked meats of any type and drinking contaminated water.

Table 39.2 Suggested treatment and prophylaxis for toxoplasmosis in HSCT recipients

Treatment	Dose
Pyrimethamine (*plus* folinic acid)	Oral, 200 mg loading dose, then 50–75 mg q.d. (folinic acid, oral or IV, 10–15 mg q.d.) + *one of the following*
Sulfadiazine	Oral, 1–1.5 g q6–8h, *OR*
Clindamycin	Oral or IV, 600 mg q6h
Prophylaxis	Dose
TMP/SMX[a,b]	1 double-strength tablet (160/800 mg)/day, 4 day × week, *OR* 2 double-strength tablets (160/800 mg)/day, 3 day × week, *OR* 1 standard-dose tablet (80/400 mg) daily, *OR*
Pyrimethamine and sulfadoxine (fansidar)[a]	2–3 tables per week
Dapsone[b]	100 mg daily
Atovaquone[b]	1500 mg daily

[a]Also effective for PJP prophylaxis, and possibly listeriosis, nocardiosis, and, in some geographic areas, partly effective in preventing gram-positive cocci and gram-negative bacillary (enterobacterial and non-glucose fermenting) infections

[b]The dose can be reduced in patients with mild renal insufficiency

39.2 Tuberculosis (TBC)

(de la Cámara et al. 2000; Cordonnier et al. 2004; Yao-Chung et al. 2016; Young and Weisdorf 2016; Beswick et al. 2018).

39.2.1 General Concepts

TBC, and especially, multidrug-resistant (MDR) TBC, continues to be a worldwide major health problem. This may surprise many EBMT HSCT physicians, who may have never seen a case of TBC.

39.2.1.1 Mycobacterium Tuberculosis

Mycobacterium tuberculosis causes nearly all cases of TBC, and these acid-fast bacilli differ from other bacteria in that they can live only in an infected human. Outside of the human body, they have a very short survival, and infection is transmitted by the inhalation of aerosolized particles from a patient. In addition, its isolation from clinical samples should never be considered as a colonization or sample contamination. TBC is not an opportunistic infection, and thus its detailed description is outside the scope of this manual.

39.2.2 Risk Factors and Incidence in HSCT

The risk of developing TBC is directly proportional to the TBC present in the geographic area of the HSCT center and the patients' residence (Fig. 39.1). A few studies have analyzed its incidence with respect to the general population, and most have found that allo-HSCT recipients have 2–10 times higher risk than the general population, while auto-HSCT recipients do not have a significantly higher risk (De la Cámara et al. 2000) (Table 39.3).

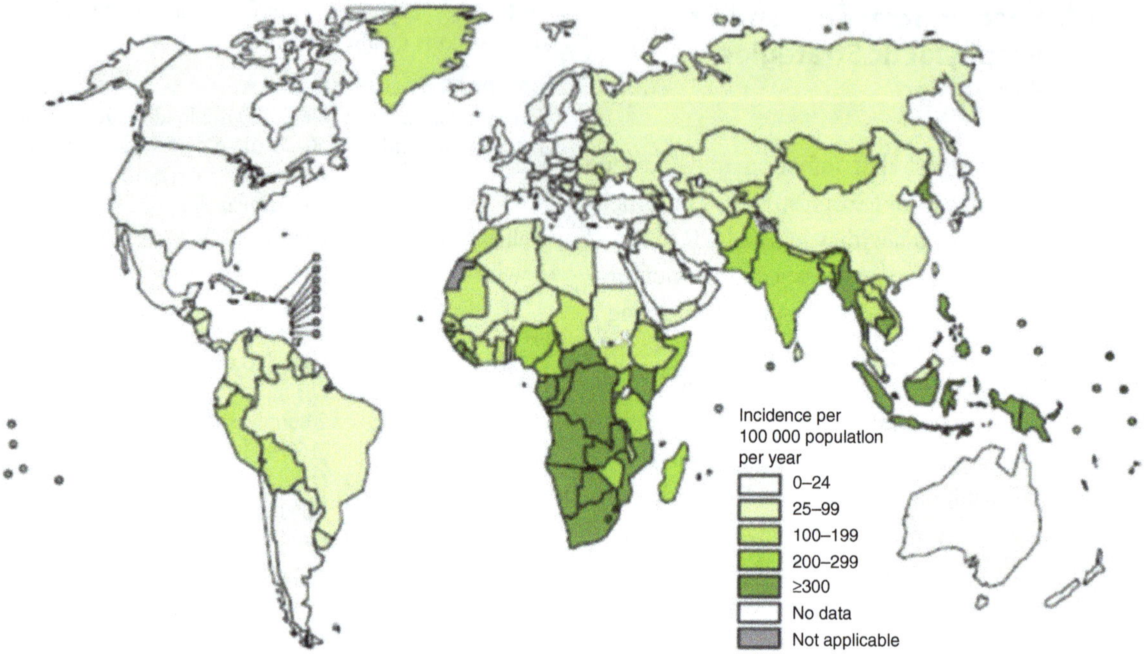

Fig. 39.1 TBC estimate incidence rate 2016 (WHO webpage)

Table 39.3 Selected case series of mycobacterial infections after HSCT before 2018

Author (year)[a]	Country	TBC/HSCT x risk with GP[b]	NTM/HSCT x risk with GP	Outcome of infection
Lee et al. (2017)	Korea	21/824 (allo) × 9.1 GP	NA	1 died
Liu et al. (2016)[c]	Taiwan	5/422 (allo)	21/422 (allo)	11 died
Beswick et al. (2018)	Canada	NA	30/1097 (allo) × 35 GP	NA
Fan et al. (2015)	Taiwan	32/1368 (allo) × 7 GP 7/672 (auto) × 2.5 GP	0	20 died
Garces-Ambrossi et al. (2005)	USA	4/577 (allo) × 10 GP	0	NA
Cordonnier et al. (2004)	Multiple (EBMT)	23/1513 (allo) 8/3012 (auto)	8	5 died
Ku et al. (2001)	Taiwan	8/255 (allo) × 13.1 GP 0/95 (auto)	0	ND
de la Cámara et al. (2000)	Spain	12/2866 (allo) × 2.2 GP 8/5147 (auto) = to GP	NA	3 died
Budak-Alpdogan et al. (2000)	Turkey	5/351 (allo) × 3.9 GP	0	No deaths
Gaviria et al. (2000)	USA	3 /6529 (3 allo)	0	No deaths
Aljurf et al. (1999)	Saudi Arabia	4/641 (allo)	0	2 died
Roy et al. (1997)	USA	2/1486 (allo) 0/755 (auto)	7/1486 (allo) 2/755 (auto)	No deaths
Martino et al. (1996, 2011)	Spain	2/698 (allo) 0/637(auto)	0	No deaths

NA Details not available in the study

[a]Not all in references

[b]x risk with GP, studies in which the relative risk of suffering TBC was compared to that in age-/sex-matched normal individuals from the general population

[c]Abstract

39.2.3 Most Common Clinical Presentations

The clinical presentation of TBC in HSCT recipients is the same as in the general population, although it may have a more rapid progression, and the ratio of pulmonary to extrapulmonary disease has been reported 34/5 to 11/10, which surely represents a publication bias, with a median of 75%/25%. The most common extrapulmonary disease is meningitis.

39.2.4 Diagnosis

Culture of even a single colony from an affected organ is diagnostic for TBC. Direct microbiologic examination for acid-fast bacilli is of course mandatory, but its sensitivity is probably low. In addition, the results of positive cultures take many days to weeks, and the use of highly sensitive and specific PCR methods is now the usual methods for the initial diagnosis.

The quantiFERON-TB Gold test is not reliable in the diagnosis of TBC in HSCT recipients due to their T-cell immunodeficiency.

39.2.5 Treatment and Prognosis

With appropriate treatment, TBC in HSCT recipients has a low attributable mortality (<30%). The author suggests that HSCT physicians contact ID physicians immediately when diagnosis of TBC is made. Empirical treatment should be started if this consultation will not be replied immediately, but herein we cannot recommend a "one fits all" drug combination, since this varies greatly according to the level of drug resistance in each geographical area.

39.2.6 Specific Screening and/or Prophylactic Strategies Available

Even in areas where TBC is endemic, pre-HSCT screening with the tuberculin skin test or the gamma-interferon quantiFERON-TB Gold test is not done in most HSCT centers. In addition, specific antibiotic prophylaxis in patients with past and cured TBC is not warranted.

Two special scenarios do, however, require contacting an ID specialist pre- or post-HSCT in order to analyze whether "prophylaxis" may be indicated, the drugs to use, and their duration:

1. Highly IS HSCT recipients or candidates who have been substantially exposed to someone with active infectious TBC
2. HSCT recipients or candidates with a positive tuberculin skin test or the gamma-interferon quantiFERON-TB Gold test who were not previously treated and have radiological evidence of TBC lung disease

39.3 Nontuberculous (or Atypical) Mycobacterial (NTM) Infections

(Cordonnier et al. 2004; Young and Weisdorf 2016; Beswick et al. 2018).

39.3.1 General Concepts

Atypical mycobacteria are fastidious microorganisms that are ubiquitous in nature and can simply colonize any body surface and secretions and often contaminate clinical samples from the environment. There are a very large number of NTM species with varying geographical distributions. However, with respect to infections in HSCT recipients, NTM can be divided into two different categories:

(1) *Mycobacterium avium-intracellulare* complex.
(2) Anonymous or atypical NTM, subdivided into the rapidly growing NTM and the slow growing NTM: the most commonly reported species from EBMT centers are *M. fortuitum, M. chelonae, M. abscessus, M. xenopi, and M. kansasii.*

39.3.2 Most Common Clinical Presentations and Risk Factor

A large number of atypical NTM infections are CVC infections, followed by skin infections. However, in patients with severe cGVHD, severe infections of any organ can occur, as well as disseminated cases. *M. avium-intracellulare* complex, on the other hand, usually causes pulmonary disease or disseminated infections, with blood cultures being positive in >50% of cases. Such infections almost always occur in severely immunocompromised allo-HSCT recipients, such as those with severe steroid-dependent cGVHD.

39.3.3 Diagnosis

Diagnosis requires isolation of a NTM from the affected organ(s). Differentiating colonization from contamination and disease can be difficult with NTM. Depending on the species, cultures can be positive in very few days or take many days, as with TBC. Thus, the use of specific PCR methods and/or special biochemical methods is now the usual method for the diagnosis of NTM infections.

39.3.4 Treatment and Prognosis

With appropriate treatment, most NTM infections have a good outcome and a low attributable mortality, although the data are very scarce (Table 39.3).

As in the case of TBC, the author suggests that HSCT physicians contact ID physicians immediately when diagnosis of NTM infection is made. In CVC infections, the catheter should probably always be removed. While awaiting for the ID specialists, empirical therapy with a macrolide (clarithromycin or azithromycin) plus moxifloxacin or levofloxacin can be started.

39.3.5 Specific Screening and/or Prophylactic Strategies Available

Screening and prophylaxis have no role in NTM infections.

39.4 Listeriosis

(Safdar et al. 2002; Boyle 2014; Martino et al. 1996).

39.4.1 General Concepts

Only one species, *Listeria monocytogenes*, produces all cases of this mostly "bacterial foodborne" infection. *L. monocytogenes* is a pseudo-"diphtheroid" gram-positive bacillus. This organism is widespread in nature and in tap water, sewage, the microbiota of pets and farm animals, and nearly all types of fresh foods. The fact that it grows well in refrigerator temperatures adds yet another variable which favors ingestion by humans, which appears to be universal worldwide. At any specific moment, 5% of healthy humans have *L. monocytogenes* in feces. With these premises, it is surprising that listeriosis is an uncommon infection in HSCT recipients.

39.4.2 Risk Factors and Incidence in HSCT

The only risk factor is the combination of ingesting colonized food or water and having a severe cellular IS.

Its incidence is unknown, and only two studies are available. At the MSKCC in New York, six cases occurred in 1315 allo-HSCT recipients from 1985 to 1997, with an incidence of 0.47% (Safdar et al. 2002). At the FHCRC in Seattle, three cases occurred among 4069 HSCT recipients (<0.1%) during the first 100 days post transplant (Boyle 2014). Finally, in our center, we have had three cases of listeriosis among 2360 adult HSCT recipients (0.1%) (Martino et al. 1996). All other information has been reported as isolated case reports.

39.4.3 Most Common Clinical Presentations

Listeriosis in HSCT recipients is almost always a sepsis syndrome with bloodstream infection, with CNS involvement in 40–60% of cases, which can present as meningitis, encephalitis, or brain abscess, and with several cases of rhombencephalitis reported (Chang et al. 1995).

39.4.4 Diagnosis

The diagnosis is made after the bacterial microbiology laboratory informs the clinicians that the patient has positive blood and/or CSF cultures for this organism. The putative source of the infection cannot be identified in outpatients.

39.4.5 Specific Screening and/or Prophylactic Strategies Available

Screening has no role in preventing listeriosis. Standard approaches to food safety handling and preparation are, of course, the main preventive measures.

The routine use of TMP/SMX prophylaxis after HSCT surely has a role in preventing listeriosis, but its low incidence makes this impossible to prove.

Cases of listeriosis in long-term inpatients should, of course, activate the rapid intervention of the hospital infection control/prevention unit in the HSCT ward.

39.4.6 Treatment and Prognosis

The treatment of choice is high-dose ampicillin (or high-dose TMP/SMX in those allergic to penicillin) combined with an aminoglycoside during 3 weeks or 6 weeks in case of CNS infection. We also recommend consultation with ID specialists.

The prognosis of listeriosis in HSCT recipients is unknown, although 20% of the reported cases died, while 10% had a CNS recurrence.

39.5 Nocardiosis

(Coussement et al. 2017; Shannon et al. 2016; Bambace et al. 2013).

39.5.1 General Concepts

Nocardia spp. (any of the dozens of currently accepted species may be involved, but most cases in Europe appear to be due to *N. asteroides*, *N. brasiliensis*, and *N. nova*) are aerobic gram-positive rods that grow in characteristic filamentous, branching chains and being acid fast, and their appearance makes them easily identifiable by microbiologists, with its acid-fast staining properties differentiating it from *Actinomyces* spp. *Nocardia* spp. grow in soil and decaying matter, and human infection usually occurs from inhalation of airborne bacilli.

39.5.2 Risk Factors and Incidence in HSCT

Nocardiosis is a late post-HSCT infection, occurring months to years after HSCT, mostly allo-HSCT. Patients usually have steroid-dependent chronic GVHD, secondary diabetes mellitus, and/or bronchiolitis obliterans or bronchiectasis from the numerous post-HSCT infections suffered. There are no specific risk factors in HSCT, although being at the right time in a place where soil-living bacilli are made massively airborne is a common-sense mechanism of infection. Similar to *M. tuberculosis*, *Nocardia* spp. do not colonize the airways.

The incidence of nocardiosis has been reported to range from 0.3 to 1.7% in allo-HSCT, although many large centers have not had a single case. In auto-HSCT the median incidence is 0%, although occasional cases have been reported and surely occur in many centers.

39.5.3 Most Common Clinical Presentations

Pulmonary infection, with its accompanying signs and symptoms, and radiologically one or more nodular lesions with a tendency to cavitate occur in 90% of patients with nocardiosis. At presentation, however, around half of the patients have disseminated disease, usually to the skin and osteoskeletal organs, but around 1/3 will have CNS involvement up front. Since CNS involvement is so common and can initially be asymptomatic, a CNS CT or MRI scan is mandatory in all HSCT recipients with pulmonary nocardiosis (in any IS host, in fact). Brain abscesses are the usual presentation, although severe hyponatremia due to SIADH is also common due to basal meningitis.

39.5.4 Diagnosis

Diagnosis, of course, requires culture of an affected organ, usually the lungs. Often, the characteristic ramified bacilli can be directly observed from sputum or a directed BAL, but culture-based diagnosis is made in at least 1/3 of the cases. This is of utmost importance, since cultures become positive at a median of 9 days after sampling but can take up to 2–4 weeks. Molecular-based methods are useful only to identify uncommon species of *Nocardia* with known multidrug resistance, but this is rarely required in clinical practice. The most common differential diagnosis is with invasive pulmonary mold infections.

39.5.5 Specific Screening and/or Prophylactic Strategies Available

Screening has no role in preventing nocardiosis, but its rapid diagnosis does have an impact on patient outcome.

The routine use of TMP/SMX prophylaxis after HSCT may prevent more cases of nocardiosis, but the 2–3-day per week schedules are not effective in preventing it. Of note, *Nocardia* spp. isolated in patients taking single-strength TMP/SMX prophylaxis 5–7 days per week have had a good in vitro susceptibility to TMP/SMX and have responded well to high doses of the drug.

39.5.6 Treatment and Prognosis

High-dose TMP/SMX is still the treatment of choice, although there have been good results with carbapenems, amikacin, second-generation cephalosporins, and/or linezolid.

When treated promptly, nocardiosis usually resolves with prolonged antibiotic therapy, but directly attributable mortality has been reported in up to 40% of cases; these are, of course, those cases that affect extremely debilitated allo-HSCT recipients due to prolonged severe GVHD and its numerous complications, as well as those with disseminated infection and extensive CNS involvement, including the brain stem. Overall mortality, however, is high, since around 40% of patients have severe coinfections when nocardiosis joins the club.

Treatment of nocardiosis usually requires at least 6 months of specific antibiotic therapy, and it is of course recommended that ID specialists are actively involved in the treatment and follow-up. Of note, most *Nocardia* isolates are susceptible to most of the too-often empirically/prophylactically used antibiotics in HSCT recipients (levofloxacin, moxifloxacin, amoxicillin-clavulanate), as well as tetracyclines and tigecycline.

Key Points

- The intense IS associated with allo-HSCT, especially when there is a chronic GVHD that requires a prolonged IST, favors the development of infections by very unusual pathogens.
- Despite its low incidence, it is necessary to know these pathologies in order to make an early diagnosis and to adapt the therapy to the causal pathogen.

References

Bambace NM, Poirier L, Cohen S, et al. Nocardiosis in allogeneic hematopoietic stem cell transplant recipients: a matched case-control study of risk factors, clinical features and outcomes. Biol Blood Marrow Transplant. 2013;19:S280.

Beswick J, Shin E, Michelis FV, et al. Incidence and risk factors for nontuberculous mycobacterial infection after allogeneic hematopoietic cell transplantation. Biol Blood Marrow Transplant. 2018;24:366–72.

Chang J, Powles R, Mehta J, et al. Listeriosis in bone marrow transplant recipients: incidence, clinical features, and treatment. Clin Infect Dis. 1995;21:1289–90.

Cordonnier C, Martino R, Trabasso P, et al. Mycobacterial infection: a difficult and late diagnosis in stem cell transplant recipients. Clin Infect Dis. 2004;38:1229–36.

Coussement J, Lebeaux D, Rouzaud C, Lortholary O. Nocardia infections in solid organ and hematopoietic stem cell transplant recipients. Curr Opin Infect Dis. 2017;30:545–51.

de la Cámara R, Martino R, Granados E, et al. Tuberculosis after hematopoietic stem cell transplantation: incidence, clinical characteristics and outcome. Spanish Group on Infectious Complications in Hematopoietic Transplantation. Bone Marrow Transplant. 2000;26:291–8.

Martino R. Toxoplasmosis after hematopoietic stem cell transplantation. In: Ljungman P, Snydman D, Boeckh M, editors. Transplant infections. Printfort: Springer; 2016. p. 773–80.

Martino R, Lopez R, Pericas R, et al. Listeriosis in bone marrow transplant recipient. Clin Infect Dis. 1996;23:419–20.

Martino R, Maertens J, Bretagne S, et al. Toxoplasmosis after hematopoietic stem cell transplantation. Clin Infect Dis. 2000;31:1188–95.

Martino R, Bretagne S, Einsele H, et al. Early detection of toxoplasma infection by molecular monitoring of toxoplasma gondii in peripheral blood samples after allogeneic stem cell transplantation. Clin Infect Dis. 2005;40:67–78.

Safdar A, Papadopoulous EB, Armstrong D. Listeriosis in recipients of allogeneic blood and marrow transplantation: thirteen year review of disease characteristics, treatment outcomes and a new association with human cytomegalovirus infection. Bone Marrow Transplant. 2002;29:913–6.

Shannon K, Pasikhova Y, Ibekweh Q, Ludlow S, Baluch A. Nocardiosis following hematopoietic stem cell transplantation. Transpl Infect Dis. 2016;18: 169–75.

Tomblyn M, Chiller T, Einsele H, et al. Guidelines for preventing infectious complications among hematopoietic cell transplantation recipients: a global perspective. Biol Blood Marrow Transplant. 2009;15: 1143–23.

Yao-Chung L, Wu C, Chien S, et al. Mycobacterial infections in adult recipients of allogeneic hematopoietic stem cell transplantation: a cohort study in a high endemic area. Blood. 2016;128:S2202.

Young JAH, Weisdorf DJ. Typical and atypical mycobacterium infections after hematopoietic stem cell or solid organ transplantation. In: Ljungman P, Snydman D, Boeckh M, editors. Transplant infections. Printfort: Springer; 2016. p. 381–96.

40 Bleeding and Thrombotic Complications

Shruti Chaturvedi, Binsah George, and Bipin N. Savani

40.1 Introduction

Bleeding and thrombotic complications are an important cause of morbidity and mortality in patients undergoing HSCT. The major thrombotic complications include venous thromboembolism, such as catheter-related thrombosis, sinusoidal obstruction syndrome (SOS), and transplant-associated thrombotic microangiopathy (TA-TMA), while bleeding can involve the GI or respiratory tracts and is most common in thrombocytopenic patients or those with GVHD.

HSCT is associated with multiple risk factors for both thrombosis and bleeding including the underlying malignancy, thrombocytopenia, high-dose MAC and immunomodulatory drugs, GVHD, infections, indwelling vascular catheters, and prolonged immobilization (Gerber et al. 2008; Chaturvedi et al. 2016; Nadir and Brenner 2007). HSCT is also associated with alterations in the coagulation system with activation of endothelium-dependent coagulation factors, increase in vWF and platelet adhesion, increased thrombin generation, decreased antithrombin levels, and decreased levels of anticoagulant proteins such as protein C (Vannucchi et al. 1994). Collectively, major patient-, disease-, and therapy-related factors contribute to hemostatic complications in HSCT patients. Thrombotic and bleeding complications in HSCT are discussed separately below.

S. Chaturvedi
Division of Hematology, Department of Medicine, Johns Hopkins Hospital, Baltimore, MD, USA

B. George · B. N. Savani (✉)
Hematology and Stem Cell Transplantation Section, Division of Hematology/Oncology, Department of Medicine, Vanderbilt University Medical Center and Veterans Affairs Medical Center, Nashville, TN, USA
e-mail: Bipin.Savani@vanderbilt.edu

40.2 Thrombotic Complications

40.2.1 Epidemiology and Risk Factors

Thromboembolic complications in HSCT recipients include venous thromboembolism (VTE), catheter-associated thrombosis (CAT), sinusoidal obstruction syndrome, and TA-TMA. VTE is the most common of these complications, and retrospective studies have reported VTE incidence as high as 4.6% over 180 days for inpatients undergoing HSCT (Gerber et al. 2008). The rate of VTE is higher with allo-HSCT than auto-HSCT and in the presence of GVHD with 1-year VTE rates of 4.8%, 6.8%, and 8.1% reported with auto-HSCT, allo-HSCT without GVHD, and allo-HSCT with GVHD, respectively (Pihusch et al. 2002). A retrospective series of 447 patients undergoing BMT reported a 5.7% incidence of VTE in the first 100 days following transplant despite being on heparin prophylaxis (100 U/kg iv daily) for hepatic SOS (Pihusch et al. 2002). Finally, Gonsalves

E. Carreras et al. (eds.), *The EBMT Handbook*, https://doi.org/10.1007/978-3-030-02278-5_40

Table 40.1 Recommendations for prophylaxis and treatment of VTE in HSCT recipients[a]

VTE prophylaxis	VTE treatment
Indications for prophylaxis – Patients with MM receiving IMiDs – During hospitalization or postoperatively, as long as platelet count is >50 × 10^9/L – Prophylaxis is not recommended in outpatients with indwelling vascular catheters *Prophylaxis strategy* – Aspirin in low-risk patients with MM receiving IMiDs – LMWH (prophylactic dose of 40 mg SC daily) for patients with MM on IMiDs and >1 risk factor for VTE – Prophylactic doses of UFH or LMWH in hospitalized patients	*General principles* – Start therapeutic doses of LMWH or IV UFH in patients who have platelet count >50 × 10^9/L and no active bleeding. UFH is preferred in case of renal impairment (GFR <30 mL/min) or high bleeding risk – Continue LMWH or transition to warfarin (if LMWH is contraindicated) for maintenance therapy – DOACs are not currently recommended in patients undergoing HSCT *Duration of anticoagulation* – *General*: 3–6 months or as long as malignancy or use of IMiDs persists, whichever is longer – *Catheter-related thrombosis*: 3 months or as long as catheter is in place *Inferior vena cava filter* Only use to patients in whom anticoagulation is contraindicated or those who develop pulmonary embolism on anticoagulation. Remove as soon as anticoagulation can be started

DOACs direct oral anticoagulants, *IMiDs* immunomodulatory drugs, *LMWH* low molecular weight heparin, *MM* multiple myeloma, *UFH* unfractionated heparin
[a]Adapted from Chaturvedi et al. (2016)

et al. reported a 1-year symptomatic VTE incidence of 3.7% in patients undergoing HSCT in an *ambulatory* care setting (Gonsalves et al. 2008).

VTE occurs most frequently following engraftment, in patient undergoing allo-HSCT, those with a history of previous VTE or GVHD (Labrador et al. 2013). The majority of VTE episodes in these studies were catheter-associated thrombosis. Cortelezzi et al. have previously reported that there was a 12% incidence of catheter-related thromboembolic complications in a cohort of 416 patients with hematologic malignancies (Cortelezzi 2005). Twenty-one percent of these patients were HSCT recipients, and 81.2% had platelet counts less than 50 × 10^9/L. There was a non-statistically significant trend toward lower rates of thrombotic complications with thrombocytopenia. Prolonged hospitalization and inherited thrombophilias (e.g., factor V Leiden, prothrombin gene mutation, protein C or S deficiency) are associated with an increased risk of thrombosis in the general population and may add to thrombosis risk in the HSCT population as well.

40.2.2 VTE Prophylaxis

40.2.2.1 Randomized Studies

Randomized studies have not evaluated empiric prophylactic anticoagulation in HSCT recipients; however, studies in patients with cancer provide the next best evidence that can be extrapolated. The PROTECHT (nadroparin versus placebo) and SAVE-ONCO (semuloparin versus placebo) trials showed a significant reduction in the relative risk of VTE with prophylactic anticoagulation in patients with cancer; however the absolute risk reduction is small, and no survival benefit has been demonstrated. The American Society of Clinical Oncology (ASCO) guidelines advise against the use of routine prophylactic anticoagulation in ambulatory patients with cancer (Lyman et al. 2015). We do not generally recommend prophylactic anticoagulation in thrombocytopenic HSCT recipients with the exception of those with multiple myeloma (MM) receiving thalidomide or lenalidomide or hospitalized patients at higher risk of thrombosis (Table 40.1).

40.2.2.2 Multiple Myeloma

Patients with MM have a high baseline risk of thrombosis of 5–10% that increases several-fold in patients being treated with the immunomodulators (IMiDs) THAL and LENA with DEX or chemotherapy. Consolidation therapy with THAL or LENA after HSCT has been shown to improve CR rates and prolong EFS and is thus rapidly becoming standard of care (McCarthy et al. 2012; Barlogie et al. 2006). In patients receiving THAL consolidation after auto-HSCT for MM, the rate of VTE was 24% and 6% in the induction and consolidation periods, respectively, despite thromboprophylaxis with low molecular weight heparin (LMWH) (Barlogie et al. 2006). McCarthy et al. reported no episodes of VTE in patients receiving consolidation therapy with LENA; however, these patients also received prophylactic anticoagulation (McCarthy et al. 2012). Based on studies showing a benefit of thromboprophylaxis in patients with newly diagnosed MM receiving LENA- or THAL-based treatment (Palumbo et al. 2011) and the ASCO recommendation for thromboprophylaxis in this population (Lyman et al. 2015), we recommend either aspirin or LMWH for lower-risk patients and LMWH for higher-risk patients receiving THAL or LENA.

40.2.2.3 Hospitalized Patients

Though there is a clear benefit of pharmacologic thromboprophylaxis in medically ill hospitalized patients (Samama et al. 1999), randomized trials have not evaluated thromboprophylaxis in HSCT patients. The potential benefit from VTE prophylaxis is proportional to VTE risk, and therefore this is particularly important in patients with reduced mobility and with a history of VTE (if not on long-term anticoagulation) due to an even higher risk of thrombosis. Our practice is to start prophylactic anticoagulation for hospitalized patients in the post transplant period once the platelet count is >50 × 10^9/L and there is no active bleeding. For very high-risk patients, anticoagulation can be considered if the platelet count is >30 × 10^9/L; however this must be balanced with the risk of bleeding.

40.2.2.4 Prophylaxis of Catheter-Related Thrombosis

HSCT patients, especially those undergoing "ambulatory" HSCT, frequently have indwelling vascular catheters with the potential of catheter-related thrombosis (CRT). Despite multiple randomized and observational studies, thromboprophylaxis for the prevention of CRT in patients with cancer remains controversial. The largest study of thromboprophylaxis in CVC randomized 1590 cancer patients undergoing chemotherapy to adjusted-dose warfarin (international normalized ratio, 1.5–2.0), fixed-dose warfarin (1 mg/day), and no prophylaxis (Young et al. 2009). Symptomatic CRT was less frequent in the patients given adjusted-dose warfarin than in those who received no prophylaxis (2.7% vs 5.9%, P = 0.019); however, both adjusted-dose and fixed-dose warfarin were significantly associated with increased risk of major bleeding (Young et al. 2009). Recent meta-analyses of randomized trials concluded that prophylactic warfarin and LMWH do not significantly reduce symptomatic CRT in patients with cancer (Akl et al. 2007). Based on the available evidence, we do not routinely recommend prophylactic anticoagulation to prevent catheter-related thrombosis.

40.2.3 VTE Diagnosis and Treatment

Venous duplex ultrasonography should be performed in patients presenting with extremity swelling, redness or tenderness, or pulmonary angiography in patients with chest pain, dyspnea, or unexplained tachycardia. A clinical assessment of bleeding risk is necessary in patients who are diagnosed with VTE. Patients with no increased risk based on bleeding history and platelet count >50 × 10^9/L should be started on therapeutic anticoagulation with either LMWH or unfractionated heparin (UFH). The use of LMWH is restricted to patients with glomerular filtration rate >30 mL/min, while UFH is used in patients with impaired renal function (glomerular filtration rate <30 mL/min) or those with high bleeding risk. Following initiation of anticoagulation with LMWH or UFH, patients may be continued on LMWH or transition to warfarin with a standard INR target of 2–3. LMWH is preferred in patients with evidence of relapsed malignancy. The direct oral anticoagulants (DOACs) have not been evaluated in HSCT recipients, and their use cannot currently be recommended outside of a research setting. The optimal duration of anticoagulation for VTE in HSCT patients has not been evaluated in prospective studies. The recommendation for patients with cancer-related VTE is anticoagulation for 3–6 months, with ongoing therapy if the malignancy persists (Lyman et al. 2015; Kearon et al. 2012). We follow an analogous strategy in HSCT patients with the caveat that extended anticoagulation is often not feasible in patients with relapsed disease and a high likelihood of disease-related or treatment-related thrombocytopenia (Table 40.1).

The use of inferior vena cava (IVC) filters should be restricted to patients with acute deep vein thrombosis and a contraindication to anticoagulation and possibly patients who develop pulmonary embolism while on therapeutic anticoagulation (Kearon et al. 2012). IVC filters should not be used for primary prophylaxis of pulmonary embolism. In patients with large, symptomatic thrombosis and severe thrombocytopenia, we sometimes follow a strategy of platelet transfusions to reach a threshold of 50×10^9/L to allow safer anticoagulation with heparin.

40.2.4 Treatment of Catheter-Related Thrombosis

The rate of PE and mortality from CRT is low, and the objectives of CRT treatment are to reduce symptoms, prevent extension into more central veins, preserve access, and prevent chronic venous stenosis. There is no evidence that removal of the catheter improves outcomes. Therefore, it is reasonable to not to remove the catheter unless it is nonfunctional, no longer needed, or may be infected. Thrombus reduction by catheter-directed thrombolysis is relatively safe and effective and may be tried in an attempt to preserve the catheter. Anticoagulation is required in patients with acute CRT regardless of whether the catheter is removed (Kearon et al. 2012; Lyman et al. 2015). We prefer LMWH, though vitamin K antagonists (VKA) may be used if LMWH is contraindicated. In a prospective study of 78 patients with CRT treated with full-dose dalteparin bridged to warfarin, there were no new thrombotic events at 3 months, and 57% of catheters were still functional (Kovacs et al. 2007). The optimum duration of anticoagulation has not been evaluated in prospective studies. Current ACCP guidelines recommend anticoagulation for 3 months or until the catheter is removed, whichever is longer (Kearon et al. 2012). Several clinicians prefer to continue anticoagulation for 1–2 weeks after the catheter is removed.

40.2.5 Sinusoidal Obstruction Syndrome (SOS)

SOS (see Chap. 49) is a life-threatening complication that presents usually within the first 45 days after HSCT with elevated serum bilirubin levels, painful hepatomegaly, and fluid retention (Carreras, 2015). Endothelial injury of the hepatic sinusoids in SOS initiates hepatocyte injury and liver failure. SOS can occur in as high as 8–13% of HSCT recipients, and mortality is in excess of 80% (Carreras, 2015). MAC, preexisting liver disease, younger age, and poor performance status are associated with increased risk of SOS (McDonald et al. 1993). Ursodeoxycholic acid is recommended as prophylaxis for SOS in patients undergoing allo-HSCT. Anticoagulation with low-dose heparin has also been studied and is sometimes prescribed to patients undergoing auto-HSCT. Defibrotide, a pro-fibrinolytic agent, is a new agent approved for the treatment of severe SOS in both children and adults and is associated with higher rates of survival than historical controls (20–30% at day 100) (Richardson et al. 2016). Defibrotide prophylaxis has been shown to have some efficacy in preventing SOS in high-risk children, but whether this benefit translates for adults is not known.

40.2.6 Transplant-Associated TMA

TA-TMA (see Chap. 42) is a heterogeneous, frequently fatal disorder that occurs within 100 days after HSCT and is caused by treatment- and disease-related endothelial damage, coagulation activation, and microvascular thrombosis (Nadir and Brenner 2007). It is characterized by thrombocytopenia, microangiopathic anemia with schistocytes on the blood smear, and varying organ impairment such as renal failure and neurological symptoms. The diagnosis can be challenging since the clinical symptoms overlap with other common complications including GVHD and infections (Rosenthal, 2016). Risk factors for developing TA-TMA include exposure to calcineurin inhibitors, high-dose chemotherapy, GVHD, infections, advanced age, female sex, and non-MAC (Elsallabi et al. 2016). Elevated levels of vWF and inflammatory mediators such as IL-1, TNF-alpha, thrombomodulin, etc. and neutrophil extracellular traps have been implicated as causing the endothelial damage in TA-TMA. Treatment of TA-TMA is mostly supportive; however, recent data show that some patients with severe TA-TMA harbor complement gene mutations and uncontrolled complement activation has been demonstrated in TA-TMA, which is a potential therapeutic target. The complement inhibitor eculizumab has been successfully used in some cases of TA-TMA (Rosenthal, 2016).

40.3 Bleeding Complications

Bleeding in HSCT recipients is closely associated with prolonged and severe thrombocytopenia. In retrospective studies, the rate of bleeding in HSCT recipients ranges from 15.2% to 27.1%, and life-threatening or fatal bleeding occurred in 1.1% to 3.6% of patients (Gerber et al. 2008; Pihusch et al. 2002, Labrador et al. 2013). Gerber et al. reported that the initiation of therapeutic anticoagulation during days 1–180 after HSCT was the strongest predictor of bleeding [OR 3.1 (95% CI 1.8–5.5)] (Gerber et al. 2008). Furthermore, GVHD [OR 2.4 (95% CI 1.1–3.3)] increased the risk of bleeding, while auto-HSCT (versus allo-HSCT) was protective [OR 0.46 (95% CI 0.33–0.64)]. Bleeding can take any form including GI hemorrhage in patients with GVHD of the gut, hemorrhagic cystitis in patients with genitourinary involvement by GVHD, viral reactivation, and alkylating agent therapy, or spontaneously. Diffuse alveolar hemorrhage (DAH) (see Chap. 52) is a devastating bleeding complication that occurs in 2–14% of HSCT recipients and presents with progressive hypoxia, pulmonary infiltrates, and bloody alveolar lavage (Nadir and Brenner 2007). DAH is more common in thrombocytopenic patients and those with acute GVHD, and the effects of inflammatory cytokines on the alveolar lining have been implicated. There are no evidence-based prophylactic and therapeutic strategies, reported mortality is around 80% (range 64% to 100%) (Afessa et al. 2002). Platelet transfusions, systemic corticosteroids, antifibrinolytics, and recombinant factor VIIa have all been used with inconsistent results. It is general practice to administer prophylactic platelet transfusions for platelet counts less than 10×10^9/L in patients undergoing myeloablative chemotherapy or HSCT, though the superiority of prophylactic over therapeutic platelet transfusions is supported by low- to moderate-grade evidence. Given the competing risks of bleeding and thrombosis, identifying patients at high risk for these outcomes can optimize strategies for prophylaxis. The timing of hemostatic complications is an important consideration since bleeding events are more likely to occur early in the post transplant course when patients are profoundly thrombocytopenic, while thrombotic events occur more frequently after hematopoietic recovery (Gerber et al. 2008; Labrador et al. 2013).

Key Points

- Hemostatic complications, including both thrombosis and bleeding, are common in HSCT recipients and contribute to morbidity and mortality.
- Indwelling vascular catheters, GVHD associated inflammation, and certain medications are important risk factors for VTE, while prolonged severe thrombocytopenia and GVHD predispose to bleeding.
- Pharmacologic thromboprophylaxis is recommended for patients with MM receiving IMiDs and hospitalized patients with platelet count >50×10^9/L, but not for routine prophylaxis of CRT.
- LMWH (or UFH) is the treatment of choice for VTE in HSCT recipients.
- Ursodiol and defibrotide are recommended for the prevention and treatment of SOS, respectively. Defibrotide may also have a role in prophylaxis of high-risk patients.

References

Afessa B, Tefferi A, Litzow MR, et al. Diffuse alveolar hemorrhage in hematopoietic stem cell transplant recipients. Am J Respir Crit Care Med. 2002;166:641–5.

Akl EA, Karmath G, Yosuico V, et al. Anticoagulation for thrombosis prophylaxis in cancer patients with central venous catheters. Cochrane Database Syst Rev. 2007;18:CD006468.

Barlogie B, Tricot G, Anaissie E, et al. Thalidomide and hematopoietic-cell transplantation for multiple myeloma. N Engl J Med. 2006;354:1021–30.

Carreras E. How I manage sinusoidal obstruction syndrome after hematopoietic stem cell transplantation. Br J Hematol. 2015;168:481–91.

Chaturvedi S, Neff A, Nagler A, et al. Venous thromboembolism in hematopoietic stem cell transplant recipients. Bone Marrow Transplant. 2016;51:473–8.

Cortelezzi A, Moia M, Falanga A, et al. Incidence of thrombotic complications in patients with hematological malignancies with central venous catheters: a prospective multicenter study. Br J Haematol 2005;129:811–7.

Elsallabi O, Bhatt VR, Dhakal P, et al. Hematopoietic stem cell transplant-associated thrombotic microangiopathy. Clin Appl Thromb Hemost. 2016;22:12–20.

Gerber DE, Segal JB, Levy MY, et al. The incidence and risk factors for venous thromboembolism (VTE) and bleeding among 1514 patients undergoing hematopoietic stem cell transplantation: implications for VTE prevention. Blood. 2008;112:504–10.

Gonsalves A, Carrier M, Wells PS, et al. Incidence of symptomatic venous thromboembolism following hematopoietic stem cell transplantation. J Thromb Haemost. 2008;6:1468–73.

Kearon C, Akl EA, Comerota AJ, et al. Antithrombotic therapy for VTE disease: antithrombotic therapy and prevention of thrombosis, 9th ed: American College of Chest Physicians Evidence-Based Clinical Practice Guidelines. Chest. 2012;141:e419S–96S.

Kovacs MJ, Kahn SR, Rodger M, et al. A pilot study of central venous catheter survival in cancer patients using low-molecular-weight heparin (dalteparin) and warfarin without catheter removal for the treatment of upper extremity deep vein thrombosis (The Catheter Study). J Thromb Haemost. 2007;5:1650–3.

Labrador J, Lopez-Anglada L, Perez-Lopez E, et al. Analysis of incidence, risk factors and clinical outcome of thromboembolic and bleeding events in 431 allogeneic hematopoietic stem cell transplantation recipients. Haematologica. 2013;98:437–43.

Lyman GH, Bohlke K, Khorana AA, et al. Venous thromboembolism prophylaxis and treatment in patients with cancer: American Society of Clinical Oncology clinical practice guideline update 2014. J Clin Oncol. 2015;33:654–6.

McCarthy PL, Owzar K, Hofmeister CC, et al. Lenalidomide after stem-cell transplantation for multiple myeloma. N Engl J Med. 2012;366:1770–81.

McDonald GB, Hinds MS, Fisher LD, et al. Veno-occlusive disease of the liver and multiorgan failure after bone marrow transplantation: a cohort study of 355 patients. Ann Intern Med. 1993;118:255–67.

Nadir Y, Brenner B. Hemorrhagic and thrombotic complications in bone marrow transplant recipients. Thromb Res. 2007;120(Suppl 2):592–8.

Palumbo A, Cavo M, Bringhen S, et al. Aspirin, warfarin, or enoxaparin thromboprophylaxis in patients with multiple myeloma treated with thalidomide: a phase III, open-label, randomized trial. J Clin Oncol. 2011;29:986–93.

Pihusch R, Salat C, Schmidt E, et al. Hemostatic complications in bone marrow transplantation: a retrospective analysis of 447 patients. Transplantation. 2002;74:1303–9.

Richardson PG, Riches ML, Kernan NA, et al. Phase 3 trial of defibrotide for the treatment of severe veno-occlusive disease and multi-organ failure. Blood. 2016;127:1656–65.

Rosenthal J. Hematopoietic stem cell transplantation-associated thrombotic microangiopathy: a review of pathophysiology, diagnosis, and treatment. J Blood Med. 2016;7:181–6.

Samama MM, Cohen AT, Darmon JY, et al. A comparison of enoxaparin with placebo for the prevention of venous thromboembolism in acutely ill medical patients. N Engl J Med. 1999;341:793–800.

Vannucchi AM, Rafanelli D, Longo G, et al. Early haemostatic alterations following bone marrow transplantation: a prospective study. Haematologica. 1994;79:519–25.

Young AM, Billingham LJ, Begum G, et al. Warfarin thromboprophylaxis in cancer patients with central venous catheters (WARP): an open-label randomised trial. Lancet. 2009;373:567–74.

41 Graft Failure

David Valcárcel and Anna Sureda

41.1 Introduction

Engraftment is defined as the first of 3 consecutive days with an absolute neutrophil count higher than 0.5 × 10^9/L (sustained >20 × 10^9/L platelets and hemoglobin >80 g/L, free of transfusion requirements).

In the setting of RIC protocols, it is also recommended to confirm the donor origin through chimerism studies.

The incidence of GF is <3–5% in the auto- and matched allo-HSCT setting, but it increases up to 10% in the cases of haploidentical or CBT.

The prognosis of graft failure (GF) is poor, and most patients die because of causes related to infections or bleeding, with an OS at 3–5 years after the diagnosis of GF less than 20%.

D. Valcárcel (✉)
Department of Hematology, Vall d'Hebron Institute of Oncology (VHIO), University Hospital Vall d'Hebron, Barcelona, Spain
e-mail: dvalcarcel@vhio.net

A. Sureda
Department of Hematology, Institut Català d'Oncologia, Barcelona, Spain

41.2 Definitions

Primary graft failure (GF)	ANC <0.5 × 10^9/L by day +28 Hemoglobin <80 g/L and platelets <20 × 10^9/L *RIC*: Confirmation of donor cell origin is required *CBT*: Up to day +42
Secondary GF	ANC <0.5 × 10^9/L *after initial engraftment* not related to relapse, infection, or drug toxicity *RIC*: Loss of donor hematopoiesis to <5%
Poor graft function	Two or three cytopenias >2 weeks, after day +28 in the presence of donor chimerism >5%
Graft rejection	GF caused by *immune rejection* of donor cells mediated by host cells

41.3 Causes and Risk Factors

The etiology of GF is multifactorial in most of the cases (Fig. 41.1, Table 41.1).

41.3.1 Donor Type, HLA Matching, and Graft Source

Classical studies showed a close relationship between the degree of HLA mismatch and the incidence of GF, but it is difficult to draw conclusions because most of them used a limited HLA matching including only low-resolution A, B, and DR locus (Anasetti et al. 1989; Petersdorf

E. Carreras et al. (eds.), *The EBMT Handbook*, https://doi.org/10.1007/978-3-030-02278-5_41

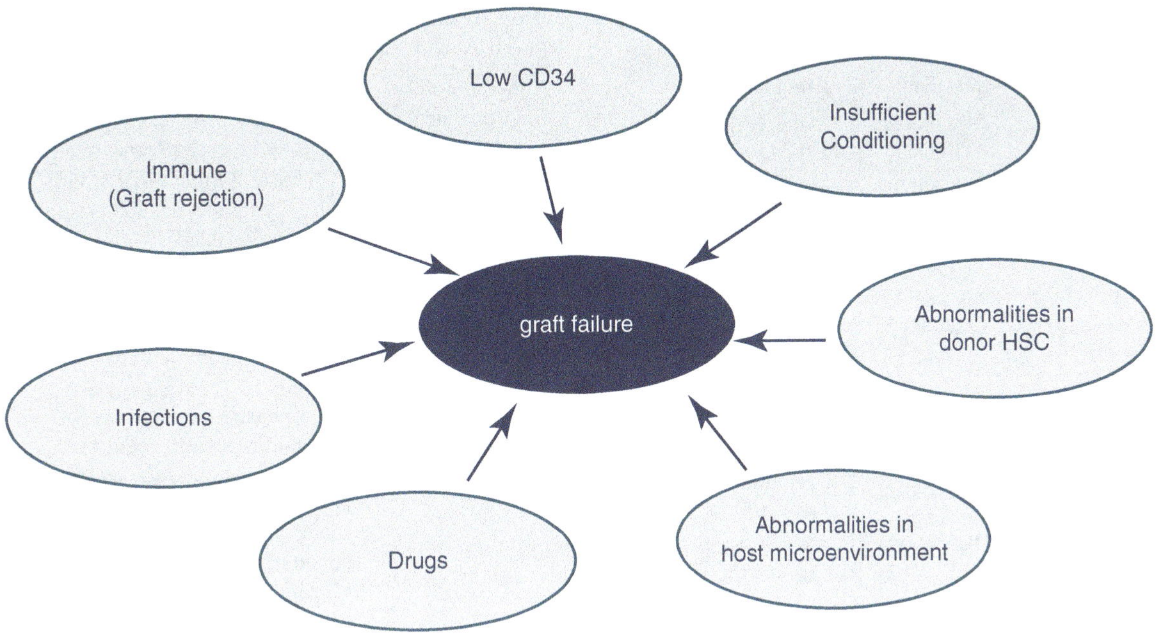

Fig. 41.1 Causes associated with the development of GF

Table 41.1 Risk factors for GF

Pre-transplant difficult to modify	Pre-transplant easy to modify	Peri-post transplant
HLA mismatches Nonmalignant disease Advanced disease Extensive marrow fibrosis extensive prior treatment Donor age Splenomegaly Iron overload HLA antibodies Transfusion history	Graft source Conditioning T-cell depletion	CD34+ cell count Viral infections GVHD Drug toxicity

et al. 2001). More recent studies, using high-resolution techniques for HLA typing and including 10–12 loci (A, B, C, DR, DQ, and DP), did not find differences in GF rates between no HLA antigen mismatch and a single HLA mismatch in both conventional MAC (Lee et al. 2007) or RIC (Passweg et al. 2011).

URD transplant was associated with a higher risk of GF (HR 1.38, $p < 0.001$ compared to HLA identical sibling) that was even higher when there were two or more mismatches (HR 1.79, $p < 0.001$) (Olsson et al. 2015).

In the haploidentical setting, the incidence of GF is around 10% which seems higher than the 3–5% currently reported MSD or URD HSCT although there are not well-designed comparative studies.

41.3.2 Graft Source and Cellular Content

BM is consistently associated with delayed neutrophil and platelet engraftment across all types of transplant; the impact on GF depends on donor type. GF incidence is not different for HLA MRD (Bensinger, 2012), but it is higher in the setting of URD (9% vs 3%, for BM and PB, respectively, $p < 0.001$) (Anasetti et al. 2012). There are no prospective randomized data either looking at MAC or RIC, but retrospective results from EBMT and CIBMTR suggest there were no differences in GF between BM and PB (less than 5% in all cases). In contrast, in a study evaluating donor characteristics, the use of BM was the only factor associated with GF after RIC (HR 2.3; $p = 0.02$) (Passweg et al. 2011).

The minimum cellular content required is still a matter of debate. Table 41.2 depicts a conservative proposal based on the literature review.

Table 41.2 Minimum cell content recommended

Progenitors	Type of transplant	Amount of cells
BM progenitors	Autologous	TNC: 2 × 10^8/kg
	Allogeneic	TNC: 3 × 10^8/kg
PB progenitors	Autologous	Minimum: CD34 >1 × 10^6/kg Optimum: CD34 >2 × 10^6/kg
	Allogeneic MAC	Minimum: CD34 >2 × 10^6/kg Optimum: CD34 >4 × 10^6/kg
	Allogeneic RIC	Minimum: CD34 >2 × 10^6/kg Optimum: CD34 4–8 × 10^6/kg
Cord blood	HLA 4–6/6	TNC >2.5–3 × 10^7/kg CD 34 >1 × 10^5/kg

TNC total nucleated cells, *MAC* myeloablative conditioning, *RIC* reduced intensity conditioning regimen

41.3.3 Anti-HLA Antibodies

The presence of donor-specific anti-HLA antibodies (DSA) is associated with higher risk of GF in the context of haploidentical CBT and URD transplants, and it may in fact translate into a reduced OS (Spellman et al. 2010; Ciurea et al. 2009; Ciurea et al. 2015). The high prevalence of anti-HLA antibodies (10–40%) (Morin-Zorman et al. 2016) and the increasing use of mismatched donors prompted the EBMT to write a set of advices and recommendations on this issue (Table 41.3) (Ciurea et al. 2018).

41.3.4 Conditioning Regimen

Increasing the intensity of MAC conditioning protocols does not reduce the incidence of GF. In contrast, RIC may be associated with a higher risk.

Although it is well accepted that TBI reduces the risk of GF, there are no comparative studies that confirm this latter point. In combination with CY, the use of full-dose TBI does not seem to reduce GF in comparison with BU. The use of ATG in the preparative regimen in combination

Table 41.3 Considerations regarding the presence of anti-HLA antibodies

Anti-HLA and DSA prevalence	Anti HLA: 10–40% DSA: 10–20%. Higher in female (increase with each pregnancy)
Detection methods	• Cell based (direct test): Donor viable lymphocytes and patient serum are needed. Complex and time-consuming technique. Low specificity and variable sensitivity (higher with flow cytometry assays than complement-based assays) • Solid phase immunoassays (virtual test): Only requires patient serum, and the technique is easy and fast. Sensitivity and specificity are intermediate/high depending on the type of assay. Modified techniques such as C4d or Cq1 assays allow to detect complement-fixing antibodies, which are at higher risk of inducing GF. These are the test most commonly used nowadays; initial DSA testing and complement assay in case of positivity are recommended • Although not well validated, the threshold of positivity for DSA can be considered >1000 and specially >5000 MFI, which is probably associated with the presence of complement binding antibodies • DSA study should be done during donor identification to select a donor and also within the month prior to transplant
Management, desensitization treatment	• No standard scheme is widely accepted; different combinations have proven to be efficacious – Ab removal: Plasmapheresis 1–4 procedures days-10 to -17 and even after transplant – Inhibition of Ab production: Rituximab 375 mg/m^2 IV days – Ab neutralization: Infusion of 20–40 platelet units selected to share donor antigens or buffy coat from 1 unit of blood, on day-1. IVIg can also be used *Avoid complement activation*: IVIg, eculizumab

DSA donor-specific antibodies, *MFI* mean fluorescence intensity, *Ab* antibodies, *IVIg* intravenous immunoglobulins with CY seems to reduce the incidence of GF in patients with aplastic anemia. Also, in aplastic anemia patients, the addition of two Gy TBI to FLU/CY did not reduce the incidence of this complication.

41.3.5 Other Factors Associated with the Development of GF

ABO mismatch: Major incompatibility was associated with primary GF (HR 1.24; $p = 0.012$).

Cryopreservation: Associated with primary GF (HR 1.43; $p = 0.013$).

Female donor to male recipient: Associated with primary GF (HR 1.28; $p = 0.001$).

Splenomegaly: Associated with primary GF in MPN (HR 3.92; $p = 0.001$) and MDS (HR 2.24; $p = 0.002$).

Use of G-CSF: Associated with reduced risk of primary GF (HR 0.36; $p < 0.001$) vs no growth factors.

Underlying disease: Nonmalignant diseases are associated with higher incidence.

Previous treatments: Impairment engraftment through the damage of marrow microenvironment. The absence of treatments may induce graft rejection.

Graft manipulation: Ex vivo TCD is associated with a higher risk of primary GF in most studies.

41.4 Management of GF

OS after GF is consistently low, even in those patients who receive a salvage transplant; thus, the most important measures should be directed to avoid graft failure GF and to identify it as soon as possible in order to adopt the measures to revert it.

41.4.1 Prevention and Early Diagnosis of GF

The identification of DSA is of utmost importance in the mismatch setting. Desensitization treatment in patients at higher risk seems reasonable. Although barely supported by well-designed studies, we would probably recommend the following measures to be adopted in patients at high risk of GF: the use of PB as stem cell source, include low dose TBI and/or ATG in the conditioning regimen, consider the use of G-CSF post transplant, and a close evaluation of engraftment including marrow chimerism studies shortly after transplant (day +14). In a single-CBT study, a level of donor chimerism in BM lower than 65% was associated with a higher risk of GF (Moscardó et al. 2009); these results cannot be directly extrapolated to other types of transplant.

Olson and colleagues developed a score to predict GF in patients at risk at day +21 post-HSCT (Olsson et al. 2015): age (<30, 1 point), Karnofsky status (<90%, 1 point), disease (MDS, 1; CLL or CML, 2; and MPN, 3 points), status (advanced, 1 point), HLA matching (mismatched, 2 points), graft (BM <2.4 × 10^8/kg, 1 point; PB, 2 points), conditioning (no TBI, 2 points), and GVHD prophylaxis (no CNI + MTX, 2 points; TCD, 3 points). A score >6 at day +21 had a positive predictive value of 28–36%, while the negative predictive value of a score <7 was 81% for GF.

41.4.2 Initial Measures

It is important to apply them as soon as GF is suspected.

- Stop as many toxic drugs as possible; treat infections; although of limited utility, it would be reasonable a trial of G-CSF.
- Adjust post transplant IS. Maintain correct IS levels in the early post transplant period. Later on, after the third/sixth month and if mixed chimerism is present, especially after a RIC transplant, a faster tapering of IST could overcome mixed chimera (in patients with SAA, it is commonly recommended to increase IST).
- Data regarding the use of TPO analogues after transplant are scarce, but the results of eltrombopag in aplastic anemia and its favorable toxicity profile would support, in our view, a trial with this drug before considering more complex and risky options as DLI or second transplant.

Table 41.4 Second allogeneic stem cell transplant in patients with GF

Author (year)	*n* patients diagnosis	Donor (same/different) source	Engraftment (median *d*)	OS
Gaziev (1999)	32 (1°, 4; 2°, 28) Thalassemia	28/4 All BM	67.7% (+19)	3 year: 60%
Guardiola (2000)	82 (1°, 7; 2°, 54) Hem Neo, AA	56/26 72 BM; 10 PB	62% (+17)	3 year: 33%
Min (2000)	20 (1°, 7; 2°, 10) Hem Neo, AA	20/0 6 BM, 14 PB	75% (NR)	3 year: 70%
Chewning (2007)	16 (1°, 11; 2°, 5) Hem Neo, FA	6/16 13 PB (8 TCD), 2 BM, 1 CB	100% (+12)	3 year: 35%
Gyurkorcza (2009)	38 (1°, 18; 2°, 20) Hem Neo, AA	14/24 36 PB, 1 BM, 1 CB	87% (+15)	4 year: 42%
Schreiber (2010)	122 (1°, 122) Hem Neo, AA	98/24 60 PB, 62 CB	66% (NR)	1 year: 11%
Remberger (2011)	20 (1°, 6; 2°, 14) Hem Neo, Non-Mal	11/9 7 PB, 11 BM, 2 CB	90% (+20)	3 year: 60%
Fuji (2012)	220 (1°, 200; 2°, 19) Hem Neo, Non-Mal	0/220 24 PB, 16 BM, 180 CB	CB 30% (21) PB-BM 70–75% (18–14)	1 year PB:58% CB: 28%
Ferrá (2014)	89 (1°, 49; 2°, 40) Hem Neo, Non-Mal	38/37 61 PB, 6 BM, 8 CB	85% (+15)	5 year: 31%

Hem Neo hematological neoplasias, *AA* aplastic anemia, *FA* Fanconi anemia, *Non-Mal* nonmalignant disorders, *PB* peripheral blood, *BM* bone marrow, *CB* cord blood, *TCD* T-cell depletion

41.4.3 DLI and CD34 Boost

DLI could be recommended if decreasing levels of donor chimerism are observed. A careful risk/benefit evaluation is warranted as this is not a risk-free approach and a high risk of development of GVHD is anticipated.

In patients with poor graft function, the use of CD34 boost can be offered. Unfortunately, it is not clear when to perform it, but probably 2–3 months without improvement after the initial measures would be a reasonable cutoff.

41.4.4 Second Transplant

The limited utility and low success of cryopreserved autologous stem cells do not allow to formally recommend to perform auto-HSC harvest in any type of transplant procedure.

Results and recommendations for second allogeneic transplantation are detailed in Tables 41.4 and 41.5.

Table 41.5 Recommendations to perform a second allogeneic HSCT as treatment for GF

Type of donor	Similar results using the same/different donor. Consider different donor if it is not associated with significant delays. Consider haploidentical donors Always avoid donors if positive DSA
Conditioning regimen	It is always required. Better RIC
Post transplant IS	It is required; CNI-based schemes are the most commonly used
Stem cell source	PB or BM show similar results and should be preferred to CB
T-cell depletion	– Avoid ex vivo T-cell depletion, especially if with immune graft rejection – In cases of poor graft function, it can be a good option as it reduces the potential risk of GVHD – ATG or alemtuzumab has been used to foster IS and also to reduce GVHD risk

DSA donor-specific antigens, *BM* bone marrow, *PB* peripheral blood

Key Points

- Graft failure is an infrequent but often fatal complication of HSCT.
- Etiology is complex and very frequently multifactorial.
- Preventive measures and early identification of potential causes in order to try to revert them are the key aspects to treat it.

References

Anasetti C, Amos D, Beatty PG, et al. Effect of HLA compatibility on engraftment of bone marrow transplants in patients with leukemia or lymphoma. N Engl J Med. 1989;320:197–204.

Anasetti C, Logan BR, Lee SJ, et al. Peripheral-blood stem cells versus bone marrow from unrelated donors. N Engl J Med. 2012;367:1487–96.

Bensinger WI. Allogeneic transplantation: peripheral blood vs bone marrow. Curr Opin Oncol. 2012;24:191–6.

Ciurea SO, de Lima M, Cano P, et al. High risk of graft failure in patients with anti-HLA antibodies undergoing haploidentical stem-cell transplantation. Transplantation. 2009;88:1019–24.

Ciurea SO, Thall PF, Milton DR, et al. Complement-binding donor-specific anti-HLA antibodies and risk of primary graft failure in hematopoietic stem cell transplantation. Biol Blood Marrow Transplant. 2015;21:1392–8.

Ciurea SO, Cao K, Fernadez-Vina M, et al. The European Society for Blood and Marrow Transplantation (EBMT) Consensus guidelines for the detection and treatment of donor-specific anti-HLA antibodies (DSA) in haploidentical hematopoietic cell transplantation. Bone Marrow Transplant. 2018;53:521–34.

Chewning JH, Castro-Malaspina H, Jakubowski A, Kernan NA, Papadopoulos EB, Small TN, et al. Fludarabine-based conditioning secures engraftment of second hematopoietic stem cell allografts (HSCT) in the treatment of initial graft failure. Biol Blood Marrow Transplant. 2007;13(11):1313–23. https://doi.org/10.1016/J.Bbmt.2007.07.006.

Ferrá C, Sanz J, Díaz-Pérez M-A, Morgades M, Gayoso J, Cabrera J-R, et al. Outcome of graft failure after allogeneic stem cell transplant: study of 89 patients. Leukemia & Lymphoma. 2014;56(3):656–62. https://doi.org/10.3109/10428194.2014.930849.

Fuji S, Nakamura F, Hatanaka K, Taniguchi S, Sato M, Mori S-I, et al. Peripheral blood as a preferable source of stem cells for salvage transplantation in patients with graft failure after cord blood transplantation: a retrospective analysis of the registry data of the Japanese Society for Hematopoietic Cell Transplantation. Biol Blood Marrow Transplant. 2012;18:1407–14.

Gaziev D, Polchi P, Lucarelli G, Galimberti M, Sodani P, Angelucci E, et al. Second marrow transplants for graft failure in patients with thalassemia. Bone Marrow Transplant. 1999;24(12):1299–306. https://doi.org/10.1038/Sj.Bmt.1702076.

Guardiola P, Kuentz M, Garban F, Blaise D, Reiffers J, Attal M, et al. Second early allogeneic stem cell transplantations for graft failure in acute leukaemia, chronic myeloid leukaemia and aplastic anaemia. French Society of Bone Marrow Transplantation. Br J Haematol. 2000;111(1):292–302.

Gyurkocza B, Cao TM, Storb RF, Lange T, Leisenring W, Franke GN, et al. Salvage allogeneic hematopoietic cell transplantation with fludarabine and low-dose total body irradiation after rejection of first allografts. Biol Blood Marrow Transplant. 2009;15(10):1314–22. https://doi.org/10.1016/j.bbmt.2009.06.011.

Lee SJ, Klein J, Haagenson M, et al. High-resolution donor-recipient HLA matching contributes to the success of unrelated donor marrow transplantation. Blood. 2007;110:4576–83.

Min CK, Kim DW, Lee JW, Min WS, Kim CC. Additional stem cell therapy for graft failure after allogeneic bone marrow transplantation. Acta Haematologica. 2000;104(4):185–92.

Morin-Zorman S, Loiseau P, Taupin JL, Caillat-Zucman S. Donor-specific anti-HLA antibodies in allogeneic hematopoietic stem cell transplantation. Front Immunol. 2016;7:1–6.

Moscardó F, Sanz J, Senent L, et al. Impact of hematopoietic chimerism at day +14 on engraftment after unrelated donor umbilical cord blood transplantation for hematologic malignancies. Haematologica. 2009;94:827–32.

Olsson RF, Logan BR, Chaudhury S, et al. Primary graft failure after myeloablative allogeneic hematopoietic cell transplantation for hematologic malignancies. Leukemia. 2015;29:1754–62.

Passweg JR, Zhang MJ, Rocha V, et al. Donor characteristics affecting graft failure, graft-versus-host disease, and survival after unrelated donor transplantation with reduced-intensity conditioning for hematologic malignancies. Biol Blood Marrow Transplant. 2011;17:1869–73.

Petersdorf EW, Hansen JA, Martin PJ, et al. Major-histocompatibility-complex class I alleles and antigens in hematopoietic-cell transplantation. N Engl J Med. 2001;345:1794–800.

Remberger M, Mattsson J, Olsson R, Ringden O. Second allogeneic hematopoietic stem cell transplantation: a treatment for graft failure. Clin Transplant. 2010;25(1):E68–76. https://doi.org/10.1111/J.1399-0012.2010.01324.X.

Schreiber J, Agovi M-A, Ho V, Ballen KK, Bacigalupo A, Lazarus HM, et al. Second unrelated donor hematopoietic cell transplantation for primary graft failure. Biol Blood Marrow Transplant. 2010;16(8):1099–106. https://doi.org/10.1016/j.bbmt.2010.02.013.

Spellman S, Bray R, Rosen-Bronson S, et al. The detection of donor-directed, HLA-specific alloantibodies in recipients of unrelated hematopoietic cell transplantation is predictive of graft failure. Blood. 2010;115:2704–8.

42 Early Complications of Endothelial Origin

Enric Carreras and Maribel Diaz-Ricart

42.1 Introduction

A group of complications that occur after transplant share several common characteristics:

(1) They appear early after HSCT (between day 0 and day +100).
(2) Their diagnosis is usually based on the presence of medical signs and symptoms, and consequently they are classified as syndromes. Their clinical manifestations are overlapping, making their differential diagnosis difficult.
(3) They seem to begin at the capillary level, in a systemic way or in one or more affected organs.
(4) If not properly treated, they can evolve into an irreversible MODS/MOF.

The animal models of SOS showed that the first morphological alterations observed occurred in endothelial cells (EC) of the hepatic sinusoids (DeLeve et al. 1996). Similarly, multiple ex vivo and in vitro studies have shown that, in auto- and allo-HSCT, there is a pro-inflammatory and prothrombotic state secondary to endothelial damage (Carreras et al. 2010; Palomo et al. 2009, 2010; Carreras and Diaz-Ricart 2011). Therefore, all these complications are nowadays grouped under the name of "early complications of endothelial origin":

- Sinusoidal obstruction syndrome (SOS) of the liver (formerly denominated VOD)
- Capillary leak syndrome (CLS)
- Engraftment and peri-engraftment syndrome (ES and peri-ES)
- Diffuse alveolar hemorrhage (DAH) (see Chap. 42)
- Thrombotic microangiopathy associated with HSCT (TA-TMA)
- Posterior reversible leukoencephalopathy syndrome (PRES)

Initially, idiopathic pneumonia syndrome (IPS) was included in this group. However, even if endothelial damage plays a role in its pathogenesis, other more relevant factors seem to be present.

Probably along the next years, GVHD will be included in this group since every day it is more evident that endothelial dysfunction is the origin and not the consequence of this complication.

E. Carreras (✉)
Spanish Bone Marrow Donor Registry, Josep Carreras Foundation and Leukemia Research Institute, Barcelona, Catalunya, Spain

Hospital Clinic Barcelona, Barcelona University, Barcelona, Catalunya, Spain
e-mail: enric.carreras@fcarreras.es

M. Diaz-Ricart
Hemostasis and Erythropathology, Hematopathology Section, Pathological Anatomy Department, CDB, Hospital Clinic, University of Barcelona, Barcelona, Spain

E. Carreras et al. (eds.), *The EBMT Handbook*, https://doi.org/10.1007/978-3-030-02278-5_42

42.2 Sinusoidal Obstruction Syndrome (See Chap. 49)

42.3 Engraftment Syndrome

42.3.1 Definition

High and well-tolerated fever of a noninfectious origin developed when the first neutrophil appears in peripheral blood indicating the engraftment. This syndrome has also been called CLS of the engraftment, autoaggression syndrome, respiratory distress of the engraftment, aseptic–septic shock, and autologous GVHD.

42.3.2 Pathogenesis

It seems to appear as a result of a systemic endothelial damage produced by the massive release of pro-inflammatory cytokines (IL-2, TNF-α, IFN-γ, IL-6), M-GSF, EPO, and products of degranulation and oxidative metabolism of neutrophils. In some cases, the concomitant administration of G-CSF, potent endothelial toxicant, contributes to its development.

42.3.3 Clinical/Biological Manifestations of ES

Around the day when engraftment starts[a]	
Classical (main criteria)	Fever ≥38.3 °C well tolerated Skin rash (>25% of body surface)[b] Pulmonary edema (non-cardiogenic) / hypoxia Sudden increase in CRP values (≥20 mg/dL)[c]
Occasional (minor criteria)	Weight gain (>2.5%) Creatinine increase (≥2 × N values) Hepatic dysfunction (bilirubin ≥2 mg/dL or AST/ALT ≥2 × N) Diarrhea[d] Encephalopathy

[a]First day with neutrophil counts greater than 0.5×10^9/L
[b]Very similar to an acute GVHD
[c]Values higher than those observed in a febrile neutropenia. Due to its recent description, this parameter is not included in the classical diagnostic criteria. The cutoff point of 6 mg/dL has a high sensitivity and specificity (90%). Additionally, CRP allows monitoring the response to the treatment since it normalizes completely in a few days (Carreras et al. 2010)
[d]At least two fluid depositions per day without microbiological documentation of infection

42.3.4 Diagnostic Criteria

Spitzer (2001)	More specific but too much complex. 3 major criteria or 2 major + 1 minor criteria within the 96 h around engraftment
Maiolino et al. (2003)	Simplest and enough specific. Noninfectious fever + another major criteria or diarrhea since 24 h before engraftment

42.3.5 Incidence and Risk Factors

ES is classically observed after autologous HSCT although it has also been described after NMA allo-HSCT (Gorak et al. 2005) and after CBT (see pre-ES).

Incidence: Ranging between 5 and 50% depending of the population analyzed and criteria used.

Most relevant *risk factors* for ES are:

- Auto-HSCT for diseases not intensively treated with chemotherapy before HSCT (AID, AL, POEMS, breast cancer, etc.)
- Intensity of the conditioning (NMA < MEL < BEAM < CY/TBI)
- In myeloma patients, previous treatment with BOR or LENA (Cornell et al. 2013)
- Use of PBSC or G-CSF

42.3.6 Prophylaxis and Treatment (Cornell et al. 2015)

Prophylaxis: Avoid the use of G-CSF after HSCT in the high-risk patients.

Treatment:

- When suspected, stop immediately G-CSF.
- If fever persists after 48 h of ATB treatment and cultures are negative, start methyl-PRD 1 mg/kg q12h (3 days) and progressive tapering in 1 week.
- When PRD is stopped, some recurrences of ES could be observed; treat again with steroids.
- With an early treatment, 90% of CR, any delay can favor the evolution to MOF.

42.4 Pre-engraftment Syndrome

ES-like was described in 2003 after CBT. Its pathogenesis is similar to ES + alloreactivity and cytokine storm (also denominated "early immune reaction" in this scenario) (Lee and Rah 2016).

Main differences with classical ES are:

- Development in the context of MAC–RIC allo-HSCT
- Earlier presentation (around day +7; up to 10–11 days before engraftment)
- Fluid retention in 30% of cases
- Higher incidence than ES (20–70% of CBT) (Lee and Rah 2016)

Patients with pre-ES have less graft failure and more GVHD without impact in TRM (Park et al. 2013).

42.5 Capillary Leak Syndrome

42.5.1 Definition

Idiopathic systemic capillary syndrome was described in healthy patients that presented episodic crisis of hypotension/hypoperfusion, hypoalbuminemia, and severe generalized edema (Clarkson disease). Usually, these manifestations could be revered with steroids, vasopressors, fluid, and colloids, but some patients could die during this recovery phase due to a cardiopulmonary failure (Druey and Greipp 2010).

Very similar episodes have also been described after the administration of IL-2, IL-4, TNF-α, GM-CSG, and G-CSF and in the context of HSCT (Nürnberger et al. 1997; Lucchini et al. 2016).

42.5.2 Pathogenesis

Many mechanisms have been suspected, but nowadays, due to the duration of the capillary leak and its reversibility, the endothelial injury seems to be the main cause for the capillary damage. The high levels of VEGF and angiopoietin-2 (potent inducers of vascular permeability) observed in these patients could play a role (Xie et al. 2012).

42.5.3 Diagnostic Criteria in the Context of HSCT (Lucchini et al. 2016)

Early after HSCT (≈days +10 to 11).

Unexplained weight gain >3% in 24 h.

Positive intake balance despite furosemide administration (at least 1 mg/kg) evaluated 24 h after its administration.

42.5.4 Incidence and Risk Factors

Mainly observed in children

True incidence unknown (variable diagnostic criteria): 5.4% in the largest series (similar incidence between MAC and RIC-HSCT)

Apparently no relationship with G-CSF administration but higher incidence among patients receiving this treatment more than 5 days.

42.5.5 Treatment and Evolution

When suspected, stop immediately G-CSF

Steroids; supportive therapy (catecholamines, colloids, and plasma)

A rapid improvement has been observed in a patient treated with bevacizumab (Yabe et al. 2010)

Sixty-seven percent of patients required ICU admittance and 47% mechanical ventilation

Fourty-seven percent reach a complete remission

TRM at day +100: 43% vs only 5% in patients w/o CLS (Lucchini et al. 2016)

42.6 Thrombotic Microangiopathy Associated with HSCT (TA-TMA)

42.6.1 Definition and Classification

TMA are a heterogeneous group of diseases characterized by microangiopathic hemolytic anemia and thrombocytopenia due to platelet clumping in the microcirculation leading to ischemic organ dysfunction. As this phenomenon could be observed in different clinical situations, a consensus on the standardization of terminology has been recently proposed by an International Working Group (Scully et al. 2017) (Fig. 42.1).

42.6.2 Pathogenesis

Like in the other vascular–endothelial syndromes after HSCT, the endothelial injury due to the action of different factors (conditioning, lipopolysaccharides, CNI, alloreactivity, GVHD) plays a crucial role in its development. Endothelial injury generates a prothrombotic and pro-inflammatory status that favors capillary occlusion.

However, unlike in other endothelial syndromes, the dysregulation of the complement system and the possible presence of specific antibodies (donor- or recipient-specific Ab, as anti-factor H Ab) could play a relevant role in some TA-TMA. The activation of the classical pathway of the complement system (by chemotherapy, infections, GVHD) and the activation of the alternative pathway (favored by a genetically determined mutation of several genes [*CFH*, *CFI*, *CFB*, *CFHR1,3,5*]) produce deposits of C4d or C5b-9 (membrane attack complex) fractions, respectively (Jodele et al. 2016b).

Recently, the two-hit hypothesis tries to unify all these pathogenetic mechanisms (Khosla et al. 2018). The first hit will be produced by the normal input signals that any EC could receive (cell interaction soluble mediators, oxygenation, hemodynamic, temperature, pH) plus predisposing risk factors as prolonged immobilization, bacterial–fungal infection, leukemia not in remission, G-CSF administration, URD HSCT, HLA mismatch, RIC (fludarabine), or high-dose BU.

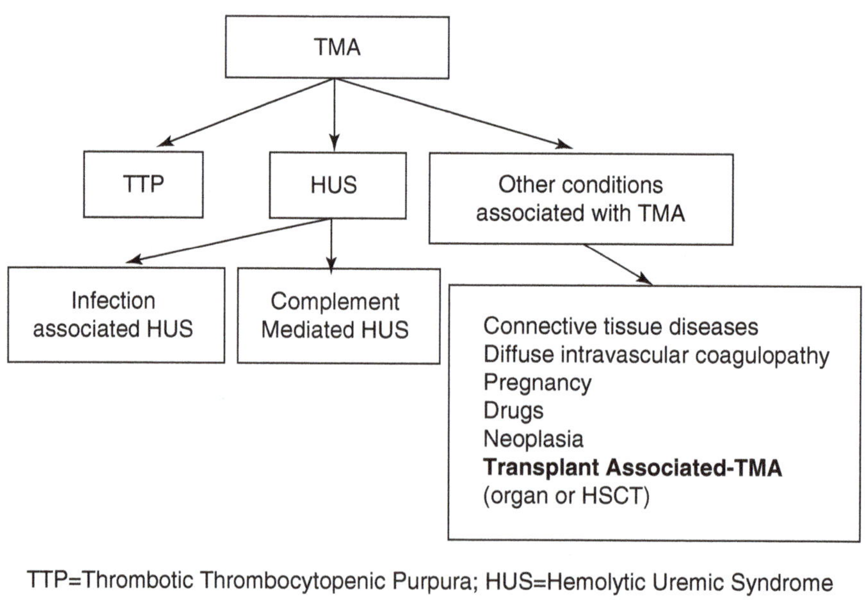

Fig. 42.1 Terminology of TMA

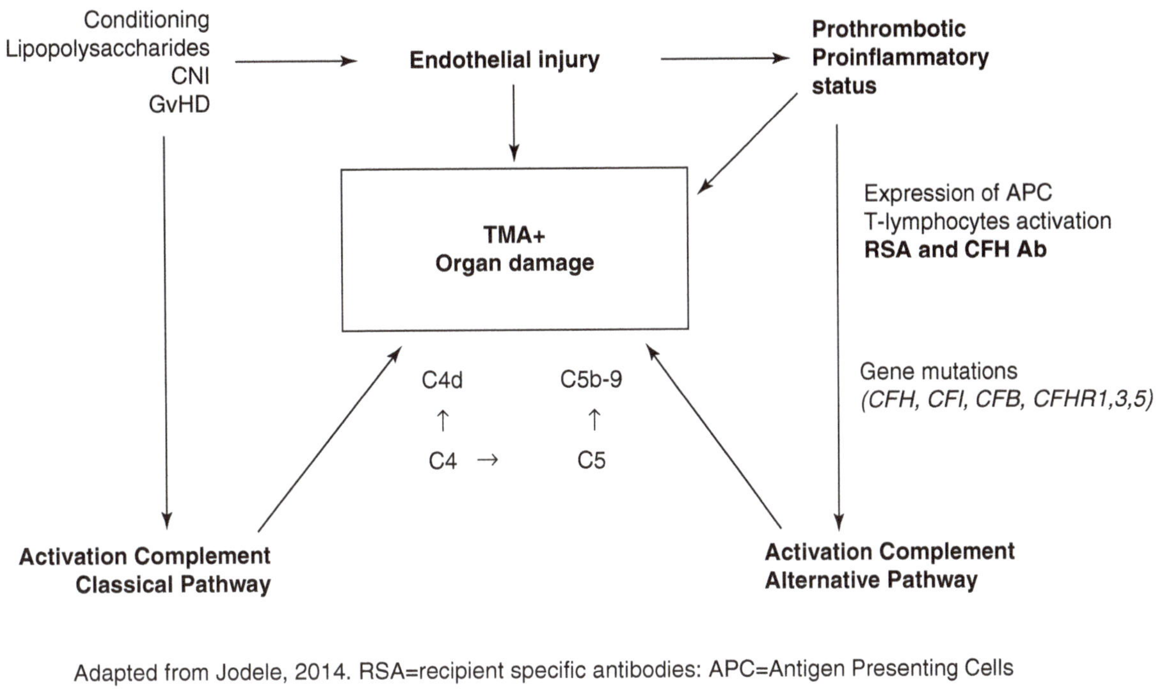

Fig. 42.2 Pathogenesis of TA-TMA

The second hit will be produced by CNI, mTOR inhibitors, severe infections, or TBI. All these events would trigger the succession of events that are observed in Fig. 42.2.

42.6.3 Clinical Manifestations

Manifestations of microangiopathic hemolytic anemia	
De novo anemia	
De novo thrombocytopenia	
Increased transfusion requirements	
Elevated LDH	
Schistocytes in the blood	
Decreased haptoglobin	
Manifestations of organ damage	
Kidney	Decreased glomerular filtration rate Proteinuria Hypertension; ≥2 medications
Lungs	Hypoxemia, respiratory distress
GI tract	Abdominal pain/GI bleeding/ileus
Central nervous system	Headaches/confusion Hallucinations/seizures

Manifestations of organ damage	
Polyserositis	Refractory pericardial/pleural effusion, and/or ascites, without generalized edema

42.6.4 Diagnostic Criteria

The gold standard for diagnosis is a biopsy of the damaged organ. However, to obtain these samples is almost impossible in these patients. Consequently, along the last years, several attempts have been carried out to reach consensus criteria for the diagnosis of this complication. The most relevant advance in this area has been to recognize some clinical data, not previously included in the diagnostic criteria, that could appear even before the classical ones and that are indicative of very bad prognosis. Unlike other TMA, the activity of ADAMTS13 never reaches levels below 5–10%.

Criteria	BMT-CTN[a]	IWG[b]	Chao[c]	Jodele[d]
Schistocytes	≥2/HPF	≥4%[e]	≥2/HPF	Yes
Elevated LDH[f]	Yes	Yes	Yes	Yes
De novo thrombocytopenia	–	Yes	Yes	Yes
Decreased Hb[g]	–	Yes	Yes	Yes
Coombs (−ve)	Yes	–	Yes	–
↓ Haptoglobin	–	Yes	Yes	–
Renal/neurological dysfunction	Yes	–	–	–
Coagulation normal	–	–	Yes	–
Proteinuria[f,h]				**±**
Hypertension[f,i]				**±**
Increased serum C5b-9 levels	–	–	–	**±**

Yes: required, ± (bold): factors not necessary for TA-TMA diagnosis, but their presence indicate a high-risk TA-TMA.
HPF high-power field
[a]Ho et al. (2005)
[b]Ruutu et al. (2007)
[c]Cho et al. (2010)
[d]Jodele et al. (2014)
[e]≥4% in 8/HPF
[f]Earlier clinical signs of TMA
[g]Or increased red cell transfusion
[h]Or protein/creatinine ratio ≥2 mg/mg
[i]Hypertension refractory to ≥2 antihypertensive drugs

42.6.5 Clinical Forms, Incidence, Risk Factors, and Prognosis

Forms: (1) TA-TMA associated to CNI—the most frequent form with good prognosis and a real incidence unknown; (2) TA-TMA not associated to CNI—bad prognosis, requiring specific measures.

Clinical manifestations: Onset day, median time day +32 to +40 (>92% before day +100).

Incidence: Unknown due to the different diagnostic criteria—literature focused on allo-HSCT, from 0.5% to 76%; EBMT survey (IWG criteria), 406 allo-HSCT, 7% (Ruutu et al. 2002); meta-analysis (variable criteria), 5423 allo-HSCT, 8.2% (George and Selby 2004); and prospective (Cho criteria), 90 allo-HSCT, 39% (Jodele et al. 2014). Similar incidence in MAC tan in RIC.

Risk factors: Use of CNI (more if associated to SIR), viral (CMV, ADV, BK virus, etc.) or fungal infection, active GVHD, URD/mismatch HSCT (probably due to more infections and GVHD), and several gene polymorphisms (predominate in non-Caucasian).

Prognosis: Despite the resolution of TA-TMA, these patients have an increased relative risk of chronic kidney disease, 4.3; arterial hypertension, 9; and TRM, 5.

42.6.6 How to Prevent/Manage TA-TMA?

Systematic screening:	LDH 3 times a week Proteinuria × 3 times per week Blood pressure (daily)	
If any data of TA-TMA evaluate:	Schistocytes in PB Quantitative proteinuria Haptoglobin and serum C5b-9 levels	
If TA-TMA criteria	w/o proteinuria and w/o increased sC5b-9	→ Stop CNI, treat any possible triggering cause (infection, GVHD)
	With proteinuria ≥30 mg/dL or increased sC5b-9	→ All the previous measures + specific treatment (see later)

42.6.7 Treatment

Supportive	Stop CNI (substitute by PRD or MMF) Treat intensively any infection, GVHD, and AHT
Therapeutic plasma exchange (TPE)	In recent prospective studies, 59–64% of CR (better if started early) In patients with Ab anti-factor H, better/good results with TPE ± RTX RTX should be administered after TPE Do not associate TPE with eculizumab
Rituximab (RTX)	Reported 12/15 responses to RTX + TPE (Uderzo et al. 2014) RTX should be administrated immediately after TPE
Defibrotide (DF)	Recent report with 46 adults and children: 77% of CR (Yeates et al. 2017)
Eculizumab	Indicated in TA-TMA with proteinuria ± > sC5b-9: 67% of responses Children could require higher doses (quantify CH50 to adjust the doses) (Jodele et al. 2015, 2016a)

CH50: Total hemolytic complement activity

Key Points

- Although endothelial dysfunction syndromes are rare, HSCT physicians should be aware of their main manifestations to establish an early diagnosis.
- Given the limited effectiveness of the available therapeutic measures, all modifiable risk factors that may favor their development should be avoided.
- Early diagnosis is essential to make effective the few available therapeutic measures.
- When one of these syndromes progresses to MOF, the prognosis is very poor.
- Even in those patients where resolution of the syndrome is achieved, the probability of survival of the procedure is clearly reduced

References

Carreras E, Fernández-Avilés F, Silva L, et al. Engraftment syndrome after auto-SCT: analysis of diagnostic criteria and risk factors in a large series from a single center. Bone Marrow Transplant. 2010;45:1417–22.

Carreras E, Diaz-Ricart M. The role of the endothelium in the short-term complications of hematopoietic SCT. Bone Marrow Transplant. 2011;46:1495–502.

Cho BS, Yahng SA, Lee SE, et al. Validation of recently proposed consensus criteria for thrombotic microangiopathy after allogeneic hematopoietic stem-cell transplantation. Transplantation. 2010;90:918–26.

Cornell RF, Hari P, Zhang MJ, et al. Divergent effects of novel immunomodulatory agents and cyclophosphamide on the risk of engraftment syndrome after autologous peripheral blood stem cell transplantation for multiple myeloma. Biol Blood Marrow Transplant. 2013;19:1368–73.

Cornell RF, Hari P, Drobyski WR. Engraftment syndrome after autologous stem cell transplantation: an update unifying the definition and management approach. Biol Blood Marrow Transplant. 2015;21:2061–8.

DeLeve LD, Wang X, Kuhlenkamp JF, et al. Toxicity of azathioprine and monocrotaline in murine sinusoidal endothelial cells and hepatocytes: the role of glutathione and relevance to hepatic venoocclusive disease. Hepatology. 1996;23:589–99.

Druey KM, Greipp PR. Narrative review: the systemic capillary leak syndrome. Ann Intern Med. 2010;153:90–8.

George JN, Selby GB. Thrombotic microangiopathy after allogeneic bone marrow transplantation: a pathologic abnormality associated with diverse clinical syndromes. Bone Marrow Transplant. 2004;33:1073–4.

Gorak E, Geller N, Srinivasan R, et al. Engraftment syndrome after nonmyeloablative allogeneic hematopoietic stem cell transplantation: incidence and effects on survival. Biol Blood Marrow Transplant. 2005;11:542–50.

Ho VT, Cutler C, Carter S, et al. Blood and marrow transplant clinical trials network toxicity committee consensus summary: thrombotic microangiopathy after hematopoietic stem cell transplantation. Biol Blood Marrow Transplant. 2005;11:571–5.

Jodele S, Davies SM, Lane A, et al. Diagnostic and risk criteria for HSCT-associated thrombotic microangiopathy: a study in children and young adults. Blood. 2014;124:645–53.

Jodele S, Laskin BL, Dandoy CE, et al. A new paradigm: diagnosis and management of HSCT-associated thrombotic microangiopathy as multi-system endothelial injury. Blood Rev. 2015;29:191–204.

Jodele S, Fukuda T, Mizuno K, et al. Variable eculizumab clearance requires pharmacodynamic monitoring to optimize therapy for thrombotic microangiopathy after hematopoietic stem cell transplantation. Biol Blood Marrow Transplant. 2016a;22:307–15.

Jodele S, Zhang K, Zou F, et al. The genetic fingerprint of susceptibility for transplant-associated thrombotic microangiopathy. Blood. 2016b;127:989–96.

Khosla J, Yeh AC, Spitzer TR, Dey BR. Hematopoietic stem cell transplant-associated thrombotic microangiopathy: current paradigm and novel therapies. Bone Marrow Transplant. 2018;53:129–37.

Lee YH, Rah WJ. Pre-engraftment syndrome: clinical significance and pathophysiology. Blood Res. 2016;51:152–4.

Lucchini G, Willasch AM, Daniel J, et al. Epidemiology, risk factors, and prognosis of capillary leak syndrome in pediatric recipients of stem cell transplants: a retrospective single-center cohort study. Pediatr Transplant. 2016;20:1132–6.

Maiolino A, Biasoli I, Lima J, et al. Engraftment syndrome following autologous hematopoietic stem cell transplantation: definition of diagnostic criteria. Bone Marrow Transplant. 2003;31:393–7.

Nürnberger W, Willers R, Burdach S, et al. Risk factors for capillary leakage syndrome after bone marrow transplantation. Ann Hematol. 1997;74:221–4.

Palomo M, Diaz-Ricart M, Carbo C, et al. The release of soluble factors contributing to endothelial activation and damage after hematopoietic stem cell transplantation is not limited to the allogeneic setting and involves several pathogenic mechanisms. Biol Blood Marrow Transplant. 2009;15:537–46.

Palomo M, Diaz-Ricart M, Carbo C, et al. Endothelial dysfunction after hematopoietic stem cell transplantation: role of the conditioning regimen and the type of transplantation. Biol Blood Marrow Transplant. 2010;16:985–93.

Park M, Lee SH, Lee YH, et al. Pre-engraftment syndrome after unrelated cord blood transplantation: a predictor of engraftment and acute graft-versus-host disease. Biol Blood Marrow Transplant. 2013;19:640–6.

Peyvandi F, Scully M, Kremer Hovinga JA, et al. Caplacizumab for acquired thrombotic thrombocytopenic purpura. N Engl J Med. 2016;374:511–22.

Ruutu T, Barosi G, Benjamin RJ, et al. Diagnostic criteria for hematopoietic stem cell transplant-associated microangiopathy: results of a consensus process by an International Working Group. Haematologica. 2007;92:95–100.

Ruutu T, Hermans J, Niederwieser D, EBMT Chronic Leukaemia Working Party, et al. Thrombotic thrombocytopenic purpura after allogeneic stem cell transplantation: a survey of the European Group for Blood and Marrow Transplantation (EBMT). Br J Haematol. 2002;118:1112–9.

Scully M, Cataland S, Coppo P, International Working Group for Thrombotic Thrombocytopenic Purpura, et al. Consensus on the standardization of terminology in thrombotic thrombocytopenic purpura and related thrombotic microangiopathies. J Thromb Haemost. 2017;15:312–22.

Spitzer TR. Engraftment syndrome following hematopoietic stem cell transplantation. Bone Marrow Transplant. 2001;27:893–8.

Uderzo CC, Jodele S, Missiry ME, et al. Transplant-associated thrombotic microangiopathy (TATMA) and consensus based diagnostic and therapeutic recommendations: which TA-TMA patients to treat and when? J Bone Marrow Res. 2014;2:152–9.

Xie Z, Ghosh CC, Patel R, et al. Vascular endothelial hyperpermeability induces the clinical symptoms of Clarkson disease (the systemic capillary leak syndrome). Blood. 2012;119:4321–32.

Yabe H, Yabe M, Koike T, et al. Rapid improvement of life-threatening capillary leak syndrome after stem cell transplantation by bevacizumab. Blood. 2010;115:2723–4.

Yeates L, Slatter MA, Bonanomi S, et al. Use of defibrotide to treat transplant-associated thrombotic microangiopathy: a retrospective study of the paediatric diseases and inborn errors working parties of the European Society of Blood and Marrow Transplantation. Bone Marrow Transplant. 2017;52:762–4.

Acute Graft-Versus-Host Disease

43

Ernst Holler, Hildegard Greinix, and Robert Zeiser

43.1 Introduction

Graft-versus-host disease (GvHD) was first recognized in murine models of HSCT, and in the absence of knowledge of the HLA system, it was termed "secondary" (secondary to recovery from irradiation damage) or "runt" disease on the basis of anorexia, reduced weight, diarrhea, ruffled fur, and eventual death. Billingham established the criteria for the occurrence of secondary disease in the 1960s, i.e.:

- The administration of a graft containing immunocompetent cells
- Immunological disparity between host and donor
- The administration of the graft to an immunosuppressed host unable to reject the graft cells

E. Holler (✉)
Clinical and Experimental HSCT, Department of Internal Medicine 3 (Haematology/Oncology), University of Regensburg, Regensburg, Germany
e-mail: ernst.holler@ukr.de

H. Greinix
Division of Hematology, Department of Internal Medicine, University Hospital Graz, Graz, Austria

R. Zeiser
Section for Tumor Immunology, Department of Hematology/Oncology, University Hospital Freiburg, University of Freiburg, Freiburg, Germany

In the human setting, we traditionally recognize two forms of GvHD, acute (aGvHD) and chronic (cGvHD). The original distinction of acute from chronic GvHD, namely, the occurrence before or after day 100 post stem cell infusion, has become blurred due to occurrence of aGvHD symptoms beyond day 100 after RIC regimens and/or after DLI (usually given after day 100). Nevertheless, the underlying combination of symptoms and signs affecting the skin, liver, and gastrointestinal tract forms a classical clinical syndrome enabling the diagnosis, and a helpful guide to the appropriate terminology is provided in Table 43.1 (Filipovich 2005).

Table 43.1 Current classification of acute and chronic GvHD

Classification	Day after SCT	Features of acute GvHD	Features of chronic GvHD
Acute GvHD	<100 days	Yes	No
– Classic acute	>100 days	Yes	No
– Persistent, recurrent, or late onset			
Chronic GvHD	No time limit	No	Yes
– Classic chronic	No time limit	Yes	Yes
– Overlap syndrome			

E. Carreras et al. (eds.), *The EBMT Handbook*, https://doi.org/10.1007/978-3-030-02278-5_43

43.2 Definition

aGvHD remains, directly or indirectly, the major cause of short-term (day 100 and 1 year) mortality after allo-HSCT. The pathophysiology of aGvHD has been attributed to a three-phase process comprising initial tissue damage from the conditioning regimen which in turn leads to activation of host antigen-presenting cells by pathogen-associated molecular patterns (PAMPs) and damage-associated molecular patterns (DAMPs) and activation and proliferation of donor T cells (afferent phase) and finally to the effector phase characterized by cytotoxic cell damage and release of inflammatory cytokines such as interleukin-1 (IL-1) and tissue necrosis factor-alpha (TNFα) that eventually produce tissue necrosis (efferent phase). The action of this pathogenetic process in the induction of aGvHD is modulated in part by the presence of cells capable of inhibiting immune response, such as T-regulatory cells (Tregs), Type 1 regulatory T cells (Tr1 cells), invariant NKT cells, and myeloid-derived suppressor cells (MDSCs) (Ferrara et al. 2009; Teshima et al. 2016).

43.3 Risk Factors

As aGvHD is a result of an alloimmune effect the major risk for occurrence is the presence of HLA disparity and increasing degrees of HLA-mismatching increase the probability of more severe disease. Other important and consistent risk factors include older patient age, the use of female donors for male recipients, prior alloimmunization of the donor, and the nature of GvHD prophylaxis. A number of publications have variously reported risk factors such as increasing donor age, increasing intensity of the preparative regimen, the use of PBSC as opposed to BM, and recipient seropositivity for CMV.

A recent study of 2941 recipients of allo-HSCT in Seattle confirmed the importance of the degree of HLA mismatching, the use of URD, and the administration of high-dose TBI in predicting the occurrence of moderate to severe aGvHD. In contrast they found that increasing donor age, cytokine-mobilized stem cells, and the use of female donors for male recipients did not impact on the likelihood of aGvHD but were associated with the occurrence of cGvHD (Flowers et al. 2011).

More recently we have begun to appreciate the importance of non-HLA genetic factors in the development of GvHD. Examples include polymorphisms in the genes encoding cytokines such as the tumor necrosis factors, the interleukins (IL-1, IL-6, and IL-10), interferon gamma (IFN-γ), and transforming growth factor-β3 (TGF-β3) and the expression of the killer cell immunoglobulin-like receptors (KIR). Interestingly one of the common features of the organs involved in aGvHD is that they are all exposed to microbial pathogens through the intestinal mucosa, epidermis, and portal circulation, and early murine studies confirmed a reduction in the severity and incidence of GvHD in animals that received antibiotic prophylaxis to "decontaminate" the GI tract or those kept in germ-free environments. This has led to the speculation that potential differences within individuals in the interactions of antigens derived from infective organisms and pathogen recognition receptors (PRR) might protect or predispose to the occurrence of GvHD. To date the most extensively studied of these receptors is N0D2 (CARD15) which detects muramyl dipeptide (MDP), a by-product of peptidoglycan, which is itself a cell wall component of most bacteria. Single nucleotide polymorphisms (SNPs) in N0D2 are present in approximately 15% of the population, and several investigators have studied their potential association with the occurrence of GvHD. Results are so far conflicting, and further work is required to determine their real significance (reviewed in Penack et al. 2010).

More recently, the availability of non-cultural methods to analyze the whole set of bacteria (called microbiota) has broadened our view as the presence of commensal microbiota and a high diversity of the patients' microbiota associated with substantial protection not only from GvHD but also from systemic and pulmonary infectious complications. The exact mechanisms of this protection need still to be defined before translation into new preventive approaches, but beneficial effects of microbial metabolites (such as short-chain fatty acids and indoles) both on epithelial integrity and on immunoregulation are likely (Shono and van den Brink 2018; Peled et al. 2016).

43.4 Diagnosis and Scoring

aGvHD is manifested by one or more of the following features: an erythematous skin reaction, cholestatic liver disease, and gastrointestinal dysfunction. The variety of presentations in each organ is provided in more detail in Table 43.2; the syndrome ranges from a mild self-limiting condition to a serious and potentially fatal disorder. Because of the complexity of care of an allo-HSCT recipient, it is often very difficult to distinguish the characteristic features of aGvHD from those of other complications such as VOD/SOS, conditioning, and general drug toxicity and infection and consequently to determine the appropriate choice of treatment.

For this reason, it is essential to establish the diagnosis by biopsy of one or more affected organs and confirmation of the characteristic histopathological features (Table 43.3). The targets of the immune response in aGvHD are the epithelial cells including basal and suprabasal cells of the epidermis, the intestinal epithelium, and the biliary duct epithelium, and the characteristic feature is identical, i.e., the presence of infiltrating immune cells close to apoptotic cells known as "satellite cell necrosis."

The first classification of aGvHD was developed by Glucksberg et al. (1974). Each organ was staged from 0 to 4 (Table 43.4), and the resultant stages were combined to provide an overall grade (Table 43.5) (Glucksberg et al. 1974). In 1994 Przepiorka et al. described the outcome of a Consensus Workshop to develop

Table 43.2 Clinical manifestations of acute GvHD

Organ	Clinical manifestation
Skin	Erythematous maculopapular rash, often initially involving the palms and soles May progress to involve the entire body surface and may be pruritic and/or painful In severe cases, bullae may form leading to desquamation
Liver	Cholestasis with or without frank jaundice Cholestatic enzymes comparatively more deranged than transaminases
Gastrointestinal (GI) tract	*Upper*: Anorexia, nausea, and vomiting *Lower*: Diarrhea, typically green and watery; in severe case diarrhea contains fresh blood and mucosa and is accompanied by abdominal cramps and, on occasion, paralytic ileus

Table 43.3 Histopathological findings in acute GvHD

Organ	Histopathological features
Skin	The diagnostic feature is a lichenoid infiltration of the upper dermis and lower epidermis with vacuolation, degeneration, and individual cell necrosis of the cells of the basal layer of the epidermis Grade I: vacuolation of epidermal basal cells Grade II: presence of individually necrotic keratinocytes Grade III: confluent areas of keratinocyte necrosis forming bullae Grade IV: sloughing of the epidermis
Liver	The most consistent histological feature is small bile duct damage, which is usually seen in association with cholestasis and is rare in other complications of HSCT The biliary epithelial cells have enlarged hyperchromatic nuclei or small pyknotic nuclei and vacuolated cytoplasm Periportal and midzone hepatocellular necrosis and minimal lymphocytic infiltrates in the portal tract Although there is a histological grading for liver histology, it has no proven prognostic value
Gastrointestinal	"Exploding crypts" within which are necrosis of individual epithelial cells at the periphery of the crypts leaving fragments of nuclear and cytoplasmatic debris Grade I: Individual cell necrosis Grade II: Loss of individual crypts Grade III: Loss of two or more adjacent crypts with ulceration Grade IV: Denudation of epithelium

Table 43.4 Staging of acute graft-versus-host disease

Stage	Skin based on maculopapular rash	Liver based on bilirubin	Gastrointestinal based on quantity of diarrhea
+	<25% of surface	34–50 μmol/L	500–1000 mL
++	25–50% of surface	51–102 μmol/L	1001–1500 mL
+++	Generalized erythroderma	103–255 μmol/L	>1500 mL
++++	Generalized erythroderma with bullae and desquamation	>255 μmol/L	Severe abdominal pain with and without ileus

Table 43.5 Overall grading of acute GvHD

Grade	
I	Skin + – ++
II	Skin + – +++, GI, and/or liver + Mild decrease in performance
III	Skin ++ – +++, GI, and/or liver ++ – +++ Marked decrease in clinical performance
IV	Skin ++ – ++++, GI, and/or liver ++ – ++++ Extreme decrease in clinical performance

an improved scoring system that retained most of the characteristics of Glucksberg but dropped the use of the clinical performance score and included upper intestinal symptoms within the definition of aGvHD (Przepiorka et al. 1995). Subsequently, the IBMTR prospectively evaluated a "severity index" against the Glucksberg criteria but were unable to identify any particular advantage for the new system (Rowlings et al. 1997). In fact, the Glucksberg score was a better predictor of survival and remains in regular use (Cahn et al. 2005). Currently, electronic applications are developed supporting accuracy of staging and grading of acute GvHD (Schoemans et al. 2018).

43.5 Epidemiology

Moderate to severe aGvHD occurs in approximately 40% of all recipients of allo-HSCT, but the precise incidence varies considerably depending predominantly on the nature of the donor and the method of GvHD prophylaxis. Without effective prophylaxis, it is an almost inevitable and frequently deleterious complication at least in unrelated matched donor and mismatched family grafts.

43.6 Prevention (Also See Chap. 25)

Grade III–IV aGvHD, especially if it turns out to be resistant to first-line treatment, has an extremely poor prognosis despite therapeutic intervention, and consequently considerable efforts are made to try and prevent its occurrence. The rationale of prophylaxis was originally directed toward prolonged IS of donor T-cell function through the peri- and post transplant administration of IS agents. Early studies identified the superiority of a combination of the CNI and CSA, with MTX over MTX alone. In practice this combination remains the most frequently used method of prophylaxis although some investigators have replaced CSA with tacrolimus (TAC) since large two phase III randomized studies reported a reduction in the incidence of grade II–IV aGvHD at 32% in recipients of sibling transplants and 56% in those who received unrelated donor grafts in patients who received TAC plus MTX compared to 44% (sibling) and 74% (unrelated) in those who were randomized to CSA and MTX. However, there was no difference in survival that could be attributed to the nature of the GvHD prevention (Ratanatharathorn et al. 1998; Nash et al. 2000). Recently, investigators have also reported the efficacy of newer agents such as mycophenolate mofetil (MMF) and sirolimus (SIR). Whereas MMF has not been tested in large randomized trials, the combination of TAC and SIR was compared with that of TAC and MTX in a phase III randomized study showing equivalent efficacy but differences in toxicity (Törlén et al. 2016).

An alternative approach to GvHD prophylaxis is to consider removal of donor T cells either ex vivo prior to infusion or in vivo before and/or after infusion using polyclonal (anti-thymocyte globulin, ATG) or MoAb. A similar effect can also be achieved by positive selection of CD34+ stem cells. These techniques, collectively known as TCD, are extremely efficient in preventing acute and chronic GvHD and were in widespread use in the 1980s and 1990s. Unfortunately, they were rapidly identified as contributing to an increased risk of infection and disease relapse and subsequently became confined to situations in which the risk of GvHD is increased, e.g., recipients of mismatched and haploidentical transplants where the risk of death from GvHD outweighs the risk of later disease recurrence. In unrelated donor SCT, polyclonal ATG has become a major player as two randomized trials showed positive effects mainly on chronic GvHD (Finke et al. 2009; Walker et al. 2016).

Recently, a prospective, double-blind phase III trial to investigate the effect of ATG in the setting of MUD HSCT showed that grade II–IV acute GvHD and moderate-severe cGvHD were lower in ATG recipients but the overall survival was lower in ATG recipients (Soiffer et al. 2017). This could be related to higher ATG levels in patients with low lymphocyte counts following TBI which might translate in subsequent infectious complications and EBV-related post transplant lymphoproliferative disease. Thus, balancing suppression of long-term GvHD versus suppressing anti-infectious defense is an ongoing challenge in GvHD (Gagelmann et al. 2017).

Other studies have explored alternative methods of aGvHD prophylaxis including the infusion of an expanded population of T-regulatory cells at the time of stem cell infusion and partial TCD such as depletion of α/β T cells or elimination of alloreactive T cells after in vitro or in vivo activation. In this context, the administration of PT-CY in order to eliminate early activated donor T cells has gained substantial interest particularly in the context of haploidentical transplantation, and further studies comparing the more complex T-cell depletion approach with the simple approach of PT-CY are currently performed (Kanakry et al. 2016).

43.7 Treatment

Grade I aGvHD, by definition affecting only the skin, can often be effectively treated with topical steroids alone. Early systemic treatment of grade I GvHD has been tested but showed no long-term advantage. More advanced grades require systemic therapy, and the mainstay of treatment remains high-dose methyl-prednisolone (or equivalent), usually at a dose of 2 mg/kg/day, continued for 7–14 days and followed by a gradual reduction in dose (Ruutu et al. 2014). Patients with mild upper GI GvHD may start on lower doses with concomitant topical treatment; higher doses of steroids resulted in more infectious complications without superior long-term response. The chance of response decreases with increasing grade of GvHD, but in general approximately 40–50% of patients will demonstrate a response. Reductions in steroid doses may be followed by an exacerbation of symptoms that can sometimes be settled by simply increasing the dose and reducing more slowly on the second occasion. Achieving a balance between the levels of IS required to control aGvHD and retaining a degree of immunocompetence against microbial infection is challenging, and viral and fungal infections are frequent complications of prolonged steroid therapy. Anti-infective prophylaxis should be considered for all such patients. Among several candidates for first-line combination treatments, the most promising combination of steroids and MMF has been taken forward to a phase III study against steroids alone but failed to show superiority for the combination again due to an increased rate of infectious complications. Thus, so far no single agent has shown superiority of results when combined with corticosteroids for first-line treatment (Martin et al. 2012; Rashidi et al. 2016).

Failure to respond to standard steroid doses (defined as progression within 3–5 days of starting treatment or an incomplete response by 7–14 days) or recurrence after initial dose reduction (steroid dependence) will necessitate second-line treatment. In this context many agents have been tried alone or in combination with corticosteroid. None have shown convincing long-term efficacy. The most frequent choice of second-line therapy involves one or more MoAb recognizing T cells or ATG. MoAb include alemtuzumab for the pan T-cell marker CD52, daclizumab, or inolimomab for the alpha subunit of the IL-2 receptor expressed on activated T cells; and infliximab and etanercept for TNF-α. These agents often result in short-term control, but durable effects are relatively infrequent, and the outcome of refractory aGvHD is dismal with approximately 80% mortality, especially if the lower GI tract is involved.

Responses have been reported with extracorporeal photopheresis administered at least twice a week on a weekly basis, and outcome seems to be superior with less toxicities occurring (Jagasia et al. 2013) (see Chap. 66).

In 2006, Ringden et al. reported the successful use of mesenchymal stromal cells (MSC) in a small group of patients with refractory severe aGvHD, and later this group described a response rate of >50% in a larger group of patients (Munneke et al. 2016). MSC exert immunosuppressive effects in a non-HLA-restricted manner and like Tregs offer interesting and novel strategies for the management of this potentially fatal complication although long-term results need to be established in future trials (Le Blanc et al. 2008).

While classical IS regimens inhibit a signal pathway or cytokine receptor, novel strategies target the signaling events downstream of cytokine receptors (e.g., Janus-activated kinase JAK 1 and 2), CD28 (e.g., Aurora kinase), cell migration (ROCK), or growth factor signaling (e.g., MEK). These inhibitors were tested in preclinical studies and showed promising activity (Hill et al. 2018). A prospective study on the JAK1 inhibitor itacitinib showed GvHD response rates of over 70%, and a retrospective survey on ruxolitinib-treated patients showed that also patients with steroid refractory GvHD may respond to JAK1/2 inhibition (Zeiser et al. 2015). The therapeutic concept of JAK1/2 inhibition is currently tested for steroid-refractory (SR) SR-aGvHD and SR-cGvHD in randomized phase III trials.

Another novel approach is infusion of alpha-1 anti-trypsin which exerts anti-inflammatory effects and stimulates regulatory T cells. Two recent phase II trials showed CR rates of 35% and OR rates of 60% of the patients on day 28 after treatment starts (Marcondes et al. 2016 Magenau et al. 2018). Vedolizumab is an antibody directed against α4/β7 integrin which is selectively expressed in the GI tract and approved for treatment of Crohn's disease. A first report indicated high response rates for SR-aGvHD (Fløisand et al. 2017). However, more recent updates indicate a high treatment-related mortality in patients receiving vedolizumab due to infections of over 70%, and the ongoing phase III trials will provide more information.

43.8 Future Perspectives: Biomarkers and Risk-Adapted Treatment

The difficulties to improve results in SR-aGvHD underline that steroid resistance might not just represent resistance of alloreactive T cells but loss of immunoregulation and tissue tolerance (Wu and Reddy 2017) which is difficult to overcome by classical immunosuppressants. Besides new approaches of modulation, potential solutions might be earlier risk adapted or even preemptive treatment strategies which require, however, reliable and reproducible identification of these patients. Recently, clinical risk scores (MacMillan et al. 2015) and novel biomarkers have been reported. The strength of these biomarkers for early identification of high-risk patients at day 7 after HSCT or at onset of GvHD has been proven in large multicenter consortia and needs now confirmation by trials on biomarker-guided treatment strategies (Vander Lugt et al. 2013; Hartwell et al. 2017; Levine et al. 2015). The strength of the current biomarkers and scores are partially explained by the fact that they identify GI GvHD as the most severe and deleterious manifestation in an early phase of the disease.

Key Points

- Acute GvHD occurs until day 100 as classical acute GvHD and beyond day 100 as delayed acute GvHD.
- As treatment options are limited beyond the use of corticosteroids, careful selection of GvHD prevention is essential.
- Besides classical IS agents like CNI, MTX or MMF, and m-ToR inhibitors, partial TCD (IV serotherapy, depletion of T-cell subpopulations, elimination of alloreactive T cells or PT-CY) are possible options for prophylaxis.
- Institutional standards of treatment and supportive care are essential.

References

Cahn JY, Klein JP, Lee SJ, et al. Prospective evaluation of 2 acute graft-versus-host (GVHD) grading systems: a joint Société Française de Greffe de Moëlle et Thérapie Cellulaire (SFGM-TC), Dana Farber Cancer Institute (DFCI), and International Bone Marrow Transplant Registry (IBMTR) prospective study. Blood. 2005;106:1495–500.

Ferrara JL, Levine JE, Reddy P, Holler E. Graft-versus-host disease. Lancet. 2009;373:1550–61.

Filipovich AH, Weisdorf D, Pavletic S, et al. National Institutes of Health consensus development project on criteria for clinical trials in chronic graft-versus-host disease: I. Diagnosis and staging working group report. Biol Blood Marrow Transplant. 2005;11:945–56.

Finke J, Bethge WA, Schmoor C, et al. Standard graft-versus-host disease prophylaxis with or without anti-T-cell globulin in haematopoietic cell transplantation from matched unrelated donors: a randomised, open-label, multicentre phase 3 trial. Lancet Oncol. 2009;10:855–64.

Fløisand Y, Lundin KEA, Lazarevic V, et al. Targeting integrin α4β7 in steroid-refractory intestinal graft-versus-host disease. Biol Blood Marrow Transplant. 2017;23:172–5.

Flowers ME, Inamoto Y, Carpenter PA, et al. Comparative analysis of risk factors for acute graft-versus-host disease and for chronic graft-versus-host disease according to National Institutes of Health consensus criteria. Blood. 2011;117:3214–9.

Gagelmann N, Ayuk F, Wolschke C, Kröger N. Comparison of different rabbit anti-thymocyte globulin formulations in allogeneic stem cell transplantation: systematic literature review and network meta-analysis. Biol Blood Marrow Transplant. 2017;23:2184–91.

Glucksberg H, Storb R, Fefer A, et al. Clinical manifestations of graft-versus-host disease in human recipients of marrow from HL-A-matched sibling donors. Transplantation. 1974;18:295–304.

Hartwell MJ, Özbek U, Holler E, et al. An early-biomarker algorithm predicts lethal graft-versus-host disease and survival. JCI Insight. 2017;2:e89798.

Hill L, Alousi A, Kebriaei P, et al. New and emerging therapies for acute and chronic graft versus host disease. Ther Adv Hematol. 2018;9:21–46.

Jagasia M, Greinix H, Robin M, et al. Extracorporeal photopheresis versus anticytokine therapy as a second-line treatment for steroid-refractory acute GVHD: a multicenter comparative analysis. Biol Blood Marrow Transplant. 2013;19:1129–33.

Kanakry CG, Fuchs EJ, Luznik L. Modern approaches to HLA-haploidentical blood or marrow transplantation. Nat Rev Clin Oncol. 2016;13:132.

Le Blanc K, Frassoni F, Ball L, Locatelli F, Developmental Committee of the European Group for Blood and Marrow Transplantation, et al. Mesenchymal stem cells for treatment of steroid-resistant, severe, acute graft-versus-host disease: a phase II study. Lancet. 2008;371:1579–86.

Levine JE, Braun TM, Harris AC, Blood and Marrow Transplant Clinical Trials Network, et al. A prognostic score for acute graft-versus-host disease based on biomarkers: a multicentre study. Lancet Haematol. 2015;2:e21–9.

MacMillan ML, Robin M, Harris AC. A refined risk score for acute graft-versus-host disease that predicts response to initial therapy, survival, and transplant-related mortality. Biol Blood Marrow Transplant. 2015;21:761–7.

Magenau JM, Goldstein SC, Peltier D, et al. α(1)-Antitrypsin infusion for treatment of steroid-resistant acute graft-versus-host disease. Blood. 2018;131:1372–9.

Marcondes AM, Hockenbery D, Lesnikova M, et al. Response of steroid-refractory acute GVHD to α1-antitrypsin. Biol Blood Marrow Transplant. 2016;22:1596–601.

Martin PJ, Rizzo JD, Wingard JR, et al. First-and second-line systemic treatment of acute graft-versus-host disease: recommendations of the American Society of Blood and Marrow Transplantation. Biol Blood Marrow Transplant. 2012;18:1150–63.

Munneke JM, Spruit MJ, Cornelissen AS, et al. The potential of mesenchymal stromal cells as treatment for severe steroid-refractory acute graft-versus-host disease: a critical review of the literature. Transplantation. 2016;100:2309–14.

Nash RA, Antin JH, Karanes C, et al. Phase 3 study comparing methotrexate and tacrolimus with methotrexate and cyclosporine for prophylaxis of acute graft-versus-host disease after marrow transplantation from unrelated donors. Blood. 2000;96:2062–8.

Peled JU, Jenq RR, Holler E, van den Brink MR. Role of gut flora after bone marrow transplantation. Nat Microbiol. 2016;1:16036. https://doi.org/10.1038/nmicrobiol.2016.36.

Penack O, Holler E, van den Brink MR. Graft-versus-host disease: regulation by microbe-associated molecules and innate immune receptors. Blood. 2010;115:1865–72.

Przepiorka D, Weisdorf D, Martin P, et al. Consensus conference on acute GVHD grading. Bone Marrow Transplant. 1995;15:825–8.

Rashidi A, DiPersio JF, Sandmaier BM, et al. Steroids versus steroids plus additional agent in frontline treatment of acute graft-versus-host disease: a systematic review and meta-analysis of randomized trials. Biol Blood Marrow Transplant. 2016;22:1133–7.

Ratanatharathorn V, Nash RA, Przepiorka D, et al. Phase III study comparing methotrexate and tacrolimus (prograf, FK506) with methotrexate and cyclosporine for graft-versus-host disease prophylaxis after HLA-identical sibling bone marrow transplantation. Blood. 1998;92:2303–14.

Rowlings PA, Przepiorka D, Klein JP, et al. IBMTR Severity Index for grading acute graft-versus-host disease: retrospective comparison with Glucksberg grade. Br J Haematol. 1997;97:855–64.

Ruutu T, Gratwohl A, de Witte T, et al. Prophylaxis and treatment of GVHD: EBMT-ELN working group recommendations for a standardized practice. Bone Marrow Transplant. 2014;49:168–73.

Schoemans HM, Goris K, Van Durm R, et al. Complications and quality of life working party of the EBMT. Accuracy and usability of the eGVHD app in assessing the severity of graft-versus-host disease at the 2017 EBMT annual congress. Bone Marrow Transplant. 2018;53:490–4.

Shono Y, van den Brink MRM. Gut microbiota injury in allogeneic haematopoietic stem cell transplantation. Nat Rev Cancer. 2018;18:283–95.

Soiffer RJ, Kim HT, McGuirk J, et al. Prospective, randomized, double-blind, phase III clinical trial of anti-T-lymphocyte globulin to assess impact on chronic graft-versus-host disease-free survival in patients undergoing HLA-matched unrelated myeloablative hematopoietic cell transplantation. J Clin Oncol. 2017;35:4003–11.

Teshima T, Reddy P, Zeiser R. Acute graft-versus-host disease: novel biological insights. Biol Blood Marrow Transplant. 2016;22:11–6.

Törlén J, Ringdén O, Garming-Legert K, et al. A prospective randomized trial comparing cyclosporine/methotrexate and tacrolimus/sirolimus as graft-versus-host disease prophylaxis after allogeneic hematopoietic stem cell transplantation. Haematologica. 2016;101:1417–25.

Vander Lugt MT, Braun TM, Hanash S, et al. ST2 as a marker for risk of therapy-resistant graft-versus-host disease and death. N Engl J Med. 2013;369:529–39.

Walker I, Panzarella T, Couban S, et al. Pretreatment with anti-thymocyte globulin versus no anti-thymocyte globulin in patients with haematological malignancies undergoing haemopoietic cell transplantation from unrelated donors: a randomised, controlled, open-label, phase 3, multicentre trial. Lancet Oncol. 2016;17:164–73.

Wu SR, Reddy P. Tissue tolerance: a distinct concept to control acute GVHD severity. Blood. 2017;129:1747–52.

Zeiser R, Burchert A, Lengerke C, et al. Ruxolitinib in corticosteroid-refractory graft-versus-host disease after allogeneic stem cell transplantation: a multicenter survey. Leukemia. 2015;29:2062–8.

44 Chronic Graft-Versus-Host Disease

Daniel Wolff and Anita Lawitschka

44.1 Introduction

Chronic GVHD (cGVHD) is the most relevant cause of late non-relapse morbidity and subsequent mortality (approximately 25%) following allo-HSCT (Grube et al. 2016). Its incidence is approximately 50% among all patients following allo-HSCT and has increased during the last two decades due to increasing patient age and increasing use of unrelated and/or mismatched donors, RIC regimens, and PBSC (Arai et al. 2015). While the incidence of cGVHD is lower (20–40%) in children, its incidence rises to 60% as age increases (Baird et al. 2010).

The *pathophysiology* of cGVHD is different from aGVHD and mainly characterized by impaired immune tolerance mechanisms affecting innate and adaptive immunity. Both autoreactive and alloreactive donor-derived T and B cells play a role (Cooke et al. 2017). Other pathophysiological factors are indirect presentations of alloantigens through antigen-presenting donor cells and mechanisms of chronic inflammation with subsequent scar formation and fibrosis. One important aspect of GVHD pathophysiology is the variability of immune reconstitution, which is age-related and dependent on thymic function and hormones. This adds to the unpredictability of the effects of transplant procedures and complications in a very heterogenous cohort of children and adolescents with malignant and nonmalignant diseases.

Known *risk factors* for adult and pediatric cGVHD are unrelated and/or mismatched donor, PBSCs as donor source, older donor age, female donor into male recipient, and the use of total body irradiation (Baird et al. 2010). By far the strongest predictor is the history and severity of acute GVHD.

In addition to the harm it causes, cGVHD also has a *protective effect*, as patients with cGVHD have lower rates of recurrence of their underlying malignant disease (Grube et al. 2016). Overall survival of patients transplanted for malignant diseases developing mild cGVHD is therefore better compared to patients without cGVHD. Even OS of patients with moderate cGVHD is not different from patients without cGVHD, as the slightly increased mortality associated with cGVHD is counterbalanced by lower disease-associated mortality (Kuzmina et al. 2012).

In contrast, the *long-term mortality* rate of patients with severe cGVHD is as high as 50% taken into account that the severity is less relevant compared to certain risk factors for mortality consisting of low platelets at diagnosis of cGVHD, the direct progression of acute GVHD into cGVHD (progressive onset), and certain organ manifestations

D. Wolff
Department of Internal Medicine III, University Hospital Regensburg, Regensburg, Germany

A. Lawitschka (✉)
St. Anna Children's Hospital, Medical University Vienna, Vienna, Austria
e-mail: anita.lawitschka@stanna.at

E. Carreras et al. (eds.), *The EBMT Handbook*, https://doi.org/10.1007/978-3-030-02278-5_44

(lung, gastrointestinal and cholestatic liver involvement) (Grube et al. 2016). One important pediatric aspect involves the high proportion (up to 50%) of nonmalignant underlying diseases as HSCT indication. While malignant diseases benefit from the graft-versus-malignancy effect induced by GVHD, it only offers harm for the nonmalignant diseases. In daily clinical routine, this fact influences GVHD prophylaxis and treatment both in regard to intensity and duration of immunosuppressants (Lawitschka et al., data of a survey by the EBMT pediatric diseases WP, submitted). However, prospective pediatric data of immune reconstitution in GVHD patients evaluating the influence of underlying diseases are scarce.

44.2 Clinical Manifestations

cGVHD usually begins between 3 months and 2 years after HSCT, but earlier onset (at least 1 month after transplantation) is possible (Jagasia et al. 2015). Besides classical manifestations, cGVHD can imitate almost any autoimmune disease, such as myasthenia gravis and myositis. As cGVHD can affect a number of organs, and patients often do not report changes until functional impairment is recognized, regular examination of all organs potentially affected is essential. The following section describes the most common clinical organ manifestations of cGVHD. In general, pediatric manifestations are similar to adult cGVHD; when indicated, specific aspects are shortly described.

44.2.1 Skin

The skin is the most frequently involved organ with different morphology, depending on the different skin layers (epidermis, cutis, subcutis, and fasciae) involved. Some manifestations may overlap with acute GVHD like erythema, maculopapular rash, and pruritus. Cutaneous cGVHD may show many different non-sclerotic and sclerotic phenotypes often simulating well-known chronic inflammatory and autoimmune diseases (Strong Rodrigues et al. 2018).

Diagnostic features of NIH-defined cGVHD include poikiloderma, lichen planus-like, lichen sclerosus-like, morphea-like, and deep sclerotic eruptions, and no biopsy is needed to confirm the diagnosis. Distinctive for cGVHD, other or common skin manifestations like depigmentation and papulosquamous lesions or ichthyosis, keratosis pilaris, pigmental changes, loss of skin appendages, and sweat impairment are not sufficient for diagnosis and require histopathological confirmation if no diagnostic signs in the skin or other organs are present (Jagasia et al. 2015).

In pediatric patients, the incidence of viral reactivation and infection seems higher (although only proven for some viruses), and therefore infection has to be ruled out. Viral skin infections can worsen or activate cGVHD (Jacobsohn 2010). Premature graying of the hair is even in small children common, possibly together with seborrheic scalp changes. Of note, if sweat glands are destroyed, this may be of importance for phototherapy because of the inability to sweat with consequent hyperthermia.

44.2.2 Eyes

cGVHD of the eyes usually manifests as keratitis sicca. In addition to atrophy of the lacrimal gland with subsequent tear deficiency (sicca syndrome), the meibomian glands and eyelids are often affected by severe blepharitis which may initially present with tearing. Around the conjunctiva there are often not only fibrotic alterations but also chronic persistent inflammation with visible erythema of the conjunctiva. As dry eye symptoms are rarely communicated by children, light sensitivity is the predominant symptom, sometimes with excessive eye rubbing. Infections have to be ruled out. Referral to a pediatric experienced ophthalmologist is recommended.

44.2.3 Oral Mucosa

Oral manifestations may appear as erythema or lichenoid changes (the latter are regarded as diagnostic) of the oral mucosa as well as ulcera and mucoceles. Sicca symptoms may result from destruction of the salivary glands. Long-term cGVHD may lead to gingivitis, periodontitis, increased tooth decay, and tooth loss. In children excessive drinking during eating may be the first symptom of oral involvement. Not only mucosal problems but abnormal teeth development (e.g., hypodontia, root malformation, enamel hypoplasia) and caries are often seen as secondary symptoms in infants.

44.2.4 Liver

Liver involvement manifests as cholestasis and may resemble primary biliary cirrhosis, but hepatitic forms with high transaminases are also possible. Other factors, such as viral infections (hepatitis A, B, C, and E, CMV, EBV, ADV, and HHV6/7), drug toxicity, or total-parenteral nutrition-related cholestasis, should be excluded, but liver biopsy may be required to confirm the diagnosis, particularly in patients with no other symptoms of cGVHD and failure to respond to initial treatment of suspected GVHD (Stift et al. 2014).

44.2.5 Gastrointestinal Tract

GI manifestations can lead to dysphagia (esophagus), nausea and vomiting (stomach), or chronic diarrhea and malabsorption syndrome (intestines, pancreas). Occasionally cGVHD may also manifest as immune-mediated pancreatitis. Of note, except esophageal involvement, intestinal involvement is regarded as manifestation of acute GVHD, and patients are therefore classified as suffering from overlap syndrome in which concomitant symptoms of chronic and acute GVHD occur.

Infections like ADV or CMV gastroenteritis, secondary gluten or lactose intolerance, pancreatic insufficiency, and drug-related side effects (e.g., mycophenolate mofetil) have to be ruled out.

Malnutition and enteral fluid and protein loss in small children require regular laboratory monitoring.

44.2.6 Genitals

The symptoms of cGVHD are similar to those of genital lichen planus which may occur in males and females. Vaginal synechiae, ulceration, and fissures can subsequently occur. Genital manifestations are often associated with oral manifestations of cGVHD. As symptoms may not be reported spontaneously, females suffering from cGVHD require regular gynecological follow-up. In girls cGVHD may manifest with vulvovaginitis, in boys with balanitis or balanoposthitis. Of note, healing may occur with fibrosis possibly leading to synechia with the risk of hematocolpos during puberty in females and of phimosis in males.

44.2.7 Lung

Pulmonary manifestations occur as progressive, irreversible obstruction (bronchiolitis obliterans) and less frequently lymphocytic alveolitis resulting in interstitial fibrosis or bronchiolitis obliterans organizing pneumonia (BOOP) (see Chap. 52).

Since the onset of pulmonary symptoms may not be symptomatic and obstruction may be irreversible, regular evaluations of a serial pulmonary function test (PFT) with body plethysmography (from the age of 4–6 years on) and diffusion capacity (usually from 8–10 years of age on) are required in asymptomatic patients.

While interstitial fibrosis is well known after lung transplant (restrictive allograft syndrome), prospective data after allogeneic HSCT are lacking, but case reports indicate that restrictive immune-mediated lung disease after allo-HSCT may occur.

Patients require follow-up by a pediatric experienced pulmonologist. Of note, the possible overlap of (1) myopathy/hypotrophy of the respiratory muscles (glucocorticoid induced, ± central obesity, and/or physical inactivity), (2) restriction of the chest wall in the context of dermal sclerosis, and (3) unproportional chest growth after TBI and/or local irradiation may contribute with a restrictive ventilator dysfunction leading to a mixed picture.

Finally, a thorough diagnostic evaluation includes a lung CT scan and a BAL to rule out viral, bacterial, fungal, and mycobacterial infections.

Coexisting IgA deficiency and chronic sinusitis or sinubronchial syndrome should be considered in the diagnostic workup (Hildebrandt et al. 2011).

44.2.8 Joints and Fasciae

cGVHD-associated fasciitis (diagnostic for cGVHD) can result in restricted mobility of joints. This can also be caused by deep cutaneous sclerosis. Moreover, rheumatoid complaints may be associated with cGVHD. In children myositis, muscle weakness, cramping, edema, and pain are quite common. However, iatrogenic glucocorticoid-induced myopathy may overlap with fasciitis. Range-of-motion (ROM) examinations are recommended at baseline and at serial intervals with the P-ROM scale providing an easy-to-apply tool. (There is a pediatric adaption, ped P-ROM; see addendum).

44.3 Diagnosis

cGVHD is diagnosed on the basis of cGVHD symptoms of eight organs, laboratory values (for hepatic manifestations), and PFTs. Each organ is graded between 0 and 3. The overall severity of cGVHD is classified as mild, moderate, or severe based on this organ-specific grading (number of organs and severity). Overall severity is calculated on the basis of the number of organs affected and the severity of their involvement. Only in case that functional involvement is solely due to none GVHD causes the impairment is not scored (Jagasia et al. 2015). Biomarkers of cGVHD are currently explored but require validation before clinical use.

44.3.1 Organ Grading of cGVHD for Adults and Children (See Annex 1 and Addendum)

44.3.2 Grading of Overall Severity of cGVHD (Jagasia et al. 2015)

Overall severity	Mild	Moderate	Severe
Number of involved organs	1–2	≥3	≥3
Severity of involved organs	Mild (excluding lung)	Mild–moderate (lung only mild)	Severe (lung moderate or severe)

If diagnostic symptoms of cGVHD are absent, histological confirmation of diagnosis may be required. This may be particularly the case in gastrointestinal, nonspecific cutaneous, hepatic, and pulmonary manifestations to rule out toxic or infectious causes or comorbidity. Clinicopathologic series indicate a significant risk for inappropriate diagnosis and subsequent treatment if diagnosis has been made solely by clinical manifestations (and lacking diagnostic symptoms) without histological confirmation.

44.4 Treatment

44.4.1 First-Line Therapy

First-line treatment (see Table 44.1) consists of steroids given alone or in combination with CNI and is based on randomized trials.

As *mild cGVHD* does not impair organ function, the use of topical IS (topical steroids, topical CNI, or phototherapy) should be considered. If this is impossible, PRD treatment at an initial dose of 0.5–1 mg/kg body weight/day is recommended. Topical IS can be used in addition to systemic IS, to improve efficacy, or to reduce systemic IS, but lack systemic efficacy.

For *moderate or severe cGVHD*, systemic treatment with PRD or methylPRD at an initial dose of 1 mg/kg body weight/day should be used. In individual cases lower doses of 0.5–1 mg/kg may be used (Jacobsohn 2010). The combination of steroids with a CNI (CSA or TAC) is particularly worth considering for severe cGVHD. Rituximab has been explored in first-line treatment of cGVHD in combination with steroids and CNI demonstrating an increased response rate on the expense of an increased risk for late infectious complications and delayed B-cell recovery. Currently, ECP and ibrutinib are evaluated in first-line treatment of cGVHD within randomized clinical trials.

As cGVHD often takes time to respond to IS treatment, response should not be assessed until at least 8 weeks have elapsed or until 3–6 months have elapsed in the presence of deep cutaneous sclerosis. Long-term IS treatment lasting at least 3–6 months is often required. Dose reduction of IS agents should be performed stepwise.

Table 44.1 First-line treatment of cGVHD

Drug	Recommendation Grade	Recommendation Evidence	Side effects in >25% patients	Response rate	Comment
Steroids	A	I	Osteoporosis, osteonecrosis, diabetes mellitus	~30–50% CR	Main drug; strategies to reduce use due to SEs very important
CNI + steroids	C-1	II	Renal toxicity, hypertension	~30–50% RC	Reduces steroid use, reduced incidence of osteonecrosis
Rituximab + steroids/CNI	C-1	III-1[12]	Increased risk for late infectious complications	~75%	Randomized data are lacking
MMF + CNI/ steroids	D	II	GI complaints, infections		No increased efficacy compared to CNI and steroids, increased risk of relapse of malignancy
Azathioprine	D	II	Cytopenia, risk of infection		Increased mortality
Thalidomide	D	II	Neurotoxicity, drowsiness, constipation		Very little effect in first-line therapy

Adapted from Wolff et al. (2011), A: should always be used; C-1: use in first-line therapy justified, D: moderate evidence of lack of efficacy or unacceptably high risks, should generally not be offered, I: evidence from ≥1 properly randomized, controlled trials, II: evidence from more than one well-planned non-randomized clinical trial, from cohort or case-controlled, analytic studies (preferably at several sites), III-1: only one non-controlled study, III-2: only one retrospective, non-controlled study or retrospective evaluation. (Evidence and recommendations graded according to the 2005 NIH Consensus), *SE* side effect, *NIH* US National Institutes of Health, *MMF* mycophenolate mofetil

Depending on the patient population, first-line therapy achieves complete remission of cGVHD in approximately 20% (adults) to 50% (children) of cases. If symptoms progress during the first 4 weeks of first-line therapy or there is no improvement in symptoms within 8–12 weeks, second-line therapy should be initiated.

44.4.2 Topical Therapy and Supportive Care

In principle, there is no difference between cGVHD treatment for children and adults. However, long-term steroid therapy in children causes major side effects in terms of growth, bone density, osteonecrosis, and organ development, making agents that reduce steroid use, entailing the use of topical drugs, particularly important. Age-based ancillary supportive care is essential in the management of pediatric cGVHD with the chance of sparing systemic therapy, often supported by highly compliant parents and/or family members as caregivers (Carpenter et al. 2015). In small children, the risk of systemic effects of topical steroid and CNI treatment must be considered. cGVHD is by itself remarkably immunosuppressive intensified by its treatment (especially high-dose corticosteroids) leading to a high risk for infections: (a) for viral reactivation like CMV, ADV, and EBV and (b) for fungal infection like candida and aspergillosis. Functional asplenia with occurrence of Howell-Jolly bodies and a higher incidence of pneumococcal sepsis has to be considered also. Breakdown of skin and mucosal barriers adds to this risk.

Revaccinations (see Chap. 29) with inactivated vaccines are strongly recommended after consolidation of cGVHD (Hilgendorf et al. 2011). Live vaccines should be avoided in this patient population. Ursodeoxycholic acid reduced liver GVHD and improved survival (Ruutu et al. 2014). Supplemental IVIG replacement is recommended in cGVHD patients with IgG <400 mg/dL or recurrent infections which is of special importance in children but does also apply to adults. In case of long-term substitution or the history of anaphylactic reactions, we prefer to substitute subcutaneously.

44.4.3 Second-Line Therapy

While first-line therapy is based on randomized trials, second-line therapy mostly is based on phase II trials, and retrospective analyses are available (see Table 44.2). In addition, because

Table 44.2 Second-line treatment of cGVHD

Drug	Recommendation		Response rate	Side effects in >25% of patients	Comments
	Grade	Evidence			
Steroids	B	III-1	n.a.	Osteoporosis, osteonecrosis, diabetes mellitus	Main drug, strategies to reduce use due to SEs very important
Ibrutinib	C-1	III-1	~50–75% ~16–25% CR	Bruising, diarrhea, infections	FDA approved in second-line treatment of cGVHD
Photophereses	C-1	II	~60–70% ~30% CR	Infections of the CVC (if applicable)	Venous access required, steroid-saving effect, good tolerability
mTOR-inh (sirolimus, everolimus)	C-1	III-1	~60% ~20% CR	TMA, hyperlipidemia, cytopenia	Increased risk of TMA when combined with CNI, regular blood levels required
MMF	C-1	III-1	~50% ~10% CR	GI SEs, risk of infection (viral) and increased risk of relapse	Steroid sparing activity
CNI	C-1	III-1	n.a.	Renal toxicity, hypertension	Reduces steroid use, regular blood levels required
MTX	C-2	III-1	~50% ~10–20% CR	Cytopenia	Best results in mucocutaneous cGVHD, reduces steroid use, contraindicated in the presence of pleural effusions or ascites
IL-2	C-2	III-1	~65% (only PR)	Fever, malaise, and fatigue	Applied in sclerodermoid skin disease
Ruxolitinib	C-2	III-1	n.a. (retrospective analysis)	Increased risk for viral reactivation, bacterial infection, hepatotoxicity	Prospective data pending
Bortezomib	C-2	III-1	n.a. for second-line Tx	Cytopenia, neuropathy	Trial was performed in first-line treatment
High-dose steroids	C-2	III-2	50–75% (only PR)	Infections	Rapid control of cGVHD
Total nodal irradiation	C-2	III-2	~50% ~25% CR	Cytopenia	Best results for fasciitis and mucocutaneous cGVHD
Hydroxychloroquine	C-2	III-2	~25% ~10% CR	GI side effects	Best results for mucocutaneous and hepatic cGVHD
Pentostatin	C-2	II	~50% ~10% CR	Cytopenia, risk of infection	Best results in children
Rituximab	C-2	II	~50% ~10% CR	Risk of infection	Effective in manifestations associated with autoAb and sclerodermoid cutaneous involvement
Imatinib	C-2	III-1	~50% ~20% CR	Fluid retention	Efficacy demonstrated mainly in sclerodermoid cGVHD and bronchiolitis obliterans
Thalidomide	C-3	II	~20–30% (only PR)	Neurotoxicity, drowsiness, constipation	Treatment for simultaneous cGVHD and recurrent multiple myeloma

(continued)

Table 44.2 (continued)

Drug	Recommendation		Response rate	Side effects in >25% of patients	Comments
	Grade	Evidence			
Azathioprine	C-3	III-1	n.a.	Cytopenia, risk of infection, secondary malignancies	Increased risk of malignant disease of the oral mucosa
Retinoids	C-3	III-2	~60% (only PR)	Skin toxicity, hyperlipidemia	Effective in sclerodermoid cutaneous involvement
Abatacept	C-3	III-2	~40%		Effective in mucocutaneous and pulmonary involvement
Regulatory T cells	C-4				Currently explored in several clinical trials
Mesenchymal stem cells	C-4	III-2	n.a.		Repetitive application required
Alemtuzumab	C-4	III-3	n.a.	Infectious risks	Last resort for refractory cGVHD
Etanercept	C-4	III-3	n.a.	Infectious risks	May be used to treat mixed acute and chronic GVHD or pulmonary or GI manifestations of cGVHD

Adapted from Wolff et al. (2011), B: should generally be used, C-1: use in second-line therapy justified, C-2: use after failure of second-line therapy justified, C-3: should only be used in specific circumstances, due to unfavorable risk profile, C-4: experimental, should only be used in clinical trials and individual cases, II: evidence from >1 well-designed clinical trial without randomization, from cohort or case-controlled analytic studies (preferable from >1 center) or from multiple time series, III-1: several reports from retrospective evaluations or small uncontrolled clinical trials, III-2: only one report from small uncontrolled clinical trial or retrospective evaluations, III-3: only case reports available, SE: side effect, n.a.: not available

the data on disease severity and patient populations are very heterogeneous (in terms of age, conditioning, and stem cell source), the published response rates cannot be fully extrapolated to the majority of patients currently treated for cGVHD. Moreover, many substances have been used almost exclusively in combination with steroids.

In general, no more than three IS agents should be combined, as combinations of more drugs often does not lead to improved efficacy but results in a significantly increased risk of side effects and infections. Because of the substantial toxicity of long-term steroid treatment, strategies for dose reduction are very important. Since no predictors of response for a single agent in individual patients are yet available, the choice of agent depends mainly on side effect profiles and patients' medical history. The response rates for specific agents range between 20% and 70% (photopheresis).

Certain drugs such as imatinib and retinoids are recommended only for manifestations associated with sclerosis (bronchiolitis obliterans [imatinib], sclerodermoid cutaneous alterations [retinoids, imatinib]), because of their specific mechanisms of action.

Response is assessed as for first-line therapy. Administration of drugs that have been shown to be ineffective should be stopped. As a rule, drugs shown to be ineffective should be tapered off stepwise with no more than one drug to be changed at a time in order to be able to evaluate their efficacy.

Appendix 1

Annex 1 - Organ Scoring of Chronic GVHD

	SCORE 0	SCORE 1	SCORE 2	SCORE 3
PERFORMANCE SCORE: **KPS ECOG LPS**	☐ Asymptomatic and fully active (ECOG 0; KPS or LPS 100%)	☐ Symptomatic, fully ambulatory, restricted only in physically strenuous activity (ECOG 1, KPS or LPS 80-90%)	☐ Symptomatic, ambulatory, capable of self-care, >50% of waking hours out of bed (ECOG 2, KPS or LPS 60-70%)	☐ Symptomatic, limited self-care, >50% of waking hours in bed (ECOG 3-4, KPS or LPS <60%)
SKIN† **SCORE %BSA**				
GVHD features to be scored by BSA: **Check all that applies:** ☐ Maculopapular rash/erythema ☐ Lichen planus-like features ☐ Sclerotic features ☐ Papulosquamous lesions or ichthyosis ☐ Keratosis pilaris-like GVHD	☐ No BSA involved	☐ 1-18% BSA	☐ 19-50% BSA	☐ >50% BSA
SKIN FEATURES SCORE:	☐ No sclerotic features		☐ **S**uperficial sclerotic features "not hidebound" (able to pinch)	**Check all that applies:** ☐ Deep sclerotic features ☐ "Hidebound" (unable to pinch) ☐ Impaired mobility ☐ Ulceration
Other skin GVHD features (NOT scored by BSA) **Check all that applies:** ☐ Hyperpigmentation ☐ Hypopigmentation ☐ Poikiloderma ☐ Severe or generalized pruritus ☐ Hair involvement ☐ Nail involvement				
☐ *Abnormality present but explained entirely by non-GVHD documented cause (specify):*				
MOUTH *Lichen planus-like features present:* ☐ **Yes** ☐ **No**	☐ No symptoms	☐ Mild symptoms **with** disease signs but not limiting oral intake significantly	☐ Moderate symptoms with disease signs **with** partial limitation of oral intake	☐ Severe symptoms with disease signs on examination **with** major limitation of oral intake
☐ *Abnormality present but explained entirely by non-GVHD documented cause (specify):*				

Annex 1 - Organ Scoring of Chronic GVHD (continued)

	SCORE 0	SCORE 1	SCORE 2	SCORE 3
EYES *Keratoconjunctivitis sicca (KCS) confirmed by Ophthalmologist:* ☐ **Yes** ☐ **No** ☐ **Not examined**	☐ No symptoms	☐ Mild dry eye symptoms not affecting ADL (requirement of lubricant eye drops ≤3 x per day)	☐ Moderate dry eye symptoms partially affecting ADL (requiring lubricant eye drops > 3 x per day or punctal plugs), **WITHOUT** new vision impairment due to KCS	☐ Severe dry eye symptoms significantly affecting ADL (special eyeware to relieve pain) **OR** unable to work because of ocular symptoms **OR** loss of vision due to KCS
☐ *Abnormality present but explained entirely by non-GVHD documented cause (specify):*				
GI TRACT ***Check all that applies:*** ☐ Esophageal web/ proximal stricture or ring ☐ Dysphagia ☐ Anorexia ☐ Nausea ☐ Vomiting ☐ Diarrhea ☐ Weight loss* ☐ Failure to thrive	☐ No symptoms	☐ Symptoms without significant weight loss* (<5%)	☐ Symptoms associated with mild to moderate weight loss* (5-15%) **OR** moderate diarrhea without significant interference of daily living	☐ Symptoms associated with significant weight loss* >15%, requires nutritional supplement for most calorie needs **OR** esophageal dilation **OR** severe diarrhea with significant interference of daily living
☐ *Abnormality present but explained entirely by non-GVHD documented cause (specify):*				
LIVER	☐ Normal total bilirubin and ALT or AP <3 x ULN	☐ Normal total bilirubin with ALT ≥3 to 5 x ULN or AP > 3 x ULN	☐ Elevated total bilirubin but ≤3 mg/dL or ALT > 5 ULN	☐ Elevated total bilirubin > 3 mg/dL
☐ *Abnormality present but explained entirely by non-GVHD documented cause (specify):*				
LUNGS** **Symptoms score**:	☐ No symptoms	☐ Mild symptoms (shortness of breath after climbing one flight of steps)	☐ Moderate symptoms (shortness of breath after walking on flat ground)	☐ Severe symptoms (shortness of breath at rest; requiring 0_2)
Lung score: FEV1 ☐	☐ FEV1≥80%	☐ FEV1 60-79	☐ FEV1 40-59%	☐ FEV1 ≤39%
Pulmonary function tests ☐ Not performed				
☐ *Abnormality present but explained entirely by non-GVHD documented cause (specify):*				

Annex 1. **Organ scoring of chronic GVHD (continued)**

	SCORE 0	SCORE 1	SCORE 2	SCORE 3
JOINTS AND FASCIA P-ROM score *(see below)* Shoulder (1-7): ___ Elbow (1-7): ____ Wrist/finger (1-7): ___ Ankle (1-4):___	☐ No symptoms	☐ Mild tightness of arms or legs, normal or mild decreased range of motion (ROM) **AND** not affecting ADL	☐ Tightness of arms or legs **OR** joint contractures, erythema thought due to fasciitis, moderate decrease ROM **AND** mild to moderate limitation of ADL	☐ Contractures **WITH** significant decrease of ROM ***AND*** significant limitation of ADL (unable to tie shoes, button shirts, dress self etc.)
☐ *Abnormality present but explained entirely by non-GVHD documented cause (specify):*				
GENITAL TRACT (*See Supplemental figure*‡) **Check all that applies** ☐ Not examined *Currently sexually active* ☐ Yes ☐ No	☐ No signs	☐ Mild signs‡ and females with or without discomfort on exam	☐ Moderate signs‡ and may have symptoms* with discomfort on exam	☐ Severe signs‡ with or without symptoms
☐ *Abnormality present but explained entirely by non-GVHD documented cause (specify):*				

Other indicators, clinical features or complications related to chronic GVHD (check all that apply and assign a score to its severity (0-3) based on its functional impact where applicable none –0,mild -1, moderate -2, severe –3)		
☐ Ascites (serositis)___	☐ Myasthenia Gravis___	
☐ Pericardial Effusion___	☐ Peripheral Neuropathy___	☐ Eosinophilia > 500µl___
☐ Pleural Effusion(s)___	☐ Polymyositis___	☐ Platelets <100,000/µl ___
☐ Nephrotic syndrome___	☐ Weight loss* without GI symptoms ___	☐ Others (specify):_______

Overall GVHD Severity *(Opinion of the evaluator)*	☐ **No GVHD**	☐ **Mild**	☐ **Moderate**	☐ **Severe**

Photographic Range of Motion (P-ROM)

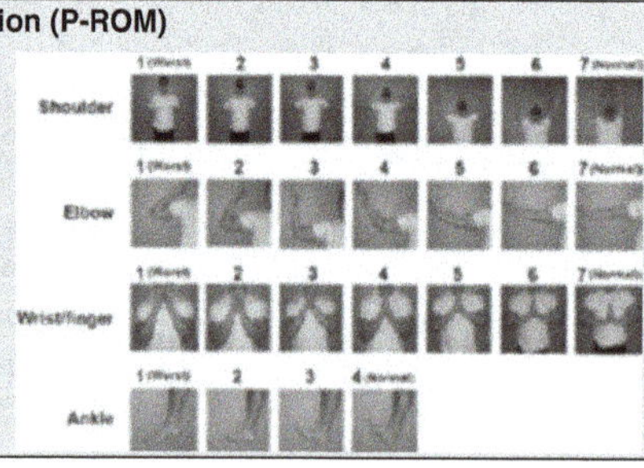

Adapted from Jagasia, 2015.

† Skin scoring should use both percentage of BSA involved by disease signs and the cutaneous features scales. When a discrepancy exists between the percentage of total body surface (BSA) score and the skin feature score, OR if superficial sclerotic features are present (Score 2), but there is impaired mobility or ulceration (Score 3), the higher level should be used for the final skin scoring.

* Weight loss within 3 months.

** Lung scoring should be performed using both the symptoms and FEV1 scores whenever possible. FEV1 should be used in the final lung scoring where there is discrepancy between symptoms and FEV1 scores.

Abbreviations: ECOG (Eastern Cooperative Oncology Group), KPS (Karnofsky Performance Status), LPS (Lansky Performance Status); BSA (body surface area); ADL (activities of daily living); LFTs (liver function tests); AP (alkaline phosphatase); ALT (alanine aminotransferase); NUL (normal upper limit).

‡ To be completed by specialist or trained medical providers (see Supplemental Figure).

Appendix 2

Diagnosis and staging cGVHD in children

Jagasia et al BBMT 2015
pediatric adaptation A. Lawitschka 11/2015

patient name

date:

patient name

►please score/check the worst manifestation
►diagnostic features are marked **bold**

classification:actual
□ feat. of acute GVHD
□ feat.of classic cGVHD
□ both

onset type ONLY at diagn.:
□ de novo
□ quiescent
□ progressive

symptoms/features	**Score 0**	**Score1**	**Score 2**	**Score 3**
KPS/LPS: %	□ asymptomatic and fully active (KPS/LPS 100%)	□ sympt., fully amb., restricted only in physically strenous activity (KPS/LPS 80-90%)	□ sympt., amb., capable of self-care, >50% of waking hours out of bed (KPS/LPS 60-70%)	□ sympt., limited self-care >50% of waking hours in bed (KPS/LPS < 60%)

SKIN

Feat. scored by BSA:	no BSA involved	1-18% BSA	19-50% BSA	> 50% BSA
□ maculopapular rash/erythema	□	□	□	□
□ **lichen planus-like features**	□	□	□	□
□ **sclerotic features:**	□	□	□	□
□ **lichen sclerosus-like**	□	□	□	□
□ **morphea-like**	□	□	□	□
□ papulosquamous lesions	□	□	□	□
□ ichthyosis	□	□	□	□
□ keratosis pilaris-like GVHD	□	□	□	□

Feat. not scored by BSA:
□ hyperpigmentation
□ hypopigmentation/ depigmentation
□ **poikiloderma**
□ severe pruritus
□ hair involvement
□ nail involvement
□ sweat impairment
□ abnormality present but explained entirely by non-GVHD cause (specify):

► feature decisive for diagnosis /scoring:

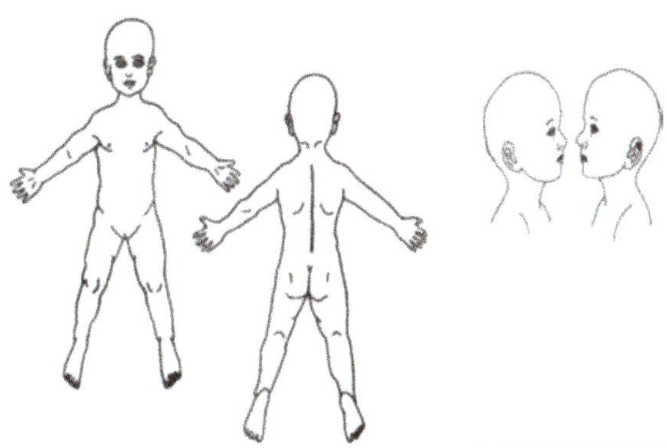

%BSA:
child: head front/back 9 / 9
back 18, chest 18,
arm left 9, arm right 9
leg left 13,5, leg right 13,5
adult: head front/back 4,5 / 4,5
back 18, chest 18
arm left 9, arm right 9
leg left 18, leg right 18
palm: 1,5

sclerotic features:	□ no sclerotic features		□ superficial sclerotic features "not hideboundʺ (able to pinch)	□ deep sclerotic features □ "hidebound" (unable to pinch) □ impaired mobility □ ulceration

MOUTH

□ erythema □ **lichen planus-like features** □ hyperkeratot. plaques □ mucoceles □ pseudomembranes □ ulcers □ mucosal atrophy □ dryness □ pain	□ no symptoms	□ mild sympt with disease signs but not limiting oral intake significantly	□ moderate sympt. with disease signs with partial limitation of oral intake	□ severe sympt. with disease signs on examination with major limitation of oral intake

□ abnormality present but explained entirely by non-GVHD cause (specify):

► feature decisive for diagnosis /scoring:

Appendix 2 - Diagnosis and staging cGVHD in children (continued)

symptoms/features	Score 0	Score1	Score 2	Score 3
EYES				
□ keratokonjunktivitis sicca (KCS) □ confirmed by opthalmologist □ dryness □ pain □ photophobia □ blepharitis □ pseudomembranes □ ulcers	□ no symptoms	□ mild dry eye sympt. not affecting ADL (requirement of lubricant eye drops ≤ 3 x per day)	□ moderate dry eye sympt. partially affecting ADL (lubricant eye drops >3 x/d or punctual plugs) without new vision impairement due to KCS	□ severe dry eye sympt. significantly affecting ADL (special eyeware to relieve pain) or unable to work because of ocular sympt or loss of vision due to KCS
□ abnormality present but explained entirely by non-GVHD cause (specify): ▸ feature decisive for diagnosis /scoring:				
GI TRACT				
□ **esophageal web/ prox stricture or ring** □ dysphagia □ abdominal pain □ anorexia □ failure to thrive □ nausea □ vomiting □ diarrhea □ weight loss ≥ 5%	□ no symptoms	□ symptoms without significant weight loss (5%)	□ sympt. associated with mild to moderate weight loss (5-15%) or moderate diarrhea without significant interference with daily living	□ symptoms associated with significant weight loss (> 15%) requires nutritional supplement for most calorie needs or esophageal dilatation or severe diarrhea with signif. Interference with daily living
□ abnormality present but explained entirely by non-GVHD cause (specify): ▸ feature decisive for diagnosis /scoring:				height: weight:
LIVER				
□ hepatic pattern **Bili:** _____ AST:_____ **ALT:** _____ GGT: _____ AP: _____	□ normal total bili and ALT or AP < 3 ULN	□ normal total bili with ALT ≥ 3-5x ULN or AP ≥ 3 x ULN	□ elevated total bili but ≤ 3 mg/dl or ALT > 5 ULN	□ elevated total bili > 3 mg/dl
□ abnormality present but explained entirely by non-GVHD cause (specify): ▸ feature decisive for diagnosis /scoring:				
LUNGS				
FEV1: _____ % MEF25:_____ % FVC: _____ % MEF50:_____ % DLCO: _____ % MEF75:_____ % RV: _____ □ RV/TLC > 120% CT:	□ no symptoms FEV1 ≥ 80%	□ mild symptoms (shortness of breath after climbing one flight of steps) FEV1 60-79%	□ moderate symptoms (shortness of breath after walking on flat ground) FEV1 40-59%	□ severe symptoms (shortness of breath at rest; requiring O2) FEV1 ≤ 39%
□ abnormality present but explained entirely by non-GVHD cause (specify): ▸ feature decisive for diagnosis /scoring:				
JOINTS AND FASCIA				
ped P-ROM score (see below) □ edema □ fasciitis □ muscle cramps □ athralgia	□ no symptoms	□ mild tightness, normal or mild ↓ of range of motion (ROM) not affecting ADL	□ tightness or joint contractures, fasciitis, moderate ↓ of ROM, mild - moderate ↓ of ADL	□ contractures, fasciitis significant ↓ of ROM, significant ↓ of ADL
□ abnormality present but explained entirely by non-GVHD cause (specify): ▸ feature decisive for diagnosis /scoring:				
GENITAL TRACT				
□ erosions, fissures □ **lichen planus-like features** □ **lichen sclerosus-like features** □ **labial/ vaginal scarring** □ **phimosis**	□ no signs	□ mild signs	□ moderate signs	□ severe signs with or without symptoms
□ abnormality present but explained entirely by non-GVHD cause (specify): ▸ feature decisive for diagnosis /scoring:				

Overall GVHD severity

□ no cGVHD

□ mild: max. score of 1 in any affected organ, max. 2 organs affected, no lung involvement

□ moderate: ≥3 organ with max score 1 or max. score of 2 in any affected organ, lung score max 1

□ severe: score 3 in any affected organ, lung score 2-3

Appendix 2 - Diagnosis and staging cGVHD in children (continued)

Other indicators, clinical features or complications related to cGVHD			**biopsy:**
check all that apply and assign a severity score (0-3) based on functional impact			organ:
☐ ascites (serositis)	☐ myasthenia gravis	☐ eosinophilia >500 /ul	GVHD confirmed?
☐ pericardial effusion	☐ peripheral neuropathy	☐ platelets <100 000/ul	
☐ pleural effusion	☐ polymyositis	☐ hypo/hyperglobulinemia	
☐ nephrotic syndrome	☐ weight loss >5% without GI sympt	☐ auto-antibodies	
☐ others (specify)	☐ diabetes		

pediatric photographic range of motion (adapted ped P-ROM):

please mark appropriate number >

shoulder: 1 (worst) 2 3 4 5 (normal)

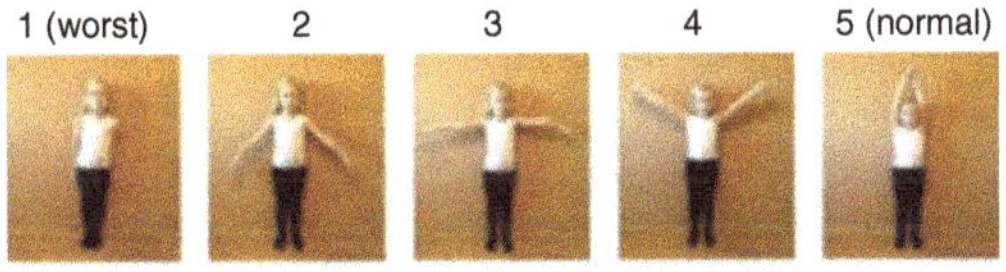

ellbow: 1 (worst) 2 3 4 (normal)

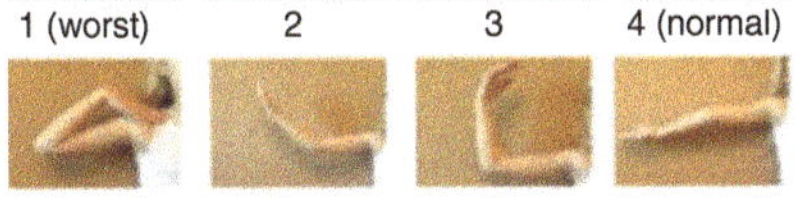

wrist / finger: 1 (worst) 2 3 4 (normal)

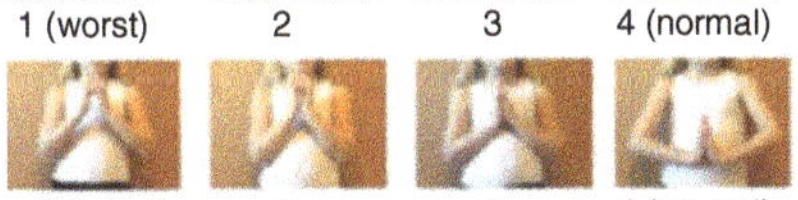

global flexion: 1 (worst) 2 3 4 (normal)

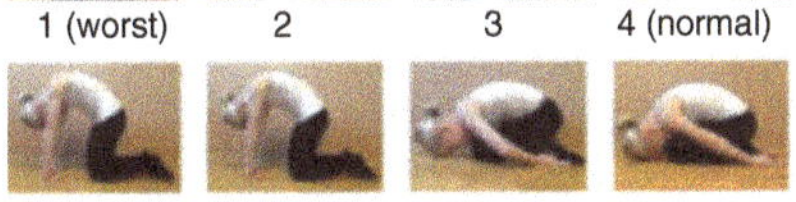

ankle: 1 (worst) 2 3 (normal)

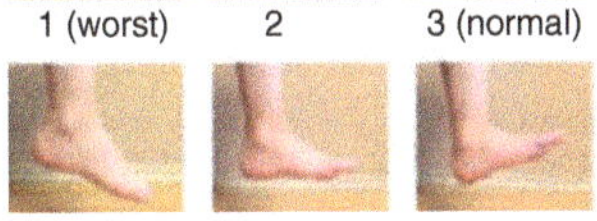

Appendix 3

Genital Tract GVHD Assessment and Scoring Form

Name:__________________________________ **Date of birth:** ________________

Assessment date: ____________

	SCORE 0	SCORE 1	SCORE 2	SCORE 3
GENITAL TRACT (male or female)	☐ No signs	☐ Mild signs and females may have symptoms* WITH discomfort on exam	☐ Moderate signs and may have symptoms* with discomfort on exam	☐ Severe signs with or without symptoms*

Currently sexually active:

☐ Yes ☐ No

Check all signs that applies:

☐ Lichen planus -like features
☐ Lichen sclerosis-like features
☐ Vaginal scarring (female)
☐ Clitoral/labial agglutination (female)
☐ Labial resorption (female)
☐ Erosions
☐ Fissures
☐ Ulcers
☐ Phimosis (male)
☐ Urethral meatusscarring/ stenosis (male)

☐ *Abnormality present but NOTthought to represent GVHD (specify cause):*

____

☐ *Abnormality thought to represent GVHD PLUSother causes(specify cause):*

____

* *Genital symptoms are not specific to cGVHD and can represent premature gonadal failure or genital tract infection.*

If a gynecologist is unavailable, external examination may be performed to determine "discomfort on exam" as follows:

a) Spread the labia majora to inspect the vulva for the above signs. Touch the vestibular gland openings (Skene's and Bartholin's), labia minora and majora gently with a qtip. Vulvar pain elicited by the gentle touch of a qtip is classified as discomfort on examination. Palpate the vaginal walls with a single digit to detect bands, shortening, narrowing or other signs of vaginal scarring.

b) If the woman is sexually active, determine whether qtip palpation or gentle palpation of scarred ridges elicits pain similar to that which the woman experiences during intercourse.

Female genitalia: Severity of signs:

1) Mild (any of the following); erythema on vulvar mucosal surfaces, vulvar lichen-planus or vulvar lichen-sclerosis.

2) Moderate (any of the following); erosive inflammatory changes of the vulvar mucosa, fissures in vulvar folds.

3) Severe (any of the following); labial fusion, clitoral hood agglutination, fibrinous vaginal adhesions, circumferential fibrous vaginal banding, vaginal shortening, synechia, dense sclerotic changes, and complete vaginal stenosis.

Male genitalia: Diagnostic features include lichen planus-like or lichen sclerosis-like features and phymosis or urethral scarring or stenosis. Severity of signs:

1) Mild: lichen planus-like feature;

2) Moderate: lichen sclerosis-like feature or moderate erythema;

3) Severe: phimosis or urethral/meatal scarring.

Biopsy obtained: ☐ **Yes** ☐ **No** **Site biopsied:**________	**GVHD confirmed by histology:** ☐ **Yes** ☐ **No**
Change from previous evaluation: ☐ **No prior or current GVHD**	☐ **Improved** ☐ **Stable** ☐ **Worse** ☐ **N/A (baseline)**

Completed by (spell out name): ______________________________

Date form completed: ______________

References

Arai S, Arora M, Wang T, et al. Increasing incidence of chronic graft-versus-host disease in allogeneic transplantation: a report from the Center for International Blood and Marrow Transplant Research. Biol Blood Marrow Transplant. 2015;21:266–74.

Baird K, Cooke K, Schultz KR. Chronic graft-versus-host disease (GVHD) in children. Pediatr Clin N Am. 2010;57:297–322.

Carpenter PA, Kitko CL, Elad S, et al. National Institutes of Health Consensus Development Project on criteria for clinical trials in chronic graft-versus-host disease: V. The 2014 Ancillary Therapy and Supportive Care Working Group Report. Biol Blood Marrow Transplant. 2015;21:1167–87.

Cooke KR, Luznik L, Sarantopoulos S, et al. The biology of chronic graft-versus-host disease: A Task Force Report from the National Institutes of Health Consensus Development Project on criteria for clinical trials in chronic graft-versus-host disease. Biol Blood Marrow Transplant. 2017;23:211–34.

Grube M, Holler E, Weber D, et al. Risk factors and outcome of chronic graft-versus-host disease after allogeneic stem cell transplantation-results from a single-center observational study. Biol Blood Marrow Transplant. 2016;22:1781–91.

Hildebrandt GC, Fazekas T, Lawitschka A, et al. Diagnosis and treatment of pulmonary chronic GVHD: report from the consensus conference on clinical practice in chronic GVHD. Bone Marrow Transplant. 2011;46:1283–95.

Hilgendorf I, Freund M, Jilg W, et al. Vaccination of allogeneic haematopoietic stem cell transplant recipients: report from the international consensus conference on clinical practice in chronic GVHD. Vaccine. 2011;29:2825–33.

Jacobsohn DA. Optimal management of chronic graft-versus-host disease in children. Br J Haematol. 2010;150:278–92.

Jagasia MH, Greinix HT, Arora M, et al. National Institutes of Health Consensus Development Project on Criteria for Clinical Trials in Chronic Graft-versus-Host Disease: I. The 2014 Diagnosis and Staging Working Group report. National Institutes of Health Consensus Development Project on Criteria for Clinical Trials in Chronic Graft-versus-Host Disease: I. Biol Blood Marrow Transplant. 2015;21:389.e1–401.e1.

Kuzmina Z, Eder S, Bohm A, et al. Significantly worse survival of patients with NIH-defined chronic graft-versus-host disease and thrombocytopenia or progressive onset type: results of a prospective study. Leukemia. 2012;26:746–56.

Ruutu T, Juvonen E, Remberger M, et al. Improved survival with ursodeoxycholic acid prophylaxis in allogeneic stem cell transplantation: long-term follow-up of a randomized study. Biol Blood Marrow Transplant. 2014;20:135–8.

Stift J, Baba HA, Huber E, et al. Consensus on the histo pathological evaluation of liver biopsies from patients following allogeneic hematopoietic cell transplantation. Virchows Arch. 2014;464:175–90.

Strong Rodrigues K, Oliveira-Ribeiro C, de Abreu Fiuza Gomes S, Knobler R. Cutaneous graft-versus-host disease: diagnosis and treatment. Am J Clin Dermatol. 2018;19:33–50.

Wolff D, Bertz H, Greinix H, et al. The treatment of chronic graft-versus-host disease: consensus recommendations of experts from Germany, Austria, and Switzerland. Dtsch Arztebl Int. 2011;108:732–40.

45 Post transplant Lymphoproliferative Syndromes

Jan Styczynski and Sebastian Giebel

45.1 Definitions

Post transplant lymphoproliferative disorders (PTLDs) constitute a heterogeneous group of lymphoproliferative diseases that occur in the setting of transplantation and result from the uncontrolled neoplastic proliferation of lymphoid or plasmacytic cells in the context of extrinsic immunosuppression after transplantation.

PTLD in HSCT setting are largely caused by latent Epstein-Barr virus (EBV, HHV-4), belonging to the herpesviruses family. It is one of the most common viruses in humans, with prevalence of 82–84% in overall population. EBV is associated with development of various diseases, which can be categorized as primary syndromes, EBV-associated tumors, and EBV-associated post transplant diseases: PTLD and other end-organ diseases (encephalitis/myelitis, pneumonitis, hepatitis, or hemophagocytic lymphohistiocytosis).

Comparably to other herpesviruses, there are two types of EBV infection: primary and recurrent. Primary EBV infection is diagnosed when EBV is detected (nucleic acid or serologically) in an EBV-naïve individual. Recurrent EBV-DNA-emia (previously: latent infection) is diagnosed by detection of EBV-DNA in the blood, in a previously infected individual.

45.2 Types of PTLD

PTLD or end-organ EBV-associated post transplant disease can be diagnosed at the probable or proven level. Probable EBV disease is diagnosed in case of significant lymphadenopathy, hepatosplenomegaly, or other end-organ manifestations (without tissue biopsy, but in the absence of other documented cause) together with high EBV-DNA-emia. Proven EBV disease (PTLD or other end-organ disease) is diagnosed in case of symptoms and/or signs from the affected organ together with the detection of EBV-encoded RNA by in situ hybridization (EBER-ISH) in a tissue specimen (immunohistochemistry for EBV proteins have good specificity but lower sensitivity; these proteins are variably expressed in PTLD biopsies). Histological WHO 2016 classification includes six types of morphological PTLD: plasmacytic hyperplasia, infectious mononucleosis-like, florid follicular hyperplasia, polymorphic, monomorphic (B-cell or T-/NK-cell types), and classical Hodgkin lymphoma PTLD.

J. Styczynski (✉)
Department of Pediatric Hematology and Oncology, Nicolaus Copernicus University Torun, Collegium Medicum, Bydgoszcz, Poland
e-mail: jstyczynski@cm.umk.pl

S. Giebel
Department of Bone Marrow Transplantation and Onco-Hematology, Maria Sklodowska-Curie Memorial Cancer Center and Institute of Oncology, Gliwice, Poland

E. Carreras et al. (eds.), *The EBMT Handbook*, https://doi.org/10.1007/978-3-030-02278-5_45

Atypical PTLD:

- EBV-negative PTLD: A growing number of cases of EBV-negative PTLD have been reported, mainly in SOT recipients. These cases tend to present later (>5 years after transplant) after transplant, and an increased risk is observed as long as 10 years after transplantation. These cases should be regarded as malignant lymphoma rather than as PTLD.
- T-lineage PTLD: T-PTLD is usually EBV-negative, and the relatively long latency between transplantation and T-PTLD onset may be explained by molecular events. The frequency of T-PTLDs ranges 4–15% of all PTLD cases. EBV is present in approximately one-third of T-PTLDs.
- Composite B-cell and T-cell lineage PTLD: Harboring both B- and T-cell clones either concurrently or successively in the same patient is extremely rare, and only a few cases have been reported in the literature, exclusively after SOT, with poor outcome.

45.3 Pathogenesis

The pathogenesis of PTLDs is a result of EBV-induced transformation of B cells in the setting of impaired anti-EBV cellular immunity due to iatrogenic IS and resulting in an outgrowth of EBV-infected B cells. GVHD prevention strategies that indiscriminately remove T cells from the graft increase the risk of PTLD.

Recurrent EBV infection preceding clinically overt PTLD is the consequence of viral latency, which is the stage in the viral life cycle in which no virions are produced, as opposed to the lytic stage. During viral latency of EBV, three associated patterns of viral protein expression, so-called latency programs, may be expressed. During infection of the B cell, these latency programs guide the B cell through the germinal center reaction pushing it toward the resting memory cell stage. Different latency proteins are implicated in EBV-driven lymphomagenesis demonstrated by the expression of a particular latency program in different lymphoma subtypes.

B cells in PTLD express a number of latency proteins which are highly immunogenic and are vigorously targeted by T lymphocytes in immunocompetent hosts. This viral gene program in EBV-PTLD is called type III of latency and is different and less immunogenic than in other EBV-related diseases with type I or II of latency.

EBV plays also an important role in pathogenesis and epidemiology of acute and chronic GVHD. As B cells also play a role in the pathophysiology of chronic GVHD, and B cells are stimulated into activity by EBV infection, and B-cell recovery occurs usually after day +100, the impact of EBV-infected B cells is stronger for development of chronic, and to less extent, acute GVHD.

45.4 Clinical Manifestations

Lymphadenopathy and fever are the most common symptoms of EBV-PTLD. Rare EBV-associated PTLD manifestations, also referred as EBV end-organ disease, include encephalitis/myelitis, pneumonitis, hepatitis, and hemophagocytic lymphohistiocytosis.

Time to PTLD	Median time of PTLD development: 2–4 months 6% PTLD cases are diagnosed within first month 90% diagnosed within first 6 months after HSCT Rarely: >5 year post-HSCT (more likely representing lymphoma)
Incidence of EBV-DNA-emia	Median: 29.4% (range: 0.1–63%) Highest in: MUD/MMUD-HSCT, haplo-HSCT without PTCy Lowest in: haplo-HSCT with PTCy (post-HSCT Cy)
Incidence of PTLD	All allo-HSCT: 3.22% MFD-HSCT: 1.16% MMFD-HSCT: 2.86% MUD-HSCT[a]: 3.97% MMUD-HSCT: 11.24% CBT: 4.06% Auto-HSCT without TCD: casuistic
Target organs	Frequently: lymph nodes Rarely: CNS, GI tract, lungs, liver

[a]Level of donor match determined locally as 8/8 or 10/10

45.5 Diagnosis

The diagnosis of EBV-PTLD must be based on symptoms and/or signs consistent with PTLD together with detection of EBV by an appropriate method applied to a specimen from the involved tissue. Definitive diagnosis of EBV-PTLD requires noninvasive and invasive techniques (biopsy and histological examination).

Noninvasive diagnostic methods

Quantitative determination of EBV-DNA-emia[a]

Imaging: CT or PET-CT[b] (for avid structures, localized in the lymph nodes, spleen, liver, GI tract, skin, lungs, bone, BM) or MRI (in CNS disease and non-avid histologies)

Invasive diagnostic methods

Biopsy of the lymph node and/or other suspected sites

Endoscopy: when GI symptoms

Histological examination

(a) Detection of viral antigens or in situ hybridization for EBER (EBV-encoded RNA) transcripts

(b) Immunohistochemistry

(c) Flow cytometry for B cell, T cell, and plasma cell lineage-specific antigens

[a]Monitoring EBV-DNA-emia: Serial quantitative measurement of EBV viral load post transplant is currently the method of choice for early detection and monitoring progression and response to treatment of EBV-PTLD. Although the value of the viral load in PTLD risk assessment is uncertain, it is recommended to begin the screening in patients with risk factors after hematological recovery and no later than 4 weeks after the day of HSCT. In EBV-DNA-negative patients, frequency of screening should be once a week, while in patients with rising EBV-DNA-emia, more frequent sampling might be considered, as the calculated doubling time for EBV might be as short as 56 h. The screening should be continued at least 4 months in high-risk patients. Longer monitoring is recommended in patients considered to have poor T-cell reconstitution, with severe GVHD, after haplo-HSCT, with the use of TCD, after conditioning with ATG/alemtuzumab, or in those having experienced an early EBV reactivation

[b]PET imaging: By definition, PTLD is a neoplastic lymphoproliferation. Malignant lymphomas have the ability to metabolize 18F-fluorodeoxyglucose (FDG), which is used by PET imaging. In most cases, PTLD has FDG-avid histology; thus FDG-PET is an important diagnostic tool for this disease

45.6 Risk Factors

Risk of development of PTLD is essentially proportional to the degree of T-cell depletion/impairment, and this should be regarded as the principal risk factor. Thus, the type of donor and type of conditioning have secondary value as risk factors. Since in HSCT setting PTLD usually originates from donor, the risk of PTLD is obviously higher when the donor is seropositive. Risk factors for PTLD in match family donor (MFD) transplants include TCD ex vivo or in vivo, EBV serology mismatch between donor and recipient, and splenectomy. ECIL-6 classified HSCT patients into three groups of the risk for EBV-PTLD: low, standard, and high risk.

Risk group	Patients
High	MUD/MMUD
	Alternative donors including CBT
	MFD-HSCT with at least one risk factor
Standard	MFD-HSCT without risk factors
	Haplo-PTCy-HSCT
Low	Auto-HSCT

45.7 Grading

No grading system currently exists for PTLD. It seems that apart from the findings from biopsy material with a histological examination; the diagnostic criteria of tissue involvement in PTLD should be consistent with those for lymphoma (the Ann Arbor and the Lugano classifications). Nowadays, the use of FDG-PET-CT has emerged as an important imaging tool for PTLD diagnosis and staging.

Possible staging of PTLD:

- Clinical end-organ staging: nodal vs. extranodal disease
- Clinical severity staging: limited (unifocal) vs. advanced (multifocal) disease
- ECIL-6 staging (based on the Lugano lymphoma classification by PET-CT imaging): limited (stages I–II), advanced forms (stages III–IV)

45.8 Treatment

45.8.1 Prevention: Donor and Recipient Issues

As EBV might be transmitted with the graft, selection of EBV-seronegative donor might be beneficial for EBV-seronegative recipient, if possible. For EBV-seropositive patients, selection of an EBV-seropositive donor might be justified, as transmission of EBV-specific CTLs outweighs the risk of transmission of EBV-positive B cells from the donor.

45.8.2 Treatment Strategies

PTLD has to be regarded as disseminated disease at diagnosis. This is because of the involvement of lymphoid tissue, which is localized throughout the whole body. Therapeutic approaches applied in the prevention and treatment of EBV-PTLD include administration of RTX, reduction of immunosuppression (RIS), use of EBV-CTL, DLI, and chemotherapy, while other methods have only historical value. No antiviral drug is currently effective against EBV. There are three major approaches to EBV infection after HSCT: *prophylaxis*, *preemptive therapy* (also known as preemptive prophylaxis), and *treatment* of established EBV-PTLD.

45.8.2.1 Prophylaxis

Prophylaxis of EBV disease is defined as drug or cellular therapy given to an asymptomatic EBV-seropositive patient to prevent EBV-DNA-emia. This strategy is administered rarely, with the use of rituximab (RTX) or EBV-CTL.

The rationale for prophylactic use of RTX before or early after allo-HSCT is B-cell depletion. Prophylactic use of post transplant RTX reduced the risk of EBV-DNA-emia, with no impact on PTLD incidence, TRM, or OS in comparison to preemptive therapy.

The prophylactic use of EBV-CTLs resulted in excellent efficacy in patients at a high-risk group for EBV-PTLD. The obstacle for the use of this approach is limited availability of CTLs for most transplant centers.

Low risk of EBV-DNA-emia and EBV-PTLD was observed after the use of PT-CY and SIR for GVHD prophylaxis.

45.8.2.2 Preemptive Therapy

Drugs or cellular therapy is given to a patient with EBV-DNA-emia in order to prevent EBV disease.

Monitoring for EBV-DNA-emia is essential in all patients with risk factors for EBV-PTLD. Significant EBV-DNA-emia without clinical symptoms of disease in high-risk patients for EBV-PTLD is usually an indication for preemptive therapy.

The goal is to obtain a negative EBV PCR or EBV-DNA-emia below the initial threshold without relapse.

Usually, EBV-DNA-emia occurs prior to the onset of clinical symptoms. There is a correlation between rising or high EBV-DNA-emia in PB and the development of EBV-PTLD, but this is not the rule.

Currently available data does not allow for the determination of an unambiguous EBV-DNA threshold value for the diagnosis of EBV-PTLD or other end-organ EBV disease in HSCT patients.

Apart from EBV-DNA value, also the kinetics of a rising EBV-DNA-emia, together with an assessment of an individual patient's immune function, are very important when appraising the need for preemptive therapy. Local experience based on correlation of clinical and laboratory data might be a rationale for center-specific cut-off value.

The primary method for preemptive therapy includes RTX, once weekly until EBV-DNA-emia negativity. Usually, 1–2 doses of RTX are sufficient. RTX should be combined with reduction of the IS (RIS), if possible. A contraindication for RIS is severe, uncontrolled acute, or chronic GVHD. This approach might have additional benefit of RTX administration, as RTX possibly reduces the risk of acute/chronic GVHD. Donor or third-party EBV-CTL is another option, although it is not widely available.

45.8.2.3 Treatment of Established EBV-PTLD

Treatment of established EBV-PTLD means therapeutic interventions for patients with probable or proven EBV disease. Due to the consequential risk of a rapidly growing high-grade lymphoid tumor, together with the potential for EBV to cause rapid MOF, therapy should be implemented as soon as possible.

For first-line therapy, three options are recommended: (a) RTX, 375 mg/m^2, once weekly; (b) RIS, if possible, usually together with administration of RTX; (c) adoptive immunotherapy with cellular therapy with in vitro generated donor or third-party EBV-CTL, if available.

For the second-line therapy, in case of RTX failure: (a) cellular therapy (non-specific DLI or specific EBV-CTLs, if available); (b) chemotherapy ± RTX. Unselected DLI from EBV-positive donor is used in order to restore broad T-cell reactivity, including EBV-specific responses.

Not recommended: IVIg, interferon, and antiviral agents should not be used for therapy of PTLD.

45.8.3 Results of Anti-EBV-PTLD Therapy

Treatment strategy	Preemptive therapy (%)	Therapy of PTLD (%)
RTX	90	65
RTX + RIS		78
EBV-CTL	94–100	71–75
RIS	68	61
DLI		58[a]
Chemotherapy		26[a]
Antivirals (cidofovir)		34[a]

RTX rituximab, *RIS* reduction of immunosuppression
[a]With other therapies

45.8.4 Treatment in CNS Disease

CNS localization of PTLD is a special form of the disease, due to the risk of neurological consequences even in case of successful eradication of EBV from CNS. No standard therapy has been accepted up to date.

Possible therapeutic options include (a) RTX, either systemic or intrathecal; in the latter case, dose of RTX was 10–30 mg in 3–10 mL saline administered weekly; (b) T-cell therapy with EBV-CTLs; (c) radiotherapy; (d) chemotherapy ± RTX according to primary CNS lymphoma protocols based on high dose of MTX ± Ara-C.

45.8.5 Criteria of Response to Therapy in EBV-PTLD

The treatment goal in EBV-PTLD setting is the resolution of all signs and symptoms of PTLD together with negative EBV-DNA-emia.

The response to RTX therapy can be identified by a decrease in EBV-DNA-emia of at least 1 log of magnitude in the first week of treatment.

Positive prognostic factors for outcome to RTX therapy include age below 30 years, underlying non-malignant disease, no acute GVHD ≥II, RIS at time of PTLD diagnosis, and decrease of viral load after 1 or 2 weeks of therapy.

Complete remission of PTLD can be defined as resolution of all symptoms of PTLD, including clearance of EBV-DNA-emia. Partial response of PTLD can be stated with the decrease of at least 50% of initial changes, including decrease of EBV-DNA-emia.

The response to therapy can be confirmed by achievement of a PET-negative complete remission for avid lymphomas and CT/MRI for non-avid histologies or CNS localization.

Key Points

- Definition: PTLD results from an uncontrolled neoplastic proliferation of lymphoid or plasmacytic cells in the context of extrinsic IS after HSCT transplantation. PTLDs in HSCT setting are largely caused by latent EBV. Risk factors for EBV-PTLD are proportional to the degree of T-cell impairment.
- Diagnosis: Should be based on invasive techniques including biopsy of the lymph node and/or other sites suspected for EBV disease. Noninvasive diagnostic methods have accessory value and include the quantitative determination of EBV-DNA-emia in blood, plasma or serum, and PET-CT/CT/MRI.
- Management strategies: Prophylaxis, preemptive treatment, and therapy of established EBV-PTLD. Therapeutic

approaches include administration of rituximab, RIS, use of EBV-CTL, or DLI and chemotherapy, while other methods have only a historical value.

- EBV-DNA-emia threshold value: No value determines diagnosis of EBV-PTLD or other end-organ EBV disease in HSCT patients. In order to initiate preemptive therapy, transplant centers should use own threshold values of EBV-DNA-emia.
- Outcome: Administration of rituximab results in a positive outcome for over 90% of patients treated preemptively and over 65% when it is used as targeted therapy for EBV-PTLD. RIS when applied in combination with rituximab: over 80%. The use of EBV-CTLs: >90% of patients treated preemptively and approximately 75% in therapy of EBV-PTLD.

Recommended References

Bollard CM, Heslop HE. T cells for viral infections after allogeneic hematopoietic stem cell transplant. Blood. 2016;127:3331–40.

Czyzewski K, Styczynski J, Krenska A, et al. Intrathecal therapy with rituximab in central nervous system involvement of post-transplant lymphoproliferative disorder. Leuk Lymphoma. 2013;54:503–6.

Dharnidharka VR, Webster AC, Martinez OM, et al. Post-transplant lymphoproliferative disorders. Nat Rev Dis Primers. 2016;2:15088.

Dierickx D, Habermann TM. Post-transplantation lymphoproliferative disorders in adults. N Engl J Med. 2018;378:549–62.

Dierickx D, Tousseyn T, Requile A, et al. The accuracy of positron emission tomography in the detection of posttransplant lymphoproliferative disorder. Haematologica. 2013;98:771–5.

Styczynski J. Managing post-transplant lymphoproliferative disorder. Expert Opin Orphan Drugs. 2017;5:19–35.

Styczynski J, Gil L, Tridello G, et al. Response to rituximab-based therapy and risk factor analysis in EBV-related lymphoproliferative disorders after hematopoietic stem cell transplantation in children and adults: a study from the Infectious Diseases Working Party of the European Group for Blood and Marrow Transplantation. Clin Infect Dis. 2013;57: 794–802.

Styczynski J, Tridello G, Gil L, et al. Impact of donor Epstein-Barr virus serostatus on the incidence of graft-versus-host disease in patients with acute leukemia after hematopoietic stem-cell transplantation: A study from the Acute Leukemia and Infectious Diseases Working Parties of the European Society for Blood and Marrow Transplantation. J Clin Oncol. 2016a;34:2212–20.

Styczynski J, van der Velden W, Fox CP, et al. Management of Epstein-Barr Virus infections and post-transplant lymphoproliferative disorders in patients after allogeneic hematopoietic stem cell transplantation: Sixth European Conference on Infections in Leukemia (ECIL-6) guidelines. Haematologica. 2016b;101:803–11.

Uhlin M, Wikell H, Sundin M, et al. Risk factors for Epstein-Barr virus-related post-transplant lymphoproliferative disease after allogeneic hematopoietic stem cell transplantation. Haematologica. 2014;99:346–52.

46 Iron Overload

Emanuele Angelucci

46.1 Introduction

Iron overload/toxicity is an unavoidable consequence in several diseases characterized by anemia and red blood cell transfusion requirement.

Our knowledge of iron pathophysiology has much improved during the last two decades, and we now recognize that iron damage is related not only to iron level "per se" but to the presence in the serum of non-transferrin forms of iron (non-transferrin bound iron = NTBI). A component of NTBI, called labile plasma iron (LPI), is a potent redox-active agent capable of permeating into cells in an uncontrolled way, thus inducing cellular iron overload and impacts the delicate equilibrium of labile cellular iron (LCI). The breakage of LCI balance catalyzes the formation of reactive oxygen species (ROS), which leads to cytotoxic cell injury (DNA damage, lipid peroxidation, protein modification, and mitochondrial damage). Iron toxicity depends on many factors in addition to the iron level: the quantity of the abovementioned toxic iron-related species, duration of exposure, individual's antioxidant genetics, and environmental factors (Coates 2014). Notably NTBI and LPI appear in the serum only when transferrin saturation exceeds 60–70% (de Swart et al. 2016) and are cheatable forms of iron.

E. Angelucci (✉)
Department of Oncology and Hematology, IRCCS Ospedale Policlinico San Martino, Genova, Italy
e-mail: emnang@tin.it

NTBI and LPI are direct markers of ongoing cellular iron accumulation and tissue damage. Their measurement is today available in selected laboratories for research purposes only. A standardization program is ongoing (de Swart et al. 2016), and hopefully NTBI and LPI assays will be available in the next future for clinical use. Transferrin saturation is at the moment a valid surrogate indicating, when exceeding 60–70%, presence of NTBI /LPI in patient serum.

Here will be discussed the impact of iron toxicity on HSCT outcome and therapeutic options (Angelucci and Pilo 2016). This chapter will be divided in three sections with the following meanings:

- *Before transplant*: any time before the starting of the conditioning regimen
- *During transplant*: from the start of conditioning regimen up to a sustained engraftment is achieved
- *After transplant*: after sustained engraftment has been achieved

46.2 Iron Overload Before HSCT (Before the Start of Conditioning)

In thalassemia it has been very well demonstrated that HSCT outcome is significantly impacted by a story of irregular chelation, presence of liver fibrosis, and hepatomegaly (Angelucci 2010).

E. Carreras et al. (eds.), *The EBMT Handbook*, https://doi.org/10.1007/978-3-030-02278-5_46

Now we can recognize that all the three risk factors are related to intensity and duration of tissue exposition to the abovementioned iron toxic-related species (Angelucci et al. 2017).

Therefore, any effort should be made to regularly suppress NTBI/LPI in the years before transplant to prevent tissue damage. This target can be achieved with early, regular, and consistent iron chelation. Thus, in any patient receiving transfusion therapy who may have an HSCT in the future, the decision starting chelation is critical and should be undertaken as soon as possible. Moreover, chelation must regular long life.

Limited data are available on the rationale for intensive pre-HSCT chelation therapy unless sufficient time is available to correct iron overload and warrant tissue lesions repair.

46.3 Iron Overload During HSCT (From the Start of Conditioning Up to Sustained Engraftment)

During conditioning regimen, a huge amount of NTBI and LPI enter the circulation due to massive erythroid marrow lysis (Dürken et al. 1997). Moreover, until the erythroid recovery begins, no iron can be released by transferrin to the erythroid system. Once erythroid recovery initiates transferrin-iron is greedily captured by the erythroid system and unbound transferrin able to receive iron from reticular endothelial system and, to a mush less extent, from storages appears in the serum. Non-transferrin-iron is uptaken by erythroid cells but is not utilized for hemoglobin synthesis (Prus and Fibach 2011).

Recent transplant animal studies demonstrated that iron toxicity could impair the hematopoietic niche by damaging hematopoietic stem cells' self-renewal potential, proliferation, differentiation, and the marrow microenvironment (Pilo and Angelucci 2018). These data suggest that iron can impact the HSC engraftment, the hemopoietic recovery, and possibly transplant outcome. From a clinical point of view, limited evidence is available. Visani and colleagues demonstrated, in an uncontrolled study, that in cases of poor and delayed engraftment, iron chelation can help in stabilizing hemopoietic engraftment (Visani et al. 2014).

Inclusion of chelation therapy during the transplant phase to suppress NTBI/LPI should be considered an experimental treatment; however, in case of slow, delayed, or incomplete marrow recovery and high transferrin saturation, chelation should be considered.

46.4 Iron Overload After HSCT (After Sustained Engraftment Has Been Achieved)

After successful transplantation, patients are usually free from transfusion support but affected by the already acquired iron overload that cannot be eliminated without active intervention. In this condition the already acquired intracellular iron overload continues to disrupt the delicate LCI equilibrium and promotes ROS generation. It has been prospectively demonstrated in transplanted thalassemia patients that elevated transferrin saturation persists indefinitely without treatment and liver disease progresses even in the absence of other comorbidities (Angelucci et al. 2002). Of course the deleterious effect can be worsened by presence of comorbidities even with low level of iron accumulation (Angelucci et al. 2002).

Therefore, even because of the results of epidemiologic studies in thalassemia (Coates et al. 2016; Puliyel et al. 2015) and in the normal population (Ellervik et al. 2011) in the post transplant setting, the target iron level should be a normal iron level. Normal transferrin saturation excluding the presence of toxic iron-reactive species should be the target level of post transplant iron removal.

Because of the acquired effective erythropoiesis, phlebotomy (Angelucci et al. 1997; Inati et al. 2017) can be an alternative to chelation. Table 46.1 reports the pros and cons for selecting phlebotomy or iron chelation for post-HSCT iron removal.

Table 46.1 Factors to be considered in selecting the appropriate post-HSCT iron removal strategy

	Phlebotomy	Chelation
Pros	– Efficient – Safe – Inexpensive – Permits complete iron removal and normalizes iron body content	– Efficient – Safe – Immediate effect on NTBI/LPI – Hospital access not required
Cons	– Requires sustained engraftment (not usable in the early post-HSCT period) – Immediate effect on NTBI/LPI still remains to be verified – Hospital access required	– Expensive – Warning of renal toxicity in the case of concomitant use of CSA – Possible increase in toxicity for low level of iron burden

Key Points

- Iron toxicity depends on the presence of free iron species: non-transferrin bound iron (NTBI) and labile plasma iron (LPI).
- Prevention of tissue damage by regularly and consistently suppressing tissue reactive iron species in the years before HSCT is the key factor to improve transplant outcome.
- Iron toxicity can impair the bone marrow microenvironment, the quantity and quality of bone marrow mesenchymal stem cells, the ratio of immature HSC, and the clonogenic capacity of hemopoietic stem and progenitor cells, thus impacting hemopoietic recovery and possibly transplant outcome.
- After successful HSCT, one should aim to achieve normal iron levels (i.e., normal transferrin saturation).

References

Angelucci E. Hematopoietic stem cell transplantation in thalassemia. Hematology Am Soc Hematol Educ Program. 2010;2010:456–62.

Angelucci E, Pilo F. Management of iron overload before, during, and after hematopoietic stem cell transplantation for thalassemia major. Ann N Y Acad Sci. 2016;1368:115–21.

Angelucci E, Muretto P, Lucarelli G, et al. Phlebotomy to reduce iron overload in patients cured of thalassemia by bone marrow transplantation. Italian Cooperative Group for Phlebotomy Treatment of Transplanted Thalassemia Patients. Blood. 1997;90:994–8.

Angelucci E, Muretto P, Nicolucci A, et al. Effects of iron overload and hepatitis C virus positivity in determining progression of liver fibrosis in thalassemia following bone marrow transplantation. Blood. 2002;100:17–21.

Angelucci E, Pilo F, Coates TD. Transplantation in thalassemia: revisiting the Pesaro risk factors 25 years later. Am J Hematol. 2017;92:411–3.

Coates TD. Physiology and pathophysiology of iron in hemoglobin-associated diseases. Free Radic Biol Med. 2014;72:23–40.

Coates TD, Carson S, Wood JC, et al. Management of iron overload in hemoglobinopathies: what is the appropriate target iron level? Ann N Y Acad Sci. 2016;1368:95–106.

de Swart L, Hendriks JCM, van der Vorm LN, et al. Second international round robin for the quantification of serum non-transferrin-bound iron and labile plasma iron in patients with iron-overload disorders. Haematologica. 2016;101:38–45.

Dürken M, Nielsen P, Knobel S, et al. Nontransferrin-bound iron in serum of patients receiving bone marrow transplants. Free Radic Biol Med. 1997;22:1159–63.

Ellervik C, Tybjærg-Hansen A, Nordestgaard BG. Total mortality by transferrin saturation levels: two general population studies and a metaanalysis. Clin Chem. 2011;57:459–66.

Inati A, Kahale M, Sbeiti N, et al. One-year results from a prospective randomized trial comparing phlebotomy with deferasirox for the treatment of iron overload in pediatric patients with thalassemia major following curative stem cell transplantation. Pediatr Blood Cancer. 2017;64:188–96.

Pilo F, Angelucci E. A storm in the niche: iron, oxidative stress and haemopoiesis. Blood Rev. 2018;32:29–35.

Prus E, Fibach E. Uptake of non-transferrin iron by erythroid cells. Anemia. 2011;2011:945289. https://doi.org/10.1155/2011/945289.

Puliyel M, Mainous AG, Berdoukas V, et al. Iron toxicity and its possible association with treatment of Cancer: Lessons from hemoglobinopathies and rare, transfusion-dependent anemias. Free Radic Biol Med. 2015;79:343–51.

Visani G, Guiducci B, Giardini C, et al. Deferasirox improves hematopoiesis after allogeneic hematopoietic SCT. Bone Marrow Transplant. 2014;49:585–7.

47 Secondary Neoplasia (Other than PTLPS)

André Tichelli

47.1 Definitions

Secondary neoplasia (SN) after HSCT includes any malignant disorder occurring after HSCT, irrespectively, if related or not to transplantation. For an individual patient, a clear relationship between HSCT and SN often cannot be provided. In this chapter, post transplant lymphoproliferative disorders are not discussed (see Chap. 45).

47.2 Types of Secondary Neoplasia After HSCT

	Therapy-related myeloid neoplasms (t-MN)[a]	Donor cell leukemia (DCL)[b]	Second solid neoplasms (SSN)[c]
Definition	t-MDS or t-AML after exposition chemo or radiation therapy	Hematologic neoplasms occurring in grafted donor cells	Solid cancers of any site and histology occurring after HSCT
Occurrence	Mainly after auto-HSCT Not excluded after allo-HSCT[d]	After allo-HSCT only	After allo-HSCT and auto-HSCT
Appearance	Within the first 10 years mainly	Variable	Increasing incidental rate with longer follow-up
Prognosis	Poor	Poor	Depends mainly on the cancer type

[a]Pedersen-Bjergaard et al. (2000); Engel et al. (2018)
[b]Sala-Torra et al. (2006); Wiseman (2011)
[c]Kolb et al. (1999); Rizzo et al. (2009)
[d]Yamasaki et al. (2017)

A. Tichelli (✉)
Department of Hematology, University Hospital Basel, Basel, Switzerland
e-mail: tichelli@datacomm.ch

E. Carreras et al. (eds.), *The EBMT Handbook*, https://doi.org/10.1007/978-3-030-02278-5_47

47.3 Pathophysiology

47.3.1 Therapy-Related Myeloid Neoplasms

t-MN are mainly associated with cytotoxic chemotherapy and radiation therapy that the patient has received either before HSCT or as conditioning. The causal role of ionizing radiation in the development of myeloid neoplasms has been demonstrated in atomic bomb survivors of Hiroshima/Nagasaki and in medical radiation workers employed before 1950.

Responsible cytotoxic drugs:

- Alkylating agents, anthracyclines, and topoisomerase II inhibitors.
- To a lesser extent antimetabolites and purines analogs.
- Controversy exists on the role of azathioprine, methotrexate, hydroxyurea, and 6-mercaptopurines used for the treatment of malignant and nonmalignant diseases.

t-MN occur mainly after auto-HSCT, where the healthy HSC has been exposed to cytotoxic effect. Rarely t-MN can be observed after allo-HSCT, despite the donor cells have not been exposed to cytotoxic agents. Persistent microchimerism with few exposed residual recipient cells may explain the development of t-MN after allo-HSCT. The incidence of t-MN after allo-HSCT might increase, since chimeric states are observed more frequently after RIC-HSCT.

Today, increasingly cytotoxic drugs are applied after the allo-HSCT, either as GVHD prophylaxis (post transplant CY) or to prevent disease recurrence (post transplant maintenance). We do not yet know whether these procedures are at risk for t-MN after allo-HSCT.

47.3.2 Donor Cell Leukemia

The cause of donor-derived hematological malignancies remains speculative. Two different mechanisms may be involved (Sala-Torra et al. 2006; Wiseman 2011):

- Malignant clone transmitted from the donor to the recipient
- Malignant transformation in the recipient

Malignant clones transferred to the recipient are mainly of lymphoid origin, observed in older donors, and may evolve into a lymphoid neoplasm in the immunosuppressed host. Myeloid clone transfer has not been reported. However, systematic NGS analysis might allow to detect myeloid clones transmitted to the recipient.

Malignant transformation in the donor cells is probably of multifactorial causes:

- Premature aging of the donor hematopoiesis in the recipient, more inclined to develop a leukemia
- Abnormal microenvironment
- Genetic predisposition
- Acquired environmental factors

47.3.3 Second Solid Neoplasms (SSN)

Little is known about pathogenesis of SSN after HSCT. An interaction between cytotoxic treatment, genetic predisposition, environmental factors, viral infections, GVHD, and its immunosuppression may play a role.

Two main types of SSN (Rizzo et al. 2009):

- Radiation-related SSN
  - Proven for thyroid, breast, and brain cancers
  - Occur after a long latency (≥10 years after radiation)
  - Is dose related
- GVHD/immunosuppression-related SSN
  - Squamous cell carcinoma of the skin and oropharyngeal area
  - Short latency
  - Can occur at different localizations

Association with viral infection

- HCV infection associated with hepatocellular cancer
- HPV associated with cervix cancer

47.4 Frequency and Risk Factors (See Table 47.1)

47.4.1 Remarks on SSN

The CI of second solid cancer is 2.2% at 10 years and 6.7% at 15 years (Rizzo et al. 2009).

Increased risk for SSN after HSCT has been demonstrated from breast, thyroid, skin, liver, lung, oral cavity and pharynx, bone and connective tissues cancers and malignant melanoma.

An individual patient can present several subsequent different SSN after HSCT. Up to five different solid cancers have been observed in a patient treated with allo-HSCT.

Table 47.1 Frequency and risk factors

Type of SN	Frequency	Risk factors
t-MN	Great variability on the CI of t-MN after auto-HSCT • In lymphoma patients between 1% at 2 years up to 24% at 43 months • Lower CI for patients treated for breast cancer, germ cell tumor, and multiple myeloma • Rare n-MN after HSCT for AID CI depends mainly on pretransplant cytotoxic therapy and the use of TBI CI of t-MN after allo-HSCT: 0.06-0.67% at 3 years[a]	• Quantity of pretransplant chemotherapy (see pathogenesis) and local radiotherapy • Conditioning with TBI • Older age at HSCT t-MN are mainly observed after HSCT for lymphoma (NHL, HL)
DCL	Rare complication, with a CI <1% at 15 years Possibly underestimated (difficulty to prove donor type of malignant cells) Could represent up to 5% of post transplant leukemia "relapses"	No clear risk factor defined (too few, heterogeneous DCL) Possible risk factors[b] • Malignant donor clone in the transplant • G-CSF therapy • In vivo T cell depletion • Multiple transplantations
SSN		
Breast, thyroid, bone, melanoma, connective tissue, brain, BCC	Breast cancer: 11% at 25 years[c] Thyroid cancer: SIR 3.2 compared to general population[d] BCC: 6.5% at 20 years[e]	Radiation before HSCT or TBI Younger age at radiation Longer follow-up Light-skinned patients (BCC)
SSC of skin, oral cavity, and esophagus	SCC of the skin: 3.4 at 20 years[f]	Chronic GVHD Prolonged GvHD therapy IS including azathioprine Male sex Unrelated with radiation At any time after HSCT
Hepatocellular carcinoma	Patients with HCV infection: CI 16% at 20 years[g]	HCV infection Cirrhosis
Lung cancer	SIR 2.59 after BuCy[h]	Conditioning with Bu-Cy Smoking prior to HCT
Cervix cancer		HPV reactivation
Melanoma		T cell depletion

BCC basal cell carcinoma of the skin, *SSC* squamous cell carcinoma, *CI* cumulative incidence, *AID* autoimmune disorders, *SIR* standardized incidence ratio
[a]Yamasaki et al. (2017)
[b]Engel et al. (2018)
[c]Friedman et al. (2008)
[d]Cohen et al. (2007)
[e]Leisenring et al. (2006)
[f]Curtis et al. (2005)
[g]Peffault de Latour et al. (2004)
[h]Majhail et al. (2011)

Colorectal cancers have not been proven to be increased after HSCT. In non-transplanted cancer patients, second colorectal cancers are increased when treated with abdominal radiation (Henderson et al. 2012; Rapiti et al. 2008; van Eggermond et al. 2017).

So far there are few long-term data on SSN after RIC. A single-center study shows an increased rate of SSC compared to MAC during the first 10 years post-HSCT (Shimoni et al. 2013). There are not yet data on CI of SSN >10 years after RIC. SSN associated with TBI conditioning (breast, thyroid) might be lower after RIC than MAC.

47.5 Screening (Majhail et al. 2012) (See Also Chap. 21)

47.5.1 Therapy-Related Myeloid Neoplasms

Annual monitoring of full peripheral blood counts during the first 10 years after auto-HSCT (most t-MN occur within 10 years after HSCT)

In case of unexpected abnormalities (increased MCV, cytopenia, dysplasia in peripheral blood, monocytosis), extended analysis of blood and bone marrow (including cytogenetics and NGS)

47.5.2 Donor Cell Leukemia

Chimerism monitoring of the malignant cells in case of "relapse" or new hematological malignancy after allo-HSCT.

Whether search of an abnormal clone in the donor should be performed in case of donor origin of the malignancy remains controversial.

47.5.3 Second Solid Cancer (Socie and Rizzo 2012)

Lifelong screening for SSN is recommended after auto-HSCT and allo-HSCT.

General recommendations are:

- During annual control, clinical screening, reviewing for possible symptoms of SSN.
- Receive at least country-specific general population recommendations for cancer screening.
- Be informed and counseled about the risk of SSN.

Specific recommendations are included in Table 47.2.

Table 47.2 Screening for secondary solid cancer after HSCT

Skin	*All patients* Encouraged to • Perform regularly genital/testicular and skin self-examination • To avoid unprotected UV skin exposure Skin examination by dermatologist every 1–2 years *Patients at risk* More frequent examination by dermatologist • After first skin cancer • Patients with chronic skin GvHD
Oral cavity and pharynx	*All patients* Examination during annual control *Patients at risk* Annual control by specialist if severe oral and pharynx GvHD Histology in case of suspicious lesion
Thyroid	*All patients* Annual thyroid palpation to identify suspicious thyroid nodules *Patients at risk* (patients at risk after TBI or local radiation) Regular thyroid ultrasound Fine needle aspiration in case of a suspicious nodule

Breast	*All patients* Discuss breast self-examination with their physician *Patients at risk* Screening mammography every 1 to 2 years starts at the age of 25 or 8 years after radiation, whichever occurs later, but not later than age of 40 years
Cervix	*All patients* Screening with pap smears every 1–3 years in women older than 21 or within 3 years of initial sexual activity, whichever occurs earlier
Lung	*All patients* Encouraged to avoid smoking and passive tobacco exposure *Patients at risk* Patients at risk (high-dose busulfan conditioning and smoking), chest CT
Liver	*Patients at risk* Patients with known HCV infection should be assessed for fibrosis/cirrhosis of the liver 8–10 years after HSCT (biopsy; fibroscan)
Colorectal	*All patients* Screening should start at age 50 in absence of a family history (first-degree relative diagnosed with colorectal cancer before age 60): annual fecal occult blood testing, sigmoidoscopy every 5 years, with fecal occult testing every 3 years, or colonoscopy every 10 years
Prostate	*All patients* No specific recommendations

47.6 Treatment

Neoplasm	Treatment
t-MN	Same treatment than de novo myeloid neoplasms Early donor search and rapid allo-HSCT[a] Decision-making including consideration of cumulative toxicity due to previous HSCT
DCL	No standard treatment Treatment depends on the nature of disease Reported treatments[b] • Retransplantation • Conventional chemotherapy • DLI • Palliation
SSN	Should be treated as de novo cancers of the same type

[a]Finke et al. (2016); Kroger et al. (2011); Metafuni et al. (2018)
[b]Engel et al. (2018)

47.7 Outcome

Neoplasm	Outcome
t-MN	Generally very poor Median survival of 6 m Identical outcome than t-MN in general
DCL	Few data available In most cases, mortality high and OS poor In a small series of 47 DCL, median survival 32.8% months Death mainly due to progression or relapse of DCL
SSN	Mainly dependent on the type of SSN[a] Favorable outcome • Thyroid, breast, prostate, melanoma, cervix Intermediate outcome • Oropharyngeal, colorectal, bladder, renal, ovarian, endometrial Poor outcome • Pancreas, lung, brain, hepatobiliary, esophageal

[a]Ehrhardt et al. (2016); Tichelli et al. (2018)

Key Points

- Three types of secondary neoplasia may occur after HSCT: therapy-related myeloid neoplasms (t-MN), mainly after autoHSCT; donor cell leukemia (DCL) after allo-HSCT; second solid neoplasia (SSN) after auto-HSCT and allo-HSCT.
- Pretreatment or conditioning with radiation and/or chemotherapy including alkylating agents, anthracyclines, and topoisomerase II inhibitors is mainly responsible for t-MN.
- DCL are extremely rare and are either transmitted from the donor or newly transformed in the host.
- Non-squamous second solid cancers (breast, thyroid, brain, etc.) are strongly related to local radiation or TBI and occur with long delay after HSCT. Squamous cell carcinoma of the skin, the oral cavity, and the pharynx is related with chronic GVHD and can occur early after HSCT.
- Outcome of t-MN is poor, and allogeneic HSCT represents the only curative treatment.
- Outcome of SSN depends mainly on the type of second cancer; second solid cancer should be treated as a de novo cancer of the same type.

References

Cohen PA, Rovelli A, Merlo DF, et al. Risk for secondary thyroid carcinoma after hematopoietic stem-cell transplantation: an EBMT late effects working party study. J Clin Oncol. 2007;25:2449–54.

Curtis RE, Metayer C, Rizzo JD, et al. Impact of chronic GVHD therapy on the development of squamous-cell cancers after hematopoietic stem-cell transplantation: an international case-control study. Blood. 2005;105:3802–11.

Ehrhardt MJ, Brazauskas R, He W, et al. Survival of patients who develop solid tumors following hematopoietic stem cell transplantation. Bone Marrow Transplant. 2016;51:83–8.

Engel N, Rovo A, Badoglio M, et al. European experience and risk factor analysis of donor cell derived leukaemia following haematopoietic cell transplantation. Leukemia. 2018;[Epub ahead of print].

Finke J, Schmoor C, Bertz H, et al. Long-term follow-up of therapy-related myelodysplasia and AML patients treated with allogeneic hematopoietic cell transplantation. Bone Marrow Transplant. 2016;51:771–7.

Friedman DL, Rovo A, Leisenring W, et al. Increased risk of breast cancer among survivors of allogeneic hematopoietic cell transplantation: a report from the FHCRC and the EBMT-Late Effect Working Party. Blood. 2008;111:939–44.

Henderson TO, Oeffinger KC, Whitton J, et al. Summaries for patients. Increased risk for gastrointestinal cancer in childhood cancer survivors. Ann Intern Med. 2012;156:1–36.

Kolb HJ, Socie G, Duell T, et al. Malignant neoplasms in long-term survivors of bone marrow transplantation. Late Effects Working Party of the European Cooperative Group for Blood and Marrow Transplantation and the European Late Effect Project Group. Ann Intern Med. 1999;131:738–44.

Kroger N, Zabelina T, van Biezen A, et al. Allogeneic stem cell transplantation for myelodysplastic syndromes with bone marrow fibrosis. Haematologica. 2011;96:291–7.

Leisenring W, Friedman DL, Flowers ME, et al. Nonmelanoma skin and mucosal cancers after hematopoietic cell transplantation. J Clin Oncol. 2006;24:1119–26.

Majhail NS, Brazauskas R, Rizzo JD, et al. Secondary solid cancers after allogeneic hematopoietic cell transplantation using busulfan-cyclophosphamide conditioning. Blood. 2011;117:316–22.

Majhail NS, Rizzo JD, Lee SJ, et al. Recommended screening and preventive practices for long-term survivors after hematopoietic cell transplantation. Bone Marrow Transplant. 2012;47:337–41.

Metafuni E, Chiusolo P, Laurenti L, et al. Allogeneic hematopoietic stem cell transplantation in therapy-related myeloid neoplasms (t-MN) of the adult: monocentric observational study and review of the literature. Mediterr J Hematol Infect Dis. 2018;e2018005:10.

Pedersen-Bjergaard J, Andersen MK, Christiansen DH. Therapy-related acute myeloid leukemia and myelodysplasia after high-dose chemotherapy and autologous stem cell transplantation. Blood. 2000;95:3273–9.

Peffault de Latour R, Levy V, Asselah T, et al. Long-term outcome of hepatitis C infection after bone marrow transplantation. Blood. 2004;103:1618–24.

Rapiti E, Fioretta G, Verkooijen HM, et al. Increased risk of colon cancer after external radiation therapy for prostate cancer. Int J Cancer. 2008;123:1141–5.

Rizzo JD, Curtis RE, Socie G, et al. Solid cancers after allogeneic hematopoietic cell transplantation. Blood. 2009;113:1175–83.

Sala-Torra O, Hanna C, Loken MR, et al. Evidence of donor-derived hematologic malignancies after hematopoietic stem cell transplantation. Biol Blood Marrow Transplant. 2006;12:511–7.

Shimoni A, Shem-Tov N, Chetrit A, et al. Secondary malignancies after allogeneic stem-cell transplantation in the era of reduced-intensity conditioning; the incidence is not reduced. Leukemia. 2013;27:829–35.

Socie G, Rizzo JD. Second solid tumors: screening and management guidelines in long-term survivors after allogeneic stem cell transplantation. Semin Hematol. 2012;49:4–9.

Tichelli A, Beohou E, Labobon M, et al. Evaluation of Second Solid Cancers after Hematopoietic Stem Cell Transplantation in European Patients. Jama Oncol. 2018;[Epub ahead of print].

van Eggermond AM, Schaapveld M, Janus CP, et al. Infradiaphragmatic irradiation and high procarbazine doses increase colorectal cancer risk in Hodgkin lymphoma survivors. Br J Cancer. 2017;117:306–14.

Wiseman DH. Donor cell leukemia: a review. Biol Blood Marrow Transplant. 2011;17:771–89.

Yamasaki S, Suzuki R, Hatano K, et al. Therapy-related acute myeloid leukemia and myelodysplastic syndrome after hematopoietic cell transplantation for lymphoma. Bone Marrow Transplant. 2017;52:969–76.

Part VI

Specific Organ Complications

Topic leaders: Grzegorz Basak and John Snowden

48 Ocular and Oral Complications

Shahrukh K. Hashmi

48.1 Ocular Complications

48.1.1 Introduction

Ocular complications in HSCT patients include both ocular GVHD- and non-GVHD-related late effects which, if left untreated, can lead to blindness. Non-GVHD associated complications include glaucoma, infections particularly (viral retinitis, fungal endophthalmitis), posterior segment abnormalities, and cataracts. Ocular GVHD is considered an umbrella term for both conjunctival disease and keratoconjunctivitis sicca, both of which can coexist simultaneously.

The World Health Organization considers blindness as one of the top causes for disability-adjusted life years, and it significantly affects the QoL. Thus, prevention and prompt management of ocular complications should be a priority of a transplant program given the morbidity associated with it.

48.1.2 Ocular GVHD

Though it is considered to be systematic disease, the pattern of isolated ocular GVHD manifesting later as GVHD in other organs is erratic (Townley et al. 2011). The 2014 NIH consensus development project on chronic GVHD does not account for therapeutic responses based mainly on patient-reported outcomes (PRO); thus the development of PRO measures (PROM) specific for ocular GVHD should be a priority of the GVHD research community. The NIH chronic GVHD consortium does recommend photoprotection, surveillance for infection, cataract formation, and increased intraocular pressure for prevention of ocular complications in GVHD—these measures should be routinely incorporated in the standard clinical practice of HSCT patients and are best achieved within the context of a multidisciplinary survivorship clinic along with ophthalmologists as part of the team.

The occurrence of ocular GVHD is variable in different series but is approximately 40 to 60% of patients receiving HSCT (Nassar et al. 2013). The risk factors for ocular GVHD include donor-recipient HLA and gender disparity (female donor to male recipient) and an older donor age.

The principles of *ocular GVHD management* include lubrication, drainage control, evaporation control, and minimization of ocular surface inflammation. The 2014 NIH chronic GVHD consensus panel has excellent recommendations for stepwise treatment of ocular GVHD which include preservative-free artificial tears for mild, topical cyclosporine or steroid eye drops for moderate/severe and oral pilocarpine or cevimeline for severe/moderate ocular GVHD, respectively (Carpenter et al.

S. K. Hashmi (✉)
Department of Adult Hematology, King Faisal Specialist Hospital and Research Center, Riyadh, Saudi Arabia

Mayo Clinic, Rochester, MN, USA
e-mail: shashmi@kfshrc.edu.sa

E. Carreras et al. (eds.), *The EBMT Handbook*, https://doi.org/10.1007/978-3-030-02278-5_48

2015). Among surgical procedures for moderate/severe ocular GVHD, punctal occlusion, superficial debridement of filamentary keratitis, and partial tarsorrhaphy have been recommended as surgeries with moderate-quality data on effectiveness. There is also some evidence on other modalities of treatment which include occlusive eye wear, lid care/warm compress/humidified environment, bandage contact lens, and gas-permeable scleral lenses. What is not clear is the optimal management algorithm for ocular GVHD with respect to medical versus surgical therapies and, within the surgical therapies, which ones would be most effective due to lack of clinical trials in this area. Thus, ocular GVHD is best managed in conjunction with ophthalmologist experienced in dealing with ocular GVHD.

In addition, special attention should be given to other risk factors for ocular complications, among which diabetes and hypertension are at the top. Thus, if a patient is on CNI or corticosteroids, then optimization of blood pressure and glycaemia control is imperative to reduce the risk of blindness due to retinopathy irrespective of the cause.

48.1.3 Posterior Segment Complications

Retinal and vitreous hemorrhages are not uncommon in HSCT patients and may happen with or without the presence of ocular GVHD (Yoo et al. 2017). This is complicated by the presence of thrombocytopenia early in transplant but also later in the course since both drugs and chronic GVHD can be associated with thrombocytopenia. Prompt referral to ophthalmologist is the key for preventing blindness; therefore, the practicing transplant clinician should have a high suspicion of retinopathy, retinal tears, or vitreous hemorrhages when a patient complains of "floaters" or just "decreased vision," which happens suddenly.

48.1.4 Ocular Infections

CMV infection is one the most widely studied ocular infections and can rapidly lead to retinitis, and since quite often IV antibiotics are required, prompt referral to ophthalmologist is mandatory. Apart from CMV, adenovirus is also a common virus and can lead to viremia if untreated. Moreover, unlike immunocompetent individuals, varicella zoster infection within hours or couple of days can lead to dissemination as well as postherpetic neuralgia, cranial nerve palsies, zoster paresis, meningoencephalitis, cerebellitis, myelopathy, and irreversible blindness.

Fungal infections in severely IS HSCT patients (particularly those on multiple IS for GVHD) can quickly lead to mortality; thus prompt referral for IV antifungals is indicated. Aspergillosis, mucormycosis, and candida have been reported in GVHD patients affecting the ocular tissues.

48.1.5 Glaucoma

Since the most common subtype of glaucoma (primary open-angle glaucoma) presents with gradual symptoms, its diagnosis is frequently missed in early phases. However, many risk factors in HSCT can predispose to glaucoma and can lead to blindness which include diabetes (allo-HSCT patients have four times higher risk of diabetes), retinopathy, and steroid use (for GVHD). Since the diagnosis of glaucoma is based in tonometry, gonioscopy, perimetry, and ophthalmoscopy, regular screening by the ophthalmologist is indicated.

48.1.6 Cataract

Cataract is the most common cause of blindness in the developed world. Risk factors in the HSCT patients include steroid use, total body irradiation, and diabetes. Since intraocular lens implantation (particularly via phacoemulsification) has become a widely performed procedure worldwide for the treatment of cataracts, early recognition and prompt treatment can help in preservation of vision. This procedure is associated with low rate of complications; however, prevention of cataracts by controlling the risk factors should be the management strategy in HSCT survivors (Table 48.1).

Table 48.1 Ocular complications of HSCT

	Risk factors/manifestations	Management	Survivorship issues
GVHD associated	– Dry eye syndrome (keratoconjunctivitis sicca)/ lacrimal gland dysfunction – Retinopathies – Cataracts – Infections	– Topical: artificial tears, steroids, CSA, scleral lenses, autologous serum, surgical procedures – Systemic: ECP, rituximab, ibrutinib	Presence of ophthalmologist in the long-term follow-up or survivorship clinic
Non-GVHD associated	– Glaucoma – Cataract – Infection – Retinal/vitreous hemorrhage	– Removal of risk factors – Surgery – Antimicrobials	

Key Points

- Ocular complications of HSCT are not restricted to GVHD, since both non-GVHD allo-HSCT and auto-HSCT recipients can suffer from cataracts, viral/fungal infections, glaucoma, and retinopathies.
- QoL compromise by ocular complications of HSCT is paramount due to ensuing blindness.
- Transplant centers should consider a close collaboration with ophthalmology teams both for treatment and preventative strategies. This could ideally be achieved in a multidisciplinary team in a long-term follow-up or a survivorship clinic.

48.2 Oral Complications

48.2.1 Introduction

Oral complications of HSCT can significantly affect the quality of the life (QoL) and can be a result of graft-versus-host-disease (GVHD) or can occur independent of it. Any oral complication, if severe, can lead to weight loss due to poor nutritional intake, mortality (especially due to cancer), aspiration pneumonia (especially in cases of oropharyngeal disorders), and psychologic sequelae (particularly disfigurement due to oral scleroderma, i.e., fish mouth) (Table 48.2).

48.2.2 Oral GVHD

Oral GVHD itself can lead to significant mortality and morbidity. GVHD-associated oral complications, e.g., mouth scleroderma, lichenification (resulting in lichenoid features and lichen planus), oral cancers, dental caries, salivary gland dysfunction (main manifestation being xerostomia), and mucoceles, are common complications of oral GVHD. In addition, avascular necrosis (AVN) of the mandible can occur as a complication of steroid therapy for GVHD (Treister et al. 2012).

The 2014 National Institutes of Health chronic GVHD consensus criteria places the scoring based on lichen-like features; however many of the associated patient-reported outcomes are not captured by this scoring system which can tremendously affect the QoL (Jagasia et al. 2015). Thus, involvement of specialists experienced in dealing with long-term HSCT complications is imperative for management of oral GVHD and its complications.

The *management of oral GVHD* requires both topical treatments and systemic therapy. Topical treatments may include local tacrolimus (i.e., protopic), PUVA, and topical steroids. Among systemic treatments for oral GVHD, extracorporeal photopheresis has one of the highest response rates, along with rituximab (Okamoto et al. 2006; Malik et al. 2014).

48.2.3 Oral Cancers

Carcinomas of the oral cavity are predominantly of squamous cell carcinoma type; however, other

Table 48.2 Oral complications of hematopoietic stem cell transplantation

	Risk factors	Management	Survivorship issues
GVHD associated	– Lichen planus – Squamous cell carcinoma – Aphthous ulcers – Fish mouth (scleroderma), carries, odynophagia, carries	– Topical: tacrolimus, steroids, PUVA – Systemic: extracorporeal photopheresis, rituximab, ibrutinib	– Presence of a dentist and/or oral surgeon in the long-term follow-up or survivorship clinic
Non-GVHD associated	– Osteonecrosis of the jaw, dysgeusia, temporomandibular joint disorders, mucositis, carries, odynophagia	Dental or oral surgery referral for corrective action; surgery in selected cases	

histologies can also manifest as oral cancers in HSCT survivors. The risks of developing oral cancers increase significantly post transplant to approximately sevenfold with the highest risk being in patients who were transplanted for bone marrow failure (BMF) syndromes especially dyskeratosis congenita and Fanconi's anemia (Rosenberg et al. 2003). Besides BMF syndromes, the most important risk factors for oral carcinomas include GVHD, radiation, and epigenetic factors (smoking). It is of utmost important that prevention strategies of oral cancers be discussed at each visit with special emphasis on smoking cessation (if applicable) and avoidance of other known risk factors, e.g., betel nut, tobacco chewing, or alcohol intake, since these are modifiable risks. Additionally, aggressive and early treatment of oral GVHD is essential to prevent this complication.

48.2.4 Non-GVHD-Associated Oral Manifestations

These include osteonecrosis of the jaw (ONJ), dysgeusia, temporomandibular disorders, gingivitis, and oral mucositis early in HSCT. Though certain symptoms like dysgeusia (Sato et al. 2017a, b) may seem trivial, they significantly affect the QoL, preservation of which is the sine qua non of managing late effects. Similarly, oral mucositis is one of the most challenging complications in early phases of HSCT with a high incidence in both reduced intensity and myeloablative regimens (Chaudhry et al. 2015). Similarly, ONJ can lead to multiple late effects of chronic pain and poor oral intake and can affect QoL tremendously (Hautmann et al. 2011). Thus, prompt referral to maxillofacial surgeon for management is imperative as soon as any symptoms start to develop.

48.2.5 Needs Provision for Oral Surgery/Dentistry in HSCT

Many experts recommend that dentistry and/or oral surgeons should be part of a multidisciplinary team managing late effects in both autologous and allogeneic HSCT survivors, and this concept was recently endorsed by the National Institutes of Health's Late Effects Initiative (Hashmi et al. 2017). Once the primary disease (for which HSCT was performed) is cured, it is essential that surveillance and preventative strategies be undertaken to alleviate the burden of comorbidities in these survivors; thus we agree that a long-term follow-up clinic should optimally have dentistry services available ad hoc if not on routine surveillance basis.

Key Points
- Oral GVHD and its associated complications can lead to significant compromise in QoL and can lead to cancers which can lead to fatal outcomes.
- Non-GVHD-associated complications also should be vigilantly dealt with as they tremendously affect QoL and include ONJ, dysgeusia, dental carries, gingivitis, and oral mucositis.
- Dentists and/or oral surgeons should ideally be a part of multidisciplinary teams of a long-term follow-up/survivorship clinic of HSCT survivors.

References

Carpenter PA, Kitko CL, Elad S, et al. National institutes of health consensus development project on criteria for clinical trials in chronic graft-versus-host disease: V. The 2014 ancillary therapy and supportive care working group report. Biol Blood Marrow Transplant. 2015;21:1167–87.

Chaudhry HM, Bruce AJ, Wolf R, et al. The incidence and outcomes of oral mucositis among allogeneic stem cell transplantation patients: a systematic review and meta-analysis. Biol Blood Marrow Transplant. 2015;21:S245–6.

Hashmi SK, Bredeson C, Duarte RF, et al. National institutes of health blood and marrow transplant late effects initiative: the healthcare delivery working group report. Biol Blood Marrow Transplant. 2017;23:717–25.

Hautmann AH, Elad S, Lawitschka A, et al. Metabolic bone diseases in patients after allogeneic hematopoietic stem cell transplantation: report from the consensus conference on clinical practice in chronic graft-versus-host disease. Transpl Int. 2011;24:867–79.

Jagasia MH, Greinix HT, Arora M, et al. National Institutes of Health consensus development project on criteria for clinical trials in chronic graft-versus-host disease: I. The 2014 diagnosis and staging working group report. Biol Blood Marrow Transplant. 2015;21:389–401.

Malik MI, Litzow M, Hogan W, et al. Extracorporeal photopheresis for chronic graft-versus-host disease: a systematic review and meta-analysis. Blood Res. 2014;49:100–6.

Nassar A, Tabbara KF, Aljurf M. Ocular manifestations of graft-versus-host disease. Saudi J Ophthalmol. 2013;27:215–22.

Okamoto M, Okano A, Akamatsu S, et al. Rituximab is effective for steroid-refractory sclerodermatous chronic graft-versus-host disease. Leukemia. 2006;20:172–3.

Rosenberg PS, Greene MH, Alter BP. Cancer incidence in persons with Fanconi anemia. Blood. 2003;101: 822–6.

Sato T, Konuma T, Miwa Y, et al. A cross-sectional study on late taste disorders in survivors of allogeneic hematopoietic cell transplantation. Ann Hematol. 2017a;96:1841–7.

Sato T, Konuma T, Miwa Y, et al. A cross-sectional study on late taste disorders in survivors of allogeneic hematopoietic cell transplantation. Ann Hematol. 2017b;96:1841–7.

Townley JR, Dana R, Jacobs DS. Keratoconjunctivitis sicca manifestations in ocular graft versus host disease: pathogenesis, presentation, prevention, and treatment. Semin Ophthalmol. 2011;26:251–60.

Treister N, Duncan C, Cutler C, Lehmann L. How we treat oral chronic graft-versus-host disease. Blood. 2012;120:3407–18.

Yoo YS, Na KS, Shin JA, et al. Posterior eye segment complications related to allogeneic hematopoietic stem cell transplantation. Retina. 2017;37:135–43.

49 Hepatic Complications

Tapani Ruutu and Enric Carreras

49.1 Introduction

The frequency and severity of TPH liver complications have decreased sharply in the last decade, with some complications that have completely disappeared, such as, for example, Candida liver abscesses. The development of more effective strategies to preventing SOS/VOD and GVHD has had a marked effect on its clinical presentation (see Chaps. 25 and 49). Finally, prophylaxis with antiviral and antifungal drugs has greatly reduced the incidence of the most common liver infections (Hockenbery et al. 2016). The major liver complications after HSCT are:

Early after HSCT (<100 days)	Late after HSCT (months-years)
SOS/VOD Acute GVHD (see Chap. 43) Acute hepatitis Pharmacological toxicity	Chronic GVHD (see Chap. 44) Autoimmune hepatitis Chronic viral hepatitis (see Chap. 38) Cirrhosis and hepatocellular carcinoma Iron overload (see Chap. 46) Other less frequent

49.2 Sinusoidal Obstruction Syndrome

49.2.1 Definition

SOS, formerly called veno-occlusive disease of the liver (VOD), is the term used to designate the symptoms and signs that appear early after HSCT because of conditioning regimen-related hepatic toxicity. This syndrome is characterized by jaundice, fluid retention, and tender hepatomegaly appearing in the first 35–40 days after HSCT (Carreras 2015).

49.2.2 Pathogenesis

The hepatic metabolism of certain drugs (e.g., CY) by the cytochrome P450 enzymatic system produces several toxic metabolites (e.g., acrolein). These toxic metabolites are converted into stable (nontoxic) metabolites by the glutathione (GSH)

T. Ruutu
Clinical Research Institute, Helsinki University Hospital, Helsinki, Finland

E. Carreras (✉)
Spanish Bone Marrow Donor Registry, Josep Carreras Foundation and Leukemia Research Institute, Barcelona, Catalunya, Spain

Hospital Clinic Barcelona, Barcelona University, Barcelona, Catalunya, Spain
e-mail: enric.carreras@fcarreras.es

E. Carreras et al. (eds.), *The EBMT Handbook*, https://doi.org/10.1007/978-3-030-02278-5_49

enzymatic system and then eliminated. When this process occurs in patients with a reduced GSH activity, caused by previous liver disease or by the action of agents such as BU, BCNU, or TBI, which consume GSH, toxic metabolites are not metabolized. Toxic metabolites are predominantly located in area 3 of the hepatic acinus (around the centrilobular veins) because this area is rich in P450 and poor in glutathione. Consequently, damage to hepatocytes and sinusoidal endothelium occurs predominantly in this zone. Many other factors (see risk factors) can also contribute to endothelial injury.

The first events after endothelial injury caused by toxic metabolites are loss of fenestrae in sinusoidal endothelial cells (SEC), formation of gaps within and between SEC, and rounding up or swelling of SEC. Consequently, red blood cells penetrate into the space of Disse and dissect off the sinusoidal lining, which embolize downstream and block the sinusoids, reducing the hepatic venous outflow and producing post-sinusoidal hypertension. The changes observed in coagulation factors in these patients seem to be a consequence of the endothelial injury and probably play a secondary role in SOS pathogenesis, despite contributing to the sinusoidal occlusion (Carreras and Diaz-Ricart 2011).

49.2.3 Clinical Manifestations of SOS

Classical manifestations	Weight gain[a]/edema/ascites/anasarca Painful hepatomegaly/jaundice Consumption of (not refractoriness to) transfused platelets[b]
Manifestations of MOF	Pleural effusion/pulmonary infiltrates Renal, cardiac, and pulmonary failure Neurological symptoms (encephalopathy, coma)

[a]Positive fluid balance not explained by excessive hydration

[b]Difficult to demonstrate by expected thrombocytopenia

49.2.4 EBMT Diagnostic Criteria for Adults (Mohty et al. 2016)

Classical SOS (Baltimore criteria)[a]	Late-onset SOS[b]
In the first 21 days after HSCT Bilirubin ≥2 mg/dL[c] and ≥ 2 of the following – Painful hepatomegaly – Weight gain >5% – Ascites	Classical SOS beyond day 21, OR Histologically proven SOS OR ≥2 of the classical criteria AND ultrasound (US) or hemodynamical evidence of SOS

[a]These symptoms/signs should not be attributable to other causes

[b]Mainly observed after conditioning including several alkylating agents (e.g., BU, MEL, or TT)

[c]Observed in almost 100% of adults but absent in up to 30% of children

49.2.5 EBMT Diagnostic Criteria for Children (Corbacioglu et al. 2018)

No limitation for time of onset of SOS[a]

The presence of two or more of the following[b]

- Unexplained consumptive and transfusion-refractory thrombocytopenia[c]
- Otherwise unexplained weight gain on 3 consecutive days despite the use of diuretics or a weight gain >5% above baseline value
- Hepatomegaly (best if confirmed by imaging) above baseline value[d]
- Ascites (ideally confirmed by imaging) above baseline value[d]
- Rising bilirubin from a baseline value on 3 consecutive days or ≥2 mg/dL within 72 h

[a]Up to 20% of children present late SOS

[b]With the exclusion of other potential differential diagnoses

[c]Weight-adjusted platelet substitution/day to maintain institutional transfusion guidelines

[d]Suggested: imaging (US, CT, or MRI) immediately before HSCT to determine baseline value for both hepatomegaly and ascites

49.2.6 Incidence

Variable depending on the diagnostic criteria used, center experience, type of patients, and year of HSCT

Author (period analyzed) (study type)	Auto-HSCT	Allo-HSCT
Coppell et al. 2010 (1979–2007) (R)	8.7%	13%
Carreras et al. (1998) (P)	3.1%	8.9%
Corbacioglu et al. 2012 (2006–2009) (P)[a]	6%	14%
Carreras et al. 2011 (1997–2008) (R)[b]	–	MAC, 8%/ RIC, 2%

R retrospective study, *P* prospective study
[a]Only children and young adolescents
[b]Only adults

49.2.7 Risk Factors for SOS

Patient-related risk factors[a,b]	
Age	Younger < **older**
Sex	Male < female
Karnofsky index	100–90 < lower than 90
Underlying disease	Nonmalignant < malignant < **some specific diseases**[c]
Status of the disease	Remission < relapse
AST level before HSCT	Normal < increased
Bilirubin level before HSCT	Normal < increased
Prior liver radiation	No < yes
Liver status	Normal < fibrosis, cirrhosis, tumor
Iron overload	Absent < present
CMV serology	Negative < positive
Prior treatment with	**Gemtuzumab or inotuzumab ozogamicin**
Concomitant drugs	**Progestogens**, azoles
Genetic factors	GSTM1-null genotype, *MTHFR* 677CC/1298CC haplotype, etc.
Transplant-related factors	
Type of HCT	Syngeneic/autologous < **allogeneic**
Type of donor	HLA-identical sibling < unrelated
Grade of compatibility	Match < minor mismatch < major mismatch
T-cell in the graft	T-cell depleted < non-T-cell depleted
Type of conditioning	NMA < RIC < TRC < **MAC**
Busulfan	IV < oral targeted < oral CY-BU < BU-CY
TBI	Fractionated < single dose Low-dose rate < high-dose rate Less than 12 Gy < more than 12 Gy Time between CY to TBI 36 h < CY to TBI 12 h
Fludarabine	Not included < included
GvHD prophylaxis	CNI (TAC < CSA) **< CNI + sirolimus**
HSCT number	First < second HSCT

Bold characters indicate the most relevant factors
[a]Many factors have been associated with an increased risk of SOS, with those in bold letters seem the most relevant
[b]Remember that the presence of several risk factors in a patient has an additive effect
[c]Due to unknown causes, some malignant or nonmalignant diseases, osteopetrosis, adrenoleukodystrophy, thalassemia, hemophagocytic lymphohistiocytosis, or neuroblastoma are associated with a higher incidence of SOS

49.2.8 How to Confirm the Diagnosis?

SOS is a syndrome and must be diagnosed clinically, but several tools can help us	
Transjugular hemodynamic study	Permits a safe measurement of the hepatic venous pressure gradient (HVPG), which evaluates the presence of intrahepatic post-sinusoidal hypertension. A HVPG >10 mmHg is highly specific (>90%) and moderately sensitive (60%) for SOS
Transvenous liver biopsies	Transvenous biopsies may be obtained during hemodynamic studies, but false-negative results could be obtained due to the patchy nature of SOS. However, biopsies carry a risk of hemorrhagic complications (e.g., into the peritoneum and biliary tract). Consequently, they are only indicated when a crucial differential diagnosis is required (e.g., SOS versus GVHD?)

Imaging techniques	They may be helpful to confirm hepatomegaly and/or ascites (relevant in overweight patients) and for the differential diagnosis. Baseline and serial US may be useful for early detection of SOS The US abnormalities observed in SOS (hepatomegaly, splenomegaly, gallbladder wall thickening, ascites) are not specific. Decrease in velocity or reversal of the portal venous flow is considered more specific for SOS but usually occurs late in the disease (reviewed in Dignan et al. 2013)
Composite biomarkers	Recently some composite markers have shown a prognostic value at day 0 (L-Ficolin, HA, VCAM-1) and at diagnosis (ST2, ANG2, L-Ficolin, HA, VCAM-1) (Akil et al. 2015)

HA hyaluronic acid, *VCAM-1* vascular cell adhesion molecule-1, *ST2* suppressor of tumorigenicity-2, *ANG2* angiopoietin-2

49.2.9 EBMT Criteria for Severity Grading

Classically the severity of SOS was stablished, prospectively, based in a mathematical model or, retrospectively, based on its evolution (resolution or not at day +100). Later, SOS may be classified as severe with the development of multiorgan failure MOF. Several systems have been proposed for early prognostication of SOS using scales, including the following elaborated by the EBMT (Mohty et al. 2016).

	Mild	Moderate	Severe	Very severe
Time since first symptoms	>7 days	5–7 days	≤4 days	Any time
Bilirubin mg/dL	≥2 to <3	≥3 to <5	≥5 to <8	≥8
Bilirubin kinetics			Doubling in 48 h	
Transaminases (× N)	≤2	>2 to ≤5	>5 to ≤8	>8
Weight gain (%)	<5	≥5 to <10[a]	≥5 to <10[a]	≥10
Renal function (× baseline at HSCT)	<1.2	≥1.2 to <1.5	≥1.5 to <2	≥2 or other data of MOF

This severity grading must be applied once SOS/VOD has been diagnosed applying the criteria mentioned in 49.2.4
Patients belong to the category that fulfills ≥2 criteria. If patients fulfill ≥2 criteria in two different categories, they should be classified in the most severe category
In the presence of two or more risk factors for SOS, patients should be in the upper grade

N normal values

[a]Weight gain ≥5% and <10% is considered as a severe SOS. However, if the patient does not fulfill other criteria for severe SOS, it is therefore considered a moderate SOS

49.2.10 Prophylaxis (Dignan et al. 2013; Carreras 2015)

Non-pharmacological measures	
Avoid modifiable risk factors: Treat Iron overload (chelation); treat viral hepatitis; delay HSCT if active hepatitis; reduce intensity of conditioning; use CY + BU instead of BU + cy; try to avoid CNI (if not possible use TAC instead CSA) for GVHD prophylaxis; avoid hepatotoxic drugs (progestogens)	
Pharmacological	*Drug (degree of recommendation)*
Not recommended	Sodium heparin (2B), low-molecular-weight heparin (2B), antithrombin III (2B), prostaglandin-1 (1B), pentoxifylline (1A)
Suggested	Ursodeoxycholic acid (2C)[a] Defibrotide: In high-risk adult patients (2B)
Recommended	Defibrotide: In high-risk children (1A) [25 mg/kg/d]

[a]In two randomized trials, UDCA reduce the incidence of SOS but in other two this effect was not observed. However, in all them, patients with UDCA have a lower TRM

49.2.11 Treatment (Degree of Recommendation) (Dignan et al. 2013; Carreras 2015)

Methylprednisolone (2C): Used by some authors. Recommended doses not defined (and range from high to low) and results difficult to analyze. Main risk: to delay treatment with defibrotide, the only agent with proved effectiveness.

Defibrotide (1B): Despite the absence of randomized studies, it is the only agent approved by FDA and EMA to treat *severe SOS* (>80% mortality). In these patients: 50% of complete remission and > 50% SRV at day +100. Early treatment strongly recommended. Dose: 6.25 mg/kg q6h in 2 h during ≥21 days, depending on the response.

49.3 Hepatitis After HSCT

Despite the reduction in the incidence of liver complications after HSCT, there remain multiple hepatic causes of elevations of serum alanine aminotransferase (ALT). In addition to the acute viral hepatitis, other noninfectious causes must be considered:

VZV, CMV, EBV, HHV-6	Infrequent (see Chap. 38)
HBV, HCV, HEV	(see Chap. 38)
Drug-induced hepatitis	Very frequent. Wide range of severity (see Sect. 49.3.1)
Hepatic GvHD	Exceptional. AST/ALT >2000 U/L usually observed in patients without or with minimal IS (or receiving DLI) (see Chaps. 43 and 44)
Autoimmune hepatitis	True autoimmune hepatitis or GVHD? Often difficult to differentiate (see Sect. 49.3.2)
Other causes	Severe SOS (see Sect. 49.2), hypoxic liver injury (septic or cardiac shock or respiratory failure), acute biliary obstruction

49.3.1 Drug Induced Hepatitis

Drug[a,b]	Comments
Thiazole antifungals[c]	Cholestatic[d] or hepatocellular hepatitis[e], liver failure
Echinocandins	Cholestatic hepatitis or mild-moderate hepatocellular hepatitis
Fluoroquinolones	Hepatocellular hepatitis
Liposomal AmB	Mild-moderate elevation of alkaline phosphatase
TMP/SMX	Hepatocellular hepatitis
CSA, tacrolimus	Cholestasis. Dose-dependent effect
Rapamycin	Hepatocellular damage, increased risk of SOS[f]
Anticonvulsants	Hepatitis, hepatocellular or cholestatic
NSAIDs	Hepatitis, hepatocellular or cholestatic
Acetaminophen	Hepatocellular hepatitis. Dose-dependent effect
Antidepressants	Hepatocellular hepatitis. Unrelated to drug dosage
Ranitidine	Cholestatic hepatitis, eosinophilic infiltration
Amoxicillin-clavulanic acid	Cholestatic and/or hepatocellular hepatitis
Antihypertensive drugs + lipid-lowering agents + oral hypoglycemics	Drugs usually associated in patients with metabolic syndrome (see Chap. 55)

AMB amphotericin B, *TMP/SMX* trimethoprim-sulfamethoxazole, *NSAID* nonsteroidal anti-inflammatory drug

[a]Other than cytostatic drugs

[b]Online resources for the consultation of toxicities and interactions: https://livertox.nlm.nih.gov

[c]Voriconazole, posaconazole

[d]Liver damage with predominant elevation of bilirubin and alkaline phosphatase

[e]Hepatic damage with predominant elevation of transaminases

[f]Especially if associated to CNI

49.3.2 Autoimmune Hepatitis (AIH)

The main problem with this hepatitis is how to differentiate them from a hepatic GVHD, since pathogenesis, clinical manifestations, and biological changes are practically identical (Dalekos et al. 2002).

	Autoimmune hepatitis	Hepatic GVHD
Jaundice	Usually mild	Various degrees
Other symptoms	Fatigue, malaise, many times asymptomatic	Hepatic tenderness, dark urine, acholic stools, anorexia, usually **GVHD in other organs**
Pathology	Inflammatory infiltrate in portal area, often penetrating lobes	Inflammatory infiltrate, **loss of small bile duct, degeneration of bile ductular epithelium**, cholestasis
Cirrhosis	May be present	Rare
>AST	Moderate to severe	Less striking

	Autoimmune hepatitis	Hepatic GVHD
>GGT	Marked	Usually normal o decreased
Auto-Ab	Type AIH-2 (**ALKM, ALC-1**)	Often found (AIH-1) (ANA, ANCA, etc.)
Response to steroids	Excellent	Depends on severity

In bold letter main differential data

49.4 Cirrhosis and Heparocellular Carcinoma

Cirrhosis[a]	– In HSCT with HBV: exceptional – In HSCT with HCV: 11% at 15 years; 20% at 20 years (Peffault de Latour et al. 2004)[b] – In HSCT with HEV: frequency not known but rapidly progressive cases have been reported (see Chap. 38) – Poorly compensated cirrhosis is a contraindication for HSCT because of the prohibitive risk of developing SOS after MAC. Even compensated cirrhosis has a high likelihood of hepatic decompensation after NMA (Hogan et al. 2004)
Carcinoma	In patients with chronic HCV: 5% at 20 years of new cases per year (Peffault de Latour et al. 2004). These patients should undergo surveillance with six monthly liver ultrasound scans according to international guidelines

[a]These data correspond to the times when new antiviral agents were not available. No updated data are available
[b]The cumulative incidence of severe liver complications in HSCT infected with the HCV was 11.7% at 20 years in multicenter cohort (Ljungman et al. 2012)

49.5 Other Less Frequent Hepatic Complications

49.5.1 Nodular Regenerative Hyperplasia

After HSCT, occasionally observed in patients with a previous SOS/VOD.

Pathogenesis: Probable consequence of changes in liver blood flow with atrophy of zone 3 of the acinus and hypertrophy of zone 1 (without fibrosis).

Clinical Manifestations: Silent evolution (occasionally increase of AP) until the appearance of portal hypertension (ascites, splenomegaly, thrombocytopenia).

Diagnosis: Investigated by imaging (primarily MRI). Liver biopsy can rule out carcinoma and cirrhosis; need for a needle biopsy (not transjugular or fine-needle biopsy).

49.5.2 Focal Nodular Hyperplasia

In one series (Sudour et al. 2009) of HSCT survivors undergoing liver MRI, these lesions were observed in 12%.

Pathogenesis: The likely cause is sinusoidal injury caused by myeloablative conditioning regimens.

Clinical Manifestations: Asymptomatic.

Diagnosis: By MRI, lesions have characteristic central scars that differentiate them from hepatocellular carcinoma and fungal lesions.

49.5.3 Idiopathic Hyperammonemia

Very rare. Observed after conditioning (Frere et al. 2000)

Diagnosis: Severe hyperammonemia (>200 μmol/L) with minimal alteration of other LFTs.

Clinical Manifestations: Lethargy, motor dyscoordination, and alkalosis.

References

Akil A, Zhang Q, Mumaw CL, et al. Biomarkers for diagnosis and prognosis of sinusoidal obstruction syndrome after hematopoietic cell transplantation. Biol Blood Marrow Transplant. 2015;21:1739–45.

Carreras E, Diaz-Ricart M. The role of the endothelium in the short-term complications of hematopoietic SCT. Bone Marrow Transplant. 2011;46:1495–502.

Carreras E, Bertz H, Arcese W. Incidence and outcome of hepatic veno-occlusive disease after blood or marrow transplantation: a prospective cohort study of the European Group for Blood and Marrow Transplantation. European Group for Blood and Marrow Transplantation Chronic Leukemia Working Party. Blood. 1998;92:3599–604.

Carreras E, Diaz-Beya M, Rosinol L, et al. The incidence of veno-occlusive disease following allogeneic hematopoietic stem cell transplantation has diminished and the outcome improved over the last decade. Biol Blood Marrow Transplant. 2011;17:1713–20.

Carreras E. How I treat sinusoidal obstruction syndrome after hematopoietic cell transplantation. Br J Haematol. 2015;168:481–91.

Coppell JA, Richardson PG, Soiffer R, et al. Hepatic veno-occlusive disease following stem cell transplantation: incidence, clinical course, and outcome. Biol Blood Marrow Transplant. 2010;16:157–68.

Corbacioglu S, Cesaro S, Faraci M, et al. Defibrotide for prophylaxis of hepatic veno-occlusive disease in paediatric haemopoietic stem-cell transplantation: an open-label, phase 3, randomized controlled trial. Lancet. 2012;379:1301–9.

Corbacioglu S, Carreras E, Ansari M, et al. Diagnosis and severity criteria for sinusoidal obstruction syndrome/veno-occlusive disease in pediatric patients: a new classification from the European society for blood and marrow transplantation. Bone Marrow Transplant. 2018;53:138–45.

Dalekos GN, Zachou K, Liaskos C, Gatselis N. Autoantibodies and defined target autoantigens in autoimmune hepatitis: an overview. Eur J Intern Med. 2002;13:293–303.

Dignan FL, Wynn RF, Hadzic N, et al. BCSH/BSBMT guideline: diagnosis and management of veno-occlusive disease (sinusoidal obstruction syndrome) following haematopoietic stem cell transplantation. Br J Haematol. 2013;163:444–57.

Frere P, Canivet JL, Gennigens C, et al. Hyperammonemia after high-dose chemotherapy and stem cell transplantation. Bone Marrow Transplant. 2000;26:343–5.

Hockenbery DM, Strasser SI, McDonald GB. Gastrointestinal and hepatic complications. In: Forman SJ, Negrin RS, Antin JH, Appelbaum FR, editors. Thomas' hematopoietic cell transplantation. 5th ed. Hoboken: Wiley; 2016. p. 1140–56.

Hogan WJ, Maris M, Storer B, et al. Hepatic injury after nonmyeloablative conditioning followed by allogeneic hematopoietic cell transplantation: a study of 193 patients. Blood. 2004;103:78–84.

Ljungman P, Locasciulli A, de Soria VG, Infectious Diseases Working Party of the European Group for Blood and Marrow Transplantation, et al. Long-term follow-up of HCV-infected hematopoietic SCT patients and effects of antiviral therapy. Bone Marrow Transplant. 2012;47:1217–21.

Mohty M, Malard F, Abecassis M, et al. Revised diagnosis and severity criteria for sinusoidal obstruction syndrome/veno-occlusive disease in adult patients: a new classification from the European Society for Blood and Marrow Transplantation. Bone Marrow Transplant. 2016;51:906–12.

Peffault de Latour R, Lévy V, Asselah T, et al. Long-term outcome of hepatitis C infection after bone marrow transplantation. Blood. 2004;103:1618–24.

Sudour H, Mainard L, Baumann C, et al. Focal nodular hyperplasia of the liver following hematopoietic SCT. Bone Marrow Transplant. 2009;43:127–32.

50 Gastrointestinal Complications

Grzegorz W. Basak

50.1 Introduction

The gastrointestinal (GI) tract is one of the systems most commonly affected by transplant complications. It is due to the high vulnerability of the gut mucosa composed of dividing cells, which are susceptible to chemotherapy-induced damage, rich vasculature, constant contact with intestinal microflora, and high content of immune-competent cells. Therefore, when evaluating symptoms from the GI system, various possible causes must be taken into account, especially drug toxicity, infections, and graft-versus-host disease. In this chapter selected GI complications most frequent after HSCT will be presented. The GI aGVHD was already discussed in Chaps. 43 and 44 and infectious causes in Chaps. 38 and 39.

50.2 Nausea/Vomiting

50.2.1 Definitions

Nausea: a disorder characterized by a queasy sensation and/or the urge to vomit.

Vomiting: a disorder characterized by the reflexive act of ejecting the contents of the stomach through the mouth.

50.2.2 Types

Acute onset: within 24 h of chemotherapy administration (peak at 4–6 h) lasting for 24–48 h.

Delayed onset: occurs more than 24 h after chemotherapy (peak at 2–3 days) lasting for prolonged period of time.

50.2.3 Pathophysiology

1. Direct activation of the vomiting center in the brain stem by chemotherapy, which triggers target organs in GI tract.
2. Damage to the GI mucosa, causing vagal stimulation and neurotransmitter (serotonin, neurokinin-1, dopamine) release causing reflexive stimulation of the vomiting center.
3. Radiotherapy-induced neurotransmitter release stimulating vomiting center concomitant with brain edema.

G. W. Basak (✉)
Department of Hematology, Oncology and Internal Medicine, Independent Public Central Clinical Hospital, Medical University of Warsaw, Warsaw, Poland
e-mail: grzegorz.basak@wum.edu.pl

E. Carreras et al. (eds.), *The EBMT Handbook*, https://doi.org/10.1007/978-3-030-02278-5_50

50.2.4 Causes

Induced directly by conditioning chemoradiotherapy
TBI, TLI, cranio-spinal irradiation
Chemotherapy drugs (NCCN 2017):
- High emetic risk (frequency > 90%): CY >1500 mg/m², BCNU >250 mg/m²
- Moderate emetic risk (frequency 30–90%): bendamustine, BU, BCNU ≤250 mg/m², CY ≤1500 mg/m², MEL
- Minimal to low emetic risk (frequency < 30%): VP, TT, FLU, MTX ≤50 mg/m²

Drugs: opioids, CNI, nystatin, AmB, voriconazole, itraconazole, TMP-SMX, MMF
GVHD
Hepatic disease: GVHD, VOD, viral hepatitis
Infection: CMV, HSV, VZV, fungal, bacterial, norovirus, rotavirus, parasites
Adrenal insufficiency
Pancreatitis

50.2.5 Diagnosis

Based on symptoms.

50.2.6 Grading (CTCAE v4.0 [NCI 2009])

Nausea	
Grade 1	Loss of appetite without alteration of eating habits
Grade 2	Oral intake decreased without significant weight loss, dehydration, or malnutrition
Grade 3	Inadequate oral caloric or fluid intake, tube feeding, TPN, or hospitalization indicated
Vomiting	
Grade 1	1–2 episodes (separated by 5 min) in 24 hs
Grade 2	3–5 episodes (separated by 5 min) in 24 h
Grade 3	≥6 episodes (separated by 5 min) in 24 h, tube feeding, TPN, or hospitalization indicated
Grade 4	Life-threatening consequences, urgent intervention indicated

50.2.7 Treatment

Prevention of nausea/vomiting is the mainstay of clinical management since treatment frequently proves ineffective. Delayed nausea should be treated with scheduled antiemetics for 2–4 days after completion of chemotherapy.

50.2.8 Prophylaxis

Choice of drugs depends on the use of drug with highest emetogenic potential (NCCN 2017):

High emetic risk	Serotonin (5-HT3 antagonist) (patients should be monitored for QT corrected prolongation) • Short-acting: ondansetron 3 × 8 mg IV on days of chemo +24–48 h, granisetron, dolasetron • Long-acting: palonosetron 0.25 mg IV, may be repeated every 3 days *Plus* Neurokinin-1 receptor antagonists, e.g., aprepitant *Plus/minus* Dexamethasone 2–10 mg IV (as required for a short duration)
Moderate emetic risk	Serotonin (5-HT3) antagonists (as above) *Plus/minus* Dexamethasone 2–10 mg IV
Low emetic risk	Serotonin (5-HT3) antagonists (short acting, as above) Metoclopramide Prochlorperazine
TBI	Serotonin (5-HT3) antagonists (short- or long-acting, as above) Dexamethasone (4 mg/d or 4 mg bid)

50.2.9 Other Nausea/Vomiting

Breakthrough treatment	Addition of a different class anti-emetic drug Prochlorperazine (10 mg IV q6h) Haloperidol (1–2 mg q4h) Metoclopramide (0.5–2 mg/kg IV q6h) Olanzapine Scopolamine transdermal patch Corticosteroids Lorazepam
Anticipatory nausea/vomiting	Prevention of nausea/vomiting by efficient prophylaxis at every treatment Strong smell avoidance Behavioral therapy Lorazepam, alprazolam

50.3 Diarrhea

50.3.1 Definitions

A disorder characterized by frequent and watery bowel movements.

50.3.2 Physiopathogeny

Depending on the cause.

50.3.3 Causes

The diarrhea in preengraftment period is most frequently caused by toxicity of conditioning. In post transplant period, aGVHD must be taken into consideration. The risk of infectious causes persists for the whole time with bacterial causes predominating relatively earlier than viral infections.

Chemotherapy and radiation therapy-related toxicity
Acute GVHD
Intestinal infections:
- *Clostridium difficile*
- Viral (CMV, VZV, rotavirus, norovirus, astrovirus, adenovirus)
- Parasitic (giardia, strongyloides, cryptosporidium)
- Fungal (candida)

Medications (antibiotics, mycophenolate mofetil, oral nutritional supplements)
Transplant-associated microangiopathy
Other: pancreatitis/pancreatic insufficiency, lactose intolerance/disaccharidase deficiency, malabsorption, inflammatory bowel disease, liver and gallbladder disease

50.3.4 Diagnosis

The standard workup for diarrhea after HSCT includes stool cultures, tests for *Clostridium difficile* toxin A and B, *Clostridium* antigen, stool and/or blood tests for viruses, and, when negative, endoscopy with biopsy for aGVHD and CMV. However, when these tests are proven negative, a broad area of causes must be considered (Robak et al. 2017).

Stool examination and microbiological workup
- *C. difficile* toxin, antigen, culture
- Parasites (giardia, strongyloides, cryptosporidium)
- Viruses (CMV, VZV, rotavirus, norovirus, astrovirus, adenovirus)
- Fungi (culture)

Sigmoidoscopy/colonoscopy ± gastroscopy
- Histopathology for GVHD, cryptosporidium, and CMV
- Viral, parasitic/bacterial cultures

Biochemistry (triglycerides, amylase, lipase),
GVHD biomarkers (calprotectin, REG3-α) (Rodriguez-Otero et al. 2012; Ferrara et al. 2011)
Ultrasound, CT (in GVHD distal ileum or proximal colon most likely involved)
Capsule endoscopy

50.3.5 Grading

When the diagnosis of gut aGVHD is established or suspected, aGVHD grading should be used as described in Chap. 43. Otherwise, (CTCAE v4.0) grading should be used (NCI 2009).

Grade 1	Increase of <4 stools per day over baseline; mild increase in ostomy output compared to baseline
Grade 2	Increase of 4–6 stools per day over baseline; moderate increase in ostomy output compared to baseline
Grade 3	Increase of ≥7 stools per day over baseline; incontinence; hospitalization indicated; severe increase in ostomy output compared to baseline; limiting self- care activities of daily living
Grade 4	Life-threatening consequences; urgent intervention indicated

50.3.6 Treatment

Targeted, according to the known or suspected cause, consider overlap with another pathology (e.g., aGVHD with gut CMV infection)
Ancillary: modification of diet
- Lactose- or gluten-free
- Restricted diet (low roughage, low residue, low or no lactose)
- Temporarily nothing per os and TPN

Avoid fluid loss and dyselectrolytemia
Monitor and replace protein losses (albumin, gamma globulin)
Loperamide 2–4 mg p.o. every 6 h if associated with toxicity of conditioning or GVHD
Octreotide

50.4 Esophagitis/Gastritis

50.4.1 Definitions/Symptoms

Heartburn and/or epigastric pain observed most frequently during conditioning and period of mucositis.

50.4.2 Causes

Mucositis, medications, altered gastric pH, peptic ulcer disease, and fungal esophagitis.

50.4.3 Diagnosis

Based on clinical symptoms ± endoscopy.

50.4.4 Treatment

Depending on the cause, elevation of the head of bed, and consideration of proton pump inhibitors and other symptomatic treatments (e.g., alginate, antacid, and topical local anesthetics, such as oxetacaine for mucositis). May require systemic analgesia if patient unable to swallow.

50.5 GI Bleeding

50.5.1 Definitions/Symptoms

May appear as melena, hematemesis or bloody stool, or emergence of normocytic anemia.

50.5.2 Causes

Thrombocytopenia, esophageal trauma, esophagitis, colitis, anal fissures or varices, viral infections, GVHD, and plasma coagulation impairment.

50.5.3 Diagnosis

Esophagogastroduodenoscopy, colonoscopy, and angioCT.

50.5.4 Treatment

Treatment of underlying disorder
Symptomatic
- Platelet transfusion to >50 × 10^9/L
- RBC transfusion
- Fresh frozen plasma, fibrinogen concentrates, vitamin K supplementation
- Octreotide
- Endoscopic cauterization or embolization

When massive blood loss
- Desmopressin
- Tranexamic acid
- Recombinant factor VII

50.6 Typhlitis

50.6.1 Definitions/Symptoms

Necrosis of usually large intestinal wall associated with chemotherapy toxicity and bacterial overgrowth.

Occurs within 30 days after HSCT, patients usually complain of pain in right lower abdominal quadrant, often with associated fever.

Additionally, nausea, emesis, increased abdominal wall tension, and watery bloody diarrhea may occur (Robak et al. 2017).

50.6.2 Causes

Toxicity/infection.

50.6.3 Diagnosis

Clinical and abdominal ultrasound or CT: bowel wall thickening usually limited to single region, e.g., ileocecal or ascending colon; may be associated with perforaton and air within intestinal wall.

50.6.4 Treatment

Antibiotics and bowel rest. Avoid surgical intervention.

50.7 Pancreatic Disease

50.7.1 Definitions/Symptoms

Pancreatic insufficiency and atrophy or acute pancreatitis.

50.7.2 Causes

Medications (prednisone, tacrolimus), stones, and pancreatic GVHD.

50.7.3 Diagnosis

Insufficiency and atrophy: low serum trypsinogen, high fecal elastase-1, and possible atrophy in imaging. Acute pancreatitis: elevated lipase and amylase, elevated fecal fat, and edema in ultrasound/CT.

50.7.4 Treatment

When insufficiency: enzyme replacement.

50.8 Chronic Esophageal GVHD

50.8.1 Definitions/Symptoms

Dysphagia to solid food, chest discomfort, and aspiration (Jagasia et al. 2015; Robak et al. 2017)

50.8.2 Diagnosis

Barium meal: mid/upper esophageal strictures, webs, rings, bullae, and desquamation. Endoscopy: as above, erythematous, friable sloughed mucosa.

50.8.3 Treatment

When severe and chronic, need serial dilations and enteral tube placement or esophagectomy.

Key Points

The workup and management of GI complications after HCT follow general medical approach; however the most frequent scenarios remain characteristic for this patient population. The most common causes include toxicity of drugs, especially those used for conditioning, infection, and/or graft-versus-host disease:

- Nausea/vomiting or diarrhea occurring before engraftment is most likely caused by toxicity of conditioning, while after engraftment, GVHD needs to be considered, especially in allo-HSCT setting.
- For the whole post transplant period, infectious causes should also be considered with bacterial or fungal causes predominating in the neutropenic period and viral reactivations/infections in the later phases.
- Importantly, inflammation caused by infection may become a trigger to GVHD, while GVHD is frequently followed by infection; therefore, overlapping scenarios always need to be taken into account.
- GI GVHD is frequently a diagnosis of exclusion (especially in patients with other overlapping causes which may impact on laboratory investigations). However, it should always be considered when symptoms persist despite extensive workup and/or directed treatment.

References

Common Terminology Criteria for Adverse Events (CTCAE). Version 4.0. Published: May 28, 2009 (v4.03: June 14, 2010) U.S. Department of Health and Human Services, National Institutes of Health, National Cancer Institute. https://www.eortc.be/services/doc/ctc/CTCAE_4.03_2010-06-14_QuickReference_5x7.pdf

Ferrara JL, Harris AC, Greenson JK, et al. Regenerating islet-derived 3-alpha is a biomarker of gastrointestinal graft-versus-host disease. Blood. 2011;118:6702–8.

Jagasia MH, Greinix HT, Arora M, et al. National Institutes of Health Consensus Development Project on Criteria for Clinical Trials in Chronic Graft-versus-Host Disease: I. The 2014 Diagnosis and Staging Working Group report. Biol Blood Marrow Transplant. 2015;21:389–401.

NCCN Clinical Practice Guidelines in Oncology (NCCN Guidelines). Antiemesis. Version 2.2017. March 28, 2017. https://www.nccn.org/professionals/physician_gls/pdf/antiemesis.pdf

Robak K, Zambonelli J, Bilinski J, Basak GW. Diarrhea after allogeneic stem cell transplantation: beyond graft-versus-host disease. Eur J Gastroenterol Hepatol. 2017;29:495–502.

Rodriguez-Otero P, Porcher R, Peffault de Latour R, et al. Fecal calprotectin and alpha-1 antitrypsin predict severity and response to corticosteroids in gastrointestinal graft-versus-host disease. Blood. 2012;119:5909–17.

51 Haemorrhagic Cystitis and Renal Dysfunction

Simone Cesaro

51.1 Haemorrhagic Cystitis

51.1.1 Introduction

Haemorrhagic cystitis (HC) is a frequent complication after HSCT. According to the time of occurrence after HSCT, HC is defined as early-onset and late-onset. Early-onset HC occurs typically during or within 48 h after the end of conditioning regimen, and it is the result of a direct toxic effect of drug metabolites and radiotherapy on the bladder mucosa. Late-onset HC usually starts around the time of the period of neutrophil engraftment (weeks 2–4) or in second-third month after HSCT (Hirsch and Pergam 2016). The concurrent presence of pro-haemorrhagic abnormalities of coagulation, severe thrombocytopenia and mucosal inflammation are predisposing factors for any type of HC.

51.1.2 Risk Factors

The main risk factor for late-onset HC is infection by polyomavirus BK (BKPyV), whereas other viruses such as ADV, CMV, and HHV6 have been rarely implicated.

BKPyV is a common cause of asymptomatic or mild flu-like infection during early infancy and childhood, and more than 90% of adults are seropositive for BKPyV. The route of transmission is not clearly defined, but it is thought to be through oral saliva or respiratory tract secretions. After the primary infection, the virus persists latently in renal tubular epithelial and urothelial cell and can replicate as the host immune control loses the capacity to mount a virus-specific T-cell response. Mild to moderate asymptomatic BKPyV viruria is seen in 5–10% of healthy individuals, especially the oldest and the pregnant women, whereas high-load BKPyV viruria is detected in 50–60% of patients who underwent an allo-HSCT due to the delayed recovery of immune responses and the use of immunosuppressive drugs.

51.1.3 Pathogenesis

The current pathogenetic model of HC following HSCT is multifactorial and includes the combined effects of the extensive cytopathic damage of bladder mucosa layer due to the high-rate replicating virus, the chemical or actinic damage induced by conditioning regimen, and the donor-cell immune alloreactivity targeting bladder mucosa (Cesaro et al. 2018). In patients receiving allogeneic HSCT, both BKPyV viruria and viremia are specific and sensitive predictive factors for BKPyV-HC: a urine BKPyV load >1 × 10^7 genomic copies/mL had a

S. Cesaro (✉)
Pediatric Hematology Oncology, Azienda Ospedaliera Universitaria Integrata, Verona, Italy
e-mail: simone.cesaro@aovr.veneto.it

E. Carreras et al. (eds.), *The EBMT Handbook*, https://doi.org/10.1007/978-3-030-02278-5_51

sensitivity of 86% and specificity of 60%, while a blood BKPyV load >1 × 10^3 genomic copies/mL had a sensitivity of 100% and a specificity of 86% for HC (Cesaro et al. 2015).

BKPyV infection develops in more than 50% of allo-HSCT in the peri-engraftment weeks, but overt HC occurs in about 20% of patients because its development is influenced by the presence of several other risk factors: the type of graft (CB and PB vs. BM); the type of donor (URD vs. MRD); the type of conditioning regimen (MAC vs. RIC); the use in the conditioning regimen of ATG, CY, or BU; the occurrence of acute GVHD grade 2–4; and, among the paediatric patients, a recipient age >7 years.

51.1.4 Diagnosis

The clinical diagnosis of BKPyV-HC is based on the presence of clinical symptoms/signs of cystitis, such as dysuria, increased urinary frequency, and lower abdominal pain, the presence of macrohaematuria, and the demonstration of BKPyV viruria, with viral loads of >7 log10 copies/mL.

The severity of haematuria is described by four categories: microscopic (grade 1), macroscopic (grade 2), macroscopic with clots (grade 3), and macroscopic with clots and renal failure secondary to urinary tract obstruction.

BKPyV viremia is often detected in patients with BKPyV-HC, and plasma viral load of >3 to 4 log10 copies/mL has been reported in more than two thirds of patients (Erard et al. 2005; Cesaro et al. 2015).

The reduction of both BKPyV viruria and BKPyV viremia has been correlated with clinical recovery from HC. Despite this, screening of asymptomatic HSCT patients at risk for BKPyV viruria and viremia remains an area of investigation and is presently not recommended since pre-emptive therapy is not established.

51.1.5 Prophylaxis

Effective preventive measures are available only for early-onset HC, and they are mainly unspecific such as *hyperhydration* and the use of *mesna* in patients who receive high dose of CY as part of the conditioning regimen. The capacity of CY and its metabolite acrolein to damage the bladder mucosa determining an inflammatory reaction is well-known, and both hyperhydration and mesna reduce the exposure of bladder mucosa to acrolein and other toxic catabolites.

In line with this, the recent increase of unmanipulated haplo-HSCT with the administration of a PT-CY as prophylaxis of GVHD has resulted in a high incidence of HC. The use of bladder irrigation through a two- or three-way urinary catheter resulted not more effective in preventing HC compared to hyperhydration, and considering its invasiveness and discomfort for the patient, its use is not recommended.

In the pathogenetic model of late-onset HC, BKPyV replication has a key role in exacerbating the damage of bladder mucosa through its cytopathic effect and in inducing the donor immune alloreactivity to target the bladder mucosa. In order to reduce BKPyV replication, *ciprofloxacin* has been used prophylactically by several authors because of the in vitro capacity of fluoroquinolones to inhibit BKPyV replication. Overall, the efficacy of ciprofloxacin was weak and limited to a reduction of BKPyV replication without significantly affecting the incidence of HC. Considering the risk of inducing bacterial resistance and the risk of tendinitis and joint damage in children, the use of fluoroquinolones is not recommended for this purpose.

51.1.6 Treatment

BKPyV replication can be controlled more effectively by *cidofovir*, a nucleotide analogue inhibiting several DNA viruses such as CMV, ADV, HHV6, HSV, HVZ, and *smallpox*. The important pharmacokinetic property of cidofovir is the long half-life of its active metabolites ranging from 15 to 65 h that allows the administration on a weekly basis. Given the significant risk of tubular nephrotoxicity, cidofovir has been used only for therapeutic purposes (Cesaro et al. 2009). The nephrotoxicity can be limited by saline hydration and by the use of probenecid that inhibits the capture and transport of cidofovir into the tubular epithelial cells of the kidney. Despite that several authors have assessed cidofovir as treatment of BKPyV-HC, there is no agreement on the optimal dose, modality of administration, and frequency of administration. Most authors use intravenous cidofovir at the dose of 3–5 mg/kg/weekly or fortnightly together with probenecid to prevent nephrotoxicity obtaining a complete clinical response in 74% of patients and at least 1 log decline in urine and blood viral loads in 38% and 84% of patients. As expected, the main adverse effect was renal toxicity with a mild to moderate increase in serum creatinine observed in 18% of the patients. The second more frequent scheme of treatment was a dose of cidofovir of 0.5–1.5 mg/kg without probenecid, administered 1–3 times a week (Ganguly et al. 2010). A complete clinical response was observed in 83% of patients, with a significant reduction of viral load in the urine and in the blood in 62% and 67% of patients, respectively. Also, with this schedule, mild to moderate renal toxicity was reported in 20% of patients. An alternative route that can reduce the risk of nephrotoxicity is the administration of *cidofovir intravesically*. Although the experience is limited to a small number of patients, the dose of 5 mg/kg/week, left in situ for 1–2 h after clamping the vesical catheter, showed an overall clinical response in 43% of patients and a virological response in about 50% (Bridges et al. 2006).

Preliminary encouraging results have also been obtained with *leflunomide*, an antimetabolite drug with immunomodulatory and antiviral activity, whereas a successful treatment has been reported anecdotal and in older series with vidarabine, oral levofloxacin, FXIII concentrate, intravesical sodium hyaluronate, and oestrogens (Cesaro et al. 2018).

The recovery from HC, whatever the cause, can benefit from treatment aiming to repair and regenerate the urothelial mucosa, such as *hyperbaric oxygen therapy* and the topical application of *fibrin glue*. Although experienced in a limited number of patients, the use of hyperbaric oxygen therapy was associated with a complete clinical response rate of 86% and a reduced urine BKPyV load in 65% of patients. The main drawback of hyperbaric oxygen is the limited availability, the requirements for dedicated hyperbaric room facilities, the risk of ear barotrauma or pressure intolerance, and claustrophobia episodes during the procedure (Zama et al. 2013; Cesaro et al. 2018). Cystoscopic application of fibrin glue to the damaged bladder mucosa to achieve haemostasis has been reported in single-centre retrospective series with a complete response rate was 83%, with most of cases resolved with just one or two applications (Tirindelli et al. 2014).

Given the important role of immune response in the pathogenesis of late-onset HC and in absence of effective antiviral drugs, innovative therapies have been trialled, such as the use of *mesenchymal stromal cells* (MSC) and adoptive immunotherapy. MSC have the potential to stimulate the tissue repairing process and exercise an immune modulatory and anti-inflammatory effect. The use of third party MSC infusion into seven patients with BKPyV-HC obtained the resolution of haematuria in five patients (Ringden et al. 2007). This approach needs to be validated further to assess the feasibility and also the safety of MSC.

Adoptive transfer of *donor-derived virus-specific T cells* (VSTs) has shown efficacy for the treatment of several viral infections although their use on a larger scale is limited by the costs, the complexity of manufacturing, the time needed to obtain the final cell product that is not suitable for the urgent treatment, and the prompt availability of a seropositive donor. The use of banked VSTs with multiple specificity obtained by a third party healthy seropositive donor cryopreserved and used as the patient developed a viral infection refractory to antiviral treatment represents a promising development. In a phase II trial, the use of VSTs directed against five viruses, CMV, EBV, ADV, HHV-6, and BKPyV, obtained an overall cumulative response rate of 92%. The virological response for BKPyV was 100%, and 13 of 14 patients treated for HC had a resolution of haematuria by 6 weeks. The infusions of VSTs resulted safe, and only 2 of 45 infusions were followed by a mild GVHD reaction (grade 1). Importantly, the functionality of VSTs persisted for up 12 weeks (Tzannou et al. 2017). These results are encouraging and support further studies.

51.2 Renal Dysfunction

Acute kidney injury (AKI) occurs in 27–66% of patients who underwent allo-HSCT mainly within the first 100 days. The incidence of AKI in less than 20% in auto-HSCT due to several reasons such as the rapid engraftment and reduced cytopenia especially with PBSC grafts, the lower incidence of infectious complications, and the absence of GVHD that can determine a renal damage directly by inducing inflammatory cytokines, CMV reactivation, diarrhoea with severe dehydration, and indirectly, through the nephrotoxicity of the drugs used to prevent or treat GVHD such as CNI and high-dose PRD (Lopes et al. 2016; Raina et al. 2017).

The diseases associated with AKI act at different renal levels: prerenal (sepsis, engraftment syndrome, SOS/VOD), renal-glomerular (transplant-associated microangiopathy), renal-tubular (acute tubular necrosis due to dehydration, sepsis, shock, engraftment syndrome, intratubular obstruction due to drugs, or tumour lysis syndrome), renal-interstitial (acute GVHD, viral infection by BKPvyV or ADV), and post-renal (obstruction by BKPyV or adenovirus cystitis, retroperitoneal fibrosis, lymphadenopathy).

Moreover, there are general favouring factors for AKI such as the presence pre-HSCT of diabetes, hypertension, and renal impairment as well as the use of nephrotoxic drugs in the conditioning regimen (ifosphamide, CY, carboplatin, cisplatin), for treatment of GVHD (MTX, CNI), for the treatment of infections (AmB, aminoglicosydes, vancomycin), and for other severe organ damages that require ICU admission and mechanical ventilation (Hingorani 2016).

Clinically, the severity of AKI is defined by the measure of serum creatinine (SCr) and urine output (UO) that permit the identification of three classes: risk of AKI (increase of SCr 1.5–2× and UO <0.5 mL/kg/h for >6 h), kidney injury (increase of SCr 2–3×, and UO < 0.5 mL/kg/h for >12 h), and kidney failure (increase of SCr >3× and UO <0.3 mL/kg/h for >24 h or anuria >12 h, or initiation of replacement therapy) (Lopes et al. 2016). AKI represents a risk factor for the development on the medium-long-term period of chronic kidney disease, especially if the acute damage is not completely resolved and proteinuria and hypertension persist and for increased of non-relapse and overall mortality (Shingai et al. 2015).

Key Points

	Early-onset HC	Late-onset HC	Comments
Incidence	<3%	7–25%	Early-onset HC is nowadays rare
Pathogenesis	Chemical or actinic damage of bladder mucosa	– BKPyV infection – Adenovirus infection – Donor alloreactivity	
Diagnosis	Macrohaematuria with dysuria, increased urinary frequency, low abdominal pain	Macrohaematuria with dysuria, increased urinary frequency, low abdominal pain, high load of BKPyV urine and/or plasma	Signs of bladder inflammation at ultrasound examination
Prevention	Hyperhydration, mesna (if CY), forced diuresis	Hyperhydration, forced diuresis	Fluoroquinolones not recommended
Therapy	– Hyperhydration – Forced diuresis – Hyperbaric O2 – Application of fibrin glue by cystoscopy	– Hyperhydration, forced diuresis – IV (or intravesical) cidofovir – Hyperbaric O2 therapy – Application of fibrin glue by cystoscopy	– Cidofovir: No agreement on dose and route of admin Limited evidence – O2 and fibrin glue limited experience
Experimental	/	– Mesenchymal cells – Virus-specific T cells	

References

Bridges B, Donegan S, Badros A. Cidofovir bladder instillation for the treatment of BK hemorrhagic cystitis after allogeneic stem cell transplantation. Am J Hematol. 2006;81:535–7.

Cesaro S, Hirsch HH, Faraci M, et al. Cidofovir for BK virus-associated hemorrhagic cystitis: a retrospective study. Clin Infect Dis. 2009;49:233–40.

Cesaro S, Tridello G, Pillon M, et al. A prospective study on the predictive value of plasma BK virus-DNA load for hemorrhagic cystitis in pediatric patients after stem cell transplantation. J Pediatric Infect Dis Soc. 2015;4:134–42.

Cesaro S, Dalianis T, Hanssen Rinaldo C, et al. ECIL guidelines for the prevention, diagnosis and treatment of BK polyomavirus-associated haemorrhagic cystitis in haematopoietic stem cell transplant recipients. J Antimicrob Chemother. 2018;73:12–21.

Erard V, Kim HW, Corey L, et al. BK DNA viral load in plasma: evidence for an association with hemorrhagic cystitis in allogeneic hematopoietic cell transplant recipients. Blood. 2005;106:1130–2.

Ganguly N, Clough LA, Dubois LK, et al. Low-dose cidofovir in the treatment of symptomatic BK virus infection in patients undergoing allogeneic hematopoietic stem cell transplantation: a retrospective analysis of an algorithmic approach. Transpl Infect Dis. 2010;12:406–11.

Hingorani S. Renal complications after hematopoietic stem cell transplantation. N Engl J Med. 2016; 374:2256–67.

Hirsch HH, Pergam SA. Human adenovirus, polyomavirus, and parvovirus infections in patients undergoing hematopoietic stem-cell transplantation. In: Forman SJ, Nagrin RS, Antin H, Appelbaum FR, editors. Thomas' hematopoietic cell transplantation. 5th ed. Hoboken: Wiley; 2016. p. 1090–104. http://www.wiley.comgoappelbaumTransplantation.

Lopes JA, Jorge S, Neves M. Acute kidney injury in HCT: an update. Bone Mmarrow Ttransplant. 2016;51:755–62.

Raina R, Herrera N, Krishnappa V, et al. Hematopoietic stem cell transplantation and kidney injury in children: a comprehensive review. Pediatr Transplant. 2017;21:e12935.

Ringden O, Uzunel M, Sundberg B, et al. Tissue repair using allogeneic mesenchymal stem cells for hemorrhagic cystitis, pneumomediastinum and perforated colon. Leukemia. 2007;21:2271–6.

Shingai N, Morito T, Najima Y, et al. Early-onset acute kidney injury a poor prognostic sign for allogeneic SCT recipients. Bone Marrow Transplant. 2015;50:1557–662.

Tirindelli MC, Flammia GP, Bove P, et al. Fibrin glue therapy for severe hemorrhagic cystitis after allogeneic hematopoietic stem cell transplantation. Biol Blood Marrow Transplant. 2014;20:1612–7.

Tzannou I, Papadopoulou A, Naik S, et al. Off-the-shelf virus specific T cells to treat BK virus, human herpes virus 6, cytomegalovirus, Epstein-Barr virus, and adenovirus infections after allogeneic hematopoietic stem cell transplantation. J Clin Oncol. 2017;35:3547–57.

Zama D, Masetti R, Vendemini F, et al. Clinical effectiveness of early treatment with hyperbaric oxygen therapy for severe late-onset hemorrhagic cystitis after hematopoietic stem cell transplantation in pediatric patients. Pediatr Transplant. 2013;17:86–91.

Check for updates

52 Noninfectious Pulmonary Complications

Enric Carreras and Kenneth R. Cooke

52.1 Introduction

Lung injury occurs frequently following HSCT and significantly contributes to morbidity and mortality in the immediate post transplant period and in the months and years that follow. It can be observed in 25–55% of recipients (Cooke and Yanik 2016).

Historically, approximately half of all pulmonary complications seen after HSCT were secondary to infection, but the judicious use of broad-spectrum antimicrobial agents has tipped the balance toward noninfectious causes.

Noninfectious lung injury following HSCT may be mediated by either immune or nonimmune mechanisms and could represent up to the 50% of noninfectious mortality after allo-HSCT.

These complications have been classified by the American Thoracic Society according to the tissue primarily injured and its etiology (Panoskaltsis-Mortari et al. 2011) (Table 52.1).

Table 52.1 Noninfectious pulmonary complications after HSCT[a]

Localization	Entity
Pulmonary parenchyma	– Acute interstitial pneumonitis[b] – Acute respiratory distress syndrome (ARDS)[b] – BCNU pneumonitis – Radiation pneumonitis – Delayed pulmonary toxicity syndrome[b] – Post-HSCT lymphoproliferative disease (see Chap. 45) – Eosinophilic pneumonia – Pulmonary alveolar proteinosis
Vascular endothelium	– Peri-engraftment respiratory distress syndrome (PERDS)[b] – Capillary leak syndrome (CLS)[b] (see Chap. 42) – Diffuse alveolar hemorrhage (DAH)[b] – Pulmonary VOD – Transfusion-assoc. acute lung injury – Pulmonary cytolytic syndrome – Pulmonary arterial hypertension – Pulmonary thromboembolism
Airway epithelium	– Cryptogenetic organizing pneumonia (COP)[b,c] – Bronchiolitis obliterans syndrome (BOS)[b]

[a]Importantly, this classification does not include the most frequent lung complication after HSCT, i.e., pulmonary edema secondary to fluid overload
[b]All these complications are categorized as IPS
[c]Formerly called bronchiolitis obliterans organizing pneumonia (BOOP)

E. Carreras (✉)
Spanish Bone Marrow Donor Registry, Josep Carreras Foundation and Leukemia Research Institute, Barcelona, Catalunya, Spain

Hospital Clinic Barcelona, Barcelona University, Barcelona, Catalunya, Spain
e-mail: enric.carreras@fcarreras.es

K. R. Cooke
Pediatric Blood and Marrow Transplantation Program, Oncology Department, Sidney Kimmel Comprehensive Cancer Center, Johns Hopkins University School of Medicine, Baltimore, MD, USA

E. Carreras et al. (eds.), *The EBMT Handbook*, https://doi.org/10.1007/978-3-030-02278-5_52

52.2 Diagnostic Methodology of Pulmonary Complications

Ideally, any respiratory/pulmonary complication observed after HSCT must be evaluated following a predetermined institutional protocol (Lucena et al. 2014), which should include:

1. Noninvasive tests: Blood samples for culture and antigen determination, sputum culture, nasopharyngeal swabs testing CMV, respiratory syncytial virus (RSV), *Legionella*, *Pneumocystis jirovecii* (PJ), parainfluenza virus (PIV), adenovirus (ADV), as well as urinary antigen tests and chest x-ray.
2. If negative → empirical treatment (variable behavior; some centers start empirical treatment before the BAL, but many others start the treatment after BAL).
3. If no response in a maximum of 2–3 days (or if galactomannan (GM) +) →
   (a) High-resolution chest-computed tomography (HRCT).
   (b) Fiber-optic bronchoscopy (FOB) including bronchial aspiration and BAL to analyze: PCR for *Legionella*, *Mycoplasma*, *Chlamydia*, herpesvirus (all), polyomavirus, ADV, parvovirus, enterovirus, and respiratory virus (RSV; influenza a, B, and C; PIV types 1–4; rhinovirus; bocavirus; metapneumovirus; and others) and GM.
4. In some selected cases, a transbronchial biopsy could be considered.

52.2.1 Results Reported Using this Methodology (Seo et al. 2015; Lucena et al. 2014; Shannon et al. 2010)

Diagnostic yield could be as high as 80%.

Sixty percent of diagnosis is achieved with noninvasive techniques.

FOB/BAL permits an etiological diagnosis in up to 78% of cases.

In suspected IPS, a BAL study may detect a pathogen in ~50% of cases.

For pathogen detection, early FOB (<5 days) offer better yield than late FOB.

The risk of complications with FOB is <5%.

52.3 Pulmonary Edema Due to Fluid Overload

Despite not being included in most classifications of pulmonary complications after HSCT, pulmonary edema (PE) as a consequence of a fluid overload (FO) is extremely frequent (Rondón et al. 2017).

Incidence	FO may be observed in up to 60% of patients in the first days after HSCT. The exact incidence of PE is not established although it could be higher than 20%
Symptoms and signs	– Weight gain, moderate breathlessness, nonproductive cough, moderate hypoxemia – Crackles and rales in both lung bases – Chest radiology with diffuse alveolar/interstitial infiltrates
Diagnosis	PE should be suspected in the context of weight gain, an increased cardiothoracic index, and crackles/rales. Though rarely necessary, the diagnosis can be confirmed by pulmonary pressure measurements
Differential diagnosis	– Heart failure (prior anthracycline toxicity or conditioning with CY) – Endothelial syndromes: SOS, CLS, ES (see Chaps. 42 and 49) – Respiratory tract infections – Post transfusion reactions
Treatment	Hydro-saline restriction, diuretics

52.4 Idiopathic Pneumonia Syndrome

52.4.1 Definition

Widespread alveolar injury in absence of active lower respiratory tract infection, cardiac or renal dysfunction, and iatrogenic fluid overload (Clark et al. 1993; Panoskaltsis-Mortari et al. 2011)

52.4.2 Clinical Manifestations

Characterized by development around day +20 after HSCT of fever and nonproductive cough, dyspnea, tachypnea, hypoxemia, rales, and diffuse alveolar or interstitial infiltrates on x-rays or CT scans.

52.4.3 Diagnosis

All of the following must be present for accepting the IPS diagnosis:

1. *Evidence of widespread alveolar injury*
   (a) Multilobar infiltrates on chest radiographs or CT
   (b) Symptoms and signs of pneumonia (cough, dyspnea, tachypnea, crackles/rales)
   (c) Evidence of abnormal pulmonary physiology
   Increased alveolar to arterial oxygen difference; need for supplemental O_2 therapy
   New or increased restrictive PFTs abnormality
2. *Absence of active lower respiratory tract infection based upon*
   (a) BAL negative for significant bacterial pathogens including acid-fast bacilli, *Nocardia*, and *Legionella* species
   (b) BAL negative for pathogenic nonbacterial microorganisms (*Note of the authors*: Most of the following diagnostic methods despite included in the initial diagnostic methodology have nowadays largely been replaced by PCR techniques)
   Routine culture for viruses and fungi
   Shell vial culture for CMV and respiratory RSV
   Cytology for CMV inclusions, fungi, and *Pneumocystis jirovecii*
   Direct fluorescence staining with antibodies against CMV, RSV, HSV, VZV, influenza virus, parainfluenza virus, adenovirus, and other organisms
   (c) Other organisms/tests to also consider:
   PCR for human metapneumovirus, rhinovirus, coronavirus, and HHV6
   PCR for *Chlamydia*, *Mycoplasma*, and *Aspergillus* spp.
   Serum and BAL fluid GM for *Aspergillus* species
   (d) Transbronchial biopsy if condition of the patient permits
3. *Absence of*
   Cardiac dysfunction, acute renal failure, or iatrogenic fluid overload as etiology for pulmonary dysfunction

52.4.4 Pathogenesis, Incidence, Presentation, and Risk Factors

Pathogenesis	The pathophysiology of IPS is complex. Data generated using experimental models support that IPS is a process in which the lung is susceptible to two distinct but interrelated pathways of immune-mediated injury: a T-cell axis and an inflammatory cytokine axis. These distinct but related pathways of inflammation culminate in the recruitment of immune cells to the lung leading to tissue damage and dysfunction (Cooke and Yanik 2016)
Incidence	– The strict methodology required to establish IPS diagnosis and the increased use of RIC have reduced its incidence of 20% to 25% observed 20 years ago (at that time IPS was called idiopathic pneumonia) – This reduction runs in parallel of the improvement in the diagnostic methodologies to detect infectious pathogens. However, the frequent absence of response to the specific treatment against a detected pathogen suggests that the true incidence of IPS may be underestimated – Nowadays: <10% of allo-HSCT (8% after MAC; 2% after RIC)
Timing	– Within first 120 days after BMT, usually observed between days +18 and +21 (20 years ago: around days +40 to +50) – Late IPS can be observed but they are exceptional (Thompson et al. 2017)
Risk factors (from Cooke and Yanik 2016)	Older age / Karnofsky index <90 / higher interval diagnosis-HSCT MAC or TBI ($\geq$12 Gy) / HLA disparity / GVHD prophylaxis with MTX Acute GVHD/previous viral infection / other malignancies than leukemia

52.4.5 Treatment and Prognosis

Supportive measures	– Supplemental O_2 therapy – Mechanical ventilation (invasive or not [high-flow nasal O_2, CPAP]) – Empiric broad-spectrum antimicrobials – Strict control of fluids balance/hemofiltration
Specific treatment	As mentioned, lung injury in IPS can occur through two pathways, the TNF-alfa/LPS dependent and IL6/IL17 dependent (Cooke and Yanik 2016); consequently, treatment options are focused in these directions • *Methyl-PDN* ≤ 2 mg/kg/d; if not clear response, consider as soon as possible: • Anti-TNFα: *Etanercept* 0.4 mg/kg twice weekly (maximum of 8 doses) + systemic steroids (2 mg/kg/d). The randomized study of etanercept + steroids vs. steroids + placebo was terminated prematurely due to slow accrual. In the limited number of patients examined, there were no differences in response rates (≈60%) at day +28. These results do not necessarily imply that this agent is not effective (lack of evidence does not imply lack of effectiveness) (Yanik et al. 2014). In a phase II trial in children, the CR rate was 71% and 1 y survival was 63% (Yanik et al. 2015). This combination has also been shown to be effective in exceptional cases of late IPS with a 42% of CR and a 2 y survival of 62% among responders (Thompson et al. 2017) • Other *investigational agents* such as – MoAb anti-IL6: Tocilizumab (experimental IPS; Varelias et al. 2015) – MoAb anti-IL17: Brodalumab (experimental IPS; Varelias et al. 2015)
Evolution	Despite the diagnosis and therapeutic advances, the mortality from IPS remains high at 59–80% at ≈2 weeks of evolution (95% if mechanical ventilation is required)

52.5 Diffuse Alveolar Hemorrhage (DAH)

Diffuse alveolar hemorrhage (DAH) is a relevant cause of acute respiratory failure that occurs in 2–14% of recipients, with similar incidence in both auto- and allo-HSCT recipients (Afessa et al. 2002a).

DAH is probably a consequence of damage to the alveolar capillary basement membrane (see Chap. 42). It is difficult to differentiate a true DAH from the alveolar hemorrhage associated with an infection (Majhail et al. 2006).

52.5.1 Clinical Aspects of DAH

Clinical manifestations	Usually observed within the first month after HSCT (a median of 23 days), often during the pre-engraftment phase; however, later onset is encountered in up to 42% of cases The clinical manifestations are those of all IPS. Hemoptysis is exceptional
Diagnosis	Based on BAL: Same criteria as IPS plus a differential characteristic; the progressive bloodier return of BAL fluid aliquots, in at least three segmental bronchi, indicating the presence of blood in the alveoli (or 20% hemosiderin-laden macrophage, although their absence does not exclude the diagnosis as it can take 72 h to appear). *Note*: DAH can have infectious or noninfectious etiologies (Majhail et al. 2006)
Risk factors	– Higher incidence after TBI and high-dose CY – Similar incidence among MAC and RIC – There is no correlation with the platelet counts
Differential diagnosis with	– Classic IPS: Very difficult, only by means of BAL. IPS usually appears after the engraftment, predominates in allo-HSCT, does not respond to steroids, and progresses to fibrosis in 85% of cases (only 15% on DAH). *Note*: Noninfectious DAH falls under the "diagnostic umbrella" of IPS (Panoskaltsis-Mortari et al. 2011) – PERDS: Almost impossible except for LBA progressively bloodier – Pulmonary hemorrhage: By FOB, no blood is seen in DAH – DAH associated with infection: Impossible without detection of the pathogen (Majhail et al. 2006)

52.5.2 Treatment and Prognosis of DAH

Treatment	– Although systematically treated with high doses of methyl-PDN (250–500 mg q6h × 5 days, followed by tapered dosage over 2–4 weeks) and aminocaproic acid (ACA), the overall response to this treatment is disappointing (Rathi et al. 2015) – A recent study seems to show that the best treatment is to use low steroid doses (≤250 mg/d) ± ACA (Rathi et al. 2015) – Factor VIIa addition does not appear to improve the results obtained with PDN (Elinoff et al. 2014) – Try to avoid mechanical ventilation by means of CPAP
Prognosis	– Poor: Overall mortality as high as 85% by day 100 (Rathi et al. 2015) – Less than 15% of patients die as a direct consequence of DAH, but the frequent evolution to MOF increases mortality to >60% (30% in auto and 70% in allo-HSCT) (Afessa et al. 2002b) – DAH that appear early after allo-HSCT (32% early vs. 70% late) or after auto-HSCT have a better prognosis (Afessa et al. 2002b; Majhail et al. 2006)

52.6 Late-Onset Noninfectious Pulmonary Complications (LONIPC)

In addition to late-onset IPS mentioned before and some other exceptional complications (thromboembolisms, pneumomediastinum), there are two forms of chronic pulmonary dysfunction commonly observed in patients surviving more than 100 days after allo-HSCT. One is an obstructive lung disease (bronchiolitis obliterans syndrome, *BOS*) and the other a restrictive lung disease (cryptogenetic organizing pneumonia, *COP*).

A recent prospective study showed that among 198 patients included after day +100, the cumulative incidence of LONIPC is 20%, and that of BOS is 11% at 3 years among allo-HSCT recipients (Bergeron et al. 2018). Another study shows the impact of these complications on 5-year survival (28% with vs. 87% w/o LONIPC) (Nishio et al. 2009).

52.6.1 Bronchiolitis Obliterans Syndrome (BOS)

Pathogenesis, timing, incidence, clinical manifestations, diagnosis, and radiology of BOS are shown in Table 52.2.

Treatment and prognosis of BOS are included in Table 52.3.

52.6.2 Cryptogenetic Organizing Pneumonia (COP)

Formerly called BOOP (bronchiolitis obliterans with organizational pneumonia). COP is a LONIPC of that is associated with restrictive pulmonary dysfunction. Reportedly, the incidence of COP among HSCT recipients is increasing due to the use of transbronchial biopsies as diagnostic tool. The greatest diagnostic challenge is the differentiation of COP from BOS (see Table 52.4) (Yoshihara et al. 2007; Cooke et al. 2017).

Table 52.2 Main clinical characteristics of BOS

Pathogenesis	The same as cGVHD but specifically involving the lung (Cooke et al. 2017). Its course may be aggravated by respiratory infections, viral infections, and gastroesophageal reflux
Timing and incidence	– Average starting period: 12 (3–24) months – Incidence: 3% at 2 years in the longest series (Arora et al. 2016); 11% in a prospective study (Bergeron et al. 2018)
Clinical manifestations	– Variable clinical course, usually insidious onset with progressive deterioration. Sometimes can present as an acute, fulminating course – Progressive breathlessness, nonproductive cough, and wheezing, although some asymptomatic cases are only detected by PFTs. – It is necessary to carry out PFT every 3 m in the first year after HSCT for an early detection[a] – In >75% of the BOS, there are chronic GVHD in other locations

(continued)

Table 52.2 (continued)

Diagnosis	• *Suspicion*: The so-called *BOS stage 0p*. More than 85% of cases can be diagnosed early by observing a 10–19% drop in the FEV1 or a reduction in FEF25–75 > 25% (Abedin et al. 2015) • *Clinical* (NIH consensus) (Chien et al. 2010; Uhlving et al. 2012) – Clinical manifestation (may be asymptomatic and only detected on PFT) + – Absence of active infection (demonstrated by BAL) + – Chronic GVHD in other locations[b] + – Obstructive alteration with air entrapment (FEV1 < 75% NV or > 10% decrease; ratio FEV1/FVC ratio < 0.7; residual volume > 120%) with nonsignificant bronchodilator test and a decreased DLCO + – Compatible radiology (see below) • *Definitive*: Histologic confirmation by thoracotomy, VATS, or transbronchial biopsy[c]
Radiology	– Chest x-ray: Normal or with signs of hyperinflation – CT scan: Radiological pattern of constrictive bronchiolitis with aerial entrapment, attenuation in mosaic, bronchiectasis and bronchial wall thickening, characteristic air trapping at exhalation

DLCO transfer capacity of CO, *FEV1* maximum expiratory volume in the first second, *FVC* forced vital capacity, *VATS* video-assisted thoracoscopic surgery

[a]Some experts consider that a 10% decrease in the FEV1 basal after HSCT should make you suspect in BOS diagnosis

[b]If the lung is the only organ with cGVHD, a biopsy is needed to confirm the diagnosis (NIH criteria)

[c]Rarely transbronchial biopsy is used (low sensitivity and low predictive value) to establish a diagnosis that is eminently clinical. If histology is available, the term bronchiolitis obliterans can be used; if not available, the process is referred to as BOS

Table 52.3 Treatment and prognosis of BOS

Treatment	*Supportive measures*: Anti-infectious prophylaxis If hypogammaglobulinemia: IVIg Treatment of gastroesophageal reflux Respiratory physiotherapy *Specific treatment* • *Prednisone*: 1–1.5 mg/kg/day, transient and unsatisfactory response in most cases. The addition of CSA, azathioprine, ATG, or photopheresis has few advantages • *Budesonide/inhaled formoterol* has been shown to be transiently effective in 60% of the patients (Bergeron et al. 2015) • *Etanercept/infliximab*: Effective in some cases (Yanik et al. 2012) • *FAM combination* therapy: Effective in disease stabilization[a]: – Fluticasone inhaled 440 mcg c/12 h (adult), 220 mcg in children + – Azithromycin 250 mg/d (adults), 5 mg/kg/d (children)[b] + – Montelukast 10 mg orally at night (adults), 5 mg (children) Two weeks before FAM increase (or start) PDN to 1 mg/kg/d, then decrease 0.25 mg/kg/d × week (Williams et al. 2015) • In BOS controlled but with a severe residual respiratory insufficiency, lung transplantation may be considered after a few years (Cheng et al. 2014)
Prognosis	– TRM is very high; 32% (18–57%) at 2 years of HSCT almost always get associated with progressive respiratory failure and opportunistic infections – SRV around 65% (4%–80%) at 2 years

[a]Fluticasone theoretically decreases the inflammatory pulmonary component; azithromycin reduces IL-8 levels and neutrophilia; and montelukast is an antagonist of the leukotriene receptors (bronchodilator)

[b]However, the ALLOZITHRO randomized trial has shown that early administration of azithromycin resulted in worse airflow decline-free survival than did placebo; the value of these findings is limited by early termination of the trial (Bergeron et al. 2017)

Table 52.4 Differential diagnosis between BOS and COP

First symptoms	BOS: >day +100 HSCT COP: Mostly in the first 100 days[a]
Incidence	BOS: 3–11% allo-HSCT (35% if cGVHD) COP: Up to 10% in URD HSCT
Clinical context	BOS: Allo-HSCT with cGVHD COP: Auto- or allo-HSCT. Almost always previous respiratory infection
Symptoms, signs	BOS: Asymptomatic, or progressive breathlessness, dry cough, wheezing. No fever, normal blood test COP: Fever, dry cough. Leukocytosis, increased CRP
Etiology	BOS: cGVHD COP: Idiopathic? Triggered by infection[b] or drugs[c]?
Pulmonary auscultation	BOS: Wheezing, hypoventilation COP: Crackles/rales
RFT	BOS: Obstructive pattern: FEV1/FVC <70%, FEV1 <75%, DLCO reduced COP: Restrictive pattern: FEV1/FVC >80%, TLC <80%, DLCO reduced
Chest radiology	BOS: Normal or airtrapping COP: Alveolar or interstitial pattern
Thoracic CT scan	BOS: Thickening of bronchial walls, bronchiectasis, air trapping on expiratory views COP: Uni- or bilateral patched bindings, glass images dull, or nodular infiltrators
BAL	BOS: Neutrophilia COP: Lymphocytosis, decreased CD4/CD8 ratio
Diagnosis	BOS: Clinical manifestations + PFTs + radiology COP: Requires lung biopsy
Response to steroids	BOS: Limited COP: Response in >80%
Prognosis	BOS: SRV <20% at 5 years if no response to steroids COP: Potentially reversible

CRP C-reactive protein
[a]If patients are adequately controlled, it is common to detect restrictive alterations before the day +100 although clinical manifestations may appear later
[b]*Mycoplasma*, *Coxiella*, *Nocardia*, and various viruses
[c]Amiodarone, bleomycin, busulfan, and cephalosporins

Key Points

- Lung injury occurs frequently following HSCT and significantly contributes to morbidity and mortality in the immediate post transplant period and in the months and years that follow. It can be observed in 25–55% of recipients.
- Noninfectious lung injury following HSCT may be mediated by either immune or nonimmune mechanisms and could represent up to the 50% of noninfectious mortality after allo-HSCT.
- Most relevant noninfectious early pulmonary complications are pulmonary edema by fluid overflow, idiopathic pneumonia syndrome, and diffuse alveolar hemorrhage, a vascular endothelial syndrome.
- The most relevant late-onset noninfectious pulmonary complications are bronchiolitis obliterans and cryptogenetic organizing pneumonia.
- All of them have specific diagnostic criteria, management, treatment, and prognosis.

References

Abedin S, Yanik GA, Braun T, et al. Predictive value of bronchiolitis obliterans syndrome stage 0p in chronic graft-versus-host disease of the lung. Biol Blood Marrow Transplant. 2015;21:1127–31.

Afessa B, Tefferi A, Litzow MR, Peters SG. Outcome of diffuse alveolar hemorrhage in hematopoietic stem cell transplant recipients. Am J Respir Crit Care Med. 2002a;166:1364–8.

Afessa B, Tefferi A, Litzow MR, et al. Diffuse alveolar hemorrhage in hematopoietic stem cell transplant recipients. Am J Respir Crit Care Med. 2002b;166:641–5.

Arora M, Cutler CS, Jagasia MH, et al. Late Acute and Chronic Graft-versus-Host Disease after Allogeneic Hematopoietic Cell Transplantation. Biol Blood Marrow Transplant. 2016;22:449–55.

Bergeron A, Chevret S, Chagnon K, et al. Budesonide/formoterol for bronchiolitis obliterans after hematopoietic stem cell transplantation. Am J Respir Crit Care Med. 2015;191:1242–9.

Bergeron A, Chevret S, Granata A, et al. Effect of azithromycin on airflow decline-free survival after allogeneic hematopoietic stem cell transplant: the ALLOZITHRO randomized clinical trial. JAMA. 2017;318:557–66.

Bergeron A, Chevret S, Peffault de Latour R, et al. Noninfectious lung complications after allogeneic haematopoietic stem cell transplantation. Eur Respir J. 2018;51(5):1702617. https://doi.org/10.1183/13993003.02617-2017.

Cheng GS, Edelman JD, Madtes DK, Martin PJ, Flowers ME. Outcomes of lung transplantation after allogeneic hematopoietic stem cell transplantation. Biol Blood Marrow Transplant. 2014;20:1169–75.

Chien JW, Duncan S, Williams KM, Pavletic SZ. Bronchiolitis obliterans syndrome after allogeneic hematopoietic stem cell transplantation-an increasingly recognized manifestation of chronic graft versus-host disease. Biol Blood Marrow Transplant. 2010;16(1 Suppl):S106–14.

Clark JG, Hansen JA, Hertz MI, et al. NHLBI workshop summary. Idiopathic pneumonia syndrome after bone marrow transplantation. Am Rev Respir Dis. 1993;147(6 Pt. 1):1601–6.

Cooke KR, Yanik GA. Lung injury following hematopoietic cell transplantation. In: Forman SJ, Negrin RS, Antin JH, Appelbaum FR, editors. Thomas' hematopoietic cell transplantation. 5th ed. Hoboken: Wiley; 2016. p. 1157–70.

Cooke KR, Luznik L, Sarantopoulos S, et al. The biology of chronic graft-versus-host disease: a task force report from the National Institutes of Health Consensus Development Project on Criteria for Clinical Trials in Chronic Graft-Versus-Host Disease. Biol Blood Marrow Transplant. 2017;23:211–34.

Elinoff JM, Bagci U, Moriyama B, et al. Recombinant human factor VIIa for alveolar hemorrhage following allogeneic stem cell transplantation. Biol Blood Marrow Transplant. 2014;20:969–78.

Lucena CM, Torres A, Rovira M, et al. Pulmonary complications in hematopoietic SCT: a prospective study. Bone Marrow Transplant. 2014;49:1293–9.

Majhail NS, Parks K, Defor TE, Weisdorf DJ. Diffuse alveolar hemorrhage and infection-associated alveolar hemorrhage following hematopoietic stem cell transplantation: related and high-risk clinical syndromes. Biol Blood Marrow Transplant. 2006;12:1038–46.

Nishio N, Yagasaki H, Takahashi Y, et al. Late-onset non-infectious pulmonary complications following allogeneic hematopoietic stem cell transplantation in children. Bone Marrow Transplant. 2009;44:303–8.

Panoskaltsis-Mortari A, Griese M, Madtes DK, et al. An official American Thoracic Society research statement: noninfectious lung injury after hematopoietic stem cell transplantation: idiopathic pneumonia syndrome. Am J Respir Crit Care Med. 2011;183:1262–79.

Rathi NK, Tanner AR, Dinh A, et al. Low-, medium- and high-dose steroids with or without aminocaproic acid in adult hematopoietic SCT patients with diffuse alveolar hemorrhage. Bone Marrow Transplant. 2015;50:420–6.

Rondón G, Saliba RM, Chen J, et al. Impact of fluid overload as new toxicity category on hematopoietic stem cell transplantation outcomes. Biol Blood Marrow Transplant. 2017;23:2166–71.

Seo S, Renaud C, Kuypers JM, et al. Idiopathic pneumonia syndrome after hematopoietic cell transplantation: evidence of occult infectious etiologies. Blood. 2015;125:3789–97.

Shannon VR, Andersson BS, Lei X, et al. Utility of early versus late fiberoptic bronchoscopy in the evaluation of new pulmonary infiltrates following hematopoietic stem cell transplantation. Bone Marrow Transplant. 2010;45:647–55.

Thompson J, Yin Z, D'Souza A, et al. Etanercept and corticosteroid therapy for the treatment of late-onset idiopathic pneumonia syndrome. Biol Blood Marrow Transplant. 2017;23:1955–60.

Uhlving HH, Buchvald F, Heilmann CJ, et al. Bronchiolitis obliterans after allo-SCT: clinical criteria and treatment options. Bone Marrow Transplant. 2012;47:1020–9.

Varelias A, Gartlan KH, Kreijveld E, et al. Lung parenchyma-derived IL-6 promotes IL-17A-dependent acute lung injury after allogeneic stem cell transplantation. Blood. 2015;125:2435–44.

Williams KM, Cheng GS, Pusic I, et al. Fluticasone, Azithromycin, and Montelukast Treatment for New-Onset Bronchiolitis Obliterans Syndrome after Hematopoietic Cell Transplantation. Biol Blood Marrow Transplant. 2016;22:710–6.

Yanik GA, Grupp SA, Pulsipher MA, et al. TNF-receptor inhibitor therapy for the treatment of children with idiopathic pneumonia syndrome. A joint Pediatric Consortium and Children's Oncology Group Study (ASCT0521). Biol Blood Marrow Transplant. 2015;21:67–73.

Yanik GA, Horowitz MM, Weisdorf DJ, et al. Randomized, double-blind, placebo-controlled trial of soluble tumor necrosis factor receptor: enbrel (etanercept) for the treatment of idiopathic pneumonia syndrome after allogeneic stem cell transplantation: blood and marrow. Biol Blood Marrow Transplant. 2014;20:858–64.

Yanik GA, Mineishi S, Levine JE, et al. Soluble tumor necrosis factor receptor: enbrel (etanercept) for sub-acute pulmonary dysfunction following allogeneic stem cell transplantation. Biol Blood Marrow Transplant. 2012;18:1044–54.

Yoshihara S, Yanik G, Cookee KR, Mineishi S. Bronchiolitis obliterans syndrome (BOS), bronchiolitis obliterans organizing pneumonia (BOOP), and other late-onset noninfectious pulmonary complications following allogeneic hematopoietic stem cell transplantation. Biol Blood Marrow Transplant. 2007;13:749–79.

Check for updates

Neurological Complications 53

Rémy Duléry

53.1 Definitions and Epidemiology

Neurological complications after HSCT are frequent and can be highly challenging to manage. The reported incidence ranges from 8% to 65%, depending on types of manifestation included, transplant setting, and patient population (Maffini et al. 2017). The severity varies widely, ranging from mild transient disorders to life-threatening illness. Main factors and causative agents include neurotoxic drugs, infectious pathogens, cerebrovascular illness, metabolic encephalopathy, and immune-mediated diseases. CNS relapse of the underlying disease, thrombotic microangiopathy (TAM), and post transplant lymphoproliferative disorder (PTLD) should also be ruled out (Table 53.1).

Neurological complications can be classified by their time of onset after HSCT. Early events are mainly due to drugs used in the conditioning regimen and IS therapy, whereas later complications are usually associated with immunodeficiency. Because clinical manifestations are often misleading and nonspecific, finding the right etiology may be long and difficult. Yet, early diagnosis and treatment are of paramount importance to reduce the risk for irreversible complications, impairment of quality of life, and transplantation-related death.

Table 53.1 Main causes of neurological complications after HSCT

	Causative agents
Drug-related	Calcineurin inhibitors (PRES) Methotrexate/cytotoxic agents (busulfan, fludarabine) Anti-infective agents Opioids, benzodiazepines
Infectious pathogens	Fungi and parasites (*Toxoplasma gondii, Aspergillus* spp., *Candida* spp., mucorales, *Cryptococcus neoformans, Histoplasma capsulatum)* Viruses (HHV6, CMV, VZV, HSV, JC virus, West Nile virus, adenovirus) Bacteria (Gram-negative rods, gram-positive *cocci, Mycobacterium tuberculosis, nocardia)*
Metabolic	Uremic encephalopathy Hepatic encephalopathy
Cerebrovascular	Hemorrhage Ischemic stroke
Immune-mediated	Demyelinating diseases Myositis Myasthenia gravis CNS chronic GVHD CRS
Thrombotic microangiopathy	Calcineurin inhibitors Infectious pathogens
Malignancies	PTLD Hematological disease relapse

R. Duléry (✉)
Hematology Department, Hôpital Saint Antoine, AP-HP, Paris, France
e-mail: remy.dulery@aphp.fr

E. Carreras et al. (eds.), *The EBMT Handbook*, https://doi.org/10.1007/978-3-030-02278-5_53

53.2 Causative Agents and Types of Neurological Complications

53.2.1 Neurotoxic Drugs

Calcineurin inhibitors (CNIs), antibiotics, antiviral drugs, and cytotoxic agents used in conditioning regimen are the most frequent causes of drug toxicity (Table 53.2). In addition, drug-drug interactions are a common cause of neurotoxicity and must be carefully checked.

53.2.1.1 Calcineurin Inhibitors

CSA and TAC are associated with neurological complications in 25% to 59% of HSCT patients (Reece et al. 1991). The clinical picture of CNI-induced neurotoxicity ranges from transient isolated symptoms to severe manifestations such as TAM (see Chap. 42) or posterior reversible encephalopathy syndrome (PRES) (Table 53.2).

Table 53.2 Neurotoxicity of the main drugs used in HSCT

Drug	Most common symptoms
Cyclosporine A	PRES, confusion, tremor, ataxia, seizures, cortical blindness
Methotrexate	Leukoencephalopathy, headache, lethargy, dysarthria
Busulfan	Seizures
Fludarabine	Acute toxic leukoencephalopathy
Thiotepa	Headache, encephalopathy, seizures, paresthesia
Rituximab	PML
Blinatumomab	Encephalopathy, headache, aphasia, ataxia, tremor, seizures
Sorafenib	PRES
Imipenem	Seizures, tremor, vertigo, paresthesia, somnolence, encephalopathy
Cefepime	Headache, paresthesia, encephalopathy
Voriconazole	Headache, seizures, vision changes, hallucinations, numbness encephalopathy
Amphotericin B	Headache, encephalopathy, numbness, vision changes
Aciclovir	Headache, tremor, dysarthria, hallucinations, encephalopathy
Foscarnet	Headache, vertigo, paresthesia, seizures, tremor, encephalopathy
Ganciclovir	Headache, numbness, tremor, seizures

PRES refers to a disorder of reversible subcortical vasogenic brain edema and is caused by endothelial injury related to abrupt blood pressure changes or direct effects of cytokines on the endothelium. It may occur in 1.6–7.2% of HSCT recipients and, if diagnosed early, is reversible after CNI withdrawal. Headache, visual disturbance, seizure, encephalopathy or focal neurologic deficit in the setting of renal failure, or blood pressure fluctuations are highly suggestive of PRES (Schmidt et al. 2016).

Although vasogenic edema can be visualized on CT in some patients, brain MRI is much more sensitive. MRI shows bilateral multifocal areas of hyperintensivity in T2-weighted sequences, especially in the white matter of parieto-occipital regions. Other variations may exist, such as superior frontal sulcus pattern of holohemispheric watershed pattern. Persistent neurological sequelae have been reported, especially if PRES is not rapidly diagnosed and treated.

53.2.1.2 MTX and Cytotoxic Agents

GVHD prophylaxis with short course of MTX may cause minor neurological disorders (lethargy, dysarthria, headache) and, very rarely, diffuse necrotizing leukoencephalopathy (Paudyal et al. 2010). BU is associated with seizure and requires preventive prophylaxis with benzodiazepines (Eberly et al. 2008). For FLU, the main neurological complication is acute toxic leukoencephalopathy. The clinical syndrome is characterized by visual disturbance, sensitive defects, and cognitive impairment.

Brain MRI shows bilateral areas of hyperintensity in T2-weighted sequences in the white matter, which differ significantly from the MRI findings seen in PRES. Classical PRES arises from subcortical white matter, whereas acute toxic leukoencephalopathy arises from periventricular white matter.

Risk factors include poor renal function, older age, fludarabine dose, previously treated CNS disease, or previous FLU-based conditioning regimen.

Outcomes are very poor with irreversible neurological sequelae and median OS of 2 months (Beitinjaneh et al. 2011).

53.2.1.3 Immunotherapy and Tyrosine Kinase Inhibitors (TKI)

Rituximab, TKI, and bispecific T-cell engaging antibodies such as blinatumomab are increasingly used after HSCT. Their neurological side effects are described in Table 53.2.

53.2.1.4 Anti-Infective Drugs

Anti-infective drugs are among the main causes of neurological complications. Dose adaptation is warranted in case of drug-drug interaction or impaired renal function. Their neurological side effects are described in Table 53.2.

53.2.2 Infectious Pathogens

Among the long list of pathogens responsible of CNS infections after HSCT, the most frequent are *Toxoplasma gondii, Aspergillus* spp., and HHV6 (Denier et al. 2006; Ogata et al. 2015). The clinical symptoms and the time of onset after HSCT may be helpful to decipher the correct diagnosis.

53.2.3 Metabolic Complications

Pharmacologic sedation with major opioids, systemic inflammatory response, and hemophagocytic lymphohistiocytosis are among the first causes to exclude in the differential diagnosis of metabolic causes of neurological dysfunction. Other causes include uremic encephalopathy—associated with CNI nephrotoxicity or TAM—and hepatic encephalopathy, associated with SOS/VOD or severe hepatic GVHD.

53.2.4 Cerebrovascular Disease

Cerebrovascular hemorrhagic or thrombotic events represent potentially lethal complications.

One of the most frequent events is subdural hematoma, which may occur in 2.6% of the patients (Colosimo et al. 2000). Risk factors for CNS hemorrhagic complications include falls, prolonged severe thrombocytopenia or refractoriness to platelet transfusions, grade III–IV GHVD, and arterial hypertension (Zhang et al. 2016). CT scans usually confirm the diagnosis but can be negative in 20–25% of the patients. Risk factors for CNS thrombotic complications include active infections, atrial fibrillation, hypercoagulative state, chronic GVHD, and corticosteroid treatment (Coplin et al. 2001).

53.2.5 Immune-Mediated Diseases

The most frequent immune-mediated neurological diseases include Guillain-Barré-like demyelinating polyneuropathy, myositis, myasthenia gravis, cytokine release syndrome (CRS), and CNS manifestations of chronic GVHD. Assigning the right diagnosis can be highly challenging and may require a neurologic consultation.

53.2.5.1 Demyelinating Polyneuropathies

Immune-mediated demyelinating polyneuropathies, which include Guillain-Barré-like syndrome, may occur in 1% of the patients, especially within the first 3 months after HSCT (Rodriguez et al. 2002). Progressive symmetrical ascending motor deficiency, numbness, hyporeflexia, and respiratory insufficiency are suggestive of Guillain-Barré-like syndromes. Lumbar puncture, MRI, and nerve conduction studies should be performed rapidly. Symptoms may resolve with polyclonal gamma globulin therapy. Rituximab may be used in unresponsive patients.

53.2.5.2 Myositis

Myositis is characterized by proximal muscle weakness, is often associated with chronic GVHD, and may occur in 2–3% of HSCT recipients (Stephenson et al. 2001). Levels of creatine phosphokinase are elevated, electromyography shows myopathic pattern, and MRI is useful to establish the diagnosis and monitor the response to treatment. Diagnosis can be proven by muscle biopsy. Patients may respond to corticosteroid therapy after 1–6 weeks of treatment.

53.2.5.3 Myasthenia Gravis

Myasthenia gravis usually occurs after the onset of GVHD in less than 1% of HSCT recipients (Lefvert and Björkholm 1987). The main symptoms include ptosis, facial weakness, diplopia, dysarthria, and dysphagia. The diagnosis is confirmed with electromyography showing a progressive decrease in the muscle action potential. Cholinesterase inhibitors and corticosteroid therapy are the treatments of choice.

53.2.5.4 Cytokine Release Syndrome

CRS can be observed after haploidentical HSCT with PT-CY and infusion of chimeric antigen receptor T (CAR T) cells or blinatumomab. CRS may cause life-threatening complications, including CNS involvement (encephalopathy, hemiparesis, ataxia, aphasia). Patients can be effectively treated with cytokine blockade using the antibodies siltuximab or tocilizumab, respectively, targeting IL-6 or the IL-6 receptor (Frey 2017).

53.2.5.5 Central Nervous System GVHD

The incidence of CNS manifestations of chronic GVHD is probably underestimated. Three main clinical manifestations have been described (Grauer et al. 2010; Saad et al. 2009). Demyelinating diseases have been reported in the cerebral white matter, optic nerve, or spinal cord. Symptoms follow a relapsing-remitting course, as observed in multiple sclerosis. The treatment consists in corticosteroid pulses. Sphingosine-1-phosphate receptor agonists, such as fingolimod, could be efficient in refractory/relapsing patients (Gauthier et al. 2018).

Vasculitis may involve small- to large-sized arterial vessels of cerebral parenchyma and meninges. Ischemic lesions, minute hemorrhages, and multifocal signal changes in the white matter can be observed on MRI. Diagnosis can be confirmed by brain biopsy, and treatment relies on corticosteroids in combination with cyclophosphamide.

Finally, patients may develop immune-mediated encephalitis. Definite diagnosis requires repeated analysis of CSF to rule out infectious encephalitis.

53.3 Diagnostic Algorithm

When faced with neurological complications following HSCT, the following ten steps can be helpful to promptly assign the correct diagnosis and start the right treatment:

1. Carefully review the medication history and search for (or exclude) metabolic disorders.
2. Are the clinical signs and/or symptoms generalized (e.g., altered consciousness, seizure) or focal (e.g., stroke, mass lesion)?
3. What is the time of onset of neurological signs and/or symptoms after HSCT?
4. Perform CT scan or MRI for ruling out PRES, encephalitis, infectious or immune parenchymal infiltrate, cerebrovascular events, or hematological disease relapse.
5. Analyze CSF for diagnosing infectious complications, Guillain-Barré-like syndrome, or underlying disease relapse.
6. Perform electroencephalography in patients with altered consciousness, hallucinations, or seizure.
7. Perform electromyography in patients with polyneuropathy or peripheral neuromuscular weakness.
8. Repeat each of the previous steps: Tests may be negative when performed early, and symptoms may evolve or fluctuate after the onset of the disease.
9. Brain or neuromuscular biopsy may be required to confirm/exclude opportunistic infections, PML, vasculitis, PTLD, or other malignancies.
10. The opinion of a neurologist at each step is highly recommended, especially for complicated clinical cases.

53.4 Conclusions

Neurological complications after HSCT, and especially allo-HSCT, are frequent and may lead to lethal complications. The main causative factors include drug-related toxicities, metabolic disorders, infections, cerebrovascular evens, immune-mediated disorders, and disease recurrence. Although their clinical diagnosis and management can be highly challenging, early treatment is extremely important to reduce mortality and improve quality of life.

Key Points

- Neurological complications after HSCT require prompt diagnosis and timely treatment to reduce post transplant mortality and improve the quality of life of the patients.
- Their etiology is often multifactorial and includes neurotoxic drugs, infectious pathogens, cerebrovascular illness, metabolic encephalopathy, and immune-mediated diseases.
- TAM, PTLD with CNS involvement, and CNS relapse of the underlying hematological disease should be included in the differential diagnosis.
- CNS manifestations of GVHD are rare and often highly challenging to manage.

References

Beitinjaneh A, McKinney AM, Cao Q, Weisdorf DJ. Toxic leukoencephalopathy following fludarabine-associated hematopoietic cell transplantation. Biol Blood Marrow Transplant. 2011;17:300–8.

Colosimo M, McCarthy N, Jayasinghe R, et al. Diagnosis and management of subdural haematoma complicating bone marrow transplantation. Bone Marrow Transplant. 2000;25:549–52.

Coplin WM, Cochran MS, Levine SR, Crawford SW. Stroke after bone marrow transplantation: frequency, aetiology and outcome. Brain. 2001;124:1043–51.

Denier C, Bourhis J-H, Lacroix C, et al. Spectrum and prognosis of neurologic complications after hematopoietic transplantation. Neurology. 2006;67:1990–7.

Eberly AL, Anderson GD, Bubalo JS, McCune JS. Optimal prevention of seizures induced by high-dose busulfan. Pharmacotherapy. 2008;28:1502–10.

Frey N. Cytokine release syndrome: who is at risk and how to treat. Best Pract Res Clin Haematol. 2017;30:336–40.

Gauthier J, Vermersch P, Chauvet P, et al. Successful treatment with fingolimod of graft-versus-host disease of the central nervous system. Blood Adv. 2018;2:10–3.

Grauer O, Wolff D, Bertz H, et al. Neurological manifestations of chronic graft-versus-host disease after allogeneic haematopoietic stem cell transplantation: report from the Consensus Conference on Clinical Practice in chronic graft-versus-host disease. Brain. 2010;133:2852–65.

Lefvert AK, Björkholm M. Antibodies against the acetylcholine receptor in hematologic disorders: implications for the development of myasthenia gravis after bone marrow grafting. N Engl J Med. 1987;317:170.

Maffini E, Festuccia M, Brunello L, et al. Neurologic complications after allogeneic hematopoietic stem cell transplantation. Biol Blood Marrow Transplant. 2017;23:388–97.

Ogata M, Fukuda T, Teshima T. Human herpesvirus-6 encephalitis after allogeneic hematopoietic cell transplantation: what we do and do not know. Bone Marrow Transplant. 2015;50:1030–6.

Paudyal B, Viets R, Skliut M. A case of low-dose oral methotrexate–induced reversible neurotoxicity. Am J Neuroradiol. 2010;31:E77.

Reece DE, Frei-Lahr DA, Shepherd JD, et al. Neurologic complications in allogeneic bone marrow transplant patients receiving cyclosporin. Bone Marrow Transplant. 1991;8:393–401.

Rodriguez V, Kuehnle I, Heslop HE, et al. Guillain-Barré syndrome after allogeneic hematopoietic stem cell transplantation. Bone Marrow Transplant. 2002;29:515–7.

Saad AG, Alyea EP, Wen PY, et al. Graft-versus-host disease of the CNS after allogeneic bone marrow transplantation. J Clin Oncol. 2009;27:e147–9.

Schmidt V, Prell T, Treschl A, et al. Clinical management of posterior reversible encephalopathy syndrome after allogeneic hematopoietic stem cell transplantation: a case series and review of the literature. Acta Haematol. 2016;135:1–10.

Stephenson AL, Mackenzie IR, Levy RD, Road J. Myositis associated graft-versus-host-disease presenting as respiratory muscle weakness. Thorax. 2001;56:82–4.

Zhang X-H, Wang Q-M, Chen H, et al. Clinical characteristics and risk factors of intracranial hemorrhage in patients following allogeneic hematopoietic stem cell transplantation. Ann Hematol. 2016;95:1637–43.

54 Skin, Hair and Musculoskeletal Complications

Francis Ayuk and Bipin N. Savani

54.1 Complications Involving the Skin and Hair

54.1.1 Introduction

Nearly every recipient of an allo-HSCT will at some stage develop complications involving the skin and hair. These complications can be grouped in drug-related toxicities and allergies, graft-versus-host disease, infections and malignant conditions.

54.1.2 Drug-Related Toxicities and Allergies

Drug-related toxicities are most often due to the conditioning regimen, antibiotics or IS agents. Presentation can vary broadly from localised erythema to epidermal necrolysis and Stevens-Johnson syndrome.

Diagnosis may be difficult because the morphological and chronological presentations of the lesions are generally non-specific. Skin biopsies and histological examination can help improve diagnostic certainty (Paun et al. 2013).

Management requires discontinuation of suspected causative agents, topical treatment with healing ointments, prevention of secondary infections and in severe cases (or when other organs are involved) systemic therapy with corticosteroids and antihistamines.

54.1.3 Graft-Versus-Host Disease

The skin is one of the most frequently affected organs in acute and chronic GVHD. Acute GVHD of the skin mainly affects the epidermis of the skin and adjacent oral, anal and genital mucosa. Chronic GVHD may affect all layers of the skin including the epidermis, dermis and subcutaneous tissue and may also manifest as skin dyspigmentation, sweat impairment, alopecia and thinning of scalp hair, hair loss in other areas (e.g. eye brows) and nail dystrophy. Chronic GVHD with sclerosis of the subcutaneous tissue including fasciae, joints and the musculoskeletal system can severely impact patients' quality of life. Sclerodermal lesions of the thorax or abdomen may impair breathing, lesions adjacent to joints may impair movement, and genital lesions may cause phimosis, vaginal scarring and narrowing of the introitus that may cause dyspareunia and even complete obliteration of the vaginal tract.

F. Ayuk (✉)
Department of Stem Cell Transplantation, University Medical Center Hamburg-Eppendorf (UKE), Hamburg, Germany
e-mail: ayuketang@uke.de

B. N. Savani
Department of Medicine, Vanderbilt University Medical Center, Nashville, TN, USA

E. Carreras et al. (eds.), *The EBMT Handbook*, https://doi.org/10.1007/978-3-030-02278-5_54

In the early "inflammatory" phase of GVHD, patients often present with oedema and discomfort which later progress to fibrosis and joint contractures. Regular survey of range of motion by patients and physicians may enable early detection of reversible lesions. Regular assessment (e.g. via questionnaire or oral interview) during routine clinical visits may encourage physicians and patients to address issues involving the genital tract, thereby enabling early detection and treatment.

General treatment and management of GVHD discussed in Chaps. 43 and 44. In patients with chronic GVHD of the skin and subcutaneous tissues, treatment is best initiated in the early phase prior to development of fibrosis and contractures, which otherwise may require protracted immunosuppression and other measures, sometimes over several years. Physiotherapy including deep myofascial massage and stretching exercises is essential to restore or maintain range of motion. In patients with genital involvement, topical treatment with immunosuppressive agents and hormones and use of vaginal dilators should be initiated early to prevent or reduce the degree of irreversible fibrosis and avoid the need for surgical intervention.

54.1.4 Infectious Complications Involving the Skin

Infection-associated skin lesions are often due to viruses. Unexplained fever and rash are more frequent in patients with HHV6 viremia compared to controls (Betts et al. 2011). Due to lack of effective prophylaxis, HHV6-related complications occur during both early and late transplant phases, while shingles (varicella zoster) are mostly seen beyond 6 months after transplant and mainly after discontinuation of prophylactic aciclovir. Other infectious conditions of the skin include fungal infections (mainly due to dermatophytes and, less frequently, *Aspergillus* or *Mucor* species) and bacterial infections. Management of infections mostly consists of systemic antiviral, antifungal or antibiotic treatment.

54.1.5 Malignant Complications of the Skin

Post transplant malignant conditions of the skin include skin cancer (basal cell carcinoma, squamous cell carcinoma and melanoma) and relapse of underlying malignant disease. BCC and SCC are much more common and have a better prognosis than melanoma. The incidence of melanoma has been reported to be higher after allo-HSCT with standardised incidence ratios ranging from 1.4 to 8.3 (Inamoto et al. 2015). Secondary cancers, risk factors and management are discussed in detail in Chap. 47.

Patients should be counselled to perform self-examination of the skin and adjacent mucosa, use adequate sun protection and avoid excessive sun exposure. Country-specific general population recommendations for screening for cancer should be adapted and modified taking increased risk of HSCT survivors into consideration.

54.2 Musculoskeletal Complications

54.2.1 Introduction

Complications involving the muscles include myopathies, myositis and cramps. Musculoskeletal complications are reported in 35% of long-term survivors 10 years after allogeneic transplantation (Syrjala et al. 2005).

54.2.2 Myopathy

The most frequent causes of myopathy early after transplant are corticosteroid therapy and inactivity. Patients report muscles weakness with no pain, and laboratory investigations show normal creatinine kinase. The proximal lower limb muscles, particularly the quadriceps muscles are most severely affected. The main risk factors include increasing dose and duration of corticosteroid therapy, older patient age and the extent and duration of inactivity, particularly when intensive care is required. Patients should receive physiotherapy as soon as corticosteroid therapy is initiated and be advised to exercise on their own. Systemic corticosteroids should be tapered or avoided when possible.

54.2.3 Myasthenia Gravis

Though rare (<1%), it has been reported after allogeneic stem cell transplantation, mostly in the context of chronic GVHD. Patients present with fatigable weakness during or after tapering of immunosuppression (Grauer et al. 2010). Diagnosis includes detection of antibodies against acetylcholine in blood. Treatment consists of cholinesterase inhibitors and IS therapies for chronic GVHD.

54.2.4 Muscle Cramps

Muscle cramps are painful and often visible contractions lasting up to 30 min. Though rarely reported, they appear to be frequent in patients with chronic GVHD (Filipovich et al. 2005); an association with chronic IS may also be possible. Magnesium deficiency and side effects of medications (e.g. ganciclovir, valganciclovir) should always be ruled out. If magnesium replacement and discontinuation of suspected causative drugs do not bring relief, treatment with, e.g., quinine or antiepileptic drugs may be considered.

54.2.5 Myositis

Myositis has been reported in up to 3% of patients after allo-HSCT. Though frequently associated with other symptoms of chronic GVHD, it can also be the sole manifestation of GVHD (Openshaw et al. 2009). Patients often present with pressure-sensitive muscle pain and increased blood creatine kinase. Management is within GVHD treatment (Couriel et al. 2002).

54.2.6 Complications Involving the Bones and Joints

The most frequent complications involving the bones and joints are chronic GVHD, avascular osteonecrosis and bone loss (osteopenia/osteoporosis). Chronic GVHD of the joints is discussed in Chap. 44.

54.2.6.1 Osteoporosis/Osteopenia

Osteopenia (defined as a T-score between −1 and −2.5) and osteoporosis (defined as a T-score less than −2.5) have been reported in about 25–50% of patients after allo-HSCT and up to 60% in patients with severe chronic GVHD (Pirsl et al. 2016). Risk factors include protracted IS, older patient age, higher cumulative corticosteroid dose (Schulte and Beelen 2004; Savani et al. 2007; Stern et al. 2001; Yao et al. 2008; Petropoulou et al. 2010; Abou-Mourad et al. 2010) and lower body weight, malnutrition, physical inactivity, female gender, higher average NIH organ score as well as higher platelet counts in patients with severe chronic GVHD (Pirsl et al. 2016).

In accordance with these risk factors, decrease in bone mineral density occurs most rapidly within the first year after transplant. If osteopenia or osteoporosis is diagnosed, endocrine causes like hyperthyroidism, hyperparathyroidism and hypogonadism need to be ruled out. Screening using dual energy X-ray absorptiometry (DEXA) is recommended 1 year after transplant and repeat measurements in patients with recognised defects (Majhail et al. 2012).

Measures to prevent bone loss include vitamin D supplementation in regions with high prevalence of vitamin D deficiency, adequate calcium intake preferable through diet and regular weight-bearing physical exercise. Beyond the above preventive measures, specific treatment of patients with severe osteopenia or osteoporosis include bisphosphonates or denosumab. Hormone replacement therapy should be considered in patients with hypogonadism. Patients should also be counselled to modify negative lifestyle factors (e.g. cease smoking) and take measures to prevent falls (e.g. physical exercise including balance training, correct visual disorders).

54.2.6.2 Avascular Necrosis

Avascular necrosis (AVN) has been reported in up to 19% of adult patients and up to 29% of patients younger than 20 years (Torii et al. 2001; Patel et al. 2008). Risk factors include GVHD, steroid therapy, microvascular changes due to GVHD and/or its therapy, younger age at transplant and TBI (Socié et al. 1997; French et al. 2008; Patel et al. 2008; Campbell et al. 2009; Jagasia et al. 2010). Patients usually present with joint pain, restricted to one or two affected joints. Though most joints can be affected, the hips are by far most frequently involved, bilateral in the majority of cases.

Screening for AVN is not recommended; however high index of suspicion and prompt MRI are necessary in symptomatic patients with risk factors, to enable early detection and intervention.

Pain relief and maintenance or restoration of patient mobility are the main aims or treatment. Discontinuation of corticosteroid and other IST should be considered where possible. Drug therapy is limited to pain relief. The role of non-surgical causative therapies, such as bisphosphonates, statins and prostacyclin analogues, is still unclear. Pressure relief by means of surgical core decompression may relief pain and slow down progression in early stages, whereby additional autologous bone marrow grafting further improves long-term outcome (Hernigou et al. 2018). In patients with late-stage disease with femoral head collapse, joint-preserving strategies are not effective, and total hip arthroplasty is the recommended long-term treatment.

References

Abou-Mourad YR, Lau BC, Barnett MJ, et al. Long-term outcome after Allo-SCT: close follow-up on a large cohort treated with myeloablative regimens. Bone Marrow Transplant. 2010;45:295–302.

Betts BC, Young JA, Ustun C, et al. Human herpesvirus 6 infection after hematopoietic cell transplantation: is routine surveillance necessary? Biol Blood Marrow Transplant. 2011;17:1562–8.

Campbell S, Sun CL, Kurian S, et al. Predictors of avascular necrosis of bone in long-term survivors of hematopoietic cell transplantation. Cancer. 2009;115:4127–35.

Couriel DR, Beguelin GZ, Giralt S, et al. Chronic graft-versus-host disease manifesting as polymyositis: an uncommon presentation. Bone Marrow Transplant. 2002;30:543–6.

Filipovich AH, Weisdorf D, Pavletic S, et al. National Institutes of Health consensus development project on criteria for clinical trials in chronic graft-versus-host disease: I. diagnosis and staging working group report. Biol Blood Marrow Transplant. 2005;11:945–56.

French D, Hamilton LH, Mattano LA, et al. A PAI-1 (Serpine1) polymorphism predicts osteonecrosis in children with acute lymphoblastic leukemia: a report from the Children's Oncology Group. Blood. 2008;111:4496–9.

Grauer O, Wolff D, Bertz H, et al. Neurological manifestations of chronic graft-versus-host disease after allogeneic haematopoietic stem cell transplantation: report from the Consensus Conference on Clinical Practice in chronic graft-versus-host disease. Brain. 2010;133:2852–65.

Hernigou P, Dubory A, Homma Y, et al. Cell therapy versus simultaneous contralateral decompression in symptomatic corticosteroid osteonecrosis: a thirty year follow-up prospective randomized study of one hundred and twenty five adult patients. Int Orthop. 2018. https://doi.org/10.1007/s00264-018-3941-8.

Inamoto Y, Shah NN, Savani BN, et al. Secondary solid cancer screening following hematopoietic cell transplantation. Bone Marrow Transplant. 2015;50:1013–23.

Jagasia S, Misfeldt A, Griffith M, Jagasia M. Age and total body irradiation in addition to corticosteroid dose are important risk factors for avascular necrosis of the bone. Biol Blood Marrow Transplant. 2010;16:1750–1.

Majhail NS, Rizzo JD, Lee SJ, et al. Recommended screening and preventive practices for long-term survivors after hematopoietic cell transplantation. Bone Marrow Transplant. 2012;47:337–41.

Openshaw H, Vogelsang GB, Pavletic SZ. Neurological manifestations of chronic graft versus host disease, chronic graft versus host disease. New York: Cambridge University Press; 2009. p. 243–51.

Patel B, Richards SM, Rowe JM, et al. High incidence of avascular necrosis in adolescents with acute lymphoblastic leukemia: a UKALL XII analysis. Leukemia. 2008;22:308–12.

Paun O, Phillips T, Fu P, Novoa RA, Honda KS, Lu KQ, Lazarus HM. Cutaneous complications in hematopoietic cell transplant recipients: impact of biopsy on patient management. Biol Blood Marrow Transplant. 2013;19(8):1204–9.

Petropoulou AD, Porcher R, Herr AL, et al. Prospective assessment of bone turnover and clinical bone diseases after allogeneic hematopoietic stem-cell transplantation. Transplantation. 2010;89:1354–61.

Pirsl F, Curtis LM, Steinberg SM, et al. Characterization and risk factor analysis of osteoporosis in a large cohort of patients with chronic graft-versus-host disease. Biol Blood Marrow Transplant. 2016;22:1517–24.

Savani BN, Donohue T, Kozanas E, et al. Increased risk of bone loss without fracture risk in longterm survivors after allogeneic stem cell transplantation. Biol Blood Marrow Transplant. 2007;13:517–20.

Schulte CM, Beelen DW. Bone loss following hematopoietic stem cell transplantation: a long-term follow-up. Blood. 2004;103:3635–43.

Socié G, Cahn JY, Carmelo J, et al. Avascular necrosis of bone after allogeneic bone marrow transplantation: analysis of risk factors for 4388 patients by the Société Francaise de Greffe de Moelle (SFGM). Br J Haematol. 1997;97:865–70.

Stern JM, Sullivan KM, Ott SM, et al. Bone density loss after allogeneic hematopoietic stem cell transplantation: a prospective study. Biol Blood Marrow Transplant. 2001;7:257–64.

Syrjala KL, Langer SL, Abrams JR, et al. Late effects of hematopoietic cell transplantation among 10-year adult survivors compared with case-matched controls. J Clin Oncol. 2005;23:6596–606.

Torii Y, Hasegawa Y, Kubo T, et al. Osteonecrosis of the femoral head after allogeneic bone marrow transplantation. Clin Orthop Relat Res. 2001;382:124–32.

Yao S, Mc Carthy PL, Dunford LM, et al. High prevalence of early-onset osteopenia/osteoporosis after allogeneic stem cell transplantation and improvement after bisphosphonate therapy. Bone Marrow Transplant. 2008;41:393–8.

Cardiovascular Diseases and Metabolic Syndrome

55

Diana M. Greenfield and John A. Snowden

55.1 Introduction

Cardiovascular disease (CVD) is a broad term covering disorders of the heart and blood vessels and includes hypertension, coronary heart disease, cerebrovascular disease, peripheral vascular disease, heart failure, rheumatic heart disease, congenital heart disease and cardiomyopathies (WHO 2017).

CVD is common; the World Health Organisation (WHO) estimates that more than 17.5 million people died of CVD such as heart attack or stroke in 2012, representing 30% of all global deaths. CVDs are the number one cause of death globally: more people die annually from CVDs than from any other cause. It is predicted that by 2030, almost 23.6 million people will die from CVDs, mainly from heart disease and stroke. These are projected to remain the single leading causes of death (WHO 2017).

D. M. Greenfield (✉)
Specialised Cancer Services, Sheffield Teaching Hospitals NHS Foundation Trust, Sheffield, UK

Department of Oncology and Metabolism, University of Sheffield, Sheffield, UK
e-mail: Diana.Greenfield@sth.nhs.uk

J. A. Snowden

Department of Haematology, Sheffield Teaching Hospitals NHS Foundation Trust, Sheffield, UK

Department of Oncology and Metabolism, University of Sheffield, Sheffield, UK

After HSCT, there is an increased incidence of CVD. Retrospective EBMT analyses have shown the cumulative incidence of a first cardiovascular event 15 years after HSCT rises to 6%. The type of transplant may be important. In the EBMT analyses, the cumulative incidence of 7.5% for the first CV event at 15 years post allo-HSCT versus 2.3% post auto-HSCT (Tichelli et al. 2007). However, in another study with a 7 year median follow-up (range 2–23.7) the 10 year cumulative incidence of ischaemic heart disease (IHD), cardiomyopathy, stroke and all-cause CV death was 3.8%, 6%, 3.5% and 3.7% respectively with similar prevalence in auto- and allo-HSCT (Chow et al. 2011).

55.2 Risk Factors

A number of pre-transplant risk factors appear to predispose to CVD (such as smoking, hypertension, dyslipidaemia, diabetes and obesity). CV toxicity of pre-transplant treatment includes anthracyclines and site-specific radiotherapy.

CV toxicity of transplant includes GVHD, and CV toxicity of post transplant treatment includes corticosteroid use and retransplant. Other contributing risk factors emerge as secondary late effects, such as hypogonadism, premature menopause and hypothyroidism (Chow et al. 2014).

E. Carreras et al. (eds.), *The EBMT Handbook*, https://doi.org/10.1007/978-3-030-02278-5_55

When risk factors combine; the term *metabolic syndrome (MetS)* is used. MetS is a cluster of interrelated factors which increase the risk of cardiovascular disease, diabetes mellitus (DM) and all-cause mortality (Alberti et al. 2009; NCEP 2002).

55.3 Metabolic Syndrome Definition

The existence of several definitions of MetS led to a harmonised definition (IDF 2006): that is, the presence of three out of five risk factors as follows:

- Abdominal obesity measured by waist circumference: With population and country specific definitions.
- Triglycerides ≥1.7 mmol/L or drug treatment for elevated levels.
- HDL-C (men) <1.0 mmol/L or drug treatment for reduced levels.
- HDL-C (women) <1.3 mmol/L or drug treatment for reduced levels.
- Blood pressure ≥130/≥85 mmHg or drug treatment for hypertension (HTN).
- Fasting glucose ≥5.6 mmol/L drug treatment for diabetes mellitus (DM).

The International Diabetes Foundation (IDF) estimates 25% of the world's population has MetS (IDF 2006).

After HSCT there is an increased incidence of MetS, with reported prevalence rates of 31–49% (Majhail et al. 2009b; McMillen et al. 2014; Oudin et al. 2015; Greenfield et al 2018). In HSCT patients, the increased incidence is accounted for by the following components:

55.3.1 Abdominal Obesity

Abdominal obesity measured by waist circumference represents fat accumulation (visceral adipose deposits) which independently confers cardiometabolic risk (Amato et al. 2013). Changes in waist circumferences are seen after HSCT with, for example, corticosteroid use and with onset of sarcopenic obesity.

55.3.2 Dyslipidaemia

Dyslipidaemia is defined by elevated levels of total cholesterol, LDL-C or triglycerides or low levels of HDL-C. Prevalence in general population is estimated at 25% in the USA (Baker et al. 2007) and in European countries (Fodor 2010; Scheidt-Nave et al. 2013; Gonzalez-Juanatey et al. 2011). Evidence suggests allo-HSCT recipients have significantly higher risk of new onset dyslipidaemia (RR2.1 CI 1.1504.65) compared with auto-HSCT (Tichelli et al. 2007) with the prevalence post HSCT estimated to be 43–73% (FACT-JACIE 2017). Factors predicting dyslipidaemia after HSCT include family history, obesity, high dose total body irradiation, grade II–IV aGvHD, cGvHD, CLD and IST use (Chow et al. 2014; Oudin et al. 2015; Kagoya et al. 2012; Blaser et al. 2012).

55.3.3 Hypertension (HTN)

Hypertension (HTN) in the general population is defined as systolic BP ≥140 mmHg or diastolic BP ≥90 mmHg but defined in context of MetS as systolic BP ≥135 mmHg or diastolic BP ≥85. HTN in people following allo-HSCT is 2.06 times (95% CI 1.39–3.04) more likely compared with sibling donors or auto-HSCT (Baker et al. 2007).

55.3.4 Insulin Resistance or Diabetes Mellitus (IR/DM)

DM is characterised by hyperglycaemia resulting from defects in insulin secretion, insulin action or both and defined as a fasting pGL ≥7 mmol/L, an HbA1C ≥6.5%, a 2 h plasma glucose ≥11.1 mmol/L during a glucose tolerance test (GTT) or a random glucose ≥11.1 mmol/L.

Both allo-HSCT and auto-HSCT recipients have been found to report DM more often than sibling donors (OR for allo-HSCT, 3.65; 95% CI, 1.82–7.32; OR for auto-HSCT: 2.03; 95% CI, 0.98–4.21) (Baker et al. 2007). High-dose corticosteroids (cumulative PRD dose of >0.25 mg/kg/day) increase the likelihood of developing DM (RR, 3.6; 95% CI, 1.7–7.5) and for having persistent DM at 2 years post-HSCT (RR, 4.1; 95% CI, 1.0–18.2) (Majhail et al. 2009a; b). TBI is also a well-evidenced risk factor (Hirabayashi et al. 2014).

55.4 Preventative Practices in the HSCT and Late Effects Clinic: A Practical Approach

Clearly HSCT clinicians cannot be expected to manage all cardiovascular risk factors and complications. The logistics would be overwhelming and the clinical expertise required to provide up-to-date management of cardiological, cerebrovascular, endocrinological and metabolic conditions lacking.

However, the fact that HSCT survivors require HSCT follow-up provides an opportunity to deliver screening for late effects and other long-term consequences of treatments. Screening for cardiovascular risk factors, including MetS and CV events, can be straightforwardly integrated into a programme of long-term and late effects follow-up.

Screening can be provided by a variety of clinicians, medical, nursing or other allied professions, depending on the model of care. If cardiovascular risk factors are detected, given the commonality, they can usually be referred back to primary care clinicians who are more experienced and frequently manage a range of long-term conditions including hypertension, glycaemic control and often have access to weight management, smoking cessation and similar relevant serves. Primary care clinicians are familiar with using risk assessment algorithms, such as the Framingham risk score (Framingham 2008) and many others which are country specific. These risk assessment tools may be useful in estimating a person's projected risk of developing CVD in the general population. They have limitations (age ethnicity, comorbid conditions) and, importantly, have not been validated in HSCT survivors and may potentially under-estimate the risk. However, it is reasonable for primary care and other clinicians to apply them until some more specific instrument is developed in HSCT survivors.

Non-acute cardiovascular problems detected in the late effects clinic can be referred back to primary care clinicians who can manage them or refer on for specialist treatment. However, there should be direct referral for clinically urgent or more serious cardiovascular problems to relevant hospital specialists, who have a state-of-the art knowledge and experience in a rapidly evolving field. Ultimately, one indispensable aspect should be close communication between all clinicians involved in the short- and long-term management of the HSCT patient, whether at primary, secondary or tertiary levels of care.

Given the specialised complexity of HSCT and its many complications, which are relatively rarely encountered by many clinicians outside of haematology, oncology and immunology, the HSCT clinic and associated late effects service can have a major role in coordinating care and facilitating communication between other relevant specialists. This aspect in underpinned by the seventh edition of the FACT-JACIE standards which feature systematic provision for late effects follow-up, including cardiovascular risk factors and complications (FACT-JACIE 2017).

For the HSCT programme and/or associated late effects clinic, Table 55.1 has been published as a guide to facilitate screening in the EBMT-CIBMTR guidelines (DeFilipp et al. 2017). This is a consensus opinion, and there is no good evidence of the safety or clinical effectiveness of these recommendations in HSCT patients, which are based on the general population. Based on the available evidence, it is important to screen for other factors in HSCT patients, including (a) personal history, (b) family history, (c) type of transplant (allo or auto), (d) use of TBI, (e) history of acute or chronic GvHD and (f) use of CNI (CSA, TAC) (DeFilipp et al. 2017).

Table 55.1 Screening guidelines for metabolic syndrome and cardiovascular risk factors for adult and paediatric patients among the general population and HSCT survivors. Taken from DeFilipp et al. 2017

	General adult population (http://www.uspreventiveservicestaskforce.org/)	Adult long-term HCT survivors Majhall et al. (2012)	General pediatric population (http://www.nhlbi.nih.gov)	Pediatric long-term HCT survivors Pulsipher et al. (2012)
Weight, height and BMI	Weight, height and BMI assessment in all adults (no specific recommendation for screening interval)	No specific recommendations	Weight, height and BMI assessment after 2 years of age (no specified screening interval)	Weight, height and BMI assessment yearly
Dyslipidemia	For persons with increased risk for coronary heart disease, assessments should begin at age 20	Lipid profile assessment every 5 years in males aged ≥35 years and females aged ≥45 years	Lipid panel between 9 and 11 years of age or earlier if family history	Lipid profile at least every 5 years; if abnormal, screen annually
	The interval for screening should be shorter for people who have lipid levels close to those warranting therapy, and longer intervals for those not at increased risk who have had repeatedly normal lipid levels	Screening should start at age 20 for anyone at increased risk (smokers, DM, HTN, BMI ≥30 kg/m² and family history of heart disease before age 50 for male relatives or before age 60 for female relatives)		
Blood pressure	Blood pressure assessment every 3–5 years in adults aged 18–39 years with normal blood pressure (<130/85 mmHg) who do not have other risk factors	Blood pressure assessment at least every 2 years	Blood pressure assessment yearly after the age of 3 years, interpreted for age/sex/height	Blood pressure assessment at each visit and at least annually
	Blood pressure assessment annually in adults aged ≥40 years and for those who are at increased risk for high blood pressure (blood pressure 130 to 139/85 to 89 mmHg, those who are overweight or obese, and African–Americans)			
Hyperglycemia	Screening for abnormal blood glucose (HbA1C, fasting plasma glucose or oral glucose tolerance test) every 3 years in adults aged 40–70 years who are overweight or obese.	Screening for type 2 DM every 3 years in adults aged ≥45 years or in those with sustained higher blood pressure (>135/80 mmHg)	Fasting glucose every 2 years after the age of 10 years in overweight children with other risk factors	Fasting glucose at least every 5 years; if abnormal, screen annually

Abbreviations: *BMI* body mass index, *DM* diabetes mellitus, *HbA1C* hemoglobin A1C, *HCT* hematopoietic cell transplantation, *HTN* hyper tension

55.5 Future Directions: Implementation, Education and Research

As survival after HSCT gradually increases, there is recognition of an impact on CVD and its risk factors, including MetS. Most research has been cross-sectional and observational. More prospective research is needed on both defining the incidence above the normal ageing population and on interventional strategies, targeting individual risk factors and/or components of the MetS. Indeed, a recent review by Armenian and colleagues (Armenian et al. 2017) provided consensus recommendations for cardiovascular disease and risk factors identifying research gaps and future study priorities to improve the long-term cardiovascular health of HSCT survivors.

Consideration of CVD and associated risk factors may also vary between indications for HSCT. For example, the most common indication for HSCT, myeloma, although mostly incurable, is now associated with relative longevity, and consideration of CV risks are relevant (Snowden et al. 2017). Likewise, new indications for HSCT, such as systemic AID, and newer techniques, such as haplo-HSCT, require individualised assessment. Whilst pharmacological, lifestyle and rehabilitation interventions are common in the general population in respect to CVD, their impact in HSCT recipients (both before and after HSCT) needs to be defined in the context of the wide range of indications and age at which patients receive their HSCT, along with the individual prognosis of each indication after successful HSCT.

Key Points

- Until more evidence is available, the best approach is to screen all patients (i.e. both autologous and allogeneic HSCT) according to international consensus guidelines (DeFilipp et al. 2017) and manage risk factors on an individual basis.
- The challenge of universal implementation of screening and management of late effects across various health services providing HSCT will be facilitated by FACT-JACIE accreditation standards.
- Systematic programmes of education and research for the development and validation of HSCT-specific care models are warranted (Battiwalla et al. 2017).

References

Alberti KG, Eckel RH, Grundy SM, et al. Harmonizing the metabolic syndrome: a joint interim statement of the International Diabetes Federation Task Force on Epidemiology and Prevention; National Heart, Lung, and Blood Institute; American Heart Association; World Heart Federation; International Atherosclerosis Society; and International Association for the Study of Obesity. Circulation. 2009;120:1640–5.

Amato MC, Guarnotta V, Giordano C. Body composition assessment for the definition of cardiometabolic risk. J Endocrinol Investig. 2013;36:537–43.

Armenian SH, Chemaitilly W, Chen M, et al. National Institutes of Health hematopoietic cell transplantation late effects initiative: the Cardiovascular Disease and Associated Risk Factors Working Group report. Biol Blood Marrow Transplant. 2017;23:201–10.

Baker KS, Ness KK, Steinberger J, et al. Diabetes, hypertension, and cardiovascular events in survivors of hematopoietic cell transplantation: a report from the bone marrow transplantation survivor study. Blood. 2007;109:1765–72.

Battiwalla M, Tichelli A, Majhail NS. Long-term survivorship after hematopoietic cell transplantation: roadmap for research and care. Biol Blood Marrow Transplant. 2017;23:184–92.

Blaser BW, Kim HT, Alyea EP, et al. Hyperlipidemia and statin use after allogeneic hematopoietic stem cell transplantation. Biol Blood Marrow Transplant. 2012;18:575–83.

Chow EJ, Baker KS, Lee SJ, et al. Influence of conventional cardiovascular risk factors and lifestyle characteristics on cardiovascular disease after hematopoietic cell transplantation. J Clin Oncol. 2014;32:191–8.

Chow EJ, Mueller BA, Baker KS, et al. Cardiovascular hospitalizations and mortality among recipients of hematopoietic stem cell transplantation. Ann Intern Med. 2011;155:21–32.

DeFilipp Z, Duarte RF, Snowden JA, et al. Complications and Quality of Life Working Party, metabolic syndrome and cardiovascular disease following hematopoietic cell transplantation: screening and preventive practice recommendations from

CIBMTR and EBMT. Bone Marrow Transplant. 2017;52:173–82.

FACT-JACIE Standards. http://www.jacie.org/7th-edition. 2017. Accessed 25 May 2018.

Fodor G. Primary prevention of CVD: treating dyslipidaemia. BMJ Clin Evid. 2010;2010:0215.

Framingham risk score. https://www.mdcalc.com/framingham-coronary-heart-disease-risk-score. 2008.

Gonzalez-Juanatey JR, Millan J, Alegria E, et al. Prevalence and characteristics of lipid abnormalities in patients treated with statins in primary and secondary prevention in Spain. DYSIS-Spain Study. Rev Esp Cardiol. 2011;64:286–94.

Greenfield DM, Salooja N, Peczynski C, et al. Metabolic syndrome is common following haematopoietic cell transplantation (HCT) and is associated with increased cardiovascular disease and second cancers: an EBMT cross-sectional non-interventional study. 2018. https://ash.confex.com/ash/2018/webprogram/Paper116533.html

Hirabayashi K, Nakazawa Y, Matsuura H, et al. Risk factors for diabetes mellitus and impaired glucose tolerance following allogeneic hematopoietic stem cell transplantation in pediatric patients with hematological malignancies. Int J Hematol. 2014;99:477–86.

International Diabetes Federation: the IDF consensus worldwide definition of the metabolic syndrome. https://www.idf.org/e-library/consensus-statements.html. 2006. Accessed 23 May 2018.

Kagoya Y, Seo S, Nannya Y, Kurokawa M. Hyperlipidemia after allogeneic stem cell transplantation: prevalence, risk factors, and impact on prognosis. Clin Transpl. 2012;26:E168–75.

Majhail NS, Challa TR, Mulrooney DA, et al. Hypertension and diabetes mellitus in adult and pediatric survivors of allogeneic hematopoietic cell transplantation. Biol Blood Marrow Transplant. 2009a;15:1100–7.

Majhail NS, Flowers ME, Ness KK, et al. High prevalence of metabolic syndrome after allogeneic hematopoietic cell transplantation. Bone Marrow Transplant. 2009b;43:49–54.

Majhail NS, Rizzo JD, Lee SJ, et al. Recommended screening and preventive practices for long-term survivors after hematopoietic cell transplantation. Biol Blood Marrow Transplant. 2012;18:348–71.

McMillen KK, Schmidt EM, Storer BE, Bar M. Metabolic syndrome appears early after hematopoietic cell transplantation. Metab Syndr Relat Disord. 2014;12:367–71.

National Cholesterol Education Program (NCEP) expert panel on detection, evaluation, and treatment of high blood cholesterol in adults (adult treatment panel III circulation. 2002.

Oudin C, Auquier P, Bertrand Y, Contet A, Kanold J, Sirvent N, et al. Metabolic syndrome in adults who received hematopoietic stem cell transplantation for acute childhood leukemia: an LEA study. Bone Marrow Transplant. 2015;50:1438–44.

Pulsipher MA, Skinner R, McDonald GB, et al. National Cancer Institute, National Heart, Lung and Blood Institute/Pediatric Blood and Marrow Transplantation Consortium First International Consensus Conference on late effects after pediatric hematopoietic cell transplantation: the need for pediatric-specific long-term follow-up guidelines. Biol Blood Marrow Transplant. 2012;18:334–47.

Scheidt-Nave C, Du Y, Knopf H, et al. Prevalence of dyslipidemia among adults in Germany: results of the German Health Interview and Examination Survey for Adults (DEGS 1). Bundesgesundheitsblatt Gesundheitsforschung Gesundheitsschutz. 2013;56:661–7.

Snowden JA, Greenfield DM, Bird JM, et al. Guidelines for screening and management of late and long-term consequences of myeloma and its treatment. Br J Haematol. 2017;176:888–907.

Tichelli A, Bucher C, Rovo A, et al. Premature cardiovascular disease after allogeneic hematopoietic stem-cell transplantation. Blood. 2007;110:3463–71.

World Health Organisation. http://www.who.int/cardiovascular_diseases/about_cvd/en/. 2017. Accessed 28 Dec 2017.

56 Endocrine Disorders, Fertility and Sexual Health

Nina Salooja, Zeev Shoham, and Jean-Hugues Dalle

Increasing numbers of HSCT are being performed annually and outcomes continue to improve. As a result, survivorship issues are assuming increasing importance. Chemotherapy and radiotherapy remain cornerstones of HSCT treatment, but whilst lifesaving, they threaten endocrine function, fertility and sexual function.

56.1 Endocrine Function

Underlying disease, pre-HSCT treatment, development of chronic GVHD and prolonged corticosteroid treatment can all contribute to the risks of endocrine dysfunction inherent from conditioning regimens used for HSCT. Systematic follow-up is important to identify and treat endocrine defects before clinical impact, and this is particularly important in children where growth and puberty are at risk.

N. Salooja (✉)
Centre for Haematology, Imperial College, London, UK
e-mail: nina.salooja@imperial.ac.uk

Z. Shoham
Department of Obstetrics and Gynecology, Kaplan Medical Center, Rehovot, Israel

J.-H. Dalle
Department of Pediatric Hematology-Immunology, Hospital Robert-Debré, Assistance Publique-Hôpitaux de Paris, Paris Diderot University, Paris, France

56.1.1 Thyroid Dysfunction

56.1.1.1 Background

The most common abnormality of thyroid function after HSCT is primary compensated hypothyroidism. This may not require treatment and commonly resolves. Overt hypothyroidism may be primary or less commonly central. Other thyroid disorders include autoimmune thyroid disease (thyroiditis, Graves' disease) and thyroid cancers (carcinomas or benign adenomas). In a single-centre study of 791 patients followed up for 38 years, new cases of thyroid dysfunction continued for 28 years after HSCT highlighting the need for indefinite follow-up (Sanders et al. 2009).

Risk factors for hypothyroidism post-HSCT include the use of TBI with single dose being associated with a five to sixfold higher risk than fractionated TBI. BU-based regimens are more likely to cause thyroid problems than those containing CY only, and patients with malignant disease (e.g. Hodgkin lymphoma) are more likely to get thyroid dysfunction than patients with non-malignant diseases (e.g. aplastic anaemia). The age of the patient is also important with younger patients at higher risk. In relation to thyroid cancer, a retrospective study which included data on >68000 patients showed that the relative risk (RR) of thyroid cancer was approximately threefold higher following HSCT than in the general population. The RR was >20 if transplanted before the age of 10 years and close to 5 if transplanted between age 11 and

E. Carreras et al. (eds.), *The EBMT Handbook*, https://doi.org/10.1007/978-3-030-02278-5_56

20 years. Female gender and GVHD were additional risk factors (Cohen et al. 2007).

56.1.1.2 Prevention/Management

Patients should have annual laboratory assessment of thyroid function. Annual clinical examination should include palpation of the thyroid gland, and there should be a low threshold for arranging a thyroid ultrasound.

56.1.2 Hypoadrenalism

56.1.2.1 Background

The main risk factor is use of glucocorticoids which lead to central corticotrophin deficiency. Adult patients receiving 5mg/day prednisolone or more or paediatric patients receiving >0.3–0.5 mg/kg/day for more than 3 months are at risk. TBI can also cause corticotrophin deficiency as can drugs. Symptoms can be non-specific including fatigue, weakness, nausea, weight loss and hypotension. Some symptoms may mimic GVHD. Diagnosis requires paired morning cortisol and ACTH levels. If the results are nonconclusive, then additional investigations should be arranged with an endocrinologist.

56.1.2.2 Prevention/Management

When confirmed hydrocortisone should be given with additional doses to cover stresses such as illness, infection or surgery. Subsequently, regular evaluation is required as it may be possible to reduce/stop medication.

56.1.3 Growth

56.1.3.1 Background

Short stature is multifactorial after transplant. It is a recognized side effect of radiation to the hypothalamic-pituitary area given in childhood, as a result of a reduction in growth hormone (GH) secretion. Radiation can also induce bone lesions. Pre-transplant cranial radiation (e.g. patients with ALL) is also relevant, and single-dose TBI rather than fractionated radiation increases the risk further.

Additional contributory factors to short stature in these patients include underlying disease (e.g. Fanconi anaemia), other hormone deficiencies (including thyroid and gonadal hormones), nutritional deficits, illness, steroids and GVHD. Male sex and young age at time of transplant are additional risk factors.

56.1.3.2 Prevention/Management

Children's growth velocity should be closely monitored with height and weight documented at each clinic visit. A possible increased risk of secondary malignancies has been described in patients receiving GH therapy after previous neoplasia; this has raised concerns regarding the use of GH in the absence of sufficient long-term follow-up data. As a consequence of this, there are currently no clear guidelines for the use of GH in these patients. A paediatric endocrinologist should be involved if growth rate is abnormal based on bone age and pubertal stage (Chow et al. 2016) and the use of GH therapy discussed for severe growth retardation (-2SD).

56.2 Gonadal Dysfunction and Infertility

56.2.1 Background

Normal reproduction in both sexes requires germ cells and an intact hypothalamic-pituitary endocrine axis. In female patients the uterus must be both receptive to implantation and capable of undergoing growth during pregnancy. Chemotherapy and radiation can lead to damage in all of these areas and compromise the likelihood of successful parenthood after HSCT. Before starting any chemoradiotherapy regimen, the potential effects on the future fertility of the patient should be considered and discussed with the patient together with a discussion of fertility-preserving strategies.

56.2.2 Gonadal Dysfunction in Women Following Chemoradiotherapy

Women are born with a finite number of eggs which can be fertilized for pregnancy and depleted over time as a result of physiological apoptosis or else menstruation. Chemoradiotherapy depletes further the number of follicles by (1) activating apoptotic pathways, (2) causing fibrosis of stromal blood vessels, (3) activating resting (antral) follicles, leading to a 'burn-out' effect (Meirow and Nugent 2001; Kalich-Philosoph et al. 2013). The degree of ovarian damage is related to the dose and type of chemotherapeutic agent used, and baseline ovarian reserve which in turn is dependent on age and previous treatment. Manifestations of premature ovarian failure range from premature menopause to varying degrees of infertility. Alkylating agents have the highest age-adjusted odds ratio of ovarian failure (Meirow 2000). A combination of BU and CY is particularly gonadotoxic to females, but younger patients who receive CY only may have some gonadal function preserved and pregnancies following CY are well described (Salooja et al. 2001). TBI is also potentially sterilizing. The estimated median lethal dose of radiation for the human oocyte is less than 2 Gy (Wallace et al. 2003). The effective sterilizing dose (ESD) decreases with increasing age, and whilst estimated as 18.4 Gy at 10 years of age, the ESD is approximately 14.3 Gy at 30 years of age, and only 6 Gy in women over age 40 (Wallace et al. 2005).

56.2.3 Gonadal Dysfunction in Men Following Chemoradiotherapy

In male patients, spermatogenesis is impaired, but testosterone levels generally remain normal because of the relative resistance of testosterone producing Leydig cells to chemoradiotherapy. As a result, secondary sexual characteristics remain normal for male patients and typically testosterone levels and luteinizing hormone (LH) levels are in the normal range. Spermatogonia are very sensitive to irradiation, and it takes approximately 2 years for sperm counts to recover to pre-irradiation levels after a single dose of 1 Gy (Meistrich and van Beek 1990). With higher doses, azoospermia persists longer or may be permanent. Following HSCT conditioned with TBI, the majority of men will be azoospermic. Chemotherapy only regimens are also associated with azoospermia but to a lesser degree (Rovo et al. 2013). Following BU, for example, approximately 50% will be azoospermic, whilst after CY alone, recovery of spermatogenesis is more frequent.

56.2.4 Uterine Dysfunction in Women After Radiation

Uterine development commences at puberty and is associated with an increase in both size and vascularity (Laursen et al. 1996). Exposure to radiation leads to reduced vascularity, fibrosis and hormone-dependent endometrial insufficiency, which subsequently lead to adverse reproductive outcomes. Increased rates of infertility, miscarriage, preterm labour, intrauterine growth retardation and low newborn birth weight have been described (Reulen et al. 2009), particularly if conception occurred within a year of radiotherapy (Fenig et al. 2001).

56.2.5 Prevention/Management of Gonadal Failure

56.2.5.1 Fertility Preservation in Males

Sperm cryopreservation is an established fertility preservation option for post-pubertal boys and men. Sperm can be used either for artificial insemination or, if the quantity and/or quality of sperm are insufficient, for intracytoplasmic sperm injections for in vitro fertilization. There is a chance of sperm recovery with time particularly if the patient was under the age of 25 years at transplant, did not have TBI and has no evidence of chronic GVHD (Rovo et al. 2013). These patients require reassessment at intervals to ascertain their fertility potential.

56.2.5.2 Fertility Preservation Techniques in Females

Gonadotropin-Releasing Hormone Agonists (GnRHa)

Despite success in animal models, the value of GnRHa to preserve ovarian function during chemotherapy in human subjects is uncertain. A Cochrane database review (2011) concluded that the use of GnRH agonists should be considered for ovarian protection in women of reproductive age who are receiving chemotherapy (Chen et al. 2011).

Embryo and Oocyte Cryopreservation

Embryo and oocyte cryopreservation are preferred methods of fertility preservation in women who require sterilizing treatment. Use of donor embryos/oocytes can also be discussed with the patient because they offer the possibility of pregnancy and parenthood albeit with a non-genetic child. Mature oocyte collection requires ovarian stimulation. These oocytes can then either be frozen or else fertilized *in vitro* before freezing. These options are not open to all patients however. Ovarian stimulation takes a minimum of 2 weeks, and this delay is prohibitive for many patients with haematological malignancies. The requirement for partner or donor sperm for embryo cryopreservation is another potential drawback; for some patients, sperm is not available, and for others the involvement of a partner/sperm donor limits future reproductive autonomy as consent from the sperm provider must be given not only at the time of cryopreservation but also at the time of reimplantation.

Ovarian Tissue Cryopreservation (OTC)

OTC is considered experimental and is not available to all patients. Nonetheless, reports of pregnancy after OTC are increasing (Van der Ven et al. 2016), and it is the only option open to prepubertal patients or to women who cannot tolerate a significant delay in treatment due to disease severity or progression. Cortical fragments containing primordial follicles with immature oocytes can be obtained by laparoscopy and cryopreserved. Ideally, ovarian tissue should be obtained before the patient has been exposed to chemotherapy, but this is not always possible and is not an absolute requirement.

A major concern reimplanting cryopreserved ovarian tissue is the possibility of reseeding the tumour. The risk depends on the individual disease. Assessment by PCR of ovarian tissue taken from patients with leukemia (CML, AML, ALL), tested positive for disease in a number of cases and assessment of tissue from mice with severe combined immunodeficiency confirmed, confirms the leukaemic potential of the tissue (Rosendahl et al. 2013). As a result, reintroduction of ovarian tissue from patients with leukemia would not currently be recommended. In the future, maturation in vitro of follicles from cryopreserved tissue may enable production of a viable disease-free alternative. In patients with lymphoma, histologically negative samples of ovarian issue have been transplanted without initiating relapse, but in some cases the follow-up time was short.

56.2.5.3 Children and Adolescents

Fertility preservation in children has been the subject of recent guidelines from the paediatric diseases working party of the EBMT (Dalle et al. 2017; Balduzzi et al. 2017). Extreme sensitivity is required, and parents have to be given complete information on the process, associated risks and success rates. For prepubertal girls, OTC is currently the only potential fertility-sparing option. In peri-pubertal boys, it is sometimes possible to extract sperm using surgery/microdissection or electroejaculation under general anaesthetic. In prepubertal males the only option is testicular tissue cryopreservation; although work in animal models is encouraging, there have been no reports to date of reimplanted testicular tissue leading to human live births.

56.2.6 Management of Pregnancy After HSCT

Most patients or their partners who conceive after HSCT have uncomplicated pregnancies. Chemoradiotherapy can potentially affect a variety of maternal organs relevant to a successful pregnancy outcome, for example, renal, cardiac and pulmonary toxicity. Patients at risk should have an expert medical review early in pregnancy and may require regular specialist monitoring throughout and review by an anaesthetist prior to delivery. Patients who have had TBI or pelvic irradiation have an increased risk of premature and small birth weight babies. Miscarriage rates are typically comparable to the background population, however, and no significant increase in congenital malformations or genetic abnormalities have so far been described when conception has taken place long after completion of therapy (Meirow and Schiff 2005; Green et al. 2009). Animal experiments suggest that most cytotoxic drugs are mutagenic and teratogenic to oocytes exposed during the maturation phase. In humans, this phase lasts approximately 6 months (Meirow and Schiff 2005), so there is a theoretical advantage to delaying conception for 6 months after completing gonadotoxic treatments.

56.3 Sexual Function

56.3.1 Background

Alterations in sexual function and sexual satisfaction are among the most common of all complications in long-term survivors of transplantation with 46% male and 80% female survivors describing sexual problems 5 years post transplant (Syrjala et al. 2008). Sexual complications in both allogeneic and autologous transplant recipients include changes in libido, dyspareunia (females) and erectile and ejaculatory dysfunction (males) (Li et al. 2015). Allogeneic recipients have additional problems linked to acute or chronic GVHD (Wong et al. 2013).

Sexuality is also affected, and this is multifactorial due to decreased self-confidence, stress, anxiety and fear of recurrence, together with a change in body image (Yi and Syrjala 2009). The sexual well-being of the survivor is also determined by their relationship with their partner (Langer et al. 2007). The partners of patients may experience a decrease in sexual desire and anxiety about initiating sexual activity with survivors. Poor communication can contribute to long-term sexual dysfunction between survivors and their partners (Hawkins et al. 2009).

56.3.2 Prevention/Management

It is important to identify relevant issues before problems with sexuality and intimacy become entrenched. It is recommended that healthcare professionals discuss sexual function with patients at 6 months, 1 year and at least annually thereafter (Majhail et al. 2012). Prompt attention should be paid to reversible risk factors such as hypogonadism or symptoms associated with urogenital GVHD so that appropriate referrals can be made to either gynaecologists or urologists. Some male patients benefit from the prescription of erectile dysfunction medication, and hormone replacement should be discussed with women prior to leaving hospital if onset of menopause is likely. Women with vaginal dryness may benefit from lubricants or topical oestrogens, and those with GVHD may benefit from topical steroids (Tirri et al. 2015). The role of vaginal dilators in preventing vaginal stenosis is not clear (Miles and Johnson 2014). It is recognized that psychological factors can play a large part in sexual dysfunction after transplant and this is relevant not only for the patient but also for the partner. For the patient it can be difficult to separate the psychological issues from coexisting physical problems, but many couples will benefit from review by a sex therapist.

References

Balduzzi A, Dalle JH, Jahnukainen K, et al. Fertility preservation issues in pediatric hematopoietic stem cell transplantation: practical approaches from the consensus of the Pediatric Diseases Working Party of the EBMT and the International BFM Study Group. Bone Marrow Transplant. 2017;52:1406–15.

Chen H, Li J, Cui T, Hu L. Adjuvant gonadotropin-releasing hormone analogues for the prevention of chemotherapy induced premature ovarian failure in premenopausal women. Cochrane Database Syst Rev. 2011;11:CD008018.

Chow EJ, Anderson L, Scott Baker K, et al. Late effects surveillance recommendations among survivors of childhood hematopoietic cell transplantation: a Children's Oncology Group Report. Biol Blood Marrow Transplant. 2016;22:782–95.

Cohen A, Rovelli A, Merlo DF, et al. Risk for secondary thyroid carcinoma after hematopoietic stem-cell transplantation: an EBMT late effects working party study. J Clin Oncol. 2007;25:2449–54.

Dalle JH, Lucchini G, Balduzzi A, et al. State-of-the-art fertility preservation in children and adolescents undergoing haematopoietic stem cell transplantation: a report on the expert meeting of the Paediatric Diseases Working Party (PDWP) of the European Society for Blood and Marrow Transplantation (EBMT). Bone Marrow Transplant. 2017;52:1029–35.

Fenig E, Mishaeli M, Kalish Y, Lishner M. Pregnancy and radiation. Cancer Treat Rev. 2001;27:1–7.

Green DM, Sklar CA, Boice JD Jr, et al. Ovarian failure and reproductive outcomes after childhood cancer treatment: results from the Childhood Cancer Survivor Study. J Clin Oncol. 2009;27:2374–81.

Hawkins Y, Ussher GE, et al. Changes in sexuality and intimacy after the diagnosis and treatment of cancer: the experience of partners in a sexual relationship with a person with cancer. Cancer Nurs. 2009;32:271–80.

Kalich-Philosoph L, Roness H, Carmely A, et al. Cyclophosphamide triggers follicle activation and "burnout"; AS101 prevents follicle loss and preserves fertility. Sci Transl Med. 2013;15:185ra62.

Langer SL, Rudd ME, Syrjala KL. Protective buffering and emotional desynchrony among spousal care givers. Health Psychol. 2007;26:635–43.

Laursen EM, Holm K, Brocks V, et al. Doppler assessment of flow velocity in the uterine artery during pubertal maturation. Ultrasound Obstet Gynecol. 1996;8:341–5.

Li Z, Mewawalla P, Stratton P, et al. Sexual health in hematopoietic stem cell transplant recipients. Cancer. 2015;121:4124–31.

Majhail NS, Rizzo D, Lee SJ, et al. Recommended screening and preventive practices for long-term survivors after hematopoietic cell transplantation. Biol Blood Marrow Transplant. 2012;18:348–71.

Meirow D, Nugent D. The effects of radiotherapy and chemotherapy on female reproduction. Hum Reprod Update. 2001;7:535–43.

Meirow D, Schiff E. Appraisal of chemotherapy effects on reproductive outcome according to animal studies and clinical data. J Natl Cancer Inst Monogr. 2005;34:21–5.

Meirow D. Reproduction post-chemotherapy in young cancer patients. Mol Cell Endocrinol. 2000;169:123–31.

Meistrich ML, van Beek MEAB. Radiation sensitivity of the human testis. Adv Radiat Biol. 1990;14:227–68.

Miles T, Johnson N. Vaginal dilator therapy for women receiving pelvic radiotherapy. Cochrane Database Syst Rev. 2014;9:CD007291.

Reulen RC, Zeegers MP, Wallace WHB, et al. Pregnancy outcomes among adult survivors of childhood cancer in the British childhood Cancer survivor study. Cancer Epidemiol Biomark Prev. 2009;18:2239–47.

Rosendahl M, Greve T, Anderson CY. The safety of transplanting cryopreserved ovarian tissue in cancer patients: a review of the literature. J Assist Reprod Genet. 2013;30:11–24.

Rovo A, Aljurf M, Chiodi S, et al. Ongoing graft-versus-host disease is a risk factor for azoospermia after allogeneic hematopoietic stem cell transplantation: a survey of the Late Effects Working Party of the European Group for Blood and Marrow Transplantation. Haematologica. 2013;98:339–45.

Salooja N, Szydlo RM, Socie G, et al. Pregnancy outcomes after peripheral blood or bone marrow transplantation: a retrospective study. Lancet. 2001;358:271–6.

Sanders JE, Paul AH, Woolfrey AE, et al. Thyroid function following hematopoietic cell transplantation in children: 30 years' experience. Blood. 2009;113: 306–8.

Syrjala KL, Kurland BF, Abrams JR, et al. Sexual function changes during the 5 years after high-dose treatment and hematopoietic cell transplantation for malignancy, with case-matched controls at 5 years. Blood. 2008;111:989–96.

Tirri BF, Hausermann P, Bertz H, et al. Clinical guidelines for gynecologic care after hematopoietic SCT. Report from the international consensus project on clinical practice in chronic GVHD. Bone Marrow Transplant. 2015;50:3–9.

Van der Ven H, Liebenthron J, Beckmann M, FertiPROTEKT network, et al. Ninety-five orthotopic transplantations in 74 women of ovarian tissue after cytotoxic treatment in a fertility preservation network: tissue activity, pregnancy and delivery rates. Hum Reprod. 2016;31:2031–41.

Wallace WH, Thomson AB, Saran F, Kelsey TW. Predicting age of ovarian failure after radiation to a field that includes the ovaries. Int J Radiat Oncol Biol Phys. 2003;62:738–44.

Wallace WHB, Thomson AB, Kelsey TW. The radiosensitivity of the human oocyte. Hum Reprod. 2003;18:117–21.

Wong FL, Francisco L, Togawa K, et al. Longitudinal trajectory of sexual functioning after hematopoietic cell transplantation: impact of chronic graft-versus-host disease and total body irradiation. Blood. 2013;122:3973–81.

Yi JC, Syrjala K. Sexuality after hematopoietic stem cell transplantation. Cancer J. 2009;15:57–64.

Part VII

Prevention and Management of Relapse

Topic leaders: Peter Bader and Nicolaus Kröger

57 Monitoring Minimal Residual Disease in ALL and AML

Peter Bader, Hermann Kreyenberg, and Gert Ossenkoppele

57.1 Monitoring MRD in ALL

Peter Bader and Hermann Kreyenberg

57.1.1 Introduction

In ALL evaluation of molecular treatment response, assessment of minimal residual disease (MRD) is a substantial independent predictor of outcome, as proven by randomized studies (Conter et al. 2010; Gökbuget et al. 2012; Bassan and Spinelli 2015). Consequently, MRD is implemented in virtually all clinical protocols in order to supplement or to redefine multifactorial risk stratification with optional customized treatment intensity. The detection of leukemic cells below the limit of classical cytomorphology is feasible either by disease-specific alterations of the immune phenotype or unique genetic features. Several competing and complementing MRD methods have been developed with preference application according to clinical protocols (Van der Velden et al. 2007; van Dongen et al. 2015).

57.1.2 MRD Assessment by IG/TCR Real-Time PCR

The discontinuous immune receptor genes provide the immune repertoire by somatic recombination of variable (V)-, diversification (D)-, and junction (J)- elements thus forming hypervariable CDR3 (complement determine region 3) regions during lymphocyte maturation. Such rearrangements can serve as clonal index of leukemia blasts originating from lymphoid precursor stages. Additionally, due to a relaxed regulatory control, leukemia blasts can harbor incomplete rearrangements and cross-lineage rearrangements and tend to accumulate simultaneously multiple rearrangements. Quantitative real-time PCR using junction complementary allele-specific oligonucleotides (ASO) frequently reaches a detection limit of 1E-05 with a quantitative range of 1E-04, is applicable to vast majority of cases, and has a high degree of standardization (Van der Velden et al. 2007).

P. Bader (✉)
Division for Stem Cell Transplantation and Immunology, University Hospital for Children and Adolescents
Goethe University Frankfurt am Main
Frankfurt Germany
e-mail: peter.bader@kgu.de

H. Kreyenberg
Division of Stem Cell Transplantation and Immunology, Center for Children and Adolescents
University Hospital Frankfurt
Frankfurt Germany

G. Ossenkoppele
Department of Hematology
Universitaire Medische Centra, VU University Medical Center
Amsterdam The Netherlands

E. Carreras et al. (eds.), *The EBMT Handbook*, https://doi.org/10.1007/978-3-030-02278-5_57

57.1.3 MRD Assessment by Fusion Gene Transcript

Most frequent recurrent reciprocal translocations are in ALL t(9;22)(q34;q11) (*BCR-ABL1*), t(12;21)(p13;q23) (*ETV6-RUNX1*), and t(4;11) (q21;q22) (*MLL-AFF1*) with age stage associated preponderance in adults, childhood, and infant ALL, respectively. Derived chimeric fusion transcripts are validated marker for MRD detection by real-time PCR with an achievable detection limit of 1E-06. The methodology has been standardized by the Europe Against Cancer (EAC) program (Gabert et al. 2003).

57.1.4 NGS (Next-Generation Sequencing)

High-throughput sequencing (HTS) of immune receptor genes by next-generation sequencing (NGS) is a novel option for MRD. This methodology provides comprehensive qualitative and quantitative information regarding clonal consistence of the diagnostic sample and shares one protocol for index determination and MRD assessment without need of individual reagents. Potential sub- and new emerging leukemic clones also are covered. PCR steps during library construction can introduce bias effecting results internal controls and normalization calculations are necessary the generated data volume is high and data interpretation demand biostatistics expertise. Due to high sample capacity, NGS favors a centralized concept and service is available to commercial providers by academic centers (Kotrova et al. 2015).

57.1.5 Flow Cytometry

MRD by multicomponent flow cytometry (MFC) distinguishes leukemia-associated immune phenotypes (LAIP) and regular cells. LAIP consists of cell lineage maturation stage-specific (backbone) markers in combination with illegitimate markers. The standard four to six color approaches have been developed simultaneously by several centers. Therefore, the applied marker panels depend on study protocol. The consistently achieved detection limit is 1E-04. Recently, increase of specificity and sensitivity was enabled by high-throughput procedures demanding eight or ten color equipment. Here the options for targeted and visualized antigens allow simultaneous visualization of all developmental lymphocyte stages serving as background to distinguish leukemic cells. The EuroFlow Consortium validated available antibody panels and controls which can be applied in a standardized way, including automated gating with supportive software, data storage and comparison, accurate quantitative result, and option for IVD development. Similar to the NGS approach, the generated data volume is high and data interpretation demands biostatistics expertise; nevertheless, the concept allows decentralized data acquisition (Pedreira et al. 2013).

57.1.6 Limitations of MRD Assessment

The determined level of MRD always is a result of complex interrelation of baseline characteristics of tumor and patient, time point of MRD evaluation, therapeutic agents, course of clearance, and degree of therapy resistance. Several measurements therefore are mandatory. Adverse circumstances for MRD assessment are clonal selection and clonal evolution, since the associated index might be missed. Potentially impacted are leukemia with initial oligoclonality as observed in approximately 15% of B-ALL and up to 1000 subclones have been reported (Wu et al. 2016). Phenotypic plasticity under treatment and massive lymphocyte regeneration can cause false negativity or positivity, a solvable problem by applying mentioned high-throughput methodologies. Achievable detection limit is correlated with cell count of sample, and aplastic samples are challenging. Finally, all methodologies use different sample preparations, and analyses refer to different units, a circumstance which interferes result comparison.

57.1.7 MRD in the Setting of HSCT

As all adult patients with ALL who relapse after initial chemotherapy have an absolute indication for allo-HSCT, pediatric patients are stratified into different treatment groups. Main prognostic determinants in these patients are the blast immune phenotype, time to relapse, and site of relapse. High-risk patients who experienced early isolated BM relapse, early relapse involving BM, and any BM relapse of T-lineage ALL have clear indication for HSCT. Intermediate-risk patients experienced early or late combined BM relapse and a late isolated BM relapse of a B-cell precursor (BCP).

ALL and very early and early isolated extramedullary relapse of either BCP-ALL or T-ALL have indication for HSCT if post induction MRD exceeds a threshold of 1E-03 (Eckert et al. 2013).

During the past decades, it could be clearly shown by several studies that the level of MRD immediately prior to transplant does have a clear prognostic impact on post-HSCT outcome (Knechtli et al. 1998). Retrospective studies in children with relapsed ALL revealed an important cutoff for post-HSCT outcome. Patients who received transplantation with an MRD load of ≥10 to 4 leukemic cells had a by far inferior prognosis than patients with lower MRD loads before transplant (Bader et al. 2009). Based on these findings, several studies are now underway investigating strategies to improve outcome in these ultrahigh-risk patients. Adaption of transplant approaches might allow successful transplantation (Leung et al. 2012).

Spinelli et al. showed that almost half of the patients with high levels of MRD before transplantation achieved molecular remission by day +100 (Spinelli et al. 2007). This finding indicates that MRD detection post transplant provides additional value to the MRD assessment prior to transplantation. It could be demonstrated in prospective clinical studies that the close monitoring of MRD by different approaches allows the prediction of relapse and may therefore form the basis of different intervention strategies making use of leukemia-specific targeted therapy (Bader et al. 2015; Balduzzi et al. 2014). Future perspectives will focus on MRD-guided intervention to prevent overt relapse (Rettinger et al. 2017).

57.2 Monitoring MRD in AML

Gert Ossenkoppele

57.2.1 Introduction

The possibility of defining residual disease far below the level of 5% leukemic cells is changing the landscape of risk classification. This so-called measurable/MRD approach at present establishes the presence of leukemia cells down to levels of $1{:}10^3$ to $1{:}10^6$ white blood cells, compared to 1:20 for morphology. Recently the ELN proposed a new response criterium: CR without minimal residual disease (CR_{MRD-}) is defined as CR with negativity for a genetic marker by RT-qPCR or CR with negativity by multicolor flow cytometry (MFC) (Döhner et al. 2017).

The reasons to apply MRD assessment in AML are (1) to provide an objective establishment of remission status; (2) to better predict outcome and guide post-remission treatment; (3) to identify early relapse as a robust post transplant surveillance, in order to enable early intervention; and (4) to be used as a surrogate endpoint to fasten drug testing and approval.

A recent ELN MRD consensus document was published with the aim to identify key clinical and scientific issues in the measurement and application of MRD in AML and to provide guidelines for the current and future use of MRD in clinical practice (Schuurhuis et al. 2018).

57.2.2 Methods for MRD Detection

57.2.2.1 MRD Detection by PCR

Real-time quantitative PCR (RT-qPCR) allows MRD detection in cases with chimeric fusion genes generated by balanced chromosomal rearrangements (Grimwade and Freeman 2014). Other genetic alterations can also be used for MRD detection including insertions/duplications, point mutations and gene overexpression. Apart from t(15;17) and *RUNX1–RUNX1T1* and *CBFB–MYH11*, currently *NPM1* is the best-validated molecular marker for MRD assessment. PCR assessment of MRD is in about 50% of patients in principle possible. The methodology has been standardized for several molecular markers for clinical implementation in the Europe Against Cancer (EAC) program (Gabert et al. 2003).

57.2.2.2 Immune MRD by Multicolor Flow Cytometry

The basic principle is to identify at diagnosis leukemia-associated immune phenotypes (LAIP). These LAIPs consist of normally occurring markers, present in aberrant combinations in AML but in very low frequencies in normal and regenerating BM. The background levels of LAIP in normal and regenerating BM levels, in particular, although low, prevent specific detection of aberrancies with sensitivities higher than 1:10,000.

If no diagnosis sample is present, one can make use of "different from normal" approach which uses a standard fixed antibody panel to recognize leukemic cells based on their difference with normal hematopoietic cells (Loken et al. 2012).

Currently, immune MRD aberrancies may be detected in over 90% of AML cases at diagnosis.

57.2.3 MRD in Clinical Studies

Despite a multitude of prognostic factors at diagnosis, the outcome of patients is still highly variable and not individually predictable. It thus seems that prognosticators at diagnosis will not enable clinicians to reach the ultimate goal of truly individualized risk assessment. Treatment parameters may be more useful (Ossenkoppele and Schuurhuis 2013).

Two large, prospective, multicenter studies have identified flow cytometry-based MRD as an independent prognostic indicator in adults with AML (Freeman et al. 2013; Terwijn et al. 2013). Flow cytometry-based MRD was assessed in a multicenter, multinational study in adults with AML between 18 and 60 years of age by HOVON/SAKK investigators (Terwijn et al. 2013). Patients were treated according to protocol, without knowledge of MRD-related data. In this study, lower levels of MRD were associated with better outcomes than higher levels, and MRD levels >0.1% of white blood cells after the second cycle of chemotherapy were associated with higher risk of relapse in multivariate analysis. The UK NCRI group assessed MRD using flow cytometry in 427 patients older than 60 years of age (Freeman et al. 2013). MRD negativity after the first cycle of chemotherapy conferred significantly better 3-year survival after CR. MRD-positive patients had increased relapses and higher risk of early relapse (median time to relapse, 8.5 v 17.1 months, respectively).

An example indicative for the usage of molecular MRD was recently published by Ivey et al. (2016) who showed in a large study by NCRI that the presence of MRD, assessed by Q-PCR of *NPM1*-mutated transcripts, provided powerful prognostic information independent of other risk factors. Persistence of *NPM1*-mutated transcripts in blood was present in 15% of the patients after the second chemotherapy cycle and was associated with a greater risk of relapse after 3 years of follow-up than was an absence of such transcripts (82% vs. 30%; hazard ratio, 4.80) and a lower rate of survival (24% vs. 75%; hazard ratio for death, 4.38).

Many other studies point in the same direction that MRD status after two cycles of chemotherapy is highly predictive independently from other prognostic factors for outcome (Hourigan et al. 2017). However surrogacy for survival has not been proven yet (Ossenkoppele and Schuurhuis 2016).

57.2.4 Pretransplant MRD

Evidence is accumulating that the presence of MRD assessed by multicolor flow cytometry immediately prior to allogeneic HCT is a strong, independent predictor of post transplant outcomes in AML (Buckley et al. 2017; Walter et al. 2015). In a recent update, Araki et al. showed that in 359 adults, the 3-year relapse rate was 67% in MRD-positive patients, compared to 22% in MRD-negative patients, resulting in OS of 26% vs. 73%, respectively (Araki et al. 2016). This applies for the myeloablative as well as for the non-myeloablative transplant setting.

Also molecular MRD as measured by RT-PCR in NPM1-mutated AML has a significant impact on outcome after allo-HSCT (Balsat et al. 2017).

Performing an allo-HSCT in case of a suboptimal reduction (<4 $\log_{10}$) of NPM1 levels after chemotherapy resulted in improved overall survival. In patients with optimal (≥4 $\log_{10}$) reduction of NPM1 levels after chemotherapy, allo-HSCT had no significant effect on survival. However, no prospective studies using MRD to guide post-remission therapy are available at the time of this publication. Regardless, it is clear that novel treatment strategies before, during, and after transplant are urgently needed to improve outcomes in AML. Thereby depth of response prior to transplant, as measured by level of MRD, has emerged as one of the most important predictors of transplant outcome. Randomized trials are warranted to determine if MRD-guided preemptive therapy is associated with improved outcome.

Currently no clinical trial including transplantation trials should be performed without including MRD assessment.

57.2.5 Future Developments

New technologies are emerging to assess MRD. Quantifying leukemic stem cells is such a promising approach (Terwijn et al. 2014; Zeijlemaker et al. 2016). Next-generation sequencing for MRD assessment can, theoretically, be applied to all leukemia-specific genetic aberrations. In a recent HOVON study, it was shown that persistence of gene mutations in CR appeared to be a highly significant independent prognostic value for relapse and overall survival (Jongen-Lavrencic et al. 2018).

Key Points

- MRD should be included in the definition of CR.
- MRD positivity is an independent predictor of relapse after chemotherapy in AML patients and a negative predictor for ALL patients.
- Pretransplant MRD positivity is highly indicative for relapse.
- MRD assessment should be implemented in every clinical trial.

References

Araki D, Wood BL, Othus M, et al. Allogeneic hematopoietic cell transplantation for acute myeloid leukemia: time to move toward a minimal residual disease-based definition of complete remission? J Clin Oncol. 2016;34:329–36.

Bader P, Kreyenberg H, Henze G, et al. Prognostic value of minimal residual disease quantification before allogeneic stem-cell transplantation in relapsed childhood acute lymphoblastic leukemia: the ALL-REZ BFM Study Group. J Clin Oncol. 2009;27:377–84.

Bader P, Kreyenberg H, Stackelberg A, et al. Monitoring of minimal residual disease after allogeneic stem-cell transplantation in relapsed childhood acute lymphoblastic leukemia allows for the identification of impending relapse: results of the ALL-BFM-SCT 2003 trial. J Clin Oncol. 2015;33:1275–84.

Balduzzi A, Di Maio L, Silvestri D, et al. Minimal residual disease before and after transplantation for childhood acute lymphoblastic leukaemia: is there any room for intervention? Br J Haematol. 2014;164:396–408.

Balsat M, Renneville A, Thomas X, et al. Postinduction minimal residual disease predicts outcome and benefit from allogeneic stem cell transplantation in acute myeloid leukemia with NPM1 mutation: a study by the acute leukemia French Association Group. J Clin Oncol. 2017;35:185–93.

Bassan R, Spinelli O. Minimal residual disease monitoring in adult ALL to determine therapy. Curr Hematol Malig Rep. 2015;10:86–95.

Buckley SA, Wood BL, Othus M, et al. Minimal residual disease prior to allogeneic hematopoietic cell transplantation in acute myeloid leukemia: a meta-analysis. Haematologica. 2017;102:865–73.

Conter V, Bartram C, Valsecchi M, et al. Molecular response to treatment redefines all prognostic factors in children and adolescents with B-cell precursor acute lymphoblastic leukemia: results in 3184 patients of the AIEOP-BFM ALL 2000 study. Blood. 2010;115:3206–14.

Döhner H, Estey E, Grimwade D, et al. Diagnosis and management of AML in adults: 2017 ELN recommendations from an international expert panel. Blood. 2017;129:424–47.

Eckert C, von Stackelberg A, Seeger K, et al. Minimal residual disease after induction is the strongest predictor of prognosis in intermediate risk relapsed acute lymphoblastic leukaemia—long-term results of trial ALL-REZ BFM P95/96. Eur J Cancer. 2013;49:1346–55.

Freeman SD, Virgo P, Couzens S, et al. Prognostic relevance of treatment response measured by flow cytometric residual disease detection in older patients with acute myeloid leukemia. J Clin Oncol. 2013;31:4123–31.

Gabert J, Beillard E, van der Velden V, et al. Standardization and quality control studies of 'real-time' quantitative reverse transcriptase polymerase chain reaction of fusion gene transcripts for residual disease detection in leukemia—a Europe Against Cancer Program. Leukemia. 2003;17:2318–57.

Gökbuget N, Kneba M, Raff T, et al. Adult patients with acute lymphoblastic leukemia and molecular failure display a poor prognosis and are candidates for stem cell transplantation and targeted therapies. Blood. 2012;120:1868–76.

Grimwade D, Freeman SD. Defining minimal residual disease in acute myeloid leukemia: which platforms are ready for prime time? Blood. 2014;124:3345–55.

Hourigan CS, Gale RP, Gormley NJ, et al. Measurable residual disease testing in acute myeloid leukaemia. Leukemia. 2017;31:1482–90.

Ivey A, Hills RK, Simpson MA, et al. Assessment of minimal residual disease in standard-risk AML. N Engl J Med. 2016;374:422–33.

Jongen-Lavrencic M, Grob T, Kavelaars F, et al. Comprehensive molecular residual disease detection of clinical value in acute myeloid leukemia. N Engl J Med. 2018;378:1189–99.

Knechtli C, Goulden N, Hancock J, et al. Minimal residual disease status before allogeneic bone marrow transplantation is an important determinant of successful outcome for children and adolescents with acute lymphoblastic leukemia. Blood. 1998;92:4072–9.

Kotrova M, Muzikova K, Mejstrikova E, et al. The predictive strength of next-generation sequencing MRD detection for relapse compared with current methods in childhood ALL. Blood. 2015;126:1045–7.

Leung W, Pui C-H, Coustan-Smith E, et al. Detectable minimal residual disease before hematopoietic cell transplantation is prognostic but does not preclude cure for children with very-high-risk leukemia. Blood. 2012;120:468–72.

Loken MR, Alonzo TA, Pardo L, et al. Residual disease detected by multidimensional flow cytometry signifies high relapse risk in patients with de novo acute myeloid leukemia: a report from Children's Oncology Group. Blood. 2012;120:1581–8.

Ossenkoppele G, Schuurhuis GJ. MRD in AML: time for redefinition of CR? Blood. 2013;121:2166–8.

Ossenkoppele G, Schuurhuis GJ. MRD in AML: does it already guide therapy decision-making? Hematology Am Soc Hematol Educ Program. 2016;2016:356–65.

Pedreira C, Costa E, Lecrevisse Q. Overview of clinical flow cytometry data analysis: recent advances and future challenges. Trends Biotechnol. 2013;31:415–25.

Rettinger E, Merker M, Salzmann-Manrique E, et al. Preemptive immunotherapy for clearance of molecular disease in childhood acute lymphoblastic leukemia after transplantation. Biol Blood Marrow Transplant. 2017;23:87–95.

Schuurhuis GJ, Heuser M, Freeman S, et al. Minimal/measurable residual disease in AML: consensus document from ELN MRD Working Party. Blood. 2018;131(12):1275–91. https://doi.org/10.1182/blood-2017-09-801498.

Spinelli O, Peruta B, Tosi M, et al. Clearance of minimal residual disease after allogeneic stem cell transplantation and the prediction of the clinical outcome of adult patients with high-risk acute lymphoblastic leukemia. Haematologica. 2007;92:612–8.

Terwijn M, van Putten WL, Kelder A, et al. High prognostic impact of flow cytometric minimal residual disease detection in acute myeloid leukemia: data from the HOVON/SAKK AML 42A study. J Clin Oncol. 2013;31:3889.

Terwijn M, Zeijlemaker W, Kelder A, et al. Leukemic stem cell frequency: a strong biomarker for clinical outcome in acute myeloid leukemia. PLoS One. 2014;9(9):e107587.

van der Velden V, Cazzaniga G, Schrauder A, et al. Analysis of minimal residual disease by Ig/TCR gene rearrangements: guidelines for interpretation of real-time quantitative PCR data. Leukemia. 2007;21:604–11.

van Dongen J, van der Velden V, Brüggemann M, Orfao A. Minimal residual disease diagnostics in acute lymphoblastic leukemia: need for sensitive, fast, and standardized technologies. Blood. 2015;125:3996–4009.

Walter RB, et al. Comparison of minimal residual disease as outcome predictor for AML patients in first complete remission undergoing myeloablative or nonmyeloablative allogeneic hematopoietic cell transplantation. Leukemia. 2015;29:137–44.

Wu J, Jia S, Wang C, et al. Minimal residual disease detection and evolved IGH clones analysis in acute B lymphoblastic leukemia using IGH deep sequencing. Front Immunol. 2016;7:403.

Zeijlemaker W, Kelder A, Oussoren-Brockhoff YJ, et al. A simple one-tube assay for immunophenotypical quantification of leukemic stem cells in acute myeloid leukemia. Leukemia. 2016;30:439–46.

58 Prevention and Treatment of Relapse by Drugs

Nicolaus Kröger

58.1 Introduction

Relapse has become the most frequent cause of treatment failure after HSCT (Horowitz et al. 2018). Because outcome after relapse remains poor, major effect is focused on prevention of relapse. Beside adoptive cell-based options, such as DLI, the availability of novel effective pharmacological compounds has opened new avenues in clinical research to use those drugs early after HSCT in order to prevent relapse (Kroger et al. 2014). The optimal pharmacological compound should have a safe toxicity profile, an antitumor effect to the underlying disease, and an immune profile which can be used to booster the graft-versus-leukemia (GVL) effect and to reduce the risk of GVHD.

58.2 Tyrosine Kinase Inhibitors (TKI) Targeting BCR/ABL

Beside a direct antitumor effect, TKIs are considered to induce also immunomodulating effects by inducing effect on T-cell cytolytic function, reducing T-cell PD-1 expression, and reducing myeloid-derived suppressor cells. TKIs targeting BCR/ABL such as *imatinib* induce more than 60% molecular remission in CML patients who relapsed after allograft. Smaller studies have investigated second-generation TKI successful as maintenance therapy after allo-HSCT for CML (Olavarria et al. 2007).

TKIs as maintenance therapy for Ph + ALL led to nonconclusive results. The CIBMTR did not find a difference in Ph + ALL patients who received post transplant TKIs regarding relapse at 3 years, while in an EBMT study, Ph + ALL patients who received TKIs post transplant had lower relapse incidence and an improved LFS. In a small randomized study comparing TKI prophylactically or preemptive in Ph + ALL, no difference in survival was observed (Pfeifer et al. 2013). In a position statement, EBMT recommended in MRD-negative patients after allo-HSCT either prophylactic or preemptive treatment (Giebel et al. 2016).

58.3 TKI Targeting FLT3-ITD

TKIs in the setting of FLT3-ITD-positive AML are of clinical relevance because a higher risk of relapse has been described for FLT3-ITD-positive patients who received allo-HSCT CR1 (30% vs. 16%). Animal experiences had shown that *sorafenib* stimulated immunogenicity by induction of IL-15 which enhanced T-cell activation and GVL effect (Mathew et al. 2018).

Midostaurin which is approved in the treatment of FLT3-positive AML has been tested in

N. Kröger (✉)
Department of Stem Cell Transplantation, University Medical Center Hamburg-Eppendorf, Hamburg, Germany
e-mail: nkroeger@uke.de

E. Carreras et al. (eds.), *The EBMT Handbook*, https://doi.org/10.1007/978-3-030-02278-5_58

a phase II study as maintenance therapy in FLT-3-ITD-positive patients with a low relapse rate at 12 months of only 9.2%. A retrospective study which compared sorafenib with a historical control showed improved outcome if TKI was used prophylactically (Brunner et al. 2016). Currently under investigation are randomized trials with *quizartinib*, *gliteritinib*, and *crenolanib*.

For relapsed FLT3-ITD-positive patients, sorafenib can induce long-lasting CR, and retrospective data show better outcome of sorafenib plus DLI in comparison to DLI alone (Mathew et al. 2018; Metzelder et al. 2012).

58.4 Checkpoint Inhibitors

Checkpoint inhibitors blocking CTLA-4 and PD-1 are now widely used in solid tumors and also in hematological malignancies such as Hodgkin's disease (Ansell et al. 2015). Because of reversal of T-cell exhaustion by checkpoint inhibitors which may enhance a graft-versus-malignancy effect, this compound has also raised interest to be investigated after HSCT. After auto-HSCT PD-1 antibody *pidilizumab* as maintenance therapy in DLBCL was well tolerated in a phase II study and *nivolumab* has shown high response rate in patients with HL who relapsed after auto-HSCT (Younes et al. 2016).

There is concern about a higher risk of GVHD after checkpoint inhibition post-allograft, but *ipilimumab* did not induce high incidence of GVHD in phase I and phase II trials although the efficacy was limited with an overall response rate of less than 30% (Davids et al. 2016). PD-1 blockade investigated in a European trial was reported for 20 patients with HL who relapsed after allograft. The remission rate was high with 95% and 30% developed GVHD which was fatal in one patient. In a similar trial including 31 lymphoma patients who relapsed after allograft, the response rate was 77%, but 54% developed acute GVHD and eight patients died from GVHD-related complications (Haverkos et al. 2017).

58.5 Hypomethylating Agents

Methylation has a crucial role in epigenetic regulation of gene expression and malignant cells using hypermethylation to switch off a variety of genes which are responsible for growth inhibition and apoptosis. DNA methyltransferase inhibitors such as *azacytidine* or *decitabine* are active in MDS and AML, and according to their toxicity profile, they can be used after allo-HSCT. Beside their effect on gene modification for differentiation and cell growth, hypomethylating agents (HMA) lead also to an upregulation of HLA and tumor-associated antigen which may be targeted by donor T cells (Hambach et al. 2009; Goodyear et al. 2010). Furthermore, CD4 and CD8 T cells were strongly suppressed by HMA while an increase of regulatory T cells has been described.

Azacytidine and decitabine either as single agent or in combination with DLI have been reported and up to 28% CR could be achieved including long-lasting remission (Schroeder et al. 2013). In a large EBMT study, an ORR of 25% with 15% CR and a 2-year OS of 12% has been reported for azacytidine in after allo-HSCT-relapsed AML/MDS patients. Overall the incidence of acute GVHD was low and the addition of DLI did not improve response or OS. Smaller studies also reported efficiency of azacytidine to convert decreasing donor cell chimerism into full donor cell chimerism (Platzbecker et al. 2012).

Treating patients with HMA prophylactically to prevent relapse has been tested (de Lima et al. 2010) and is currently investigated in prospective randomized clinical trials.

58.6 Immunomodulating Drugs (IMiDs)

After auto-HSCT *thalidomide* has been tested alone and with glucocorticoids as maintenance to prevent relapse/progression. Most of these phase III trials demonstrated an improved PFS or EFS with variable improvement in OS, but due to toxicity, the drug has not become a standard care of treatment (Barlogie et al. 2008; Spencer et al. 2009). *Lenalidomide* is approved as maintenance therapy since a significant improvement in PFS has been shown in two randomized trials and improved OS on one randomized trial (McCarthy et al. 2012; Attal et al. 2012). A meta-analysis with data from three large studies (CALGB 100104, IFM-05-02, and GIMEMA RV-MM-PI-209) demonstrated an OS and a PFS benefit for lenalidomide maintenance. However, an increased risk of secondary primary malignancies was observed after lenalidomide maintenance therapy.

After allo-HSCT a stimulation of T cells has been shown for thalidomide, but second-generation IMiDs such as lenalidomide and *pomalidomide* are even more potent stimulation of T-cell-mediated immunity. IMiDs also stimulate the innate immune system including γ/δ-T cells and NK T cells. While after thalidomide even if combined with DLI, no increased GVHD risk was observed (Kroger et al. 2004). Because of the stronger T-cell stimulation, lenalidomide given early post-allo-HSCT can cause severe GVHD (Sockel et al. 2012), but starting with a low dose of only 5 mg and given the drug after discontinuation of IS reduces the risk of GVHD markedly (Wolschke et al. 2013).

Overall, IMiDs are potent agents for preventing relapse after auto-HSCT, but their use post-allo-HSCT remains to be defined primarily due to the increased risk of GvHD.

58.7 Proteasome Inhibitors

Proteasome inhibitors are mainly used as induction therapy prior auto-HSCT. Some studies investigated proteasome inhibitors as maintenance therapy after auto-HSCT to reduce the risk of relapse. In a prospective study, *bortezomib* as maintenance therapy was superior to thalidomide particularly in patients with renal insufficiency and high-risk cytogenetics t(4;14) or del(17q) (Goldschmidt et al. 2018).

Bortezomib after allo-HSCT was tested so far only in smaller studies with acceptable rates of GVHD (Caballero-Velazquez et al. 2013), and novel proteasome inhibitors such as *ixazomib* are currently tested as maintenance therapy after allografting in MM.

58.8 Monoclonal Antibodies

Most studies of maintenance therapy with MoAb have been conducted after auto-HSCT. While maintenance therapy after autograft with anti-CD20 antibody *rituximab* failed to demonstrate an advantage for DLBCL with respect to RFS and OS (Gisselbrecht et al. 2012) for follicular lymphoma, an improved PFS but not an improvement in OS has been reported in a randomized study (Pettengell et al. 2013). An improved PFS and OS with rituximab as maintenance therapy has recently been shown for mantle cell lymphoma after auto-HSCT (Le Gouill et al. 2017).

After allo-HSCT for DLCBL, rituximab maintenance therapy did not improve overall survival (Glass et al. 2014). Anti-CD30 antibody drugs conjugate *brentuximab vedotin* as maintenance therapy after auto-HSCT for HL did improve PFS but not OS (Moskowitz et al. 2015).

Anti-CD22-conjugated antibody *inotuzumab ozogamicin* has been approved for relapsed ALL and has shown also activity in patients with ALL who relapsed after HSCT (Kantarjian et al. 2016), but the risk of SOS/VOD is about 11% and up to 22% for those who underwent allo-HSCT after inotuzumab ozogamicin.

Bispecific antibodies such as CD19-directed CD3 T-cell-engaged *blinatumomab* are active in relapsed and refractory ALL and also in MRD positive ALL and has been investigated successfully in combination with DLI after relapse post-allo-HSCT (Ueda et al. 2016).

58.9 Histone Deacetylase Inhibition (HDACI)

Histone deacetylation is a crucial mechanism of epigenetic modulation and HDACI promotes gene expression by unwinding of histone-bound DNA. Since HDACI reduces inflammatory cytokines and increases T-regulatory cells, the drug was also used for GVHD prevention in a phase I/II study (Choi et al. 2014). *Panobinostat* was tested in two trials as maintenance therapy after allo-HSCT in AML/MDS with or without (Bug et al. 2017) DLI resulting in an encouraging

1-year RFS of 66% in combination with DLI and 2-year RFS of 74% if used as single agent. This agent will now be tested as maintenance therapy in a prospective randomized phase III trial.

Incorporating novel agents into a transplant concept is an exciting new field of investigation, because in many cases, auto-HSCT alone does not lead to cure. To reduce the risk of relapse, well-designed clinical trial with novel agents is necessary.

Key Points

- Outcome after relapse to allogeneic stem cells remains poor and major efforts should focus on prevention of relapse.
- Beside adoptive cell-based options such as DLI, the availability of novel effective pharmacological compounds has opened new avenues in clinical research, mainly:
  - Tyrosine kinase inhibitors (TKI) targeting BCR/ABL.
  - TKI targeting FLT3-ITD (sorafenib, midostaurin, quizartinib, gliteritinib, crenolanib).
  - Checkpoint inhibitors (pidilizumab, nivolumab, ipilimumab).
  - Hypomethylating agents (azacytidine, decitabine).
  - Immunomodulating drugs (thalidomide, lenalidomide, pomalidomide).
  - Proteasome inhibitors (bortezomib, ixazomib).
  - Antibodies (rituximab, brentuximab vedotin, inotuzumab ozogamicin, blinatumomab).
  - Histone deacetylase inhibition (panobinostat).
- The optimal pharmacological compound should have a safe toxicity profile, an antitumor effect to the underlying disease, and an immune profile which can be used to booster the GVL effect and to reduce the risk of GVHD.

References

Ansell SM, Lesokhin AM, Borrello I, et al. PD-1 blockade with nivolumab in relapsed or refractory Hodgkin's lymphoma. N Engl J Med. 2015;372:311–9.

Attal M, Lauwers-Cances V, Marit G, et al. Lenalidomide maintenance after stem-cell transplantation for multiple myeloma. N Engl J Med. 2012;366:1782–91.

Barlogie B, Pineda-Roman M, van Rhee F, et al. Thalidomide arm of Total therapy 2 improves complete remission duration and survival in myeloma patients with metaphase cytogenetic abnormalities. Blood. 2008;112:3115–21.

Brunner AM, Li SL, Fathi AT, et al. Haematopoietic cell transplantation with and without sorafenib maintenance for patients with FLT3-ITD acute myeloid leukaemia in first complete remission. Br J Haematol. 2016;175:496–504.

Bug G, Burchert A, Wagner EM, et al. Phase I/II study of the deacetylase inhibitor panobinostat after allogeneic stem cell transplantation in patients with high-risk MDS or AML (PANOBEST trial). Leukemia. 2017;31:2523–5.

Caballero-Velazquez T, Lopez-Corral L, Encinas C, et al. Phase II clinical trial for the evaluation of bortezomib within the reduced intensity conditioning regimen (RIC) and post-allogeneic transplantation for high-risk myeloma patients. Br J Haematol. 2013;162:474–82.

Choi SW, Braun T, Chang L, et al. Vorinostat plus tacrolimus and mycophenolate to prevent graft-versus-host disease after related-donor reduced-intensity conditioning allogeneic haemopoietic stem-cell transplantation: a phase 1/2 trial. Lancet Oncol. 2014;15:87–95.

Davids MS, Kim HT, Bachireddy P, et al. Ipilimumab for patients with relapse after allogeneic transplantation. N Engl J Med. 2016;375:143–53.

de Lima M, Giralt S, Thall PF, et al. Maintenance therapy with low-dose azacitidine after allogeneic hematopoietic stem cell transplantation for recurrent acute myelogenous leukemia or myelodysplastic syndrome: a dose and schedule finding study. Cancer. 2010;116:5420–31.

Giebel S, Czyz A, Ottmann O, et al. Use of tyrosine kinase inhibitors to prevent relapse after allogeneic hematopoietic stem cell transplantation for patients with Philadelphia chromosome-positive acute lymphoblastic leukemia: a position statement of the Acute Leukemia Working Party of the European Society for Blood and Marrow Transplantation. Cancer. 2016;122:2941–51.

Gisselbrecht C, Schmitz N, Mounier N, et al. Rituximab maintenance therapy after autologous stem-cell transplantation in patients with relapsed CD20(+) diffuse large B-cell lymphoma: final analysis of the collaborative trial in relapsed aggressive lymphoma. J Clin Oncol. 2012;30:4462–9.

Glass B, Hasenkamp J, Wulf G, et al. Rituximab after lymphoma-directed conditioning and allogeneic stem-cell transplantation for relapsed and refractory aggressive non-Hodgkin lymphoma (DSHNHL R3): an open-label, randomised, phase 2 trial. Lancet Oncol. 2014;15:757–66.

Goldschmidt H, Lokhorst HM, Mai EK, et al. Bortezomib before and after high-dose therapy in myeloma: long-term results from the phase III HOVON-65/GMMG-HD4 trial. Leukemia. 2018;32:383–90.

Goodyear O, Agathanggelou A, Novitzky-Basso I, et al. Induction of a CD8+ T-cell response to the MAGE cancer testis antigen by combined treatment with azacitidine and sodium valproate in patients with acute myeloid leukemia and myelodysplasia. Blood. 2010;116:1908–18.

Hambach L, Ling KW, Pool J, et al. Hypomethylating drugs convert HA-1-negative solid tumors into targets for stem cell-based immunotherapy. Blood. 2009;113:2715–22.

Haverkos BM, Abbott D, Hamadani M, et al. PD-1 blockade for relapsed lymphoma post-allogeneic hematopoietic cell transplant: high response rate but frequent GVHD. Blood. 2017;130:221–8.

Horowitz M, Schreiber H, Elder A, et al. Epidemiology and biology of relapse after stem cell transplantation. Bone Marrow Transplant. 2018. https://doi.org/10.1038/s41409-018-0171-z.

Kantarjian HM, DeAngelo DJ, Stelljes M, et al. Inotuzumab ozogamicin versus standard therapy for acute lymphoblastic leukemia. N Engl J Med. 2016;375:740–53.

Kroger N, Shimoni A, Zagrivnaja M, et al. Low-dose thalidomide and donor lymphocyte infusion as adoptive immunotherapy after allogeneic stem cell transplantation in patients with multiple myeloma. Blood. 2004;104:3361–3.

Kroger N, Stubig T, Atanackovic D. Immune-modulating drugs and hypomethylating agents to prevent or treat relapse after allogeneic stem cell transplantation. Biol Blood Marrow Transplant. 2014;20:168–72.

Le Gouill S, Thieblemont C, Oberic L, et al. Rituximab after autologous stem-cell transplantation in mantle-cell lymphoma. N Engl J Med. 2017;377:1250–60.

Mathew NR, Baumgartner F, Braun L, et al. Sorafenib promotes graft-versus-leukemia activity in mice and humans through IL-15 production in FLT3-ITD-mutant leukemia cells. Nat Med. 2018;24:282–91.

McCarthy PL, Owzar K, Hofmeister CC, et al. Lenalidomide after stem-cell transplantation for multiple myeloma. N Engl J Med. 2012;366:1770–81.

Metzelder SK, Schroeder T, Finck A, et al. High activity of sorafenib in FLT3-ITD-positive acute myeloid leukemia synergizes with allo-immune effects to induce sustained responses. Leukemia. 2012;26:2353–9.

Moskowitz CH, Nademanee A, Masszi T, et al. Brentuximab vedotin as consolidation therapy after autologous stem-cell transplantation in patients with Hodgkin's lymphoma at risk of relapse or progression (AETHERA): a randomised, double-blind, placebo-controlled, phase 3 trial. Lancet. 2015;385:1853–62.

Olavarria E, Siddique S, Griffiths MJ, et al. Post transplantation imatinib as a strategy to postpone the requirement for immunotherapy in patients undergoing reduced-intensity allografts for chronic myeloid leukemia. Blood. 2007;110:4614–7.

Pettengell R, Schmitz N, Gisselbrecht C, et al. Rituximab purging and/or maintenance in patients undergoing autologous transplantation for relapsed follicular lymphoma: a prospective randomized trial from the lymphoma working party of the European Group for Blood and Marrow Transplantation. J Clin Oncol. 2013;31:1624–30.

Pfeifer H, Wassmann B, Bethge W, et al. Randomized comparison of prophylactic and minimal residual disease-triggered imatinib after allogeneic stem cell transplantation for BCR-ABL1-positive acute lymphoblastic leukemia. Leukemia. 2013;27:1254–62.

Platzbecker U, Wermke M, Radke J, et al. Azacitidine for treatment of imminent relapse in MDS or AML patients after allogeneic HSCT: results of the RELAZA trial. Leukemia. 2012;26:381–9.

Schroeder T, Frobel J, Cadeddu RP, et al. Salvage therapy with azacitidine increases regulatory T cells in peripheral blood of patients with AML or MDS and early relapse after allogeneic blood stem cell transplantation. Leukemia. 2013;27:1910–3.

Sockel K, Bornhaeuser M, Mischak-Weissinger E, et al. Lenalidomide maintenance after allogeneic HSCT seems to trigger acute graft-versus-host disease in patients with high-risk myelodysplastic syndromes or acute myeloid leukemia and del(5q): results of the LENAMAINT trial. Haematologica. 2012;97:e34–5.

Spencer A, Prince HM, Roberts AW, et al. Consolidation therapy with low-dose thalidomide and prednisolone prolongs the survival of multiple myeloma patients undergoing a single autologous stem-cell transplantation procedure. J Clin Oncol. 2009;27:1788–93.

Ueda M, de Lima M, Caimi P, et al. Concurrent blinatumomab and donor lymphocyte infusions for treatment of relapsed pre-B-cell ALL after allogeneic hematopoietic cell transplant. Bone Marrow Transplant. 2016;51:1253–5.

Wolschke C, Stubig T, Hegenbart U, et al. Postallograft lenalidomide induces strong NK cell-mediated antimyeloma activity and risk for T cell-mediated GvHD: results from a phase I/II dose-finding study. Exp Hematol. 2013;41:134–42.e3.

Younes A, Santoro A, Shipp M, et al. Nivolumab for classical Hodgkin's lymphoma after failure of both autologous stem-cell transplantation and brentuximab vedotin: a multicentre, multicohort, single-arm phase 2 trial. Lancet Oncol. 2016;17:1283–94.

59 Delayed Transfer of Immune Cells or the Art of Donor Lymphocyte Infusion

J. H. Frederik Falkenburg, Christoph Schmid, Hans Joachim Kolb, Franco Locatelli, and Jürgen Kuball

59.1 Biology of Donor Lymphocyte Infusion (DLI)

59.1.1 Diversity of Lymphocyte Subsets Used for DLI

In the context of an allogeneic HSCT, the interplay between host and donor immune cells is considered to be the primary mechanism responsible for graft-versus-leukemia (GVL) reactivity and also able to mediate GVHD (Kolb et al. 2004). The tissue specificity of the immune response determines the balance between GVL and GVHD, as well as tropism of GVHD. The main population for success and failure of HSCT and DLIs originates from αβT cells. However, other subsets are also key modulators of efficacy, e.g., NK cells most likely provide acute control of leukemia and of infections like CMV. However, NK cells become rapidly educated over time (Orr and Lanier 2010) and lose their antileukemia activity. Other subsets, like γδT cells, appear to have a more prolonged antileukemia effect (Handgretinger and Schilbach 2018) and are also helpful in controlling CMV reactivation (Scheper et al. 2013; de Witte et al. 2018). NKT cells, like regulatory T cells, have been mainly reported to influence GVHD effects. While an increase in NKT cells in the graft associates with a reduced GVHD incidence (Malard et al. 2016), depletion of T regulatory T cells in DLI improves GVL effects, although it augments the risk of GVHD (Maury et al. 2010). Thus, lymphocyte infusions as part of the graft at the time of transplantation, or delayed as DLI, have multiple effector cells that need to be considered in terms of different alloreactive effects.

J. H. Frederik Falkenburg
Department of Hematology, Leiden University Medical Center, Leiden, The Netherlands

C. Schmid
Klinikum Augsburg, University of Munich, Munich, Germany

H. J. Kolb
Department of Hematology-Oncology Immunology Infectious Diseases, Klinikum München-Schwabing, Munich, Germany

F. Locatelli
Department of Pediatric Hematology and Oncology, IRCCS Bambino Gesù Children's Hospital, Rome, Italy

Department of Pediatric Science, University of Pavia, Pavia, Italy

J. Kuball (✉)
Department of Hematology, UMC, Utrecht, The Netherlands

Laboratory of Translational Immunology, UMC, Utrecht, The Netherlands
e-mail: J.H.E.Kuball@umcutrecht.nl

E. Carreras et al. (eds.), *The EBMT Handbook*, https://doi.org/10.1007/978-3-030-02278-5_59

59.1.2 Naïve αβT Cell: Host Dendritic Cell (DC) Interaction as a Key Driver of Immune Response

Since in the context of HLA-matched transplantation, most alloreactive αβT cells are present within the naïve repertoire of the donor, recipient-derived dendritic cells (DC) play an essential role in provoking the αβT cell immune response (Stenger et al. 2012). DC are key players in provoking appropriate T cell activation, and because DC are derived from the hematopoietic system, an immune response of donor origin targeting DC from the recipient will likely result in an immune response against recipient hematopoietic cells, including the malignant population, and therefore give rise to GVL. The level of cross-reactivity against antigens broadly expressed on non-hematopoietic cells will determine the likelihood and severity of GVHD. DCs are present in the lympho-hematopoietic system but also with relatively high frequencies in the target tissues of GVHD. At the time of transplant, all DCs are of recipient origin. When activated by danger signals provoked by tissue damage and pathogens, DCs will present endogenous antigens, as well as cross-present antigens derived from the non-hematopoietic tissues and pathogens. Therefore, in T-cell-replete HSCT, it is difficult to dissect the GVL and GVHD effects (Boelens et al. 2018; Admiraal et al. 2017).

Consequently, many current transplantation techniques deplete immune cells from the graft and administer DLIs at later time points as standard part of the transplantation regimen. Both a complete immune depletion by selection of CD34-positive stem cells (Pasquini et al. 2012) and partial depletion of alloreactive T-cells through PT-CY (Mielcarek et al. 2016) are used. This upfront T-cell depletion associates with a lower risk of GVHD and allows very early DLIs for the majority of patients (e.g., 100 days after HSCT) and an improved segregation of GVL and GVHD effects. More recent transplantation strategies better consider the sophisticated variety of immune cells. These novel strategies utilize either a selective depletion of αβT cell (Locatelli et al. 2017) or naïve subsets (Bleakley et al. 2015) to abrogate GVHD, while maintaining early immune surveillance directed against infections as well as leukemia.

59.1.3 Diversity of Immune Repertoires and Potential Impact on Interventions

After HSCT, the αβ and γδTCR repertoire is reconstituted out of the graft of the donor, which contains in T-cell-replete transplantations between 5×10^7 and 1×10^9 T cells/kg (Czerw et al. 2016). Of the T cells, the γδT cells are the first to reach normal numbers, followed by the CD8+ αβT cells and finally the CD4+ αβT cells which do not reach normal levels within the first year after HSCT (Kanakry et al. 2016). It is important to note that numerical reconstitution of the T cells does not mean that the diversity of the repertoire is already normalized, reflected by the clinical observations that patients are highly vulnerable to many infections for years after HSCT. (van Heijst et al. 2013; Ravens et al. 2018).

Factors that influence the T-cell repertoire reconstitution after HSCT include the source of the graft and occurrence of infectious challenges such as CMV and EBV, GVHD, and cellular interventions such as DLI. The repertoire of αβT cells after HSCT has been studied extensively in different HSCT settings. Six months after HSCT, the αβTCR repertoire is still very restricted when compared to that of healthy individuals. A cord blood graft leads to a greater diversity of the αβTCR repertoire at 6 and 12 months, compared to other graft sources (van Heijst et al. 2013). Even 2–5 years after HSCT, the repertoire is still not as diverse as in healthy individuals (Kanakry et al. 2016; van Heijst et al. 2013). CMV reactivation shapes the repertoire in such a way that a marked contraction of the diversity is observed (Kanakry et al. 2016; van Heijst et al. 2013; Suessmuth et al. 2015). GVHD has been associated with both an increased (van Heijst et al. 2013) and a decreased diversity (Yew et al. 2015). We favor the hypothesis that selective GVL reactivity is associated with lower diversity, lower magnitude, and relatively tissue-specific recognition of hematopoiesis by alloreactive αβT cells (van Bergen et al. 2017). Less is known about the diversity of the γδTCR repertoire after HSCT. The repertoire of the γδT cells seems to be established quite early, at 30–60 days after HSCT. CMV reactivation promotes a massive expansion of a few γδT cell clonotypes (mainly belonging to the δ1 subset), which leads to a so-called repertoire focusing (Ravens et al. 2018). Within this context, it is reasonable to argue that the administration of a DLI might in the future depend not only on the type of the disease or timing but also on the size of the αβ and γδT cell repertoire observed at a given time point.

59.2 Guidelines for Prophylactic and Preemptive DLI as Well as DLI After Relapse

59.2.1 General Considerations

Currently, neither the diversity of the TCR repertoire nor the infusion of subsets of lymphocytes is used to guide or fine-tune the intervention DLI in daily practice. To prevent relapse of the underlying disease, timing and dosing of non-manipulated DLI after HSCT can be used to relatively skew the immune response toward GVL reactivity, as tissue damage after transplantation is gradually repaired and the donors' DCs steadily replace the recipients' DCs within the first 6 months after HSCT. Therefore, the magnitude and diversity of the interplay between host and donor immune subsets will progressively diminish. This is evidenced by the clinical observation that when the interval between HSCT and the infusion of DLI increases, the total number of αβT cells that can be administered without induction of severe GVHD will increase from less than 10^5/kg after 3 months, to more than 10^6/kg at 6 months (Table 59.1) (Yun and Waller 2013). Main prerequisite at the time of DLI is therefore also the absence of tissue damage and inflammatory circumstances, thus a lack of GVHD and uncontrolled infections.

59.2.2 Timing, Dosing, and Frequency of DLI

The following recommendations refer to the infusion of non-manipulated donor cells after no or in vivo T-cell-depleted transplantation from matched sibling or unrelated donors in patients with acute leukemia or MDS, which is the most frequently studied scenario. Further aspects, which may modify these recommendations, are discussed below. With respect to the indication of DLI for prevention of overt hematological relapse, two situations are distinguished. Furthermore, DLIs can be given within the context for overt relapses.

59.2.2.1 Prophylactic DLI

A prophylactic DLI *is* applied in patients with a high-risk of relapse, but at a stage when there is no evidence of the underlying disease. Usually, prophylactic DLIs are given starting from day +90 or +100 after HSCT, provided that the patient is off IS and free of GVHD for about 1 month. CD3+ doses used for the first infusion depend on donor type and timing and vary between 1×10^5/kg patient and 1×10^6/kg (Table 59.1). In the absence of GvHD, most groups have given prophylactic DLIs as single-shot intervention, but also repetitive DLIs are reported (Table 59.1; Tsirigotis et al. 2016; Jedlickova et al. 2016).

Table 59.1 Timing and dosing of prophylactic and preemptive DLI[a]

	Timing	Related	Unrelated	Haplo
Preemptive and prophylactic[b]	3 months	$1–5 \times 10^5$/kg	1×10^5/kg	
	6 months	1×10^6/kg	1×10^6/kg	1×10^4/kg
Relapse in combination with chemotherapy[c]	After chemotherapy	1×10^7/kg	1×10^7/kg	

Level C evidence

[a]A DLI can be repeated at 1-log higher 6–8 weeks after the first DLI, when, e.g., MRD is still present and no GVHD is observed. GVHD as endpoint of repetitive DLIs for preemptive DLIs is in the era of MRD monitoring no longer recommended

[b]Tsirigotis et al. (2016)

[c]Schmid et al. (2012)

59.2.2.2 Preemptive DLI

DLIs are administered preemptively, i.e., in case of persistent MRD or when the first signs of relapse are observed, like MRD positivity or a decreasing donor chimerism. For persisting MRD, either the same initial cell dosages as for prophylactic DLI are used, followed by repetitive DLIs in 4–12 weeks' intervals, using an escalated dose schedule and increasing the cell dosages by five to tenfold at each infusion. Alternatively, five to tenfold higher initial cell doses are used in the preemptive situation as compared to prophylaxis. A total of three to four DLIs may be administered, and subsequent infusions are mostly taken from the same apheresis as the first but are frozen in the previously planned dosages. Occurrence of GVHD after DLI will result in no further DLI administration. For reappearance of MRD or mixed chimerism, obviously timing of DLI depends on the occurrence of these circumstances.

59.2.2.3 Overt Relapses

For overt relapses a combination of DLI with chemotherapy is mandatory (Schmid et al. 2012), and cell doses used in that situation are usually one order of magnitude higher than in the prophylactic or preemptive situation (1×10^7/kg). In particular in acute leukemia, DLI alone may not be the preferred strategy for treatment of relapse. Repetitive DLIs can be considered after overt relapses based, e.g., on MRD positivity 6–8 weeks after DLI.

59.2.3 Factors that May Influence Timing, Dosing, and Frequency of DLI

59.2.3.1 MRD

Six weekly scheduled DLI with escalating doses until the first signs of GVHD as described above might no longer be necessary in the era of molecular disease monitoring. A MRD-driven strategy with more time between DLIs (8–12 weeks) might still allow for control of the hematological malignancy while avoiding long-term side effects like chronic GVHD. An alternative is the infusion of donor αβT cells engineered with a suicide gene. The thymidine kinase (TK) suicide gene has received conditional approval by EMA (Chabannon et al. 2018), and a novel safety switch (inducible caspase-9) characterized by lack of immunogenicity and rapid mechanism of action is under investigation (Zhou et al. 2014).

59.2.3.2 Impact of Underlying Disease

The different underlying diseases might require different doses, considering their sensitivity to a DLI-mediated GvL effect. The relapse workshop of the National Cancer Institute has proposed an estimate of the sensitivity of different diseases to DLI (Alyea et al. 2010). Accordingly, sensitivity is regarded as high for CML, myelofibrosis, and low-grade NHL; intermediate for AML, MDS, multiple myeloma, and Hodgkin's disease; and low for ALL and DLBCL.

59.2.3.3 Donor Origin

Dosage of DLI can under certain circumstances relate to the origin of the donor (Table 59.1). There is no consensus as to whether the dose between an unrelated and a related donor needs to differ. Similarly, cells doses in the haploidentical setting are unclear. More importantly and not well understood, but of greater impact, is most likely the processing of the DLI product with higher potency of freshly infused DLI when compared to frozen DLIs or DLIs used from the mobilized stem cell product due to different viabilities and compositions (Lemieux et al. 2016).

59.2.3.4 Combination with Other Drugs

DLIs are used in many diseases in combination with specific drugs targeting molecular aberrations of the underlying malignancy and/or acting via immune-modulating activities. However, the early administration of LENA after transplantation has been associated with a high incidence of GVHD (Kneppers et al. 2011), indicating that doses of DLI can also critically depend on the co-administration of drugs. Combinations with interferon-α and GM-CSF have also been reported as successful intervention to enhance the GVL effect (Dickinson et al. 2017). Other drugs currently explored are AZA, HDAC inhibitors (Bug et al. 2017), and Flt3-

inhibiting TKI (Mathew et al. 2018), and dosage and timing of combined DLIs might be guided by the experience from prophylactic and preemptive DLIs but need to be carefully monitored.

Key Points
- DLIs are used prophylactically or as preemptive treatment of a persistent MRD.
- DLIs in combination with chemotherapy can be used to treat overt relapse after HSCT.
- Despite the wide use of DLI, it is challenging to provide specific guidelines for dosing and timing of DLIs, and there is no consensus on how to precisely administer them.
- Strict institutional guidelines and rigorous reporting on details of DLI like processing, timing, dosing, intervals, and combination with immune-modulating drugs are therefore needed, and the new cellular therapy registry of EBMT is designed to allow for analysis of daily practice and its impact on clinical outcome in years to come.

References

Admiraal R, Nierkens S, de Witte MA, et al. Association between anti-thymocyte globulin exposure and survival outcomes in adult unrelated haemopoietic cell transplantation: a multicentre, retrospective, pharmacodynamic cohort analysis. Lancet Haematol. 2017;4:e183–e91.

Alyea EP, DeAngelo DJ, Moldrem J, et al. NCI First International Workshop on the Biology, Prevention and Treatment of Relapse after Allogeneic Hematopoietic Cell Transplantation: report from the committee on prevention of relapse following allogeneic cell transplantation for hematologic malignancies. Biol Blood Marrow Transplant. 2010;16:1037–69.

Bleakley M, Heimfeld S, Loeb KR, et al. Outcomes of acute leukemia patients transplanted with naive T cell-depleted stem cell grafts. J Clin Invest. 2015;125:2677–89.

Boelens JJ, Admiraal R, Kuball J, Nierkens S. Fine-tuning antithymocyte globulin dosing and harmonizing clinical trial design. J Clin Oncol. 2018;36:1175–6.

Bug G, Burchert A, Wagner EM, et al. Phase I/II study of the deacetylase inhibitor panobinostat after allogeneic stem cell transplantation in patients with high-risk MDS or AML (PANOBEST trial). Leukemia. 2017;31:2523–5.

Chabannon C, Kuball J, Bondanza A, et al. Hematopoietic stem cell transplantation in its 60s: a platform for cellular therapies. Sci Transl Med. 2018;10:eaap9630.

Czerw T, Labopin M, Schmid C, et al. High CD3+ and CD34+ peripheral blood stem cell grafts content is associated with increased risk of graft-versus-host disease without beneficial effect on disease control after reduced-intensity conditioning allogeneic transplantation from matched unrelated donors for acute myeloid leukemia: an analysis from the Acute Leukemia Working Party of the European Society for Blood and Marrow Transplantation. Oncotarget. 2016;7:27255–66.

de Witte MA, Sarhan D, Davis Z, et al. Early reconstitution of NK and gammadelta T cells and its implication for the Design of Post-Transplant Immunotherapy. Biol Blood Marrow Transplant. 2018;24:1152–62.

Dickinson AM, Norden J, Li S, et al. Graft-versus-leukemia effect following hematopoietic stem cell transplantation for leukemia. Front Immunol. 2017;8:496.

Handgretinger R, Schilbach K. The potential role of gammadelta T cells after allogeneic HCT for leukemia. Blood. 2018;131:1063–72.

Jedlickova Z, Schmid C, Koenecke C, et al. Long-term results of adjuvant donor lymphocyte transfusion in AML after allogeneic stem cell transplantation. Bone Marrow Transplant. 2016;51:663–7.

Kanakry CG, Coffey DG, Towlerton AM, et al. Origin and evolution of the T cell repertoire after posttransplantation cyclophosphamide. JCI Insight. 2016;1(5):e86252.

Kneppers E, van der Holt B, Kersten MJ, et al. Lenalidomide maintenance after nonmyeloablative allogeneic stem cell transplantation in multiple myeloma is not feasible: results of the HOVON 76 trial. Blood. 2011;118:2413–9.

Kolb HJ, Schmid C, Barrett AJ, Schendel DJ. Graft-versus-leukemia reactions in allogeneic chimeras. Blood. 2004;103:767–76.

Lemieux J, Jobin C, Simard C, Neron S. A global look into human T cell subsets before and after cryopreservation using multiparametric flow cytometry and two-dimensional visualization analysis. J Immunol Methods. 2016;434:73–82.

Locatelli F, Merli P, Pagliara D, et al. Outcome of children with acute leukemia given HLA-haploidentical HSCT after alphabeta T-cell and B-cell depletion. Blood. 2017;130:677–85.

Malard F, Labopin M, Chevallier P, et al. Larger number of invariant natural killer T cells in PBSC allografts correlates with improved GVHD-free and progression-free survival. Blood. 2016;127:1828–35.

Mathew NR, Baumgartner F, Braun L, et al. Sorafenib promotes graft-versus-leukemia activity in mice and humans through IL-15 production in FLT3-ITD-mutant leukemia cells. Nat Med. 2018;24: 282–91.

Maury S, Lemoine FM, Hicheri Y, et al. CD4+CD25+ regulatory T cell depletion improves the graft-versus-tumor effect of donor lymphocytes after allogeneic hematopoietic stem cell transplantation. Sci Transl Med. 2010;2:41ra52.

Mielcarek M, Furlong T, O'Donnell PV, et al. Posttransplantation cyclophosphamide for prevention of graft-versus-host disease after HLA-matched mobilized blood cell transplantation. Blood. 2016;127:1502–8.

Orr MT, Lanier LL. Natural killer cell education and tolerance. Cell. 2010;142:847–56.

Pasquini MC, Devine S, Mendizabal A, et al. Comparative outcomes of donor graft CD34+ selection and immune suppressive therapy as graft-versus-host disease prophylaxis for patients with acute myeloid leukemia in complete remission undergoing HLA-matched sibling allogeneic hematopoietic cell transplantation. J Clin Oncol. 2012;30:3194–201.

Ravens S, Schultze-Florey C, Raha S, et al. Human gammadelta T cells are quickly reconstituted after stem-cell transplantation and show adaptive clonal expansion in response to viral infection. Nat Immunol. 2017;18:393–401.

Scheper W, van Dorp S, Kersting S, et al. GammadeltaT cells elicited by CMV reactivation after allo-SCT cross-recognize CMV and leukemia. Leukemia. 2013;27:1328–38.

Schmid C, Labopin M, Nagler A, et al. Treatment, risk factors, and outcome of adults with relapsed AML after reduced intensity conditioning for allogeneic stem cell transplantation. Blood. 2012;119:1599–606.

Stenger EO, Turnquist HR, Mapara MY, Thomson AW. Dendritic cells and regulation of graft-versus-host disease and graft-versus-leukemia activity. Blood. 2012;119:5088–103.

Suessmuth Y, Mukherjee R, Watkins B, et al. CMV reactivation drives posttransplant T-cell reconstitution and results in defects in the underlying TCRbeta repertoire. Blood. 2015;125:3835–50.

Tsirigotis P, Byrne M, Schmid C, et al. Relapse of AML after hematopoietic stem cell transplantation: methods of monitoring and preventive strategies. A review from the ALWP of the EBMT. Bone Marrow Transplant. 2016;51:1431–8.

van Bergen CA, van Luxemburg-Heijs SA, de Wreede LC, et al. Selective graft-versus-leukemia depends on magnitude and diversity of the alloreactive T cell response. J Clin Invest. 2017;127:517–29.

van Heijst JW, Ceberio I, Lipuma LB, et al. Quantitative assessment of T cell repertoire recovery after hematopoietic stem cell transplantation. Nat Med. 2013;19:372–7.

Yew PY, Alachkar H, Yamaguchi R, et al. Quantitative characterization of T-cell repertoire in allogeneic hematopoietic stem cell transplant recipients. Bone Marrow Transplant. 2015;50:1227–34.

Yun HD, Waller EK. Finding the sweet spot for donor lymphocyte infusions. Biol Blood Marrow Transplant. 2013;19:507–8.

Zhou X, Di Stasi A, Tey SK, et al. Long-term outcome after haploidentical stem cell transplant and infusion of T cells expressing the inducible caspase 9 safety transgene. Blood. 2014;123:3895–905.

60 Cellular Therapy with Engineered T Cells, Efficacy and Side Effects

Attilio Bondanza, Chiara Bonini, Boris Fehse, and Michael Hudecek

60.1 Introduction

The cellular basis of cancer immune surveillance, already hypothesized in ancient times, was only demonstrated with the advent of HSCT. Indeed, the discovery of the nature of GVHD and its anti-leukemic effects (Weiden et al. 1979) were followed by the first successful attempts of adoptive immunotherapy using donor leukocytes (Kolb et al. 1990).

To address the significant GVHD risk associated with allogeneic T cells, several approaches of T-cell manipulation were developed and tested (Table 60.1). Some of these strategies rely on the genetic manipulation of T cells. First, suicide gene therapy approaches were established to promote GVL and immune reconstitution while controlling GVHD.

More recently, strategies based on the genetic transfer of tumor-specific T-cell receptors (TCRs) or chimeric antigen receptors (CARs) were developed to improve antitumor efficiency of T cells. This chapter provides an overview of this vastly evolving area.

60.2 Suicide Gene Therapy

The transfer of a suicide gene into donor lymphocytes was designed and tested at preclinical and clinical level in the 1990s, with the aim of transferring the entire donor T-cell repertoire, inclusive of cancer and infectious specificities, to transplanted patients, while enabling the selective elimination of the transferred lymphocytes in case of GVHD (Bonini et al. 1997). The first suicide gene, and to date the most extensively tested in clinical trials, is thymidine kinase of herpes simplex virus (HSV-TK). HSV-TK expression confers selective sensitivity to the antiviral drug ganciclovir. Upon gene transfer, HSV-TK is stably expressed by donor T lymphocytes not interfering with their functionality. However, when

A. Bondanza
Innovative Immunotherapies Unit, Division of Immunology, Transplantation and Infectious Diseases, University Vita-Salute San Raffaele and Ospedale San Raffaele Scientific Institute, Milan, Italy

C. Bonini (✉)
Experimental Hematology Unit, Division of Immunology, Transplantation and Infectious Diseases, University Vita-Salute San Raffaele and Ospedale San Raffaele Scientific Institute, Milan, Italy
e-mail: bonini.chiara@hsr.it

B. Fehse
Research Department Cell and Gene Therapy, Department of Stem Cell Transplantation, University Medical Centre Hamburg-Eppendorf, Hamburg, Germany

M. Hudecek
Medizinische Klinik und Poliklinik II, Universitätsklinikum Würzburg, Würzburg, Germany

E. Carreras et al. (eds.), *The EBMT Handbook*, https://doi.org/10.1007/978-3-030-02278-5_60

Table 60.1 T-cell-based cellular therapy approaches to increase GVL/GVI while taming GVHD

Strategy	Mechanism of action	References
Infusions of pathogen (i.e., CMV, EBV)-specific T cells	Isolation and infusion of T cells specific for opportunistic pathogens, to control post transplant infectious morbidity and mortality	Riddell et al. (1992), Rooney et al. (1995), Koehne et al. (2003)
Infusions of T cells depleted of alloreactive specificities	In vitro activation of host-reactive T cells followed by their depletion, infusion of remaining cells with the aim of promoting immune reconstitution with a reduced GVHD risk	André-Schmutz et al. (2002), Hartwig et al. (2008), Mielke et al. (2008)
Infusions of regulatory T cells	Isolation and/or expansion T-cell subsets with regulatory properties to promote immune reconstitution with a reduced GVHD risk	Groux et al. (1997), Chen et al. (2003), Trenado et al. (2004), Brunstein et al. (2011), Di Ianni et al. (2011), Bacchetta et al. (2014)
Infusion of T cells depleted of regulatory T cells	Infusion of T cells depleted of regulatory T cells to increase the antileukemic activity of DLI	Maury et al. (2010)
Infusions of leukemia-specific T cells	Isolation and infusion of T cells specific for leukemia-associated antigens to boost the GVL potency of DLI	Warren et al. (2010), Bornhauser et al. (2011), Chapuis et al. (2013), Comoli et al. (2017)
Infusion of alpha/beta depleted T cells	Infusion of a graft in vitro depleted of conventional alpha/beta T cells, thus enriched of gammadelta T cells, endowed with antitumor activity and a low GVHD potential	Lang et al. (2015), Airoldi et al (2015), Mashan et al. (2016)
Infusion naïve-depleted T cells	Infusion of donor T-cell subsets in vitro depleted of naïve cells, with the aim of promoting immune reconstitution with a reduced GVHD risk	Bleakley (2015)
Infusions of CIK	Infusions of in vitro activated donor CIK cells to promote GVL and reduce the risk of GVHD	Introna (2007), Introna (2010)
Suicide gene therapy	Donor lymphocytes are genetically engineered to express a suicide gene and then infused after HSCT to promote GVT and immune reconstitution while selectively controlling GVHD with the prodrug-mediated activation of the suicide gene	Bonini et al. (1997), Ciceri, Bonini et al (2009), Di Stasi et al. (2011), Zhan et al. (2013), Oliveira et al. (2015)
CAR/TCR T cells	Lymphocytes are genetically engineered to express a chimeric antigen receptor (CAR) or a T-cell receptor (TCR) that confers to T cells specificity for an antigen expressed by cancer cells	Kochenderfer et al. (2010), Porter et al. (2011), Brentjens et al. (2013), Morgan et al. (2006), Robbins et al. (2011)

CIK-cytokine-activated killer

exposed to ganciclovir, highly proliferating HSV-TK expressing T cells (TK-cells) will die in a dose-dependent manner. Thus, if ganciclovir is administered during GVHD to patients treated with TK-cells, activated, highly proliferating alloreactive TK-cells will be eliminated. The HSV-TK/ganciclovir suicide system proved highly effective in controlling GVHD in several transplant settings (Table 60.2), including haploidentical HSCT (haplo-HSCT). After TCD haplo-HSCT, the infusion of TK-cells promoted broad and rapid immune reconstitution that, being associated to GVHD control, has led to abrogation of late transplant-related mortality (Ciceri et al. 2009). Overall, clinical results obtained with TK-cells led to their conditional approval by EMA in 2016, thus representing the first genetically engineered medicinal product approved for

Table 60.2 Clinical trials of TK-suicide gene therapy in allogeneic HSCT

Clinical application (references)	Suicide gene/ marker gene	Disease indication	Patients treated	T cells infused/ kg	Clinical response (no. patients)	Incidence of aGvHD/ chronic no. pts (grade)	CR of aGvHD and cGVHD to GCV
To treat disease relapse occurring after HLA-identical allo-HSCT[a]	HSV-TK/ΔLNGFr HSV-TK/NeoR	AML, CML, CMML, MM, NHL (adults) AML, CML, NHL (adults)	28 34	10^6–10^8 10^6–10^8	15[b] 9[b]	6 (I–III) 2 (I)	5/5[c] 1/1
Day 0 in TCD allo-HSCT[d]	HSV-TK/NeoR	ALL, AML, CML, MDS, NHL, WD (adults)	15		5[b]	6 (II–III)	6/6
Day 60 in TCD allo-HSCT[e]	HSV-TK/ΔLNGFr	AML, ALL, MDS, CML (adults)	9		7[f]	3 (I–II)	1/1
Day 42 in TCD haplo-HSCT[g]	HSV-TK/ΔLNGFr	AML, MDS, NHL (adults)	40	10^6–10^7	29[h]	12 (I–IV)	11/11[i]
Day 1 in TCD haplo-HSCT[j]	HSV-TK-CD34 fusion gene	FA, ID, MDS (pediatrics)	3	10^4–10^5	3/3[h]	1	–
Day 30–90 in TCD haplo-HSCT[k]	iCasp9/ΔCD19[l]	MDS, AML, ALL (pediatrics)	10	10^6–10^7	10[h] [5[b]]	4 (I–II)	4/4
Day 13 after alpha/beta depleted haplo-HSCT[m]	iCasp9/ΔCD19	ALL (adult)	1		1	1(I)	0
Total			140		79 (56%)	35	28/28 (100%)

GCV ganciclovir, *Ne* not evaluable
[a]Bonini et al. (1997), Ciceri et al. (2007), Onodera et al. (2008), Champlin et al. (1999), Munshi et al. (1997)
[b]Clinical outcome is measured as clinical response of the malignant disease
[c]One patient with GVHD achieved CR after GCV administration and immunosuppressive drugs
[d]Tiberghien et al. (2001) and Fehse et al. (2004)
[e]Weissinger et al. (2011, 2014)
[f]One patient with GVHD achieved CR after administration of GCV and steroids
[g]Bonini et al. (2007), Ciceri, Bonini et al. (2009), and Lupo-Stanghellini (2017)
[h]Clinical outcome is measured in terms of T-cell immune reconstitution (evaluated as more than 100 circulating CD3+ T lymphocytes/μL) and pathogen-specific immunocompetence
[i]Four patients with GVHD achieved CR after administration of GCV and short-course low-dose steroids; two patients with GVHD achieved CR after GCV administration and IS
[j]Zhan et al. (2013)
[k]Di Stasi et al. (2011) and Zhou et al. (2014)
[l]T cells were genetically engineered and depleted of host-reactive specificities before infusion
[m]Elshoury et al. (2017)

cancer patients in Europe. Although when infused after haplo-HSCT TK-cells could be detected for more than 14 years (Oliveira et al. 2015), their persistence might be limited when cells are infused to immunocompetent patients, due to the viral origin of HSV-TK and to its subsequent immunogenicity in humans.

Alternative suicide genes were designed and tested in clinical trials (Table 60.2). iCasp9, in particular, is an innovative suicide gene based on human components and thus with a reduced risk of immunogenicity that was recently proposed and successfully tested in clinical trials (Table 60.2) (Di Stasi et al. 2011; Zhou et al. 2014). Overall, more than half of the patients who had received suicide gene-expressing donor T cells experienced a clinical benefit in terms of immune reconstitution and GVL (Table 60.2). Of notice, all cases of GVHD were completely controlled by the suicide gene/prodrug systems (Table 60.2).

60.3 CAR-T Cells

60.3.1 CAR-T Cells, Clinical Efficacy

CARs are designer molecules comprised of several components: an extracellular antigen-binding domain, usually the variable light and heavy chains of a MoAb (scFv); a spacer and transmembrane region that anchors the receptor on the T-cell surface and provides the reach and flexibility necessary to bind to the target epitope; and an intracellular signaling module, most commonly CD3 zeta and one or more costimulatory domains that mediate T-cell activation after antigen binding, resulting in selective tumor cell killing.

The most advanced clinical development is the use of CARs specific for the B-lineage marker CD19. Several groups have demonstrated that CD19 CAR-T cells are able to induce durable complete remissions in patients with chemotherapy- and radiotherapy-refractory B-cell ALL, NHL, and CLL (Maude et al. 2014; Park et al. 2018; Turtle et al. 2017).

With longer follow-up, resistance mechanisms to CD19 CAR-T-cell therapy have become apparent, including the development of leukemia cell variants that lost their CD19 antigen expression, particularly in ALL. Several mechanisms may contribute to the development of this phenotype including lymphoid-to-myeloid transdifferentiation, selection of pre-existing CD19-low/CD19-negative leukemia clones, and emergence of clones that lost the specific epitope targeted by the CD19-CAR due to alternative splicing (Gardner et al. 2016; Sotillo et al. 2015; Ruella and June 2016). In ALL, CD19-low/CD19-negative leukemia cells may still express CD20, CD22, and/or CD123 that are being pursued as rescue antigens. A recent study highlighted the potential to re-induce remissions in patients that had relapsed with CD19-low/CD19-negative leukemia and subsequently received CD22 CAR-T cells (Fry et al. 2018). Unfortunately, CD22 itself is prone to internalization and downregulation, and indeed a significant proportion of patients experienced successive CD22-low/CD22-negative leukemia relapse. At present, combinatorial targeting of CD19 with either CD20, CD22, or CD123 is being explored, either through bispecific CAR constructs with two scFvs *in cis* or through co-expression of two CAR constructs in the same T cells (Zah et al. 2016).

Clinical results obtained with CAR-T cells (Table 60.3) led to recent FDA approval of two CD19 CAR-T-cell products for the treatment of ALL and NHL. Both products are manufactured by viral gene transfer and made headlines due to their considerable market price and the complex logistics behind this treatment. This involves harvesting the patient's T cells at a leukapheresis center, shipping to a centralized manufacturing facility to perform CAR gene transfer and T-cell expansion and return shipment of the cryopreserved cell product. There is a recent increase in the use of exportable manufacturing devices that are anticipated to provide on-site, point-of-care CAR-T cell manufacture to reduce costs and wait-time.

Another clinical proof-of-concept for CAR-T-cell therapy has been obtained in MM. The lead antigen for CAR-T cells in multiple myeloma is B-cell maturation antigen (BCMA). A recent clinical trial with BCMA-specific CAR-T cells has highlighted their therapeutic potential with several PRs and CRs (Ali et al. 2016), and additional data from ongoing trials continue to emerge. Also, with BCMA, antigen downregulation and the emergence of myeloma cell variants with antigen loss were described, underscoring the need to explore additional target antigens, e.g., SLAMF7 (Gogishvili et al. 2017), CD44v6 (Casucci et al. 2013), and CD38 (Mihara et al. 2009).

60.3.2 Side Effects and Their Management

Results from pioneering clinical studies investigating CAR-T cells in patients with hematologi-

Table 60.3 Clinical trials with CAR-T cells

Clinical application (reference)	Antigen	No. of pat	Clinical response	Toxicity	No. of T cells (infused/kg BW)	CAR design	Gene transfer vector	Safety technology
ALL[a]	CD19	30	90% CR 79% MRD	B-cell aplasia CRS Neurotoxicity	0.76–20 x 10^6	FMC63 scFv CD8 alpha spacer 4-1BB costim	Lentivirus	None
ALL[b]	CD19	16	88% CR 75% MRD	B-cell aplasia CRS Neurotoxicity	3 x 10^6	SJ25C1 scFv CD28 ECD spacer CD28 costim	Retrovirus	None
ALL[c]	CD19	29	93% CR 86% MRD	B-cell aplasia CRS Neurotoxicity	2 x 10^5 to 2 x 10^7	FMC63 scFv IgG4 Hinge spacer 4-1BB costim	Lentivirus	EGFRt depletion marker
NHL/CLL[d]	CD19	15	53% CR 26% PR	B-cell aplasia CRS Neurotoxicity	1–5 x 10^6	FMC63 scFv CD28 ECD spacer CD28 costim	Retrovirus	None
NHL/CLL[e]	CD19	32	50% CR 72% ORR	B-cell aplasia CRS Neurotoxicity	2 x 10^5 to 2 x 10^7	FMC63 scFv IgG4 Hinge spacer 4-1BB costim	Lentivirus	EGFRt depletion marker
CLL[f]	CD19	20	21% CR 53% PR	B-cell aplasia CRS Neurotoxicity	2 x 10^5 to 2 x 10^7	FMC63 scFv IgG4 Hinge spacer 4-1BB costim	Lentivirus	EGFRt depletion marker
MM[g]	CD19	10	1CR 2PR	B-cell aplasia CRS (mild)	1–5 x 10^7 (total)	FMC63 scFv CD8 alpha spacer 4-1BB costim	Lentivirus	None
MM[h]	BCMA	12	1 CR 1 PR 2 VGPR	Hematologic (Cytopenia) CRS Neurotoxicity	0.3–3 x 10^6	C11D5.3 scFv CD28 ECD spacer CD28 costim	Retrovirus	None

ALL acute lymphoblastic leukemia, *NHL* non-Hodgkin lymphoma, *CLL* chronic lymphocytic leukemia, *MM* multiple myeloma, *BCMA* B-cell maturation antigen, *CR* complete remission, *MRD* minimal residual disease, *PR* partial remission, *VGPR* very good partial remission, *CRS* cytokine release syndrome, *kg* kilogram, *BW* body weight, *scFv* single-chain variable fragment, *costim* costimulatory domain, *IgG* immunoglobulin G, *ECD* extracellular domain, *EGFRt* epidermal growth factor receptor (Wang 2011)

[a]Maude et al. (2014)
[b]Davila et al. (2014)
[c]Turtle et al. (2016)
[d]Kochenderfer et al. (2015)
[e]Turtle et al. (2016)
[f]Turtle et al. (2017)
[g]Garfall et al. (2015)
[h]Ali et al. (2016)

cal cancers highlight the frequent occurrence of severe adverse reactions, which in some cases were fatal. The most obvious toxicity by CAR-T cells is the elimination of lineage cells expressing the target antigen of choice. For example, profound and, in some cases, long-lasting B-cell aplasia was observed after the infusion of CD19 CAR-T cells in patients with ALL, NHL, and CLL (Maude et al. 2014; Park et al. 2018; Turtle et al. 2017). By analogy, BCMA CAR-T cells are expected to induce plasma cell ablation in MM patients. The depletion of antibody-producing cells, or their precursors, in turn causes hypogammaglobulinemia, requiring constant supplementation with immunoglobulins.

Besides these expected on-target/off-tumor effects, a new class of on-target/on-tumor adverse reactions is represented by the cytokine release syndrome (CRS) and by neurotoxicity. CRS is initiated by CAR-T cell recognition of tumor cells, igniting the release of massive amounts of inflammatory cytokines, possibly by recruiting cells of the innate immunity. A master cytokine of the CRS is IL-6, as demonstrated by prompt and often complete response to the anti-IL-6 receptor monoclonal antibody tocilizumab. CRS symptoms range from high fever, headache, and myalgia to life-threatening cardiocirculatory and renal insufficiency. Clinical data reported so far utilize three slightly different systems for severity grading, which makes it difficult to draw meaningful comparisons in CRS liability between CAR-T-cell trials (Table 60.4). Nonetheless, there is generalized consensus on the fact that severe CRS is more frequent in ALL compared to NHL and that high tumor burden is an important risk factor.

Differently from CRS, the pathophysiology of neurotoxicity by CAR-T cells remains an uncharted territory and decisively worthy of further research, given its highly dismal prognosis, as demonstrated by several cases of lethal cerebral edema. Initially thought to be caused by tumor recognition by CAR-T cells within the brain, neurotoxicity is now recognized to be independent from leukemic localization to the CNS. Moreover, unresponsiveness to tocilizumab suggests that excessive IL-6 signaling may not be sufficient to explain neurotoxicity and that additional pharmacological measures should be investigated.

60.4 TCR Gene Transfer and Future Perspectives

In contrast to CARs that only bind surface molecules, TCRs recognize small pieces (peptides) derived from any cellular protein and presented by MHC molecules. Since the vast majority of tumor-specific/associated antigens are expressed intracellularly, they will only be addressable by TCRs, but not CARs. Moreover, therapeutically relevant cancer-driver mutations in most cases happen in intracellular proteins (e.g., signal transducers).

At the same time, the advantage of TCRs represents a major hurdle for broad clinical application: Any transgenic TCR only functions in the context of one specific HLA complex. Thus, in order to offer TCR-T-cell therapy to virtually all candidate patients, for each antigen a whole set of active TCRs will have to be established for different HLA molecules.

Table 60.4 CRS severity scoring systems

	Penn scale	CTCAE	Lee (2014)
Grade 1	Mild reaction treated with antipyretics and/or antiemetics	Mild reaction, no treatment needed	– Non-life-threatening reaction responsive to symptomatic treatment
Grade 2	Moderate reaction requiring hospitalization and IV therapy (no fluid resuscitation)	Moderate reaction responsive to symptomatic treatment within 24 h	– Moderate reaction requiring oxygen <40%, fluid resuscitation, or low-dose pressors – Any G2 organ toxicity
Grade 3	Severe reaction requiring high-flow oxygen or noninvasive lung ventilation, fluid resuscitation, or low-dose pressors	Prolonged reaction nonresponsive to symptomatic treatment	– Severe reaction requiring oxygen >40%, high-dose pressors – Any G3 organ toxicity
Grade 4	Life-threatening reaction requiring high-dose pressors and/or mechanical ventilation	Life-threatening reaction, pressor, or ventilator requirement	– Life-threatening reaction requiring mechanical ventilation – Any G4 organ toxicity

The first TCR gene therapies were applied to melanoma patients (MART-1 antigen), but meanwhile many cancers have been addressed. Based on their almost complete absence in adult tissues, cancer/testis antigens (MAGE, NY-ESO1) represent particularly promising targets. Many studies showed significant antitumor activity, but on-target as well as off-target activities were associated with severe side effects, including mortality (Morris and Stauss 2016).

Genome editing has been proposed to improve efficacy and decrease side effects of TCR gene therapy. Editing might be used to knock out the endogenous TCR to increasing expression of the transgenic one and decreasing the mispairing risk between endogenous and transgenic TCR chains (potentially leading to autoreactive T cells) (Provasi et al. 2012). Moreover, targeted integration in the TCR locus can improve long-term expression of transgenic TCRs (Eyquem et al. 2017).

In conclusion, T-cell therapies have become a promising novel anticancer weapon. Their broad application will require (1) identification of additional targets, (2) availability of TCRs against established targets for many HLA molecules, and (3) improved methods for large-scale GMP production. All these points will become particularly relevant in concepts addressing multiple tumor neoantigens to decrease the likelihood of escape (Tran et al. 2017).

Key Points

- The cellular basis of cancer immune surveillance was demonstrated with the discovery of the nature of GVHD and its antileukemic effects.
- This observation was followed by the first successful attempts of adoptive immunotherapy using DLI to promote GVL.
- Several approaches of T-cell manipulation have been developed and tested to reduce the GVHD risk associated with allogeneic T cells. These strategies rely on the genetic manipulation of T cells or the use of suicide gene therapy.
- More recently, strategies based on the genetic transfer of tumor-specific T-cell receptors (TCRs) or chimeric antigen receptors (CARs) were developed to improve antitumor efficiency of T cells.

References

Ali SA, Shi V, Maric I, et al. T cells expressing an anti-B-cell maturation antigen chimeric antigen receptor cause remissions of multiple myeloma. Blood. 2016;128:1688–700.

Bonini C, Ferrari G, Verzeletti S, et al. HSV-TK gene transfer into donor lymphocytes for control of allogeneic graft-versus-leukemia. Science. 1997;276:1719–24.

Casucci M, Nicolis di Robilant B, Falcone L, et al. CD44v6-targeted T cells mediate potent antitumor effects against acute myeloid leukemia and multiple myeloma. Blood. 2013;122:3461–72.

Ciceri F, Bonini C, Stanghellini MT, et al. Infusion of suicide-gene-engineered donor lymphocytes after family haploidentical haemopoietic stem-cell transplantation for leukaemia (the TK007 trial): a non-randomised phase I–II study. Lancet Oncol. 2009;10:489–500.

Di Stasi A, Tey SK, Dotti G, et al. Inducible apoptosis as a safety switch for adoptive cell therapy. N Engl J Med. 2011;365:1673–83.

Eyquem J, Mansilla-Soto J, Giavridis T, et al. Targeting a CAR to the TRAC locus with CRISPR/Cas9 enhances tumour rejection. Nature. 2017;543:113–7.

Fry TJ, Shah NN, Orentas RJ, et al. CD22-targeted CAR T cells induce remission in B-ALL that is naive or resistant to CD19-targeted CAR immunotherapy. Nat Med. 2018;24:20–8.

Gardner R, Wu D, Cherian S, et al. Acquisition of a CD19-negative myeloid phenotype allows immune escape of MLL-rearranged B-ALL from CD19 CAR-T-cell therapy. Blood. 2016;127:2406–10.

Gogishvili T, Danhof S, Prommersberger S, et al. SLAMF7-CAR T cells eliminate myeloma and confer selective fratricide of SLAMF7+normal lymphocytes. Blood. 2017;130:2838–47.

Kolb HJ, Mittermüller J, Clemm C, et al. Donor leukocyte transfusions for treatment of recurrent chronic myelogenous leukemia in marrow transplant patients. Blood. 1990;76:2462–5.

Maude SL, Frey N, Shaw PA, et al. Chimeric Antigen Receptor T Cells for Sustained Remissions in Leukemia. N Engl J Med. 2014;371:1507–17.

Mihara K, Yanagihara K, Takigahira M, et al. Activated T-cell-mediated immunotherapy with a chimeric receptor against CD38 in B-cell non-Hodgkin lymphoma. J Immunother. 2009;32:737–43.

Morris EC, Stauss HJ. Optimizing T-cell receptor gene therapy for hematologic malignancies. Blood. 2016;127:3305–11.

Oliveira G, Ruggiero E, Stanghellini MT, et al. Tracking genetically engineered lymphocytes long-term reveals the dynamics of T cell immunological memory. Sci Transl Med. 2015;7:317ra198.

Park JH, Rivière I, Gonen M, et al. Long-term follow-up of CD19 CAR therapy in acute lymphoblastic leukemia. N Engl J Med. 2018;378:449–59.

Provasi E, Genovese P, Lombardo A, et al. Editing T cell specificity towards leukemia by zinc finger nucleases and lentiviral gene transfer. Nat Med. 2012;18:807–15.

Ruella M, June CH. Chimeric antigen receptor T cells for B cell neoplasms: choose the right CAR for you. Curr Hematol Malig Rep. 2016;11:368–84.

Sotillo E, Barrett DM, Black KL, et al. Convergence of acquired mutations and alternative splicing of CD19 enables resistance to CART-19 immunotherapy. Cancer Discov. 2015;5:1282–95.

Tran E, Longo DL, Urba WJ. A milestone for CAR T cells. N Engl J Med. 2017;377:2593–6.

Turtle CJ, Hay KA, Hanafi LA, et al. Durable molecular remissions in chronic lymphocytic leukemia treated with CD19-specific chimeric antigen receptor-modified T cells after failure of ibrutinib. J Clin Oncol. 2017;35:3010–20.

Weiden PL, Flournoy N, Thomas ED, et al. Antileukemic effect of graft-versus-host disease in human recipients of allogeneic-marrow grafts. N Engl J Med. 1979;300:1068–73.

Zah E, Lin MY, Silva-Benedict A, et al. T cells expressing CD19/CD20 bispecific chimeric antigen receptors prevent antigen escape by malignant B cells. Cancer Immunol Res. 2016;4:498–508.

Zhou X, Di Stasi A, Tey SK, et al. Long-term outcome after haploidentical stem cell transplant and infusion of T cells expressing the inducible caspase 9 safety transgene. Blood. 2014;123:3895–905.

61 Mechanisms of Immune Resistance

Luca Vago and Francesco Dazzi

61.1 Introduction

It is widely accepted that the curative potential of allo-HSCT for malignant diseases relies on the transfer of healthy donor immune cells capable of recognizing transplantation antigens on residual tumor cells (graft versus leukemia, GvL) and eliminating them. However, as extensively documented in solid cancers, if tumor eradication is incomplete, the prolonged immune pressure selectively allows immune-resistant subclones to survive (Schreiber et al. 2011). There is growing evidence that such an "immunoediting" also accounts for relapse after HSCT. Malignant cells evade GvL either by reducing their immunogenicity and conveying inhibitory signals to the donor immune system (intrinsic evasion) or through the microenvironment (extrinsic evasion).

L. Vago
Unit of Immunogenetics, Leukemia Genomics and Immunobiology, Hematology and Bone Marrow Transplantation Unit, IRCCS San Raffaele Scientific Institute, Milano, Italy

F. Dazzi (✉)
School of Cancer and Pharmacological Sciences, King's College London, London, UK
e-mail: francesco.dazzi@kcl.ac.uk

61.2 Mechanisms of Immune Evasion

61.2.1 Mechanisms Intrinsic to the Malignant Clone

A remarkable example of tumor-intrinsic mechanism of immune evasion is the *genomic loss of the mismatched HLA haplotype* frequently documented in leukemia relapses after T-cell-replete HSCT from HLA haploidentical family donors (Vago et al. 2009). In this setting, donor T cells mount a vigorous alloreactive response against the incompatible HLA molecules, and this reaction is not only responsible for a significant risk of severe GvHD but also a major contributor to the GvL effect. Yet, this strong and selective immune pressure is easily overturned by tumor cells which, by losing the allogeneic HLA haplotype, find a means to avoid recognition and re-emerge. "HLA-loss" variants account for up to one third of relapses after HLA-haplo-HSCT (Crucitti et al. 2015) and have been described also in the setting of HSCT from partially HLA-incompatible URD, although their actual frequency in this setting is yet to be determined (Waterhouse et al. 2011). The documentation of HLA loss at relapse has an important clinical impact, because IS withdrawal or administration of DLI would be much less effective against these diseases variants (Tsirigotis et al. 2016).

Another evidence that supports "leukemia immunoediting" is the occurrence of *isolated*

E. Carreras et al. (eds.), *The EBMT Handbook*, https://doi.org/10.1007/978-3-030-02278-5_61

extramedullary relapses after allo-HSCT or even more frequently after DLI. These relapses may occur, but not necessarily, in immunological sanctuaries, including the CNS. Although to date the biological drivers of extramedullary relapses remain unknown, some studies have suggested a link with immune-related factors such as chronic GvHD (Solh et al. 2012; Harris et al. 2013).

A number of studies have highlighted a further strategy by which hematological cancers can evade immune control, whereby they express large numbers of *molecules capable of dampening immune responses* such as programmed death-ligand (PD-L)1. The expression of these inhibitory ligands significantly increases at relapses after allo-HSCT. This observation provides a rationale for the use of "checkpoint blockade" to restore immune control at relapse. Initial experience in patients with relapsed lymphoma or extramedullary leukemia with anti-PD1 and anti-cytotoxic T-lymphocyte-associated antigen (CTLA)-4 MOAb is very promising (Davids et al. 2016; Herbaux et al. 2017). However, the risks of triggering life-threatening GvHD remain to be quantified.

61.2.2 Mechanisms Extrinsic to the Leukemic Cells

The alternative, but not mutually exclusive, strategy by which malignant cells enact evasion from immune cell recognition relies on hijacking the stem cell niches in which normal HSC self-renew and differentiate. By doing this, malignant cells create a *tumor microenvironment* (TME) that has profound consequences on disease progression and relapse. The initial studies conducted on solid tumors have shown that the TME consists of two major cellular populations that alone or in combination drive resistance to conventional therapies and suppress antitumor immune responses. The first group comprises a diverse and heterogeneous group of myeloid-derived cells which, according to a yet unresolved debate on their nomenclature, can be generally classified as tumor-associated monocytes/macrophages (TAM) and myeloid-derived suppressor cells (MDSC) (Bronte et al. 2016). The IS activity of these cells is mediated by factors that include nitric oxide synthase-2 (NOS-2), arginase-1, heme oxygenase-1 (HO-1), interleukin (IL)-10, transforming growth factor (TGF)-β, and prostaglandin E2 (PGE2). All these molecules also favor the recruitment of regulatory T cell (Tregs) that eventually contribute to the inhibition of antitumor $CD8^+$ T-cell and natural killer cell effector function (Ostuni et al. 2015). Although most of these mechanisms have been initially demonstrated in solid tumors, there is consistent evidence that they are also involved in hematological malignancies. High-risk AML can actually behave as MDSC by upregulating NOS and suppressing T-cell responses (Mussai et al. 2013). The presence of MDSC in AML has later been confirmed and also identified in multiple myeloma whereby they protect malignant cells through MUC1 oncoprotein (Bar-Natan et al. 2017; Pyzer et al. 2017).

The second cellular group consists of an equally heterogeneous population of mesenchymal origin, variously referred to as *mesenchymal stromal cells* (MSC) or *cancer-associated fibroblasts* (CAF) (Raffaghello and Dazzi 2015). Regardless of their developmental heterogeneity, they all play a similar role by protecting the malignant cells from cytotoxic agents and immune responses. In the bone marrow, MSC protect CML and AML cells from imatinib and Ara-C via the CXCR4-CXCL12 axis (Vianello et al. 2010).

Much information has been provided about the *IS activity of MSC* that is exerted in a non-antigen-specific fashion (Jones et al. 2007). One of the primary direct mechanisms responsible for this involves the expression of indoleamine 2-3 dioxygenase-1 (IDO-1), which consumes the essential amino acid tryptophan. Additional IS mechanisms include the release of suppressive factors such as TGF-β1, hepatocyte growth factor, PGE2, soluble human leukocyte antigen G, and TNF-α stimulated gene 6 protein (TSG-6). However, more recent data have highlighted the important contribution of tissue-resident monocytes/macrophages in delivering a more sustainable IS effect (Cheung and Dazzi 2018).

Finally, the role of *Tregs* in generating immune resistance has been much discussed. While there is plenty of data indicating how these cells exert a very negative impact on the outcome of solid tumors, data in preclinical models of allogeneic HSCT have suggested that Tregs may selectively inhibit GvHD without compromising GvL (Edinger et al. 2003). In contrast, clinical data suggest to consider Treg levels post transplant with caution (Nadal et al. 2007).

Key Points

- Leukemia can counteract the beneficial graft-versus-leukemia effects post transplant.
- This is effected either by changes in the tumor cells which make them evade immune recognition or by instructing different components of the microenvironment to deliver in situ immunosuppression.

References

Bar-Natan M, Stroopinsky D, Luptakova K, et al. Bone marrow stroma protects myeloma cells from cytotoxic damage via induction of the oncoprotein MUC1. Br J Haematol. 2017;176:929–38.

Bronte V, Brandau S, Chen S-H, et al. Recommendations for myeloid-derived suppressor cell nomenclature and characterization standards. Nat Commun. 2016;7:12150.

Cheung TS, Dazzi F. Mesenchymal-myeloid interaction in the regulation of immunity. Semin Immunol. 2018;35:59–68.

Crucitti L, Crocchiolo R, Toffalori C, et al. Incidence, risk factors and clinical outcome of leukemia relapses with loss of the mismatched HLA after partially incompatible hematopoietic stem cell transplantation. Leukemia. 2015;29:1143–52.

Davids MS, Kim HT, Bachireddy P, et al. Ipilimumab for patients with relapse after allogeneic transplantation. N Engl J Med. 2016;375:143–53.

Edinger M, Hoffmann P, Ermann J, et al. CD4+CD25+ regulatory T cells preserve graft-versus-tumor activity while inhibiting graft-versus-host disease after bone marrow transplantation. Nat Med. 2003;9:1144–50.

Harris AC, Kitko CL, Couriel DR, et al. Extramedullary relapse of acute myeloid leukemia following allogeneic hematopoietic stem cell transplantation: incidence, risk factors and outcomes. Haematologica. 2013;98:179–84.

Herbaux C, Gauthier J, Brice P, et al. Efficacy and tolerability of nivolumab after allogeneic transplantation for relapsed Hodgkin lymphoma. Blood. 2017;129:2471–8.

Jones S, Horwood N, Cope A, Dazzi F. The antiproliferative effect of mesenchymal stem cells is a fundamental property shared by all stromal cells. J Immunol. 2007;179:2824–31.

Mussai F, De Santo C, Abu-Dayyeh I, et al. Acute myeloid leukemia creates an arginase-dependent immunosuppressive microenvironment. Blood. 2013;122:749–58.

Nadal E, Garin M, Kaeda J, et al. Increased frequencies of CD4(+) CD25(high) T(regs) correlate with disease relapse after allogeneic stem cell transplantation for chronic myeloid leukemia. Leukemia. 2007;21:472–9.

Ostuni R, Kratochvill F, Murray PJ, Natoli G. Macrophages and cancer: from mechanisms to therapeutic implications. Trends Immunol. 2015;36:229–39.

Pyzer AR, Stroopinsky D, Rajabi H, et al. MUC1-mediated induction of myeloid-derived suppressor cells in patients with acute myeloid leukemia. Blood. 2017;129:1791–801.

Raffaghello L, Dazzi F. Classification and biology of tumour associated stromal cells. Immunol Lett. 2015;168:175–82.

Schreiber RD, Old LJ, Smyth MJ. Cancer immunoediting: integrating immunity's roles in cancer suppression and promotion. Science. 2011;331:1565–70.

Solh M, DeFor TE, Weisdorf DJ, Kaufman DS. Extramedullary relapse of acute myelogenous leukemia after allogeneic hematopoietic stem cell transplantation: better prognosis than systemic relapse. Biol Blood Marrow Transplant. 2012;18:106–12.

Tsirigotis P, Byrne M, Schmid C, et al. Relapse of AML after hematopoietic stem cell transplantation: methods of monitoring and preventive strategies. A review from the ALWP of the EBMT. Bone Marrow Transplant. 2016;51:1431–8.

Vago L, Perna SK, Zanussi M, et al. Loss of mismatched HLA in leukemia after stem-cell transplantation. N Engl J Med. 2009;361:478–88.

Vianello F, Villanova F, Tisato V, et al. Bone marrow mesenchymal stromal cells non-selectively protect chronic myeloid leukemia cells from imatinib-induced apoptosis via the CXCR4/CXCL12 axis. Haematologica. 2010;95:1081–9.

Waterhouse M, Pfeifer D, Pantic M, et al. Genome-wide profiling in AML patients relapsing after allogeneic hematopoietic cell transplantation. Biol Blood Marrow Transplant. 2011;17:1450–9.

62 Regulatory Aspects of ATMP Versus Minimally Manipulated Immune Cells

Eoin McGrath and Christian Chabannon

Under current European regulations, hematopoietic cellular therapies fall under two categories: stem cell transplants and advanced therapy medicinal products (ATMPs). Routinely administered auto- and allo-HSCT—including subsequent peripheral blood allogeneic mononuclear cells (DLI)—undergo non-substantial manipulations following cell procurement and before being administered to the recipient.

Cell processing is performed in facilities termed tissue establishments (TEs) under the EU Tissues and Cells Directive (see https://ec.europa.eu/health/blood_tissues_organs/tissues_en. Accessed 20 Feb 2018), and these are authorized by national and/or regional competent authorities (CA). TEs usually operate on a relatively small scale, serving the clinical program(s) in their immediate vicinity although some national or regional services may support a more extensive network of clinical programs. The combination of a clinical department(s) with a collection and a processing facility represents the core structure for a transplant program that applies for the JACIE accreditation (see Chap. 5). Such an organization leaves room for significant procedural and organizational variations, many driven by local or national factors, despite all attempts from the various professional associations to harmonize practices through surveys, the publication of guidelines, and regularly revised standards for these therapies, e.g., FACT-JACIE International Standards for Hematopoietic Cellular Therapies (see www.jacie.org. Accessed 19 Feb 2018).

ATMPs represent a new category of medicinal products defined in EU Regulation 1394/2007 (see http://eur-lex.europa.eu/LexUriServ/LexUriServ.do?uri=OJ:L:2007:324:0121:0137:en:PDF. Accessed 20 Feb 2018). ATMPs—known in the USA as human cells, tissues, and cellular- and tissue-based products (HCT/Ps) regulated under Section 351 of the PHS Act and/or the FD&C Act (see https://www.fda.gov/biologicsbloodvaccines/tissuetissueproducts/regulationoftissues/ucm150485.htm. Accessed 21 Feb 2018)—are subdivided in four categories, of which two are relevant in the context of hematopoietic cellular therapies: somatic cell therapy medicinal products (SCTMP) and gene therapy medicinal products (GTMP). Examples of SCTMP include ex vivo expanded autologous or allogeneic stem cells (de Lima et al. 2012; Delaney et al. 2010), mesenchymal stem cells (Le Blanc et al. 2008), and allogeneic T lymphocytes depleted of alloreactive T cells (Andre-Schmutz et al. 2002). Examples of GTMP

E. McGrath
European Society for Blood and Marrow Transplantation (EBMT), Barcelona, Spain

C. Chabannon (✉)
Institut Paoli-Calmettes, Centre de Lutte Contre le Cancer, Marseille, France

Université d'Aix-Marseille, Marseille, France

Inserm BCT-1409, Centre d'Investigations Cliniques en Biothérapies, Marseille, France
e-mail: chabannonc@ipc.unicancer.fr

E. Carreras et al. (eds.), *The EBMT Handbook*, https://doi.org/10.1007/978-3-030-02278-5_62

include allogeneic T cells engineered to express a suicide gene (Ciceri et al. 2009), autologous or allogeneic CAR-T cells (Schuster et al. 2017; Neelapu et al. 2017), and autologous CD34+ cells genetically engineered to express a mini-globin gene and designed to treat inherited β-globin disorders (Cavazzana-Calvo et al. 2010; Ribeil et al. 2017).

The regulation was designed in part to foster the competitiveness of European pharmaceutical companies in this emerging field, but the number of ATMPs that have received a centralized marketing authorization remains relatively low and with poor overall commercial success so far. In the HSCT field, it was not until 2015 that an ATMP of interest reached the market with authorization given for Zalmoxis® (allogeneic T cells engineered to express a suicide gene). Production, distribution, and administration of ATMPs imply a totally different organization than that used for HSCT, with manufacturing at a central facility in compliance with good manufacturing practices (GMP) (Wang and Rivière 2016, 2017), a version of which was recently released by the European Medicines Agency (EMA) to specifically deal with manufacturing of ATMPs (see https://ec.europa.eu/health/sites/health/files/files/eudralex/vol-4/2017_11_22_guidelines_gmp_for_atmps.pdf. Accessed 19 Feb 2018). Since a majority of the ATMPs that progress to authorization or at least to clinical trials are manufactured from autologous mononuclear cells, starting material is currently procured by hospital- or blood bank-operated apheresis facilities creating a peculiar situation in which a product starts under one regulation—Tissues and Cells Directive—before passing to another, ATMP Regulation, and where a hospital acts as a service provider to industry, an interaction that requires further definition of the respective responsibilities and liabilities.

Publication of Regulation 1394/2007 created a situation in which some cell- or tissue-based therapeutic products that were previously prepared and delivered through an organization similar to that for cell transplants were classified as ATMPs. This had a limited impact in the field of hematopoietic cellular therapies, although some cell-based products such as allogeneic T cells with specific anti-CMV activity engineered through the gamma-catch technology (Feuchtinger et al. 2010) were affected. In recognizing that many potential ATMP were used for limited numbers of patients and with no commercial motivation, Regulation 1394/2007 created the so-called hospital exemption (HE) under Article 28 exempting from authorization requirements those ATMPs manufactured in hospitals, universities, or start-up companies where the medicine is prescribed for individual patients under the care of a medical practitioner. This manufacture should occur on a non-routine basis according to specific quality standards (GMP) (Vives et al. 2015), and the ATMP should be used in a hospital and only within the same member state. National authorities oversee the approval of HE products which has resulted in significant variations between member states in how it is applied and which has led to criticism from both industry and academia that it is unclear and inconsistent.

Access to ATMPs including cellular therapies is likely to be a particular challenge for patients, healthcare professionals, and national health systems due to their expected high costs. Even access to decades-old HSCT remains strongly associated with higher-income countries (Gratwohl et al. 2015). One potential effect of limited access could be the so-called stem cell tourism whereby patients with the means travel to centers outside their own countries for care and who may be vulnerable to false promises or may not have access to all of the information needed to make this important decision. The International Society for Cellular Therapy (ISCT) leads the publication of patient advice and other documentation on this phenomenon (see http://www.celltherapysociety.org/page/UCT. Accessed 21 Feb 2018).

Academic facilities including stem cell transplant practitioners at large should strive to remain active players in the development of ATMPs. Academia remains very active in the early phases of clinical trials designed to evaluate innovative SCTMP and GTMP as potential complements, substitutes, or bridges to historical forms of hematopoietic cell transplants (Pearce et al. 2014). One recent study calculated that only 20% of CAR T cell trials are sponsored by pharmaceutical industry (Hartmann et al. 2017). Many public institutions have invested significant resources to upgrade their processing facilities to GMP-compliant levels thus allowing for small-scale manufacturing of experimental medicinal products to support phase I and possibly phase II studies, often with the hope that industry will take over in case that promising results warrant further development (de Wilde et al. 2016a). Furthermore, academia has to become a proactive stakeholder in the regulatory area by engaging with the authorities, sharing their know-how, and voicing their opinion (de Wilde et al. 2016b).

The field is moving at a fast pace. So far, there has been proof of concept that tissue-based or cell-based medicinal products can be manufactured by a "conventional" pharmaceutical company (Locke et al. 2017), although with continued reliance on critical contributions from academic facilities, e.g., basic science and provision of starting materials. Some of these innovative medicinal products have remarkable clinical efficacy for severe or debilitating diseases although sometimes at the expense of equally remarkable toxicity. However, a commercial ATMP "hit" is still to emerge which could explain why the CAR-T cell field is being highly scrutinized by clinicians, regulators, and industry after the first two marketing authorizations for CAR-T cell therapies were granted by FDA in the USA in 2017 and by EMA in the EU in August 2018. These developments carry many regulatory and operational uncertainties including the very sustainability of how academic facilities currently deliver HSCT, but availability of this new category of innovative medicinal products offers new hopes to patients. Their therapeutic pathway is likely to become increasingly complex (Chabannon et al. 2015) and will require long-term follow-up for evidence of sustained clinical efficacy and detection of late adverse effects (see http://www.ema.europa.eu/ema/index.jsp?curl=pages%2Fregulation%2Fgeneral%2Fgeneral_content_000658.jsp&mid=WC0b01ac0580961211). Academia through continental registries such as EBMT will continue to play a key role with data and know-how that will be very useful not just for researchers but also for industry, healthcare regulators, and payers.

Key Points

- In this chapter, we review the fast-evolving regulatory framework that leads to the coexistence of two categories of hematopoietic cell-based therapeutics.
- Innovative and industry-manufactured somatic cell therapy or gene therapy medicinal products are now entering the field at an accelerating pace and will complete or compete with traditional HSCT practices in the near future.
- We describe the organizational consequences for academic facilities of this historical shift that brings new opportunities to patients and practitioners in the field.

References

Andre-Schmutz I, Le Deist F, Hacein-Bey-Abina S, et al. Immune reconstitution without graft-versus-host disease after haemopoietic stem-cell transplantation: a phase 1/2 study. Lancet. 2002;360:130–7.

Cavazzana-Calvo M, Payen E, Negre O, Wang G, Hehir K, Fusil F, et al. Transfusion independence and HMGA2 activation after gene therapy of human beta-thalassaemia. Nature. 2010;467:318–22.

Chabannon C, Hildebrandt M, Scheding S, Humpe A, Lowdell M, Slaper-Cortenbach I. Regulation of advanced therapy medicinal products will affect the practice of haematopoietic SCT in the near future: a perspective from the EBMT cell-processing committee. Bone Marrow Transplant. 2015;50:321–3.

Ciceri F, Bonini C, Stanghellini MT, Bondanza A, Traversari C, Salomoni M, et al. Infusion of suicide-gene-engineered donor lymphocytes after family haploidentical haemopoietic stem-cell transplantation for leukaemia (the TK007 trial): a non-randomised phase I-II study. Lancet Oncol. 2009;10:489–500.

de Lima M, McNiece I, Robinson SN, et al. Cord-blood engraftment with ex vivo mesenchymal-cell coculture. N Engl J Med. 2012;367:2305–15.

de Wilde S, Guchelaar HJ, Herberts C, Lowdell M, Hildebrandt M, Zandvliet M, et al. Development of cell therapy medicinal products by academic institutes. Drug Discov Today. 2016a;21:1206–12.

de Wilde S, Veltrop-Duits L, Hoozemans-Strik M, Ras T, Blom-Veenman J, Guchelaar HJ, et al. Hurdles in clinical implementation of academic advanced therapy medicinal products: a national evaluation. Cytotherapy. 2016b;18:797–805.

Delaney C, Heimfeld S, Brashem-Stein C, et al. Notch-mediated expansion of human cord blood progenitor cells capable of rapid myeloid reconstitution. Nat Med. 2010;16:232–6.

Feuchtinger T, Opherk K, Bethge WA, et al. Adoptive transfer of pp65-specific T cells for the treatment of chemorefractory cytomegalovirus disease or reactivation after haploidentical and matched unrelated stem cell transplantation. Blood. 2010;116:4360–7.

Gratwohl A, Pasquini MC, Aljurf M, et al. One million haemopoietic stem-cell transplants: a retrospective observational study. Lancet Haematol. 2015;2:e91–100.

Hartmann J, Schussler-Lenz M, Bondanza A, Buchholz CJ. Clinical development of CAR T cells-challenges and opportunities in translating innovative treatment concepts. EMBO Mol Med. 2017;9:1183–97.

Le Blanc K, Frassoni F, Ball L, et al. Mesenchymal stem cells for treatment of steroid-resistant, severe, acute graft-versus-host disease: a phase II study. Lancet. 2008;371:1579–86.

Locke FL, Neelapu SS, Bartlett NL, et al. Phase 1 results of ZUMA-1: a multicenter study of KTE-C19 anti-CD19 CAR T cell therapy in refractory aggressive lymphoma. Mol Ther. 2017;25:285–95.

Neelapu SS, Locke FL, Bartlett NL, et al. Axicabtagene ciloleucel CAR T-cell therapy in refractory large B-cell lymphoma. N Engl J Med. 2017;377:2531–44.

Pearce KF, Hildebrandt M, Greinix H, Scheding S, Koehl U, Worel N, et al. Regulation of advanced therapy medicinal products in Europe and the role of academia. Cytotherapy. 2014;16:289–97.

Ribeil JA, Hacein-Bey-Abina S, Payen E, et al. Gene therapy in a patient with sickle cell disease. N Engl J Med. 2017;376:848–55.

Schuster SJ, Svoboda J, Chong EA, Nasta SD, Mato AR, Anak O, et al. Chimeric antigen receptor T cells in refractory B-cell lymphomas. N Engl J Med. 2017;377:2545–54.

Vives J, Oliver-Vila I, Pla A. Quality compliance in the shift from cell transplantation to cell therapy in non-pharma environments. Cytotherapy. 2015;17:1009–14.

Wang X, Rivière I. Clinical manufacturing of CAR T cells: foundation of a promising therapy. Mol Ther Oncolytics. 2016;3:16015. https://doi.org/10.1038/mto.2016.15.

Wang X, Riviere I. Genetic engineering and manufacturing of hematopoietic stem cells. Mol Ther Methods Clin Dev. 2017;5:96–105.

Part VIII

Specific Modalities of HSCT and Management

Topic leaders: Andrew Gennery, Anna Sureda and Arjan Lankester

At-Home HSCT

63

Francesc Fernandez-Avilés
and Gonzalo Gutiérrez-García

63.1 Autologous HSCT

63.1.1 Introduction

Toxicity and mortality associated with auto-HSCT have been reduced, and outpatient parenteral antimicrobial treatment has been proven feasible and safe, thanks to modern CVC and infusion devices. These advances have led to the development of outpatient auto-HSCT programs, and several studies have demonstrated their feasibility and safety.

There are various reasons for transferring the support of the neutropenic phase of auto-HSCT to the ambulatory setting, including patient preference, reduced exposure to hospital microorganisms, better use of hospital resources, and cost-saving issues (Meisenberg et al. 1997). In this model, however, patients experience time-consuming daily travel to the outpatient clinic for blood tests and physician checkups. "Hospital at home" is an alternative, designed to reduce hospital outpatient admissions by providing hospital equivalent care to patients in the home setting (Westermann et al. 1999; Fernández Avilés et al. 2006).

63.1.2 Ambulatory Auto-HSCT Models

Complete outpatient program (Holbro et al. 2013)	
Conditioning regimen, HPC and management of the aplastic phase	Outpatient clinics
Delayed admission (Anastasia et al. 2009)	
Conditioning regimen and HPC infusion	Inpatient
Management of the aplastic phase	Early discharge (+1) and readmission (+5)
Mixed inpatient-outpatient (Morabito et al. 2002)	
Conditioning regimen	Outpatient clinics
HPC infusion	Inpatient
Management of the aplastic phase	Outpatient clinics
Early discharge outpatient (Martino et al. 2014)	
Conditioning regimen and HPC infusion	Inpatient
Management of the aplastic phase	Outpatient clinics
Early discharge at home (Fernández Avilés et al. 2006)	
Conditioning regimen and HPC infusion	Inpatient
Management of the aplastic phase	At home

F. Fernandez-Avilés (✉) · G. Gutiérrez-García
Department of Hematology, Bone Marrow Transplantation Unit, Hospital Clínic de Barcelona, Universitat de Barcelona, Barcelona, Catalunya, Spain
e-mail: ffernand@clinic.cat

E. Carreras et al. (eds.), *The EBMT Handbook*, https://doi.org/10.1007/978-3-030-02278-5_63

63.1.3 Inclusion Criteria for Ambulatory Auto-HSCT

Patient	– Age ≤65 years – ECOG ≤2 – Normal cardiac, lung, liver, and renal function – Recent documented infection with a proven secondary prophylaxis – Absence of refractoriness to platelet transfusion – Signed written informed consent
Transplant Center	– Outpatient clinics available 24 h per day or bed reserved in the transplant unit – Dedicated phone line 24h × 365 days to allow patients or their caregivers to contact an expert physician of the transplant team
Disease	– CR or PR before the auto-HSCT – No symptomatic advanced disease
Caregiver	Availability of a suitable caregiver 24 h per day, 7 days a week
Home	– Clean house – Travel time from home to the hospital less than 60 min at rush hours

63.1.4 General Recommendations for At-Home Auto-HSCT

Dose of CD34+ cells, use of G-CSF after HPC infusion, primary antimicrobial prophylaxis, and supportive care (hydration, management of emesis and metabolic disorders, analgesic therapy, and transfusion of blood products) should not differ from that recommended for conventional auto-HSCT. All these treatments can routinely be performed at home or in outpatient clinic.

63.1.5 Most Frequent Reasons for Readmission (Ordered by Frequency)

Persistent fever >38 °C without identified infectious focus

Severe oral mucositis or gastrointestinal toxicity (WHO grade III or IV) with insufficient liquid intake

Severe sepsis with organic failure

Request of the patient (psychological distress) or loss of caregiver support

63.1.6 Treatment of Fever in At-Home Setting

If fever occurs, the patient should be evaluated quickly by an expert hematologist on call. The use of empiric antibacterial treatment should follow guidelines/recommendations for patients with hematologic malignancies and neutropenic fever. IV antibiotics should be preferred and chosen in the light of clinical and laboratory findings. After at least 6 h monitoring, hemodynamically stable patients without relevant clinical problems may be followed at home. Table 63.1 shows the different empiric antibiotic therapy that could be used at home.

63.1.7 Incidence of Readmission in Outpatient and At-Home Auto-HSCT

The incidence of readmissions is closely related to the experience of the group of professionals in outpatient or at-home management of complications and by the support infrastructure available in the hospital.

Table 63.1 Empirical antibiotic therapy

Patients not receiving prophylaxis with quinolones
Levofloxacin (PO or IV)
Moxifloxacin PO
Ciprofloxacin PO associated or not to amoxicillin/clavulanate
Ciprofloxacin PO associated or not to linezolid PO
Patients receiving prophylaxis with quinolones
IV ceftriaxone or piperacillin/tazobactam[a] or meropenem[b] associated to teicoplanin IV[c] if intense oral mucositis
If there is a high suspicion of CVC infection, add teicoplanin and an anti-GNB such as amikacin IV and evaluate the CVC withdrawal
If allergic to beta-lactam: quinolones PO/IV associated with teicoplanin IV and amikacin IV

[a]Stable at room temperature so it can be administered at home by electronic intermittent infusion pump

[b]Accurate refrigeration to achieve adequate stability for home administration

[c]The first option at home would be teicoplanin once daily instead of vancomycin IV (twice a day). Other alternatives rarely necessary in the context of auto-HSCT are daptomycin IV or linezolid PO

In patients with *MM*, usually conditioned with MEL, the lowest readmission rates have been reported (between 10 and 20%) due to the low organic toxicity (Martino et al. 2016). They are clearly the best option when considering starting an outpatient or at-home auto-HSCT program.

In patients with *NHL or HL* usually conditioned with a more toxic regime (BEAM or BEAC), there is a significantly higher readmission rate, between 30 and 90%, according to the series (Faucher et al. 2012; Scortechini et al. 2014).

In the *hospital clinic* at-home auto-HSCT experience, the low rate of febrile neutropenia is achieved, thanks to the intensification of antibiotic prophylaxis (ceftriaxone in MM and piperacillin/tazobactam in NHL and LH patients), and the successful control of fever at home resulted in an overall readmission rate significantly lower (8.5%) in a series of 325 patients.

63.1.8 Quality of Life

The data published are limited and contradictory. Thus, (Summers et al. 2000) reported significantly higher scores for emotional well-being and global QOL in outpatients, while (Martino et al. 2018) indicated that the outpatient model neither improves nor impairs global patient QOL on the first 30 days after auto-HSCT. In this sense (Schulmeister et al. 2005) reported that the QOL decreased immediately post treatment but then increased to above pretreatment levels by 6 months. A good clinical outcome following auto-HSCT was associated with better QOL and greater satisfaction with care.

63.1.9 Cost Data

The study of "real" costs of these ambulatory/domiciliary auto-HSCT programs is still to be carried out. In the absence of well-designed studies aimed at evaluating the "real" savings achieved with outpatient/at-home auto-HSCT programs, some authors cite direct savings between 10% and 50% (Meisenberg et al. 1998; Fernández Avilés et al. 2006; Holbro et al. 2013), especially influenced by the release of hospital beds and low readmission rates.

63.2 Allogeneic HSCT

63.2.1 Introduction

The consolidation of ambulatory auto-HSCT modalities as a safe and potentially cost-saving procedure and the introduction of NMA and RIC conditioning chemotherapies minimizing toxicity have allowed the development of allo-HSCT ambulatory programs. Indeed, the main relevant results with this type of modality have shown a safe profile in terms of lower rate of infection and GVHD improving QOL, conditions that should expand the development of ambulatory modalities into the allo-HSCT setting (Svahn et al. 2002). However, after two decades of the first ambulatory allo-HSCT program, the experience with this modality is limited to few BMT groups.

63.2.2 Ambulatory Allo-HSCT Models

Complete outpatient program (McDiarmid et al. 2010)	
Conditioning regimen and HPC infusion	Outpatient clinics
Management of the aplastic phase	
Mixed inpatient-outpatient (Solomon et al. 2010)	
Conditioning regimen	Outpatient clinic
HPC infusion	Inpatient
Management of the aplastic phase	Outpatient clinic
Early discharge at home (Ringdén et al. 2018)	
Conditioning regimen and HPC infusion	Inpatient
Management of the aplastic phase	At home

63.2.3 Inclusion Criteria for At-Home Allo-HSCT Patients

Inclusion criteria for at-home allo-HSCT patients: Specifically, apply similar conditions as an at-home auto-HSCT.

63.2.4 General Recommendations for At-Home Allo-HSCT

Apply whole hints described for auto-HSCT. Moreover, strictly frequent dosage of IS (2–3 times per week) is recommended. Monitoring of CMV and *Aspergillus* should not differ from that recommended for conventional allo-HSCT. Primary prophylaxis for *Aspergillus* is not established but is strongly suggested.

63.2.5 Which Readmission Criteria?

Which readmission criteria? Apply similar conditions for ambulatory auto-HSCT plus evidence of GVHD grades II–IV.

63.2.6 Treatment of Fever in At-Home Setting

Treatment of fever in at-home setting: See at-home auto-HSCT.

63.2.7 Incidence of Readmission in Outpatient and At-Home Allo-HSCT

Readmission rate is high (50–80%, according to the series) mainly due to organ toxicity associated with the preparative regimen in MAC with TBI and use of MTX or CY-PT such as GVHD prophylaxis.

The incidence of infection rate is lower than inpatient modality (15–30%, according to the series). Particularly, the incidence of *Aspergillus* or other mold infections was low (0–7%, according to series).

Severe GVHD is a low frequent cause of readmission in the first 30 days.

This incidence is related to the experience of the group of professionals and by the support infrastructure available in the hospital. In our experience, only 1 of the 28 patients (3.6%) required hospital readmission.

63.2.8 Quality of Life and Cost

The limited experience seems to show that at-home allo-HSCT modality improves nutrition/caloric intake, physical activity, and welfare of self that probably help to recover quickly and reduce toxicity, minimizing infection risk and GVHD (Svahn et al. 2008; Ringdén et al. 2013). Nevertheless, it is difficult to determine that these measures impact on a reduction of the total cost taking into account that the readmission rate is high and that most experiences include pre-planned booking of inpatient beds.

Key Points
- At home auto-HSCT is feasible and safe with a good selection of patients.
- At home auto-HSCT is cost-effective considering the patient setting, not analyzed in the context of the whole hospital budged.
- MM is the best indication for at-home auto-HSCT.
- With an adequate selection of patients, at-home allo-HSCT is feasible and safe.
- Allo-HSCT performed with the use of NMA and RIC conditioning regimens is the best option due to their inherent low organic toxicity.

References

Anastasia A, Giglio F, Mazza R, et al. Early discharge after high-dose melphalan and peripheral blood stem cell reinfusion in patients with hematological and non-hematological disease. Leuk Lymphoma. 2009;50:80–4.

Faucher C, Le Corroller Soriano AG, Esterni B, et al. Randomized study of early hospital discharge following autologous blood SCT: medical outcomes and hospital costs. Bone Marrow Transplant. 2012;47:549–55.

Fernández Avilés F, Carreras E, Urbano-Ispizua A, et al. Case-control comparison of at home to total hospital care for autologous stem-cell transplantation for hematologic malignancies. J Clin Oncol. 2006;24:4855–61.

Holbro A, Ahmad I, Cohen S, et al. Safety and cost-effectiveness of outpatient autologous stem cell transplantation in patients with multiple myeloma. Biol Blood Marrow Transplant. 2013;19:547–51.

Martino M, Montanari M, Ferrara F, et al. Very low rate of re-admission after an early discharge outpatient model for autografting in multiple myeloma patients: an Italian multi-center retrospective study. Biol Blood Marrow Transplant. 2014;20:1026–32.

Martino M, Lemoli RM, Girmenia C, et al. Italian consensus conference for the outpatient autologous stem cell transplantation management in multiple myeloma. Bone Marrow Transplant. 2016;51:1032–40.

Martino M, Ciavarella S, De Summa S, et al. A comparative assessment of quality of life in patients with multiple myeloma undergoing autologous stem cell transplantation through an outpatient and inpatient model. Biol Blood Marrow Transplant. 2018;24:608–13.

McDiarmid S, Hutton B, Atkins H, et al. Performing allogeneic and autologous hematopoietic SCT in the outpatient setting: effects on infectious complications and early transplant outcomes. Bone Marrow Transplant. 2010;45:1220–6.

Meisenberg BR, Miller WE, McMillan R, et al. Outpatient high-dose chemotherapy with autologous stem-cell rescue for hematologic and nonhematologic malignancies. J Clin Oncol. 1997;15:11–7.

Meisenberg BR, Ferran K, Hollenbach K, et al. Reduced charges and costs associated with outpatient autologous stem cell transplantation. Bone Marrow Transplant. 1998;21:927–32.

Morabito F, Martino M, Stelitano C, et al. Feasibility of a mixed inpatient-outpatient model of peripheral blood stem cell transplantation for multiple myeloma. Haematologica. 2002;87:1192–9.

Ringdén O, Remberger M, Holmberg K, et al. Many days at home during neutropenia after allogeneic hematopoietic stem cell transplantation correlates with low incidence of acute graft-versus-host disease. Biol Blood Marrow Transplant. 2013;19:314–20.

Ringdén O, Sadeghi B, Moretti G, et al. Long-term outcome in patients treated at home during the pancytopenic phase after allogeneic haematopoietic stem cell transplantation. Int J Hematol. 2018;107:478–85.

Schulmeister L, Quiett K, Mayer K. Quality of life, quality of care, and patient satisfaction: perceptions of patients undergoing outpatient autologous stem cell transplantation. Oncol Nurs Forum. 2005;32:57–67.

Scortechini I, Montanari M, Mancini G, Inglese E, Calandrelli M, Chiarucci M, Offidani M, Capelli D, Gini G, Poloni A, Mancini S, Raggetti G, Leoni P, Olivieri A. Conditioning regimen with BCNU, etoposide, cytarabine and melphalan plus amifostine for outpatient autologous stem cell transplant: feasibility and outcome in 97 patients with lymphoma. Leuk Lymphoma. 2014;55:1657–60.

Solomon SR, Matthews RH, Barreras AM, et al. Outpatient myeloablative allo-SCT: a comprehensive approach yields decreased hospital utilization and low TRM. Bone Marrow Transplant. 2010;45:468–75.

Summers N, Dawe U, Stewart DA. A comparison of inpatient and outpatient ASCT. Bone Marrow Transplant. 2000;26:389–95.

Svahn BM, Remberger M, Myrback KE, et al. Home care during the pancytopenic phase after allogeneic hematopoietic stem cell transplantation is advantageous compared with hospital care. Blood. 2002;100:4317–24.

Svahn BM, Remberger M, Heijbel M, et al. Case-control comparison of at-home and hospital care for allogeneic hematopoietic stem-cell transplantation: the role of oral nutrition. Transplantation. 2008;85:1000–7.

Westermann AM, Holtkamp MMJ, Linthorst GAM, et al. At home management of aplastic phase following high-dose chemotherapy with stem-cell rescue for hematological and non-hematological malignancies. Ann Oncol. 1999;10:511–7.

64 Umbilical Cord Blood Transplantation in Children and Adults

Jaime Sanz, Paul Veys, and Vanderson Rocha

64.1 Introduction

Umbilical cord blood transplantation (UCBT) from unrelated donors is a suitable option of HSCT for patients in whom it is indicated, and a suitable related or unrelated BM or PB donor is not available in due time.

Since the 1990s, the majority of UCBT have been performed in children, but the number in adults was growing steadily. In fact, since 2004 the number of UCBT in adults registered in Eurocord was higher than in children. However, a certain decline in the UCBT activity has been observed over the last few years, which is mainly due to an increasing activity of partially matched related (haploidentical) HSCT. It should be noted that, although both options compete in the same niche, their comparative data are very limited and randomized studies are not yet available. As far as we know, two phase III randomized studies are currently ongoing to compare UCBT and haplo-HSCT in the RIC and MAC setting (NCT0159778 and NCT02386332, respectively).

64.2 Potential Advantages and Disadvantages of UCBT

UCBT versus BMT/PBSCT	
Advantages	Disadvantages
• Expanded access to transplant[a] – Higher availability of donor[a] – Faster search and shorter time to transplant[a] – Greater HLA disparity allowed with low incidence of GVHD[a] • Lower risk of transmission of viral infections • More versatile transplant planning[a] • No risk of donor refusal • No risk to the donor	• Slower engraftment • Higher risk of non-immunological rejection (graft failure) • Remote possibility of transmission of a genetic disease[b] • Greater delay in immune reconstitution • No possibility of donor lymphocyte infusion[b]

[a]Advantages shared with haplo-HSCT
[b]Disadvantages not shared with haplo-HSCT

Similar to UCBT, haplo-HSCT can also be used on an urgent basis and extends donor availability to the vast majority of patients. In addition,

J. Sanz (✉)
Department of Medicine, University Hospital La Fe, University of Valencia, Valencia, Spain
e-mail: sanz_jai@gva.es

P. Veys
Great Ormond Street Hospital (GOSH) for Children NHS Foundation Trust, and University College London GOSH Institute of Child Health, London, UK

V. Rocha
Hospital de Clinicas, Hematology, Transfusion and Cell Therapy Service, University of São Paulo, Sao Paulo, Brazil

Churchill Hospital, NHS-BT, Oxford University, Oxford, UK

E. Carreras et al. (eds.), *The EBMT Handbook*, https://doi.org/10.1007/978-3-030-02278-5_64

haplo-HSCT allows a DLI if necessary. Unfortunately, comparative data of these two approaches are limited and inconclusive (Brunstein et al. 2011; Ruggeri et al. 2015), and randomized studies are still lacking.

64.3 Indications

Except for some patients with severe BMF, such as aplastic anemia and paroxysmal nocturnal hemoglobinuria, UCBT in adults is performed almost exclusively in patients with malignant hematological diseases. However, UCBT in children has been used for many other nonmalignant diseases, including primary immunodeficiency diseases and inherited metabolic disorders (see Eurocord experience in Table 64.1).

The American Society for Blood and Marrow Transplantation (ASBMT), EBMT, and British Society of Blood and Marrow Transplantation (BSBMT) have recently published their respective guidelines that include recommendations for transplant indications in children and adults. It should be noted that the ASBMT did not differentiate recommendations for transplant indications based on donor source (i.e., MRD, URD, UCB, or haploidentical donor) or graft source (i.e., BM, PBSC, or UCB). This is in contrast to guidelines published by the EBMT and BSBMT.

Table 64.1 Distribution by diseases of UCBT registered in Eurocord (1994–2017)

	Children (n = 4128) n (%)	Adults (n = 3733) n (%)
Malignant disorders	2569 (62)	3609 (97)
– AML	761 (18)	1504 (40)
– ALL	1329 (32)	706 (19)
– MDS/MPS	367 (9)	703 (19)
– Lymphoid mature disorders	86 (2)	544 (15)
– Plasma cell disorders	0 (0)	114 (3)
– Others	26 (1)	38 (1)
Nonmalignant disorders	1559 (38)	124 (3)
– Primary immunodeficiencies	588 (14)	6 (0.1)
– Inborn errors of metabolism	423 (10)	9 (0.1)
– Bone marrow failure syndromes	318 (8)	104 (3)
– Histiocytic disorders	180 (4)	1 (0.1)
– Others	50 (0.1)	4 (0.1)

AML acute myeloid leukemia, *ALL* acute lymphoblastic leukemia, *MDS* myelodysplastic syndrome

64.4 Approaches to Improve Outcomes After UCBT

Apart from refining criteria for UCB unit selection and optimization of conditioning regimens, several strategies have been developed aiming to shorten the time to engraftment and decrease NRM.

Approaches to improve outcomes of UCBT	Expert point of view
(a) Refining criteria for UCB unit selection	See Chap. 18 of banking, processing, and procurement of cord blood cells
(b) Optimization of conditioning regimens	Specific conditioning regimen can influence transplant outcomes. See Sect. 64.5
(c) Strategies aiming to shorten the time to engraftment	To date none of these strategies have consistently shown to improve outcomes over single unmanipulated UCBT
1. Double UCBT	– In children, two randomized trials have demonstrated no benefit and increased risk of GVHD (Wagner et al. 2014; Michel et al. 2016) – In adults, retrospective studies showed no advantage when single-unit with TNC dose >2.5 × 10^7/kg available (Scaradavou et al. 2013)
2. Co-infusion with third-party cells	Has consistently demonstrated benefit to accelerate hematopoietic recovery. No proved benefit on NRM or survival (Sanz et al. 2017)
3. Ex vivo expansion of UCB cells	Promising early studies showing fast engraftment with different expansion techniques. No comparative studies or long-term data (Mehta et al. 2017)
(d) Improvement of supportive measures	Supportive care to prevent or treat opportunistic infections until neutrophil and immune recovery has occurred which is critical in UCBT. See Sect. 64.7

64.5 Conditioning Regimens

The selection of conditioning regimen for HSCT, including UCBT, should take into account the risk of toxicity and the risk of graft failure and relapse in malignant diseases. In UCBT, given the relatively lower cell dose (T-cells and CD34+ cells) and the use of HLA-mismatched grafts, graft failure is of particular concern, especially in adults. The choice of the conditioning regimen is as important as the graft characteristics and can influence transplant outcomes (Ruggeri et al. 2014).

In fact, specific conditioning regimens seem to tolerate infusion of lower cell doses in the graft (Sanz et al. 2013). A comprehensive and exhaustive review of MAC and non-MAC/RIC regimens in the UCBT setting has recently been published (Ross and Gutman 2017).

The Sorror comorbidity index may be a helpful tool to choose the appropriate conditioning intensity for a given patient. Some conditioning regimens options of varying intensity are to be considered:

Myeloablative conditioning regimens (MAC)	
Chemotherapy-based	
• Adults: TBF regimen (Sanz et al. 2012)	TT 10 mg/kg + IV BU 9.6 mg/kg + FLU 150 mg/m^2 + ATG 6 mg/kg
• Children: FTT regimen (Hough et al. 2016)	TREO 30–42 g/m^2 + FLU 150 mg/m^2 + TT 10 mg/kg
• BF regimen (Admiraal et al. 2015)	BU (PK guided) + FLU 160 mg/m^2 + ATG 19 mg/kg
TBI-based	
• TCF regimen (Barker et al. 2005)	TBI 13.2 Gy + CY 120 mg/kg + FLU 75 mg/m^2
Medium-intensity conditioning regimens (MIDI)	
• MIDI regimen (Barker et al. 2017)	TT 10 mg/kg + CY 50 mg/kg + FLU 150 mg/m^2 + TBI 4 Gy
Reduced-intensity conditioning regimens (RIC)	
• rTCF regimen (Brunstein et al. 2007)	TBI 2 Gy + CY 50 mg/kg + FLU 200 mg/m^2 ± ATG

64.6 GVHD Prophylaxis

The most important advantage of UCB over unrelated donor grafts is the capability to tolerate HLA disparities and facilitate a low incidence of chronic GVHD. However, acute GVHD is still one of the most important contributors to morbidity and mortality. Different GVHD prophylaxis regimens have been explored with no evidence of benefit of any specific strategy. MTX is generally not recommended to avoid myelotoxicity and delayed neutrophil recovery although it is widely used in Asia. The most frequently used regimen worldwide is the combination of CNI for 6–9 months with MMF for 2–6 months.

The use of in vivo TCD with ATG is controversial. ATG in the conditioning regimen has been used to enhance myeloid engraftment as well as to prevent GVHD. Its use has been associated with reduced rates of GVHD. However, although there is no evidence of a negative impact on NRM (Ponce et al. 2015), there is a concern of impaired immune reconstitution and increased viral infections (Chiesa et al. 2012). Recent data suggest that safety of ATG can be improved by adjusting dose with ATG pharmacokinetics (Admiraal et al. 2016).

64.7 Supportive Care

The supportive measures described below are not intended to be recommendations but only to be taken into account and to consider their use in the context of each institution's own experience and epidemiology. The most common measures are described merely as a guide since they have a very variable level of evidence (see Table 64.2).

Table 64.2 Prophylaxis, monitoring, and treatment options to be considered for infections in UCBT

Prophylaxis	Monitoring	Treatment
Supportive measures for bacterial infections		
Levofloxacin or ciprofloxacin	Surveillance cultures to detect colonization with MDR gram-negative bacteria	Empirical antibacterial therapy according to institutional epidemiologic patterns
Supportive measures for fungal infections		
Mold-covering azole	Galactomannan and beta-D-glucan assays[a]	Liposomal AmB, azoles, and/or echinocandins (according to previous prophylaxis)
Supportive measures for viral infections		
CMV: letermovir	(qPCR) Weekly on days 0–100 and then as clinically indicated	Ganciclovir, valganciclovir, foscarnet
HHV-6: none	(qPCR) as clinically indicated	Ganciclovir, valganciclovir, foscarnet
Adenovirus: none	(qPCR) weekly on days 0–100 and then as clinically indicated[b]	Cidofovir
EBV: none	(qPCR) weekly on days 0–100 and then as clinically indicated[c]	Preemptive rituximab
Supportive measures for protozoal infections		
Pneumocystis: co-trimoxazole, pentamidine, or atovaquone	–	Co-trimoxazole, pentamidine, or atovaquone
Toxoplasmosis: co-trimoxazole, atovaquone, or pyrimethamine	–	Co-trimoxazole, atovaquone, or pyrimethamine

MDR multidrug-resistant, *AmB* amphotericin B, *qPCR* quantitative PCR

[a]Both have been included as microbiological criteria in the definitions of invasive fungal infections by the European Organization for Research and Treatment of Cancer (EORTC) and the Mycoses Study Group (MSG)

[b]Specially in children

[c]Reduced-intensity conditioning and ATG are risk factors for EBV-PTLD

Table 64.3 Expected results overall survival at 2 years after UCBT

Adults	2-years OS (%)	Children	2-years OS (%)
Outcomes according to DRI		Malignant disorders	49 ± 1
Low	55 ± 3	Acute leukemia	52 ± 1
Intermediate	47 ± 1	MDS	55 ± 3
High	27 ± 2	Lymphoproliferative disorders	55 ± 3
Very high	19 ± 3	Nonmalignant disorders	63 ± 1
Disease-specific outcomes		Inborn error of metabolism	70 ± 2
Acute leukemia	37 ± 1	Hemoglobinopathies	68 ± 9
MDS/MPS	32 ± 2	Primary immunodeficiency	68 ± 2
Lymphoproliferative disorders	45 ± 2	Histiocytic disorders	60 ± 4
Plasma cell disorder	37 ± 5	BMF syndrome	52 ± 3

DRI disease risk index, *MDS* myelodysplastic syndrome, *MPS* myeloproliferative syndrome, *OS* overall survival, *MDS* myelodysplastic syndrome, *BMF* bone marrow failure

64.8 Results (See Table 64.3)

UCBT outcomes have improved in more recent years, probably explained by better patient and CBU selection, improved conditioning, and supported care. Registry data also showed important center effect with superior survival obtained in experienced centers. Eurocord recently updated clinical results.

Multiple retrospective studies have demonstrated that UCBT offers similar long-term outcomes compared with the gold standard of HLA-matched URD transplants in patients with hematologic malignancies, both in children and adults (Eapen et al. 2007; Brunstein et al. 2010; Atsuta et al. 2012). Interestingly, UCBT seems to offer a potent antileukemic efficacy, through yet unknown mechanisms. A recent report that needs to be validated suggested a markedly reduced relapse rate after UCBT as compared to URD transplantation in patients transplanted with MRD (Milano et al. 2016).

Key Points

- UCB remains a rapidly available and valuable source of stem cells for HSCT.
- In the absence of a fully matched donor available at an appropriate time, similar outcomes are achieved with CBT, MMURD, and haplo-HSCT approaches in the pediatric and adult setting.
- CBT may reduce relapse following HSCT for AML.
- There is a much room for improvement in the field and important progresses are expected in the near future. Decrease in NRM should be the number one goal in future research.
- Strategies to enhance engraftment and, more importantly, approaches to improve immune reconstitution, such as appropriate ATG dosing, are warranted.

References

Admiraal R, Lindemans CA, van Kesteren C, et al. Excellent T-cell reconstitution and survival depend on low ATG exposure after pediatric cord blood transplantation. Blood. 2016;128:2734–41.

Admiraal R, van Kesteren C, Jol-van der Zijde CM, et al. Association between anti-thymocyte globulin exposure and CD4+ immune reconstitution in paediatric haemopoietic cell transplantation: a multicentre, retrospective pharmacodynamic cohort analysis. Lancet Haematol. 2015;2:e194–203.

Atsuta Y, Morishima Y, Suzuki R, et al. Comparison of unrelated cord blood transplantation and HLA-mismatched unrelated bone marrow transplantation for adults with leukemia. Biol Blood Marrow Transplant. 2012;18:780–7.

Barker JN, Kurtzberg J, Ballen K, et al. Optimal practices in unrelated donor cord blood transplantation for hematologic malignancies. Biol Blood Marrow Transplant. 2017;23:882–96.

Barker JN, Weisdorf DJ, DeFor TE, Blazar BR, McGlave PB, Miller JS, Verfaillie CM, Wagner JE. Transplantation of 2 partially HLA-matched umbilical cord blood units to enhance engraftment in adults with hematologic malignancy. Blood. 2005;105:1343–7.

Brunstein CG, Barker JN, Weisdorf DJ, et al. Umbilical cord blood transplantation after nonmyeloablative conditioning: impact on transplantation outcomes in 110 adults with hematologic disease. Blood. 2007;110:3064–70.

Brunstein CG, Fuchs EJ, Carter SL, et al. Alternative donor transplantation after reduced intensity conditioning: results of parallel phase 2 trials using partially HLA-mismatched related bone marrow or unrelated double umbilical cord blood grafts. Blood. 2011;118:282–8.

Brunstein CG, Gutman JA, Weisdorf DJ, et al. Allogeneic hematopoietic cell transplantation for hematologic malignancy: relative risks and benefits of double umbilical cord blood. Blood. 2010;116:4693–9.

Chiesa R, Gilmour K, Qasim W, et al. Omission of in vivo T-cell depletion promotes rapid expansion of naive CD4+ cord blood lymphocytes and restores adaptive immunity within 2 months after unrelated cord blood transplant. Br J Haematol. 2012;156:656–66.

Eapen M, Rubinstein P, Zhang MJ, et al. Outcomes of transplantation of unrelated donor umbilical cord blood and bone marrow in children with acute leukaemia: a comparison study. Lancet. 2007;369:1947–54.

Hough R, Danby R, Russell N, et al. Recommendations for a standard UK approach to incorporating umbilical cord blood into clinical transplantation practice: an update on cord blood unit selection, donor selection algorithms and conditioning protocols. Br J Haematol. 2016;172:360–70.

Mehta RS, Dave H, Bollard CM, et al. Engineering cord blood to improve engraftment after cord blood transplant. Stem Cell Investig. 2017;4:41.

Michel G, Galambrun C, Sirvent A, et al. Single- vs double-unit cord blood transplantation for children and young adults with acute leukemia or myelodysplastic syndrome. Blood. 2016;127:3450–7.

Milano F, Gooley T, Wood B, et al. Cord-blood transplantation in patients with minimal residual disease. N Engl J Med. 2016;375:944–53.

Ponce DM, Eapen M, Sparapani R, et al. In vivo T cell depletion with myeloablative regimens on outcomes after cord blood transplantation for acute lymphoblastic leukemia in children. Biol Blood Marrow Transplant. 2015;21:2173–9.

Ross K, Gutman J. Cord blood transplantations. New York: Springer; 2017.

Ruggeri A, Labopin M, Sanz G, et al. Comparison of outcomes after unrelated cord blood and unmanipulated haploidentical stem cell transplantation in adults with acute leukemia. Leukemia. 2015;29:1891–900.

Ruggeri A, Sanz G, Bittencourt H, et al. Comparison of outcomes after single or double cord blood transplantation in adults with acute leukemia using different types of myeloablative conditioning regimen, a retrospective study on behalf of Eurocord and the Acute Leukemia Working Party of EBMT. Leukemia. 2014;28:779–86.

Sanz J, Boluda JCH, Martín C, et al. Single-unit umbilical cord blood transplantation from unrelated donors in patients with hematological malignancy using busulfan, thiotepa, fludarabine and ATG as myeloablative conditioning regimen. Bone Marrow Transplant. 2012;47:1287–93.

Sanz J, Kwon M, Bautista G, et al. Single umbilical cord blood with or without CD34+ cells from a third-party donor in adults with leukemia. Blood Adv. 2017;1:1047.

Sanz J, Wagner JE, Sanz MA, et al. Myeloablative cord blood transplantation in adults with acute leukemia: comparison of two different transplant platforms. Biol Blood Marrow Transplant. 2013;19:1725–30.

Scaradavou A, Brunstein CG, Eapen M, et al. Double unit grafts successfully extend the application of umbilical cord blood transplantation in adults with acute leukemia. Blood. 2013;121:752–8.

Wagner JE, Eapen M, Carter S, et al. One-unit versus two-unit cord-blood transplantation for hematologic cancers. N Engl J Med. 2014;371:1685–94.

Haploidentical HSCT

65

Fabio Ciceri, Andrea Bacigalupo, Arjan Lankester, and Alice Bertaina

65.1 Introduction

Haploidentical hematopoietic stem cell transplantation (haplo-HSCT) is now considered a clinical therapeutic option in patients candidate to allo-HSCT. Primary prevention and treatment of GvHD have been a major challenge in this peculiar major HLA-mismatched setting. Two main platforms have been developed: ex vivo TCD and unmanipulated graft transplantation. Overall, the primary objective of a stable haploidentical hematopoietic engraftment at a low GvHD rate resulted feasible in both platforms in a significant proportion of patients undergoing haplo-HSCT for any clinical indication.

The great interest in transplantation from haploidentical donors arises from the immediate availability of a suitable one-haplotype mismatched donor for virtually all patients in the appropriate timing. In the absence of a HLA full-matched donor, alternative family haploidentical donors have been intensively investigated in the past decade.

Primary prevention and treatment of GvHD have been a major challenge in this peculiar HLA-mismatched setting of HSCT. Two main clinical platforms have been developed: ex vivo TCD and more recently unmanipulated graft transplantation.

65.2 Ex Vivo TCD Platforms

The physical removal of donor T-cells from the graft has been pioneered by the group of Perugia in the late 1990s (Aversa et al. 1998). The original concept was to prevent GvHD through a graft with a T-cell content not exceeding a total T-cell graft dose of 1×10^4/kg of recipient body weight.

65.2.1 Positive CD34 Selection

The most experienced ex vivo manipulation has been the positive selection of CD34+ cells realized by CliniMACS® CD34 System Miltenyi,

F. Ciceri (✉)
IRCCS San Raffaele Scientific Institute, University Vita-Salute San Raffaele, Milan, Italy
e-mail: ciceri.fabio@hsr.it

A. Bacigalupo
Istituto di Ematologia, Fondazione Polclinico Universitario A. Gemelli, Universita' Cattolica del Sacro Cuore, Roma, Italy

A. Lankester
Department of Pediatrics, Section Immunology, Hematology and Stem Cell Transplantation, Leiden University Medical Center, Leiden, Netherlands

A. Bertaina
Division of Stem Cell Transplantation and Regenerative Medicine, Department of Pediatrics, School of Medicine, Stanford University, Stanford, CA, USA

E. Carreras et al. (eds.), *The EBMT Handbook*, https://doi.org/10.1007/978-3-030-02278-5_65

providing a TCD graft with high cell dose of CD34+ cells starting from G-CSF-mobilized PBSC graft of family haploidentical donors (Aversa et al. 1998; Ciceri et al. 2008; Reisner et al. 2011). This profound TCD graft required the development of conditioning regimens aimed at a maximal host IS through the use of ATG, full-dose TBI, and the combination of intensive IS, FLU, and TT.

Despite the application of intensive immunoablative regimens, the rate of graft rejection has been 10–15% requiring a salvage subsequent second HSCT providing an overall engraftment rate >95%. According to the primary objective, ex vivo TCD by CD34+ selection allows a stable engraftment with a GvHD rate <10% in the absence of any additional post transplant IST.

Unfortunately, this intense graft TCD translated into a slow post transplant immune recovery with a prolonged and profound T-cell lymphopenia (Reisner et al. 2011; Perruccio et al. 2005). In this clinical platform, TRM have been observed in a significant proportion of recipients (Ciceri et al. 2008). Leading causes of deaths reported were opportunistic infections occurring even as late as 1-year post transplant in the absence of GvHD and any IST. The improvement of post transplant immune reconstitution while controlling GvHD prompted the concurrent development of several additional strategies of cell therapy (Perruccio et al. 2005; Di Ianni et al. 2011; Ciceri et al. 2009). Particularly in the pediatric population, virus-specific T-cells have been a promising tool (Leen 2009); Feucht 2015). Donor T-cells genetically modified to express HSV-thymidine kinase suicide gene (Zalmoxis®) have been recently registered by the European Medicines Agency as adjunctive therapeutic tool post haploidentical HSCT.

65.2.2 CD3/CD19 Negative Selection

A partial T-cell depletion less profound than CD34+ selection can be provided by alternative selections, such as CD3/CD19 negative selection. The CliniMACS CD3/CD19 Product Line was developed for the simultaneous depletion of unwanted T- and B-cells in combination with the CliniMACS System. This approach keeps stem and progenitor cells untouched and leaves immune effector cells, such as NK cells and dendritic cells, in the cellular product (Bethge et al. 2006; Federmann et al. 2011; Federmann et al. 2012). Starting from G-CSF-mobilized PBSC in adults, grafts contained a median of 7.0×10^6 CD34+ cells/kg, 4.2×10^4 CD3+ T-cells/kg, and 2.7×10^7 CD56+ cells/kg; incidence of grade II–IV acute GVHD and chronic GVHD was 46% and 18%, respectively, requiring the post transplant use of a CNI as additional GvHD prophylaxis in adult patients.

65.2.3 TCRα/β and CD19 Depletion

More recently, Miltenyi developed CliniMACS TCRα/β and CD19-depleted stem cell grafts from haploidentical donors for HSCT in children and adults. The ex vivo protocol has been designed to selectively remove donor T-cells with TCRα/β that are recognized to mediate GvHD. Preliminary clinical experience in children showed a very low rate of skin GvHD and no visceral acute or chronic GVHD (Bertaina et al. 2014; Li Pira et al. 2016).

Overall, ex vivo TCD is a platform clinically useful to provide hematopoietic engraftment with low GvHD in haploidentical setting. Furthermore, the different cell population selection in the graft provides a unique clinical setting to dissect the biology of different immune cells as NK, TCRα/β, and TCRγ/δ T-cells in the clinical post transplant immune reconstitution and antitumor and immune protective in vivo effects (Ruggeri et al. 2002; Aversa et al. 2005; Locatelli et al. 2013).

65.2.4 Regulatory T-Cells

The Perugia group has recently presented a variation of ex vivo TCD, with the addition of regulatory T-cells, followed by mature T-cells (Martelli et al. 2014): preferential migration of regulatory T-cells to the lymph nodes, but not the bone marrow, prevents GvHD (in the lymph nodes) and allows, at the same time, a strong graft versus leukemia (in the bone marrow). The result is an extremely low incidence of leukemia relapse (Martelli et al. 2014).

65.3 Unmanipulated Haploidentical HSCT

The number of unmanipulated HLA haploidentical transplants has been rapidly increasing over the past 15 years (Passweg et al. 2012), due to the successful prevention of two major problems: lethal GvHD and graft rejection. There are currently three main platforms to perform unmanipulated haplo-HSCT (Fig. 65.1).

65.3.1 Anti-thymocyte Globulin (ATG) Based

In 2006 the Chinese group led by Dao-Pei Lu compared the outcome of 158 leukemia patients grafted from HLA-identical siblings with 135 leukemia patients grafted from HLA-haplotype mismatch family members, after a MAC regimen (Lu et al. 2006; Fig. 65.1: ATG-based; GBM + GPB + CSA + MMF + MTX). The results were surprising, with the OS and DFS identical for both groups. The conditioning therapy consisted of Ara-C (4 g/m^2/day, on days −10 to −9), BU (4 mg/kg/day, orally on days −8 to −6 before January 2008 and 3.2 mg/kg/day, IV on days −8 to −6 after January 2008), CY (1.8 g/m^2/day, on days −5 to −4), 1-(2-chloroethyl)-3-(4-methylcyclohexyl)-1-nitrosourea (Me-CCNU) (250 mg/m^2, once on day −3), and ATG (2.5 mg/kg/day, rabbit; Sanofi Genzyme, France, days −5 to −2).

All patients received CSA, MTX, and MMF; the HLA-mismatch group received in addition ATG (Lu et al. 2006). The graft source was a combination of G-CSF (G)-mobilized bone marrow (G-BM) and G-mobilized PB. The cohort in HLA-haplotype mismatch group had a higher risk of acute GvHD (P = 0.02) and of TRM (P = 0.05), but OS was comparable (P = 0.6). This was the first report on a large number of family mismatched grafts, showing survival identical to sibling HLA-matched grafts, and this led to the emergence of other programs.

Another group of Chinese investigators developed an ATG-based program with unmanipulated G-BM alone (Ji et al. 2005; Fig. 65.1, G-BM + CSA + MMF + MTX + basiliximab). They included intensive GvHD prophylaxis with ATG,

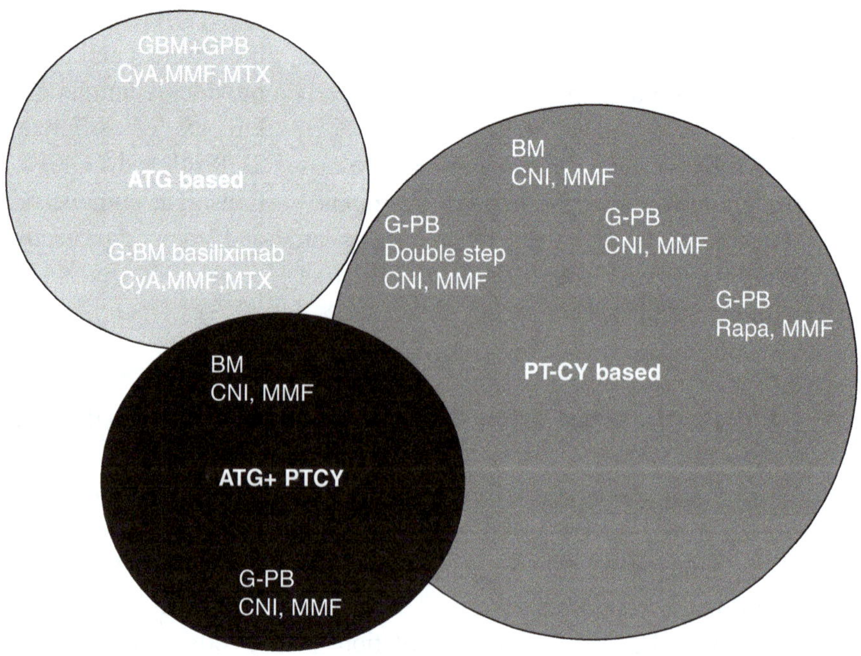

Fig. 65.1 Different modalities of haplo-HSCT. See text for details abbreviations: *ATG* anti-thymocyte globulin, *GBM* G-CSF-mobilized bone marrow, *MTX* methotrexate, *PT-CY* post transplant cyclophosphamide, *CNI* calcineurin inhibitor, *MMF* mycophenolate, *Rapa* rapamycin

CSA, MTX, and MMF with the addition of basiliximab, an anti-CD25 antibody. The same GvHD prophylaxis has been reported by an Italian consortium (Di Bartolomeo et al. 2010): acute GvHD grade II–IV and III–IV was, respectively, 24% and 5%, which is extremely low for family HLA-haplotype mismatch, T-cell-replete transplants. The TRM was not negligible, being 30% for "standard" and 45% for "high-risk" patients (Di Bartolomeo et al. 2010). Overall 3-year survival was 54% for standard and 33% for high-risk patients. Di Bartolomeo et al. used for most patients a conditioning regimen combining TT, IV BU, and FLU (TBF), originally described by Sanz and coworkers for cord blood transplants (Sanz et al. 2012).

65.3.2 Post transplant Cyclophosphamide (PT-CY) Based

The use of PT-CY on day +3 and +4 after an unmanipulated haplo-HSCT has been pioneered by the Baltimore group. It is based on the idea that high-dose CY (50 mg/kg) will kill alloreactive T-cells proliferating on day +3 and +4 after the transplant, whereas stem cells would be protected because they are not proliferating and with a high concentration of aldehyde dehydrogenase.

In 2001, the Baltimore group published their first clinical study and showed that PT-CY was able to protect patients from GvHD after haplo-HSCT (Luznik et al. 2001). Again, this was not picked up immediately, not until 2008 when a joint Baltimore Seattle study showed that haplo-HSCT in Hodgkin's lymphoma (HL) produces DFS superior to sibling or unrelated transplants (Chiusolo et al. 2018): not only GvHD could be prevented, but GvL seemed superior, at least in patients with HL.

There have been numerous variations of the Baltimore protocol (Fig. 65.1) with use of G-PB instead of BM, rapamycin, and MMF, instead of a CNI (Figs. 65.2 and 65.3), the use of a MAC regimen instead of the NMA regimen of Baltimore.

All these platforms seem to achieve a high rate of engraftment, but severe acute GvHD can vary from as low as 3% to as high as 30%. A modified PT-CY regimen has recently been reported in patients with AML (Chiusolo et al. 2018): in this multicenter retrospective study on 150 patients, CSA was administered on day 0, MMF on day +1, and PT-CY on days +3 and +5 (Fig. 65.1). The MA regimen consisted mainly of TBF: the rate of leukemia relapse was extremely low in remission patients (Chiusolo et al. 2018). The major difference here lies in the CSA given before PT-CY and in the two doses of PT-CY spaced on days +3 and +5. It should be noted that this regimen is safe when using BM as a stem cell source, with acute GvHD III–IV rates of 3%; however, it is not known what the outcome would be with PB as a stem cell source, since CSA will protect some

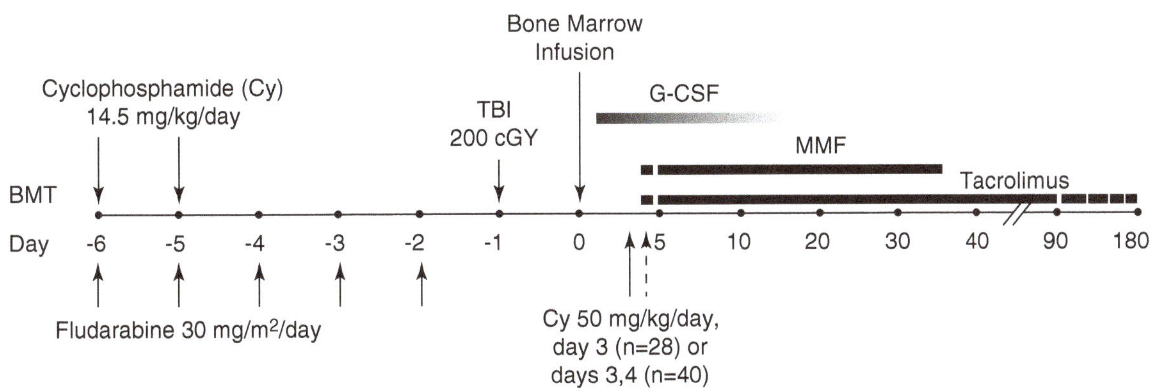

Fig. 65.2 The original Baltimore protocol consisting of CY 14.5 mg/kg × 2, fludarabine 30 mg/m^2 × 5, and total body irradiation (TBI) 2 Gy day −1. CY 50 mg/kg days +3 and +4 and CSA, MMF starting day +5. GCSF starts on day +6. From Luznik et al. (2001)

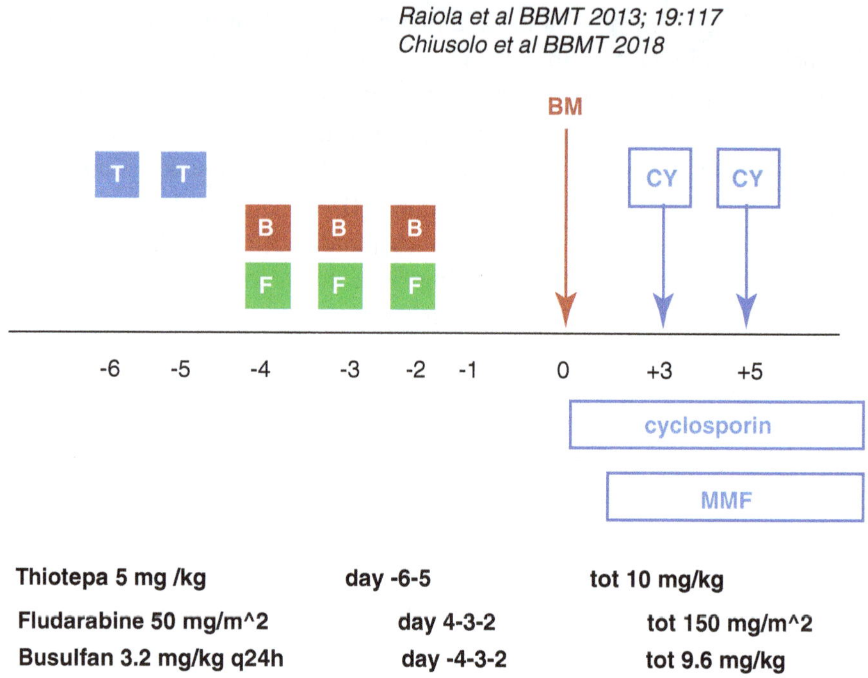

Fig. 65.3 Modified PT-CY regimen. Thiotepa (T), busulfan (B), and fludarabine (F) followed by unmanipulated haploidentical BM. Cyclosporin on day 0, mycophenolate on day +1, and CY 50 mg/kg on days +3 and +5

T-cells from PT-CY purging, and these may produce a beneficial GvL effect but also cause detrimental GvHD.

65.3.3 ATG + PT-CY

Some centers are combining the two basic platforms (PT-CY and ATG) and early results seem promising. The Baltimore group is using this combination for patients with sickle cell disease, in the attempt of avoiding GvHD completely. Also, the group in Saint-Antoine, Paris, is using a combination of ATG 2.5 mg/kg and PT-CY, CSA, and MMF for patients with acute leukemia undergoing a MAC haplo-HSCT (Duléry et al. 2018).

65.4 Other Relevant Aspects of Haplo-HSCT

65.4.1 Choice of the Best Haploidentical Donor

The EBMT ALWP has established younger donor age and kinship, as a major determinant of outcome for leukemia patients grafted from haploidentical donor (Canaani et al. 2018).

The Beijing group has confirmed younger age to be relevant, using their ATG-based platform together with a mismatch for non-inherited maternal antigen (NIMA) (Wang et al. 2014).

The age, CMV status, and ABO matching are general rules which should always be considered: a CMV+ patient should be grafted with a CMV+ donor, if available, and a CMV- patient with a CMV− donor.

Table 65.1 summarizes the most relevant general and immunologic criteria for donor selection in haplo-HSCT.

Table 65.1 Criteria for donor selection

(a) Immunologic criteria (only in malignancies)
1. Presence of NK alloreactivity (KIR/KIR-L mismatch in GvH direction)
2. Larger size of NK alloreactive subset
3. KIR haplotype
4. Higher B content value in B haplotype donors
5. Presence of educated KIR2DS1 in case of C2+ patient
6. Higher % NK cells and T lymphocytes

(b) General criteria
7. Donor/recipient HCMV serology
8. Donor age
9. Donor sex
10. Donor/recipient body weight

65.4.1.1 Natural Killer (NK)

Natural killer (NK) cells are the first post-HSCT cellular population, reconstituting antiviral and antitumor activity. In this setting, donor NK cell inhibitory receptors mismatched for cognate HLA class I ligands play a key role in the graft-versus-leukemia (GVL) effect. Remarkably, these cells may be uniquely poised to enhance GVL without eliciting GvHD because healthy non-hematopoietic tissues lack activating receptor ligands present on tumor cells.

Over 20 years ago, Moretta et al. 1995 described the concept of NK cells' alloreactivity, showing that defined NK cell subsets were able to kill in vitro allogeneic lymphoblasts. (Ruggeri et al. 2016) first reported the positive impact of KIR ligand-mismatched donor NK cell alloreactivity after TCD haplo-HSCT resulting in a lower risk of relapse and a better OS in adult with AML. Of note, only patients receiving a transplant from a donor who showed NK cell alloreactivity against recipient cells displayed an efficient GVL effect. This happens, for example, in the presence of a KIR-HLA-I (KIR-L) mismatch in the donor-versus-recipient direction. Thus, in donor/patient pairs with KIR-HLA-I mismatch, the event-free survival (EFS) rate was 60%, while in the absence of such mismatch, it was less than 5%.

However, the contribution of NK cell alloreactivity on HSCT outcome is still controversial due to different evaluation criteria, the nature of KIR/KIR ligand genetic combinations studied, and NK cell repertoire size. Given the central role of NK cell alloreactivity in preventing leukemia relapse, in the setting of haplo-HSCT, it is crucial to determine in different potential donors if alloreactive NK cells are present and the size of such alloreactive populations. More recently, in addition to the flow analysis of the alloreactive NK cell populations, other selection criteria have been added (Table 65.1). Among these, the presence of a KIR B haplotype has been shown to be associated with a relevant improvement of the survival in both adult AML and pediatric ALL.

While the antileukemic activity of NK cells and the role of KIR are well known and established by several groups, their impact in preventing graft failure and/or infections in patients affected by nonmalignant disorders remains unclear.

65.4.2 Comparison of ATG-Based Versus PT-CY-Based Platforms

The EBMT Acute Leukemia Working Party has compared these two platforms in a recent study (Ruggeri et al. 2017). In a Cox analysis, ATG-based haplo grafts had a higher risk of failure, in terms of LFS (RR 1.48, $p = 0.03$), GvHD relapse-free survival (RR 1.45, $p = 0.03$), and OS (HR 1.43, $p = 0.06$): there was for all end points a very strong center effect ($p < 0.001$), suggesting that a learning curve is required for optimal results in haplo-HSCT.

65.4.3 Bone Marrow or Peripheral Blood

There are now two studies comparing BM versus PB for unmanipulated haplo-HSCT: the EBMT study (Ruggeri et al. 2018) shows increased GvHD II–IV and III–IV with PB, same chronic GvHD, same relapse, and same 2-year OS (55% and 56%). The CIBMTR shows increased GvHD II–IV, but not III–IV with PB grafts, increased chronic GvHD, and reduced relapse (Bashey et al. 2017): survival at 2 years also in this study is quite similar, 54% vs 57%.

Key Points

- Following the pioneering work of the Perugia group, HLA-haplotype mismatch family transplants are rapidly increasing in numbers, due to improved platforms in both TCD, as well as unmanipulated grafts, with encouraging results in most centers.
- This is true with different stem cell sources, different conditioning regimens, and different GvHD prophylaxes:

in one word, there is more than one way to perform haplo-HSCT.

- One important question is how haplo-HSCT compare with unrelated donor grafts, and to answer this question, randomized trials have been designed and are about to start.
- One should consider that HLA-haplotype mismatch transplants remain an alternative donor procedure and should be regarded as such: complications, including blood stream infections, invasive fungal disease, viral infections, GvHD, and toxicity may occur with significant frequency and expose the patients to the risk of TRM. For this reason, HLA-haplotype mismatch grafts, whether TCD or unmanipulated, should be performed in centers with expertise in MUD or CB HSCT and should follow clinical protocols.

So, it seems that one can use both stem cell sources, with some difference in the short term (more GvHD with PB) and perhaps some differences in the long term (cGvHD and relapse): at the end survival seems comparable.

References

Aversa F, Tabilio A, Velardi A, et al. Treatment of high risk acute leukemia with T-cell-depleted stem cells from related donors with one fully mismatched HLA haplotype. N Engl J Med. 1998;339:1186–93.

Aversa F, Terenzi A, Tabilio A, et al. Full haplotype-mismatched hematopoietic stem-cell transplantation: a phase II study in patients with acute leukemia at high risk of relapse. J Clin Oncol. 2005;23:3447–54.

Bashey A, Zhang MJ, McCurdy SR, et al. Mobilized peripheral blood stem cells versus unstimulated bone marrow as a graft source for T-cell–replete haploidentical donor transplantation using post-transplant cyclophosphamide. J Clin Oncol. 2017;35:3002–9.

Bertaina A, Merli P, Rutella S, et al. HLA-haploidentical stem cell transplantation after removal of αβ+ T and B cells in children with nonmalignant disorders. Blood. 2014;124:822–6.

Bethge WA, Haegele M, Faul C, et al. Haploidentical allogeneic hematopoietic cell transplantation in adults with reduced-intensity conditioning and CD3/CD19 depletion: fast engraftment and low toxicity. Exp Hematol. 2006;34:1746–52.

Canaani J, Savani BN, Labopin M, et al. Donor age determines outcome in acute leukemia patients over 40 undergoing haploidentical hematopoietic cell transplantation. Am J Hematol. 2018;93:246–53.

Chiusolo P, Bug G, Olivieri A, et al. A modified post-transplant cyclophosphamide regimen, for unmanipulated haploidentical marrow transplantation, in acute myeloid leukemia: a multicenter study. Biol Blood Marrow Transplant. 2018;24:1243–9.

Ciceri F, Labopin M, Aversa F, Acute Leukemia Working Party (ALWP) of European Blood and Marrow Transplant (EBMT) Group, et al. A survey of fully haploidentical hematopoietic stem cell transplantation in adults with high-risk acute leukemia: a risk factor analysis of outcomes for patients in remission at transplantation. Blood. 2008;112:3574–81.

Ciceri F, Bonini C, Stanghellini MT, et al. Infusion of suicide-gene-engineered donor lymphocytes after family haploidentical haemopoietic stem-cell transplantation for leukaemia (the TK007 trial): a non-randomised phase I-II study. Lancet Oncol. 2009;10:489–500.

Di Bartolomeo P, Santarone S, De Angelis G, et al. Unmanipulated bone marrow transplantation from haploidentical related donors for patients with high risk hematologic malignancies. Blood. 2010;116:2350.

Di Ianni M, Falzetti F, Carotti A, et al. Tregs prevent GvHD and promote immune reconstitution in HLA-haploidentical transplantation. Blood. 2011;117:3921–8.

Duléry R, Ménard AL, Chantepie S, et al. Sequential conditioning with thiotepa in T cell- replete hematopoietic stem cell transplantation for the treatment of refractory hematologic malignancies: comparison with matched related, haplo-mismatched, and unrelated donors. Biol Blood Marrow Transplant. 2018;24(5):1013–21.

Federmann B, Hägele M, Pfeiffer M, et al. Immune reconstitution after haploidentical hematopoietic cell transplantation: impact of reduced intensity conditioning and CD3/CD19 depleted grafts. Leukemia. 2011;25:121–9.

Federmann B, Bornhauser M, Meisner C, et al. Haploidentical allogeneic hematopoietic cell transplantation in adults using CD3/CD19 depletion and reduced intensity conditioning: a phase II study. Haematologica. 2012;97:1523–31.

Feucht J, Opherk K, Lang P, et al. Adoptive T-cell therapy with hexon-specific Th1 cells as a treatment of refractory adenovirus infection after HSCT. Blood. 2015;125:1986–94.

Ji S-Q, Chen H-R, Yan H-M, et al. Anti-CD25 monoclonal antibody (basiliximab) for prevention of graft-versus-host disease after haploidentical bone marrow transplantation for hematological malignancies. Bone Marrow Transplant. 2005;36:349–54.

Leen AM, Christin A, Myers GD, et al. Cytotoxic T lymphocyte therapy with donor T cells prevents and treats adenovirus and Epstein-Barr virus infections after haploidentical and matched unrelated stem cell transplantation. Blood. 2009;114:4283–92.

Li Pira G, Malaspina D, Girolami E, et al. Selective depletion of αβ T cells and B cells for human leukocyte antigen-haploidentical hematopoietic stem cell transplantation. A three-year follow-up of procedure efficiency. Biol Blood Marrow Transplant. 2016;22:2056–64.

Locatelli F, Pende D, Mingari MC, et al. Cellular and molecular basis of haploidentical hematopoietic stem cell transplantation in the successful treatment of high-risk leukemias: role of alloreactive NK cells. Front Immunol. 2013;4:15.

Lu D-P, Dong L, Wu T, et al. Conditioning including antithymocyte globulin followed by unmanipulated HLA-mismatched/haploidentical blood and marrow transplantation can achieve comparable outcomes with HLA-identical sibling transplantation. Blood. 2006;107:3065–73.

Luznik L, Jalla S, Engstrom LW, et al. Durable engraftment of major histocompatibility complex-incompatible cells after nonmyeloablative conditioning with fludarabine, low-dose total body irradiation, and posttransplantation cyclophosphamide. Blood. 2001;98:3456–64.

Martelli MF, Di Ianni M, Ruggeri L, et al. HLA-haploidentical transplantation with regulatory and conventional T-cell adoptive immunotherapy prevents acute leukemia relapse. Blood. 2014;124:638–44.

Moretta A, Sivori S, Vitale M, et al. Existence of both inhibitory (p58) and activatory (p50) receptors for HLA-C molecules in human natural killer cells. J Exp Med. 1995;182:875–84.

Passweg JR, Baldomero H, Gratwohl A, European Group for Blood and Marrow Transplantation (EBMT), et al. The EBMT activity survey: 1990–2010. Bone Marrow Transplant. 2012;47:906–23.

Perruccio K, Tosti A, Burchielli E, et al. Transferring functional immune responses to pathogens after haploidentical hematopoietic transplantation. Blood. 2005;106:4397–06.

Reisner Y, Hagin D, Martelli M. Haploidentical hematopoietic transplantation: current status and future perspectives. Blood. 2011;118:6006–17.

Ruggeri L, Capanni M, Urbani E, et al. Effectiveness of donor natural killer cell alloreactivity in mismatched hematopoietic transplants. Science. 2002;295:2097–100.

Ruggeri L, Mancusi A, Urbani E, Velardi A. Identifying NK alloreactive donors for haploidentical hematopoietic stem cell transplantation. Methods Mol Biol. 2016;1393:141–5.

Ruggeri A, Sun Y, Labopin M, et al. Post-transplant cyclophosphamide versus anti-thymocyte globulin as graft-versus-host disease prophylaxis in haploidentical transplant. Haematologica. 2017;102:401–10.

Ruggeri A, Labopin M, Bacigalupo A, et al. Bone marrow versus mobilized peripheral blood stem cells in haploidentical transplants using posttransplantation cyclophosphamide. Cancer. 2018;124:1428–37.

Sanz J, Boluda JCH, Martín C, et al. Single-unit umbilical cord blood transplantation from unrelated donors in patients with hematological malignancy using busulfan, thiotepa, fludarabine and ATG as myeloablative conditioning regimen. Bone Marrow Transplant. 2012;47:1287–93.

Wang Y, Chang YJ, Xu LP, et al. Who is the best donor for a related HLA haplotype-mismatched transplant? Blood. 2014;124:843–50.

66 Photopheresis in Adults and Pediatrics

Hildegard Greinix

66.1 Introduction

Extracorporeal photopheresis (ECP) is a leukapheresis-based treatment that has been used during the last decades by many clinicians. Based on results of a prospective, multicenter, international clinical trial in patients with cutaneous T-cell lymphoma (CTCL), ECP was approved by the FDA as the first cellular immunotherapy for cancer in 1988 (Edelson et al. 1987). During the last decades, ECP has been investigated worldwide for prevention and treatment of a variety of T-cell-mediated diseases including acute and chronic GvHD, solid organ and tissue transplantation, systemic sclerosis, systemic lupus erythematodes, and Crohn's disease (Knobler et al. 2014). Administering ECP to patients suffering of these diseases revealed promising results both in prospective and retrospective single and multicenter clinical studies. Despite its frequent use, the mode of action of ECP remains elusive including reduction of pro-inflammatory cytokines and induction of anti-inflammatory cytokines and modulation of immune cell populations.

H. Greinix (✉)
Division of Hematology, Medical University of Graz, Graz, Austria
e-mail: hildegard.greinix@medunigraz.at

66.2 Technical Aspects

During ECP the patient's blood is collected via an antecubital vein or via a permanent catheter, and the white blood cells are separated from the red blood cells and plasma by centrifugation in a device that is specifically constructed for the procedure (Knobler et al. 2014; Schoonemann 2003). Collected mononuclear cells (MNCs) using either continuous or discontinuous cell separators are then exposed ex vivo to a photosensitizing agent, 8-methoxypsoralen (8-MOP), which is added directly to the buffy coat/plasma fraction followed by photoactivation with ultraviolet A (UV-A) irradiation and then reinfusion of the photoactivated product (Schoonemann 2003).

ECP has originally been developed as a single procedure which combines the separation of the MNCs from the whole blood with irradiation of the 8-MOP-treated leukapheresis products within a single machine ("closed system of ECP"). The "offline technique" (two-step method) of ECP treatment includes as the first step cell separation with a standard blood cell separator that can also be used for the collection of peripheral blood stem cells. The apheresis product is transferred into another disposable, 8-MOP is added, and irradiation is performed with a separate machine at a dosage of 2 J/cm^2. After irradiation transfusion of the treated cells is carried out manually by a standard transfusion set. Both ECP techniques have demonstrated clinical efficacy, but almost all clinical studies have been performed with the single

E. Carreras et al. (eds.), *The EBMT Handbook*, https://doi.org/10.1007/978-3-030-02278-5_66

ECP technique, and studies comparing both systems are almost completely lacking (Schoonemann 2003; Andreu et al. 1994; Brosig et al. 2016).

66.3 Results of ECP in Acute GvHD

To date, no consensus on the optimal choice of agents for salvage therapy of steroid-refractory acute GvHD has been reached, and treatment choices are based on physician's experience, risk of toxicity and potential exacerbation of pre-existing comorbidity, interactions with other agents, and ease of use (Martin et al. 2012). During the last years, more and more HSCT centers have administered ECP to patients with steroid-refractory acute GvHD. Results of larger prospective studies on the use of ECP in this indication are shown in Table 66.1. The intensified schedule of ECP with two to three treatments per week on a weekly basis significantly improved response rates in patients with GI involvement and grade IV acute GvHD (Greinix et al. 2006).

In a systematic review of prospective studies including 6 studies with 103 patients given ECP for steroid-refractory acute GvHD, an overall response rate (ORR) of 69% was achieved including ORR for skin, liver, and GI involvement of 84%, 55%, and 65%, respectively (Abu-Dalle et al. 2014). Compared to anticytokine treatment, administration of ECP for steroid-refractory acute GvHD not only achieved significantly higher ORR (66% vs 32%) and CR (54% vs 20%), but ECP was also an independent predictor of response and survival and was associated with significantly lower NRM and superior survival in steroid-refractory grade II acute GvHD (Jagasia et al. 2013). Compared to other IST, ECP has an excellent safety profile with limited toxicity concerns, no increased concerns for viral reactivations, and no documented interaction with other drugs (Martin et al. 2012).

66.4 Results of ECP in Chronic GvHD

Although many therapeutic options have been reported for salvage treatment of steroid-refractory chronic GvHD, no single class of IS agent has been established as standard therapy (Wolff et al. 2011). ECP represents a frequently used therapeutic approach for treatment of chronic GvHD patients failing corticosteroids (Table 66.2) (Knobler et al. 2014; Wolff et al. 2011; Greinix et al. 1998; Flowers et al. 2008; Jagasia et al. 2009; Greinix et al. 2011). Most of the clinical experience in ECP treatment of steroid-refractory chronic GvHD patients is based on retrospective analyses with consistently high response rates in up to 80% of patients with cutaneous manifestations and substantial improvement in sclerodermatous skin involvement (Knobler et al. 2014; Wolff et al. 2011).

Table 66.1 Results of second-line treatment of acute GvHD using extracorporeal photopheresis

Author (year)	No. of patients	CR skin no. (%)	CR liver no. (%)	CR gut no. (%)	OS%
Salvaneschi (2001)	9	6/9 (67)	1/3 (33)	3/5 (60)	67
Dall'Amico (2002)	14	10/14 (71)	4/7 (57)	6/10 (60)	57
Messina et al. (2003)	33	25/33 (76)	9/15 (60)	15/20 (75)	69 at 5 y
Greinix et al. (2006)	59	47/57 (82)	14/23 (61)	9/15 (60)	47 at 5 y
Garban (2005)	12	8/12 (67)	0/2 (0)	2/5 (40)	42
Kanold (2007)	12	9/10 (90)	5/9 (56)	5/6 (83)	75 at 8.5 m
Calore (2008)	15	12/13 (92)		14/14 (100)	85 at 5 y
Perfetti (2008)	23	15/23 (65)	3/11 (27)	8/20 (40)	48 at 37 m
Gonzalez-Vicent (2008)	8	8/8 (100)	2/2 (100)	4/7 (57)	38
Perotti (2010)	50	39/47 (83) (1)	16/24 (67) (1)	8/11 (73) (1)	64 at 1 y
Jagasia (2013)	57	38/57 (67) (1)	38/57 (67) (1)	38/57 (67) (1)	59 at 2 y
Calore (2015)	72	50/64 (78)	10/12 (84)	42/55 (76)	71 at 5 y

Abbreviations: *No* number, *CR* complete resolution, *OS* overall survival, *y* years, *m* months
Results were provided as complete and partial resolution.

Table 66.2 Results of use of extracorporeal photopheresis in chronic GvHD

Author (year)	No of patients	CR/PR skin (%)	CR/PR liver (%)	CR/PR oral (%)	ORR (%)
Greinix et al. (1998)	15	80	70	100	na
Salvaneschi (2001)	14	83	67	67	64
Messina (2003)	44	56	60	–	57
Seaton (2003)	28	48	32	21	36
Apisarnthanarax (2003)	32	59	0	na	56
Foss (2005)	25	64	0	46	64
Rubegni (2005)	32	81	77	92	69
Greinix (2006)	47	93	84	95	83
Couriel (2006)	71	57	71	78	61
Kanold (2007)	15	75	82	86	50
Perseghin (2007)	25	67	67	78	73
Flowers (2008)	48	40	29	53	40
Jagasia (2009)	43				65
Perotti (2010)	23	96	100	80	69
Dignan (2012)	82	92	na	91	74
Greinix (2011)	29	31	50	70	na
Del Fante (2012)	102	na	na	na	81
Ussowicz (2013)	13	67	89	86	69
Hautmann (2013)	32	59	100	60	44
Dignan (2014)	38	65	-	29	50

Abbreviations: *No* number, *CR* complete resolution, *PR* partial resolution, *ORR* overall response rate, *na* not available

In a multicenter, randomized, controlled, prospective phase II study of ECP in 95 patients with steroid-refractory/dependent/intolerant chronic GvHD, significantly more patients in the ECP arm achieved a complete or partial response of cutaneous manifestations ($p < 0.001$) as well as a 50% reduction in steroid dose and at least a 25% decrease in total skin score ($p = 0.04$) by week 12 (Greinix et al. 1998). A steroid-sparing effect of ECP has also been reported by other investigators (Knobler et al. 2014; Wolff et al. 2011; Flowers et al. 2008; Jagasia et al. 2009).

In a systematic review of prospective studies on the use of ECP in patients with chronic GvHD, an ORR of 71% in cutaneous, 62% in GI, 58% in hepatic, 63% in oral mucosal, and 45% in musculoskeletal manifestations of chronic GvHD was reported (Abu-Dalle et al. 2014). Rate of IS discontinuation was 23% and ECP was tolerated excellently. In another meta-analysis high response rates in cutaneous and extracutaneous manifestations of chronic GvHD including 48% of responses in lung involvement were confirmed (Del Fante et al. 2016). The ECP schedule in chronic GvHD is empirical ranging from multiple treatments per week on a weekly basis to two treatments biweekly and in case of response prolongation of the treatment interval to 4–6 weeks, respectively. No clear association between ECP dose intensity and response has been reported. Higher response rates were achieved in steroid-refractory patients given ECP earlier in the course of their disease (Malik et al. 2014; Messina et al. 2003). Improvements in quality of life and survival in ECP responders have been reported (Knobler et al. 2014; Wolff et al. 2011; Greinix et al. 1998; Malik et al. 2014; Messina et al. 2003).

ECP is a safe and efficacious treatment for patients with chronic GvHD with steroid-sparing capacity. Transient hypotension during treatment and mild anemia and/or thrombocytopenia have been reported as side effects of ECP. Prospective clinical studies are warranted to assess the efficacy of ECP in well-defined cohorts of chronic GvHD patients treated earlier in the course of their disease. Recently, Jagasia and colleagues reported first results of a randomized, controlled, multicenter study in NIH-defined moderate/severe chronic GvHD patients given ECP in the study arm in combination with standard of care IS (Jagasia et al. 2017). Besides an ORR of 74%, and thus, a promising efficacy ECP demonstrated to be safe and tolerated well.

66.5 Conclusions

ECP has been used for over 30 years in the treatment of CTCL, acute and chronic GvHD, and solid organ transplant rejection. Multiple scientific organizations recommend its use due to ECP's efficacy and excellent safety profile (Knobler et al. 2014). Due to the lack of interactions with other agents and the avoidance of general IS, ECP compares favorably with other IS strategies, supporting its increasingly frequent use as second-line therapy of steroid-refractory/dependent acute and chronic GvHD. Of note, the corticosteroid-sparing potential of ECP has been confirmed in numerous retrospective and prospective studies and translates into immediate clinical benefit for patients with GvHD as well as a reduction of transplant-associated morbidity and mortality.

No general recommendation can be made on treatment schedule due to missing evidence. Ideally, ECP treatment should be initiated as early as possible after the indication is confirmed. Especially in patients with steroid-refractory acute GvHD, earlier treatment onset and an intensified weekly ECP schedule resulted in improved response rates and patients' outcome. Prospective studies on the use of ECP as upfront treatment in GvHD are warranted as well as its investigation for prophylactic/preemptive use during allo-HSCT.

Key Points

- ECP is a safe and efficacious adjunct therapy of steroid-refractory acute and chronic GvHD.
- Results in upfront therapy of chronic GvHD are promising.

References

Abu-Dalle I, Reljic T, Nishihori T, et al. Extracorporeal photopheresis in steroid-refractory acute or chronic graft-versus-host disease: Results of a systematic review of prospective studies. Biol Blood Marrow Transplant. 2014;20:1677–86.

Andreu G, Leon A, Heshmati F, et al. Extracorporeal photochemotherapy: evaluation of two techniques and use in connective tissue disorders. Transfus Sci. 1994;15:443–54.

Apisarnthanarax N, Donato M, Korbling M, et al. Extracorporeal photopheresis therapy in the management of steroid-refractory or steroid-dependent cutaneous chronic graft-versus- host disease after allogeneic stem cell transplantation: feasibility and results. Bone Marrow Transplant. 2003;31:459–65.

Brosig A, Hähnel V, Orsó E, et al. Technical comparison of four different photopheresis systems. Transfusion. 2016;56:2510–9.

Calore E, Calo A, Tridello G, et al. Extracorporeal photochemotherapy may improve outcome in children with acute GVHD. Bone Marrow Transplant. 2008;42:421–5.

Calore E, Marson P, Pillon M, et al. Treatment of acute graft-versus-host disease in childhood with extracorporeal photochemotherapy/photopheresis: the Padova experience. Biol Blood Marrow Transplant. 2015;21:1963–72.

Couriel DR, Hosing C, Saliba R, et al. Extracorporeal photochemotherapy for the treatment of steroid-resistant chronic GVHD. Blood. 2006;107:3074–80.

Dall'Amico R, Messina C. Extracorporeal photochemotherapy for the treatment of graft-versus-host disease. Ther Apher. 2002;6:296–304.

Del Fante C, Galasso T, Bernasconi P, et al. Extracorporeal photopheresis as a new supportive therapy for bronchiolitis obliterans syndrome after allogeneic stem cell transplantation. Bone Marrow Transplant. 2016;51:728–31.

Dignan FL, Greenblatt D, Cox M, et al. Efficacy of bimonthly extracorporeal photopheresis in refractory chronic mucocutaneous GVHD. Bone Marrow Transplant. 2012;47:824–30.

Dignan FL, Aguilar S, Scarisbrick JJ, et al. Impact of extracorporeal photopheresis on skin scores and quality of life in patients with steroid-refractory chronic GVHD. Bone Marrow Transplant. 2014;49:704–8.

Edelson R, Berger C, Gasparro F, et al. Treatment of cutaneous T-cell lymphoma by extracorporeal photochemotherapy. Preliminary results. N Engl J Med. 1987;316:297–303.

Flowers MED, Apperley J, von Besien K, et al. A multicenter prospective phase 2 randomized study of extracorporeal photopheresis for treatment of chronic graft-versus-host disease. Blood. 2008;112:2667–74.

Foss FM, DiVenuti GM, Chin K, et al. Prospective study of extracorporeal photopheresis in steroid-refractory or steroid-resistant extensive chronic graft-versus-host disease: analysis of response and survival incorporating prognostic factors. Bone Marrow Transplant. 2005;35:1187–93.

Garban F, Drillat P, Makowski C, et al. Extracorporeal chemophototherapy for the treatment of graft-versus-host disease: hematologic consequences of short-term, intensive courses. Haematologica. 2005;90:1096–101.

Greinix HT, Volc-Platzer B, Rabitsch W, et al. Successful use of extracorporeal photochemotherapy in the treatment of severe acute and chronic graft-versus-host disease. Blood. 1998;92:3098–104.

Greinix HT, Knobler RM, Worel N, et al. The effect of intensified extracorporeal photochemotherapy on long-term survival in patients with severe acute graft-versus-host disease. Haematologica. 2006;91: 405–8.

Greinix HT, van Besien K, Elmaagacli AH, et al. Progressive improvement in cutaneous and extracutaneous chronic graft-versus-host disease after a 24-week course of extracorporeal photopheresis–results of a crossover randomized study. Biol Blood Marrow Transplant. 2011;17:1775–82.

Gonzalez-Vicent M, Ramirez M, Perez A, et al. Extracorporeal photochemotherapy for steroid-refractory graft-versus-host disease in low-weight pediatric patients. Immunomodulatory effects and clinical outcome. Haematologica. 2008;93:1278–80.

Hautmann AH, Wolff D, Hahn J, et al. Extracorporeal photopheresis in 62 patients with acute and chronic GVHD: Results of treatment with the COBE Spectra system. Bone Marrow Transplant. 2013;48: 439–45.

Jagasia MH, Savani BN, Stricklin G, et al. Classic and overlap chronic graft-versus-host disease (cGVHD) is associated with superior outcome after extracorporeal photopheresis (ECP). Biol Blood Marrow Transplant. 2009;15:1288–95.

Jagasia M, Greinix H, Robin M, et al. Extracorporeal photopheresis versus anticytokine therapy as a second-line treatment for steroid-refractory acute GVHD: a multicentre comparative analysis. Biol Blood Marrow Transplant. 2013;19:1124–33.

Jagasia M, Greinix H, Scheid C, et al. A randomized controlled study of extracorporeal photopheresis (ECP) therapy with UVADEX (methoxsalen) for National Institutes of Health (NIH)-graded moderate to severe chronic graft-versus-host disease (cGvHD). Blood. 2017;130:1970.

Kanold J, Merlin E, Halle P, et al. Photopheresis in pediatric graft-versus- host disease after allogeneic marrow transplantation: clinical practice guidelines based onfield experience and review of the literature. Transfusion. 2007;47:2276–89.

Knobler R, Berlin G, Calzavara-Pinton P, et al. Guidelines on the use of extracorporeal photopheresis. JEADV. 2014;28(Suppl 1):1–37.

Malik MI, Litzow M, Hogan W, et al. Extracorporeal photopheresis for chronic graft-versus-host disease: a systematic review and meta-analysis. Blood Res. 2014;49:100–6.

Martin PJ, Rizzo JD, Wingard JR, et al. First-and second-line systemic treatment of acute graft-versus-host disease: recommendations of the American Society of Blood and Marrow Transplantation. Biol Blood Marrow Transplant. 2012;18:1150–63.

Messina C, Locatelli F, Lanino E, et al. Extracorporeal photochemotherapy for paediatric patients with graft-versus-host disease after haematopoietic stem cell transplantation. Br J Haematol. 2003;122:118–27.

Perfetti P, Carlier P, Strada P, et al. Extracorporeal photopheresis for the treatment of steroid refractory acute GVHD. Bone Marrow Transplant. 2008;42:609–17.

Perotti C, Del Fante C, Tinelli C, et al. Extracorporeal photochemotherapy in graft- versus-host disease: a longitudinal study on factors influencing the response and survival in pediatric patients. Transfusion. 2010;50:1359–69.

Perseghin P, Galimberti S, Balduzzi A, et al. Extracorporeal photochemo-therapy for the treatment of chronic graft-versus-host disease: Trend for a possible cell dose-related effect? Ther Apher Dial. 2007;11:85–93.

Rubegni P, Cuccia A, Sbano P, et al. Role of extracorporeal photochemotherapy in patients with refractory chronic graft-versus-host disease. Br J Haematol. 2005;130:271–5.

Salvaneschi L, Perotti C, Zecca M, et al. Extracorporeal photochemotherapy for treatment of acute and chronic GVHD in childhood. Transfusion. 2001;41:1299–305.

Schoonemann F. Extracorporeal photopheresis technical aspects. Transfus Apher Sci. 2003;28:51–61.

Seaton ED, Szydlo RM, Kanfer E, et al. Influence of extracorporeal photopheresis on clinical and laboratory parameters in chronic graft-versus-host disease and analysis of predictors of response. Blood. 2003;102:1217–23.

Ussowicz M, Musiał J, Mielcarek M, et al. Steroid-sparing effect of extracorporeal photopheresis in the therapy of graft-versus-host disease after allogeneic hematopoietic stem cell transplantation. Transplant Proc. 2013;45:3375–80.

Wolff D, Schleuning M, von Harsdorf S, et al. Consensus conference on clinical practice in chronic GVHD: second-line treatment of chronic graft-versus-host disease. Biol Blood Marrow Transplant. 2011;17:1–17.

67 Overweight and Obese Patients

Claudia Langebrake

67.1 Introduction

"More obese people in the world than underweight" was the headline on BBC News on April 1, 2016. This statement is based on a study comparing the prevalence of BMI categories of more than 19.2 million adult participants in 186 of 200 countries (N. C. D. Risk Factor Collaboration 2016). Comparing the age-standardised mean BMI by country in 1975 and 2014, there is a significant increase in both men (21.7 vs 24.2 kg/m^2) and women (22.1 vs 24.4 kg/m^2). Looking for the proportion of overweight in selected industrialised countries, it is estimated that the prevalence of overweight and obesity in the USA will exceed 70% in 2020, followed by England and Australia. Korea, France and Italy are projected to have less than 50% of the population being overweight (Lyman and Sparreboom 2013).

Obesity is associated with a significant increase in morbidity (including metabolic diseases and cancer) and mortality. It has been estimated that worldwide 481,000 (3.6%) of all new cancer cases in 2012 were attributable to excess body mass index (BMI) (Arnold et al. 2015).

C. Langebrake (✉)
Department of Stem Cell Transplantation and Hospital Pharmacy, University Medical Centre Hamburg-Eppendorf, Hamburg, Germany
e-mail: c.langebrake@uke.de

67.1.1 Definitions and Size Describers of Obesity

Classification of overweight and obesity is usually based on BMI that is calculated using height and weight of an individual. The World Health Organization (WHO), defines adults according to their BMI as:

- Normal weight with 18.5–24.9 kg/m^2
- Overweight with 25–29.9 kg/m^2
- Obese with ≥30 kg/m^2

However, one has to keep in mind that although BMI has been shown to correlate with SC fat (but not with percentage body fat), in individuals with greater muscle mass, women or the elderly, BMI might not be the best describer, as muscle mass is more dense than fat mass. In those people, percent body fat would better describe body composition, but direct measurement is usually not readily available as it requires advanced technical equipment (e.g. hydrodensitometry, skinfold measurement, bioelectrical impedance analysis or dual-energy X-ray absorptiometry) (Hanley et al. 2010). As a consequence, indirect measures of body composition, like BMI or ideal body weight (IBW), remain the standard, as they are easy to calculate.

E. Carreras et al. (eds.), *The EBMT Handbook*, https://doi.org/10.1007/978-3-030-02278-5_67

67.2 Influence of Overweight and Obesity on the Pharmacokinetics of Drugs

Obesity is associated with physiological changes that can alter the pharmacokinetic parameters of many drugs (Hanley et al. 2010; Green and Duffull 2004; Han et al. 2007; Alobaid et al. 2016). Observed physiological changes in obese patients influencing pharmacokinetic behaviour of drugs and resulting consequences for drug dosing are summarised in Table 67.1.

Nevertheless, it has to be kept in mind that the effects of physiological changes are usually drug specific and that for the majority of drugs both pharmacokinetic and clinical data in obese patients are sparse. Due to unusual distribution processes, the kinetics of drugs is difficult to predict in obese patients.

The impact of obesity on GFR as well as on tubular secretion is not completely understood. Discrepant results regarding GFR in obese as compared with normal-weight individuals might be explained by estimating GFR using serum creatinine, as no instrument has been validated for obesity. Especially, if using weight-based formulas like the widespread Cockroft-Gault formula, GFR will be overestimated if total body weight is used, but underestimated if ideal body weight is used. But also the use of weight-independent formulas, as MDRD (Modification of Diet in Renal Disease) or CKD-EPI (Chronic Kidney Disease Epidemiology Collaboration), which has been shown to result in more reliable estimates, has limitations: As the GFR is provided in ml/min/1.73 m^2, the possibly incorrect calculation of body surface area in the obese might negatively influence the results.

Taken together, there is only limited evidence-based information about drug clearance in obese patients due to restrictions of clinical trials and the lack of pharmacokinetic (PK) analyses. It is important to remember that there is no single-size descriptor for all drugs.

Table 67.1 Physiological changes in obese individuals influencing pharmacokinetics of drugs

	Changes in obese patients	Consequences for drug dosing
Absorption	– Increased gastrointestinal blood flow – Accelerated gastric emptying	– Only little data on oral bioavailability – For a couple of drugs including CSA, midazolam or propranolol, no differences in oral bioavailability have been observed
Distribution	– Hydrophilic drugs: Vd is similar in normal-weight and obese patients – Moderate or high lipophilic drugs: significant differences in Vd – Tissue blood flow may be reduced – Obesity does not appear to have impact on plasma protein binding	– Vd is important for the determination of a loading dose, in order to achieve a rapid and adequate exposition – Vd changes are drug specific (attributable to the physicochemical properties of the drug)
Clearance (renal and hepatic)	– Altered hepatic blood flow – TBW-proportional increase in phase II metabolism – GFR and renal perfusion similar, but imprecision in GFR estimation (see text above) – Obese individuals exhibit higher absolute drug clearance – Clearance does not increase linearly with TBW – Clearance and lean body weight are linearly correlated	– Elimination of hydrophilic and extensively renally cleared drugs mainly depends upon renal function – No apparent relationship between lipophilicity and clearance mechanism – Essential parameter to determine maintenance dose – Physicochemical attributes of drugs have little impact on clearance

GFR glomerular filtration rate, *TBW* total body weight, *Vd* volume of distribution

67.3 Recommendations for Drug Dosing

Besides the above-described physicochemical attributes and pharmacokinetic (PK) properties, recommendations from the literature and plasma concentration monitoring are important to determine drug dosing in morbidly obese patients (Hanley et al. 2010; Green and Duffull 2004; Han et al. 2007).

67.3.1 Which Weight to Use for Calculation?

For some drugs, the use of adjusted ideal body weight (AIBW) resulted in similar drug exposure in obese as compared to normal-weight patients (Pai and Bearden 2007; Polso et al. 2014; Bearden and Rodvold 2000): This is, for example, true for aminoglycosides, acyclovir (Turner et al. 2016) or liposomal AmB. AIBW is calculated by adding 25–40% of the difference between total body weight (TBW) and IBW to the IBW. This method is also well examined using population PK models for busulfan (Nguyen et al. 2006). On the other hand, initial vancomycin dosing should be based on TBW with subsequent therapeutic drug monitoring (Polso et al. 2014; Rybak et al. 2009). However, for many drugs the optimal basis for dose calculation has still to be determined.

67.3.2 Impact on Drug Dosing of Chemotherapy

The majority of dosing recommendations in obese patients exist for antimicrobial drugs (Alobaid et al. 2016; Pai and Bearden 2007; Polso et al. 2014; Bearden and Rodvold 2000; Falagas and Karageorgopoulos 2010) and for conventional chemotherapy (Griggs et al. 2012). The American Society of Clinical Oncology (ASCO) published the following main statements in 2012 guidelines:

- Dose should be selected according to body surface area (BSA) using actual body weight.
- Dose reductions should be based on toxicity and comorbidities independent of the obesity status.
- There is no evidence that obese patients experience increased toxicity when actual weight is used for calculation of chemotherapy.

However, some limitations have to be kept in mind, as (1) there are no RCTs comparing actual body weight with other adjusted dosing approaches in obese patients, (2) recommendations are based on subgroup analyses of obese patients from RCTs or observational studies using actual versus adjusted weight calculation and (3) there are no recommendations for HSCT conditioning.

One case report described drug dosing morbidly of an obese patient undergoing allo-HSCT (Langebrake et al. 2011). Here it was observed that for hydrophilic and extensively renally cleared drugs, standard dosages for adult patients or dosing based on ideal body weight can be used. For more lipophilic drugs like CSA or digitoxin, it could be shown that after achieving sufficient plasma levels using high initial doses, maintenance doses similar to those used in normal-weight patients are sufficient. Monitoring of plasma concentrations is highly recommended for drugs with a narrow therapeutic index.

67.3.3 Preparative Regimens Prior to HSCT

In patients undergoing auto- or allo-HSCT, specific features and purposes have to be taken into account. In auto-HSCT, high-dose chemotherapy aims to reduce tumour burden, while in allo-HSCT, therapeutic effect is based on donor immune cells and myeloablation.

The ASBMT reviewed the current published literature on dosing of pharmacologic agents used for HCT preparative regimens in obese patients in 2014. They concluded that dose adjustments were usually performed empirically or have been extrapolated from published data in non-transplant patients. Therefore, evidence for clear standards or dosing guidelines are currently not available as there are insufficient data to determine optimal drug dosing in obese patients undergoing HSCT (Bubalo et al. 2014). Nevertheless, consensus dosing recommendations were given (see Table 67.2).

Recently, the approach to use AIBW-based BSA for dose calculation of MEL prior to auto-HSCT has been shown to be non-inferior as compared to the nonobese population in terms of 3-year event-free survival (Shultes et al. 2018).

Even for ATG, TBW for dose calculation is recommended by ASBMT. However, from a PK point of view, it would be more reasonable to use the IBW, as ATG has a volume of distribution that is almost equal to the whole blood volume. Recently, it has been proposed to rather base ATG dosing on absolute lymphocyte count, as this is the target of ATG (Kennedy et al. 2018).

Reports of obese patients undergoing HCT are challenging to interpret because of the heterogeneity of obesity definitions, underlying diseases, graft sources and chemotherapy regimens employed. Compared with normal-weight patients, it appears that obese patients undergoing allo-HSCT have a higher risk of non-relapse mortality and inferior survival, whereas those receiving auto-HSCT appear to have equivalent outcomes. Another important limitation for interpretation of published data is that there is no consistent standard for calculating chemotherapy dose in this group. Therefore, it is recommended that future studies utilise more consistent and biologically relevant definitions of obesity and that the PK and pharmacodynamics of specific conditioning regimens be studied (Weiss et al. 2013). In clinical practice, about 80% of HSCT centres routinely perform dose adjustment for obesity; however, the methods used for determining the weight for chemotherapy calculation are different among the transplant centres (Shem-Tov et al. 2015).

Table 67.2 Overview of volume of distribution

Drug	Vd[a]	Recommendation (ASBMT 2014) Bubalo et al. (2014)
Alemtuzumab	Low	Flat dosing
Amsacrine	High	n.a.
ATG	Low	TBW (for mg/kg)
Busulfan	Medium	– AIBW25 in adults (obese and nonobese) for mg/kg – TBW (for BSA) – PK targeting for regimens >12 mg/kg PO equivalent
Carboplatin	Low	TBW (for BSA)
Carmustine	High	TBW (for BSA), unless >120% IBW, then AIBW25
Clofarabine	High	TBW (for BSA)
Cyclophosphamide	Medium	– 200 mg/kg: lesser of IBW or TBW – 120 mg/kg: either IBW or TBW until >120% IBW and then dose based on AIBW25 (former is preferred for adults, latter for children)
Cytarabine	High	TBW (for BSA)
Etoposide	Low-medium	– AIBW25 for mg/kg – TBW (for BSA)
Fludarabine	High	TBW (for BSA)
Melphalan	Medium	TBW (for BSA)
Pentostatin	Medium	TBW (for BSA)
Thiotepa	Medium	TBW (for BSA), unless >120% IBW, then AIBW40 for BSA
Treosulfan	Medium	n.a.

[a]*Vd* volume of distribution (low, <0.3 L/kg; medium, 0.3–1.5 L/kg; high, >1.5 L/kg), and recommendations for dose calculation for adults according to ASBMT. *AIBW25* adjusted ideal body weight 25%, *AIBW40* adjusted ideal body weight 40%, *BSA* body surface area, *IBW* ideal body weight, *n.a.* not available, *PO* per os, *TBW* total body weight

Key Points

- Obesity is associated with a significant increase in morbidity (including metabolic diseases and cancer) and mortality.
- Indirect measures of body composition, like BMI or ideal body weight, remain the standard, as they are easy to calculate.
- There is only limited evidence-based information about drug clearance in obese patients due to restrictions of clinical trials and the lack of pharmacokinetic analyses.
- Evidence for clear standards or dosing guidelines are currently not available as there are insufficient data to determine optimal drug dosing in obese patients undergoing HSCT.
- Despite that, in clinical practice, about 80% of HSCT centres routinely perform dose adjustment for obesity. However, the methods used for determining the weight for chemotherapy calculation are different among the transplant centres.

References

Alobaid AS, Wallis SC, Jarrett P, et al. Effect of obesity on the pharmacokinetics of antimicrobials in critically ill patients: a structured review. Int J Antimicrob Agents. 2016;47:259–68.

Arnold M, Pandeya N, Byrnes G, et al. Global burden of cancer attributable to high body-mass index in 2012: a population-based study. Lancet Oncol. 2015;16:36–46.

Bearden DT, Rodvold KA. Dosage adjustments for antibacterials in obese patients: applying clinical pharmacokinetics. Clin Pharmacokinet. 2000;38:415–26.

Bubalo J, Carpenter PA, Majhail N, et al. Conditioning chemotherapy dose adjustment in obese patients: a review and position statement by the American Society for Blood and Marrow Transplantation practice guideline committee. Biol Blood Marrow Transplant. 2014;20:600–16.

Falagas ME, Karageorgopoulos DE. Adjustment of dosing of antimicrobial agents for bodyweight in adults. Lancet. 2010;375:248–51.

Green B, Duffull SB. What is the best size descriptor to use for pharmacokinetic studies in the obese? Br J Clin Pharmacol. 2004;58:119–33.

Griggs JJ, Mangu PB, Temin S, Lyman GH, et al. Appropriate chemotherapy dosing for obese adult patients with cancer: American Society of Clinical Oncology clinical practice guideline. J Clin Oncol. 2012;30:1553–61.

Han PY, Duffull SB, Kirkpatrick CM, Green B. Dosing in obesity: a simple solution to a big problem. Clin Pharmacol Ther. 2007;82:505–8.

Hanley MJ, Abernethy DR, Greenblatt DJ. Effect of obesity on the pharmacokinetics of drugs in humans. Clin Pharmacokinet. 2010;49:71–87.

Kennedy VE, Chen H, Savani BN, et al. Optimizing antithymocyte globulin dosing for unrelated donor allogeneic hematopoietic cell transplantation based on recipient absolute lymphocyte count. Biol Blood Marrow Transplant. 2018;24:150–5.

Langebrake C, Bernhardt F, Baehr M, et al. Drug dosing and monitoring in obese patients undergoing allogenic stem cell transplantation. Int J Clin Pharm. 2011;33:918–24.

Lyman GH, Sparreboom A. Chemotherapy dosing in overweight and obese patients with cancer. Nat Rev Clin Oncol. 2013;10:451–9.

N. C. D. Risk Factor Collaboration. Trends in adult body-mass index in 200 countries from 1975 to 2014: a pooled analysis of 1698 population-based measurement studies with 19.2 million participants. Lancet. 2016;387:1377–96.

Nguyen L, Leger F, Lennon S, Puozzo C. Intravenous busulfan in adults prior to haematopoietic stem cell transplantation: a population pharmacokinetic study. Cancer Chemother Pharmacol. 2006;57:191–8.

Pai MP, Bearden DT. Antimicrobial dosing considerations in obese adult patients. Pharmacotherapy. 2007;27:1081–91.

Polso AK, Lassiter JL, Nagel JL, et al. Impact of hospital guideline for weight-based antimicrobial dosing in morbidly obese adults and comprehensive literature review. J Clin Pharm Ther. 2014;39:584–608.

Rybak M, Lomaestro B, Rotschafer JC, et al. Therapeutic monitoring of vancomycin in adult patients: a consensus review of the American Society of Health-System Pharmacists, the Infectious Diseases Society of America, and the Society of Infectious Diseases Pharmacists. Am J Health Syst Pharm. 2009;66:82–98.

Shem-Tov N, Labopin M, Moukhtari L, et al. Chemotherapy dose adjustment for obese patients undergoing hematopoietic stem cell transplantation: a survey on behalf of the Acute Leukemia Working Party of the European Society for Blood and Marrow Transplantation. Oncologist. 2015;20:50–5.

Shultes KC, Arp C, Stockerl-Goldstein K, et al. Impact of dose-adjusted melphalan in obese patients undergoing autologous stem cell transplantation. Biol Blood Marrow Transplant. 2018;24:687–93.

Turner RB, Cumpston A, Sweet M, et al. Prospective, controlled study of acyclovir pharmacokinetics in obese patients. Antimicrob Agents Chemother. 2016;60:1830–3.

Weiss BM, Vogl DT, Berger NA, et al. Trimming the fat: obesity and hematopoietic cell transplantation. Bone Marrow Transplant. 2013;48:1152–60.

68 HSCT in Elderly Patients

Rafael F. Duarte and Isabel Sánchez-Ortega

68.1 Introduction

The hematological malignancies which are the most common indications for auto- and allo-HSCT (e.g., AML/MDS, NHL, MM, and others) are diagnosed at a median age greater than 65 years old. Thus, if classical chronological age exclusion criteria were followed, a majority of patients with these malignancies would not be offered a HSCT, despite it being their treatment of choice and in many cases their only curative option (Sureda et al. 2015). While elderly patients are more likely to face toxic effects from HSCT, this risk must be considered and balanced against the poor outcome of transplant candidates with these malignancies who do not proceed to HSCT.

68.2 HSCT Activity in Elderly Patients

Auto- and allo-HSCT annual activity continues to steadily increase in Europe and worldwide with no signs of saturation (Gratwohl et al. 2015). Specifically, in elderly patients, HSCT activity at EBMT centers has increased markedly in the past two decades. Auto-HSCT activity in patients ≥65 years old increased from 3.4% (443 out of 13,163 autologous HSCT) in 2000 to 9.8% (2444 out of 23,883 auto-HSCT) in 2014 (Sánchez-Ortega et al. 2016). Allo-HSCT activity in patients ≥65 years old increased from <1% (37 out of 6413 allo-HSCT) in 2000 to 6.7% (1057 out of 16,765 allogeneic HSCT) in 2014 (Basak et al. 2016). In the USA, over 50% of auto-HSCT for lymphomas and MM were performed in patients over 60 years old and 12% in patients ≥70 years old in 2015 (D'Souza and Zhu 2016). The number of patients aged ≥60 undergoing allo-HSCT doubled in 2007–2013 compared to 2000–2006 (D'Souza and Zhu 2016), and US allografts for patients ≥70 years rose tenfold over the past decade, with AML as the leading indication (Muffly et al. 2016).

Improvements in supportive care, HSC mobilization, and the use of RTC and RIC regimens have contributed to the increase in HSCT activity overall and, in particular, to the increase of HSCT activity rates in elderly patients. With sustained improvement in these areas, and as the population ages, these numbers will only continue to increase.

68.3 HSCT Outcomes in Elderly Patients

Compared to younger adults, elderly patients may have higher overall rates of transplant failure. Potential comorbidities, impaired health,

R. F. Duarte (✉)
Hospital Universitario Puerta de Hierro Majadahonda, Madrid, Spain
e-mail: rduarte.work@gmail.com

I. Sánchez-Ortega
Institut Català d'Oncologia Hospitalet, Barcelona, Spain

E. Carreras et al. (eds.), *The EBMT Handbook*, https://doi.org/10.1007/978-3-030-02278-5_68

and performance status could lead to higher transplant-related morbidity and mortality. In addition, malignancies in elderly patients often have more adverse disease features (e.g., higher-risk cytogenetics and molecular patterns in AML/MDS patients) and may have been treated less aggressively prior to HSCT, which may potentially also increase the risk of disease relapse.

Historically, HSCT outcome analysis in elderly patients has been limited by the fact that these patients are underrepresented in clinical trials and the majority of data come from relatively small series and subgroup analyses of small subsets of elderly patients in larger disease-specific studies including adults of all ages. More recently, HSCT outcomes of elderly patients are being analyzed specifically and have reported feasibility and safety of autologous HSCT in MM patients >65 years (Winn et al. 2015), in selected populations of elderly patients with R/R DLBCL (Chihara et al. 2014), and in R/R HL in patients ≥60 years of age (Martínez et al. 2017). Prospective studies addressing the value of allogeneic HSCT compared to non-transplant approaches are limited and generally restricted to patients <65 years old. Interestingly, several large series in AML/MDS patients reported that NRM and OS were negatively affected by KPS <80–90% but not by chronological age (Heidenreich et al. 2017; McClune et al. 2010). Despite significantly poorer outcomes in older patients, additional trials have also not shown a significant impact of advanced age on major outcomes including NRM (Sorror et al. 2011; Chevallier et al. 2012).

The largest experience reported to date on auto- and allo-HSCT outcomes in elderly patients comes from two EBMT studies including a total of 21,390 auto-HSCT and 6046 allo-HSCT in patients ≥65 years old between 2000 and 2014 (Basak et al. 2016; Sánchez-Ortega et al. 2016). Patient numbers and key HSCT outcomes overall and by age group are presented in Table 68.1.

These studies confirm the feasibility of auto- and allo-HSCT in elderly patients, with acceptable NRM and OS at 1 and 3 years. Multivariate analyses in both studies showed that performance status (i.e., Karnofsky score) had a more significant independent impact on patient outcomes than chronological age. Thus, these data in a large cohort of elderly patients strongly suggest that age per se should not be an exclusion criterion to consider HSCT in this population. Undoubtedly, this is presumably a highly selected fraction of elderly patients considered for auto- and allo-HSCT. Nevertheless, this further endorses the need to assess comorbidity and frailty beyond age in older HSCT candidates to improve outcomes further.

Table 68.1 HSCT outcomes in elderly patients: EBMT experience[a]

Type of HSCT	All cases ≥65 years	Group I 65–69 years	Group II ≥70 years
Autologous, *n*	21,390	17,531	3859
– NRM year 1	4.9%	4.6%	5.9%
– OS year 1	87%	88%	83%
– OS year 3	67%	69%	61%
Allogeneic, *n*	6046	4914	1132
– NRM year 1	27%	26%	29%
– OS year 1	57%	57%	53%
– OS year 3	39%	40%	35%

n number of cases
[a]Basak et al. (2016) and Sánchez-Ortega et al. (2016)

68.4 Assessment of Elderly Candidates for HSCT

In addition to the elements already discussed in Chap. 11 for younger patients, the evaluation and counseling of elderly patients as candidates for auto- and allo-HSCT require the evaluation of additional health domains of interest in patients of advanced age. The following tables address general principles and considerations for evaluation and counseling of these patients, discuss the issue of patient frailty beyond age and comorbidities, and describe the key elements of a multidimensional geriatric assessment in this population.

68.4.1 General Principles and Considerations for Elderly HSCT Candidates

- HSCT decision *should not be driven by chronological age* but by a broader multidimensional assessment including fitness, comorbidities, physiologic reserve, and frailty.
- Elderly patients require *information and counseling in plain language* regarding the HSCT process, donor sources, specific protocol, timeline, risks, benefits, and outcomes.
- They also need information regarding patients' *quality of life outcomes, caregivers, and psychosocial needs*, for which social workers and other support staff will be needed.
- A *multidisciplinary individualized assessment* is required to appropriately address the multidimensional nature of the evaluation of elderly patients.
- Fit older transplant candidates should follow the *same indications for auto- and allo-HSCT as younger adults*.
- In the case of allo-HSCT, particular consideration to *RIC and NMA regimens* is essential, and donor selection must take into account the *age of the donor*, as donor older age may associate with impaired outcomes.
- Outcome analysis in elderly patients may require the use of *clinically relevant composite endpoints* that, beyond survival, incorporate quality of life, good overall mental and physical condition, and freedom from severe complications.

68.4.2 Frailty in Elderly HSCT Candidates

- Frailty is a term used to describe a multidimensional syndrome of loss of physiologic reserves (energy, physical ability, cognition, health) that leads to vulnerability.
- The ability to measure frailty in elderly patients is useful clinically.
- Although it appears to be a valid construct to assess elderly patients, how exactly to define it remains unclear. There is a large abundance of possible scales to measure frailty, which likely reflects uncertainty about the term and its components.
- A. Hedge et al. have recently reported on frailty as the missing piece of pre-HSCT assessment (Hegde and Murthy 2018). Data shows that the prevalence of frailty prior to HSCT in patients ≥50 years old is higher than in the general geriatric population at around 25%. Importantly, age has no effect on prevalence of frailty.
- Frailty is associated with poorer OS even after adjusting for age and HCT-CI and may be associated as well with an increased incidence of disease relapse (Muffly et al. 2014, Hegde and Murthy 2018).

68.4.3 Geriatric Assessment for Elderly HSCT Candidates

68.4.3.1 General Concept

- The geriatric assessment is a multidimensional, multidisciplinary assessment designed to evaluate an older person's functional ability, physical health, cognition, mental health, and socioenvironmental circumstances (Artz 2016).
- The goal of geriatric assessment in this context would be to capture vulnerability pre-HSCT to help deciding on patient suitability for the procedure, as well as to individualize post-HSCT support strategies to prevent complications and reduce transplant-associated morbidity and mortality (Artz 2016).

68.4.3.2 Elements Involved in Elderly HSCT Candidates

- Ensure appropriate performance status (Karnofsky score ≥80).
- Rule out significant comorbidities by the HCT-CI (Sorror et al. 2005), as their prevalence increases with age.
- Assess the modified EBMT (Armand et al. 2014) and the revised PAM scores (Au et al. 2015), as global prognostic models that incorporate both NRM and disease factors.

- Measure functional status by self-reported function and performance-based testing (ability to perform tasks necessary to live independently in the community [i.e., shopping, food preparation, housekeeping, telephone, laundry, transportation and driving, manage finances and medication, number of times a patient can rise from the chair (i.e., timed up and go), gait speed, 6-min walk test, hand grip strength, or provocative cardiopulmonary testing], polypharmacy requirements).
- Cognitive function: if necessary, perform neuropsychological testing and/or consult geriatrics.
- Psychosocial evaluation (assessment of social support, availability of a caregiver, financial matters, psychological disturbances, etc.).
- Nutritional status and weight loss.
- Biomarkers to characterize physiologic age (serum C-reactive protein, ferritin, serum albumin, or protein biomarkers panels in development).

68.4.3.3 Scales

- No standard geriatric assessment scales have been validated for HSCT.
- Most scales available for geriatric assessment in cancer patients are complex and time-consuming, which limits its use in daily practice.
- The Geriatric Assessment in Hematology (GAH) scale is a brief, comprehensive geriatric assessment scale designed and validated for older patients diagnosed with hematological malignancies (MDS, AML, MM, and CLL) (Bonanad et al. 2015).
- The GAH scale includes 30 items grouped into 8 pre-defined dimensions (number of drugs, gait speed, mood, activities of daily living, subjective health status, nutrition, mental status, and comorbidities) and requires a relatively short period of time to be administered in routine clinical practice (10–12 min).
- Thus, the GAH scale could be an interesting tool to assess elderly patients with hematological malignancies who are being considered for transplantation. However, it still needs to be validated in the setting of HSCT.

Key Points

- HSCT activity in elderly patients has increased markedly in the past two decades and is predicted to continue to increase as the population ages, with a sustained improvement in HSCT methodology and care.
- Auto- and allo-HSCT in elderly patients is feasible and has acceptable outcomes.
- Age should not be an exclusion criterion per se to consider elderly patients for HSCT.
- Assessing comorbidity is essential in older HSCT candidates, but adjusting only for comorbidity may not identify frail patients vulnerable to adverse outcomes.
- Frailty is a multidimensional syndrome of loss of physiologic reserves (energy, physical ability, cognition, health) that leads to vulnerability, is higher in HSCT recipients than the general geriatric population, and associates with poorer HSCT outcome.
- Geriatric assessment is a multidimensional, multidisciplinary assessment designed to evaluate an older person's functional ability, physical health, cognition, mental health, and socioenvironmental circumstances.
- The goal of geriatric assessment in HSCT would be to capture vulnerability to pre-HSCT to help deciding on patient suitability for the procedure and to adapt post-HSCT support strategies to improve outcomes.
- Currently, there are no standard geriatric assessment scales validated for HSCT. The GAH scale has been described and validated in elderly patients with hematological malignancies, is relatively simple to apply in clinical practice, and may be a candidate scale for elderly HSCT candidates, validation pending.

References

Armand P, Kim HT, Logan BR, et al. Validation and refinement of the disease risk index for allogeneic stem cell transplantation. Blood. 2014;123:3664–71.

Artz AS. Biologic vs physiologic age in the transplant candidate. Hematology Am Soc Hematol Educ Program. 2016;2016:99–105.

Au BK, Gooley TA, Armand P, et al. Reevaluation of the pretransplant assessment of mortality score after allogeneic hematopoietic transplantation. Biol Blood Marrow Transplant. 2015;21:848–54.

Basak GW, Sánchez-Ortega I, Beohou E, et al. Allogeneic hematopoietic cell transplantation in elderly patients aged 65 and older: a retrospective analysis by the complications and quality of life working party of the EBMT. Blood. 2016;128:681.

Bonanad S, De la Rubia J, Gironella M, et al. Development and psychometric validation of a brief comprehensive health status assessment scale in older patients with hematological malignancies: the GAH scale. J Geriatr Oncol. 2015;6:353–61.

Chevallier P, Szydlo RM, Blaise D, et al. Reduced-intensity conditioning before allogeneic hematopoietic stem cell transplantation in patients over 60 years: a report from the SFGM-TC. Biol Blood Marrow Transplant. 2012;18:289–94.

Chihara D, Izutsu K, Kondo E, et al. High-dose chemotherapy with autologous stem cell transplantation for elderly patients with relapsed/refractory diffuse large B cell lymphoma: a nationwide retrospective study. Biol Blood Marrow Transplant. 2014;20:684–9.

D'Souza A, Zhu X. Current uses and outcomes of hematopoietic cell transplantation (HCT): CIBMTR summary slides. 2016. Available at http://www.cibmtr.org.

Gratwohl A, Pasquini MC, Aljurf M, et al. One million haematopoietic stem-cell transplants: a retrospective observational study. Lancet Haematol. 2015;2:e91–100.

Hegde A, Murthy HS. Frailty: the missing piece of the pre-hematopoietic cell transplantation assessment? Bone Marrow Transplant. 2018;53:3–10.

Heidenreich S, Ziagkos D, de Wreede LC, et al. Allogeneic stem cell transplantation for patients age >/= 70 years with myelodysplastic syndrome: a retrospective Study of the MDS Subcommittee of the Chronic Malignancies Working Party of the EBMT. Biol Blood Marrow Transplant. 2017;23:44–52.

Martínez C, Jorge AS, Pereira A, Hodgkin Lymphoma Subcommittee of Spanish Group of Lymphoma and Bone Marrow Transplantation (GELTAMO), et al. Comorbidities, not age, are predictive of survival after autologous hematopoietic cell transplantation for relapsed/refractory Hodgkin's lymphoma in patients older than 50 years. Ann Hematol. 2017;96:9–16.

McClune BL, Weisdorf DJ, Pedersen TL, et al. Effect of age on outcome of reduced-intensity hematopoietic cell transplantation for older patients with acute myeloid leukemia in first complete remission or with myelodysplastic syndrome. J Clin Oncol. 2010;28:1878–87.

Muffly LS, Kocherginsky M, Stock W, et al. Geriatric assessment to predict survival in older allogeneic hematopoietic cell transplantation recipients. Haematologica. 2014;99:1373–9.

Muffly L, Pasquini MC, Martens M, et al. Increasing use of allogeneic hematopoietic cell transplantation (HCT) in patients age 70 years and older: a CIBMTR study of trends and outcomes. Bone Marrow Transplant. 2016;22:S68–9.

Sánchez-Ortega I, Basak G, Beohou E, et al. Performance status drives the impact of age on the outcomes of autologous hematopoietic cell transplantation in elderly patients aged 65 and older: a retrospective analysis by the Complications and Quality of Life Working Party of the EBMT. Blood. 2016;128:678.

Sorror ML, Maris MB, Storb R, et al. Hematopoietic cell transplantation (HCT)-specific comorbidity index: a new tool for risk assessment before allogeneic HCT. Blood. 2005;106:2912–9.

Sorror ML, Sandmaier BM, Storer BE, et al. Long-term outcomes among older patients following nonmyeloablative conditioning and allogeneic hematopoietic cell transplantation for advanced hematologic malignancies. JAMA. 2011;306:1874–83.

Sureda A, Bader P, Cesaro S, et al. Indications for allo- and auto-SCT for haematological diseases, solid tumours and immune disorders: current practice in Europe, 2015. Bone Marrow Transplant. 2015;50:1037–56.

Winn AN, Shah GL, Cohen JT, et al. The real world effectiveness of hematopoietic transplant among elderly individuals with multiple myeloma. J Natl Cancer Inst. 2015;107:1–6.

Part IX

Indications and Results

Topic leaders: Rafael Duarte and Nicolaus Kröger

Acute Myeloid Leukemia in Adults

69

Jurjen Versluis, Jan J. Cornelissen, Charles Craddock, Miguel Á. Sanz, Jonathan Canaani, and Arnon Nagler

69.1 AML in CR1

Jurjen Versluis, Jan J. Cornelissen

69.1.1 Definition, Subtypes

AML is a malignancy of hematopoietic immature precursors (myeloblasts) that accumulate in the BM at the expense of their normal counterparts. AML is diagnosed by cytomorphology if more than 20% myeloblasts are present in the BM or PB. In addition, immunophenotyping and cytogenetic and molecular characterization are used to identify a number of AML subtypes.

The WHO defines seven major subtypes of AML based largely on genetic, morphological, and cytochemical characteristics of the disease, whereas the most recent update (2016) included a new category termed "myeloid neoplasms with germ line predisposition" (Arber et al. 2016). In addition, risk classification is increasingly done according to the latest European LeukemiaNet (ELN) recommendations, whereby three risk groups are distinguished, including favorable risk, intermediate risk, and adverse risk, largely based on pretreatment cytogenetic abnormalities and aberrations in the *NPM1, FLT3, CEBPA, RUNX1, ASXL1,* and *TP53* genes (Dohner et al. 2017).

69.1.2 Clinical Presentation

The median age at diagnosis is approximately 70 years, and the annual age-standardized incidence rate varies between 3 and 4 cases per 100,000. Patients with AML may present with symptoms such as fatigue and loss of appetite, whereas lymphadenopathy and hepatosplenomegaly may be found by physical examination. Analysis of blood work often reveals thrombocytopenia, anemia, and/or neutropenia. In some patients a serious bleeding diathesis can occur, particularly in the early phase of treatment, because the leukemic blasts are able to activate the coagulation cascade as well as cause hyperfibrinolysis. This particularly occurs in patients with acute promyelocytic leukemia (APL).

J. Versluis · J. J. Cornelissen
Department of Hematology, Erasmus Medical Center Cancer Institute, Rotterdam, The Netherlands

C. Craddock
Centre for Clinical Haematology, Queen Elizabeth Hospital, Birmingham, UK

M. Á. Sanz
Department of Hematology, University Hospital La Fe, University of Valencia, Valencia, Spain

J. Canaani · A. Nagler (✉)
Hematology and BMT Division, Chaim Sheba Medical Center, Tel-Hashomer, Israel
e-mail: Arnon.Nagler@sheba.health.gov.il

E. Carreras et al. (eds.), *The EBMT Handbook*, https://doi.org/10.1007/978-3-030-02278-5_69

69.1.3 First-Line Treatment

Achievement and maintenance of complete remission (CR) are crucial in younger AML patients aged below 60 years, but treatment may largely fail because of relapse from CR rather than primary resistance or treatment-related mortality (TRM).

With modern supportive care, TRM rates average <5%. For 30 years standard induction treatment (to produce CR) has consisted of 7–10 days of the antimetabolite cytosine arabinoside (Ara-C) and 3 days of an anthracycline (i.e., daunorubicin or idarubicin). CR rates with standard induction estimate between 70 and 90%. Favorable-risk patients may experience relatively good outcome with overall survival rates of approximately 60%, whereas outcome for patients with intermediate-risk and adverse-risk AML remains unsatisfactory.

Following the introduction of targeted therapies in other malignancies including TKI in CML, studies to evaluate targeted treatment in AML were initiated 5–10 years ago, and a large randomized study in patients with *FLT3* AML demonstrated a survival benefit for younger AML patients treated with the kinase inhibitor midostaurin in conjunction with intensive induction and consolidation chemotherapy (Stone et al. 2017). That study led to the approval of midostaurin, which has now become standard of care in AML patients with mutated *FLT3*. The ability of the pretreatment features such as incorporated in the ELN risk classification to predict outcome is important to direct treatment decisions; however probably more prognostically important than the pretreatment features is response to treatment (CR vs. lesser degrees of "response") and especially presence, in hematological remission, of "minimal residual disease" (MRD) as assessed by flow cytometry or molecular testing in patients with abnormalities such as mutated *NPM1*.

Allo-HSCT clearly reduces relapse rates but is associated with TRM (see sect. 69.1.4). Patients who do not qualify for HSCT are usually offered intensive consolidation chemotherapy based on high-dose cytarabine (HDAC). The dose of Ara-C has been a subject of study and intense debate questioning the application of dosages exceeding 2 g/m^2, which is now generally considered the upper dose (Lowenberg 2013). Induction chemotherapy in younger patients may include the 3 + 7 scheme, whereas older patients may not tolerate intensive induction therapy and therefore are considered for non-intensive induction. However, it should be noted that also patients above the age of 60 years without comorbidities and no organ dysfunctions may be candidates for intensive therapy, which has been demonstrated to result in superior outcome (Lowenberg et al. 2009). Nevertheless, with a median age of approximately 70 years, most older patients are offered non-intensive therapy. With regard to non-intensive therapy, low-dose cytarabine (LDAC) is generally preferred over best supportive care (BSC) (Burnett et al. 2007). More recently, demethylation agents were compared with LDAC or BSC in older patients with AML and/or MDS, and both azacitidine (AZA) and decitabine showed a modest survival advantage. Although these agents resulted in a small improvement in overall survival, they may be preferred over LDAC or BSC in patients who cannot tolerate intensive induction therapy. At present the demethylating agents are predominantly used in those patients with myelodysplastic features.

69.1.4 HSCT and AML Risk Categories

69.1.4.1 ELN Risk Categories

Previously, conventional cytogenetics and mutations of *NPM1*, *FLT3*-ITD, and *CEBPA* were included in the ELN 2010 risk classification of AML patients (Dohner et al. 2010). The current ELN 2017 risk classification has added mutations in three genes including *RUNX1*, *ASXL1*, and *TP53* (Table 69.1) (Dohner et al. 2017). Similar to the previous risk classification, the ELN 2017 AML risk classification is advocated to be used for risk-stratifying AML and to a risk-adapted treatment approach of patients with AML. Such a risk-adapted treatment approach of patients with AML depends on the risk of relapse of the underlying AML but also on the risk of TRM associated with the applied post-remission treatment. The application of MRD, detected by either multiparametric

Table 69.1 Risk-adapted post-remission treatment for patients with AML in first CR[a]

AML risk classification[b]	MRD status[c]	Preferred post-remission treatment
Favorable		
t(8;21)(q22;q22.1); *RUNX1-RUNX1T1*	Negative	Chemotherapy/auto-HSCT
inv(16)(p13.1q22) or t(16;16)(p13.1;q22); *CBFB-MYH11*		
Mutated *NPM1* without *FLT3*-ITD or with *FLT3*-ITD^{low}	Positive	Allo-HSCT[d], (unless excessive TRM can be predicted)
Biallelic mutated *CEBPA*		
Intermediate		
Mutated *NPM1* and *FLT3*-ITD^{high}	Negative	Allo-HSCT[d] (if acceptable risk of TRM; alternative, chemo/auto-HSCT)
Wild-type *NPM1* without *FLT3*-ITD or with *FLT3*-ITD^{low} (without adverse risk genetic lesions)		
t(9;11)(p21.3;q23.3); *MLLT3-KMT2A*	Positive	Allo-HSCT[e]
Cytogenetic abnormalities not classified as favorable or adverse		
Adverse		
t(6;9)(p23;q34.1); *DEK-NUP214*	Negative	Allo-HSCT[e]
t(v;11q23.3); *KMT2A* rearranged		
t(9;22)(q34.1;q11.2); *BCR-ABL1*	Positive	Allo-HSCT[e]
inv(3)(q21.3q26.2) or t(3;3)(q21.3;q26.2); *GATA2, MECOM(EVI1)*		
−5 or del(5q); −7; −17/abn(17p)		
Complex karyotype, monosomal karyotype		
Wild-type *NPM1* and *FLT3*-ITD^{high}		
Mutated *RUNX1*		
Mutated *ASXL1*		
Mutated *TP53*		

[a]Adapted from Cornelissen et al. 2012a, b), Table 4
[b]Adapted from Dohner et al. (2017), Table 5
[c]Detected with multiparametric flow cytometry or with for qPCR specific markers
[d]Allo-HSCT using HLA-identical sibling or 10/10 MUD donors
[e]Allo-HSCT using HLA-identical sibling, MUD, umbilical cord blood, or haploidentical donors

flow cytometry or quantitative PCR for specific molecular markers, may further improve AML risk classifications. MRD may be detected at time points early after induction treatment to assess the remission status of the AML but also after PRT to detect imminent relapse. Consequently, MRD negativity was introduced as an endpoint in patients with a hematological CR (Dohner et al. 2017).

69.1.4.2 Transplant Risk Categories

The risk-adapted approach of patients with AML in first CR should also include the assessment of TRM for each individual patient. TRM may be attributed to GVHD, infectious complications, organ toxicity, and other causes (Gooley et al. 2010). A number of parameters may relate to allo-HSCT-related TRM, including the procedure (e.g., conditioning regimen, application of TCD), donor characteristics (e.g., HLA-matching), and recipient features (e.g., age and comorbidity). The risk of mortality may be quantified by composite risk scores, which have been established to predict for TRM and overall outcome.

Two generally approved transplant risks were developed and validated, including the EBMT risk score (Gratwohl et al. 1998) and the hematopoietic cell transplantation-comorbidity index (HCT-CI) (Sorror et al. 2005). The EBMT risk score is based on patient and transplantation characteristics, which was developed in CML patients and subsequently validated in other patient groups including AML (Gratwohl et al. 2009). The HCT-CI originated from the Charlson comorbidity index and consists of 17 comorbidities which contribute to a cumulative score (Sorror et al. 2005). The HCT-CI was extensively validated and has been continuously being refined including age, disease status, or biomarkers

(Sorror et al. 2007, 2014). Other groups have also developed predictive models for TRM modifying the weights of the EBMT risk score and the HCT-CI (Barba et al. 2010), whereas others combined transplant-related parameters and patient characteristics (Parimon et al. 2006; Barba et al. 2014; Shouval et al. 2015).

A more sophisticated, machine-based learning model was developed by the EBMT-acute leukemia working party (ALWP) based on 10 variables, which resulted in an alternating decision tree model highly predicting for mortality at 100 days and at 2 years (Shouval et al. 2015).

However, with the introduction of RIC, allo-HSCT is increasingly being applied as post-remission treatment for older or less fit patients with comorbidities. Several groups have reported less predictive power of the EBMT-score and the HCT-CI in these subgroups of patients as a number of comorbidities are less strongly associated with mortality after RIC than after MAC (Gratwohl et al. 2009; Barba et al. 2010; Barba et al. 2014). The EBMT-ALWP has developed an integrated score based on the EBMT risk score and the HCT-CI with increased predictive power in the setting of RIC allo-HSCT (Versluis et al. 2015). The lack of predictive power of the established risk scores and the development of a refined and dedicated model emphasize that prediction of TRM requires a continued reassessment of risk scores in specific patient groups.

69.1.5 HSCT in First-Line AML Treatment: A Risk-Adapted Approach

AML risk classifications are being used for tailoring patients' optimal post-remission treatment, which may include allo-HSCT, auto-HSCT, and continued chemotherapy. Allo-HSCT is the most optimal post-remission treatment for the prevention of relapse due to a potent GVL effect, which has been demonstrated to be exerted irrespective of underlying AML cytogenetic subcategories and MRD status (Cornelissen et al. 2012b; Versluis et al. 2017a). However, absolute estimates of relapse incidence differ and may reflect molecular or cytogenetic differences resulting in resistance of the AML. Although the GVL effect of allo-HSCT is unequivocally present in patients with AML in first CR, concurrent TRM may compromise overall outcome, especially in AML patients with a relatively low incidence of relapse. Thus, a risk-adapted approach of post-remission treatment for patients with AML in first CR should include an assessment of the TRM risk profile in addition to leukemia characteristics and MRD (Cornelissen et al. 2012a; Cornelissen and Blaise 2016). Table 69.1 summarizes a risk-adapted approach based on the latest ELN AML risk classification, MRD status, and the risk for TRM. The risk for TRM should be preferably assessed with dedicated scores for specific subgroups of patients. Patients with MRD are considered high-risk for relapse and preferably receive an allo-HSCT in first CR, unless excessive NRM may be predicted.

Allo-HSCT is generally not being indicated in patients with a favorable AML risk profile; for those patients auto-HSCT or continued chemotherapy may be preferred (Dohner et al. 2017; Cornelissen et al. 2012a; Cornelissen and Blaise 2016). However, favorable-risk patients with persistent MRD may receive an allo-HSCT, especially those patients with a low risk for TRM.

Results of allo-HSCT compared with auto-HSCT or chemotherapy have yielded contradicting results in intermediate-risk patients, especially taking molecular markers into account (Koreth et al. 2009; Schlenk et al. 2008; Rollig et al. 2015; Stelljes et al. 2014; Versluis et al. 2017b). Assessment of the MRD status is strongly advocated for patients with an intermediate-risk AML. Allo-HSCT may be applied in patients with intermediate-risk AML with MRD after induction chemotherapy, except for patients with a high risk for TRM. Allo-HSCT is also preferred for patients with intermediate-risk MRD-negative AML, but auto-HSCT or chemotherapy may be considered when the predicted risk for TRM is high.

Adverse-risk patients with MRD should be transplanted with an allografted as soon as a hematological CR is obtained. Adverse-risk patients without MRD still have a significant risk of relapse and may also receive an allo-HSCT, although patients with a very high risk for TRM may alternatively receive autologous HSCT or a third cycle of chemotherapy.

69.2 Allo-HSCT in Advanced AML

Charles Craddock

69.2.1 Introduction

Allo-HSCT plays an increasingly important role in the management of AML in adults (Cornelissen et al. 2012a). The advent of RIC regimens coupled with increased donor availability has dramatically increased the number of patients in whom allo-HSCT can be contemplated.

At the same molecular characterization at diagnosis coupled with measurable MRD quantitation after induction, chemotherapy has considerably improved our ability to predict relapse risk in patients treated with intensive chemotherapy (IC) alone permitting accurate identification of allo-mandatory patients.

As a result, allo-HSCT in patients with AML in CR1 is an increasingly important personalized component of the treatment algorithm. At the same time, transplantation is also emerging as an important, potentially curative treatment modality in patients with advanced AML.

The increasingly important role of allo-HSCT in the management of AML mandates the development of novel strategies with the potential to improve transplant outcome. Although the last three decades has witnessed a substantial reduction in TRM, the risk of disease relapse post transplant remains stubbornly high and now represents the major cause of treatment failure in patients allografted for AML. There is consequently an urgent requirement to develop novel strategies with the potential to reduce the risk of disease recurrence.

69.2.2 The Role of Allo-HSCT in the Management of AML Beyond CR1

While a small proportion of patients with AML in CR2 achieve long-term survival if treated with salvage chemotherapy alone, compelling data identify allo-HSCT as the preferred curative option (Gale et al. 1996). Long-term survival rates in the region of 30–50% have been reported after both transplantation from either a matched sibling or MUD (Tauro et al. 2005). Encouraging results are also reported in patients transplanted using CBU with a good total nucleated cell dose and, more recently, haploidentical donors. In patients who have achieved a morphological CR2, it is wise to proceed immediately to transplant, providing the patient is fit and a donor has been identified and there is no evidence supporting further courses of chemotherapy prior to transplantation.

While a rigorous comparison of MAC and RIC regimens has not been performed in fit patients under the age of 50, a MAC regimen should probably be preferred. Retrospective studies have demonstrated that auto-HSCT can achieve comparable results to those observed with an allogeneic donor in adults with AML associated with a CBF abnormality, and this can represent an important treatment option in patients with comorbidities or in the absence of a well-matched donor (Gorin et al. 2008), particularly if both the patient and stem cell graft are MRD negative.

Ten to forty percent of adults with newly diagnosed AML fail to achieve a morphological CR after two courses of induction chemotherapy (Ferguson et al. 2016). Factors determining refractoriness to induction therapy include patient age and the presence of an adverse risk karyotype. Although recognized as one of the most important causes of treatment failure, it is perhaps surprising that there is no consensus definition of primary refractory AML (PREF AML). While the International Working Group (IWG) and the European LeukemiaNet (ELN) define resistant disease as persistent leukemic blasts following one course of induction chemotherapy in either the PB or the BM in a patient alive 7 days or more following treatment (Cheson et al. 2003; Dohner et al. 2010), most transplant studies instead have classified PREF AML as a failure to achieve a morphological CR after two induction courses.

The UK NCRI group recently studied more than 8000 patients with the aim of more precisely defining a measure of chemo-refractoriness. Patients with greater than 15% residual blasts or less than a 50% proportional reduction in blast count after the first course of induction chemotherapy were observed to have similar outcomes to patients who fail to achieve a morphological CR after two courses. Such patients were observed to possess genuinely chemo-refractory disease with long-term survival rates <10% if treated with chemotherapy alone (Ferguson et al. 2016). In contrast, patients who fulfilled either definition of refractory disease achieved long-term survival rates in the region of 25–30% after allo-HSCT.

Evidence that allo-HSCT can deliver long-term survival in a significant proportion of patients with PREF AML has been accumulating over the last decade and represents an important advance in management of this sizeable patient population for whom no other effective therapy exists (Craddock et al. 2011; Todisco et al. 2017; Brissot et al. 2017). Nonetheless outcomes in patients allografted for PREF AML remain unsatisfactory, and both TRM and disease relapse continue to represent significant barriers to long-term survival. There is also a lack of clarity concerning which patients with PREF AML are the most likely to benefit from transplantation. Outcome is clearly superior in patients who proceed swiftly to transplant after no more than two courses of IC, and relapse appears to be lower in those with a lower burden of disease at the time of transplantation. Importantly the impact of presentation karyotype and genotype on remains undetermined although some studies, perhaps unsurprisingly, identify worse outcome in patients with a complex karyotype. It is therefore important that further studies examining the impact of presentation karyotype, mutational status, and pre-transplant disease load on outcome after allo-HSCT are prioritized. What is incontrovertible however is that adults with high-risk AML should undergo an urgent search for sibling and URD at presentation so that transplant can be swiftly scheduled if the patients are refractory to chemotherapy.

The optimal conditioning regimen in patients with PREF AML remains a matter of conjecture. While MAC regimens should be preferred in fit patients under the age of 50, encouraging results have also been reported using the sequential FLAMSA regimen which incorporates additional tumor debulking, using Ara-C and amsacrine, prior to a FLU-based RIC regimen (Schmid et al. 2006). Importantly this schedule also incorporates early administration of DLI, at day +120, in patients with no evidence of active GVHD.

69.2.3 Strategies to Prevent Disease Relapse in Patients Allografted for AML

Disease relapse remains the major cause of treatment failure in patients allografted for AML (Cornelissen et al. 2012b). Despite substantial progress in reducing the toxicity of allo-HSCT, the risk of disease recurrence remains stubbornly high, and novel strategies with the potential to reduce the risk of disease recurrence are urgently required (Craddock et al. 2018). Key to the development of effective new interventions is an understanding of both the clinical factors determining disease relapse and an improved understanding of the biology of disease recurrence (Ossenkoppele et al. 2016). In addition to the impact of presentation karyotype, next-generation sequencing (NGS) studies have identified molecular determinants of disease relapse post transplant (Lindsley et al. 2017). Retrospective studies have also demonstrated that pre-transplant MRD is an important predictor of disease relapse after allo-HSCT, although confirmation of these data in prospective trials is still lacking (Walter et al. 2011).

The risk of disease relapse also appears to be impacted by the conditioning regimen, and retrospective studies consistently demonstrate an increased risk of recurrence in patients transplanted using a RIC regimen although recent prospective randomized trials have yielded conflicting data (Fasslrinner et al. 2018; Kroger et al. 2017; Scott et al. 2017). Finally, the intensity of post transplant IS is also a critical factor influencing relapse risk consistent with the exertion of a potent GVL effect in patients allografted for AML (Bacigalupo et al. 1991; Craddock et al. 2010).

A number of novel approaches toward reducing post transplant relapse are currently undergoing evaluation. Firstly, quantitation of pre-transplant MRD status, using immunophenotypic or molecular methodologies, can identify patients with a higher risk of relapse and has resulted in exploration of approaches which reduce the pre-transplant MRD status as a means of improving transplant outcome. Pivotal to the implementation of such strategies are reproducible and accurate measurements of pre-transplant MRD status, and of note novel NGS technologies with improved sensitivity are emerging (Jongen-Lavrencic et al. 2018). Secondly, identification of the optimal conditioning regimen remains key to optimizing transplant outcome. One of the most important considerations in interpretation of comparisons of MAC and RIC regimens will be whether pre-transplant MRD influences patient outcome in a regimen-dependent manner.

Finally, there is increasing interest in the elective administration of pharmacological agents or cellular therapies post transplant. A number of agents are currently under evaluation as post transplant maintenance strategies including targeted therapies such as Flt3 inhibitors or agents with a broader antileukemic activity including demethylating agents such as AZA or checkpoint inhibitors (Craddock et al. 2016; Soiffer et al. 2018). In the future it is likely that the choice of maintenance strategies will be informed by a greater understanding of the biology of disease recurrence. In this context it is of interest that a significant number of patients who relapse post-allograft demonstrate loss or acquisition of candidate driver mutations at the time of relapse (Quek et al. 2016).

69.3 Practical Issues in Allo-HSCT for AML

Jonathan Canaani, Arnon Nagler

69.3.1 Stem Cell Source (See Also Chaps. 14 and 15)

One of the fundamental issues in the initial decision-making for transplantation physicians is the optimal source for procuring the stem cells for transplant. Whereas the initial methodology for donor stem cell procurement involved direct BM harvesting, the introduction of PBSC mobilization more than two decades ago into routine clinical practice has shifted the field toward the latter approach. Indeed, it has been estimated that PBSC is used in more than 75% of allo-HSCT (per National Marrow Donor Program data; http://www.marrow.org).

Whether PBSC are preferable to BM harvesting as the stem cell source for patients with AML is still an open question; however there are several noteworthy facts which need to be mentioned. In patients receiving grafts from MSD, early publications suggested superior engraftment rates in PBSC concomitant to an increased risk of acute and chronic GVHD in some of the studies (Couban et al. 2002). A phase 3 study was conducted by the BMT CTN randomized patients with various myeloid malignancies (including 261 AML patients) to receive PBSC versus BM harvested cells from MUD (Anasetti et al. 2012). The results of this pivotal study revealed comparable rates of survival and relapse between both groups with increased rates of graft failure in the bone marrow group counterbalanced by an increased likelihood of chronic GVHD in the PBSC group. Two analyses from the EBMT and the CIBMTR in the RIC setting also confirmed the absence of a survival difference for either approach (Nagler et al. 2012; Eapen et al. 2015). Thus, it seems reasonable to conclude that at present both stem cell sources are acceptable options to use in AML patients.

69.3.2 Best Donor (See Also Chap. 12)

AML patients referred to transplant are currently candidates for several potential donor sources including HLA MSD, HLA MUD, UCB grafts, and haploidentical donors. Indeed, the rapid evolution of the field of HSCT is possibly best exemplified by the potential donor pool which has expanded from the initial requirement for an HLA-matched sibling to include also MUD, UCB grafts, and more recently also use of haploidentical donors. While MSD and MUD remain the preferred donor source in most clinical settings (Schlenk et al. 2010), the accumulating experience with UCB and haplo donors provides a much-needed donor resource for those patients lacking suitable MSD or MUD donors, a need especially evident in minority populations.

The original pediatric experience with UCB has been successfully translated into adult transplantation protocols both in the RIC and MAC settings (Oran et al. 2011). Published data from a joint CIBMTR/EBMT retrospective study comparing UCB and MUD transplants in over 1500 acute leukemia patients suggested equivalent LFS rates in both groups (Eapen et al. 2010). Of note, UCB patients in this study had higher TRM rates but a lower incidence of acute and chronic GVHD. Interestingly, an analysis in high-risk AML patients who underwent either RIC UCB transplant or RIC MSD/MUD revealed that the incidence of relapse was more than doubled in the UCB group (Devillier et al. 2014), while a CIBMTR/Eurocord retrospective study of patients over the age of 50 showed that UCB transplant is feasible in this age group albeit at the price of an increased rate of TRM and lower LFS rate (Weisdorf et al. 2014). Whether a two-unit UCB transplant is superior to a one-unit UCB transplant is not entirely clear at this point; however a randomized study conducted in pediatric and adolescent patients indicates similar survival and relapse rates between both groups in addition to improved rates of grade III/IV acute and extensive chronic GVHD in those patients receiving a single unit of UCB (Wagner Jr. et al. 2014).

The inherent benefit in using haplo donors is the near-universal availability of several potential donors which could be either siblings, parents, or children dependent on the patient's age. The initial experience with this approach was limited by a substantial component of TRM due to the slow kinetics of immune reconstitution resulting in infectious complications as well as graft rejection (Ciurea et al. 2015). A significant breakthrough was realized with the advent of novel IS modulation approaches such as PT-CY-based (Robinson et al. 2016) and ATG-based protocols (Chang et al. 2014), which via selective in vivo TCD have achieved acceptable rates of engraftment. An evolving body of literature suggests comparable outcomes between haplo transplantation and transplantation from partially HLA MMUD and possibly MUD and MSD as well (Bashey et al. 2013). In conclusion, when available, MSD and 10/10 HLA MUD remain the first choice for donors. For patients lacking MSD/MUD, both UCB and haplo donors are reasonable alternative donor sources.

69.3.3 **Conditioning** (See Also Chap. 13)

The ideal conditioning regimen for patients with AML is a yet unsettled question in the field of transplantation. Yet, the pivotal point to initially consider when deciding on a specific conditioning regimen is whether the patient would be eligible to receive MAC or rather RIC. For younger (less than 45 years of age for most MAC candidates) and fit patients, MAC is the preferred choice given its superior antileukemia activity shown in previous studies (Martino et al. 2013) and especially in light of the recent data presented by the BMT CTN 0901 trialists underscoring the marked relapse-free survival advantage experienced by MAC patients compared to RIC patients (67% vs. 47%) (Scott et al. 2017).

From a toxicity standpoint, older patients derive the most benefit from RIC resulting in more favorable NRM and TRM rates. Notably, the incidence of GVHD, late infectious complications, and CMV reactivation is comparable between MAC and RIC, while the incidence of acute transplant complications (i.e., SOS/VOD, mucositis, IPS, and hemorrhagic cystitis) is more common in MAC and provides the advantage NRM for RIC (Sengsayadeth et al. 2015).

69.3.4 **Graft Versus Host Disease Prophylaxis** (See Also Chap. 25)

Up to 70% of transplanted patients will experience acute GVHD to some extent, and these patients are at a significant risk of morbidity and mortality resulting from this severe inflammatory reaction. Thus, from a therapeutic standpoint, prophylaxis of acute GVHD is one of the crucial intervention points during the process of allo-HSCT. In current practice standard prophylaxis regimens for acute GVHD comprise the dual use of a CNI, namely, CSA or TAC, added to MTX or MMF for the first 180 days following transplantation (Ruutu et al. 2014). Published data from studies conducted two decades ago suggested that TAC/MTX was superior to CSA/MTX in terms of acute GHVD, however this did not translate into a survival advantage, and in fact the latter regimen may be more commonly used among transplant centers (Nash et al. 2000). MMF, an inosine monophosphate dehydrogenase inhibitor, is not often used in the MAC setting, and currently its role is mostly limited to CBT and non-MAC-HSCT. SIR (rapamycin) was evaluated in several phase I/II with non-heterogeneous patient cohorts which limited interpretation of its efficacy; however a phase III BMT CTN study did not show an improvement in the incidence of GVHD over MTX (Cutler et al. 2014).

Whereas the abovementioned therapeutic modalities are quite adept at prevention of acute GVHD, preventing chronic GVHD is still a major challenge with these agents, and thus more specialized strategies to mitigate GVHD have been attempted including TCD accomplished using either ex vivo (via positive selection of CD34-positive cells or through negative depletion of specific T cell subsets) (Saad and Lamb 2017) or in vivo methodologies (by use of TCD drugs such as ALEM or ATG). Recent publications from several phase III studies clearly demonstrate using ATG was beneficial for patients with acute leukemia as well as other hematological malignancies (Kroger et al. 2016). Ex vivo TCD is a promising approach and has been shown to be effective for GVHD prophylaxis in smaller trials (Pasquini et al. 2012), although wider application of this methodology will require further data.

69.4 Acute Promyelocytic Leukemia

Miguel Á. Sanz

69.4.1 Concept and Incidence

APL is a subtype of AML with peculiar clinical and morphological characteristics that presents a specific genetic alteration, the t (15; 17), with its corresponding molecular counterpart, the rearrangement *PML-RARA*, which confer a particular sensitivity to all-*trans* retinoic acid (ATRA) and arsenic trioxide (ATO). It also highlights the presence of a hemorrhagic diathesis associated with a peculiar coagulopathy, which causes a high incidence of hemorrhagic complications at presentation and early during the induction treatment.

APL accounts for 10–15% of AML.

69.4.2 Diagnosis

69.4.2.1 Morphology, Immunophenotyping, and Other Features

M3 typical (hypergranular)	M3 variant (microgranular)
Morphology	
• Cytoplasm with dense granulation. Frequent Auer rods • Reniform or bilobed nucleus	• Cytoplasm with fine granulation or hypogranular. Less frequent Auer rods • Reniform nucleus, bi- or multilobed
Immunophenotyping	
HLA-DR^{-}/CD34^{-}/CD33^{+a}/CD13^{+b}/CD15$^{-/+}$	HLA-DR$^{\pm}$/CD34$^{\pm}$/CD33^{+a}/CD9^{+}/CD2$^{\pm}$/CD13^{+b}/CD56$^{\pm}$
Other associated features	
• Most frequently, low WBC counts • Less frequently, BCR3 isoform	• Most frequently, high WBC counts • Most frequently, BCR3 isoform

[a]Intense and homogeneous expression
[b]Heterogeneous expression

69.4.2.2 Genetic Diagnosis

Conventional cytogenetics t(15;17)(q22;q21)	
Pros	– Very specific
	– Detects additional anomalies in 30% (+8 the most frequent)
Cons	– Low sensitivity (80%)
	– Inadequate, bad metaphases or normal karyotype (false negative) in 20%
FISH *PML-RARA*	
Pros	– Very specific and rapid
Cons	– Not very sensitive and does not provide information about the isoform
RT-PCR	
Pros	– Very specific, rapid, and sensitive
	– Identifies the isoform, which allows MRD monitoring
Cons	– Occasional artifacts and contaminations
Immunostaining with anti-PML antibody (PG-M3)	
Pros	– Very specific, rapid, and cheap
	– Characteristic microspeckled pattern by indirect immunofluorescence
Cons	– Does not provide information about the isoform

69.4.2.3 Other Rearrangements of the RARA Gene on Chromosome 17

Chromosomal abnormality	*RARA* rearrangement
• t(11;17) (q23;q21)	• *PLZF/RARA* (poorly responsive to ATRA)
• t(17;17) (q21;q21)	• *STAT5b/RARA* (poorly responsive to ATRA)
• t(11;17) (q23;q21)	• *KMT2a/RARA* (ATRA sensitivity unknown)
• t(5;17) (q35;q21)	• *NPM/RARA* (ATRA sensitivity unknown)
• t(11;17) (q13;q21)	• *NuMA1-RARA* (ATRA sensitivity unknown)
• t(17;17)(q21;q24)	• *PRKAR1A/RARA* (ATRA sensitive)
• t(X;17)(p11;q21	• *BCOR/RARA* (ATRA sensitive in two cases)
• t(4;17) (q12;q21)	• *FIP1L1/RARA* (ATRA sensitivity unknown)
• t(2;17) (q32;q21)	• *OBFC2A/RARA* (ATRA sensitive in one case)
• t(3;17) (q26;q21)	• *TBLR1/RARA* (insensitive to ATRA)
• t(7;17) (q11;q21)	• *GTF2I/RARA (*ATRA sensitive)
• t(1;17) (q42;q21)	• *IRF2BP2/RARA* (ATRA sensitive)

69.4.3 First-Line Treatment

The European LeukemiaNet (ELN) recommendations in 2009 already recognized the promising results reported in several non-randomized studies using ATRA plus ATO, with or without minimal use of chemotherapy, but the standard of care was still considered the combination of ATRA plus anthracycline-based chemotherapy (Sanz et al. 2009). However recent findings have led to modify this recommendation.

The long-term results of a non-randomized study (Abaza et al. 2017) and two recently reported randomized clinical trials (Lo-Coco et al. 2013; Burnett et al. 2015), comparing the efficacy and safety of ATRA plus ATO versus the standard ATRA plus chemotherapy approach, strongly support the former combination as the new standard of care for patients with low-to-intermediate-risk APL with WBC counts lower than 10×10^9/L at presentation. Nevertheless, in countries where chemotherapy is more affordable than ATO, the classical combination of ATRA and chemotherapy is still an acceptable option. For high-risk patients, however, there are two valid options, either ATRA plus chemotherapy or ATRA plus ATO with a certain amount of cytoreductive chemotherapy, at least during the induction phase.

HSCT is never indicated in patients in CR1, except for the small fraction of patients with persistent RQ-PCR positivity of *PML-RARA* after consolidation (<1%), given the poor prognosis of this subset of patients. HSCT is also indicated in APL patients who relapse and achieve second or subsequent CR.

69.4.4 Salvage Therapy

Apart from patients with MRD positivity at the end of consolidation (molecular persistence), there is a general agreement that patients with the more common molecular or hematological relapse later on require immediate additional treatment, including HSCT. Salvage treatment should be given to attempt to achieve molecular remission as a bridge to HSCT. Salvage treatment with ATRA plus ATO is recommended when ATRA plus chemotherapy has been previously used front-line, whereas ATRA plus chemotherapy would be the option when front-line therapy was ATRA plus ATO.

The use of gemtuzumab ozogamicin may also be considered in both situations, but always as a bridge to HSCT. Based on recent studies, (Yanada et al. 2013; Holter Chakrabarty et al. 2014; Lengfelder et al. 2015) auto-HSCT should be considered the first choice for eligible patients achieving second molecular remission. Patients unsuitable for HSCT and those with a very prolonged CR1 can be managed with some type of continuation therapy which would be chosen taking into account previous treatments and clinical condition.

Allo-HSCT should be reserved for patients with high risk of relapse and low risk of TRM but also as a second option, for those who relapse after an auto-HSCT.

69.4.5 Indications of HSCT

HSCT is never indicated in patients in CR1, except for those patients who do not achieve molecular remission at the end of consolidation (<1%). Indications of HSCT and other recommendations for patients in whom HSCT is indicated are summarized in Table 69.1.

69.4.6 Main Series Reported on HSCT in APL

There are no randomized trials to evaluate the efficacy and safety of the different modalities of HSCT in refractory/relapsed APL. The data come mostly from retrospective studies comparing historical cohorts from registries (Tables 69.2 and 69.3).

Table 69.2 Indications of HSCT in patients with APL

	Auto-HSCT	Allo-HSCT
Not indicated	CR1 in molecular remission	CR1 in molecular remission
Indicated	≥CR2, but in molecular remission	– ≥CR2 with *PML-RARA* (+) after salvage therapy – ≥CR2 if an auto-HSCT has failed previously – ≥CR2 in patients with high risk of relapse and low risk of TRM
Salvage therapy as a bridge to HSCT	Attempt to achieve molecular remission with ATRA plus ATO in patient who relapsed after ATRA plus chemotherapy as front-line therapy, whereas ATRA plus chemotherapy is the option when patients relapse after ATRA plus ATO	Attempt to achieve molecular remission with ATRA plus ATO in patient who relapsed after ATRA plus chemotherapy as front-line therapy, whereas ATRA plus chemotherapy is the option when patients relapse after ATRA plus ATO
Conditioning regimen	Either for use in AML, preferably containing HDAC (e.g., BEA (Gondo et al. 1997): BU/VP/Ara-C)	Either for use in AML
Cell source	Mobilized peripheral blood	Mobilized peripheral blood
Indication of CNS prophylaxis	ITT with MTX, hydrocortisone, and Ara-C, especially in those who presented relapse in CNS	ITT with MTX, hydrocortisone, and Ara-C, especially in those who presented relapse in CNS
Maintenance therapy post-HSCT	Not proven, but conceivable that ATO + ATRA may be effective	Not proven, but conceivable that ATO + ATRA may be effective
Molecular monitoring	Recommended by RQ-PCR at least every 3 months for 2–3 years	Recommended by RQ-PCR at least every 3 months for 2–3 years

Table 69.3 Main series reported on HSCT in APL

Group and reference	Patients	Type of study	Main conclusions
European APL Group (Thomas et al. 2000)	33	– Retrospective – Inclusion of patients from the pre-ATRA era	– Higher morbidity and TRM with allo-HSCT – Short follow-up
EBMT (Sanz et al. 2007)	332	– Retrospective – Only patients of the pre-ATRA era	– Higher TRM but lower relapse rate with allo-HSCT compared with auto-HSCT – Similar EFS
Japan Adult Leukemia Study Group (Yanada et al. 2013)	35	– Prospective, phase II, multicenter – Salvage therapy with ATO+Ida, followed by ATO x 2, HDAC, and auto-HSCT	– Outstanding efficacy and feasibility of the sequential treatment featuring ATO and auto-HSCT for relapsed APL
IBMTR (Holter Chakrabarty et al. 2014)	294	– Retrospective – Only patients of the pre-ATRA era	– Auto-HSCT yields superior OS for APL in CR2
ELN registry (Lengfelder et al. 2015)	155	– Retrospective – Salvage therapy with ATO±ATRA for induction and consolidation followed by auto- or allo-HSCT	– Good but similar results with allo- and auto-HSCT – Unfavorable prognostic impact of PML-RAR positivity at time of HSCT even in the allogeneic setting

References

Abaza Y, Kantarjian H, Garcia-Manero G, et al. Long-term outcome of acute promyelocytic leukemia treated with all-trans-retinoic acid, arsenic trioxide, and gemtuzumab. Blood. 2017;129:1275–83.

Anasetti C, Logan BR, Lee SJ, et al. Peripheral-blood stem cells versus bone marrow from unrelated donors. N Engl J Med. 2012;367:1487–96.

Arber DA, Orazi A, Hasserjian R, et al. The 2016 revision to the World Health Organization classification of myeloid neoplasms and acute leukemia. Blood. 2016;127:2391–405.

Bacigalupo A, Van Lint MT, Occhini D, et al. Increased risk of leukemia relapse with high-dose cyclosporine A after allogeneic marrow transplantation for acute leukemia. Blood. 1991;77:1423–8.

Barba P, Pinana JL, Martino R, et al. Comparison of two pretransplant predictive models and a flexible HCT-CI using different cut off points to determine low-, intermediate-, and high-risk groups: the flexible HCT-CI Is the best predictor of NRM and OS in a population of patients undergoing allo-RIC. Biol Blood Marrow Transplant. 2010;16: 413–20.

Barba P, Martino R, Perez-Simon JA, et al. Combination of the Hematopoietic Cell Transplantation Comorbidity Index and the European Group for Blood and Marrow Transplantation score allows a better stratification of high-risk patients undergoing reduced-toxicity allogeneic hematopoietic cell transplantation. Biol Blood Marrow Transplant. 2014;20:66–72.

Bashey A, Zhang X, Sizemore CA, et al. T-cell-replete HLA-haploidentical hematopoietic transplantation for hematologic malignancies using post-transplantation cyclophosphamide results in outcomes equivalent to those of contemporaneous HLA-matched related and unrelated donor transplantation. J Clin Oncol. 2013;31:1310–6.

Brissot E, Labopin M, Stelljes M, et al. Comparison of matched sibling donors versus unrelated donors in allogeneic stem cell transplantation for primary refractory acute myeloid leukemia: a study on behalf of the Acute Leukemia Working Party of the EBMT. J Hematol Oncol. 2017;10:130.

Burnett AK, Milligan D, Prentice AG, et al. A comparison of low-dose cytarabine and hydroxyurea with or without all-trans retinoic acid for acute myeloid leukemia and high-risk myelodysplastic syndrome in patients not considered fit for intensive treatment. Cancer. 2007;109:1114–24.

Burnett AK, Russell NH, Hills RK, et al. Arsenic trioxide and all-trans retinoic acid treatment for acute promyelocytic leukaemia in all risk groups (AML17): results of a randomised, controlled, phase 3 trial. Lancet Oncol. 2015;16:1295–305.

Chang YJ, Wang Y, Huang XJ. Haploidentical stem cell transplantation for the treatment of leukemia: current status. Expert Rev Hematol. 2014;7:635–47.

Cheson BD, Bennett JM, Kopecky KJ, et al. Revised recommendations of the International Working Group for diagnosis, standardization of response criteria, treatment outcomes, and reporting standards for therapeutic trials in acute myeloid leukemia. J Clin Oncol. 2003;21:4642–9.

Ciurea SO, Zhang MJ, Bacigalupo AA, et al. Haploidentical transplant with posttransplant cyclophosphamide vs matched unrelated donor transplant for acute myeloid leukemia. Blood. 2015;126:1033–40.

Cornelissen JJ, Blaise D. Hematopoietic stem cell transplantation for patients with AML in first complete remission. Blood. 2016;127:62–70.

Cornelissen JJ, Gratwohl A, Schlenk RF, et al. The European LeukemiaNet AML Working Party consensus statement on allogeneic HSCT for patients with AML in remission: an integrated-risk adapted approach. Nat Rev Clin Oncol. 2012a;9:579–90.

Cornelissen JJ, Breems D, van Putten WL, et al. Comparative analysis of the value of allogeneic hematopoietic stem-cell transplantation in acute myeloid leukemia with monosomal karyotype versus other cytogenetic risk categories. J Clin Oncol. 2012b;30:2140–6.

Couban S, Simpson DR, Barnett MJ, et al. A randomized multicenter comparison of bone marrow and peripheral blood in recipients of matched sibling allogeneic transplants for myeloid malignancies. Blood. 2002;100:1525–31.

Craddock C, Nagra S, Peniket A, et al. Factors predicting long-term survival after T-cell depleted reduced intensity allogeneic stem cell transplantation for acute myeloid leukemia. Haematologica. 2010;95:989–95.

Craddock C, Labopin M, Pillai S, et al. Factors predicting outcome after unrelated donor stem cell transplantation in primary refractory acute myeloid leukaemia. Leukemia. 2011;25:808–13.

Craddock C, Jilani N, Siddique S, et al. Tolerability and clinical activity of post-transplantation azacitidine in patients allografted for acute myeloid leukemia treated on the RICAZA Trial. Biol Blood Marrow Transplant. 2016;22:385–90.

Craddock C, Hoelzer D, Komanduri KV. Current status and future clinical directions in the prevention and treatment of relapse following hematopoietic transplantation for acute myeloid and lymphoblastic leukemia. Bone Marrow Transplant. 2018. https://doi.org/10.1038/s41409-018-0203-8.

Cutler C, Logan B, Nakamura R, et al. Tacrolimus/sirolimus vs tacrolimus/methotrexate as GVHD prophylaxis after matched, related donor allogeneic HCT. Blood. 2014;124:1372–7.

Devillier R, Harbi S, Furst S, et al. Poor outcome with nonmyeloablative conditioning regimen before cord blood transplantation for patients with high-risk acute myeloid leukemia compared with matched related or unrelated donor transplantation. Biol Blood Marrow Transplant. 2014;20:1560–5.

Dohner H, Estey EH, Amadori S, et al. Diagnosis and management of acute myeloid leukemia in adults:

recommendations from an international expert panel, on behalf of the European LeukemiaNet. Blood. 2010;115:453–74.

Dohner H, Estey E, Grimwade D, et al. Diagnosis and management of AML in adults: 2017 ELN recommendations from an international expert panel. Blood. 2017;129:424–47.

Eapen M, Rocha V, Sanz G, et al. Effect of graft source on unrelated donor haemopoietic stem-cell transplantation in adults with acute leukaemia: a retrospective analysis. Lancet Oncol. 2010;11:653–60.

Eapen M, Logan BR, Horowitz MM, et al. Bone marrow or peripheral blood for reduced-intensity conditioning unrelated donor transplantation. J Clin Oncol. 2015;33:364–9.

Fasslrinner F, Schetelig J, Burchert A, et al. Long-term efficacy of reduced-intensity versus myeloablative conditioning before allogeneic haemopoietic cell transplantation in patients with acute myeloid leukaemia in first complete remission: retrospective follow-up of an open-label, randomised phase 3 trial. Lancet Haematol. 2018;5:e161–9.

Ferguson P, Hills RK, Grech A, et al. An operational definition of primary refractory acute myeloid leukemia allowing early identification of patients who may benefit from allogeneic stem cell transplantation. Haematologica. 2016;101:1351–8.

Gale RP, Horowitz MM, Rees JK, et al. Chemotherapy versus transplants for acute myelogenous leukemia in second remission. Leukemia. 1996;10:13–9.

Gondo H, Harada M, Miyamoto T, et al. Autologous peripheral blood stem cell transplantation for acute myelogenous leukemia. Bone Marrow Transplant. 1997;20:821–6.

Gooley TA, Chien JW, Pergam SA, et al. Reduced mortality after allogeneic hematopoietic-cell transplantation. N Engl J Med. 2010;363:2091–101.

Gorin NC, Labopin M, Frassoni F, et al. Identical outcome after autologous or allogeneic genoidentical hematopoietic stem-cell transplantation in first remission of acute myelocytic leukemia carrying inversion 16 or t(8;21): a retrospective study from the European Cooperative Group for Blood and Marrow Transplantation. J Clin Oncol. 2008;26:3183–8.

Gratwohl A, Hermans J, Goldman JM, et al. Risk assessment for patients with chronic myeloid leukaemia before allogeneic blood or marrow transplantation. Chronic Leukemia Working Party of the European Group for Blood and Marrow Transplantation. Lancet. 1998;352:1087–92.

Gratwohl A, Stern M, Brand R, et al. Risk score for outcome after allogeneic hematopoietic stem cell transplantation: a retrospective analysis. Cancer. 2009;115:4715–26.

Holter Chakrabarty JL, Rubinger M, Le-Rademacher J, et al. Autologous is superior to allogeneic hematopoietic cell transplantation for acute promyelocytic leukemia in second complete remission. Biol Blood Marrow Transplant. 2014;20:1021–5.

Jongen-Lavrencic M, Grob T, Hanekamp D, et al. Molecular minimal residual disease in acute myeloid leukemia. N Engl J Med. 2018;378:1189–99.

Koreth J, Schlenk R, Kopecky KJ, et al. Allogeneic stem cell transplantation for acute myeloid leukemia in first complete remission: systematic review and meta-analysis of prospective clinical trials. JAMA. 2009;301:2349–61.

Kroger N, Solano C, Bonifazi F. Antilymphocyte globulin for chronic graft-versus-host disease. N Engl J Med. 2016;374:1894–5.

Kroger N, Iacobelli S, Franke GN, et al. Dose-reduced versus standard conditioning followed by allogeneic stem-cell transplantation for patients with myelodysplastic syndrome: a prospective randomized phase III study of the EBMT (RICMAC Trial). J Clin Oncol. 2017;35:2157–64.

Lengfelder E, Lo-Coco F, Adès L, et al. Arsenic trioxide-based therapy of relapsed acute promyelocytic leukemia: registry results from the European LeukemiaNet. Leukemia. 2015;29:1084–91.

Lindsley RC, Saber W, Mar BG, et al. Prognostic mutations in myelodysplastic syndrome after stem-cell transplantation. N Engl J Med. 2017;376:536–47.

Lo-Coco F, Avvisati G, Vignetti M, et al. Retinoic acid and arsenic trioxide for acute promyelocytic leukemia. N Engl J Med. 2013;369:111–21.

Lowenberg B. Sense and nonsense of high-dose cytarabine for acute myeloid leukemia. Blood. 2013;121:26–8.

Lowenberg B, Ossenkoppele GJ, van Putten W, et al. High-dose daunorubicin in older patients with acute myeloid leukemia. N Engl J Med. 2009;361:1235–48.

Martino R, de Wreede L, Fiocco M, et al. Comparison of conditioning regimens of various intensities for allogeneic hematopoietic SCT using HLA-identical sibling donors in AML and MDS with <10% BM blasts: a report from EBMT. Bone Marrow Transplant. 2013;48:761–70.

Nagler A, Labopin M, Shimoni A, et al. Mobilized peripheral blood stem cells compared with bone marrow from HLA-identical siblings for reduced-intensity conditioning transplantation in acute myeloid leukemia in complete remission: a retrospective analysis from the Acute Leukemia Working Party of EBMT. Eur J Haematol. 2012;89:206–13.

Nash RA, Antin JH, Karanes C, et al. Phase 3 study comparing methotrexate and tacrolimus with methotrexate and cyclosporine for prophylaxis of acute graft-versus-host disease after marrow transplantation from unrelated donors. Blood. 2000;96:2062–8.

Oran B, Wagner JE, DeFor TE, Weisdorf DJ, Brunstein CG. Effect of conditioning regimen intensity on acute myeloid leukemia outcomes after umbilical cord blood transplantation. Biol Blood Marrow Transplant. 2011;17:1327–34.

Ossenkoppele GJ, Janssen JJ, van de Loosdrecht AA. Risk factors for relapse after allogeneic transplantation in acute myeloid leukemia. Haematologica. 2016;101:20–5.

Parimon T, Au DH, Martin PJ, Chien JW. A risk score for mortality after allogeneic hematopoietic cell transplantation. Ann Intern Med. 2006;144:407–14.

Pasquini MC, Devine S, Mendizabal A, et al. Comparative outcomes of donor graft CD34+ selection and immune suppressive therapy as graft-versus-host disease prophylaxis for patients with acute myeloid leukemia in complete remission undergoing HLA-matched sibling allogeneic hematopoietic cell transplantation. J Clin Oncol. 2012;30:3194–201.

Quek L, Ferguson P, Metzner M, et al. Mutational analysis of disease relapse in patients allografted for acute myeloid leukemia. Blood Adv. 2016;1:193–204.

Robinson TM, O'Donnell PV, Fuchs EJ, Luznik L. Haploidentical bone marrow and stem cell transplantation: experience with post-transplantation cyclophosphamide. Semin Hematol. 2016;53:90–7.

Rollig C, Bornhauser M, Kramer M, et al. Allogeneic stem-cell transplantation in patients with NPM1-mutated acute myeloid leukemia: results from a prospective donor versus no-donor analysis of patients after upfront HLA typing within the SAL-AML 2003 trial. J Clin Oncol. 2015;33:403–10.

Ruutu T, Gratwohl A, de Witte T, et al. Prophylaxis and treatment of GVHD: EBMT-ELN working group recommendations for a standardized practice. Bone Marrow Transplant. 2014;49:168–73.

Saad A, Lamb LS. Ex vivo T-cell depletion in allogeneic hematopoietic stem cell transplant: past, present and future. Bone Marrow Transplant. 2017;52:1241–8.

Sanz MA, Labopin M, Gorin NC, et al. Hematopoietic stem cell transplantation for adults with acute promyelocytic leukemia in the ATRA era: a survey of the European Cooperative Group for Blood and Marrow Transplantation. Bone Marrow Transplant. 2007;39:461–9.

Sanz MA, Grimwade D, Tallman MS, et al. Management of acute promyelocytic leukemia: recommendations from an expert panel on behalf of the European LeukemiaNet. Blood. 2009;113:1875–91.

Schlenk RF, Dohner K, Krauter J, et al. Mutations and treatment outcome in cytogenetically normal acute myeloid leukemia. N Engl J Med. 2008;358:1909–18.

Schlenk RF, Dohner K, Mack S, et al. Prospective evaluation of allogeneic hematopoietic stem-cell transplantation from matched related and matched unrelated donors in younger adults with high-risk acute myeloid leukemia: German-Austrian trial AMLHD98A. J Clin Oncol. 2010;28:4642–8.

Schmid C, Schleuning M, Schwerdtfeger R, et al. Long-term survival in refractory acute myeloid leukemia after sequential treatment with chemotherapy and reduced-intensity conditioning for allogeneic stem cell transplantation. Blood. 2006;108:1092–9.

Scott BL, Pasquini MC, Logan BR, et al. Myeloablative versus reduced-intensity hematopoietic cell transplantation for acute myeloid leukemia and myelodysplastic syndromes. J Clin Oncol. 2017;35:1154–61.

Sengsayadeth S, Savani BN, Blaise D, Malard F, Nagler A, Mohty M. Reduced intensity conditioning allogeneic hematopoietic cell transplantation for adult acute myeloid leukemia in complete remission - a review from the Acute Leukemia Working Party of the EBMT. Haematologica. 2015;100:859–69.

Shouval R, Labopin M, Bondi O, et al. Prediction of allogeneic hematopoietic stem-cell transplantation mortality 100 days after transplantation using a machine learning algorithm: A European Group for Blood and Marrow Transplantation Acute Leukemia Working Party Retrospective Data Mining Study. J Clin Oncol. 2015;33:3144–51.

Soiffer RJ, Davids MS, Chen YB. Tyrosine kinase inhibitors and immune checkpoint blockade in allogeneic hematopoietic cell transplantation. Blood. 2018;131:1073–80.

Sorror ML, Maris MB, Storb R, et al. Hematopoietic cell transplantation (HCT)-specific comorbidity index: a new tool for risk assessment before allogeneic HCT. Blood. 2005;106:2912–9.

Sorror ML, Sandmaier BM, Storer BE, et al. Comorbidity and disease status based risk stratification of outcomes among patients with acute myeloid leukemia or myelodysplasia receiving allogeneic hematopoietic cell transplantation. J Clin Oncol. 2007;25:4246–54.

Sorror ML, Storb RF, Sandmaier BM, et al. Comorbidity-age index: a clinical measure of biologic age before allogeneic hematopoietic cell transplantation. J Clin Oncol. 2014;32:3249–56.

Stelljes M, Krug U, Beelen DW, et al. Allogeneic transplantation versus chemotherapy as postremission therapy for acute myeloid leukemia: a prospective matched pairs analysis. J Clin Oncol. 2014;32:288–96.

Stone RM, Mandrekar SJ, Sanford BL, et al. Midostaurin plus chemotherapy for acute myeloid leukemia with a FLT3 mutation. N Engl J Med. 2017;377:454–64.

Tauro S, Craddock C, Peggs K, et al. Allogeneic stem-cell transplantation using a reduced-intensity conditioning regimen has the capacity to produce durable remissions and long-term disease-free survival in patients with high-risk acute myeloid leukemia and myelodysplasia. J Clin Oncol. 2005;23:9387–93.

Thomas X, Dombret H, Cordonnier C, et al. Treatment of relapsing acute promyelocytic leukemia by all-trans retinoic acid therapy followed by timed sequential chemotherapy and stem cell transplantation. APL Study Group. Acute promyelocytic leukemia. Leukemia. 2000;14:1006–13.

Todisco E, Ciceri F, Boschini C, et al. Factors predicting outcome after allogeneic transplant in refractory acute myeloid leukemia: a retrospective analysis of Gruppo Italiano Trapianto di Midollo Osseo (GITMO). Bone Marrow Transplant. 2017;52:955–61.

Versluis J, Labopin M, Niederwieser D, et al. Prediction of non-relapse mortality in recipients of reduced intensity conditioning allogeneic stem cell transplantation with AML in first complete remission. Leukemia. 2015;29:51–7.

Versluis J, Kalin B, Zeijlemaker W, et al. Graft-versus-leukemia effect of allogeneic stem-cell transplantation and minimal residual disease in patients with acute myeloid leukemia in first complete remission. JCO Precis Oncol. 2017a. https://doi.org/10.1200/PO.17.00078.

Versluis J, In't Hout FE, Devillier R, et al. Comparative value of post-remission treatment in cytogenetically normal AML subclassified by NPM1 and FLT3-ITD allelic ratio. Leukemia. 2017b;31:26–33.

Wagner JE Jr, Eapen M, Carter S, et al. One-unit versus two-unit cord-blood transplantation for hematologic cancers. N Engl J Med. 2014;371:1685–94.

Walter RB, Gooley TA, Wood BL, et al. Impact of pre-transplantation minimal residual disease, as detected by multiparametric flow cytometry, on outcome of myeloablative hematopoietic cell transplantation for acute myeloid leukemia. J Clin Oncol. 2011;29:1190–7.

Weisdorf D, Eapen M, Ruggeri A, et al. Alternative donor transplantation for older patients with acute myeloid leukemia in first complete remission: a center for international blood and marrow transplant research-eurocord analysis. Biol Blood Marrow Transplant. 2014;20:816–22.

Yanada M, Tsuzuki M, Fujita H, et al. Phase 2 study of arsenic trioxide followed by autologous hematopoietic cell transplantation for relapsed acute promyelocytic leukemia. Blood. 2013;121:3095–102.

70 Acute Myeloid Leukemia in Children

Brenda E. S. Gibson, Martin G. Sauer, and Persis Amrolia

70.1 Introduction

The outcome for children with acute myeloid leukemia (AML) has serially improved over the past three decades with an overall survival (OS) of 70–75% and event-free survival (EFS) of 60–65% widely reported. Much of this improvement is due to better supportive care, optimization of intensity of treatment including employment of Haematopoietic Stem Cell Transplantation (HSCT) in 1st complete remission (CR1) and better salvage in 2nd complete remission (CR2).

Whilst the majority of children (>90%) achieve CR, the relapse rate (RR) in CR1 remains unacceptably high at 30–35%, albeit varying by risk group. This global relapse risk has not improved significantly over the past three decades, and relapse remains the commonest cause of death.

B. E. S. Gibson (✉)
Haematology Department, Royal Hospital for Children, University of Glasgow, Glasgow, UK
e-mail: brenda.gibson@ggc.scot.nhs.uk

M. G. Sauer
Pediatric Hematology, Oncology and Blood Cell Transplantation, Medizinische Hochschule Hannover, Hannover, Germany

P. Amrolia
Department of Bone Marrow Transplant, Great Ormond St Children's Hospital, London, UK

HSCT, compared to chemotherapy as consolidation treatment, reduces the relapse risk in CR1 in all risk groups. However, this reduction in relapse risk has not always translated into an improvement in OS due to the treatment related mortality (TRM). The challenge is to identify children with a relapse risk in CR1, which is sufficiently high, to absorb the TRM and balance the risk in favour of HSCT. It is particularly important to establish the benefit of HSCT across all risk groups and within rare subtypes of AML associated with a poor outcome when treated with chemotherapy alone and not to assume that these children will benefit from HSCT. This will require evaluation by clinical trials which in turn will require international collaboration. Particularly worthy of consideration when weighing the benefits of transplantation in children are the associated late effects.

It is accepted that HSCT offers children with relapsed AML, who achieve a CR2, their only chance of long-term survival, and that some children with relapsed/refractory disease may benefit from HSCT.

70.2 Prognostic Factors and Indications

70.2.1 First Complete Remission

Consolidation therapy with allogeneic HSCT in CR1 of paediatric AML has been shown

E. Carreras et al. (eds.), *The EBMT Handbook*, https://doi.org/10.1007/978-3-030-02278-5_70

consistently to reduce the relapse risk through a GVL effect, which is stronger in AML than ALL.

Historically, HSCT trials employed a biological randomisation with children who had a matched sibling donor (MSD) receiving a HSCT as consolidation therapy and those without a MSD receiving consolidation chemotherapy. Improvements in HLA typing and donor selection have made HSCT an option for the majority of patients. Historical trials reported a reduction in RR which was counterbalanced by an increased TRM and better salvage for those who received chemotherapy only in CR 1 (Stevens et al. 1998; Woods et al. 2001; Lie et al. 2003). However, delaying transplant to CR2 carries risk. The mortality rate for reinduction after relapse is high, and those patients who do not achieve CR2 may be denied the opportunity of HSCT.

The criteria for transplanting patients have evolved from transplanting patients irrespective of risk group, to transplanting all patients other than those with good-risk cytogenetics (about 80% of all patients), to the current practice of restricting transplant to those with poor-risk (PR) cytogenetics (about 30% of all patients). These are the patients believed to be at the highest risk of relapse and therefore those most likely to benefit from HSCT in CR1 in an era of low TRM. There is no universal agreement on how high-risk (HR) disease should be defined. Different criteria have been, and continue to be, used by different national groups to define high risk. A combination of cytogenetics/molecular aberrations, which are currently considered to be the strongest indicator of outcome, and the presence of minimal residual disease (MRD), which may be assessed by morphology, flow cytometry or RT-PCR assessments of fusion transcripts, is evolving.

The percentage increase in disease free survival (DFS) or decrease in cumulative incidence of relapse (CIR) which would support HSCT as the best option in CR1 is undefined. This has been set at 10% in adults (Cornelissen et al. 2012), but the improved salvage after relapse and greater toll from late effects in children suggests that the bar should be set higher.

70.2.1.1 Cytogenetics

The cytogenetic abnormalities most commonly considered indicative of high risk of relapse include monosomy 7, monosomy 5/5q-, abnormal 12p, inv(3)/t(3;3)/abn (3q), CBFA2T3-GLIS2, t(4;11), t(5;11), t(6;11), t(10;11), t(6;9) ,t(9;22), t(7;12), t(11;17), t(8;16), t(3;5) and complex karyotype. There is not complete consensus between national groups, and, in particular, not all agree that abnormalities of 3q, t (6; 11) and complex (4 or more) are poor risk. Most consider a *FLT3-ITD* mutation (approximately 12% of children with AML) to be HR. However, some groups require the absence of good-risk cytogenetics, whilst other groups restrict this to *FLT3 ITD-WT1* mutations or base the risk on the allelic ratio (>0.4). The development of next-generation FLT3 inhibitors may challenge the role of HSCT in *FLT3-ITD*-mutated patients. A number of more recently recognised poor-risk cytogenetic abnormalities are cryptic, and it is expected that more cryptic abnormalities will be identified and that the list of poor-risk cytogenetic abnormalities may change with time. Currently poor-risk cytogenetics comprise about 25–30% of all AML in children.

An OS in excess of 70% is reported for HR patients after HSCT, although the definition of HR is not uniform. However, a combined COG and CIBMTR review of 233 children with AML between 1989 and 2006 with HR cytogenetics (-7, 7q-, -5, 5q-, abn 3q, t (6; 9), complex karyotype) reported no benefit for HSCT over chemotherapy. 123 children received chemotherapy, 55 a matched related donor (MRD) HSCT and 55 an unrelated donor (URD) HSCT. The 5-year OS from the time of consolidation or conditioning was similar: chemotherapy 43%, MRD 46% and URD 50% ($p = 0.99$).

The pattern of failure differed: CIR at 5 years 61% vs. 51% vs. 30% for chemotherapy, MRD and URD, respectively ($p < 0.001$), and TRM 7%, 13% and 23%, respectively ($p = 0.005$). HR was defined by cytogenetics alone and did not include FLT3 mutational or MRD status (Kelly et al. 2014). The benefit for HSCT in a number of poor-risk cytogenetic subgroups has not been proven and must not be assumed.

Whilst HSCT is generally directed at patients defined as HR by cytogenetic abnormalities, a meta-analysis of MRC and POG trials of HSCT vs. chemotherapy showed that only intermediate-risk patients, where risk was defined by cytogenetics and poor morphological response to treatment, benefited from transplant (OS 61% vs. 51%). There was no advantage for HSCT in patients with poor-risk cytogenetics; however there were too few patients in the poor-risk group to make firm conclusions (Horan et al. 2008).

70.2.1.2 Minimal Residual Disease Assessment (See Chap. 57)

MRD is variably employed in risk stratification to direct patients to HSCT. It has been shown to be strongly predictive of outcome, and whilst it is commonly used to intensify treatment in poor responders, it may equally identify those with poor-risk cytogenetic aberrations who have a favourable early response and may not require HSCT. Currently multidimensional flow (MDF) cytometry is most commonly employed either by measuring leukemia aberrant immunophenotype (LAIP) or a "different from normal" phenotype. The discretionary level is 0.1%, and the most commonly used time point is post course 2. Alternatively, discretionary levels of 0.1% or 1% post course 1 are used by some groups to guide patients to HSCT in CR1. About 20% of patients with a MRD level <0.1% after course 1 will relapse, which implies that genetic aberrations may influence relapse more than MRD. Similarly, 30% of patients with a MRD level of >0.1% after course 1 will remain in remission. MDF cytometry is sensitive to a level of 0.1–0.01% and applicable in 90% of patients with AML.

Molecular MRD may be more sensitive and informative but data is limited. It is not commonly used outwith acute promyelocytic leukemia (APL), but our understanding and employment of molecular MRD may change with experience. MRD assessment by reverse transcription PCR (RT-PCR) for fusion transcripts has a sensitivity level of 0.01–001% and is applicable in approximately 50% of patients. The generally accepted discriminatory level is a greater than three-log reduction in transcript levels.

The relative significance of cytogenetics/ molecular aberrations and MRD status may evolve. Digital PCR and next-generation sequencing may be more sensitive but remain in the research arena. Similarly, leukemia stem cell monitoring may be more informative (Schuurhuis et al. 2018).

The main benefit of measuring MRD by any methodology is that it may allow the tailoring of the intensity of treatment. Thirty one of 267 (12%) children treated on NOPHO-AML 20024 were defined as poor responders—15% blasts morphologically after course 1 or 5% blasts after course 2. These patients had time-intensive chemotherapy followed by HSCT in 25 of 31 with a donor. The 3-year probability of survival for these HR patients was 70%. Patients classified as intermediate risk (defined as 5–14.9% blasts after course 1) had a significantly inferior EFS compared to HR patients. Both groups had time-intensive chemotherapy, but only HR patients proceeded to HSCT (Wareham et al. 2013; Abrahamsson et al. 2011).

The level of MRD after course 1 of chemotherapy in children treated on AIEOP 2002/01 correlated with outcome. At 8 years the outcomes for the 125 children in morphological remission with MRD level post course 1 of <0.1% vs. ≥0.1% was DFS 73.1% vs. 35.2% ($p < 0.01$), OS 82.2% vs. 51.6% ($p = 0.0005$) and CIR 23.5 % vs. 62.8% ($p = 0.0005$). Post course 2, the outcomes at 8 years for MRD of <0.1% vs. ≥0.1% was DFS 68.4% vs. 21.9% ($p < 0.01$), OS 77.1% vs. 55.5% ($p = 0.0275$) and CIR 31.6 % vs. 73.9% ($p = 0.00078$).

Thirty-six patients had a MRD level of ≥0.1% at the end of course 1:13 achieved a MRD <0.1% after course 2, and their DFS was 45.4% vs. 22.8 % for patients with persisting MRD ≥0.1% ($p = 0.037$). Therefore, patients who achieve a level of MRD <0.1% after course 2 but who were MRD positive (>0.1%) after course 1 remain at higher risk of relapse and have a poorer outcome compared to those who are MRD negative after course 1. This suggests that not only clearance of MRD but additional effective treatment is required to improve outcome (Buldini et al. 2017; Loken et al. 2012).

St Jude's AML 02 study showed no difference in OS between HR patients undergoing HSCT compared to those who received chemotherapy. When the analysis was restricted to HR patients defined by MRD >1% after induction 1, the OS for HSCT was 43% vs. 23% for chemotherapy: $p = 0.14$ (Rubnitz et al. 2010). Whilst the difference was not statistically significant, this may have been limited by low patient numbers.

There is no advantage for HSCT in CR1 for patients with good-risk cytogenetics—t (8; 21), inv (16), normal karyotype with NPM1 and normal karyotype with biallelic CEBPA. Some groups include t(1;11) (q21; q23) in the good-risk cytogenetic group.

The benefit of HSCT in CR1 for patients with intermediate-risk cytogenetics is less clear, and these may be the patients without PR cytogenetics but with a poor early response to chemotherapy in whom MRD can identify those at high risk of relapse. There is no role for HSCT in CR1 of APL or DS AML. HSCT for patients with Fanconi anaemia and MDS/AML and those with JMML are discussed elsewhere.

70.2.2 Second Complete Remission

Patients with relapsed AML have a dismal prognosis with chemotherapy alone, and it is generally accepted that they should proceed to transplant in CR2. The chance of achieving a second CR after relapse is dependent on the length of CR1: CR1 <1 year vs. CR >1 year is 50% vs. 75% with an overall CR rate of 60%, OS for CR <1 year 26% vs. 45% CR >1 year, $p < 0.001$ (Kaspers et al. 2013). Prognostically significant are the time to relapse, cytogenetics, no HSCT in CR1 and the speed of response to reinduction. Cytogenetics are strong prognostic indicators in relapse as in de novo disease with patients with CBF leukemias fairing the best: CBF leukemias vs. others—OS 67% vs. 31%, $p < 0.001$.

70.2.3 Refractory Disease

It has long been accepted that a poor morphological response >5% blasts at day 15 or resistant disease after course 1 or 2 has a poor outcome with chemotherapy alone. If CR cannot be achieved, the outlook is poor, but aggressive chemotherapy followed by HSCT may benefit some patients. Residual disease/MRD positivity pre-HSCT increases the risk of relapse post-HSCT, but the susceptibility of AML to GVL does not preclude transplant. MRD status just prior to HSCT is an important prognostic indicator.

A small study reported a 5-year OS of 80.4% for children with <0.01% MRD ($n = 27$), 66.7% for those with 0.01–5% MRD ($n = 9$) and 58.3% for those with >5% MRD (Leung et al. 2012). It is not clear what level of disease should preclude HSCT.

The role of transplant in CR1, CR2 and refractory disease may change with time if new effective chemotherapy agents become available.

70.3 Conditioning Regimens

No advantage has been shown for total body irradiation (TBI) in AML and chemotherapy-only regimens should be used. Adult data from the CIBMTR demonstrated improved non relapse mortality (NRM), OS and DFS in patients with AML transplanted using IV Busulfan (Bu) with therapeutic drug monitoring (TDM) compared with TBI (Copelan et al. 2013). Myeloablative conditioning (MAC) regimens are most commonly used, but a number of reduced toxicity conditioning (RTC) regimens are being tested. There is no proven "best" chemotherapy conditioning regimen, though MAC regimens with Bu and cyclophosphamide (Cy) with TDM of Bu levels are currently the standard of care. A retrospective EBMT study of Bu, Cy and Melphalan (Mel) (enhanced MAC) in paediatric AML in CR1 suggested improved RR and Leukemia free survival (LFS) compared with BuCy, but the majority of patients receiving BuCy on this study did not undergo TDM (Lucchini et al. 2017). Moreover, whilst this regimen is well tolerated in children under the age of 12 years, it is associated with non-acceptable TRM rates between 20 and 30% in teenagers and should therefore be avoided or used with caution in this group (Sauer et al. 2017). There is an increasing body of experience with MAC Bu and

Fludarabine (Flu), which is well tolerated, but no randomised comparisons are available to determine relative anti-leukaemic activity of BuFlu vs BuCy (Harris et al. 2018). Replacing Bu with Treosulfan (Treo) to reduce toxicity whilst maintaining efficacy is being tested and given in combination with Cy (TreoCy) or with Flu and Thiotepa (FTT). The choice of conditioning regimen is a balance between efficacy and toxicity. Comorbidity; pretreatment with drugs which may contribute to toxicity, i.e. gemtuzumab and VOD/SOS, age and HLA disparity may influence the choice of conditioning regimen. Comorbidity or heavy previous treatment may indicate a reduced intensity conditioning (RIC) with BuFlu or FluMel. Targeted Bu levels will differ between MAC, RTC and RIC. Patient toxicities may suggest avoidance of specific agents. Newer regimens which include clofarabine are also being tested.

A retrospective comparison of RIC (39) vs. MAC (141) in matched patients has reported no difference in a-GVHD, c-GVHD, TRM, LFS and OS. The OS was 45% vs. 48%, $p = 0.99$; RR 39% vs. 39%, $p = 0.95$; and TRM 16% vs. 16%, $p = 0.73$. However, about 50% of MAC used TBI, whilst BuCy was the commonest chemotherapy regimen. Patients who received a RIC had had more pre-HSCT morbidity. The performance score influenced OS, LFS and CIR (Bitan et al. 2014). The current paediatric AML protocol MyeChild01 is prospectively comparing MAC BuCy with a reduced toxicity BuFlu regimen.

70.4 Donor Selection Hierarchy and Stem Cell Source

70.4.1 Autologous HSCT

There is no evidence from a number of studies and meta-analysis that auto-HSCT is superior to intensive chemotherapy as consolidation therapy and it is now not employed. AML 2002/01 study reported a DFS of 73% for allo-HSCT in HR patients compared to 63% for auto-HSCT, p-ns. The CIR was 17% vs. 28% in favour of allo-HSCT, $p = 0.043$. There was no difference in TRM at 7% for both groups at 8 years (Locatelli et al. 2015).

70.4.2 Allogeneic HSCT

The choice of donor for allo-HSCT is based on HLA compatibility and CMV status. Outcomes are similar for MSD and well matched unrelated donors (UDs). The degree of mismatch which is acceptable depends on the risk of relapse and CR status. Mismatched unrelated donor (MMUD) or cords and haplo-HSCT are generally reserved for very HR disease or early relapses.

Patients and their siblings should be tissue-typed at diagnosis. In the absence of a HLA matched family donor (MFD), an URD and cord blood unit (CBU) search should be initiated as soon as possible after induction course 1 for patients with intermediate or PR cytogenetics. Donors should be selected using the selection hierarchy of the national group. Medium-/high-resolution typing is required for adult URD (HLA A, B, C, HLA-DRB1 and HLA-DQB1) and unrelated cords (HLA A, B, C and DR loci).

The risk of relapse does not just direct the need for transplant but the HLA discrepancy which is acceptable. MFD or well-MUD should be identified for CR1 patients, whilst mismatched donors (8/10 MMUD), cords (4/8 MMUCB) or haplo-HSCT should be reserved for very high-risk disease, CR2 or refractory disease.

For family/unrelated donors, BM is the preferred stem cell source, but the use of PBSC is permissible and is more commonly used. The use of PBSC from mismatched donors should be avoided wherever possible.

In the UK, serotherapy is only given to patients transplanted from unrelated donors, 9/10 mismatched family donors or 5/8 matched cords blood units, but not to patients receiving grafts from matched family donors or 6–8/8 unrelated cord blood units. Other European groups only employ T-cell depletion in mismatched donors (MMUD).

70.5 GVHD Prophylaxis

All patients should receive immunosuppression (IS) with ciclosporin (CSA). Most, but not all, national groups add short-course methotrexate (MTX) for all patients. Patients receiving grafts from a mismatched donor or those in whom the stem cell source is PBSC or unrelated cord blood should receive prophylaxis in addition to CSA with either mycophenolate mofetil (MMF) or short-course MTX. In adult AML, increased exposure to CSA was associated with increased relapse and decreased survival (Craddock et al. 2010), supporting early withdrawal of IS where possible. In the absence of GVHD, MMF can be stopped at day 28 post transplant, and CSA tailed over 4–6 weeks from day 60 (MFD), day 100 (MUD) or earlier if mixed chimerism is detected in the whole blood.

70.6 Donor Lymphocyte Infusions (DLI)

The evidence of benefit for DLI is weak. Rettinger et al. investigated the use of pre-emptive immunotherapy with reduction of IS and low-dose DLI in patients with paediatric AML developing mixed chimerism (MC) after HSCT for AML; 6/13 patients with MC who received immunotherapy remained in long-term CR, whereas all 7 patients with MC who did not receive immunotherapy relapsed (Rettinger et al. 2017). Based on these limited data, our practice is to use pre-emptive immunotherapy in patients with confirmed MC (defined as >1% autologous cells in the whole blood on two occasions 1 week apart) without active acute GVHD >Grade 1 or chronic GVHD in the first-year post transplant. If patients are still receiving IS, this should be discontinued and chimerism reassessed a month later. In patients already off IS, chimerism should be reassessed a month off IS. If mixed chimerism persists, DLI should be given to recipients of MFD or MUD. DLI is not recommended in the context of 9/10 mismatched donor HSCT. The DLI cell dose administered is dependent on the donor source and the timing post transplant. In the future, the use of pre-emptive DLI is likely to be based on detection of flow or molecular MRD in the bone marrow.

70.7 Management of Relapse Post transplant

For selected patients who relapse late (>1 year) post first HSCT and respond to reinduction chemotherapy, a second transplant may be curative with survival rates of 24–35% reported (Yaniv et al. 2018; Uden et al. 2017). DLI is of limited efficacy in frank relapse post transplant except if a further remission can be achieved (Schmid et al. 2007; Kolb et al. 1995).

Interestingly, CR has been seen in cutaneous (but not bone marrow) relapse of AML post transplant with the checkpoint inhibitor ipilimumab (Davids et al. 2016). Novel agents targeting specific pathways, e.g. FLT 3 inhibition, have met with limited success to date. Treatment options for patients who relapse early after transplant are challenging, and at present, for the majority of such patients, we recommend symptom care or enrolment in a clinical trial. Antibody-drug conjugates, bispecific T-cell-engaging antibodies and chimeric antigen receptor (CAR) T cells under development may be tested in such patients in the future (Table 70.1).

Table 70.1 Donor and source for HSCT: the hierarchy of the UK

Choice	Family donor	Unrelated donor	Unrelated cord
1st	MFD (BM, PBSC, CB)		
2nd		10/10 MUD 9/10 1DQ MMUD	8/8 MUCB (total nucleated cell (TNC >3 × 10^7/kg)
3rd	9/10 MMFD	9/10 (other) MMUD	5–7/8 MMUCB (TNC >3 × 10^7/kg)[a]

MFD matched family donor, *MUD* matched unrelated donor, *MMUD* mismatched unrelated donor, *MUCB* matched unrelated cord blood, *MMFD* mismatched family donor, *MMUCB* mismatched unrelated cord blood

[a]For unrelated cord blood, a single cord is used if the cryopreserved TNC dose is >3 × 10^7/kg. If <3 × 10^7/kg, a double cord transplant is preferred

Key Points

- There is increasing evidence that patients with cytogenetic or molecular high-risk features may benefit from HSCT in CR1. About 30% of children fall into this risk group. A TRM below 10% should be achievable.
- A matched family or unrelated donor is considered the optimal donors and the bone marrow the preferred stem cell source. Mismatched donors may be considered appropriate for patients with poorly responding disease.
- Children who achieve CR2 after first relapse have a bleak prognosis without HSCT.
- MAC, TBI-free, conditioning is recommended for patients transplanted in CR1 and CR2, and to date the standard regimen had been BuCy.
- Novel conditioning regimens incorporating TREO or clofarabine are being explored, and these need to be compared with BuCy in prospective, randomised studies.
- Relapse after HSCT in CR1 is associated with a very poor outcome and not curable without a second HSCT. TRM for second HSCTs exceeds 30% which might favour the use of a RIC in this setting. The prevention of relapse remains the major challenge.

References

Abrahamsson J, Forestier E, Heldrup J, et al. Response-guided induction therapy in pediatric acute myeloid leukemia with excellent remission rate. J Clin Oncol. 2011;29:310–5.

Bitan M, He W, Zhang MJ, et al. Transplantation for children with acute myeloid leukaemia: a comparison of outcomes with reduced intensity and myeloablative regimens. Blood. 2014;123:1615–20.

Buldini B, Rizzati F, Masetti R, et al. Prognostic significance of flow-cytometry evaluation of minimal residual disease in children with acute myeloid leukaemia treated according to the AIEOP-AML 2002/01 study protocol. Br J Haematol. 2017;177:116–26.

Copelan EA, Hamilton BK, Avalos B, et al. Better leukaemia-free and overall survival in AML in first remission following cyclophosphamide in combination with Busulfan compared with TBI. Blood. 2013;122:3863–70.

Cornelissen JJ, Gratwohl A, Schlenk RF, et al. The European LeukaemiaNet AML Working Party consensus statement on allogeneic HSCT for patients with AML in remission: an integrated–risk adapted approach. Nat Rev Clin Oncol. 2012;9: 579–90.

Craddock C, Nagra S, Peniket A, et al. Factors predicting long-term survival after T-cell depleted reduced intensity allogeneic stem cell transplantation for acute myeloid leukaemia. Haematologica. 2010;95:989–95.

Davids MS, Kim HT, Bachireddy P, et al. Ipilimumab for patients with relapse after allogeneic transplantation. N Engl J Med. 2016;375:143–53.

Harris AC, Boelens JJ, Ahn KW, et al. Comparison of pediatric allogeneic transplant outcomes using myeloablative Busulfan with cyclophosphamide or fludarabine. Blood Adv. 2018;2:1198–206.

Horan JT, Alonzo TA, Lyman GH, et al. Impact of disease risk on efficacy of matched related bone marrow transplantation for pediatric acute myeloid leukaemia; the Children's Oncology Group. J Clin Oncol. 2008;26:5797–801.

Kaspers GL, Zimmermann M, Reinhardt D, et al. Improved outcome in pediatric relapsed acute myeloid leukaemia: results of a randomised trial on liposomal daunorubicin by the International BFM Study Group. J Clin Oncol. 2013;31:599–607.

Kelly MJ, Horan JT, Alonzo TA, et al. Comparable survival for pediatric acute myeloid leukaemia with poor-risk cytogenetics following chemotherapy, matched related donor or unrelated donor transplantation. Pediatr Blood Cancer. 2014;61:269–75.

Kolb HJ, Schattenberg A, Goldman JM, et al. Graft-versus-leukemia effect of donor lymphocyte transfusions in marrow grafted patients. European Group for Blood and Marrow Transplantation Working Party Chronic Leukemia. Blood. 1995;86:2041–50.

Leung W, Pui CH, Coustan-Smith E, et al. Detectable minimal residual disease before hematopoietic cell transplantation is prognostic but does not preclude cure for children with very –high-risk leukaemia. Blood. 2012;120:468–72.

Lie SO, Abrahamsson J, Clausen N, et al. Treatment stratification based on initial in vivo response in acute myeloid leukaemia in children without Down's syndrome: results of NOPHO-AML trials. Br J Haematol. 2003;122:217–25.

Locatelli F, Masetti R, Rondelli R, et al. Outcome of children with high –risk acute myeloid leukaemia given autologous or allogeneic hematopoietic cell transplantation in the AIEOP AML-2002/01 study. Bone Marrow Transplant. 2015;50:181–8.

Loken MR, Alonzo TA, Pardo L, et al. Residual disease detected by multidimensional flow cytometry signifies high relapse risk in patients with de novo acute myeloid leukaemia: a report from Children's Oncology Group. Blood. 2012;120:1581–8.

Lucchini G, Labopin M, Beohou E, et al. Impact of conditioning regimen on outcomes for children with acute myeloid leukaemia undergoing transplantation in first complete remission. an analysis on behalf of the Pediatric Disease Working Party of the European Group for Blood and Marrow Transplantation. Biol Blood Marrow Transplant. 2017;23:467–74.

Rettinger E, Merker M, Salzmann-Manrique E, et al. Preemptive immunotherapy for clearance of molecular disease in childhood acute lymphoblastic leukaemia after transplantation. Biol Blood Marrow Transplant. 2017;23:87–95.

Rubnitz JE, Inaba H, Dahl G, et al. Minimal residual disease – directed therapy for childhood acute myeloid leukaemia; results of the AML 02 multicentre trial. Lancet Oncol. 2010;11:543–52.

Sauer MG, Lang P, Albert M, et al. AML SCT-BFM 2007: results of the prospective hematopoietic stem cell transplantation (HSCT) trial of the Berlin-Frankfurt-Münster (BFM) Study Group for children with very high risk acute myeloid leukemia. Blood. 2017;130(Suppl 1):599.

Schmid C, Labopin M, Nagler A, et al. Donor lymphocyte infusion in the treatment of first hematological relapse after allogeneic stem-cell transplantation in adults with acute myeloid leukaemia: a retrospective risk factors analysis and comparison with other strategies by the EBMT Acute Leukaemia Working Party. Clin Oncol. 2007;25:4938–45.

Schuurhuis GJ, Heuser M, Freeman S, et al. Minimal/measurable residual disease in AML: a consensus document from the European leukemiaNet MRD working party. Blood. 2018;131:1275–91.

Stevens RF, Hann IM, Wheatley K, Gray RG. Marked improvements in outcome with chemotherapy alone in paediatric acute myeloid leukaemia: results of the United Kingdom Medical Research Council's 10th AML trial. MRC Childhood Leukaemia Working Party. Br J Haematol. 1998;101:130–40.

Uden T, Bertaina A, Abrahamsson J, et al. Outcome of children relapsing after first allogeneic hematopoietic stem cell transplantation for pediatric acute myeloid leukemia: a retrospective I-BFM analysis of 336 children between 2005 and 2016. Blood. 2017;130(Suppl 1):272.

Wareham NE, Heilmann C, Abrahamsson J, et al. Outcome of poor response paediatric AML using early SCT. Eur J Haematol. 2013;90:187–94.

Woods WG, Neudorf S, Gold S, et al. A comparison of allogeneic bone marrow transplantation, autologous bone marrow transplantation, and aggressive chemotherapy in children with acute myeloid leukaemia in remission. Blood. 2001;97:56–62.

Yaniv I, Krauss AC, Beohou E, et al. Second hematopoietic stem cell transplantation for post-transplantation relapsed acute leukaemia in children: a retrospective EBMT-PDWP Study. Biol Blood Marrow Transplant. 2018;24(8):1629–42.

71 Acute Lymphoblastic Leukemia in Adults

Matthias Stelljes and David I. Marks

71.1 Definition and Epidemiology

ALL is a malignant transformation and proliferation of lymphoid progenitor cells in the bone marrow, blood, and extramedullary sites. While 80% of ALL occurs in children, it represents a devastating disease in adults. The incidence of ALL is bimodal, with the first peak occurring in childhood and a second peak occurring around 50 years. The estimated overall incidence of ALL and lymphoblastic lymphoma in Europe is 1.28 per 100,000 individuals annually, with significant age-related variations (0.53 at 45–54 years, ~1.0 at 55–74 years, and 1.45 at 75–99 years) (Terwilliger and Abdul-Hay 2017).

71.2 Diagnosis

Typical but nonspecific clinical manifestations of patients with ALL are constitutional symptoms, bleeding, infections, and/or bone pain, with less than 10% of individuals having symptomatic CNS involvement at diagnosis (Lazarus et al. 2006). Mature B-cell ALL can also present as an extramedullary (e.g., GI or testicular involvement) disease. Mediastinal mass with wheezing and stridor can be a presenting feature of T-lineage ALL. For diagnostic purposes, the addition of flow cytometry to the morphologic identification of neoplastic lymphoblasts is essential for classification of ALL.

71.3 Classification

In 1997, the WHO proposed a composite classification in attempt to account for morphology and cytogenetic profile of the leukemic blasts and identified three types of ALL: B-lymphoblastic, T-lymphoblastic, and Burkitt cell leukemias. Later revised in 2008, Burkitt cell leukemia was eliminated as it is no longer seen as a separate entity from Burkitt lymphoma, and B-lymphoblastic leukemia was divided into two subtypes: B-ALL with recurrent genetic abnormalities and B-ALL not otherwise specified. B-ALL with recurrent genetic abnormalities is further delineated based on the specific chromosomal rearrangement present. In 2016, two new provisional entities were added to the list of recurrent genetic abnormalities, and hypodiploid was redefined as either low hypodiploid (<40 chromosomes) or hypodiploid with *TP53* mutations.

M. Stelljes (✉)
Department of Hematology and Oncology, University Hospital of Münster, University of Münster, Münster, Germany
e-mail: matthias.stelljes@ukmuenster.de

D. I. Marks
Department of Haematology and BMT, Bristol Haematology and Oncology Centre, Bristol, UK

E. Carreras et al. (eds.), *The EBMT Handbook*, https://doi.org/10.1007/978-3-030-02278-5_71

71.4 Risk Factors

Historically, age and white blood cell count at the time of diagnosis have been used to risk stratify patients. Increasing age portends a worse prognosis. Patients over 55 years have particularly poor outcomes, with only 10–15% long-term survival (Rowe et al. 2015). In most studies the cut point for high-risk ALL has been 30 × 10^9/L for B-cell precursor ALL and 100 × 10^9/L for T-cell precursor ALL, respectively.

According to the maturation marker profile measured by *immunophenotyping*, both entities, B- and T-cell precursor ALL, can be classified as less mature ALL, which are associated with an inferior prognosis compared to the more mature subtypes. In B-lineage ALL, the most important markers for subclassification are CD19, CD20, CD22, CD24, and CD79a. The earliest B-lineage markers are CD19, CD22 (membrane and cytoplasm), and CD79a. A positive reaction for any two of these three markers, without further differentiation markers, identifies pro-B ALL. The early T-cell precursor ALL is a subtype of high-risk ALL defined by reduced expression of T-cell markers (CD1a, CD8, and CD5) and aberrant expression of myeloid or stem cell markers (Chiaretti et al. 2014).

Cytogenetics represents an important part of ALL classification (Moorman et al. 2007). Probably the most well-known aberration in acute leukemia, associated with a high-risk disease, is Philadelphia chromosome-positive ALL. This aberration is present in approximately 20% to 30% of adults with ALL. It can be detected as the translocation t(9;22)(q34;q11) by conventional karyotyping including FISH and/or by detection of the *BCR-ABL1* rearrangement by PCR. In addition, aberrations like t(4;11)(q21;q23) or *MLL* rearrangements at 11q23 and hypodiploidy/low hypodiploidy (and the strictly related near-triploid group) fall also into the poor-risk cytogenetic category, with an overall disease-free survival rate of about 25%. The prognostic relevance of a complex karyotype (five or more chromosomal aberrations) in ALL remains controversial among different study groups.

Most ALL cases harbor multiple somatic *genetic alterations* in addition to gross chromosomal alterations. Chromosomal rearrangements and aneuploidy are early events in leukemogenesis, with DNA copy number alterations and sequence mutations acquired subsequently. Genes encoding transcriptional regulators of lymphoid development are among the most frequently mutated genes, particularly in B-linage ALL. Several key genetic alterations may be associated with an inferior outcome, e.g., the IKZF1 alterations with treatment failure (Dhedin et al. 2015). However, these findings have to be verified in further prospective trials.

Persistence of *MRD* after induction/early consolidation, between weeks 4 and 22 and with a level $\geq 10^{-4}$, indicates intrinsic drug resistance (Holowiecki et al. 2008). MRD is evaluable using either multichannel flow cytometry or the real-time quantitative polymerase chain reaction (RQ-PCR). Aberrant phenotypes are identified on the basis of different combinations and/or asynchronous expression and/or variable intensity staining of several antigens. PCR targets are fusion genes associated with chromosomal abnormalities (e.g., BCR-ABL, MLL-AF4) or rearranged immunoglobulin or T-cell receptor sequences (TCR β, γ, δ, IgH, IgK-Kde) unique to each patient with ALL. A MRD level exceeding 10^{-4} after 2–3 months of treatment is an indicator for a high-risk disease, whereas an increase above 10^{-3} represents a very high risk for relapse (Bruggemann et al. 2010).

71.5 Prognostic Factors Used to Indicate Allo-HSCT in CR1

Although data from prospective randomized studies are lacking and are most likely impossible to obtain due to the small numbers in some subgroups, some patient–/disease-related risk factors might be an indication for an allo-HSCT in the first remission.

Prognostic factor	Indication of allo-HSCT if
Age	>40 years
High WBC count at diagnosis	>30 × 10^9/L in BCP-ALL >100 × 10^9/L in T-ALL
Poor-risk cytogenetics	Ph chromosome t(4;11)(q21;q23) t(8;14)(q24.1;q32) Complex karyotype Low hypodiploidy/near triploidy

Prognostic factor	Indication of allo-HSCT if
ALL subtypes with poor prognosis	Early T-cell precursor ALL (Ph-like ALL) (limited data, pending trials)
High-risk genetics	IKZF1 deletion in B precursor ALL (NOTCH1/FBXW7; N/K-RAS; PTEN genetics in T-ALL (Trinquand et al. 2013)) (limited data, pending trials)
Failure to attain CR	Within 4 weeks of therapy
Minimal residual disease	$>1 \times 10^{-4}$ after two courses of therapy Reappearance of MRD marker (no MRD marker at initial diagnosis)

71.6 First-Line Treatment

The first-line chemotherapy usually consists of induction, treatment intensification/consolidation, and long-term maintenance, with CNS prophylaxis given at intervals throughout therapy. The goal of induction therapy is to achieve CR remission and to restore normal hematopoiesis. The backbone of induction therapy typically includes VCR, PRD, and an anthracycline with or without L-asp and CY.

Intensive postremission consolidation therapies improve outcome. Most study groups recommend six to eight courses, two to four of which contain high-dose MTX, Ara-C, and L-asp, and one to two represent reinduction blocks.

Postremission consolidation is most often followed by long-term maintenance with daily oral mercaptopurine and weekly MTX for 2 years or longer, sometimes with periodic applications of, e.g., VCR, PRD, or other drugs (Bassan and Hoelzer 2011).

The addition of RTX to the induction and consolidation therapy for patients with B-precursor ALL (Maury et al. 2016), as well as imatinib for patients with Ph-positive ALL (Fielding et al. 2014), has significantly improved the outcome in these subgroups.

These modern regimens usually allow remission rates of 90% and more in patients with standard-risk ALL. However, in patients of older age (e.g., >45 years) treated with pediatric-inspired protocols, significantly higher rate of chemotherapy-related events compared to younger patients occurs, and response rates decrease.

The introduction of novel agents like nelarabine for patients with T-precursor ALL and blinatumomab and inotuzumab ozogamicin for B-precursor ALL, as part of the frontline therapy, is currently being evaluated in prospective trials.

71.7 Second-Line Treatment

While 85–90% of patients go into remission after induction therapy, there are subsets that are refractory to induction therapy. In addition, many of the patients with complete remission will have a relapse, and only approximately 30–50% will have disease-free survival lasting 3 years or longer. Conventional standard chemotherapy regimens for adults with relapsed or refractory B-cell ALL are associated with rates of CR of 31–44% when they are the first salvage therapy administered after an early relapse and 18–25% when they are the second salvage therapy (Gokbuget et al. 2016). Because CR is typically a prerequisite for subsequent allo-HSCT, the low rates of CR associated with conventional chemotherapy regimens mean that few adults with relapsed or refractory (R/R) B-cell ALL (5–30%) proceed to HSCT, which is considered to be the main goal after salvage treatment because it is the only potentially curative treatment option.

Recently, two randomized trials comparing conventional salvage regimens with novel immunotherapy-based therapies, the Tower trial (Kantarjian et al. 2017) with blinatumomab (targeting CD19) and the INO-VATE ALL trial (Kantarjian et al. 2016) with inotuzumab ozogamicin (targeting CD22), demonstrated significantly higher remission rates (up to 80%) for patients with R/R B-precursor ALL treated with either antibody-based therapy. Moreover, these novel treatments showed a favorable toxicity profile compared to conventional chemotherapies and allowed the treatment, of many of the patients, in an outpatient setting. Both trials defined a new standard therapy option in patients with R/R B-precursor ALL. Conventional chemotherapy might be still a reasonable option in patients with late relapse. However, with regard to treatment toxicity and option of outpatient treatment, antibody-based therapies should be discussed with the patients, if available.

In patients with R/R Ph + ALL, usually treated with imatinib as part of the first-line treatment, molecular testing of mutations leading to the resistance to particular tyrosine kinase inhibitors (TKIs) should be performed. According to these results, a second-generation TKI (e.g., dasatinib or ponatinib) should be chosen as salvage therapy.

Anti-CD19 chimeric antigen receptor (CAR)-expressing T cells have proved extremely effective against R/R B precursor ALL, at least in children and young adult patients with up to 70–90% response rates reported (Maude et al. 2018; Park et al. 2018). With lacking comparative trials, highly selected patients, and a clinically relevant toxicity profile (e.g., severe cytokine release syndrome, neurotoxicity, and long-lasting B-cell depletion), CAR-T cells have to be evaluated in further prospective trials.

Despite advantages in the treatment of B-precursor ALL, treatment options for patients with R/R T-precursor ALL are limited. So far, there is no agreed standard of care in adults with relapsed T-cell ALL. Standard chemotherapy regimens such as FLAG (FLU, Ara-C, and G-CSF) ± idarubicin only result in 30% to 40% response rates with 6 months median OS in responders. Nelarabine as monotherapy or in combination with other chemotherapeutic agents has shown promising response rates and is a reasonable option (Gokbuget et al. 2011(Gokbuget et al. 2011)).

Patients with persisting MRD or reappearance of their MRD marker without evidence of a hematological relapse have usually an indication for an allo-HSCT. However, treatment of MRD prior to transplant to potentially optimize outcome after HSCT should be discussed for patients in case of high/increasing MRD and particularly for those with an option for a targeted therapy (e.g., change of TKI therapy in patients with Ph + ALL of blinatumomab).

71.8 Autologous HSCT

71.8.1 Indication

Auto-HSCT is not considered a standard therapy for adult ALL. Optional for patients with MRD-negative high-risk ALL, not eligible for allo-HSCT.

71.8.2 Conditioning

Fractionated TBI (e.g., 6 × 2 Gy) in combination with CY and/or VP.

71.8.3 Results

In some trials, patients excluded from allo-HSCT were randomly assigned between chemotherapy and auto-HSCT. In one of the largest studies, chemotherapy proved superior, while a marginal superiority of auto-HSCT was ascertained in high-risk patients in another (Goldstone et al. 2008). In a European retrospective analysis on auto-HSCT, a cohort of patients who were MRD negative had a significantly better survival compared to those being MRD positive. Results of another retrospective study comparing auto- and allo-HSCT for adults with Philadelphia-positive ALL in first complete molecular remission showed similar survival rates for both groups (higher rate of relapse after auto-HSCT and higher rates of death in remission after allo-HSCT).

It remains a matter of debate if the MRD-negative patients in these retrospective trials would have shown similar results with conventional chemotherapy. The value of high-dose therapy, particularly in ALL patients being early MRD negative after induction therapy, has to be evaluated in prospective trials.

71.9 Allogeneic HSCT

71.9.1 Indication

Standard therapy for patients with high-risk ALL in CR1 (see Sect. 71.5) and standard therapy for patients with subsequent remission after induction failure or relapsed ALL (Dhawan and Marks 2017). Optional for patients with standard-risk ALL in CR1 and unexpectable treatment-related toxicities (e.g., prolonged severe cytopenia), which preclude continuation of conventional therapy. Optional for patients with refractory/active ALL (Pavlu et al. 2017).

71.9.2 Conditioning

For fit patients <45 years and no relevant comorbidities, preferable fractionated TBI (cumulative dose of 12–13 Gy) in combination with CY or

VP (Marks et al. 2006); alternative BU (preferable IV BU targeted plasma-drug level monitoring) in combination with CY. For patients aged 45 years and older, dose-adapted/dose-reduced conditioning should be considered. So far, no standard regimen has been established. Reasonable options are TBI-based therapies (e.g., 8 Gy TBI in combination with FLU or CY) and MEL-, BU-, or TREO-based conditioning regimes.

Especially patients transplanted beyond first remission are at risk for severe transplant-related toxicities with cumulative incidence of death in remission exceeding 30% and more. Consequently, dose-reduced conditioning regimes should be discussed in patients being in a MRD-negative subsequent remission after treatment with novel antibody-based salvage therapies. Moreover, conditioning therapies associated with significant toxicities (e.g., SOS/VOD for patients treated with inotuzumab ozogamic) must be avoided (Kebriaei et al. 2018).

71.9.3 Donor

MSD, HLA-MUD (at least matched for HLA-A, HLA-B, HLA-C, and DR), HLA-MMUD, haploidentical donor. In patients with HLA-MMUD, a transplant with UCB (Marks et al. 2014) or from haploidentical donor (Santoro et al. 2017) may be the better choice, particularly in those cases with >1 HLA-antigen-mismatched donor (Figs. 71.1 and 71.2).

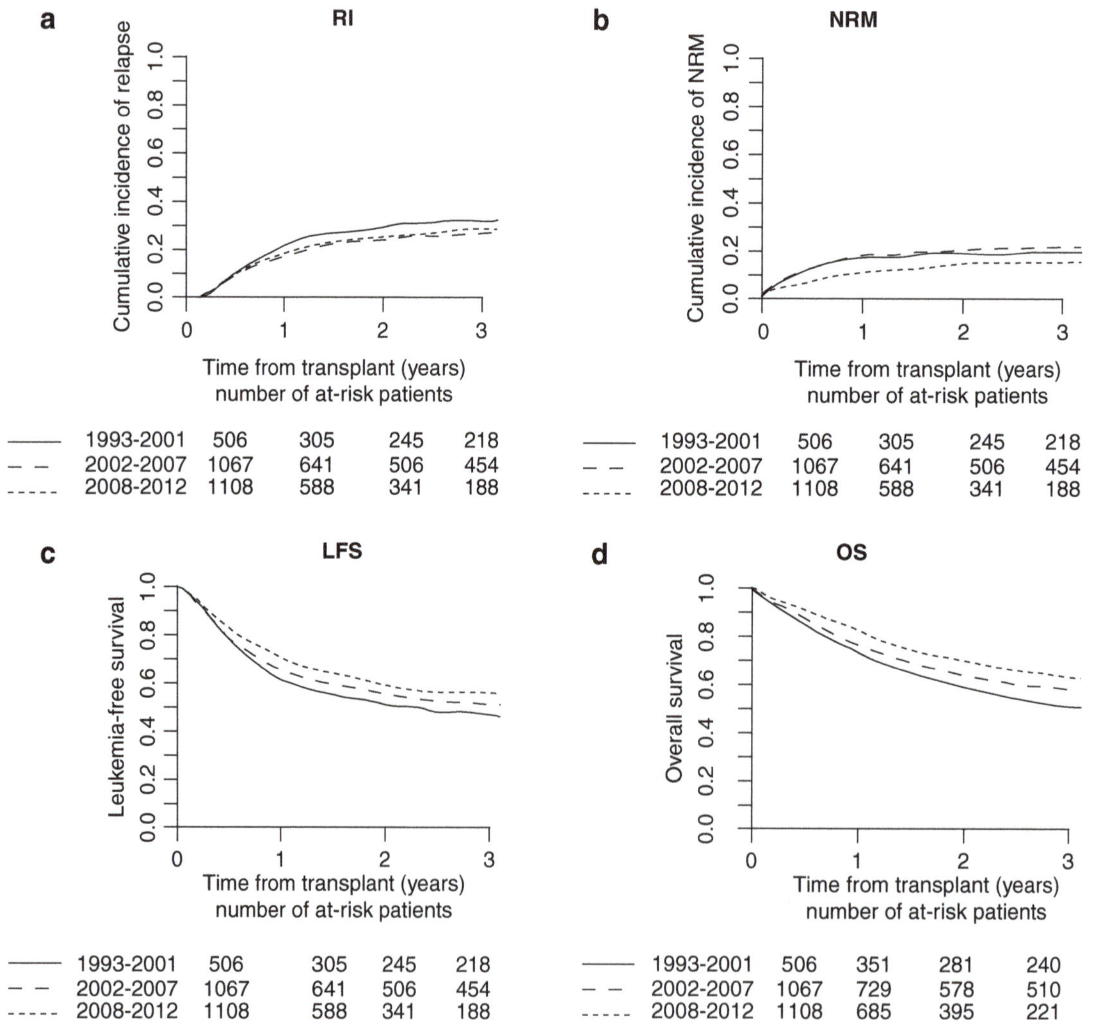

Fig. 71.1 Outcome of *matched sibling donor*—HSCT adults with ALL in CR1. Changes over time in the period 1993–2012. (**a**) Relapse incidence (RI), (**b**) non-relapse mortality (NRM), (**c**) leukemia-free survival (LFS), (**d**) overall survival (OS) (Giebel et al. 2017)

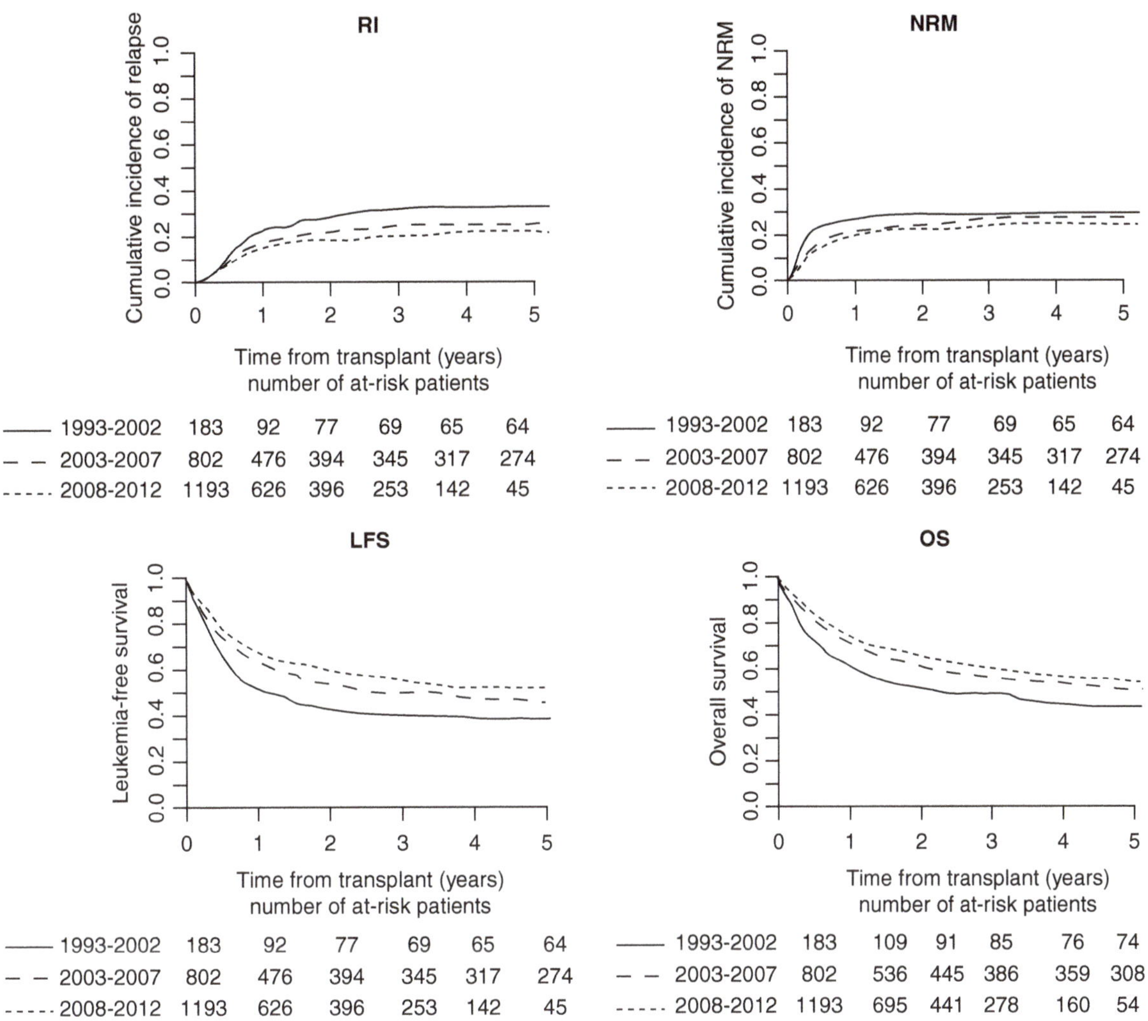

Fig. 71.2 Outcome of *matched sibling donor*—hematopoietic cell transplantation for adults with acute lymphoblastic leukemia (ALL) in first complete remission (CR1). Changes over time in the period 1993–2012. (**a**) Relapse incidence (RI), (**b**) non-relapse mortality (NRM), (**c**) leukemia-free survival (LFS), (**d**) overall survival (OS) (Giebel et al. 2017)

71.9.4 Stem Cell Source

Most likely no relevant difference with regard to GvHD between BM and PBSC as transplant source from an unrelated donor when ATG is part of the conditioning. Faster engraftment and low risk of graft failure with PBSC.

71.9.5 GvHD Prophylaxis

CSA + MTX or CSA + MMF are standard options. ATG should be considered in all patients receiving an allograft from an URD and can be discussed in patients transplanted from an MSD. For haplo-HSCT, using T cell replete allografts combined with post transplant cyclophosphamide (to eliminate alloreactive T cells while sparing other T cells, leading to faster immune reconstitution) is an established option.

71.9.6 Maintenance

For patients with Ph + ALL, maintenance with TKI after allo-HSCT should be applied as a prophylactic or preemptive therapy. At least in patients with B-precursor ALL and positive findings for MRD after allo-HSCT, preemptive therapies with antibodies/antibody-drug conjugates or CAR-T cells are valuable options to be evaluated in prospective trials.

Key Points

Allo-HSCT indicated in	– CR1: high-risk ALL[a] – >CR1: all patients with no contraindication for allogeneic HSCT	
Donor	MSD > MUD > MMUD > Haplo	
Conditioning	– <45 years: TBI/CY; TBI/VP; IV BU/CY. TBI probable associated with lower relapse rates, TBI dose for patients <45 years: cumulative 12–13 Gy – >44 years (or <45 + contraindication for MAC) FLU/IV BU; FLU/MEL; FLU/TBI 8 Gy; FLU/TREO[b]	
Source of SC	PB/BM	
GvHD Proph.	CSA + MTX or CSA + MMF (ATG in MUD or MMUD, consider ATG in MRS)	
Maintenance	Consider TKI in case of Ph + ALL	
TRM	CR1 (age 18–55 year)	MSD: 11–24% (2 year) MUD: 18–29% (2 year)
	CR1 (age >60 year)	MSD: approx. 23% (3 year) MUD: approx. 24% (3 year)
REL	CR1 (age 18–55 year)	MSD: 23–32% (2 year) MUD: 14–21% (2 year)
	CR1 (age >60 year)	MSD: approx. 47% (3 year) MUD: approx. 35% (3 year)
OS	CR1 (age 18–55 year)	MSD: 60–76% (2 year) MUD: 62–70% (2 year)
	CR1 (age >60 year)	MSD: approx. 39% (3 year) MUD: approx. 46% (3 year)
	>CR1[c]	MSD: 8–60% MUD: 10–50%

[a]Definition of "high risk" differs between study groups; most important risk factors: persisting MRD after two courses of therapy, high-risk cytogenetic, early T-cell precursor ALL

[b]For patients treated with inotuzumab ozogamicin, avoid regimens associated with SOS/VODS

[c]Data beyond CR1 are very limited

References

Bassan R, Hoelzer D. Modern therapy of acute lymphoblastic leukemia. J Clin Oncol. 2011;29:532–43.

Bruggemann M, Schrauder A, Raff T, et al. Standardized MRD quantification in European ALL trials: proceedings of the Second International Symposium on MRD assessment in Kiel, Germany, 18-20 September 2008. Leukemia. 2010;24:521–35.

Chiaretti S, Zini G, Bassan R. Diagnosis and subclassification of acute lymphoblastic leukemia. Mediterr J Hematol Infect Dis. 2014;6:e2014073.

Dhawan R, Marks DI. Who should receive a transplant for acute lymphoblastic leukaemia? Curr Hematol Malig Rep. 2017;12:143–52.

Dhedin N, Huynh A, Maury S, et al. Role of allogeneic stem cell transplantation in adult patients with Ph-negative acute lymphoblastic leukemia. Blood. 2015;125:2486–96.

Fielding AK, Rowe JM, Buck G, et al. UKALLXII/ECOG2993: addition of imatinib to a standard treatment regimen enhances long-term outcomes in Philadelphia positive acute lymphoblastic leukemia. Blood. 2014;123:843–50.

Giebel S, Labopin M, Socie G, et al. Improving results of allogeneic hematopoietic cell transplantation for adults with acute lymphoblastic leukemia in first complete remission: an analysis from the Acute Leukemia Working Party of the European Society for Blood and Marrow Transplantation. Haematologica. 2017;102:139–49.

Gokbuget N, Basara N, Baurmann H, et al. High single-drug activity of nelarabine in relapsed T-lymphoblastic leukemia/lymphoma offers curative option with subsequent stem cell transplantation. Blood. 2011;118:3504–11.

Gokbuget N, Dombret H, Ribera JM, et al. International reference analysis of outcomes in adults with B-precursor Ph-negative relapsed/refractory acute lymphoblastic leukemia. Haematologica. 2016;101:1524–33.

Goldstone AH, Richards SM, Lazarus HM, et al. In adults with standard-risk acute lymphoblastic leukemia, the greatest benefit is achieved from a matched sibling allogeneic transplantation in first complete remission, and an autologous transplantation is less effective than conventional consolidation/maintenance chemotherapy in all patients: final results of the International ALL Trial (MRC UKALL XII/ECOG E2993). Blood. 2008;111:1827–33.

Holowiecki J, Krawczyk-Kulis M, Giebel S, et al. Status of minimal residual disease after induction predicts outcome in both standard and high-risk Ph-negative adult acute lymphoblastic leukaemia. The Polish Adult Leukemia Group ALL 4-2002 MRD Study. Br J Haematol. 2008;142:227–37.

Kantarjian H, Jabbour E, Topp S. Blinatumomab for acute lymphoblastic leukemia. N Engl J Med. 2017; 376:e49.

Kantarjian HM, DeAngelo DJ, Stelljes M, et al. Inotuzumab Ozogamicin versus Standard Therapy for Acute Lymphoblastic Leukemia. N Engl J Med. 2016;375:740–53.

Kebriaei P, Cutler C, de Lima M, et al. Management of important adverse events associated with inotuzumab ozogamicin: expert panel review. Bone Marrow Transplant. 2018;53:449–56.

Lazarus HM, Richards SM, Chopra R, et al. Central nervous system involvement in adult acute lymphoblastic leukemia at diagnosis: results from the international ALL trial MRC UKALL XII/ECOG E2993. Blood. 2006;108:465–72.

Marks DI, Forman SJ, Blume KG, et al. A comparison of cyclophosphamide and total body irradiation with etoposide and total body irradiation as conditioning regimens for patients undergoing sibling allografting for acute lymphoblastic leukemia in first or second complete remission. Biol Blood Marrow Transplant. 2006;12:438–53.

Marks DI, Woo KA, Zhong X, et al. Unrelated umbilical cord blood transplant for adult acute lymphoblastic leukemia in first and second complete remission: a comparison with allografts from adult unrelated donors. Haematologica. 2014;99: 322–8.

Maude SL, Laetsch TW, Buechner J, et al. Tisagenlecleucel in children and young adults with B-cell lymphoblastic leukemia. N Engl J Med. 2018;378:439–48.

Maury S, Chevret S, Thomas X, et al. Rituximab in B-lineage adult acute lymphoblastic leukemia. N Engl J Med. 2016;375:1044–53.

Moorman AV, Harrison CJ, Buck GA, et al. Karyotype is an independent prognostic factor in adult acute lymphoblastic leukemia (ALL): analysis of cytogenetic data from patients treated on the Medical Research Council (MRC) UKALLXII/Eastern Cooperative Oncology Group (ECOG) 2993 trial. Blood. 2007;109(8):3189–97.

Park JH, Riviere I, Gonen M, et al. Long-term follow-up of CD19 CAR therapy in acute lymphoblastic leukemia. N Engl J Med. 2018;378:449–59.

Pavlu J, Labopin M, Zoellner AK, et al. Allogeneic hematopoietic cell transplantation for primary refractory acute lymphoblastic leukemia: A report from the Acute Leukemia Working Party of the EBMT. Cancer. 2017;123:1965–70.

Rowe JM, Buck G, Burnett AK, et al. Induction therapy for adults with acute lymphoblastic leukemia: results of more than 1500 patients from the international ALL trial: MRC UKALL XII/ECOG E2993. Blood. 2015;106:3760–7.

Santoro N, Ruggeri A, Labopin M, et al. Unmanipulated haploidentical stem cell transplantation in adults with acute lymphoblastic leukemia: a study on behalf of the Acute Leukemia Working Party of the EBMT. J Hematol Oncol. 2017;10:113.

Terwilliger T, Abdul-Hay M. Acute lymphoblastic leukemia: a comprehensive review and 2017 update. Blood Cancer J. 2017;7:e577.

Trinquand A, Tanguy-Schmidt A, Ben Abdelali R, et al. Toward a NOTCH1/FBXW7/RAS/PTEN-based oncogenetic risk classification of adult T-cell acute lymphoblastic leukemia: a Group for Research in Adult Acute Lymphoblastic Leukemia study. J Clin Oncol. 2013;31:4333–42.

72 Acute Lymphoblastic Leukemia in Children and Adolescents

Christina Peters, Franco Locatelli, and Peter Bader

72.1 Introduction

Although the majority of children and adolescents with acute lymphoblastic leukemia (ALL) are curable with current chemotherapy regimens, poor outcome persists in some individuals (Eckert et al. 2011; von Stackelberg et al. 2011; Schrappe et al. 2012). Allo-HSCT is the most established treatment to control leukemia by means of the GVL effect. During the last decade, it was demonstrated in prospective trials that HSCT from HLA-MSD and from HLA-MURD results in similar outcomes.

Standardized MAC for paediatric patients with high relapse risk produced a low incidence of TRM and effective control of leukemia (Mann et al. 2010; Pulsipher et al. 2011; Peters et al. 2015). Currently, also HSCT from HLA haplo-identical family donors or mismatched CB gives promising results (Rocha et al. 2009; Luznik et al. 2012; Ruggeri et al. 2012; Berger et al. 2016; Klein et al. 2017; Locatelli et al. 2017).

To offer the patients the best available treatment options, a close collaboration between international therapy study groups and transplant consortia are necessary. This is realized within the big treatment consortia for childhood leukemia (e.g. IBFM-SG, IntReALL, NOPHO, UKALL, AIEOP, FRALLE and others) and the paediatric transplant community (e.g. EBMT-PD WG, IBFM-SC SCT, GETMON, GITMO). The study groups for ALL treatment evaluate outcome according to their chemotherapy protocols and stratify patients to relapse standard-risk, medium-risk and high-risk groups. In contrast to adult patients, only patients with high-relapse risk are eligible for allo-HSCT to protect children from the potential long-term consequences of myeloablation and GVHD.

72.2 Prognostic Factors and Indications for HSCT

HSCT indications have to be defined prospectively and must be re-evaluated and reconfirmed at intervals dependent on modifications and improvements in non-transplant approaches for both front-line and relapse protocols. Some risk factors conveying a dismal prognosis in childhood

C. Peters (✉)
Stem Cell Transplantation Unit, St. Anna Children's Hospital, Vienna, Austria
e-mail: christina.peters@stanna.at

F. Locatelli
Department of Pediatric Hematology and Oncology, IRCCS Bambino Gesù Children's Hospital, Rome, Italy

Department of Pediatric Science, University of Pavia, Pavia, Italy

P. Bader
Division for Stem Cell Transplantation and Immunology, University Hospital for Children and Adolescents, Goethe University Frankfurt am Main, Frankfurt, Germany

E. Carreras et al. (eds.), *The EBMT Handbook*, https://doi.org/10.1007/978-3-030-02278-5_72

ALL can be identified even at diagnosis (Moorman 2016; O'Connor et al. 2018). Additionally, response to induction treatment measured by MRD has a strong predictive value and defines nowadays many indications or HSCT (Bader et al. 2009; Conter et al. 2010; Schrappe et al. 2011; Eckert et al. 2013).

72.2.1 Indications: CR1

Only patients with high-risk cytogenetic features or insufficient response to chemotherapy are eligible for HSCT in first remission. In contrast to earlier recommendations, for these patients a MSD and a MURD and for the highest relapse category also mismatched donors are an option (Table 72.1).

72.2.2 Indications: CR2 and Later

All patients with relapse of T-ALL and patients who relapse during or within 6 months of cessation of chemotherapy (very early and early relapse) have a dismal prognosis when treated with conventional chemotherapy. Allo-HSCT from any donor type is the contemporary standard approach (Table 72.2).

If patients achieve a third or higher remission, allo-HSCT should be considered if the physical state allows such a procedure. Patient not in morphological remission should not receive allografts except in extraordinary experimental situations.

72.3 Donor Selection and Stem Cell Source

OS and incidence of NRM have constantly improved; however it has been shown that in children, a BMT from a HLA-identical sibling results in quicker myeloid engraftment, immunoreconstitution and less severe infections and should be therefore the preferred option (Peters et al. 2015). As only 25% of patients have a MSD, HSCT from other donors is the most applied method. Several groups have demonstrated that HSCT from unrelated donors, identified by HLA high-resolution typing and matching, has similar outcome results as MSD-HSCT (Zhang et al. 2012; Fagioli et al. 2013; Burke et al. 2015).

Table 72.1 Indications for allogeneic HSCT in CR1 according to AIEOP-BFM ALL 2009-trial

		PCR-MRD results[a]				
				MRD-HR		
		MRD-SR	MRD-MR[b]	MRD TP2 ≥ 10^{-3} to <10^{-2}	MRD TP2 ≥ 10^{-2}	No MRD result
Criteria hierarchical	No CR d33	No[c]	MMD	MMD	MMD	MMD
	t(4;11)[d]	No	MD	MD	MMD	MD
	Hypodiploidy < 44 chromosomes[e]	No	MD	MD	MMD	MD
	PPR + T-ALL	No	No	MD	MMD	MD
	None of the above features[f]	No	No	MD	MMD	No

PPR Prednisone Poor Response on day 8, *NRd33* No Remission day 33 *MRD*Minimal Residual Disease, *no* Allo HSCT not indicated, *MD* Permitted donor: HLA-matched sibling or non-sibling donor, *MMD* Permitted donor: HLA-matched or HLA-mismatched donor

[a]FCM-MRD results have no impact on the allo-HSCT indication

[b]Including MRD-MR SER (MRD TP1 ≥ 10^{-3} and TP2 $10^{-4/-5}$)

[c]Non-remission in patients with this rare constellation should be due to extramedullary disease. Allo-HSCT indication in these cases should be discussed with the national study coordinator

[d]Independent of prednisone response

[e]The finding of exactly 44 chromosomes qualifies for HR treatment but has no impact on allo-HSCT indication

[f]Including patients with 44 chromosomes

Table 72.2 Indication for HSCT according to IntReALL SR 2010 and HR protocol criteria

Relapse risk group	Phenotype	Time of relapse	Site of relapse	MRD-status	Donor type
Very High	T-ALL	Any time	I-BM, C-BM, I-EM		MSD, MD, MMD
	Non-T-ALL				
		Very early	I-BM, C-BM, I-EM		
		Early	I-BM, C-BM	PR, ND	
High	Non-T-ALL				MSD, MD
		Late	I-BM, C-BM	PR, ND	
		Early	C-BM	GR	
			I-EM		
		Late	I-BM	PR, ND	
			C-BM	ND	

I-BM isolated bone marrow, *C-BM* combined bone marrow and extramedullary site, *I-EM* isolated extramedullary, *MRD: GR* good response as defined by the specific chemotherapy-protocol, *PR* poor response, *ND* not detectable.

Table 72.3 Matching criteria according to HLA typing/matching and stem cell source for children and AYAs with ALL

MSD	HLA-genotypically matched sibling, or 10/10 allelic match (if parental haplotypes unknown)	BM, PBSC
MSD	6/6 or 8/8, 5/6 or 7/8[a]	CB
MD	9/10 or 10/10 allelic matched related or unrelated	BM, PBSC
MD	5–6/6 unrelated or 6–7-8/8 unrelated	CB
MMD	Less than 9/10 matched	BM, PBSC
MMD	Less than 5/6 or 6/8 UCB	CB

MSD matched sibling donor, *MD* matched donor, *MMD* mismatched donor.

[a]4 digits high-resolution typing recommended also for CB matching definition.

Several methods were developed to overcome the HLA barriers. Today it is not clearly proven whether HSCT from HLA-mismatched CB, TCD (alpha-beta depleted, CD34+ selected or CD3/CD19 depleted) haplo-identical grafts or PT-CY approaches will result in the best outcome (Lang and Handgretinger 2008; Smith et al. 2009; Ruggeri et al. 2014; Locatelli et al. 2017) (Tables 72.3 and 72.4).

72.4 Conditioning Regimen

Most children receive a MAC. This consists either of TBI and VP and/or CY or—especially for children below 4 years of age—of BU-/FLU-

Table 72.4 Donor hierarchy—further selection criteria

Variable/ order	Priority
CMV-status	
Patient CMV IgG positive	
1	Donor CMV IgG positive
2	Donor CMV IgG negative
Patient CMV IgG negative	
1	Donor CMV IgG negative
2	Donor CMV IgG positive
Gender	
Female patient	
1	Male or female (preferentially not allo-immunized by prior pregnancy) donor
Male patient	
1	Male Donor
2	Female (preferentially not allo-immunized by prior pregnancy) donor
Age	
1	Younger donor if body weight enables sufficient SC harvest
2	Older donor
Stem cell source	
HSCT from MSD or MD	
1	Bone marrow
2	PPBSC (CAVE: adjust GvHD-prophylaxis for matched siblings)
2	Cord blood with sufficient cell number (>3 × 10^7 NC/kg)
HSCT from MMD: possible options	
	BM, 8/10 matches, unmanipulated
	PBSC, haploidentical, CD3/CD19 depleted, α/β depleted
	CB, sufficient stem cell dose
	PBSC, haploidentical, CD34+ selection
	PT-CY

containing regimen, often combined with TT. An increasing use is recognized for TREO which results also in myeloablation but seems to have less toxic side effects (Wachowiak et al. 2011; Boztug et al. 2015; Lee et al. 2015; Peters et al. 2015).

To reduce acute organ toxicity, the interval between the end of the last chemotherapy and the start of conditioning is 3 or at most 6 weeks. If infection or toxicity requires a delay of conditioning, patients receive risk-adjusted chemotherapy to bridge the time until transplantation. Currently, a multinational trial comparing TBI/VP with either FLU/TT/BU or FLU/TT/TREO investigates in a randomized study the value of both conditioning regimens (FORUM study: allogeneic HSCT for children and AYAs with ALL comparing TBI with myeloablative chemoconditioning) (Willasch et al. 2017).

72.5 GVHD Prophylaxis

Children transplanted with BM from matched sibling donors might benefit from an augmented GVL effect if only single and short GVHD prophylaxis is given (Locatelli et al. 2000). However careful monitoring and rapid treatment intervention are crucial to prevent severe GVHD. After HSCT from non-sibling donors, a combination of CNI and ATG with or without short MTX is given in most patients (Veys et al. 2012; Peters et al. 2015).

72.6 Post-transplant Follow-Up and Interventions

72.6.1 Mixed Chimerism (MC) and MRD

Mixed chimerism (MC) and MRD strongly predict risk for relapse in children (Bader and Kreyenberg 2015).

Preemptive immunotherapy, e.g. withdrawal of IS or DLI guided by chimerism and MRD monitoring, can prevent impending relapse. However, the dynamic of leukaemic reappearance hampers the final success of these methods. Therefore, new post-transplant intervention strategies with less risk for severe complications like bi-specific antibodies or CAR-T-cell interventions may expedite the control of impending relapse (Handgretinger et al. 2011; Maude et al. 2018).

72.6.2 Children with Ph+

Children with Ph + should receive post-transplant TKIs: Whether the prophylactic approach (all Ph + patients will receive TKIs) or a preemptive therapy (only patients with a Ph + signal peri-HSCT) is more effective has to be prospectively proven (Schultz et al. 2010; Bernt and Hunger 2014). Both TKI options are currently under investigation.

72.6.2.1 The Amended EsPhALL Recommendation

Administration of imatinib prophylaxis post HSCT when more than 50,000 platelets are reached. Duration, 365 days after HSCT.

72.6.2.2 TKI According to MRD Result

Administration of imatinib post HSCT for all MRD-positive patients until two negative results are achieved. FACS- and PCR-MRD analyses are accepted.

72.7 Results

Figure 72.1 shows the event-free survival (EFS), overall survival (OS), relapse incidence (RI) and non-relapse mortality (NRM) of the prospective international multicentre trial comparing MSD with MURD (Peters et al. 2015).

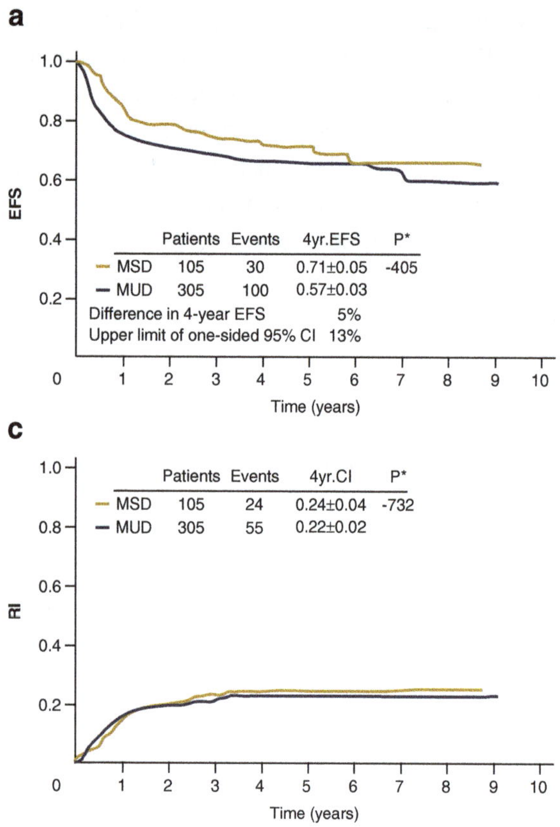

Fig. 72.1 Four-year event-free survival (EFS), overall survival (OS), relapse incidence (RI) and non-relapse mortality (NRM) of the prospective international multicentre trial comparing sibling donors with matched unrelated donors – the ALL-SCT-BFM-2003 trial on behalf of the BFM Study Group, the IBFM Study Group and the EBMT Paediatric Diseases Working Party (Peters et al. 2015)

Key Points

- Only children and adolescents with very high or high relapse risk should be candidates for allo-HSCT. The definition of relapse risk depends on the leukaemic phenotype, response to chemotherapy and—if applicable—time and site of relapse.
- MRD levels during chemotherapy but also pre- and post-HSCT are powerful predictors for outcome after HSCT.
- Patients who are not in morphological remission before conditioning should not undergo allogeneic HSCT except in extraordinary situations.
- MAC is recommended for children with ALL. Whether TBI is necessary to control leukemia is subject of a prospective randomized EBMT/IBFM trial.

References

Bader P, Kreyenberg H, Henze GH, et al. Prognostic value of minimal residual disease quantification before allogeneic stem-cell transplantation in relapsed childhood acute lymphoblastic leukemia: the ALL-REZ BFM Study Group. J Clin Oncol. 2009;27:377–84.

Bader P, Kreyenberg H, von Stackelberg A, et al. Monitoring of minimal residual disease after allogeneic stem-cell transplantation in relapsed childhood acute lymphoblastic leukemia allows for the identification of impending relapse: results of the ALL-BFM-SCT 2003 trial. J Clin Oncol. 2015;33:1275–84.

Berger M, Lanino E, Cesaro S, et al. Feasibility and outcome of haploidentical hematopoietic stem cell transplantation with post-transplant high-dose cyclophosphamide for children and adolescents with hematologic malignancies: an AIEOP-GITMO Retrospective Multicenter Study. Biol Blood Marrow Transplant. 2016;22:902–9.

Bernt KM, Hunger SP. Current concepts in pediatric Philadelphia chromosome-positive acute lymphoblastic leukemia. Front Oncol. 2014;4:54.

Boztug H, Zecca M, Sykora KW, et al. EBMT paediatric diseases working party. Treosulfan-based conditioning regimens for allogeneic HSCT in children with acute lymphoblastic leukemia. Ann Hematol. 2015;94:297–306.

Burke MJ, Verneris MR, Le Rademacher J, et al. Transplant outcomes for children with t cell acute lymphoblastic leukemia in second remission: a report from the center for international blood and marrow transplant research. Biol Blood Marrow Transplant. 2015;21:2154–9.

Conter V, Bartram CR, Valsecchi MG, et al. Molecular response to treatment redefines all prognostic factors in children and adolescents with B-cell precursor acute lymphoblastic leukemia: results in 3184 patients of the AIEOP-BFM ALL 2000 study. Blood. 2010;115:3206–14.

Eckert C, Flohr T, Koehler R, et al. Very early/early relapses of acute lymphoblastic leukemia show unexpected changes of clonal markers and high heterogeneity in response to initial and relapse treatment. Leukemia. 2011;25:1305–13.

Eckert C, von Stackelberg A, Seeger K, et al. Minimal residual disease after induction is the strongest predictor of prognosis in intermediate risk relapsed acute lymphoblastic leukemia - long-term results of trial ALL-REZ BFM P95/96. Eur J Cancer. 2013;49:1346–55.

Fagioli F, Quarello P, Zecca M, et al. Hematopoietic stem cell transplantation for children with high-risk acute lymphoblastic leukemia in first complete remission: a report from the AIEOP registry. Haematologica. 2013;98:1273–81.

Handgretinger R, Zugmaier G, Henze G, et al. Complete remission after blinatumomab-induced donor T-cell activation in three pediatric patients with post-transplant relapsed acute lymphoblastic leukemia. Leukemia. 2011;25:181–4.

Klein OR, Buddenbaum J, Tucker N, et al. Nonmyeloablative haploidentical bone marrow transplantation with post-transplantation cyclophosphamide for pediatric and young adult patients with high-risk hematologic malignancies. Biol Blood Marrow Transplant. 2017;23:325–32.

Lang P, Handgretinger R. Haploidentical SCT in children: an update and future perspectives. Bone Marrow Transplant. 2008;42(Suppl 2):S54–9.

Lee JW, Kang HJ, Kim S, et al. Favorable outcome of hematopoietic stem cell transplantation using a targeted once-daily intravenous busulfan-fludarabine-etoposide regimen in pediatric and infant acute lymphoblastic leukemia patients. Biol Blood Marrow Transplant. 2015;21:190–5.

Locatelli F, Bruno B, Zecca M, et al. Cyclosporin A and short-term methotrexate versus cyclosporin A as graft versus host disease prophylaxis in patients with severe aplastic anemia given allogeneic bone marrow transplantation from an HLA-identical sibling: results of a GITMO/EBMT randomized trial. Blood. 2000;96:1690–7.

Locatelli F, Merli P, Pagliara D, et al. Outcome of children with acute leukemia given HLA-haploidentical HSCT after alphabeta T-cell and B-cell depletion. Blood. 2017;130:677–85.

Luznik L, O'Donnell PV, Fuchs EJ. Post-transplantation cyclophosphamide for tolerance induction in HLA-haploidentical bone marrow transplantation. Semin Oncol. 2012;39:683–93.

Mann G, Attarbaschi A, Schrappe M, et al. Improved outcome with hematopoietic stem cell transplantation in a poor prognostic subgroup of infants with mixed-lineage-leukemia (MLL)-rearranged acute lymphoblastic leukemia: results from the Interfant-99 Study. Blood. 2010;116:2644–50.

Maude SL, Laetsch TW, Buechner J, et al. Tisagenlecleucel in children and young adults with b-cell lymphoblastic leukemia. N Engl J Med. 2018;378:439–48.

Moorman AV. New and emerging prognostic and predictive genetic biomarkers in B-cell precursor acute lymphoblastic leukemia. Haematologica. 2016;101:407–16.

O'Connor D, Enshaei A, Bartram J, et al. Genotype-specific minimal residual disease interpretation improves stratification in pediatric acute lymphoblastic leukemia. J Clin Oncol. 2018;36:34–43.

Peters C, Schrappe M, von Stackelberg A, et al. Stem-cell transplantation in children with acute lymphoblastic leukemia: A prospective international multicenter trial comparing sibling donors with matched unrelated donors-The ALL-SCT-BFM-2003 trial. J Clin Oncol. 2015;33:1265–74.

Pulsipher MA, Peters C, Pui CH. High-risk pediatric acute lymphoblastic leukemia: to transplant or not to transplant? Biol Blood Marrow Transplant. 2011;17(Suppl 1):S137–48.

Rocha V, Kabbara N, Ionescu I, et al. Pediatric related and unrelated cord blood transplantation for malignant diseases. Bone Marrow Transplant. 2009;44:653–9.

Ruggeri A, Michel G, Dalle JH, et al. Impact of pretransplant minimal residual disease after cord blood transplantation for childhood acute lymphoblastic leukemia in remission: an Eurocord, PDWP-EBMT analysis. Leukemia. 2012;26:2455–61.

Ruggeri A, Labopin M, Sormani MP, et al. Engraftment kinetics and graft failure after single umbilical cord blood transplantation using a myeloablative conditioning regimen. Haematologica. 2014;99:1509–15.

Schrappe M, Valsecchi MG, Bartram CR, et al. Late MRD response determines relapse risk overall and in subsets of childhood T-cell ALL: results of the AIEOP-BFM-ALL 2000 study. Blood. 2011;118:2077–84.

Schrappe M, Hunger SP, Pui CH, et al. Outcomes after induction failure in childhood acute lymphoblastic leukemia. N Engl J Med. 2012;366:1371–81.

Schultz KR, Prestidge T, Camitta B. Philadelphia chromosome-positive acute lymphoblastic leukemia in children: new and emerging treatment options. Expert Rev Hematol. 2010;3:731–42.

Smith AR, Baker KS, Defor TE, et al. Hematopoietic cell transplantation for children with acute lymphoblastic leukemia in second complete remission:

similar outcomes in recipients of unrelated marrow and umbilical cord blood versus marrow from HLA matched sibling donors. Biol Blood Marrow Transplant. 2009;15:1086–93.

Veys P, Wynn RF, Ahn KW, et al. Impact of immune modulation with in vivo T-cell depletion and myleoablative total body irradiation conditioning on outcomes after unrelated donor transplantation for childhood acute lymphoblastic leukemia. Blood. 2012;119:6155–61.

von Stackelberg A, Volzke E, Kuhl JS, et al. Outcome of children and adolescents with relapsed acute lymphoblastic leukemia and non-response to salvage protocol therapy: a retrospective analysis of the ALL-REZ BFM Study Group. Eur J Cancer. 2011;47:90–7.

Wachowiak J, Sykora KW, Cornish J, et al. Treosulfan-based preparative regimens for allo-HSCT in childhood hematological malignancies: a retrospective study on behalf of the EBMT pediatric diseases working party. Bone Marrow Transplant. 2011;46:1510–8.

Willasch A, Peters C, Sedlacek P, et al. Myeloablative conditioning for first allogeneic hematopoietic stem cell transplantation in children with all: total body irradiation or chemotherapy? - a multicenter EBMT-PDWP Study. Blood. 2017;130:911.

Zhang MJ, Davies SM, Camitta BM, et al. Comparison of outcomes after HLA-matched sibling and unrelated donor transplantation for children with high-risk acute lymphoblastic leukemia. Biol Blood Marrow Transplant. 2012;18:1204–10.

Check for updates

73 Myelodysplastic Syndromes

Marie Robin and Theo de Witte

73.1 Introduction

Myelodysplastic syndromes (MDS) are a heterogeneous group of clonal stem cell disorders characterized by hypercellular bone marrow, peripheral cytopenias, and dysplastic features in blood and bone marrow. The clinical progression of these diseases varies from an indolent course, over a number of years, to a more rapid transition into secondary AML. MDS is mainly diagnosed in elderly patients, with an annual incidence of 4.9/100,000, but this increases to between 20 and 50 cases per 100,000 persons annually after the age of 60. The current WHO classification (2016) distinguishes various MDS subtypes, which are detailed in Table 73.1 (Arber et al. 2016).

Due to the variable course the disease may take, a number of different *risk-scoring systems* have been developed. The most frequently used of these is the International Prognostic Scoring System (IPSS), introduced by Greenberg et al. (1997) (Table 73.2) and revised in 2012 (Greenberg et al. 2012) (Table 73.3). As a result, intensive treatment strategies are predominantly applied in patients with intermediate and higher-risk MDS. The importance of transfusion dependency is included in a WHO classification-based prognostic scoring system (WPSS) (Della Porta et al. 2015). The role of somatic mutations has been explored recently, highlighting the prognostic role of mutations. *SF3B1* mutations are commonly associated with refractory anemia with ringed sideroblasts and expected survival of more than 10 years. Poor prognostic mutations, such as *TP53* mutations, occur mainly in patients with higher-risk MDS and confer a higher risk of transition to acute leukemia (Makishima et al. 2017). In the setting of allo-HSCT, both somatic mutations and cytogenetic characteristics conserve their prognostic impacts after transplantation, and this aspect will be discussed further hereafter.

Allo-HSCT is increasingly performed, with 940 MDS patients transplanted in 2004 and 2646 patients transplanted in 2015 (EBMT registry). This increase is due to rising numbers of transplants in older patients (>60 years), from 22% of all transplants in 2004 to 44% in 2015, and more MURD, from 37% of all transplants in 2004 to 58% in 2015. The increasing use of unmanipulated haplo-HSCT using intensified IS therapy may also lead to a greater proportion of related donors in future.

M. Robin (✉)
Department of Hematology – Transplantation, Hôpital Saint-Louis, Assistance Publique Hôpitaux de Paris, Paris, France
e-mail: marie.robin@sls.aphp.fr

T. de Witte
Tumor Immunology, Radboud Institute for Molecular Life Sciences, Radboud University Medical Center, Nijmegen, Netherlands

E. Carreras et al. (eds.), *The EBMT Handbook*, https://doi.org/10.1007/978-3-030-02278-5_73

Table 73.1 World Health Organization classification (2016 revision) of MDS

Name	Dysplastic lineage	Cytopenia[a]	RS as % BME	BM and PB blasts, Auer rods (AR)	Cytogenetics[b]
MDS with single-lineage dysplasia (MDS-SLD)	1	1 or 2	<15%/<5%[b]	BM < 5%, PB < 1%, no AR	Any
MDS with multilineage dysplasia (MDS-MLD)	2 or 3	1–3	<15%/<5%[c]	BM < 5%, PB < 1%, no AR	Any
MDS with ring sideroblasts (MDS-RS)					
— MDS-RS SLD — MDS-RS-MLD	1 2–3	1 or 2 1–3	≥15%/>5%[c] ≥15%/>5%[c]	BM < 5%, PB < 1%, no AR	Any
MDS with isolated del(5q)	1–3	1–2	None or any	BM < 5%, PB < 1%, no AR	Del(5q)[d]
MDS with excess blasts (MDS-EB)					
— MDS-EB1	0–3	1–3	None or any	BM 5–9% or PB 2–4%, no AR	Any
— MDS-EB2	0–3	1–3	None or any	BM 10–19% or PB 5–19%, or AR	Any
MDS, unclassifiable (MDS-U)					
— With 1% blood blasts	1–3	1–3	None or any	BM < 5%, PB = 1%, no AR	Any
— With SLD and pancytopenia	1	3	None or any	BM < 5%, PB < 1%, no AR	Any
— Based on defining cytogenetic	0	1–3	<15%	BM < 5%, PB < 1%, no AR	Defining abnormality
Refractory cytopenia in childhood	1–3	1–3	None	BM < 5%, PB < 2%	Any

BM bone marrow, *PB* peripheral (blood) blast, RS as %BME, ring sideroblasts as a % of marrow erythroid elements
[a]Cytopenia defined as hemoglobin <10 g/dL, platelet count <100 g/L, absolute neutrophil count <1.8 g/L
[b]Cytogenetics by conventional karyotype analysis
[c]If *SF3B1* is present
[d]Alone or with one additional abnormality except −7 or del(7q)

Table 73.2 "Classic IPSS"

Points	*0*	*0.5*	*1*	*1.5*	2
Marrow blast	<5	5–10	>10	11–20	21–30
Cytogenetic[a]	Good	Intermediate	Poor		
Cytopenia[b]	0–1	2/3			
Risk	*Low*	*Intermediate-1*	*Intermediate-2*	*High*	
Number of points	0	0.5–1	1.5 or more		
Median OS (years)	5.7	3.5	1.2	0.4	
Median time to 25% AML transformation in years	9.4	3.3	1.1	0.2	

OS overall survival
[a]*Good*, normal, -Y, del(5q), del(20q); *poor*, complex karyotype (three or more abnormalities) or chromosome 7 anomalies; *intermediate*, other abnormalities
[b]Cytopenia was defined as follows: hemoglobin <10 g/dL, platelet <100 g/L, absolute neutrophil count <1 g/L

73.2 Indication of HSCT in MDS and Timing to Transplant

HSCT is an established procedure for MDS leading to long-term survival. The indications for HSCT may change following the introduction of new treatment strategies, and the HSCT approach itself has consistently evolved over time. TRM should always be balanced against the benefits associated with HSCT. Comparisons of several transplant and non-transplant cohorts show a gain in life expectancy in patients, with higher risks if they receive an allo-HSCT at MDS diagnosis, while in lower-risk MDS patients, a survival

Table 73.3 "Revised IPSS"

Points	*0*	*0.5*	*1*	*1.5*	*2*	*3*	*4*
Marrow blast	<3		3–4		5–10	11–20	
Cytogenetic[a]	Very good		Good		Intermediate	Poor	Very poor
Cytopenia[b]	No	Mild	Moderate	Severe anemia			
Risk	*Very low*	*Low*	*Intermediate*	*High*	*Very high*		
Number of points	≤ 1.5	2–3	4–4.5	5–6	>6		
Median OS (years)	8.8	5.3	3	1.6	0.8		
Median time to 25% AML transformation in years		10.8	3.2	1.4	0.73		

[a]Cytogenetics: *very good*, -Y, del(11q); *good*, normal, del(5q), del(12p), del(20q), double including del(5q); intermediate, del(7q), −8, −19, i(17q), any other single or double independent clones; *poor*, −7, inv.(3)/t(3q)/del(3q), double including −7/del(7q), complex, 3 abnormalities; *very poor*, complex, > 3 abnormalities
[b]cytopenia, *mild cytopenia*, platelet count <100 g/L or neutrophil count <0.8 g/L; *moderate cytopenia*, hemoglobin <10 g/dL but >10 g/dL, platelet count <50 g/L; *severe anemia*, hemoglobin <8 g/dL

advantage can be seen if HSCT is deferred (Cutler et al. 2004; Koreth et al. 2013; Della Porta et al. 2017; Robin et al. 2015). An international expert panel has also confirmed the indication of HSCT in higher-risk patients as well as lower-risk patients with specific poor prognostic features, including genetic alterations, failure to respond to usual treatment, life-threatening cytopenias, and high-intensity transfusions (de Witte et al. 2017). Figures 73.1 and 73.2 summarize transplant indications in MDS patients.

73.3 Post-HSCT Outcomes

Several recent registry studies including cytogenetic classification have reported outcomes for transplanted MDS patients (Table 73.4). Overall survival (OS) ranged from 35 to 50%, NRM from 30 to 40%, and relapse rates from 15 to 30%. Lower-risk MDS patients had better prognoses, and the EBMT cohort of low and intermediate-1 MDS patients showed that OS could reach 57%, with relapse incidence at 16% after 7 years (Robin et al. 2017a). Patients with poor and very poor risk cytogenetic characteristics, including monosomal karyotypes, were associated with poor outcomes. FAB classification, age, platelet count, stage at time of transplantation, and hematopoietic cell transplant-comorbidity index (HCT-CI) were prognostic clinical risk factors. Somatic mutations, i.e., *TP53, TET2, ASXL1, RUNX1*, and *RAS* pathways mutations, have been reported to be prognostic independent factors in several reports (Bejar et al. 2014; Della Porta et al. 2016; Lindsley et al. 2017; Yoshizato et al. 2017).

Due to the increase in patient age, transplantation results in these patients should be highlighted, as outcomes seem to be highly impacted by performance status and HCT-CI (McClune et al. 2010; Lim et al. 2010). The EBMT recently published two studies focusing on transplants in elderly patients. The first study included 1333 MDS patients above the age of 55, transplanted between 1998 and 2006 (Lim et al. 2010). Four-year OS was 31%, with NRM of 36%. The second study reported 313 MDS patients above the age of 70, transplanted between 2000 and 2013 (Heidenreich et al. 2017). The study findings showed 3-year OS of 34% and NRM of 42% confirming that transplant was feasible in this category of patients.

73.4 Alternative Donors and Donor Choice

In recent EBMT studies, HSCT from an URD did not appear to be a mortality risk factor compared with HSCT using MSD (Onida et al. 2014; Koenecke et al. 2015). Saber et al., on behalf of

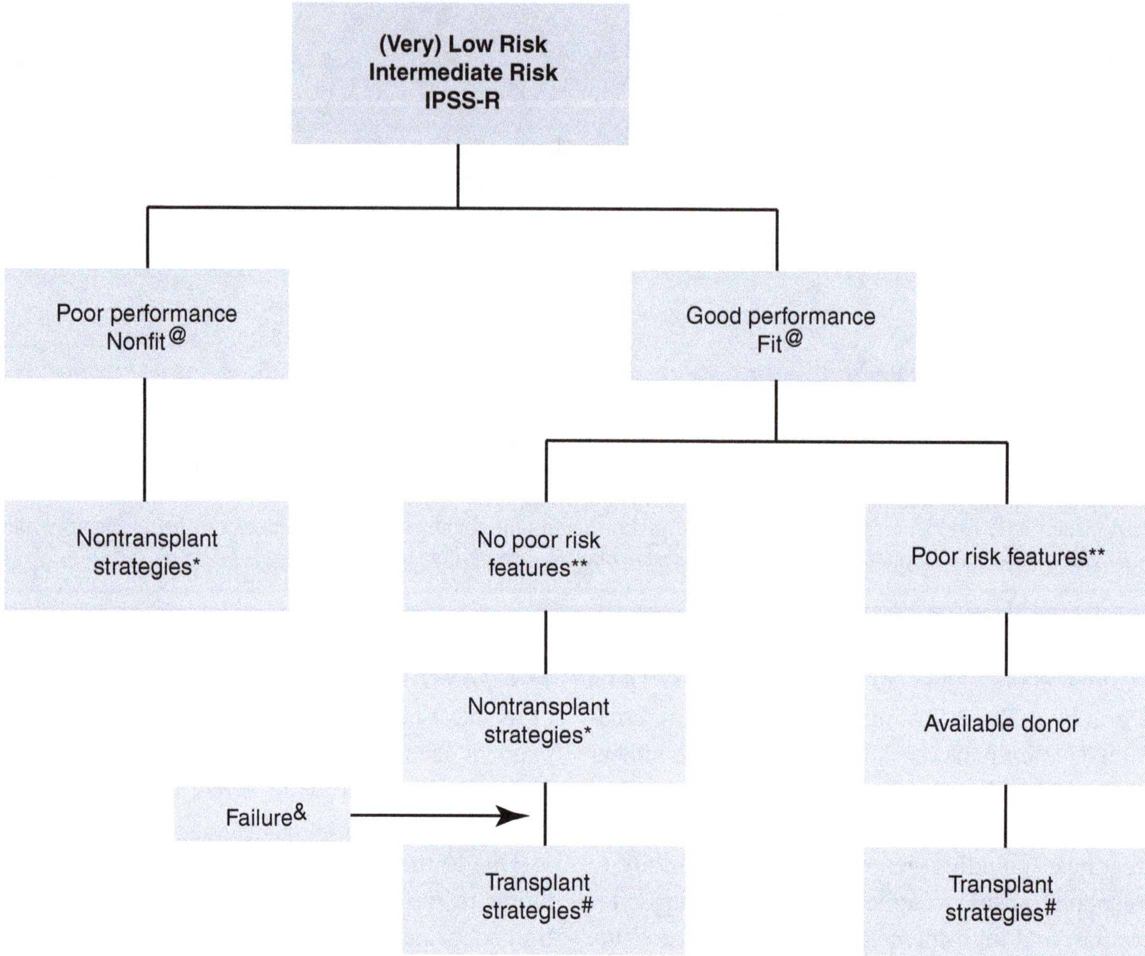

Fig. 73.1 Therapeutic flow chart for adult MDS patients with (very) low-risk or intermediate-risk IPSS-R scores @ indicates nonfit (patients with multiple comorbidities and/or poor performance) or fit (patients with no comorbidities and good performance status). * indicates nontransplant strategies according to most recent versions published by international MDS expert groups, including ELN and NCCN. & indicates failure of nontransplant strategies. ** indicates poor-risk features (defined as poor-risk cytogenetic characteristics, persistent blast increase [>50% or with >15% BM blasts], life-threatening cytopenias, high transfusion intensity >2 units per months for 6 months; molecular testing should be seriously considered, in case of absence of poor-risk cytogenetic characteristics or persistent blast increase). # indicates transplant strategies (all forms of HSCT, for details of the donor selection, type of conditioning, and post transplant strategies, see text; no upper age limit if patients are fit, without serious comorbidity, and with good Karnofsky status)

the CIBMTR, reported the results of HSCT in 701 MDS patients according to donor type: MRD, MUD (8 out of 8 high-resolution HLA compatibilities), and MMUD (Saber et al. 2012). Multiple-variable analysis showed that NRM was significantly lower with the use of MRDs compared with other donors, but that treatment failure (death or relapse) was similar to MUD, while it was significantly higher in patients transplanted from a MMUD (Saber et al. 2012).

The EBMT group reported outcomes for 631 MDS patients transplanted with a MUD (n = 379), a MMUD (n = 107), or a MMUCB (n = 129) (Robin et al. 2014). Patients transplanted with a MUD had better outcomes for OS, relapse-free survival, and NRM, while patients transplanted from MMUDs had similar outcomes, with a trend to a better DFS for MMUD compared with UCB. Recommendations are to choose an HLA-matched related or unrelated

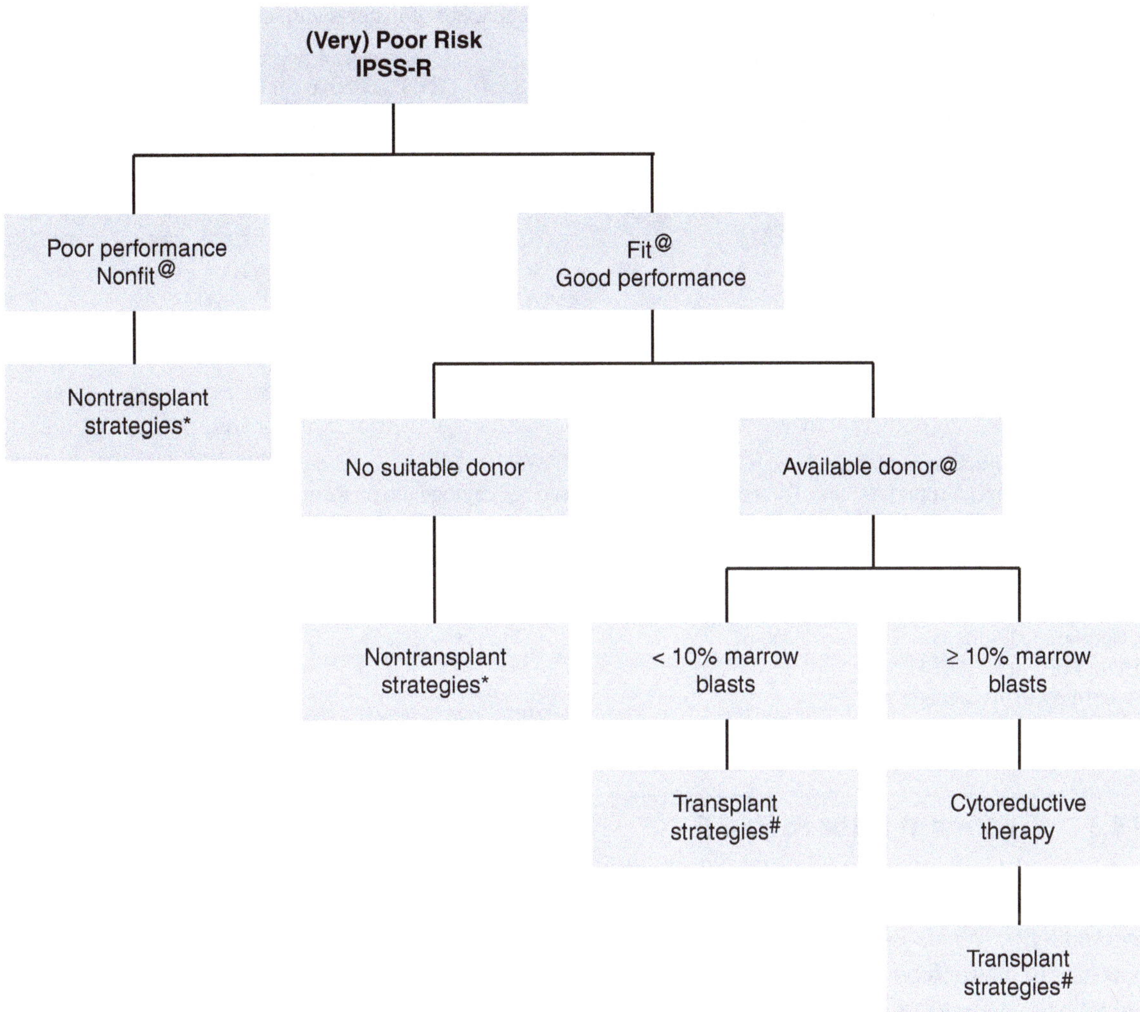

Fig. 73.2 Therapeutic flow chart for adult MDS patients with poor IPSS-R scores. @ indicates nonfit (patients with multiple comorbidities and/or poor performance) or fit (patients with no comorbidities and good performance status). * indicates nontransplant strategies according to most recent versions published by international MDS expert groups, including ELN and NCCN. & indicates failure of nontransplant strategies. ** indicates poor-risk features (defined as poor-risk cytogenetic characteristics, persistent blast increase [>50% or with >15% BM blasts], life-threatening cytopenias, high transfusion intensity >2 units per months for 6 months; molecular testing should be seriously considered, in case of absence of poor-risk cytogenetic characteristics or persistent blast increase). # indicates transplant strategies (all forms of HSCT, for details of the donor selection, type of conditioning, and post transplant strategies, see text; no upper age limit if patients are fit, without serious comorbidity,and with good Karnofsky status)

donor as both kinds of donor may lead to similar outcomes (Bowen 2017).

HSCT from haplo-identical related donors has been revisited due to new GVHD prophylaxis strategies, including the use of PT-CY. Little data has been published on MDS patients, although results in patients with other diseases are very promising (Bashey et al. 2013; Ciurea et al. 2015). A recent EBMT study reported 234 patients transplanted from haplo-donors between 2007 and 2014. Although NRM was relatively high, results were encouraging, with better results using PT-CY and RIC (Robin et al. 2017b). A recent issue is the impact of donor age on post transplant outcomes, suggesting that outcomes may be better with younger donors (Kollman et al. 2016; Kröger et al. 2013). This is particularly relevant in MDS, where both recipients and related donors are typically old.

Table 73.4 Patient outcomes in recent studies, including a large number of patients with cytogenetic data

HSCT centers; HSCT periods	Number of patients	Median age	RI	NRM	OS	RFS	Mortality risk factors in multiple-variable analysis
FHCRC[a] 1980–2010	1007	45	25	40	38	35	Blast count, CG, non-MAC, AML transformation, age, platelet count, HLA MM
EBMT[b] 1981–2006	523	43	25	36	43	38	CG, disease stage at HSCT, age, FAB, TCD[g]
EBMT[c] 1981–2012	903	50	36	33	36	32	Age, FAB, CG
SFGM-TC[d] 1999–2009	367	54	31–50	21–>31	32–>53		CG, marrow blast %, TBI in regimen, donor type
GITMO[e] 2000–2011	519	48	16–>41[f]	27–>35[f]	48–>15[f]		IPSS, HCT-CI, CG, disease stage at HSCT, donor type

FHCRC Fred Hutchinson Cancer Research Center, *SFGM-TC* Société Francophone de greffe de moelle et de thérapie cellulaire, *GITMO* Gruppo Italiano Trapianto di Midollo Osseo, *CG* cytogenetics, *RI* relapse incidence, *TBI* total body irradiation in conditioning regimen
[a]Deeg et al. (2012)
[b]Onida et al. (2014)
[c]Koenecke et al. (2015)
[d]Gauthier et al. (2015)
[e]Della Porta et al. (2014)
[f]According to cytogenetic risk
[g]Was assessed only in "untreated RA/RARS" because there were no prognostic factors in this group

73.5 Treatment Prior to HSCT

No randomized studies have compared pre-graft cytoreduction versus upfront transplants in MDS patients. Because hypomethylating agents (HMA) have been reported to improve survival in MDS patients, they are routinely used before considering a transplant procedure, leading to a delay in transplantation. It is very difficult from registry data to gain real insight into the risks or benefits of treatment with HMA. International guidelines generally recommend that patients with more than 10% marrow blast should receive cytoreductive treatment, which can be either intensive chemotherapy or HMA (de Witte et al. 2017b; Malcovati et al. 2013). The EBMT group reported that refractoriness to pre-graft treatment is associated with poor outcomes, confirming a French retrospective study (Potter et al. 2016; Damaj et al. 2012).

73.6 Preparative Regimen

The use of RIC regimens for HSCT has raised considerable interest. Multiple centers have developed novel RIC regimens that have reduced NRM and morbidity and subsequently expanded the curative potential of HSCT to older individuals who have historically not been considered to be HSCT candidates.

The EBMT group has compared outcomes for MDS patients treated by RIC or MAC (Martino et al. 2006; Martino et al. 2017). Studies show that relapse rates increased after RIC, while NRM was higher after MAC, in line with the findings of another study (Scott et al. 2006). Subsequent research by the EBMT group reported outcomes for 878 MDS or AML patients transplanted with less than 10% marrow blasts and classified according to the intensity of conditioning regimen considering four groups: non-MAC, RIC, standard regimen and hyperintensive regimen (Martino et al. 2013). OS after 7 years was 29, 53, 56, and 51%, respectively, for each regimen, with a disadvantage for the non-MAC. An EBMT prospective study comparing the use of RIC (FLU/BU) and MAC (CY/BU) in patients with MDS or secondary AML was published recently (Kröger et al. 2017). Multivariable analysis failed to show any impact of the regimen intensity in NRM, relapse, and RFS, while there was an advantage for RIC in OS, after adjustment for cytogenetics, performance status, and disease stage. The BMT-CTN performed a prospective study on 272 patients with MDS or AML who were randomized between RIC and MAC. There was no difference in OS between the two groups, despite a higher relapse rate after RIC (Scott et al. 2017).

A novel RIC sequential regimen consisting of FLU 30 mg/m², Ara-C 2 g/m², and amsacrine 100 mg/m² (FLAMSA), followed 3 days later by 4 Gy TBI and CY 80–120 mg/kg showed promising results (Schmid et al. 2005; Schmid et al. 2006). Prospective randomized trials comparing sequential regimens with other regimens are ongoing.

73.7 Post-HSCT Treatment

MDS patients with relapse after HSCT are often refractory to treatment, or not fit enough to be treated. A German group recently reported outcomes for AML ($n = 124$) and MDS ($n = 28$) patients treated with AZA and DLI (Schroeder et al. 2015). The main risk factors for treatment response were molecular relapse only or marrow blast <13%. In these cases, OS was more than 60%, although it was below 10% in high-risk patients. An EBMT study of 181 patients treated with AZA for post transplant relapse of MDS confirmed that lower blast counts upon relapse and relapsing more than 6 months after HSCT were both good prognostic factors (Craddock et al. 2016a, b). In this study, the addition of DLI did not modify outcomes. Another EBMT study on cellular therapy after relapse (DLI or second transplant) showed that a second allo-HSCT performed in CR may rescue patients with relapse after initial HSCT, especially if they have no previous history of GVHD, and in cases where they may be transplanted from a new donor (Schmid et al. 2018). The French SFGM-TC group recently reported 147 MDS patients relapsing after transplant (Guieze et al. 2016). Only patients who received "cellular therapy" (DLI or second SCT) were able to achieve long-term survival (32% versus 6% for chemotherapy alone).

Other strategies involve preventive or preemptive treatment after transplantation to avoid morphological relapse. Preemptive strategies based on underlying risk or monitoring of minimal residual disease may be of use in these patients who present a high risk of post transplant relapse (Platzbecker et al. 2012). Although relapse remains the most common cause of transplant failure, particularly in patients with high-risk features, novel strategies such as the preemptive use of AZA or DLI may be effective in improving historically poor outcomes. Preventive post transplant treatment testing demethylating agents early after transplantation have also been reported in small prospective studies (de Lima et al. 2010; Pusic et al. 2015; Craddock et al. 2016a, b). This kind of treatment appears to be especially useful in patients with higher-risk MDS.

Key Points

- Allo-HSCT is the treatment of choice for all patients with (very) poor-risk MDS, or intermediate patients with high-risk features, who are fit enough to be considered for transplantation.
- Delayed HSCT is associated with reduced chances of prolonged relapse-free survival. Also, patients with less advanced MDS categories may benefit from deferred HSCT after they develop poor-risk features.
- Allo-HSCT outcomes have improved progressively in recent years, mainly due to a gradual reduction in non-relapse mortality. Reduced-intensity conditioning (RIC) regimens have extended the use of allo-HSCT to older patients, including those entering their eighth decade.
- However, a number of questions remain to be resolved by prospective studies, such as the choice of donor, including haplo-identical donors, the role of post transplant treatment, and the timing of transplantation in patients with lower-risk MDS.

References

Arber DA, Orazi A, Hasserjian R, et al. The 2016 revision to the World Health Organization classification of myeloid neoplasms and acute leukemia. Blood. 2016;127:2391–405.

Bashey A, Zhang X, Sizemore CA, et al. T-cell-replete HLA-haploidentical hematopoietic transplantation for hematologic malignancies using post-transplantation cyclophosphamide results in outcomes equivalent to those of contemporaneous HLA-matched related and unrelated donor transplantation. J Clin Oncol. 2013;31:1310–6.

Bejar R, Stevenson KE, Caughey B, et al. Somatic mutations predict poor outcome in patients with myelodysplastic syndrome after hematopoietic stem-cell transplantation. J Clin Oncol. 2014;32:2691–8.

Ciurea SO, Zhang M-J, Bacigalupo AA, et al. Haploidentical transplant with posttransplant cyclophosphamide vs matched unrelated donor transplant for acute myeloid leukemia. Blood. 2015;126:1033–40.

Craddock C, Jilani N, Siddique S, et al. Tolerability and clinical activity of post-transplantation azacitidine in patients allografted for acute myeloid leukemia treated on the RICAZA trial. Biol Blood Marrow Transplant. 2016a;22:385–90.

Craddock C, Labopin M, Robin M, et al. Clinical activity of azacitidine in patients who relapse after allogeneic stem cell transplantation for acute myeloid leukemia. Haematologica. 2016b;101:879–83.

Cutler CS, Lee SJ, Greenberg P, et al. A decision analysis of allogeneic bone marrow transplantation for the myelodysplastic syndromes: delayed transplantation for low-risk myelodysplasia is associated with improved outcome. Blood. 2004;104:579–85.

Damaj G, Duhamel A, Robin M, et al. Impact of azacitidine before allogeneic stem-cell transplantation for myelodysplastic syndromes: a study by the Societe Francaise de Greffe de Moelle et de Therapie-Cellulaire and the Groupe-Francophone des Myelodysplasies. J Clin Oncol. 2012;30:4533–40.

de Lima M, Giralt S, Thall PF, et al. Maintenance therapy with low-dose azacitidine after allogeneic hematopoietic stem cell transplantation for recurrent acute myelogenous leukemia or myelodysplastic syndrome: a dose and schedule finding study. Cancer. 2010;116:5420–31.

de Witte T, Bowen D, Robin M, et al. Use of hematopoietic cell transplantation for patients with myelodysplastic syndrome and chronic myelomonocytic leukemia. Blood. 2017;129:1753–62.

de Witte T, Bowen D, Robin M, et al. Allogeneic hematopoietic stem cell transplantation for MDS and CMML: recommendations from an international expert panel. Blood. 2017b;129:1753–62.

Deeg HJ, Scott BL, Fang M, et al. Five-group cytogenetic risk classification, monosomal karyotype, and outcome after hematopoietic cell transplantation for MDS or acute leukemia evolving from MDS. Blood. 2012;120:1398–408.

Della Porta MG, Tuechler H, Malcovati L, et al. Validation of WHO classification-based Prognostic Scoring System (WPSS) for myelodysplastic syndromes and comparison with the revised International Prognostic Scoring System (IPSS-R). A study of the International Working Group for Prognosis in Myelodysplasia (IWG-PM). Leukemia. 2015;29:1502–13.

Della Porta MG, Alessandrino EP, Bacigalupo A, et al. Predictive factors for the outcome of allogeneic transplantation in patients with MDS stratified according to the revised IPSS-R. Blood. 2014;123:2333–42.

Della Porta MG, Gallì A, Bacigalupo A, et al. Clinical effects of driver somatic mutations on the outcomes of patients with myelodysplastic syndromes treated with allogeneic hematopoietic stem-cell transplantation. J Clin Oncol. 2016;34(30):3627–37. https://doi.org/10.1200/JCO.2016.67.3616.

Della Porta MG, Jackson CH, Alessandrino EP, et al. Decision analysis of allogeneic hematopoietic stem cell transplantation for patients with myelodysplastic syndrome stratified according to the revised International Prognostic Scoring System. Leukemia. 2017;31:2449–57.

Gauthier J, Damaj G, Langlois C, et al. Contribution of revised International Prognostic Scoring System cytogenetics to predict outcome after allogeneic stem cell transplantation for myelodysplastic syndromes: a study from the French Society of Bone Marrow Transplantation and Cellular Therapy. Transplantation. 2015;99:1672–80.

Greenberg P, Cox C, LeBeau MM, et al. International scoring system for evaluating prognosis in myelodysplastic syndromes. Blood. 1997;89:2079–88.

Greenberg PL, Tuechler H, Schanz J, et al. Revised international prognostic scoring system for myelodysplastic syndromes. Blood. 2012;120:2454–65.

Guieze R, Damaj G, Pereira B, et al. Management of myelodysplastic syndromes relapsing after allogeneic hematopoietic stem-cell transplantation: a study by the SFGM-TC. Biol Blood Marrow Transplant. 2016;22:240–7.

Heidenreich S, Ziagkos D, de Wreede LC, et al. Allogeneic stem cell transplantation for patients age ≥ 70 years with myelodysplastic syndrome: a retrospective study of the MDS subcommittee of the chronic malignancies working party of the EBMT. Biol Blood Marrow Transplant. 2017;23:44–52.

Koenecke C, Gohring G, de Wreede LC, et al. Impact of the revised International Prognostic Scoring System cytogenetics and monosomal karyotype on outcome after allogeneic stem cell transplantation for myelodysplastic syndromes and secondary acute myeloid leukemia evolving from myelodysplastic syndromes: a retrospective multicenter study of the European Society of Blood and Marrow Transplantation. Haematologica. 2015;100:400–8.

Kollman C, Spellman SR, Zhang M-J, et al. The effect of donor characteristics on survival after unrelated donor transplantation for hematologic malignancy. Blood. 2016;127:260–7.

Koreth J, Pidala J, Perez WS, et al. Role of reduced-intensity conditioning allogeneic hematopoietic stem-cell transplantation in older patients with de novo myelodysplastic syndromes: an international collaborative decision analysis. J Clin Oncol. 2013;31:2662–70.

Kröger N, Zabelina T, de Wreede L, et al. Allogeneic stem cell transplantation for older advanced MDS patients: improved survival with young unrelated donor in comparison with HLA-identical siblings. Leukemia. 2013;27:604–9.

Kröger N, Iacobelli S, Franke G-N, et al. Dose-reduced versus standard conditioning followed by allogeneic stem-cell transplantation for patients with myelodysplastic syndrome: a prospective randomized phase III study of the EBMT (RICMAC Trial). J Clin Oncol. 2017;35:2157–64.

Lim Z, Brand R, Martino R, et al. Allogeneic hematopoietic stem-cell transplantation for patients 50 years or older with myelodysplastic syndromes or secondary acute myeloid leukemia. J Clin Oncol. 2010;28:405–11.

Lindsley RC, Saber W, Mar BG, et al. Prognostic mutations in myelodysplastic syndrome after stem-cell transplantation. N Engl J Med. 2017;376:536–47.

Makishima H, Yoshizato T, Yoshida K, et al. Dynamics of clonal evolution in myelodysplastic syndromes. Nat Genet. 2017;49:204–12.

Malcovati L, Hellstrom-Lindberg E, Bowen D, et al. Diagnosis and treatment of primary myelodysplastic syndromes in adults: recommendations from the European LeukemiaNet. Blood. 2013;122:2943–64.

Martino R, Iacobelli S, Brand R, et al. Retrospective comparison of reduced-intensity conditioning and conventional high-dose conditioning for allogeneic hematopoietic stem cell transplantation using HLA-identical sibling donors in myelodysplastic syndromes. Blood. 2006;108:836–46.

Martino R, de Wreede L, Fiocco M, et al. Comparison of conditioning regimens of various intensities for allogeneic hematopoietic SCT using HLA-identical sibling donors in AML and MDS with <10% BM blasts: a report from EBMT. Bone Marrow Transplant. 2013;48:761–70.

Martino R, Henseler A, van Lint M, et al. Long-term follow-up of a retrospective comparison of reduced-intensity conditioning and conventional high-dose conditioning for allogeneic transplantation from matched related donors in myelodysplastic syndromes. Bone Marrow Transplant. 2017;52:1107–12.

McClune BL, Weisdorf DJ, Pedersen TL, et al. Effect of age on outcome of reduced-intensity hematopoietic cell transplantation for older patients with acute myeloid leukemia in first complete remission or with myelodysplastic syndrome. J Clin Oncol. 2010;28:1878–87.

Onida F, Brand R, van Biezen A, et al. Impact of the International Prognostic Scoring System cytogenetic risk groups on the outcome of patients with primary myelodysplastic syndromes undergoing allogeneic stem cell transplantation from human leukocyte antigen-identical siblings: a retrospective analysis of the European Society for Blood and Marrow Transplantation-Chronic Malignancies Working Party. Haematologica. 2014;99:1582–90.

Platzbecker U, Wermke M, Radke J, et al. Azacitidine for treatment of imminent relapse in MDS or AML patients after allogeneic HSCT: results of the RELAZA trial. Leukemia. 2012;26:381–9.

Potter VT, Iacobelli S, van Biezen A, et al. Comparison of Intensive Chemotherapy and Hypomethylating Agents before Allogeneic Stem Cell Transplantation for Advanced Myelodysplastic Syndromes: A Study of the Myelodysplastic Syndrome Subcommittee of the Chronic Malignancies Working Party of the European Society for Blood and Marrow Transplant Research. Biol Blood Marrow Transplant. 2016;22:1615–20.

Pusic I, Choi J, Fiala MA, et al. Maintenance Therapy with Decitabine after Allogeneic Stem Cell Transplantation for Acute Myelogenous Leukemia and Myelodysplastic Syndrome. Biol Blood Marrow Transplant. 2015;21:1761–9.

Robin M, Ruggeri A, Labopin M, et al. Comparison of Unrelated Cord Blood and Peripheral Blood Stem Cell Transplantation in Adults with Myelodysplastic Syndrome after Reduced-Intensity Conditioning Regimen: A Collaborative Study from Eurocord (Cord blood Committee of Cellular Therapy & Immunobiology Working Party of EBMT) and Chronic Malignancies Working Party. Biol Blood Marrow Transplant. 2014;21:489–95.

Robin M, Porcher R, Ades L, et al. HLA-matched allogeneic stem cell transplantation improves outcome of higher risk myelodysplastic syndrome A prospective study on behalf of SFGM-TC and GFM. Leukemia. 2015;29:1496–501.

Robin M, Porcher R, Zinke-Cerwenka W, et al. Allogeneic haematopoietic stem cell transplant in patients with lower risk myelodysplastic syndrome: a retrospective analysis on behalf of the Chronic Malignancy Working Party of the EBMT. Bone Marrow Transplant. 2017a;52:209–15.

Robin M, Porcher R, Ciceri F, et al. Haploidentical transplant in patients with myelodysplastic syndrome. Blood Adv. 2017b;1:1876–83.

Saber W, Opie S, Rizzo JD, et al. Outcomes after matched unrelated donor versus identical sibling hematopoietic cell transplantation in adults with acute myelogenous leukemia. Blood. 2012;119:3908–16.

Schmid C, de Wreede LC, van Biezen A, et al. Outcome after relapse of myelodysplastic syndrome and secondary acute myeloid leukemia following allogeneic stem cell transplantation: a retrospective registry analysis on 698 patients by the Chronic Malignancies Working Party of the European Society of Blood and Marrow Transplantation. Haematologica. 2018;103:237–45.

Schmid C, Schleuning M, Ledderose G, et al. Sequential regimen of chemotherapy, reduced-intensity conditioning for allogeneic stem-cell transplantation, and prophylactic donor lymphocyte transfusion in high-risk acute myeloid leukemia and myelodysplastic syndrome. J Clin Oncol. 2005;23:5675–87.

Schmid C, Schleuning M, Schwerdtfeger R, et al. Long-term survival in refractory acute myeloid leukemia after sequential treatment with chemotherapy and reduced-intensity conditioning for allogeneic stem cell transplantation. Blood. 2006;108:1092–9.

Schroeder T, Rachlis E, Bug G, et al. Treatment of acute myeloid leukemia or myelodysplastic syndrome relapse after allogeneic stem cell transplantation with azacitidine and donor lymphocyte infusions--a retrospective multicenter analysis from the German Cooperative Transplant Study Group. Biol Blood Marrow Transpl. 2015;21:653–60.

Scott BL, Sandmaier BM, Storer B, et al. Myeloablative vs nonmyeloablative allogeneic transplantation for patients with myelodysplastic syndrome or acute myelogenous leukemia with multilineage dysplasia: a retrospective analysis. Leukemia. 2006;20:128–35.

Scott BL, Pasquini MC, Logan BR, et al. Myeloablative versus reduced-intensity hematopoietic cell transplantation for acute myeloid leukemia and myelodysplastic syndromes. J Clin Oncol Off J Am Soc Clin Oncol. 2017;35:1154–61.

Yoshizato T, Nannya Y, Atsuta Y, et al. Genetic abnormalities in myelodysplasia and secondary acute myeloid leukemia: impact on outcome of stem cell transplantation. Blood. 2017;129:2347–58.

74 Pediatric MDS Including Refractory Cytopenia and Juvenile Myelomonocytic Leukemia

Charlotte M. Niemeyer

74.1 Introduction

For pediatric patients with MDS and 2–19% blasts in the PB or 5–19% blasts in the BM, the same diagnostic criteria utilized for adults with MDS with excess blasts (MDS-EB) are applied (WHO). Some cases with 20–30% blasts may also have slowly progressive disease, may lack clinical features of acute leukemia, and thus behave more like MDS than AML. These cases of MDS-EB in transformation (MDS-EB-t) together with cases of MDS-EB account for approximately a quarter of all childhood MDS.

In the large cohort of children with MDS-EB/MDS-EB-t of the European Working Group of MDS in Childhood (EWOG-MDS), allo-HSCT with a full MAC consisting of the combination of BU/CY/MEL resulted in an OS at 5 years of 63%, with NRM and relapse contributing equally to treatment failure (Strahm et al. 2011). The update shows that the outcome for patients who received a graft from either a MSD or an UD matched for 9/10 or 10/10 HLA-loci by using high-resolution typing is superimposable (Locatelli and Strahm 2018). Because patients ≥12 years of age had a high risk of NRM, EWOG-MDS recommends an intensified GVHD prophylaxis (CSA + MTX) for older patients transplanted from a MSD (see http://ewog-mds.org). The presence of a structurally complex karyotype was found to be strongly associated with poor prognosis (Göhring et al. 2010).

74.2 Refractory Cytopenia of Childhood (RCC)

Most children and adolescents with MDS present with RCC, a provisional MDS entity characterized by persistent cytopenia and <5% blasts in the BM and <2% blasts in the PB (Baumann et al. 2017). BM biopsy shows considerable hypocellularity in about 80% of RCC cases. Most of these children with RCC have a normal karyotype and a low risk of progression to MDS-EB, while about 10–15% display an abnormal karyotype with monosomy 7, del(7q), or ≥2 aberrations.

It recently became evident that approximately half of all pediatric patients with primary MDS and monosomy 7 or del(7q) have GATA2 deficiency or SAMD9/SAMD9L syndrome (Wlodarski et al. 2016). Most of these children present as RCC. Since the presence of monosomy 7 is correlated with a high risk of progression to more advanced MDS, patients with monosomy 7 should generally receive HSCT as soon as possible. For RCC with monosomy 7, del(7q), or ≥2 aberrations, MAC is recommended. EWOG-MDS currently advocates a TREO-based regimen which results in prompt initial engraft-

C. M. Niemeyer (✉)
Department of Pediatrics and Adolescent Medicine, University Medical Center, Freiburg, Germany
e-mail: charlotte.niemeyer@uniklinik-freiburg.de

E. Carreras et al. (eds.), *The EBMT Handbook*, https://doi.org/10.1007/978-3-030-02278-5_74

ment with a low incidence of secondary graft failure and an OS of approx. 90% (see http://ewog-mds.org). Historical data with a BU/CY have provided an OS of approx. 75%, NRM being the major cause of treatment failure (Starý and Locatelli 2005).

In the absence of monosomy 7, RCC patients with mild cytopenia (no transfusion dependency for red cells or platelets and an absolute neutrophil count of ≥1 × 10^9/L) may have a stable course of disease and therefore qualify for a watch-and-wait strategy. For patients with more pronounced cytopenia, treatment is stratified according to cellularity.

In normo- or hypercellular RCC, a MAC regimen like that described for monosomy 7 may be utilized irrespective of karyotype. In patients with hypocellular BM, Fanconi anemia and dyskeratosis congenita should be excluded by chromosomal breakage and telomere length/molecular studies, respectively.

HSCT with a RIC is the treatment of choice for hypocellular RCC and normal karyotype (Inagaki et al. 2015; Strahm et al. 2007). HSCT with a preparative regimen of TT/FLU (Strahm et al. 2007) resulted in an OS of 94% and EFS of 88% (Strahm et al. 2017). However, approx. 10% of patients experience primary and secondary graft failure requiring a stem cell boost and/or second HSCT. Thus, EWOG-MDS currently recommends a preparative regimen of TREO/FLU aiming at an improved rate of engraftment (see http://ewog-mds.org). With a very low risk of disease recurrence, GVHD should be avoided; thus, BM is the preferred stem cell source combined with an effective GVHD prophylaxis (Locatelli and Strahm 2018). In the absence of a suitable donor, IST with horse ATG and CSA may be a therapeutic option in patients with hypocellular RCC and the absence of poor-risk karyotype (Yoshimi et al. 2014).

74.3 Juvenile Myelomonocytic Leukemia (JMML)

JMML is a unique clonal hematopoietic disorder of early childhood with myeloproliferative and myelodysplastic features (Locatelli and Niemeyer 2015). Splenomegaly, leukocytosis, monocytosis, and myeloid and/or erythroid precursors on PB smear are noted in close to all cases. Age ≥ 2 years, platelet count <40 × 10^9/L, and a high hemoglobin F are poor prognostic factors.

JMML is characterized by hyperactivation of the RAS signal transduction pathway. About 90% of patients harbor molecular alteration in 1 of 5 genes (*PTPN11*, *NRAS*, *KRAS*, *NF1*, *CBL*) which define genetically and clinically distinct JMML subtypes. PTPN11-, NRAS-, and KRAS-mutated JMMLs are characterized by heterozygous somatic gain-of-function mutations in non-syndromic children, while JMML in neurofibromatosis type 1 (NF1) and JMML in children with CBL syndrome are characterized by germline RAS disease (RASopathy) and acquired biallelic inactivation of the respective tumor suppressor gene in hematopoietic cells.

JMML with somatic *PTPN11* mutations is a rapidly fatal disorder unless the patient undergoes HSCT. HSCT in JMML patients with *PTPN11* mutations is followed by a significantly higher relapse rate when compared to patients of the other JMML genetic subtypes. Like *PTPN11*-mutated disease, JMML in patients with *NF1* is fatal in the absence of HSCT.

Children with somatic heterozygous *KRAS* mutations (14%) often have a clinically particular aggressive form of disease. Close to all of these children require prompt HSCT. *NRAS*-associated JMML (16%) displays a great clinical diversity. While a considerable percentage of patients transplanted for JMML with *NRAS* mutations relapse after HSCT, others survive in the absence of HSCT with persistence of *NRAS* mutation but slowly regressing disease. Clinically these patients are well and show a normal or only slightly elevated HbF. Molecular studies suggest that children with *NRAS* mutation and spontaneous regression have a low methylation profile and no subclonal mutations.

The vast majority of children with *CBL*-mutated JMML myeloproliferation is self-limiting with splenomegaly decreasing over years without HSCT. In the absence of one of the five canonical RAS pathway alterations, rare mutations in other RAS genes and non-JMML myeloproliferative disorders need to be excluded. Most of these cases require HSCT.

In JMML, allo-HSCT, either from a histocompatible sibling or from an HLA-matched/1-antigen-disparate URD, results in a DFS of 52% (Locatelli et al. 2005). Disease recurrence is the most important cause of failure, occurring with a cumulative incidence of 35%. UCBT is a suitable option for children lacking an HLA-compatible relative (Locatelli et al. 2013). Standard preparative regimen consists of BU/CY/MEL (Locatelli et al. 2005; Dvorak et al. 2018). While intensive chemotherapy prior to transplantation is generally not followed by durable responses, azacitidine might be an attractive option to bridge to HSCT (Cseh et al. 2015).

Key Points

- Most children and adolescents with MDS present with refractory cytopenia of childhood (RCC). In RCC, bone marrow cells often show a normal karyotype, and there is a low risk of progression to MDS-EB. In the presence of mild cytopenia and a hypocellular marrow, a watch-and-wait strategy may be appropriate; if HSCT is required, a preparative regimen with TREO/FLU results in prompt engraftment.
- In RCC with monosomy 7, del(7q), or ≥2 aberrations and in normo- or hypercellular RCC with any karyotype, MAC HSCT is recommended.
- JMML is characterized by hyperactivation of the RAS signal transduction pathway. About 90% of patients harbor molecular alteration in 1 of 5 genes (*PTPN11*, *NRAS*, *KRAS*, *NF1*, *CBL*) which define genetically and clinically distinct JMML subtypes.
- JMML with somatic *PTPN11* mutations is a rapidly fatal disorder in the absence of HSCT. Patients with *KRAS* mutations often have a clinically particular aggressive disease. *NRAS*-associated JMML displays a great clinical diversity, some patients have a slowly regressing disease in the absence of HSCT, while others relapse post HSCT. Most *CBL*-mutated JMML patients have a self-limiting myeloproliferation.
- The standard preparative regimen for HSCT in JMML consists of BU/CY/MEL.

References

Baumann I, Niemeyer CM, Bennett JM. Juvenile myelomonocytic leukaemia. In: Swerdlow SH, Campo E, Harris NL, et al., editors. WHO classification of tumors of haematopoietic and lymphoid tissues. Lyon: International Agency for Research on Cancer (IARC); 2017. p. 103–6.

Cseh A, Niemeyer CM, Yoshimi A, et al. Bridging to transplant with azacitidine in juvenile myelomonocytic leukemia: a retrospective analysis of the EWOG-MDS study group. Blood. 2015;125:2311–3.

Dvorak CC, Satwani P, Stieglitz E, et al. Disease burden and conditioning regimens in ASCT1221, a randomized phase II trial in children with juvenile myelomonocytic leukemia: A Children's Oncology Group study. Pediatr Blood Cancer. 2018;65:e27034.

Göhring G, Michalova K, Beverloo HB, et al. Complex karyotype newly defined: the strongest prognostic factor in advanced childhood myelodysplastic syndrome. Blood. 2010;116:3766–9.

Inagaki J, Fukano R, Kurauchi K, et al. Hematopoietic stem cell transplantation in children with refractory cytopenia of childhood: single-center experience using high-dose cytarabine containing myeloablative and aplastic anemia oriented reduced-intensity conditioning regimens. Biol Blood Marrow Transplant. 2015;21:565–9.

Locatelli F, Nollke P, Zecca M, et al. Hematopoietic stem cell transplantation (HSCT) in children with juvenile myelomonocytic leukemia (JMML): results of the EWOG-MDS/EBMT trial. Blood. 2005;105:410–9.

Locatelli F, Crotta A, Ruggeri A, et al. Analysis of risk factors influencing outcomes after cord blood transplantation in children with juvenile myelomonocytic leukemia: a EUROCORD, EBMT, EWOG-MDS, CIBMTR study. Blood. 2013;122:2135–41.

Locatelli F, Niemeyer CM. How I treat juvenile myelomonocytic leukemia. Blood. 2015;125:1083–90.

Locatelli F, Strahm B. How I treat myelodysplastic syndromes of childhood. Blood. 2018;131:1406–14.

Starý J, Locatelli F. Niemeyer CM; European Working Group on Myelodysplastic Syndrome (EWOG-

MDS) and Pediatric Diseases Working Party of the EBMT. Stem cell transplantation for aplastic anemia and myelodysplastic syndrome. Bone Marrow Transplant. 2005;35(Suppl 1):S13–6.

Strahm B, Locatelli F, Bader P, et al. Reduced intensity conditioning in unrelated donor transplantation for refractory cytopenia in childhood. Bone Marrow Transplant. 2007;40:329–33.

Strahm B, Nöllke P, Zecca M, EWOG-MDS study group, et al. Hematopoietic stem cell transplantation for advanced myelodysplastic syndrome in children: results of the EWOG-MDS 98 study. Leukemia. 2011;25:455–62.

Strahm B, Albert M, Bierings M, et al. EWOG-MDS study SCT RC RIC 06: Reduced intensity conditioning for children and adolescents with refractory cytopenia of childhood. Bone Marrow Transplant. 2017;52:S103.

Wlodarski MW, Hirabayashi S, Pastor V, et al. EWOG-MDS. Prevalence, clinical characteristics, and prognosis of GATA2-related myelodysplastic syndromes in children and adolescents. Blood. 2016;127:1387–97.

Yoshimi A, van den Heuvel-Eibrink MM, Baumann I, et al. Comparison of horse and rabbit antithymocyte globulin in immunosuppressive therapy for refractory cytopenia of childhood. Haematologica. 2014;99:656–63.

75 Myelodysplastic/ Myeloproliferative Neoplasms

Francesco Onida and Yves Chalandon

75.1 Definition, Epidemiology, Diagnosis, and Classification

The myelodysplastic syndrome-myeloproliferative neoplasms (MDS/MPNs) are a heterogeneous group of hematologic malignancies characterized by dysplastic and myeloproliferative clinical, laboratory, and morphological overlapping features, both in marrow and in blood. The MDS/MPN category, recently updated by the last revision to the WHO classification of myeloid neoplasms and acute leukemia (Arber et al. 2016), includes chronic myelomonocytic leukemia (CMML), atypical chronic myelogenous leukemia (aCML), juvenile myelomonocytic leukemia (JMML), MDS/MPN with ringed sideroblasts and thrombocytosis (MDS/MPN-RS-T), as well as unclassifiable forms of mixed myelodysplastic/myeloproliferative disorders (MDS/MPN-U) (Table 75.1).

While JMML affects only children from birth up to 14 years of age (median age at diagnosis 2 years), with an estimated incidence of approximately 1.2 cases per million annually (Chang et al. 2014), adulthood MDS/MPN are typically diagnosed in elderly age with CMML being definitely the most frequent subtype (incidence of around 1 case/100,000 inhabitants per year, median age 70 years) (Solary 2014). Being very uncommon, data concerning the incidence of aCML, MDS/MPN-RS-T, and MDS/MPN-U are currently unknown.

75.2 Risk Factors and Prognostic Index

The clinical course of MDS/MPN varies from an indolent course over several years for a minor fraction of patients with CMML and MDS/MPN-RS-T to a more rapid progression with dismal prognosis and frequent transformation into secondary acute myeloid leukemia in the preponderance of patients with CMML and in the vast majority of patients with aCML and MDS/MPN-U, for whom allo-HSCT still represents the only curative option (Onida and Beran 2008; Onida 2017). Alike, long-term survival in the greater part of children with JMML may only be achieved by means of allo-HSCT.

CMML is highly heterogeneous, with clinical and hematological characteristics varying from mainly myelodysplastic to predominantly myeloproliferative. Based on marrow and peripheral blood blast percentage, the last WHO classification recognized three disease subtypes

F. Onida
Department of Hematology, Fondazione IRCCS Ca' Granda Ospedale Maggiore Policlinico, University of Milan, Milan, Italy

Y. Chalandon (✉)
Department of Oncology, Hematology Division, Hôpitaux Universitaires de Genève, University of Geneva, Geneva, Switzerland
e-mail: yves.chalandon@hcuge.ch

E. Carreras et al. (eds.), *The EBMT Handbook*, https://doi.org/10.1007/978-3-030-02278-5_75

Table 75.1 Classification and diagnostic criteria of MDS/MPNs

Disease	Blood findings	Bone marrow findings
Chronic myelomonocytic leukemia (CMML)	Monocytes ≥1 × 10^9/L, (≥10% of the WBC) <20% blasts (1)	<20% blasts[a] Dysplasia in one or more myeloid lineages[b] *No evidence of BCR/ABL1, PDGFRA, PDGFRB, or FGFR1 rearrangement or PCM1-JAK2*
Atypical chronic myelogenous leukemia (aCML)	Leukocytosis due to increased numbers of neutrophils with IMC, ≥10% of WBC Basophils <2%, Monocytes <10% <20% blasts Dysgranulopoiesis	<20% blasts Dysgranulopoiesis Hypercellularity, with granulocytic proliferation and granulocytic dysplasia, ± dysplasia in the erythroid and megakaryocytic lineages *No evidence of BCR/ABL1, PDGFRA, PDGFRB, or FGFR1 rearrangement or PCM1-JAK2*
Juvenile myelomonocytic leukemia (JMML)[c]	Monocytes ≥1 × 10^9/L, (≥10% of the WBC count); <20% blasts	<20% blasts *The absence of BCR/ABL1 rearrangement*[d]
MDS/MPN with ringed sideroblasts and thrombocytosis (MDS/MPN-RS-T)	Anemia, ≥15% ring sideroblasts, platelet count ≥450 × 10^9/L <1% blasts	Erythroid lineage dysplasia with or without multilineage dysplasia, <5% blasts The presence of a *SF3B1* mutation or, in its absence, no history of recent cytotoxic or growth factor therapy that could explain the MD/MP features *No rearrangement of BCR/ABL1, PDGFRA, PDGFRB, FGFR1, or PCM1-JAK2. No (3;3)(q21;q26), inv(3)(q21q26) or del(5q)*
MDS/MPN unclassifiable (MDS/MPN-U)[e]	<20% blasts	<20% blasts

IMC immature myeloid cells (promyelocytes, myelocytes, metamyelocytes)
[a]Including monoblasts and promonocytes
[b]If myelodysplasia is absent or minimal but other requirements are met, an acquired clonal cytogenetic or molecular genetic abnormality should be identified, or a nonreactive monocytosis persisting at least 3 months should be observed
[c]Splenomegaly is a mandatory feature
[d]Plus genetic abnormality (at least one) or additional criteria (Arber et al. 2016—Table 14)
[e]Myeloid neoplasms with mixed proliferative and dysplastic features that do not meet the criteria for CMML, aCML, JMML, or MDS/MPN-RS-T are classified as MDS/MPN-U

(CMML-0, CMML-1, and CMML-2), associated to a corresponding decreasing life expectations (Arber et al. 2016). Over the latest years, a number of disease-specific prognostic systems have been developed in CMML in order to allow the best treatment strategy allocation (Onida 2017a). The most recent ones are listed in Table 75.2.

Atypical CML, also named as BCR-ABL-negative CML, is a rare hematologic malignancy with an overall dismal prognosis (median 24 months). Age, hemoglobin level, and leukocyte count have been identified as variables with independent prognostic significance, allowing the stratification of two groups with significantly different life expectations. Likewise, for MDS/MPN-RS-T, three risk categories of patients were recently differentiated by a Mayo Clinic prognostic model including molecular investigations (Table 75.2).

With regard to the JMML, acquisitions from modern genetic studies assign uncommon treatment indication in patients with germ line PTPN11 and CBL mutations, who frequently experience spontaneous disease regression. In contrast, patients with neurofibromatosis type 1, somatic *PTPN11*, *KRAS*, and most of those with *NRAS* mutations require early allo-HSCT as a result of rapidly progressive disease (Hasle 2016).

MDS/MPN-U is the most heterogeneous and the least well-characterized entity, with no currently recognized specific molecular findings. Some description of the biological and clinical characteristics have been recently reported in two series (DiNardo et al. 2014; Wang et al. 2014),

Table 75.2 Prognostic systems in MDS/MPN

MDS/MPN	Prognostic model	Variables included [score]	Risk groups	Median OS (months)
CMML	GFM (Itzykson et al. 2013)	Age > 65 years [2] WBC >15 × 10^9/L [3] PLT <100 × 10^9/L [2] Anemia (F < 10 g/dL, M < 11 g/dL) [2] *ASXL1* mutation [2]	Low (score ≤ 4) Intermediate (score = 5–7) High (score ≥ 8)	Not reached 38.5 14.4
	CPSS (Such et al. 2013)	WBC ≥13 x 10^9/L [1] WHO CMML-2 subtype [1] CMML-specific CG[a] inter/high [1/2] Transfusional dependency [1]	Low (score = 0) Intermediate-1 (score = 1) Intermediate-2 (score = 2–3) High (score = 4–5)	72 31 13 5
	MMM (Patnaik et al. 2014)	Hb <10 g/dL [2] AMC >10 x 10^9/L [2] Circulating IMC >0% [2] PLT <100 x 10^9/L [1.5] *ASXL-1* Mut (frameshift/ nonsense) [1.5]	Low (score = 0) Intermediate-1 (score = 1.5–2) Intermediate-2 (score = 2.5–4.5) High (score ≥ 5)	97 59 31 16
	CPSS-Mol (Elena et al. 2016)	WBC ≥13 x 10^9/L [1] BM blasts ≥5% [1] Genetic risk group[b] [score 0 to 3] Transfusional dependency [1]	Low (score = 0) Intermediate-1 (score = 1) Intermediate-2 (score = 2–3) High (score ≥ 4)	Not reached 64 37 18
aCML	MDACC (Onida et al. 2002)	Age > 65 years [1] Hb ≤10 g/dL [1] WBC >50 x 10^9/L [1]	Low (score = 0–1) High (score = 2–3)	38 9
MDS/ MPN-RS-T	Mayo (Patnaik et al. 2016)	Hb <10 g/dL [1] CG abnormalities [2] ASXL-1 mutation [1] SETBP1 mutation [1]	Low (score = 0) Intermediate (score = 1) High (score ≥ 2)	80 42 11

[a]CMML-specific cytogenetic risk classification, low, normal, and isolated –Y; intermediate, other abnormalities; and high, trisomy 8, complex karyotype (≥3 abnormalities), and abnormalities of chromosome 7
[b]genetic risk group, CMML-specific cytogenetic risk classification + *ASXL1/NRAS/SETBP1* mutation (score = 1)/*RUNX1* mutation (score = 2)

with median survival of 12.4 and 21.8 months, respectively, and possible association of thrombocytosis with a more favorable outcome.

75.3 Pretransplantation Treatment

For this rare group of diseases, there are only few prospective studies on therapy, most being either retrospective analyses or case reports, making it difficult to give recommendations. In general, because apart from allo-HSCT no therapy has been shown to modify the disease course, pretransplantation treatments point toward symptom control rather than the achievement of disease remission (Odenike et al. 2015).

75.3.1 CMML

In general, treatment strategies in patients with CMML with symptomatic or progressive disease are based on the dysplastic versus proliferative features and the percentage of marrow blasts (Onida et al. 2013). In the presence of rising leukocytosis and/or organ infiltration (mostly splenomegaly) with low marrow blast percentage, hydroxyurea (HU) remains the drug of choice. Patients showing high blast percentages may be bridged to transplant through AML-like induction chemotherapy or by means of hypomethylating agents (HMAs), with a reported 20–50% overall response rate. In a recent retrospective study including a relatively small number of patients, HMAs have been suggested to increase progression-free survival (PFS) through the reduction of post-transplantation relapse rate (Kongtim et al. 2016). Treatment strategies based on the combination of HMAs with other agents (e.g., lenalidomide) and the advent of new targeted therapies such as JAK2 inhibitors or poly(ADP-ribose) polymerase (PARP) inhibitors may further increase the response rate leading to an overall improvement of post-transplantation outcomes.

75.3.2 aCML

Due to its absolute rarity in patients having no age or comorbidity barrier to allo-HSCT, no consensus subsists on to whether any pretransplant treatment may have an impact on post-transplantation outcome and what kind of therapy should be best used. Control of leukocytosis is generally achieved with cytoreductive agents such as HU or IFN-α immunomodulation. Chemotherapy induction treatment is preferred when facing high blast count in advanced disease phases or in patients showing AML transformation.

Some efficacy of decitabine and of ruxolitinib single agent has also been reported, whereas a phase II trial of AZA and ruxolitinib in combination in a series of 35 MDS/MPN patients showed promising activity, with an overall response rate of 57% according to the 2015 international consortium response criteria for MDS/MPN (Savona et al. 2015), even though median survival of the few aCML included patients ($n = 4$) was only 8 months (Assi et al. 2018). According to the most recent discovery, *SETBP1* and *ETNK1* mutations are present in 15–32% and up to 10% of aCML patients, respectively, whereas *JAK2* mutation is rare (0–7%), and *CSF3R* mutations are only occasionally observed. Even though in the near future these findings may influence therapeutic approaches by means of evolving targeted therapies, currently allo-HSCT remains the only treatment strategy with established curative potential in eligible patients (Dao et al. 2017).

75.3.3 JMML

For JMML patients the possible therapeutic interventions prior to transplantation are rather scarce. Different chemotherapeutic agents have been used prior to transplant, but there is no consensus on to whether there should be any pre-transplant therapy and what type should be given. HMAs may have potential activity (Cseh et al. 2015), but data are too few to make any recommendation. Other potentially active agents include JAK, MEK, and SRC inhibitors, but clinical trial with these drugs is still on their way.

75.3.4 MDS/MPN-RS-T

MDS/MPN-RS-T generally represents the disease entity associated with the best prognosis among overlap syndromes, with a median survival of about 6 years (Broseus et al. 2012). Guidelines for disease management are not formally recognized, and treatment strategies are generally extrapolated from low-risk MDS and MPN, with adjusted individual management depending on presenting problems. While lenalidomide has been occasionally reported to reduce transfusion need, antiplatelet and cytoreductive treatments are often required due to the high risk of thrombosis. Based on the different gene mutations possibly involved (*SF3B1*, *JAK2*, *TET2*, *DNMT3A*), attentiveness in targeted therapies is developing.

75.3.5 MDS/MPN-U

MDS/MPN-U is a very rare and heterogeneous disease entity, with no consensus on which therapy (if any) should be given for patients candidate to allo-HSCT. Augmented leukocyte proliferation is generally managed by means of cytoreductive agents such as HU or through immunomodulation with IFNα, while HMAs as well as lenalidomide may represent an option in case of prevailing cytopenias. JAK inhibitors are also potential therapeutic options, either alone or in combination with HMAs (Assi et al. 2018). When patients are progressing to AML transformation, induction chemotherapy should be used as a bridge to allo-HSCT.

75.4 Autologous HSCT

Because the harvesting of polyclonal hematopoietic progenitor cells is not feasible through the currently available treatment options, autologous HSCT is currently not a recommended strategy in MDS/MPN.

75.5 Allogeneic HSCT

Currently still representing the only curative strategy, the role of allo-HSCT in adult MDS/MPN patients remains controversial mainly due to the lack of prospective studies, being therefore generally considered a possible treatment option for eligible patients with high-risk diseases.

In *CMML* benefits and risks of allo-HSCT have been analyzed retrospectively in various series, with different characteristics at transplant and much variable outcomes described (Table 75.3). Recent recommendations from an international expert panel agreed to limit indication for allo-HSCT in CMML patients classified in the intermediate-2 and high-risk CPSS categories (de Witte et al. 2017), representing the preferred treatment modality for younger patients with acceptable comorbidity index (Patnaik et al. 2015).

Table 75.3 Summary of selected studies on allo-HSCT in CMML

Author (year)	Pt N.	Median age (range)	Disease type/ stage	Donor type	Conditioning (MAC vs RIC)	TRM/relapse rate	Survival outcome
Kröger et al. (2002)	50	44 (19–61)	CMML-1 = 28 CMML-2 = 17 Missing = 5	MRD = 43 MUD = 7	MAC = 50 RIC = 0	TRM = 52% RR = 28%	OS (5y) = 21% DFS (5y) = 18%
Eissa et al. (2011)	85	51 (1–69)	CMML-1 = 57 CMML-2 = 26	MRD = 38 MUD = 47	MAC = 58 RIC = 27	TRM (10y) = 35% RR (10y) = 27%	OS (10y) = 40% DFS (10y) = 40%
Park et al. (2013)	73	53 (27–66)	CMML-1 = 24 CMML-2 = 26 Missing = 23	MRD = 41 MUD = 32	MAC = 30 RIC = 43	TRM = 35% RR = 35%	OS (3y) = 32% DFS (3y) = 29%
Symeonidis et al. (2015)	513	53 (18–75)	CMML-1 = 87 CMML-2 = 32 s-AML = 95 Missing = 299	MRD = 285 MUD = 228	MAC = 249 RIC = 226	TRM (4y) = 41% RR (4y) = 32%	OS (4y) = 33% DFS (4y) = 27%
Kongtim et al. (2016)	83	57 (18–78)	CMML-1/2 = 47 sAML = 36	MRD = 30 MUD = 47 MMR = 6	MAC = 64 RIC = 19	TRM (3y) = 31% RR (3y) 33%	OS (3y) = 35% DFS (3y) = 34%
Liu et al. (2017)	209	57 (23–74)	CMML-1 = 140 CMML-2 = 52 Missing = 17	MRD = 73 MUD = 127 MMUD = 9	MAC = 105 RIC = 99 Missing = 5	TRM (5y) = 28% RR (5y) = 52%	OS (5y) = 30% DFS (5y) = 20%
Itonaga et al. (2018)	159	54 (16–75)	Not reported	MRD = 51 MUD (BM) = 66 Cord = 30 MMR = 12	MAC = 92 RIC = 67	TRM = 28% RR = 39%	OS (3y) = 33%

As *aCML* is extremely rare in people younger than 65 years, outcome after allo-HSCT has been described only in small single-institution series. A 5-years OS and RFS of 51% and 36%, respectively, were recently reported by the EBMT-CMWP in a retrospective analysis of 42 patients transplanted between 1997 and 2006. With a RR of 40%, a better OS was recognized in young patients with low EBMT risk score (Onida et al. 2017).

With regard to *JMML*, 5-years OS and EFS out of 100 patients transplanted 1993 through 2002 within the EWOG-MDS/EBMT trial were 64% and 52%, respectively, with a 5-years TRM of 13% (Locatelli et al. 2005). Overall, younger age, male sex, low HbF, and low BM blast percentage were associated to better survival. Early disease recurrence was the major cause of treatment failure, irrespective of donor type (sibling vs unrelated vs CB). Although both acute and chronic GvHD are associated with a lower relapse risk, DLI in JMML relapse is mostly unsuccessful. In contrast, a second HSCT with the same or an alternative donor may cure about 30% of the patients (Locatelli and Niemeyer 2015).

In *MDS/MPN-RS-T* allo-HSCT is generally not indicated, being reserved for patients developing refractory cytopenias or accelerated/blastic transformation (Sharma et al. 2017), whereas eligible patients with MDS/MPN-U should always be considerate as potential candidate for allo-HSCT due to the general dismal prognosis.

75.6 Source of HSC

No impact of HSC source on the transplant outcome has been observed in the largest CMML series reported by the EBMT-CMWP (Symeonidis et al. 2015). This was in contrast to the CIBTMR study, in which the survival was statistically better with PBMC than with BM, with no clear explanation outside the small proportion of BM transplants (16%) (Liu et al. 2017). The source of stem cell is therefore left open, but PBSC may potentially be preferred to decrease the risk of graft failure and the relapse risk, particularly with the use of RIC.

In the pediatric population, the majority of transplantation are done with BM, mainly due to the potential of decreasing the incidence of GVHD. In the largest series of JMML patients reported, BM was the stem cell source in 79% with no significant difference on the outcome in comparison to PBSC (Locatelli et al. 2005).

For aCML, MDS/MPN-RS-T, and MDS/MN-U, data are too scarce to make clear recommendations.

75.7 Conditioning and GvHD Prophylaxis

In MDS/MPN patients, the choice of conditioning regimen depends on many different conditions, the major ones being comorbidities, patient age, disease phase at transplant, type of donor, and HSC source. In the two largest retrospective series of CMML patients (Symeonidis et al. 2015; Liu et al. 2017), MAC and RIC were almost equal in proportion, with no outcome difference. Likewise, in the largest reported series of aCML patients, conditioning intensity had no impact on the outcome (MAC were used in 76%). Noteworthy, an improved outcome following a combined fractionated 6–8 Gray TBI/FLU conditioning regimen was recently reported in advanced CMML (Radujkovic et al. 2017).

In general, for young patients (<60 years), with a HSCT-CI (Sorror et al. 2005) less than 2, MAC regimens such as BU-CY, TT/BU/FLU (TBF), or the reduced-toxicity FLU/BUx4 (FB4) may be advisable, particularly in the proliferative variant of CMML and in other MDS/MPN with predominant proliferative features, whereas a RIC regimen such as BU/FLU or reduced TBF may be preferred for patients with older age or comorbidities and for patients undergoing transplant with disease remission following pretransplant treatment.

Facing an aggressive disease in a very young population, MAC regimens are generally preferred in JMML. In the biggest series published, the conditioning included CT, BU and MEL (Locatelli et al. 2005), with a 5-years OS of 64%. More recently, a conditioning containing BU,

FLU, and MEL showed promising results, with more than 50% of patients in remission after alternative donor transplantation (Yabe et al. 2015). Based on those data, the recommended conditioning for JMML patients should rely on the backbone of BU and MEL with either CY or FLU.

75.8 Maintenance/Post transplant Strategies

As disease recurrence represents the major cause of transplant failure in MDS/MPN, there is a growing interest toward post transplant strategies, although few data are currently available in this particular setting.

Indirect evidence of a graft versus CMML by a reduced incidence of relapse in patients with GvHD has been recently reported (Itonaga et al. 2018). Some effect of DLI has also been reported in patients with relapsing CMML and low disease burden.

With more molecular markers potentially available, cell therapy-based interventions may be planned on the base of residual or increasing MRD.

Potential interest both as preemptive and as maintenance strategy derive from the use of post transplant HMAs, alone or in combination with DLI, as reported in AML and MDS.

The use of lenalidomide and checkpoint inhibitors, but also JAK2 or PARP inhibitors, alone or even in combination, together with post transplant targeted therapies represents areas of growing interest under development.

References

Arber DA, Orazi A, Hasserjian R, Thiele J, Borowitz MJ, Le Beau MM, Bloomfield CD, Cazzola M, Vardiman JW. The 2016 revision to the World Health Organization classification of myeloid neoplasms and acute leukemia. Blood. 2016;127:2391–405.

Assi R, Kantarjian HM, Garcia-Manero G, et al. A phase II trial of ruxolitinib in combination with azacytidine in myelodysplastic syndrome/myeloproliferative neoplasms. Am J Hematol. 2018;93:277–85.

Broseus J, Florensa L, Zipperer E, et al. Clinical features and course of refractory anemia with ring sideroblasts associated with marked thrombocytosis. Haematologica. 2012;97:1036–41.

Chang TY, Dvorak CC, Loh ML. Bedside to bench in juvenile myelomonocytic leukemia: insights into leukemogenesis from a rare pediatric leukemia. Blood. 2014;124:2487–97.

Cseh A, Niemeyer CM, Yoshimi A, et al. Bridging to transplant with azacitidine in juvenile myelomonocytic leukemia: a retrospective analysis of the EWOG-MDS study group. Blood. 2015;125:2311–3.

Dao KT, Tyner JW, Gotlib J. Recent Progress in chronic neutrophilic leukemia and atypical chronic myeloid leukemia. Curr Hematol Malig Rep. 2017;12:432–41.

de Witte T, Bowen D, Robin M, et al. Allogeneic hematopoietic stem cell transplantation for MDS and CMML: recommendations from an international expert panel. Blood. 2017;129:1753–62.

DiNardo CD, Daver N, Jain N, et al. Myelodysplastic/myeloproliferative neoplasms, unclassifiable (MDS/MPN, U): natural history and clinical outcome by treatment strategy. Leukemia. 2014;28:958–61.

Eissa H, Gooley TA, Sorror ML, et al. Allogeneic hematopoietic cell transplantation for chronic myelomonocytic leukemia: relapse-free survival is determined by karyotype and comorbidities. Biol Blood Marrow Transplant. 2011;17:908–15.

Elena C, Gall A, Such E, et al. Integrating clinical features and genetic lesions in the risk assessment of patients with chronic myelomonocytic leukemia. Blood. 2016;128:1408–17.

Hasle H. Myelodysplastic and myeloproliferative disorders of childhood. Hematology Am Soc Hematol Educ Program. 2016;1:598–604.

Itonaga H, Aoki K, Aoki J, et al. Prognostic impact of donor source on allogeneic hematopoietic stem cell transplantation outcomes in adults with chronic myelomonocytic leukemia: a Nationwide retrospective analysis in Japan. Biol Blood Marrow Transplant. 2018;24:840–8.

Itzykson R, Kosmider O, Renneville A, et al. Prognostic score including gene mutations in chronic myelomonocytic leukemia. J Clin Oncol. 2013;31:2428–36.

Kongtim P, Popat U, Jimenez A, et al. Treatment with hypomethylating agents before allogeneic stem cell transplant improves progression free survival for patients with chronic myelomonocytic leukemia. Biol Blood Marrow Transplant. 2016;22:47–53.

Kröger N, Zabelina T, Guardiola P, et al. Allogeneic stem cell transplantation of adult chronic myelomonocytic leukaemia. A report on behalf of the Chronic Leukaemia Working Party of the European Group for Blood and Marrow Transplantation (EBMT). Br J Haematol. 2002;118:67–73.

Liu HD, Ahn KW, Hu ZH, et al. Allogeneic hematopoietic cell transplantation for adult chronic myelomonocytic leukemia. Biol Blood Marrow Transplant. 2017;23:767–75.

Locatelli F, Nöllke P, Zecca M, et al. European working group on childhood MDS; European Blood and Marrow Transplantation Group. Hematopoietic stem cell transplantation (HHSCT) in children with juvenile myelomonocytic leukemia (JMML): results of the EWOG-MDS/EBMT trial. Blood. 2005;105:410–9.

Locatelli F, Niemeyer CM. How I treat juvenile myelomonocytic leukemia. Blood. 2015;125:1083–90.

Odenike O, Onida F, Padron E. Myelodysplastic syndromes and myelodysplastic/myeloproliferative neoplasms: an update on risk stratification, molecular genetics, and therapeutic approaches including allogeneic hematopoietic stem cell transplantation. Am Soc Clin Oncol Educ Book. 2015;35:e398–412.

Onida F, Ball G, Kantarjian HM, et al. Characteristics and outcome of patients with Philadelphia chromosome negative, bcr/abl negative chronic myelogenous leukemia. Cancer. 2002;95:1673–84.

Onida F, Beran M. Diagnosis and management of chronic myelomonocytic leukemia. Curr Hematol Malig Rep. 2008;3:31–6.

Onida F, Barosi G, Leone G, et al. Management recommendations for chronic myelomonocytic leukemia: consensus statements from the SIE, SIES, GITMO groups. Haematologica. 2013;98:1344–52.

Onida F. Models of prognostication in chronic myelomonocytic leukemia. Curr Hematol Malig Rep. 2017;12:513–21.

Onida F, de Wreede LC, van Biezen A, et al. Allogeneic stem cell transplantation in patients with atypical chronic myeloid leukaemia: a retrospective study from the chronic malignancies working Party of the European Society for Blood and Marrow Transplantation. Br J Haematol. 2017;177:759–65.

Park S, Labopin M, Yakoub-Agha I, et al. Allogeneic stem cell transplantation for chronic myelomonocytic leukemia: a report from the Societe Francaise de Greffe de Moelle et de Therapie Cellulaire. Eur J Haematol. 2013;90:355–64.

Patnaik MM, Itzykson R, Lasho T, et al. ASXL1 and SETBP1 mutations and their prognostic contribution in chronic myelomonocytic leukemia: a two-center study of 466 patients. Leukemia. 2014;28:2206–12.

Patnaik MM, Lasho TL, Finke CM, et al. Predictors of survival in refractory anemia with ring sideroblasts and thrombocytosis (RARS-T) and the role of next-generation sequencing. Am J Hematol. 2016;91:492–8.

Patnaik MM, Wassie EA, Padron E, et al. Chronic myelomonocytic leukemia in younger patients: molecular and cytogenetic predictors of survival and treatment outcome. Blood Cancer J. 2015;5:e280.

Radujkovic A, Hegenbart U, Müller-Tidow C, et al. High progression-free survival after reduced intensity total body irradiation-based conditioning in patients allografted for chronic myelomonocytic leukemia (CMML). Blood. 2017;130:4571.

Savona MR, Malcovati L, Komrokji R, et al. An international consortium proposal of uniform response criteria for myelodysplastic/myeloproliferative neoplasms (MDS/MPN) in adults. Blood. 2015;125:1857–65.

Sharma P, Shinde SS, Damlaj M, et al. Allogeneic hematopoietic stem cell transplant in adult patients with myelodysplastic syndrome/myeloproliferative neoplasm (MDS/MPN) overlap syndromes. Leuk Lymphoma. 2017;58:872–81.

Solary E. Chronic Myelomonocytic Leukemia (CMML). Atlas Genet Cytogenet Oncol Haematol. 2014;18:50–2.

Sorror ML, Maris MB, Storb R, et al. Hematopoietic cell transplantation (HSCT)-specific comorbidity index: a new tool for risk assessment before allogeneic HSCT. Blood. 2005;106:2912–9.

Such E, Germing U, Malcovati L, et al. Development and validation of a prognostic scoring system for patients with chronic myelomonocytic leukemia. Blood. 2013;121:3005–15.

Symeonidis A, van Biezen A, de Wreede L, et al. Achievement of complete remission predicts outcome of allogeneic haematopoietic stem cell transplantation in patients with chronic myelomonocytic leukaemia. A study of the Chronic Malignancies Working Party of the European Group for Blood and Marrow Transplantation. Br J Haematol. 2015;171:239–46.

Wang SA, Hasserjian RP, Fox PS, et al. Atypical chronic myeloid leukemia is clinically distinct from unclassifiable myelodysplastic/myeloproliferative neoplasms. Blood. 2014;123:2645–51.

Yabe M, Ohtsuka Y, Watanabe K, et al. Transplantation for juvenile myelomonocytic leukemia: a retrospective study of 30 children treated with a regimen of busulfan, fludarabine, and melphalan. Int J Hematol. 2015;101:184–90.

76 Myeloproliferative Neoplasms

Nicolaus Kröger and Yves Chalandon

76.1 Primary and Post ET/PV Myelofibrosis

Nicolaus Kröger

76.1.1 Definition and Risk Scores

Polycythemia vera (PV) and essential thrombocythemia (ET) have a favorable outcome without need for allo-HSCT unless the disease progressed to post-ET/PV myelofibrosis or secondary AML (Lussana et al. 2014).

Primary myelofibrosis (PMF) or post-ET/PV myelofibrosis is one of the Philadelphia-negative myeloproliferative neoplasms (MPN) with worst survival which is approximately 6 years. Allo-HSCT can cure a substantial number of patients but is still not universally applicable due to toxicity which leads to therapy-related morbidity and mortality.

N. Kröger (✉)
Department of Stem Cell Transplantation
University Medical Center Hamburg-Eppendorf
Hamburg Germany
e-mail: nkroeger@uke.de

Y. Chalandon (✉)
Department of Oncology, Hematology Division
Hôpitaux Universitaires de Genève,
University of Geneva
Geneva Switzerland
e-mail: yves.chalandon@hcuge.ch

76.1.2 Transplant Results in Myelofibrosis

In the late 1980s and the early 1990s, the feasibility of allo-HSCT for myelofibrosis could be shown in small reports. One multicenter report described in a retrospective study with MAC in relatively young patients (median age 42 years) with a NRM of 27% and a 9% incidence of graft failure. The OS and PFS was 47% and 39% at 5 years (Guardiola et al. 1999). A single-center study from Seattle included 104 patients most of whom received allo-HSCT after MAC, and NRM at 5 years of 34% and OS at 7 years of 61% were reported (Deeg et al. 2003).

The evidence of graft-versus-myelofibrosis effect was documented by responses to DLI after failure of allo-HSCT (Byrne et al. 2000). RIC for myelofibrosis was investigated in two prospective studies. The EBMT published results of 103 patients who received a BU/FLU-based RIC followed by related or unrelated HSCT. The median age was 55 years, and the NRM at 1 year was 16%. Cumulative incidence of relapse was 22% at 3 years. PFS and OS at 5 years were 51% and 67%, respectively. Advanced age and HLA-mismatched donor were independent predictive factors for reduced survival (Kroger et al. 2009). A recent update of the study after a median follow-up of 60 months showed an 8-year OS of 65% with stable plateau. Five-year DFS was 40%, and 5-year cumulative incidence of relapse/progression was 28% with 3-year NRM of 21%.

The Myeloproliferative Disorders Research Consortium performed also a prospective phase II trial including 66 patients with primary or post-ET/PV myelofibrosis investigating a reduced

E. Carreras et al. (eds.), *The EBMT Handbook*, https://doi.org/10.1007/978-3-030-02278-5_76

conditioning regimen with MEL/FLU. With a median follow-up of 25 months, OS was 75% in the sibling group and only 32% in the unrelated group due to a higher NRM in the URD group (59% vs. 22%) (Rondelli et al. 2014). Other studies using RIC or MAC confirmed the curative effect of allo-HSCT irrespectively of the intensity of the conditioning (summarized in Kröger et al. 2015a).

76.1.3 Disease-Specific Risk Factors

Patients with PMF or post-ET/PV myelofibrosis have a median survival of approximately 6 years, but survival varies from less than 2 to more than 15 years. Risk scores (see Table 76.1) such as IPSS (Cervantes et al. 2009), dynamic IPSS (DIPSS) (Passamonti et al. 2010), or DIPSS plus (Gangat et al. 2011) are currently used in clinical practice to determine the prognosis of patients with PMF. More recently molecular markers have been introduced into the PMF risk score, (Guglielmelli et al. 2018) and a specific score for post-ET/PV myelofibrosis has been proposed (Passamontiet al. 2017; Kroger et al. 2015a). The EBMT/ELN consensus paper recommended allo-HSCT for patients less than 70 years with an estimated median survival of less than 5 years. This would include patients with IPSS or DIPSS intermediate-2 and high risk and is based on a comparison between transplanted and non-transplanted patients in the pre-ruxolitinib era (Kroger et al. 2015a, b). Patients with intermediate-1 risk can be considered for allo-HSCT if other high-risk features such as *ASXL1* mutation, more than 2% peripheral blasts, refractory transfusion-dependent anemia, or adverse cytogenetics according to DIPSS plus are present (Kroger et al. 2015a).

76.1.4 Transplant-Specific Risk Factors

In most of the transplant studies, alternative donors were associated with a worse outcome independent of disease-specific risk factors. CBT resulted in a high risk of graft failure (Robin et al. 2014). Haplo-identical donor with PT-CY as GVHD prophylaxis is currently under investigation, but more recent EBMT data reported a 5-year survival of only 38% (Raj et al. 2016).

The intensity of the conditioning regimen has not been investigated within prospective studies, but retrospective comparisons of MAC and RIC preparative regimens resulted in similar outcome. Because of the reduced toxicity and a generally older age of patients with myelofibrosis, RIC regimens are currently used more frequently and account for about two-thirds of allotransplants for myelofibrosis reported to the EBMT registry.

Table 76.1 Prognosis risk scores for myelofibrosis

Score	Adverse factors (puntos)	Risk group and median SRV
IPSS	Age > 65 years (1 p) Constitutional symptoms (1 p) Hb <100 g/L (1 p) Leucocytes >25 × 10^9/L (1 p) Blasts in PB ≥1% (1 p)	Low (0 p), 11.3 years Intermediate-1 (1 p), 7.9 years Intermediate-2 (2 p), 4 years High (3–5 p), 2.3 years
DIPSS	Age > 65 years (1 p) Constitutional symptoms (1 p) Hb <100 g/L (2 p) Leucocytes >25 × 10^9/L (1 p) Blasts in PB ≥1% (1 p)	Low (0 p), not reached Intermediate-1 (1–2 p):,14.2 years Intermediate-2 (3–4 p), 4 years High (5–6 p), 1.5 years
DIPSS plus	DIPSS Int-1 (1 p) DIPSS Int-2 (2 p) DIPSS High (3 p) Platelets <100 × 10^9/L (1 p) Transfusion requirement (1 p) Unfavorable karyotype[a] (1 p)	Low (0 p), 15.4 years Intermediate-1 (1 p), 6.5 years Intermediate-2 (2–3 p), 2.9 years High (4–6 p), 1.3 years

DIPSS: https://qxmd.com/calculate/dipss-prognosis-in-myelofibrosis
DIPSS-plus: https://qxmd.com/calculate/dipss-plus-score-for-prognosis-in-myelofibrosis
[a]+8; −7/7q-; −5/5q-; i17q; 12p-; rearrangement 11q23

76.1.5 Patient-Specific Risk Factors

Age is a significant patient-specific risk factor for outcome after allo-HSCT (Scott et al. 2012; Kroger et al. 2015a). Besides age, comorbidities and geriatric assessments (see Chap. 11) also impact on outcome after allo-HSCT but have not been studied especially in myelofibrosis patients to date.

76.1.6 Role of Splenectomy and JAK Inhibition

Splenomegaly is a hallmark of myelofibrosis and may have an impact on engraftment and graft function after HSCT. Splenectomy is an option to reduce spleen size prior to transplantation, but high morbidity and even mortality have been reported (Tefferi et al. 2000). Spleen irradiation to reduce spleen size has been reported successfully in single cases prior to conditioning. Since ruxolitinib is approved for myelofibrosis, the drug can be used prior to transplantation to improve constitutional symptoms and to reduce spleen size. The European LeukemiaNet and the European Society for Blood and Marrow Transplantation recommend the use of ruxolitinib at least 2 months prior to HSCT and a careful weaning prior to conditioning to avoid the rebound phenomenon. More recent data suggest better outcome after HSCT if patients received transplant after responding to ruxolitinib rather than postponing the transplant until ruxolitinib failure (Shanavas et al. 2016).

76.1.7 Impact of Molecular Remission

About 90% of myelofibrosis patients harbor one of the driver mutations JAK2V617F, calreticulin (CALR), or MPL which are used to monitor MRD in PB by highly sensitive qPCR or digital PCR to determine molecular remission (Wolschke et al. 2017). In a retrospective single center experience, no achievement of molecular remission on day 180 post-allograft was associated with a significant higher incidence of a subsequent clinical relapse. Due to a graft-versus-myelofibrosis effect, donor lymphocyte infusion has been successfully applied in patients with residual to induce a molecular remission (Fig. 76.1).

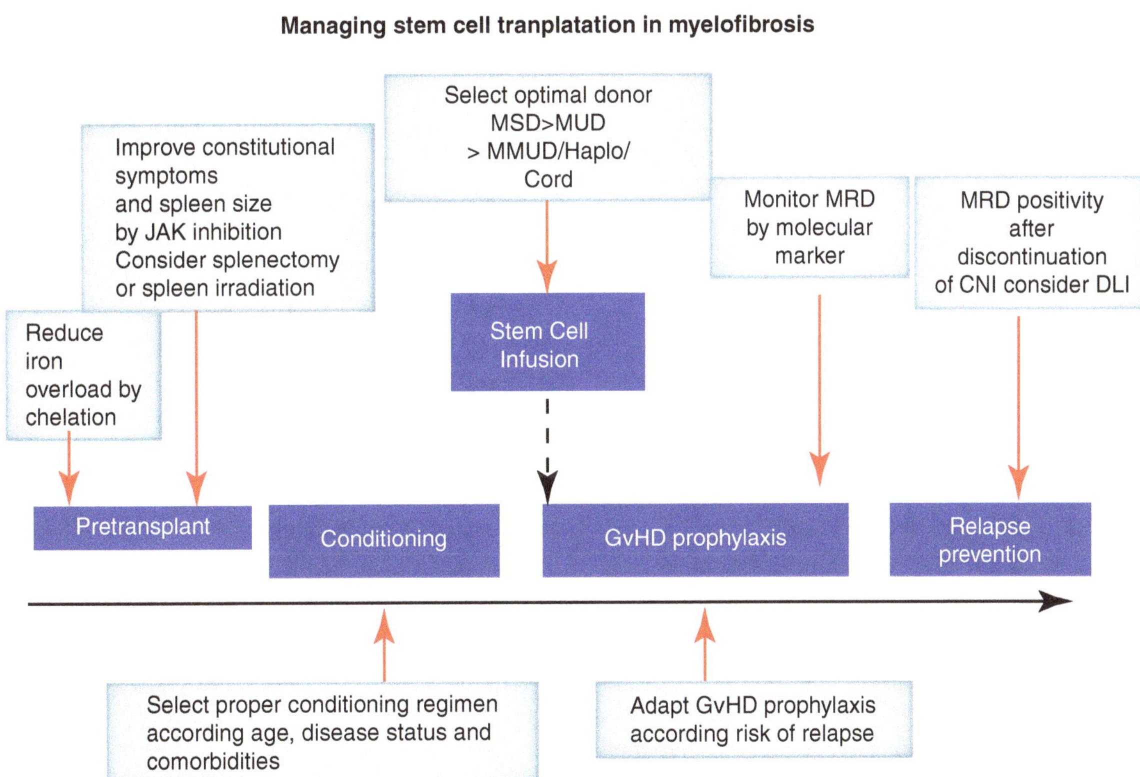

Fig. 76.1 *MSD* matched sibling donor, *MUD* matched unrelated donor, *MMUD* mismatched unrelated donor, *MRD* minimal residual disease, *CNI* calcineurin inhibitor, *GVHD* graft-versus-host disease

Furthermore, BM fibrosis is another hallmark of the disease, with rapid regression after allo-HSCT suggesting that fibrogenesis is a highly dynamic process (Thiele et al. 2005). Systematic investigations have shown that about 60% of the patients have a complete or nearly CR of BM fibrosis on day+100, and the percentage of patients increased to 90% at day+180. Notably, those patients with a rapid resolution of BM fibrosis had the best long-term outcome.

Key Points

- Primary or post-ET/PV myelofibrosis can only be cured by allo-HSCT which can induce molecular remission and resolution of bone marrow fibrosis.
- Indication for allo-HSCT is recommended for patients younger than 70 years and a median survival expectation of less than 5 years such as risk score intermediate or high risk according to DIPPS or intermediate-1 risk with additional risk factors.
- Splenectomy prior to transplant is not recommended, but patients with large spleen may benefit from JAK inhibitor treatment prior to transplantation.
- Major risk factors for worse outcome are advanced age and not fully HLA-matched donor.

76.2 Chronic Myeloid Leukemia

Yves Chalandon

76.2.1 Definition, Epidemiology, Diagnosis, and Classification

Chronic myeloid leukemia (CML) is a clonal myeloproliferative disorder of the HSC. CML was the first leukemia described and the first to be characterized by a consistent chromosomal aberration, the 22q- or "Philadelphia" (Ph) chromosome, later identified as a reciprocal translocation, t(9;22), encoding the BCR-ABL oncoprotein.

CML is the most common of the myeloproliferative disorders. The incidence is 0.4–1.75 per 100,000 population per year, and it increases with age (Höglund et al. 2015). The disease can occur at any age, but the median age at presentation ranges between 45 and 55 years. There is a slight male predominance, with a male to female ratio of 1.3:1.

CML present initially as an indolent or chronic phase (CP), easily controlled with treatment. The natural history continues with a bi- or triphasic stage, becoming more aggressive through accelerated phase (AP) and then blast crisis (BC) or directly from CP to BC.

76.2.2 Risk Factors and Prognostic Index

Several multivariate-derived prognostic models and staging have been proposed to help define individual prognosis and allow assigning patients to different strategies of therapy based on risks. The most commonly used are the Sokal and Hasford one (Sokal et al. 1984; Hasford et al. 1998).

The benefit of allo-HSCT is that it can provide cure, but the clear disadvantage is its association with considerable morbidity and mortality, which typically occur early post procedure. Outcome can be improved by better selection of those most likely to benefit. In this context the EBMT developed a risk score for patients with CML, based on five variables: donor type, disease phase, recipient age, donor/recipient gender combination, and interval from diagnosis to transplant, which together results in a score of 0–7 (see risk factors in Chap. 11) (Gratwohl et al. 1998).

Results of transplant are now highly predictable based on these five factors. It is worth remembering that the EBMT or "Gratwohl" score was developed in the mid-1990s and was based on 3142 patients transplanted between 1989 and 1996 (Fig. 76.2a). With overall improvements in supportive care, it would be reasonable to expect that a similar analysis performed on patients transplanted more recently would demonstrate improved results across all-risk scores. However, the analysis is complicated by the change in approach to management of CML. During the period of the original analysis, allo-HSCT was the treatment of choice for all patients. Since 2000

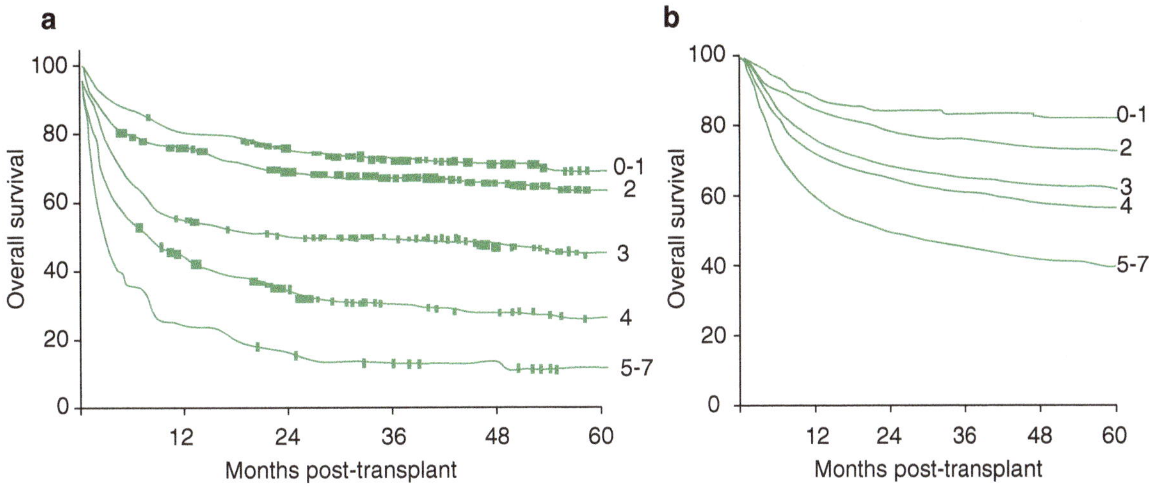

Fig. 76.2 (**a**) OS of CML patients after allo-HSCT according to EBMT risk score. Original curves published in 3142 patients transplanted between 1989 and 1996. Modified from (Gratwohl et al. 1998). (**b**) OS curves supplied by Mrs. Linda Koster for the EBMT CMWP and based on 3497 patients transplanted from 2007 to 2017

allo-HSCT has been replaced by tyrosine kinase inhibitors (TKI) as frontline therapy, and hence the reasons for patients coming to transplant are not always clear from registry data. Although this should be compensated by the use of factors such as age at transplant, disease phase, and time from diagnosis to transplant, some caution should be exercised in the interpretation of more recent results. Having said this, the analysis has been repeated recently for 3497 patients transplanted from 2007 to 2017 and confirmed improved outcome of 5-year OS across all-risk scores by 11–26% (Fig. 76.2b). Although these pretransplant factors are known to affect outcome in all diseases, it is worth focusing specifically on the impact of disease phase in CML, in particular because one of the few problems of TKI therapy is that within the cohort of patients receiving transplants, the proportion transplanted in or after blast crisis has increased over time (Table 76.2).

Table 76.2 Change in proportion of patients transplanted in each disease phase from 2007 to 2017

Year of transplant	1st CP Number (% total)	AP Number (% total)	≥2CP Number (% total)	BC Number (% total)
2007	164 (50)	49 (15)	82 (25)	34 (10)
2008	134 (45)	34 (12)	84 (28)	44 (15)
2009	133 (41)	46 (14)	92 (28)	53 (16)
2010	128 (36)	57 (16)	106 (30)	65 (18)
2011	148 (49)	50 (15)	86 (26)	46 (14)
2012	127 (46)	34 (12)	74 (27)	42 (15)
2013	136 (44)	41 (13)	78 (25)	54 (18)
2014	138 (43)	48 (15)	75 (24)	57 (18)
2015	137 (44)	43 (14)	73 (23)	62 (20)
2016	111 (42)	30 (11)	70 (26)	55 (21)
2017	74 (36)	20 (10)	68 (33)	45 (22)

Data provided by Mrs. Linda Koster on behalf of the EBMT CMWP

Allografts for CML were initially restricted to patients in AP, and improvements in survival came only when transplant was performed in the CP. Data of 138 patients with CML transplanted between 1978 and 1982 and reported to the IBMTR showed 3-year survivals of 63%, 36%, and 12% for patients transplanted in the CP, AP, and BC, respectively. The probability of relapse for those transplanted in CP was 7% (Speck et al. 1984). The effect of disease phase on the outcome of transplantation has not changed over the years. To optimize the effect of allo-HSCT for a patient who has progressed to blast crisis, a second CP should be achieved using TKI and/or conventional combination chemotherapy.

76.2.3 Pretransplantation Treatment

Early descriptions of therapy included radiotherapy, introduced at the beginning of the twentieth century and later oral chemotherapy, in particular BU and hydroxycarbamide. These approaches could control the signs and symptoms of CML in chronic phase but could not prevent its inevitable transformation into a rapidly fatal chemoresistant blastic disease. The first treatment that eradicated the Ph-positive clone and induced cure was BMT, initially described in syngeneic twins and soon followed by procedures involving HLA-matched siblings and later URD. Transplantation, once the treatment of choice for this disease, has been relegated to second-, third-, and even fourth-line treatment in parallel with the development of the TKI. As more potent TKI move to first-line therapy, patients destined to respond poorly to these drugs are identified earlier, and transplant will return to use as an earlier line strategy.

76.2.4 Autologous HSCT

Autologous HSCT for CML started about at the same time as allo-HSCT in the late 1970s early 1980s in Europe with the goal to set up the clock to early phase with high-dose therapy followed by reinfusion of autologous HSC. However, following the introduction of targeted therapy with TKI, the number of auto-HSCT in Europe has decreased rapidly, with only 0–4 per year between 2012 and 2016 as per the EBMT registry data. Auto-HSCT is currently not a recommended strategy in CML; however, it should be mentioned that due to the lack of randomized studies, the potential role of autologous HSCT for CML remains unknown.

76.2.5 Allogeneic HSCT

76.2.5.1 Indication

Although the introduction of TKI in the early 2000s dramatically changed the therapeutic strategy for CML, allo-HSCT has still a place, offering a very long-term PFS. This is particularly true as the leukemic quiescent stem cells are not dependent on BCR-ABL signaling for survival, and therefore those cells are not targeted by TKIs leading to a proportion of patients who will relapse or will have resistant disease despite TKI treatment. With extended follow-up, it appears that some 60% of patients can achieve excellent long-term disease control on imatinib, and a small proportion may even be able to stop treatment without experiencing disease recurrence. Approximately half of this group will achieve or regain remission on one of the second-generation TKI (2ndGTKI), bosutinib, dasatinib, and nilotinib, or third-generation TKI (3rdGTKI) ponatinib which is the only one that is effective against T315I mutation.

The efficacy of 2ndGTKI has led to their use as first-line therapy, and recently completed phase III studies suggest that approximately 80% of patients will achieve complete cytogenetic remissions within the first year, compared to 65% on imatinib. Based on these results, dasatinib and nilotinib have both been licensed for use in newly diagnosed patients. However, allo-HSCT remains the therapy of choice for advanced phase CML as well as for those with CP who failed to respond, develop TKI-resistant mutations, and lose an established response and/or are intolerant of the drug.

The time to proceed to transplant remains controversial. This is particularly true for the substantial number of patients being started on 2ndGTKI as first-line therapy, who, in case of resistance, progression, or relapse, may be rescued with either another 2ndGTKI or 3rdGTKI, and then the question to proceed to transplant immediately or wait for another progression and third-line therapy rescue before to have allo-HSCT is a matter of debate. This is less true for those who are failing third-line therapy or have T315I mutation for whom allo-HSCT is recommended.

A number of national and international study groups are now reporting that long-term response to imatinib and 2ndGTKI can be predicted by the rate of fall of BCR-ABL transcript levels (as measured by RQ-PCR at 3 and 6 months). It is therefore possible to identify the patient destined for transplant within the first year of diagnosis while still in CP and return to a more measured approach to transplant. Recently the CMWP of the EBMT analyzed the data of patients transplanted for CML in the 3rdGTKI era that showed that the number of TKI given prior to allo-HSCT seems not to impact on the outcome; however, the stage of the disease as well as the performance status of patients did have an important impact (Chalandon et al. 2018). It is therefore very important to try to keep patients in first CP and avoid progression, even for those rescued to second or more CP after having progressed to advanced phase, as the results after transplantation are worse in this category. Allo-HSCT is also recommended for patients with BC after debulking with second or 3rdGTKI plus induction chemotherapy. For AP CML patients, this should be individualized, but the search for a donor and referral to a transplant center should be done rapidly, and transplant should be initiated after obtaining a new response to TKI for those progressing from CP to AP under therapy as their outcome is not good without allo-HSCT.

76.2.5.2 Source of SC

About two-thirds of the transplantation done nowadays for CML use PBSC as source of HSC (Chalandon et al. 2018); this is close to what is seen in other hematological malignancies (Holtick et al. 2014). It appears that there is no difference in general outcome depending on the stem cell source, although BM seems to have a decrease incidence on chronic GvHD and its severity. The source of stem is therefore left open, but PBSC may potentially be preferred to decrease the risk of graft failure and the relapse risk in more advanced disease, particularly with the use of RIC.

76.2.5.3 Conditioning and GvHD Prophylaxis

For CML patients, the best conditioning regimen as well as the best GvHD prophylaxis remains to be determined. Regarding the MAC, CY combined either with BU or TBI is still the one that has shown the best overall long-term survival (Copelan 2006). RIC that has been introduced later to offer transplantation to older patients or with more comorbidities did not show improved outcome over MAC, particularly in relation with a higher incidence of relapse with RIC (Kebriaei et al. 2007; Chalandon et al. 2018). Therefore, for elderly patients or those with comorbidities, RIC (FLU with BU or MEL) will be the choice, and for the others, particularly with advanced phases in order to control better the disease, MAC should be proposed.

For GvHD prophylaxis, CSA combined with short course MTX seems also to remain the standard for allo-HSCT for CML (Copelan 2006). In order to reduce the incidence and severity of GvHD, TCD was introduced in the 1980s; however, there was an increase of relapse rate (Apperley et al. 1986). This led to many groups abandoning the use of TCD in sibling allografts for CML and often also in URD procedures. Others continued with its use and have reported good outcomes in sibling transplants, particularly following the introduction of DLI. In a small series of 23 CML patients with a median age of 36 years (range 18–58 years) transplanted with sibling donors and MAC between 1998 and 2016 at the University Hospital of Geneva using partial TCD with Campath-1H (alemtuzumab), the 15-year OS and LFS was 95% using the strategy of escalating doses DLI for early molecular relapses with a low incidence of acute and chronic GvHD (Chalandon, unpublished data).

76.2.5.4 Post transplant Strategies

After allo-HSCT, rising or persistently high levels of BCR-ABL1 mRNA can be detected prior to cytogenetic or hematological relapse. Low or falling BCR-ABL1 transcript levels are associated with continuous remission, while high or rising transcript levels predict relapse. Therefore monitoring BCR-ABL1 post-allo-HSCT for CML is of utmost importance, even in the long term, due to relapses that have occurred up to more than 15 years post-HSCT.

Many CML patients will remain RQ-PCR positive during the first 3 months after allo-HSCT, especially in the era of RIC or using TCD. In patients who are at least 4 months post-allo-HSCT, one working definition of molecular relapse is one of the following:

(a) BCR-ABL/ABL1 ratio higher than 0.02% in three samples a minimum of 4 weeks apart.
(b) Clearly rising BCR-ABL/ABL1 ratio in three samples a minimum of 4 weeks apart with the last two higher than 0.02%.
(c) BCR-ABL/ABL1 ratio higher than 0.05% in two samples a minimum of 4 weeks apart (Kaeda et al. 2006).

Administration of DLI can re-induce remission in 60–90% of patients with CML transplanted in, and relapsing in CP. The use of escalating doses in case of persistent disease reduces the risk of GvHD

(Mackinnon et al. 1995). An EBMT study showed 69% 5-year survival in 328 patients who received DLI for relapsed CML. DLI-related mortality was 11%, and disease-related mortality was 20%. Some form of GvHD was observed in 38% of patients. Risk factors for developing GvHD after DLI were T-cell dose at first DLI, time interval from transplant to DLI and donor type. In a time-dependent multivariate analysis, GvHD after DLI was associated with a 2.3-fold increase in risk of death as compared with patients without GvHD (Chalandon et al. 2010).

With the advent of TKI, the CML post transplant interventions are more complexes but give more opportunities to rescue patients. It is possible to combine DLI and TKI for relapsing patients; however, the best order (TKI first, DLI first, or both combined) has not yet been defined. The CMWP of the EBMT reported 431 patients with CML relapses post-allo-HSCT who received TKI either alone (55%) or in combination with DLI (14.5% before, 4.4% at the same time, and 26% after TKI). Only 42% of the patient obtained either a complete molecular (17.7%), cytogenetic (4.4%), or hematological (20.2%) remission with a 5-year OS of 60% and of 47% for RFS (Chalandon et al. 2017). This rather low response rate may be in relation with the fact that 235 patients were transplanted for advanced phases (AP, BC or > CP1).

Key Points

- With the advent of targeted therapy, allo-HSCT use has decreased; however, it is of importance to monitor closely patients who are under TKI and avoid that they progress to advanced phase (AP or BC) as the outcome after transplant is better for CP1 as compared to all other conditions.
- Allo-HSCT should be considered for patient with BC after their return to CP, for those progressing from CP to AP and for the one in CP after failure of third-line therapy or with T315I mutation.

References

Apperley JF, Jones L, Hale G, et al. Bone marrow transplantation for patients with chronic myeloid leukaemia: T-cell depletion with Campath-1 reduces the incidence of graft-versus-host disease but may increase the risk of leukaemic relapse. Bone Marrow Transplant. 1986;1:53–66.

Byrne JL, Beshti H, Clark D, et al. Induction of remission after donor leucocyte infusion for the treatment of relapsed chronic idiopathic myelofibrosis following allogeneic transplantation: evidence for a 'graft vs. myelofibrosis' effect. Br J Haematol. 2000;108:430–3.

Cervantes F, Dupriez B, Pereira A, et al. New prognostic scoring system for primary myelofibrosis based on a study of the International Working Group for Myelofibrosis Research and Treatment. Blood. 2009;113:2895–901.

Chalandon Y, Passweg JR, Schmid C, et al. Outcome of patients developing GVHD after DLI given to treat CML relapse: a study by the Chronic Leukemia Working Party of the EBMT. Bone Marrow Transplant. 2010;45:558–64.

Chalandon Y, Iacobelli S, Hoek J et al. Use of first or second generation TKI for CML after allogeneic hematopoietic stem cell transplantation: a study by the CMWP of the EBMT. EBMT annual meeting, Marseille, France, 2017.

Chalandon Y, Sbianchi G, Hoek J et al. Allogeneic stem cell transplantation in patients with CML-CP in the era of third generation tyrosine kinase inhibitors: a study by the CMWP of the EBMT. EBMT annual meeting, Lisbon, Portugal, 2018.

Copelan EA. Hematopoietic stem-cell transplantation. N Engl J Med. 2006;354:1813–26.

Deeg HJ, Gooley TA, Flowers ME, et al. Allogeneic hematopoietic stem cell transplantation for myelofibrosis. Blood. 2003;102:3912–8.

Gangat N, Caramazza D, Vaidya R, et al. DIPSS plus: a refined Dynamic International Prognostic Scoring System for primary myelofibrosis that incorporates prognostic information from karyotype, platelet count, and transfusion status. J Clin Oncol. 2011;29:392–7.

Gratwohl A, Hermans J, Goldman JM, et al. Risk assessment for patients with chronic myeloid leukaemia before allogeneic blood or marrow transplantation. Chronic Leukemia Working Party of the European Group for Blood and Marrow Transplantation. Lancet. 1998;352:1087–92.

Guardiola P, Anderson JE, Bandini G, et al. Allogeneic stem cell transplantation for agnogenic myeloid metaplasia: a European Group for Blood and Marrow Transplantation, Societe Francaise de Greffe de Moelle, Gruppo Italiano per il Trapianto del Midollo Osseo, and Fred Hutchinson Cancer Research Center Collaborative Study. Blood. 1999;93:2831–8.

Guglielmelli P, Lasho TL, Rotunno G, et al. MIPSS70: mutation-enhanced International Prognostic Score

System for transplantation-age patients with primary myelofibrosis. J Clin Oncol. 2018;36:310–8.

Hasford J, Pfirrmann M, Hehlmann R, et al. A new prognostic score for survival of patients with chronic myeloid leukemia treated with interferon alfa. Writing Committee for the Collaborative CML Prognostic Factors Project Group. J Natl Cancer Inst. 1998;90:850–8.

Hoglund M, Sandin F, Simonsson B. Epidemiology of chronic myeloid leukaemia: an update. Ann Hematol. 2015;94(Suppl 2):S241–7.

Holtick U, Albrecht M, Chemnitz JM, et al. Bone marrow versus peripheral blood allogeneic haematopoietic stem cell transplantation for haematological malignancies in adults. Cochrane Database of Syst Rev. 2014;4:CD010189.

Kaeda J, O'Shea D, Szydlo RM, et al. Serial measurement of BCR-ABL transcripts in the peripheral blood after allogeneic stem cell transplantation for chronic myeloid leukemia: an attempt to define patients who may not require further therapy. Blood. 2006;107:4171–6.

Kebriaei P, Detry MA, Giralt S, et al. Long-term follow-up of allogeneic hematopoietic stem-cell transplantation with reduced-intensity conditioning for patients with chronic myeloid leukemia. Blood. 2007;110:3456–62.

Kroger N, Giorgino T, Scott BL, et al. Impact of allogeneic stem cell transplantation on survival of patients less than 65 years of age with primary myelofibrosis. Blood. 2015b;125:3347–50.

Kroger N, Holler E, Kobbe G, et al. Allogeneic stem cell transplantation after reduced-intensity conditioning in patients with myelofibrosis: a prospective, multicenter study of the Chronic Leukemia Working Party of the European Group for Blood and Marrow Transplantation. Blood. 2009;114:5264–70.

Kroger NM, Deeg JH, Olavarria E, et al. Indication and management of allogeneic stem cell transplantation in primary myelofibrosis: a consensus process by an EBMT/ELN international working group. Leukemia. 2015a;29:2126–33.

Lussana F, Rambaldi A, Finazzi MC, et al. Allogeneic hematopoietic stem cell transplantation in patients with polycythemia vera or essential thrombocythemia transformed to myelofibrosis or acute myeloid leukemia: a report from the MPN Subcommittee of the Chronic Malignancies Working Party of the European Group for Blood and Marrow Transplantation. Haematologica. 2014;99:916–21.

Mackinnon S, Papadopoulos EB, Carabasi MH, et al. Adoptive immunotherapy evaluating escalating doses of donor leukocytes for relapse of chronic myeloid leukemia after bone marrow transplantation: separation of graft-versus-leukemia responses from graft-versus-host disease. Blood. 1995;86:1261–8.

Passamonti F, Cervantes F, Vannucchi AM, et al. A dynamic prognostic model to predict survival in primary myelofibrosis: a study by the IWG-MRT (International Working Group for Myeloproliferative Neoplasms Research and Treatment). Blood. 2010;115:1703–8.

Passamonti F, Giorgino T, Mora B, et al. A clinical-molecular prognostic model to predict survival in patients with post polycythemia vera and post essential thrombocythemia myelofibrosis. Leukemia. 2017;31:2726–31.

Raj K, Olavarria E, Eikema D-J, et al. Family mismatched donor transplantation for myelofibrosis: a retrospective analysis of the EBMT chronic leukaemia working party. Blood. 2016;128:4655.

Robin M, Giannotti F, Deconinck E, et al. Unrelated cord blood transplantation for patients with primary or secondary myelofibrosis. Biol Blood Marrow Transplant. 2014;20:1841–6.

Rondelli D, Goldberg JD, Isola L, et al. MPD-RC 101 prospective study of reduced-intensity allogeneic hematopoietic stem cell transplantation in patients with myelofibrosis. Blood. 2014;124:1183–91.

Scott BL, Gooley TA, Sorror ML, et al. The Dynamic International Prognostic Scoring System for myelofibrosis predicts outcomes after hematopoietic cell transplantation. Blood. 2012;119:2657–64.

Shanavas M, Popat U, Michaelis LC, et al. Outcomes of allogeneic hematopoietic cell transplantation in patients with myelofibrosis with prior exposure to Janus kinase 1/2 inhibitors. Biol Blood Marrow Transplant. 2016;22:432–40.

Sokal JE, Cox EB, Baccarani M, et al. Prognostic discrimination in "good-risk" chronic granulocytic leukemia. Blood. 1984;63:789–99.

Speck B, Bortin MM, Champlin R, et al. Allogeneic bone-marrow transplantation for chronic myelogenous leukaemia. Lancet. 1984;1:665–8.

Tefferi A, Mesa RA, Nagorney DM, Schroeder G, Silverstein MN. Splenectomy in myelofibrosis with myeloid metaplasia: a single-institution experience with 223 patients. Blood. 2000;95:2226–33.

Thiele J, Kvasnicka HM, Dietrich H, et al. Dynamics of bone marrow changes in patients with chronic idiopathic myelofibrosis following allogeneic stem cell transplantation. Histol Histopathol. 2005;20:879–89.

Wolschke C, Badbaran A, Zabelina T, et al. Impact of molecular residual disease post allografting in myelofibrosis patients. Bone Marrow Transplant. 2017;52:1526–9.

Severe Aplastic Anemia and PNH

77

Régis Peffault de Latour, Antonio Risitano, and Carlo Dufour

77.1 Definition and Epidemiology

Severe aplastic anemia (SAA) is an autoimmune disorder (AID) due to the attack of autoreactive cytotoxic T lymphocytes to the hematopoietic component of the bone marrow. The triggering antigen is so far unknown. The incidence of SAA is about 2.34/million in Europe and the United States and threefold higher in East Asia, with two age peaks of incidence (in young adults and in the elderly) (Young and Kaufman 2008).

Paroxysmal nocturnal hemoglobinuria (PNH) is another bone marrow failure syndrome (BMFS) which is often embedded with SAA. PNH is a more heterogeneous disease since its clinical presentation includes hemolytic anemia and thrombophilia in addition to bone marrow failure.

R. P. de Latour
French Reference Center for Aplastic Anemia and Paroxysmal Nocturnal Hemoglobinuria, Saint-Louis Hospital, Paris, France

Assistance Publique–Hôpitaux de Paris, Saint-Louis Hospital, Paris, France

University Paris VII, Denis Diderot, Paris, France

A. Risitano
Department of Clinical Medicine and Surgery, Federico II University of Naples, Naples, Italy

C. Dufour (✉)
Hematology Unit, G. Gaslini Research Children Hospital, Genoa, Italy
e-mail: carlodufour@gaslini.org

77.2 Diagnosis and Indication for Treatment for SAA

SAA is usually diagnosed in the setting of pancytopenia and a hypocellular BM. Diseases such as myelodysplasia, myelofibrosis, hypocellular acute leukemia, inherited BMF such as Fanconi's anemia (FA), or telomeropathies need to be excluded. Cytogenetic abnormalities can be found in up to 10% of true SAA (Rovo et al. 2016; Barone et al. 2015).

There is a close relationship between PNH and acquired SAA with a concomitant diagnosis in 40% of cases. SAA is diagnosed when marrow hematopoietic cellularity is <30%, and two of three of the following criteria are met: absolute neutrophil count $<0.5 \times 10^9/L$, absolute reticulocyte count $<60 \times 10^9/L$, and platelet count $<20 \times 10^9/L$ (Camitta et al. 1976).

Treatment requires careful planning and may be prolonged. A watch and wait strategy is often used initially if there is milder pancytopenia. Conversely, in case of transfusion requirement or if the criteria for SAA are met, treatment should begin with no delay. Prior to treatment the patient should be stable clinically with control of bleeding and infections. Once the diagnosis is confirmed, and the disease severity is assessed, family HLA-typing and matched unrelated donor search should be done in the work-up phase. In the absence of sign of intravascular hemolysis, patient's treatment algorithm is similar with or without PNH.

E. Carreras et al. (eds.), *The EBMT Handbook*, https://doi.org/10.1007/978-3-030-02278-5_77

77.3 Treatment of SAA

77.3.1 First Line Treatment for SAA

The choice of first-line treatment depends on the age of the patient and the availability of an HLA MSD (Fig. 77.1). The standard first-line treatments for a newly diagnosed patient with SAA are HSCT from a HLA-identical sibling donor or IS therapy (IST) using a combination of horse ATG and CSA (ATG + CSA). Early bone marrow HSCT after a conditioning regimen with CY, ATG, and GVHD prophylaxis combining CSA and MTX promotes excellent engraftment (95%) and OS (90% at 2 years) (Bacigalupo et al. 2012; Peffault de Latour 2016). This approach enabled also a very good long-term outcome with a rather limited number of late effects consisting in avascular necrosis, endocrine dysfunctions, and very rare secondary malignancy (Konopacki et al. 2012). However, toxicity related to transplantation as well as increased risk of GvHD is still a problem for patients older than 40 years of age and for those with high comorbidity index (Marsh et al. 2011).

For these categories first-line IS with horse ATG + CSA is recommended. This combination showed both in prospective controlled studies (Scheinberg et al. 2011; Marsh et al. 2012) and in real-life surveys (Peffault de Latour et al. 2018) a response rate of about 60%. Frontline IST provided similar findings in children and adolescents (Dufour et al. 2014; Dufour et al. 2015a). After IST, responders might experience relapse (20–30%), CSA dependence (20–30%), or long-term clonal evolution (PNH, MDS, or AML) (Scheinberg and Young 2012), justifying regular follow-up and bone marrow evaluation every 12–18 months.

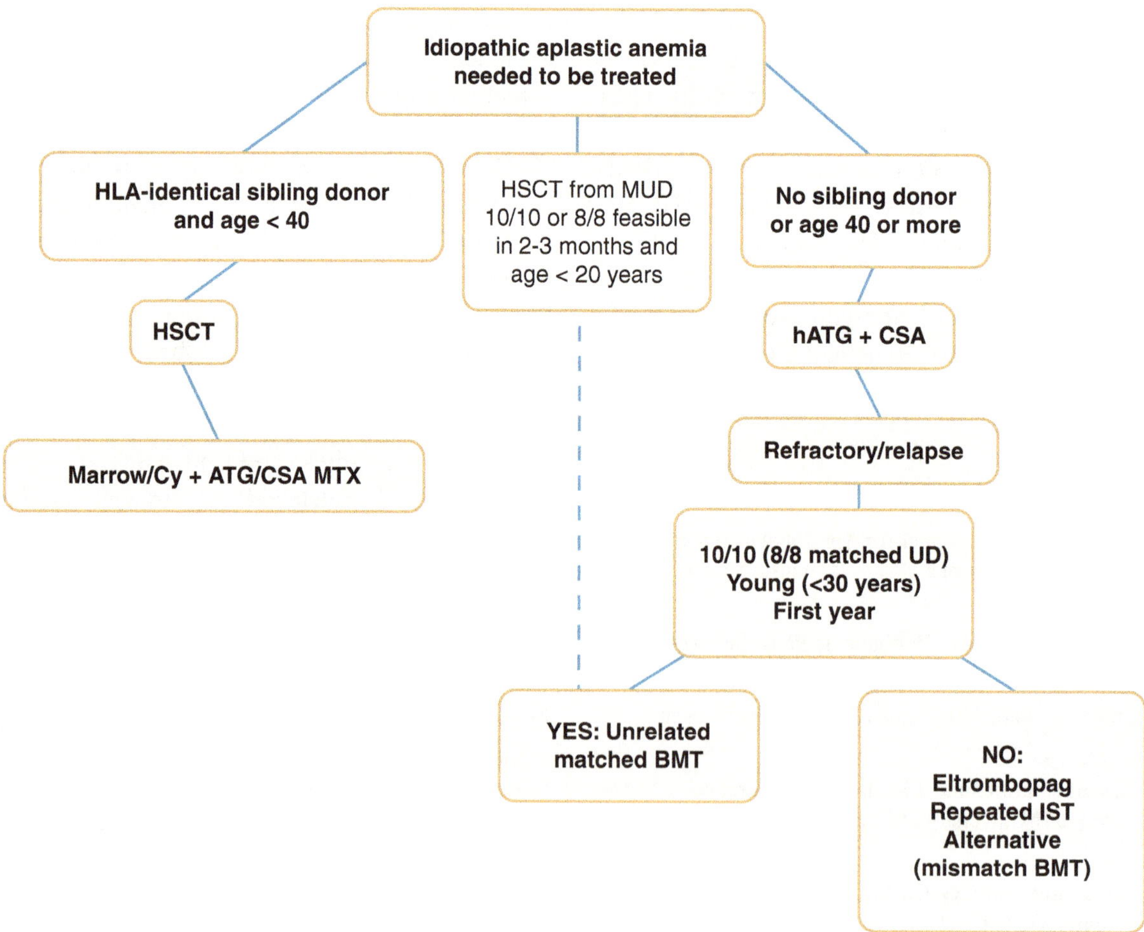

Fig. 77.1 Treatment algorithm of SAA in 2019

77.3.2 Second-Line Treatment for SAA

The choice of second-line treatment is also driven by age, by comorbidities, and by the presence of a matched related (MRD) or unrelated donor (MUD):

- In older patients with a MRD and confirmed refractory SAA, HSCT should be considered in the absence of significant comorbidities.
- In younger patients with a MUD and refractory or relapsed SAA, HSCT is recommended. Results of MUD HSCT have improved to such an extent that OS of idiopathic SAA are not statistically inferior to MRD transplants (Bacigalupo et al. 2015). This improvement has been largely attributed to better donor selection through allele matching, progress in supportive care, prophylaxis of GVHD, incorporation of FLU in conditioning regimens, and the addition of low-dose TBI. Recently some factors were found to positively affect OS after MUD HSCT including age ≤ 30 years, transplant within the first year after diagnosis (Devillier et al. 2016), use of BM vs PB, and CMV status (Bacigalupo et al. 2015).
- For patients older than 30 years, monotherapy with eltrombopag, an oral thrombopoietin-receptor agonist, produced in prospective studies in refractory patients an overall response of 40% with trilineage responses in some cases (Olnes et al. 2012; Desmond et al. 2014). A retrospective French study found similar results on patients with relapsed/refractory SAA. The overall rates of red blood cell and platelet transfusion independence were 7%, 33%, 46%, and 46 at 1, 3, and 6, months and last follow-up, respectively. No clonal evolution has been documented so far (Lengline et al. 2018). Other second-line options for patients not eligible to HSCT and who relapse or do not respond to frontline IST are a second course of ATG (rabbit) + CSA and alemtuzumab offering a response rate of 65% (Scheinberg et al. 2006) and 37% (Scheinberg and Young 2012), respectively.

77.3.3 Emerging Strategies for SAA

77.3.3.1 Eltrombopag Added to the Standard Horse ATG + CSA First Line Treatment

Many efforts to improve results of the standard treatment with horse ATG and CSA have failed since 40 years (Scheinberg 2012). Excellent results obtained with eltrombopag in monotherapy in refractory patients prompted American colleagues from the NIH to test if the addition of eltrombopag to standard IST as the first treatment for SAA would have increased the rate of CR and improved the long-term outcome. In the best cohort (eltrombopag associated to ATG and CSA from day 1), complete and overall response rates at 6 months were 58% and 94%, respectively. After a median follow-up of 2 years, survival rate is 97% (Townsley et al. 2017). Rates of relapse and clonal evolution were similar to historical experience. Whether eltrombopag might substantially improve horse ATG + CSA platform is at the moment under investigation through a large, randomized, controlled, prospective European trial on behalf of the SAA working party of the EBMT (RACE trial; ClinicalTrials.gov number, NCT02099747).

77.3.3.2 Up-Front Matched Unrelated Donor Transplantation

Although pediatric patients respond better to IST, the long-term risks of relapse, CSA dependence, and clonal evolution are high (Dufour et al. 2014). UK investigators reported an excellent estimated 5-year FFS of 95% in 44 consecutive children who received a 10-antigen (HLA-A, HLA-B, HLA-C, HLA-DRB1, HLA-DQB1) MUD HSCT; 40 of these children had previously failed IST. HSCT conditioning was with FLU, CY, and campath (FCC) (Samarasinghe and Webb 2012). Because of those excellent results, up-front MUD HSCT became an attractive first-line option in children. Between 2005 and 2014, a UK cohort of 29 consecutive children with idiopathic SAA received UD HSCTs (including five patients with 1 Ag mismatched transplants) as first-line therapy after conditioning with FCC. Results were excellent, with OS and EFS of 96% and 92%, respectively, low GVHD rates, and only one death (from idiopathic pneumonia) (Dufour et al. 2015b). This cohort was then compared with historical matched controls who had received (1) first-line MRD HSCT, (2) first-line IST with horse ATG + CSA, and (3) MUD HSCT post-IST failure as second-line therapy. Outcomes for the up-front unrelated cohort were similar to MRD HSCT and superior to IST and UD HSCT post-IST failure. Similar results were observed in another pediatric study (Choi et al. 2017).

Currently a North American study aims to compare outcomes of children with SAA treated de novo with IST vs MUD HSCT (ClinicalTrials.gov number NCT02845596). While waiting the results of this trial, if a 10/10 MUD is available and the transplant appears feasible within 2–3 months since diagnosis, this type of HSCT has become a reasonable frontline option for young patients in many centers. Another option is to perform MUD HSCT early after failure of frontline IST within 4–6 months since diagnosis. This is why MUD donor search should be started at diagnosis in young patients who lack a MRD.

77.3.3.3 Alternative Donor Transplantation in SAA

Alternative HSCTs (MMURD, CB, and haplo-family donors) are possible for individuals with no suitable MUD. Alternative HSCTs may be curative, but the risks of graft rejection, infectious complications, and GVHD are higher than those for MRD or MUD HSCT. Patient age, comorbidities, and alternative HSCT specificities are thus important issues in the decision-making process. Age and comorbidities are the first barriers to this type of procedure. Most numerous cohorts (>50 patients) tend to mainly include pediatric patients. In older studies long-term OS of about 60% (Yagasaki et al. 2011; Horan et al. 2012; Peffault de Latour et al. 2011)) compared to 5-year OS seen in refractory patients receiving only supportive care (Valdez et al. 2011). More recent studies with shorter follow-up showed OS and EFS >80% in unmanipulated haplo-HSCT with a high rate of cGVHD greater than 30% (Xu et al. 2016, 2017).

Based on this, alternative HSCT can be considered a salvage option that needs to be carefully balanced with best supportive care. The latter might be preferable for patients with comorbidities or advanced age (> 40 years or older) because of lower risks.

77.4 Treatment of PNH

Clinical presentation of PNH is extremely heterogeneous, including a variable combination of bone marrow failure, hemolytic anemia, and thromboembolism (Peffault de Latour et al. 2008). These clinical manifestations may change during the disease course of each individual patient so that the treatment of PNH should target the specific clinical presentation (Risitano 2017).

The treatment of marrow failure in PNH parallels that of SAA, and it has been described above; indeed, the presence of a PNH clone does not change the treatment algorithm of SAA.

In contrast, the treatment of complement-mediated hemolytic anemia and of thromboembolic PNH is based on complement inhibition through the anti-C5 MoAb eculizumab. Eculizumab has proven to be effective in inhibiting intravascular hemolysis of PNH, leading to hemoglobin stabilization and transfusion independency in about half of patients (Hillmen et al. 2006; Brodsky et al. 2008). This dramatic effect on intravascular hemolysis, eventually resulting in improved quality of life, is also associated with a significant reduction of the risk of thromboembolic complications (Hillmen et al. 2007). Notably, eculizumab treatment leads to a significant improvement of overall survival of PNH patients, as documented by two independent long-term retrospective studies showing 5-year survival rates >90% (Kelly et al. 2011; Loschi et al. 2016). Based on this, eculizumab is currently the standard of care for all PNH patients presenting with symptomatic hemolytic and/or thromboembolic disease; occasionally, when this occurs concomitantly with a BMF, the anticomplement treatment may be considered also in combination with IST (i.e., sequential or concomitant treatment) (Pagliuca et al. 2018).

77.4.1 Emerging Strategies for PNH

Even if currently available anticomplement treatment addresses most clinical needs of patients with hemolytic (and thrombotic) PNH, a number of novel strategies of complement modulation are in their preclinical or clinical development (Risitano and Marotta 2016). These strategies may target specific unmet clinical needs pertaining PNH patients. Novel anti-C5 agents (either MoAb, small molecules or small interfering RNA) may represent an improvement of current eculizumab, mostly in terms of patient comfort due to long-lasting activity (with longer dosing interval) and/or self-administration (usually SC). In addition, a novel class of compounds targeting early steps of the complement cascade at the level of C3 or even upstream (inhibitors of complement factor B and factor B) may anticipate a better efficacy in terms of hematological response, due to possible effect on C3-mediated extravascular hemolysis. Ongoing clinical trials will reveal whether any of this strategy may lead to change in the standard of care of anticomplement treatment of hemolysis (and thrombophilia) of PNH patients (Risitano and Marotta 2018).

Key Points

- SAA is usually diagnosed in the setting of pancytopenia and a hypocellular BM when other diseases, especially inherited BMF such as Fanconi's anemia or telomeropathy, have been excluded.
- The preferred treatment of SAA is HSCT from HLA-identical sibling donor. Transplantation from a MUD may be considered for patients without a sibling donor after failure of IS therapy or up front in younger ≤20 years if feasible in 2–3 months since diagnosis.
- Eltrombopag might substantially change in the coming years the standard horse ATG + CSA platform.
- The role of alternative donor HSCT needs further validation to enter the current clinical practice.

References

Bacigalupo A, Boyd A, Slipper J, et al. Foscarnet in the management of cytomegalovirus infections in hematopoietic stem cell transplant patients. Expert Rev AntiInfect Ther. 2012;10:1249–64.

Bacigalupo A, Socié G, Hamladji RM, et al. Current outcome of HLA identical sibling versus unrelated donor transplants in severe aplastic anemia: an EBMT analysis. Haematologica. 2015;100:696–702.

Barone A, Lucarelli A, Onofrillo D, et al. Diagnosis and management of acquired aplastic anemia in childhood. Guidelines from the Marrow Failure Study Group of the Pediatric Haemato-Oncology Italian Association (AIEOP). Blood Cells Mol Dis. 2015;55:40–7.

Brodsky RA, Young NS, Antonioli E, et al. Multicenter phase III study of the complement inhibitor eculizumab for the treatment of patients with paroxysmal nocturnal hemoglobinuria. Blood. 2008;114:1840–7.

Camitta BM, Thomas ED, Nathan DG, et al. Severe aplastic anemia: a prospective study of the effect of early marrow transplantation on acute mortality. Blood. 1976;48:63–70.

Choi YB, Yi ES, Lee JW, et al. Immunosuppressive therapy versus alternative donor hematopoietic stem cell transplantation for children with severe aplastic anemia who lack an HLA-matched familial donor. Bone Marrow Transplant. 2017;52:47–52.

Desmond R, Townsley DM, Dumitriu B, et al. Eltrombopag restores trilineage hematopoiesis in refractory severe aplastic anemia that can be sustained on discontinuation of drug. Blood. 2014;123:1818–25.

Devillier R, Dalle JH, Kulasekararaj A, et al. Unrelated alternative donor transplantation for severe acquired aplastic anemia: a study from the French Society of Bone Marrow Transplantation and Cell Therapies and the EBMT Severe Aplastic Anemia Working Party. Haematologica. 2016;101:884–90.

Dufour C, Pillon M, Passweg J, et al. Outcome of aplastic anemia in adolescence: a survey of the Severe Aplastic Anemia Working Party ofthe European Group for Blood and Marrow Transplantation. Haematologica. 2014;99:1574–81.

Dufour C, Pillon M, Sociè G, et al. Outcome of aplastic anaemia in children. A study by the severe aplastic anaemia and paediatric disease working parties of the European group blood and bone marrow transplant. Br J Haematol. 2015a;169:565–73.

Dufour C, Veys P, Carraro E, et al. Similar outcome of upfront-unrelated and matched sibling stem cell transplantation in idiopathic paediatric aplastic anemia. A study on behalf of the UK BMT WP, Paediatric Diseases and Severe Aplastic Anemia Working Party of EBMT. Br J Haematol. 2015b;171:585–94.

Hillmen P, Young NS, Schubert J, et al. The complement inhibitor eculizumab in paroxysmal nocturnal hemoglobinuria. N Engl J Med. 2006;355:1233–43.

Hillmen P, Muus P, Duhrsen U, et al. Effect of the complement inhibitor eculizumab on thromboembolism in patients with paroxysmal nocturnal hemoglobinuria. Blood. 2007;110:4123–8.

Horan J, Wang T, Haagenson M, et al. Evaluation of HLA matching in unrelated hematopoietic stem cell transplantation for nonmalignant disorders. Blood. 2012;120:2918–24.

Kelly RJ, Hill A, Arnold LM, et al. Long-term treatment with eculizumab in paroxysmal nocturnal hemoglobinuria: sustained efficacy and improved survival. Blood. 2011;117:6786–92.

Konopacki J, Porcher R, Robin M, et al. Long-term follow up after allogeneic stem cell transplantation in patients with severe aplastic anemia after cyclophosphamide plus antithymocyte globulin conditioning. Haematologica. 2012;97:710–6.

Lengline E, Drenou B, Peterlin P, et al. Nationwide survey on the use of eltrombopag in patients with severe aplastic anemia: a report on behalf of the French Reference Center for Aplastic Anemia. Haematologica. 2018;103:212–20.

Loschi M, Porcher R. Barraco et al. Impact of eculizumab treatment on paroxysmal nocturnal hemoglobinuria: A treatment versus no-treatment study. Am J Hematol. 2016;91:366–70.

Marsh JC, Gupta V, Lim Z, et al. Alemtuzumab with fludarabine and cyclophosphamide reduces chronic graft-versus-host disease after allogeneic stem cell transplantation for acquired aplastic anemia. Blood. 2011;118:2351–7.

Marsh JC, Bacigalupo A, Schrezenmeier H, et al. Prospective study of rabbit antithymocyte globulin and cyclosporine for aplastic anemia from the EBMT Severe Aplastic Anaemia Working Party. Blood. 2012;119:5391–6.

Olnes MJ, Scheinberg P, Calvo KR, et al. Eltrombopag and improved hematopoiesis in refractory aplastic anemia. N Engl J Med. 2012;367:11–9.

Pagliuca S, Risitano AM, De Fontbrune FS, et al. Combined intensive immunosuppression and eculizumab for aplastic anemia in the context of hemolytic paroxysmal nocturnal hemoglobinuria: a retrospective analysis. Bone Marrow Transplant. 2018;53:105–7.

Peffault de Latour R, Mary JY, Salanoubat C, et al. Paroxysmal nocturnal hemoglobinuria: natural history of diseases ubcategories. Blood. 2008;112:3099–106.

Peffault de Latour R, Purtill D, Ruggeri A, et al. Influence of nucleated cell dose on overall survival of unrelated cordbloodtransplantation for patients with severe acquired aplastic anemia: a study by eurocordand the aplastic anemia working party of the European group for blood and marrow transplantation. Biol Blood Marrow Transplant. 2011;17:78–85.

Peffault de Latour R. Transplantation for bone marrow failure: current issues. Hematology Am Soc Hematol Educ Program. 2016;2016(1):90–8.

Peffault de Latour R, Tabrizi R, Marcais A, et al. Nationwide survey on the use of horse antithymocyte globulins (ATGAM) in patients with acquired aplastic anemia: A report on behalf of the French Reference Center for Aplastic Anemia. Am J Hematol. 2018;93:635–42.

Risitano AM, Marotta S. Therapeutic complement inhibition in complement-mediated hemolytic anemias: Past, present and future. Semin Immunol. 2016;28:223–40.

Risitano AM. In: Aljurf M, Gluckman E, Dufour C, editors. Congenital and acquired bone marrow failure. New York: Elsevier Inc; 2017. p. 153–64.

Risitano AM, Marotta S. Toward complement inhibition 2.0: Next generation anticomplement agents for paroxysmal nocturnal hemoglobinuria. Am J Hematol. 2018;93:564–77.

Rovo A, et al. Current approach for the diagnosis of Aplastic Anemia. Curr Drug Targets. 2016;17:1.

Samarasinghe S, Webb DK. How I manage aplastic anaemia in children. Br J Haematol. 2012;157:26–40.

Scheinberg P, Nunez O, Young NS. Retreatment with rabbit anti-thymocyte globulin and cyclosporin for patients with relapsed or refractory severea plastic anaemia. Br J Haematol. 2006;133:622–7.

Scheinberg P, Nunez O, Weinstein B, et al. Horse versus rabbit antithymocyte globulin in acquired aplastic anemia. N Engl J Med. 2011;365:430–8.

Scheinberg P, Young NS. How I treat acquired aplastic anemia. Blood. 2012;120:1185–96.

Scheinberg P. Aplastic anemia: therapeutic updates in immunosuppression and transplantation. Hematology Am Soc Hematol Educ Program. 2012;2012:292–300.

Townsley DM, Scheinberg P, Winkler T, et al. Eltrombopag added to standard immunosuppression for aplastic anemia. N Engl J Med. 2017;376:1540–50.

Valdez JM, Scheinberg P, Nunez O, et al. Decreased infection-related mortality and improved survival in severe aplastic anemia in the past two decades. Clin Infect Dis. 2011;52:726–35.

Xu LP, Wang SQ, Wu DP, et al. Haplo-identical transplantation for acquired severe aplastic anaemia in a multicentre prospective study. Br J Haematol. 2016;175:265–74.

Xu LP, Zhang XH, Wang FR, et al. Haploidentical transplantation for pediatric patients with acquired severe aplastic anemia. Bone Marrow Transplant. 2017;52:381–7.

Yagasaki H, Kojima S, Yabe H, et al. Acceptable HLA-mismatching in unrelated donor bone marrow transplantation for patients with acquired severe aplastic anemia. Blood. 2011;118:3186–90.

Young NS, Kaufman DW. The epidemiology of acquired aplastic anemia. Haematologica. 2008;93:489–92.

Fanconi's Anemia and Other Hereditary Bone Marrow Failure Syndromes

78

Cristina Díaz de Heredia, Marc Bierings, Jean-Hugues Dalle, Francesca Fioredda, and Brigitte Strahm

78.1 Introduction

Inherited bone marrow failure syndromes (IBMFS) are a heterogeneous group of rare blood disorders due to hematopoiesis impairment, with different clinical presentations and pathogenic mechanisms. Some patients present congenital malformations, may progress through clonal evolution (MDS and acute leukemia), and are at risk of solid tumors at early ages. The number of involved genes rises annually; comprehensive next-generation sequencing analyses improve diagnostic accuracy. HSCT is an option for these congenital disorders. However, it should be well understood that it will only improve the hematopoietic defect and not cure the congenital malformations or lower the risk of solid tumors. Moreover, the HSCT procedure per se may increase this risk. Consequently, the decision to transplant a patient should be taken by a multidisciplinary team. HSCT must be performed at specialized centers owing to patient susceptibilities to toxicity and the need for specific management during and after the procedure. The general recommendations for management of IBMFS are included in the key points at the end of the chapter.

78.2 Fanconi's Anemia

78.2.1 Pathogenesis and Principal Clinical Features

Fanconi's anemia (FA) is the most common IBMFS with an estimated incidence of 1/200,000. FA is a disorder of DNA damage repair, leading to increased chromosomal breakage in diagnostic assays. Twenty underlying genes have been identified. The presentation is variable with somatic abnormalities in 70% of patients, marrow failure, and a highly increased risk of malignancies (MDS, leukemia, head and neck cancer, gynecological cancers) at an early age. Patients can be

C. Díaz de Heredia (✉)
Department of Pediatric Hematology and Oncology and HSCT, Hospital Universitari Vall d'Hebron, Barcelona, Spain
e-mail: crdiaz@vhebron.net

M. Bierings
Pediatric Hematology and HSCT Division, Wilhelmina Kinderziekenhuis, Utrecht, Netherlands

J.-H. Dalle
HSCT Programme, Hemato Immunology Department, Hôpital Robert Debré Université Paris 7 - Denis Diderot, Paris, France

F. Fioredda
Hematology Unit, Istituto Giannina Gaslini, Genoa, Italy

B. Strahm
Department of Pediatrics and Adolescent Medicine Division of Pediatric Hematology and Oncology, Medical Center Faculty of Medicine, University of Freiburg, Freiburg im Breisgau, Germany

E. Carreras et al. (eds.), *The EBMT Handbook*, https://doi.org/10.1007/978-3-030-02278-5_78

identified at adult age, e.g., in cases of (familial) pancytopenia, myelodysplasia, or unexpected severe toxicity of treatment. FA patients are highly susceptible to chemotherapy and irradiation-induced damage such as mucositis.

78.2.2 Indications of HSCT

Indications for transplant include marrow failure (transfusion dependency or severe neutropenia) and myelodysplasia/leukemia. Since transplantation implies exposure to chemo/radiotherapy and since the outcome is dependent on age at transplant, the decision to proceed to transplant should be individualized and discussed with experts in the field.

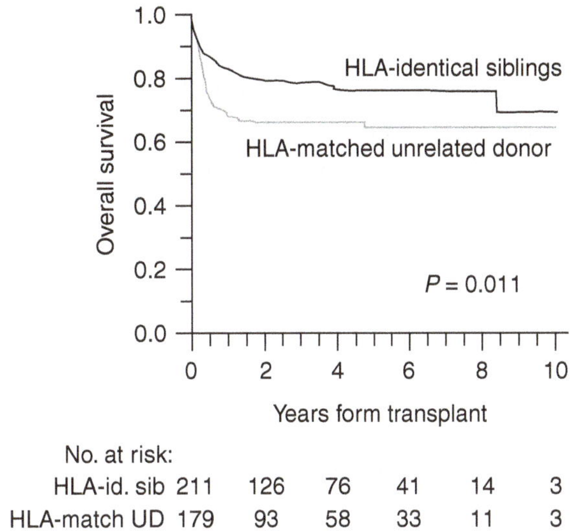

Fig. 78.1 OS for Fanconi's anemia according to the type of donor: transplant period 2000–2009. The EBMT experience. Peffault de Latour R. Blood 2013; 122: 4279–86

78.2.3 Specific Considerations for Conditioning Regimen

Conditioning regimens should be adapted for FA patients, with reduced doses of many cytotoxic drugs and irradiation. Current conditioning regimens generally contain FLU (cumulative dose 150 mg/m^2), in combination with reduced doses of CY (up to 50 mg/kg cumulative) and/or low-dose TBI (100–300 cGy) in the case of unrelated donors. For adults no clear recommendations can be given at this point.

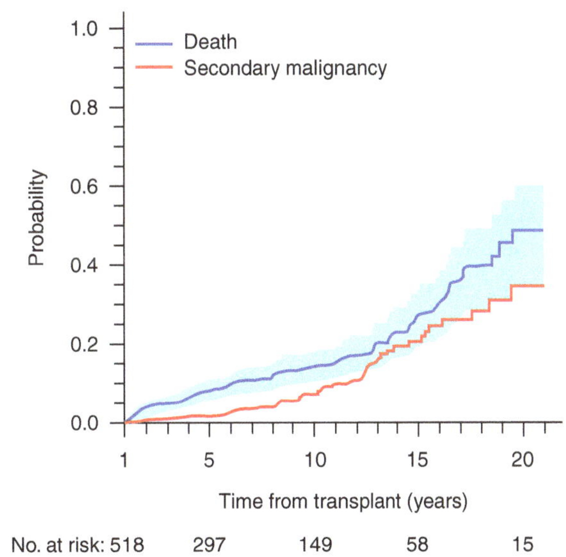

Fig. 78.2 Fanconi's anemia: probability of death and secondary malignancies post transplant. The EBMT experience. Peffault de Latour R. Blood 2013; 122: 4279–86

78.2.4 Results

Current results of transplant for marrow failure in children with FA show survival rates depending on donor type ranging from 50% to more than 90%. Factors influencing outcome include age at transplant, sibling donor availability, and the use of FLU in the conditioning regimen. A EBMT study of the period 2000–2009 reported 78% and 65% OS at 5-year post transplant for MSD and MUD, respectively (Fig. 78.1).

Clonal disease and adult age at transplant remain a challenge. Both TRM and relapse of malignant disease contribute to these generally poor results.

78.2.5 Recommendations for Long-Term Follow-Up

After transplant, the risk of secondary malignancies is high (Fig. 78.2). Patients should be carefully monitored for head-neck malignancies (regular ear, nose, and throat specialist checks for early signs of malignant transformation, and women undergo gynecological checkups and screening for breast cancer with ultrasound and MRI) and other manifestations of FA (e.g., endocrinopathies such as thyroid dysfunction, diabetes, growth problems, and early menopause). As more FA patients survive into adulthood, specialist multidisciplinary teams taking care of these complex patients are needed.

78.3 Dyskeratosis Congenita

78.3.1 Pathogenesis and Principal Clinical Features

Dyskeratosis congenita (DC) is a multisystemic disorder characterized by the nail dystrophy, skin pigment alteration and oral leukoplakia triad frequently associated with bone marrow failure and organ involvement (pulmonary fibrosis, liver, neurological and gastrointestinal abnormalities, ocular impairment and cancer predisposition). The causative mechanism of the disease is abnormal telomere shortening due to a defect in one of the genes encoding for the telomerase-shelterin complex. Bone marrow failure is the main cause of death, although pulmonary fibrosis, liver cirrhosis, and cancer significantly contribute to morbidity and mortality. Androgens have shown some effect on hematopoiesis and lung function.

78.3.2 Indications for Transplant

HSCT is the only curative option for bone marrow failure in DC. Organ dysfunction is not corrected by HSCT and limits its indication by negatively affecting outcome. HSCT is not indicated as a preemptive measure but is recommended in cases of progressive marrow failure without significant organ dysfunction.

78.3.3 Specific Considerations for Donor Selection and Conditioning Regimen

MSD are the donors of choice; MUD and mismatched related donors are associated with inferior outcomes. Given tissue "fragility," a reduced intensity combination containing fludarabine would be preferable to myeloablative regimen. A thorough evaluation of organ status is recommended prior to transplant.

78.3.4 Results

Five- and 10-year survival is 57% and 23%, respectively. Age >20 years at HSCT, HSCT before 2000 and alternative donor transplant were poor prognostic markers. Patients transplanted after 2000 had improved early survival to 70% at 5-year post transplant.

78.3.5 Specific Recommendations for Long-Term Follow-Up

Since HSCT may increase the risk of secondary malignancies in these patients, long-term follow-up is mandatory.

78.4 Severe Congenital Neutropenia and Shwachman-Diamond Syndrome

78.4.1 Pathogenesis and Principal Clinical Features

The term "severe congenital neutropenia" (SCN) covers a group of inherited disorders characterized by a persistent absolute neutrophil count (ANC) below 0.5×10^9/L and early onset of severe infections. To date, 24 distinct genes have been associated with SCN which may manifest as an isolated disorder or associated with various extra-hematologic features.

The most common form (60%) of genetic neutropenia is due to mutations in the *ELANE* gene. Shwachman-Diamond syndrome (SDS) caused by a mutation of *SDSB* gene is the most common form of neutropenia associated with extra-hematologic features (exocrine pancreas deficiency, metaphyseal dysplasia, mental retardation, cardiomyopathy, and immune dysfunction).

The underlying pathogenic mechanism of most genetic SCN is accelerated apoptosis of promyelocytes causing blockage of neutrophil maturation. In SDS, the defect in the SBDS protein causes abnormal ribosomal assembly and inadequate maintenance of the stromal microenvironment.

The SCN clinical phenotype consists of predisposition to severe infections. The use of G-CSF improved the prognosis of the disease which had been lethal in almost 50% of cases. The aim of treatment is to maintain protective neutrophil values (between 1.0 and 5.0×10^9/L) that are usually achieved with G-CSF doses of 3–5 µg/kg/day. Patients requiring G-CSF between 10 and 15 µg/kg/day are defined as "poor responders," whereas those requiring >20 µg/kg/day are considered "non-responders."

Another feature of SCN is its tendency to transform into MDS/AL. The overall cumulative incidence of MDS/AL is 10.8% and 22% after 15–20 years of G-CSF treatment according to the French and International Severe Chronic Neutropenia Registries, respectively. In SDS the cumulative incidence is between 18% and 36% at 20–30 years.

78.4.2 Indications for Transplant

The definitive cure of the hematologic defect is HSCT. Given the non-negligible mortality rate, indications are limited to patients with MDS/AL and absent or poor response to G-CSF. For SDS the indications for transplant are worsening cytopenias with increased transfusion dependence and transformation into MDS/AL.

78.4.3 Specific Considerations for Conditioning Regimen

A MAC regimen is considered appropriate in SCN, while a RIC is more indicated in SDS owing to possible secondary organ dysfunction (e.g., heart disease).

78.4.4 Results

OS has been assessed at 82% with TRM of 17% in the largest cohort (136 patients) described. Better results have been obtained in patients under 10 years of age, in those transplanted after 2000 and in cases of MSD transplants.

78.5 Diamond-Blackfan Anemia

78.5.1 Pathogenesis and Principal Clinical Features

Diamond-Blackfan anemia (DBA) is a rare IBMFS caused by heterozygous mutations in ribosomal genes. No genetic aberration is identified in approximately 30% of patients. Patients usually present with transfusion-dependent macrocytic anemia at birth or in early infancy. Mild neutropenia and progressive thrombocytopenia have been observed in the course of the disease. Despite various possible physical abnormalities (short stature, abnormal thumbs, cleft palate, heart defects, urogenital malformations), the non-hematologic phenotype is usually rather subtle in around 50% of patients. Patients with DBA are at increased risk of developing hematologic (AML/MDS) and non-hematologic malignancies (osteosarcoma, colon cancer).

After the first year of life, at least two trials of steroid therapy are recommended; around 60% of the patients are responders. Patients <12 months of age or those who are steroid non-responders are treated with red blood cell (RBC) transfusions. Iron chelation is essential to prevent organ damage from iron overload. About 20% of patients become transfusion independent with no further treatment (spontaneous remission).

78.5.2 Indications for Transplant

HSCT is the only cure for hematologic manifestations. Indications are non-response to steroids, steroid dependency at a dose ≥0.3 mg/kg/day, transfusion dependency, alloimmunization to

RBC, progressive pancytopenia, or MDS/AML. Published data indicate that HSCT should be performed before the age of 10 years; however, an earlier time point might be preferable to avoid iron overload. Indications must be evaluated taking into account the alternative approach with RBC transfusions combined with rigorous iron chelation.

78.5.3 Specific Considerations for Donor Selection and Conditioning Regimen

HSCT from a MSD including cord blood has resulted in OS >80% and is recommended for all indications. Sibling donors should be carefully assessed to rule out silent carrier status. Recent reports described improved outcome of MUD HSCT with OS ranging from 70 to 85% (Strahm, EBMT abstract 2018). By contrast, data supporting HSCT from mismatched donors as standard procedure are insufficient. The majority of transplants reported were performed with myeloablative conditioning. Based on available data, a standard regimen including FLU and BU or TREO is recommended.

78.5.4 Specific Recommendations for Long-Term Follow-Up

Long-term care for patients being transplanted for DBA should focus on the management of iron overload. Depending on its extent, phlebotomies and/or iron chelation therapy might be indicated. Furthermore, patients and physicians should be aware of the increased risk of malignancies (especially osteosarcoma, colon cancer).

78.6 Congenital Amegakaryocytic Thrombocytopenia

78.6.1 Pathogenesis and Principal Clinical Features

Congenital amegakaryocytic thrombocytopenia (CAMT) is a rare IBMFS caused by mutations in the gene coding for the thrombopoietin receptor *MPL*. Patients usually present with thrombocytopenia at birth or within the first year of life. Most patients develop hypocellular bone marrow and progress to pancytopenia early in the course of disease. Clonal evolution with acquired chromosomal aberrations and the development of myelodysplastic syndromes are very rare events. Characteristic non-hematologic manifestations of the disease have not been described.

78.6.2 Indications for Transplant

HSCT is the only curative treatment and should be offered to all patients with transfusion-dependent thrombocytopenia, pancytopenia, or clonal evolution.

78.6.3 Specific Considerations for Donor Selection and Conditioning Regimen

HSCT from a MSD is the preferred option, and successful transplants from heterozygous-related donors have been reported. HSCT from MUD (≥ 9/10) is an acceptable alternative. Successful HSCT from mismatched family donors or mismatched unrelated cord blood donors have been reported. However, these should preferentially be performed in clinical trials.

In view of a considerable graft failure rate, a MAC with FLU in combination with TREO or BU is preferred. However, there have been reports of successful engraftment after a RIC, and this might be considered in cases with severely hypocellular bone marrow in the absence of clonal aberrations and alloimmunization to platelet transfusions.

78.6.4 Results

Five-year overall survival was 77% with TRM of 12.6% in a retrospective EBMT study. However, this series included HSCT performed over a period of 26 years with a variety of donors, regimens, and stem cell sources, with no difference in outcome.

Key Points

Patient	– Evaluate carefully hematologic and extra-hematologic manifestations of the disease prior to transplant
Donor	– The best donor is MSD; however, it is mandatory to test the genetic defect in the donor since some IBMFS may present different clinical and hematologic expression in members of the same family – Consider MUD in case of no appropriate MSD – Mismatched related and UD and unrelated CB only in experienced centers and preferentially in clinical trials
Source of stem cells	BM is the best source of stem cells Matched related CB is a good option PB is associated with higher risk of cGVHD and should be avoided
Cell dose	It is important for graft failure prevention: NC > 3 × 10^8/kg recipient bw for BM NC > 3 × 10^7/kg recipient bw for related CB NC > 4 × 10^7/kg recipient bw for unrelated CB
Conditioning regimen	MAC or RIC depending on the type of IBMF Irradiation should be avoided owing to the known risk of cancer Patients with Fanconi's anemia and dyskeratosis congenita must receive a RIC
GVHD prophylaxis	GVHD must be avoided Include two immunosuppressive drugs Serotherapy for UD transplants
Long-term follow-up	– It is mandatory owing to high risk of secondary malignancies, extra-hematologic manifestations and iron overload – Patients should be followed-up by a multidisciplinary team

Recommended References

Ayas M, Saber W, Davies SM, et al. Allogeneic hematopoietic stem cell transplantation for Fanconi anemia in patients with pre-transplantation cytogenetic abnormalities, myelodysplastic syndrome or acute leukemia. J Clin Oncol. 2013;31:1669–76.

Ballmaier M, Germeshausen M. Congenital amegakaryocytic thrombocytopenia: clinical presentation, diagnosis, and treatment. Semin Thromb Hemost. 2011;37:673–81.

Barbaro P, Vedi A. Survival after hematopoietic stem cell transplant in patients with dyskeratosis congenita: a systematic review of the literature. Biol Blood Marrow Transplant. 2016;22:1152–8.

Benajiba L, Salvado C, Dalle JH, et al. HLA-matched related donor HSCT in Fanconi anemia patients conditioned with cyclophosphamide and fludarabine. Blood. 2015;125:417–8.

Bizzetto R, Bonfim C, Rocha V, et al. Outcomes after related and unrelated umbilical cord blood transplantation for hereditary bone marrow failure syndromes other than Fanconi anemia. Haematologica. 2011;96:134–41.

Dalle JH, Fahd M, et al. Allogeneic stem cell transplantation in amegacaryocytosis: results of a retrospective study in EBMT centers. Biol Blood Marrow Transplant. 2014;20:S81–2.

Donadieu J, Beaupain B, Fenneteau O, et al. Congenital neutropenia in the era of genomics: classification, diagnosis, and natural history. Br J Haematol. 2017;79:557–74.

Dufour C. How I manage patients with Fanconi anaemia. Br J Haemat. 2017;178:32–47.

Fagioli F, Quarello P, Zecca M, et al. Haematopoietic stem cell transplantation for diamond Blackfan anaemia: a report from the Italian association of Paediatric Haematology and oncology registry. Br J Haematol. 2014;165:673–81.

Fioredda F, Iacobelli S, van Biezen A, et al. Severe aplastic anemia the inborn error and the pediatric disease working parties of the European Society for Blood and Bone Marrow Transplantation (EBMT) and stem cell transplant for Immunodeficiencies in Europe (SCETIDE). Stem cell transplantation in severe congenital neutropenia: an analysis from the European Society for Blood and Marrow Transplantation. Blood. 2015;126:1885–92.

Frangoul H, Keates-Baleeiro J, Calder C, et al. Unrelated bone marrow transplant for congenital amegakaryocytic thrombocytopenia: report of two cases and review of the literature. Pediatr Transplant. 2010;14:E42–5.

Knight S, Vulliamy T, Copplestone A, et al. Dyskeratosis congenita (DC) registry: identification of new features of DC. Br J Haematol. 1998;103:990–6.

Mahadeo KM, Tewari P, Parikh SH, et al. Durable engraftment and correction of hematological abnormalities in children with congenital amegakaryocytic thrombocytopenia following myeloablative umbilical cord blood transplantation. Pediatr Transplant. 2015;19:753–7.

Meerpohl JJ, Kartal BME, et al. Stem cell transplantation in diamond-Blackfan Anaemia: a retrospective analysis. Bone Marrow Transplant. 2009;43:S76.

Mugishima H, Ohga S, Ohara A, et al. Hematopoietic stem cell transplantation for diamond-Blackfan anemia: a report from the aplastic anemia Committee of the Japanese Society of pediatric hematology. Pediatr Transplant. 2007;11:601–7.

Muraoka K, Ischii E. IharaK et al. successful bone marrow transplantation in a patient with c-mpl-mutated congenital amegakaryocytic thrombocytopenia from a carrier donor. Pediatr Transplant. 2005;9:101–3.

Peffault de Latour R, Peters C, Gibson B, et al. On behalf of the pediatric working Party of the European Group for blood and marrow transplantation and the severe aplastic anemia working Party of the European Group for blood and marrow transplantation. Recommendations on hematopoietic stem cell transplantation for inherited bone marrow failure syndromes. Bone Marrow Transplant. 2015;50:1168–72.

Peffault de Latour R, Porcher R, Dalle JH, et al. Allogeneic hematopoietic stem cell transplantation in Fanconi anemia: the European Group for Blood and Marrow Transplantation experience. Blood. 2013;122:4279–86.

Rosenberg PS, Zeidler C, Bolyard AA, et al. Stable long-term risk of leukaemia in patients with severe congenital neutropenia maintained on G-CSF therapy. Br J Haematol. 2010;150:196–9.

Savage SA, Dufour C. Classical inherited bone marrow failure syndromes with high risk for myelodysplastic syndrome and acute myelogenous leukemia. Semin Hematol. 2017;54:105–14.

Vlachos A, Muir E. How I treat diamond-Blackfan anemia. Blood. 2010;116:3715–23.

Woods G, Bajwa RP, Rose MJ, et al. Reduced intensity transplantation for congenital amegakaryocytic thrombocytopenia: report of a case and review of the literature. Pediatr Transplant. 2014;18:E31–4.

79 Hemoglobinopathies (Sickle Cell Disease and Thalassemia)

Barbara Cappelli, Eliane Gluckman, Khaled Ghanem, and Miguel R. Abboud

79.1 HSCT for Sickle Cell Disease

Barbara Cappelli and Eliane Gluckman

79.1.1 Definition and Epidemiology

Sickle cell disease (SCD) is the most common inherited hemoglobinopathy worldwide. It results from a single-nucleotide substitution that leads to a propensity toward hemoglobin polymerization and sickling of red blood cells. Sickle cell disease is characterized by anemia, ongoing hemolysis, and acute and chronic vaso-occlusive complications affecting multiple organs. SCD affects over 100,000 Americans, and it occurs in about one in 500 African-American births and in one in every 1000–1400 Hispanic-American births (NIH 2014; Piel et al. 2013).

The implementation of newborn screening, penicillin prophylaxis, vaccination programs, narcotics, chronic transfusions, hydroxyurea, and the early detection of cerebral vasculopathy with transcranial Doppler (TCD) have improved the perspective for children with SCD (Angelucci et al. 2014; Yawn et al. 2014; Ware et al. 2016; Bernaudin et al. 2016).

79.1.2 Allo-HSCT with an HLA Identical Sibling

HSCT remains the only curative therapy for SCD (Angelucci et al. 2014; Arnold et al. 2016; Gluckman et al. 2017). The goal when performing HSCT is to replace the patient's marrow with genetic functional cells before major organ dysfunction and complications (Bernaudin et al. 2007). Some of the most common indications for HSCT are listed in Table 79.1 (Angelucci et al. 2014; Bernaudin et al. 2016).

B. Cappelli
Eurocord-Monacord, Centre Scientifique de Monaco, Monaco, Monaco

E. Gluckman (✉)
Eurocord, Department of Hematology, Hospital Saint Louis, University Paris-Diderot, Paris, France
e-mail: eliane.gluckman@aphp.fr

K. Ghanem
BASMA Pediatric Oncology Unit, Al Bairouni Hospital, Damascus, Syria

M. R.Abboud
Department of Pediatrics and Adolescent Medicine, American University of Beirut Medical Center, Beirut, Lebanon

E. Carreras et al. (eds.), *The EBMT Handbook*, https://doi.org/10.1007/978-3-030-02278-5_79

Several barriers prevent HSCT widespread application including lack of a suitable donor, lack of information, and limited understanding of HSCT. Moreover, HSCT encompasses a risk of early- and late-onset regimen-related toxicities, rejection, and mortality. Nevertheless, the annual number of transplants have been increasing and has quadrupled in the last decade (CIBMTR personal communication). The first successful HLA identical HSCT was performed in a patient affected by both SCD and AML in 1984 (Johnson et al. 1984). After that, many groups have described a series of patients transplanted from an HLA identical sibling with an OS that varies between 91 and 100% and EFS that varies between 73 and 100% (Bernaudin et al. 2007; Walters et al. 2016). Recently, 1000 HLA identical transplants, performed between 1986 and 2013 and reported to EBMT, Eurocord, and the CIBMTR, have been published with a 5-year EFS and OS of 91.4% (95% CI 89.6–93.3%) and 92.9% (95% CI 91.1–94.6%), respectively. The EFS and OS were both lower with increasing age, EFS was higher for transplantations performed after 2006, and OS was lower for peripheral blood transplant recipients (Fig. 79.1) (Gluckman et al. 2017).

Table 79.1 Indications for HSCT in SCD patients

Age <16 years	
HLA identical sibling donor	
One or more of the following complications:	Stroke or central nervous system event lasting >24 h
	Sickle lung disease
	Sickle nephropathy
	Retinopathy
	Osteonecrosis
	Red-cell alloimmunization
	Acute chest syndrome
	Recurrent priapism
	Recurrent vaso-occlusive painful episodes
	Failure to benefit or unable or unwilling to continue supportive care therapy including hydroxyurea
	Impaired neuropsychological function with abnormal cerebral MRI and angiography
	Abnormal transcranial Doppler velocities

Modified from (Angelucci et al. 2014)

79.1.3 Indications

Indication for HSCT for "less severe patients" before significant organ damage has occurred is open to discussion. In fact, on one hand, it would be better to transplant them early in order to pre-

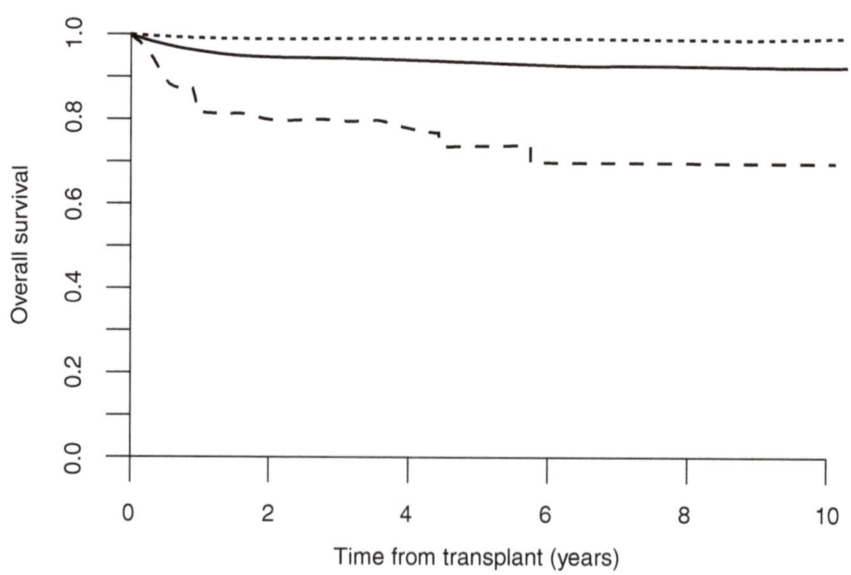

number of at-risk patients

— BM	839	673	546	446	383	322	262	215	177	152	120
- - PB	73	49	41	33	28	24	14	10	9	7	5
···· CB	88	81	70	60	47	37	29	27	24	17	13

Fig. 79.1 Overall survival according to stem cell source on 1000 SCD patients transplanted from an HLA identical sibling (Gluckman et al. 2017)

vent early organ damage secondary to SCD, avoid SCD complications in childhood, and achieve better HSCT outcomes secondary to less pre-HSCT organ damage and alloimmunization and, on the other hand, it could be considered to wait to perform an HSCT for the establishment of new available SCD supportive cares (new medications other than hydroxyurea), promising curative therapies (gene therapy), and advances in HSCT technology, others may be available. Nevertheless, it has been demonstrated that patients transplanted at a young age have a better 3-year OS and 3-year EFS, with lower incidence of aGvHD and cGvHD (Gluckman et al. 2017). These findings outline the importance of early referral to HSCT for SCD patients.

79.1.4 Conditioning

To date, a myeloablative conditioning regimen (especially with BU/CY + ATG) is the gold standard for HLA identical sibling HSCTs (EFS: 73–96%, OS: 91–100%) despite the risk of long-term transplant-related toxicity (Bernaudin et al. 2007; Walters et al. 2016). A conditioning regimen including FLU and BU has been used but with high GvHD risk; therefore, it should be considered to add ATG to the conditioning regimen to lower the GvHD risk in these patients.

A RIC regimen has been explored to decrease toxicity and allow a stable, mixed chimerism. The aim of a tailored conditioning regimen in children is to preserve fertility, whereas in adults is to reduce toxicity in severely compromised patients due to their underlying disease. Several reduced intensity conditioning regimens (FLU/MEL + ALEM +/− TT or ALEM + TBI 300 cGy +/− PT-CY or FLU/CY or TBI 300 cGy +/− ATG) have been used in many small patient series but with high degree of graft rejection (Talano and Cairo 2015; Arnold et al. 2016). Thus, recently, encouraging outcomes and low early- and long-term toxicity have been confirmed by other groups after FLU-based RIC regimens (Bhatia et al. 2014). Lately, 13 high-risk patients conditioned with a chemotherapy-free regimen (ALEM-TBI 300 cGy) have shown a 92% DFS and 100% OS (Saraf et al. 2016).

Moreover, a prospective multicenter trial comparing allogeneic matched related HSCT after a RIC regimen, with standard of care in adolescents and adults with severe SCD, has shown encouraging preliminary results (Dhedin et al. 2016).

Despite MAC dosing in the conditioning regimens, a mixture of both donor and recipient hematopoietic cells (mixed donor chimerism) can be consistently observed in approximately 10–20% of these children (Bernaudin et al. 2007; Walters et al. 2016). Interestingly, this mixed chimeric state with the presence of both recipient and donor blood cells is sufficient to direct bone marrow to preferentially produce donor-type hemoglobin (rather than abnormal hemoglobin of the recipient), and red cells revert the SCD phenotype, and minimize the risk of GVHD, confirming the therapeutic efficacy of mixed chimerism for hemoglobinopathies. New studies on mixed chimerism are ongoing.

79.1.5 Alternative Donors

Finding a potential MUD is based on the ethnic and racial background; for SCD patients the probability for an 8/8 HLA MUD or CB donor is less than 18%. Nevertheless, some small series of patients using URD have been published, but for now relapse rate and GvHD risk remain unacceptable (Justus et al. 2015).

Strategies that explore the use of mismatched related (haplo) donors are ongoing (Dallas et al. 2013; Talano and Cairo 2015). Recently promising results of CD3+/CD19+ depleted T-cell haplo-HSCT after TREO/FLU/TT + ATG have been shown to be safe and efficient with a low incidence of GvHD in advanced stage SCD (Foell et al. 2017).

Moreover, new strategies using gene therapy have been recently published with encouraging results (Ribeil et al. 2017), and the use of gene editing is being explored for this single-mutation disease (Canver and Orkin 2016).

79.2 Thalassemia

Khaled Ghanem and Miguel R. Abboud

79.2.1 Introduction

The outcome of thalassemia major (TM, transfusion-dependent thalassemia) has improved dramatically over the past two decades due to improvements in supportive care and iron chelation therapy (Taher et al. 2018). Life expectancy for TM patients exceeds 40 years, and it is no longer significantly different from the life expectancy of thalassemia intermedia patients, in developed countries (Vitrano et al. 2017).

Match family donor (MFD) allo-HSCT is currently considered the only curative standard therapeutic approach for TM, which despite holding its own risks, could release the patient from lifelong treatments, and possible iron accumulation complications. Despite encouraging results of gene therapy, its use is currently limited to clinical trials.

79.2.2 Best Transplant Candidates

In late 1990s, the Pesaro group has proposed a risk classification for pediatric patients undergoing MFD HSCT for TM (Lucarelli et al. 1998). The classification depended on three risk factors (Table 79.2) and was validated in the pediatric population; however, it did not predict risk in adult patients (Angelucci et al. 2017). Limitations to this risk stratification include the interobserver variability regarding hepatomegaly and the lack of clear definition of adequate iron chelation. The Pesaro classification is applicable in the setting of best medical care. In developing countries, where medical care might not be optimal, a very-high-risk group was identified in Pesaro class 3 patients if liver size is >5 cm below the costal margin and if the patient age is >7 years (Mathews et al. 2007). The EBMT has recently identified the age of 14 years as the oldest age for optimal outcome in MFD HSCT for TM (Baronciani et al. 2016).

Table 79.2 Pesaro classifications for risk assessment prior to HSCT for TM (Lucarelli et al. 1998)

Risk factor	Class 1	Class 2 (min. 1, max. 2)	Class 3
Inadequate chelation	×	×/✓	✓
Hepatomegaly >2 cm	×	×/✓	✓
Portal fibrosis	×	×/✓	✓

Accurate assessment of iron content in the liver and heart is crucial before proceeding to transplant. No consensus is currently available regarding the best method of iron content assessment in both organs. Serum ferritin level might not reflect accurately the severity of iron overload. Liver biopsy is the gold standard; however, it carries the risks of the invasive procedure. Transient elastography (FibroScan) and T2 MRI have been shown to be reliable noninvasive methods to predict liver fibrosis secondary to iron overload, for TM patients who are candidates to HSCT (Hamidieh et al. 2014; Hamidieh et al. 2015).

79.2.3 Conditioning Regimens

The use of the myeloablative BU and CY as the conditioning regimen for HSCT for TM has been the standard practice, due to the increased marrow activity and the allo-sensitization in heavily transfused patients (Lucarelli et al. 1990). However, this regimen was associated with hepatic and cardiac toxicity due to the iron overload and the toxic hepatic and cardiac effects of BU and CY, respectively.

ATG or ALEM have been added in some protocols to the conditioning regimen to prevent GvHD and enhance engraftment (Law et al. 2012; Mohty 2012). Despite being effective with low incidence of infections, the use of these agents is still debatable.

In an attempt to reduce the extramedullary toxicity of BU and CY, a non-myeloablative regimen of TREO/FLU/TT has been used with encouraging results (Bernardo et al. 2012). Defibrotide has been used successfully to prevent SOS/VOD in patients with TM undergoing

HSCT with conditioning regimen containing IV BU (Cappelli et al. 2009). The use of BU pharmacokinetics was associated with better engraftment and less toxicity (Gaziev et al. 2010); however, these studies are available in limited number of institutions worldwide.

79.2.4 Alternative Donors

79.2.4.1 Matched Unrelated Donors (MUD)

In case MFD is not available, the discovery of high-resolution HLA typing techniques made the performance of successful MUD transplant possible. The probability of finding a matched unrelated donor varies between 50% in Caucasians to less than 10% in some minorities (Rocha and Locatelli 2008). With the use of BU, CY, TT, and FLU as conditioning regimen and ATG, MMF, and short-course MTX as GvHD prophylaxis, the outcome of PBSC MUD in TM was comparable to MFD HSCT in regard to OS, TRM, TFS, and aGvHD (Li et al. 2012).

79.2.4.2 Unrelated Umbilical Cord

The use of unrelated umbilical cord as a source of stem cells for HSCT in TM is hampered by the high incidence of graft failure due to the low stem cell dose. The graft failure rate could be as high as 57% (Ruggeri et al. 2011). This could be partially overcome by the use of double UCB units. The 5-year overall and thalassemia-free survival rates were 88.3 and 73.9%, respectively, when using two units instead of one if no single units included more than 25×10^6 total nucleated cells/kg of recipient weight. Other strategies to overcome the main barrier of low cell dose include co-transplantation of third-party mesenchymal stromal or TCD haploidentical cells (Kwon et al. 2014; Kim et al. 2004).

79.2.4.3 Haploidentical HSCT

Due to the low probability of finding a MUD in some ethnicities and the previously mentioned issues with umbilical-cord transplant, new strategies have been evolved to develop an effective and safe haploidentical transplant procedure for TM patients. The use of TCD graft was associated with high rate of infections and increased risk of graft failure due to allo-sensitization and hyperactive marrow (Gaziev et al. 2000). This was overcome by pretransplant over-transfusion and immunosuppressive therapy and post transplant infusion of transduced donor T-cells with gene-inducible caspase-9 (Bertaina et al. 2017). The use of T-cell replete grafts is still under investigation to explore the best strategy to prevent GvHD.

79.2.5 Mixed Chimerism

The incidence of mixed chimerism after HSCT for TM was reported to be around 12%. the risk of graft rejection in patients with mixed chimerism was high only if mixed chimerism had been observed within two months post-transplant. Most cases with late persistent mixed chimerism evolved into either stable chimerism or complete engraftment and did not require additional PRBC transfusion support (Andreani et al. 2000).

79.2.6 Post transplant Iron Chelation

Iron overload remains a problem after HSCT, and most investigators rely on phlebotomy to decrease excessive iron stores. In a recent phase II, multicenter, single-arm trial, deferasirox at a dose of 20 mg/kg/day, starting after a minimum of 6 months of transplant, and continued for 1 year, was safe and associated with decreased burden of iron overload after transplant (serum ferritin, liver, and cardiac iron content by MRI) (Yesilipek et al. 2018).

Key Points

- HLA identical sibling HSCT is an established treatment option for SCD.
- HSCT should be performed as early as possible, preferably at pre-school age, and BU, CY, and ATG should be used as conditioning regimen.
- Match family donor allo-HSCT is currently considered the only curative standard therapeutic approach for thalassemia major, which despite holding its own risks, could release the patient from lifelong treatments and possible iron accumulation complications.
- Despite encouraging results of gene therapy, its use in TM is currently limited to clinical trials.

References

Andreani M, Nesci S, Lucarelli G, et al. Long-term survival of ex-thalassemic patients with persistent mixed chimerism after bone marrow transplantation. Bone Marrow Transplant. 2000;25:401–4.

Angelucci E, Matthes-Martin S, Baronciani D, et al. EBMT Inborn Error and EBMT Paediatric Working Parties. Hematopoietic stem cell transplantation in thalassemia major and sickle cell disease: indications and management recommendations from an international expert panel. Haematologica. 2014;99:811–20.

Angelucci E, Pilo F, Coates TD. Transplantation in thalassemia: Revisiting the Pesaro risk factors 25 years later. Am J Hematol. 2017;92:411–3.

Arnold SD, Bhatia M, Horan J, Krishnamurti L. Haematopoietic stem cell transplantation for sickle cell disease - current practice and new approaches. Br J Haematol. 2016;174:515–25.

Baronciani D, Angelucci E, Potschger U, et al. Hemopoietic stem cell transplantation in thalassemia: a report from the European Society for Blood and Bone Marrow Transplantation Hemoglobinopathy Registry, 2000-2010. Bone Marrow Transplant. 2016;51:536–41.

Bernardo ME, Piras E, Vacca A, et al. Allogeneic hematopoietic stem cell transplantation in thalassemia major: results of a reduced-toxicity conditioning regimen based on the use of treosulfan. Blood. 2012;120:473–6.

Bernaudin F, Socie G, Kuentz M, et al. SFGM-TC. Long-term results of related myeloablative stemcell transplantation to cure sickle cell disease. Blood. 2007;110:2749–56.

Bernaudin F, Verlhac S, Arnaud C, et al. Long-term treatment follow-up of children with sickle cell disease monitored with abnormal transcranial Doppler velocities. Blood. 2016;127:1814–22.

Bertaina A, Pitisci A, Sinibaldi M, Algeri M. T Cell-Depleted and T Cell-Replete HLA-Haploidentical Stem Cell Transplantation for Non-malignant Disorders. Curr Hematol Malig Rep. 2017;12:68–78.

Bhatia M, Jin Z, Baker C, et al. Reduced toxicity, myeloablative conditioning with BU, fludarabine, alemtuzumab and SCT from sibling donors in children with sickle cell disease. Bone Marrow Transplant. 2014;49:913–20.

Canver MC, Orkin SH. Customizing the genome as therapy for the beta-hemoglobinopathies. Blood. 2016;127:2536–45.

Cappelli B, Chiesa R, Evangelio C, et al. Absence of VOD in paediatric thalassaemic HSCT recipients using defibrotide prophylaxis and intravenous Busulphan. Br J Haematol. 2009;147:554–60.

Dallas MH, Triplett B, Shook DR, et al. Long-term outcome and evaluation of organ function in pediatric patients undergoing haploidentical and matched related hematopoietic cell transplantation for sickle cell disease. Biol Blood Marrow Transplant. 2013;19:820–30.

Dhedin N, de la Fuente J, Bernaudin F, et al. Haploidentical Bone Marrow Transplant with Post-Transplant Cytoxan Plus Thiotepa Improves Donor Engraftment in Patients with Sickle Cell Anemia: Results of an International Multicenter Learning Collaborative Trial. Blood. 2016;128:1233. (ASH Abstract).

Foell J, Pfirstinger B, Rehe K, et al. Haploidentical stem cell transplantation with CD3(+)-/CD19(+)- depleted peripheral stem cells for patients with advanced stage sickle cell disease and no alternative donor: results of a pilot study. Bone Marrow Transplant. 2017;52:938–40.

Gaziev D, Galimberti M, Lucarelli G, et al. Bone marrow transplantation from alternative donors for thalassemia: HLA-phenotypically identical relative and HLA-nonidentical sibling or parent transplants. Bone Marrow Transplant. 2000;25:815–21.

Gaziev J, Nguyen L, Puozzo C, et al. Novel pharmacokinetic behavior of intravenous busulfan in children with thalassemia undergoing hematopoietic stem cell transplantation: a prospective evaluation of pharmacokinetic and pharmacodynamic profile with therapeutic drug monitoring. Blood. 2010;115:4597–604.

Gluckman E, Cappelli B, Bernaudin F, et al. Sickle cell disease: an international survey of results of HLA-identical sibling hematopoietic stem cell transplantation. Blood. 2017;129:1548–56.

Hamidieh AA, Moeininia F, Tayebi S, et al. Efficacy of hepatic T2* MRI values and serum ferritin concentration in predicting thalassemia major classification for hematopoietic stem cell transplantation. Pediatr Transplant. 2015;19:301–6.

Hamidieh AA, Shazad B, Ostovaneh MR, et al. Noninvasive measurement of liver fibrosis using transient elastography in pediatric patients with major thalassemia who are candidates for hematopoietic stem cell transplantation. Biol Blood Marrow Transplant. 2014;20:1912–7.

Johnson FL, Look AT, Gockerman J, et al. Bone-marrow transplantation in a patient with sickle-cell anemia. N Engl J Med. 1984;311:780–3.

Justus D, Perez-Albuerne E, Dioguardi J, et al. Allogeneic donor availability for hematopoietic stem cell transplantation in children with sickle cell disease. Pediatr Blood Cancer. 2015;62:1285–7.

Kim DW, Chung YJ, Kim TG, et al. Cotransplantation of third-party mesenchymal stromal cells can alleviate single-donor predominance and increase engraftment from double cord transplantation. Blood. 2004;103:1941–8.

Kwon M, Bautista G, Balsalobre P, et al. Haplo-cord transplantation using CD34+ cells from a third-party donor to speed engraftment in high-risk patients with hematologic disorders. Biol Blood Marrow Transplant. 2014;20:2015–22.

Law J, Cowan MJ, Dvorak CC, et al. Busulfan, fludarabine, and alemtuzumab as a reduced toxicity regimen for children with malignant and nonmalignant diseases improves engraftment and graft-versus-host disease without delaying immune reconstitution. Biol Blood Marrow Transplant. 2012;18:1656–63.

Li C, Wu X, Feng X, et al. A novel conditioning regimen improves outcomes in beta-thalassemia major patients using unrelated donor peripheral blood stem cell transplantation. Blood. 2012;120:3875–81.

Lucarelli G, Galimberti M, Giardini C, et al. Bone marrow transplantation in thalassemia. The experience of Pesaro. Ann N Y Acad Sci. 1998;850:270–5.

Lucarelli G, Galimberti M, Polchi P, et al. Bone marrow transplantation in patients with thalassemia. N Engl J Med. 1990;322:417–21.

Mathews V, George B, Deotare U, et al. A new stratification strategy that identifies a subset of class III patients with an adverse prognosis among children with beta thalassemia major undergoing a matched related allogeneic stem cell transplantation. Biol Blood Marrow Transplant. 2007;13:889–94.

Mohty M. A bit of antithymocyte globulin can take you a long way! Bone Marrow Transplant. 2012;47:617–8.

National Heart, Lung, and Blood Institute. Evidence-based management of sickle cell disease. Expert Panel Report. Bethesda: National Heart, Lung, and Blood Institute; 2014. https://www.nhlbi.nih.gov/sites/www.nhlbi.nih.gov/files/sicklecell-disease-report.pdf.

Piel FB, Hay SI, Gupta S, et al. Global burden of sickle cell anaemia in children under five, 2010-2050: modelling based on demographics, excess mortality, and interventions. PLoS Med. 2013;10:e1001484.

Ribeil JA, Hacein-Bey-Abina S, Payen E, et al. Gene Therapy in a Patient with Sickle Cell Disease. N Engl J Med. 2017;376:848–55.

Rocha V, Locatelli F. Searching for alternative hematopoietic stem cell donors for pediatric patients. Bone Marrow Transplant. 2008;41:207–14.

Ruggeri A, Eapen M, Scaravadou A, et al. Umbilical cord blood transplantation for children with thalassemia and sickle cell disease. Biol Blood Marrow Transplant. 2011;17:1375–82.

Saraf SL, Oh AL, Patel PR, et al. Nonmyeloablative Stem Cell Transplantation with Alemtuzumab/Low-Dose Irradiation to Cure and Improve the Quality of Life of Adults with Sickle Cell Disease. Biol Blood Marrow Transplant. 2016;22:441–8.

Taher AT, Weatherall DJ, Cappellini MD. Thalassaemia. Lancet. 2018;391:155–67.

Talano JA, Cairo MS. Hematopoietic stem cell transplantation for sickle cell disease: state of the science. Eur J Haematol. 2015;94:391–9.

Vitrano A, Calvaruso G, Lai E, et al. The era of comparable life expectancy between thalassaemia major and intermedia: Is it time to revisit the major-intermedia dichotomy? Br J Haematol. 2017;176:124–30.

Walters MC, De Castro LM, Sullivan KM, et al. Indications and results of HLA-identical sibling hematopoietic cell transplantation for sickle cell disease. Biol Blood Marrow Transplant. 2016;22:207–11.

Ware RE, Davis BR, Schultz WH, et al. Hydroxycarbamide versus chronic transfusion for maintenance of transcranial doppler flow velocities in children with sickle cell anaemia-TCD With Transfusions Changing to Hydroxyurea (TWiTCH): a multicentre, open-label, phase 3, non-inferiority trial. Lancet. 2016;387:661–70.

Yawn BP, Buchanan GR, Afenyi-Annan AN, et al. Management of sickle cell disease: summary of the 2014 evidence-based report by expert panel members. JAMA. 2014;312:1033–48.

Yesilipek MA, Karasu G, Kaya Z, et al. A Phase II, Multicenter, Single-Arm Study to Evaluate the Safety and Efficacy of Deferasirox after Hematopoietic Stem Cell Transplantation in Children with beta-Thalassemia Major. Biol Blood Marrow Transplant. 2018;24:613–8.

Multiple Myeloma

80

Joan Bladé, Benedetto Bruno, and Mohamad Mohty

80.1 Definition, Epidemiology, and Diagnosis

Multiple myeloma (MM) consists of a malignant proliferation of BM plasmatic cells (BMPCs), which produce a monoclonal protein that can be found in serum and/or urine, resulting in skeletal involvement, hypercalcemia, anemia, renal function impairment, and/or soft-tissue plasmacytomas. The cause is unknown.

The annual incidence is four per 100,000. It represents 1% of all malignant diseases and about 15% of all hematological malignancies. The median age at diagnosis is between 65 and 70 years. Only 15% and 2% are younger than 50 and 30 years, respectively.

The diagnosis of symptomatic MM requires the presence of clonal BMPCs, usually >10%, or plasmacytoma, the presence of serum and/or urine M-protein (except in the uncommon nonsecretory) and related organ or tissue impairment (end-organ damage, including bone lesions). In the absence of organ damage, the presence of >60% BMPCs, a serum-free light-chain (FLC) ratio >100 or the presence of more than one focal lesion at the MRI defines symptomatic MM requiring therapy.

80.2 Risk Stratification

The International Staging System (ISS), based on the serum beta2-microglobulin and albumin levels discriminates three prognostics subgroups:

- Stage I (beta2-m <3.5 mg/L and albumin >3.3 g/dL),
- Stage III (beta2-m >5.5 mg/L) and
- Stage II (all remaining cases).

FISH can identify the following poor cytogenetic findings: t(4;14), t(14;16), and/or del 17p which account for about 25% of patients with MM, the remaining 75% having a so-called standard risk. High LDH, the presence of hematogenous extramedullary disease, and the coexistence of plasma cell leukemia are also poor prognostic indicators. A revised ISS incorporating cytogenetics and LDH have been developed as follows:

J. Bladé
Amyloidosis and Myeloma Unit, Department of Hematology, Hospital Clinic of Barcelona, IDIBAPS, Barcelona, Spain

B. Bruno
Department of Oncology, AOU Città della Salute e della Scienza, University of Torino, Torino, Italy

Department of Molecular Biotechnology and Health Sciences, AOU Città della Salute e della Scienza, University of Torino, Torino, Italy

M. Mohty (✉)
Department of Clinical Hematology and Cellular Therapy, Hospital Saint-Antoine, Sorbonne University, Paris, France
e-mail: mohamad.mohty@inserm.fr

E. Carreras et al. (eds.), *The EBMT Handbook*, https://doi.org/10.1007/978-3-030-02278-5_80

- R-ISS I: ISS I, standard-risk cytogenetics and normal LDH,
- R-ISS III: ISS III, plus high-risk cytogenetics or high LDH and
- R-ISS II: all remaining cases.

An ultra-high-risk group, accounting for 5–7% of patients eligible for auto-HSCT and who received bortezomib-based regimens, with a median OS of less than 2 years, has been recognized (ISS III and high-risk cytogenetics or high LDH).

80.3 First-Line Treatment (Induction Prior to Auto-HSCT)

Conventional chemotherapy (VAD, VBMCP/VBAD, CY/DEX) or the doublets thalidomide (THAL)/DEX or bortezomib (BOR)/DEX results in 10% CR pre-auto-HSCT, 25–35% CR post-auto-HSCT and in 5–10% in continued CR beyond 10 years from HSCT.

The triplets combining BOR/DEX with an immunomodulatory drug (IMiD), thalidomide (VTD), or lenalidomide (VRD) result in a pre-auto-HSCT CR of 20–35%, and a post-auto-HSCT CR of 45–55%. However, there is not enough follow-up to determine the proportion of patients in continued CR >10 years beyond auto-HSCT.

The results of BOR-based triplets PAD and VCD (including Adriamycin or CY), widely used in Europe, are inferior to the reported with the combination of proteasome inhibitors plus IMiDs. Although most groups administer four induction cycles, the dose intensity and the induction exposure with an increased depth of response overtime and with higher CR rates pre- and post-auto-HSCT with six cycles have been observed with both VTD and VRD. The potential benefit of adding a MoAb, particularly daratumumab, to VTD or VRD is being investigated.

80.4 Criteria of Response and Progression

Complete remission (CR): negative serum and urine immunofixation, less than 5% BMPCs and no soft-tissue plasmacytomas.

Stringent CR: as above plus normal free light-chain ratio and absence of clonal plasma cells.

Very good partial response (VGPR): 90% or more decrease in the serum M-protein and urine M-protein <100 mg/24 h.

Partial response (PR): 50% or more decrease in the serum M-protein, 90% or more decrease in urine M-protein or to <200 mg/24 h plus 50% or more decrease in soft-tissue plasmacytomas.

Progressive disease (PD) requires one or more of the following: increase in 25% or more from nadir in serum M-protein (absolute increase of at least 0.5 g/dL), urine M-protein (absolute increase of at least 200 mg/24 h), BMPC (absolute increase of at least 10%), soft-tissue plasmacytomas, and development of new bone lesions, soft-tissue plasmacytomas, or hypercalcemia.

80.5 High-Dose Therapy (HDT), Consolidation, and Maintenance

Auto-HSCT remains the standard of care for young and fit MM patients. MEL 200 mg/m^2 (MEL-200) is the standard high-dose regimen, and the source of PBS. The addition of BOR peritransplant, as well as other attempts, is of no benefit. MEL-140 plus IV BU vs. MEL-200 is being investigated. The increase in the CR with HDT is 15–20%.

Recent trials have shown that early transplant is superior to delayed (at relapse) auto-HSCT, even in the era of novel agents.

It seems that patients with high-risk cytogenetics are the most likely to benefit from tandem auto-HSCT.

The TRM with auto-HSCT is very low (1–2%), the best reported median PFS is 50–56 months and the expected median OS of 8–10 years. The proportion of patients operationally cured (i.e., in continued CR beyond 10 years) with the current regimens is still unknown.

Although the results of post transplant consolidation are controversial, it seems to be a promising approach and usually recommended by experts. Post-auto-HSCT maintenance with lenalinomide (LENA) has been recently approved. The optimal maintenance duration based on sequential MRD studies, as well as whether or not the association of other drugs such as glucocorticoids, proteasome inhibitors or MoAb can be of benefit, is currently investigated.

80.6 Treatment at Relapse After Auto-HSCT

There is a consensus that a rescue or salvage auto-HSCT could be tried when the response duration to the first transplant in longer than 18–24 months. Such rescue transplant should only be performed in patients with sensitive disease, so prior salvage chemotherapy is needed. The components of the initial therapy, depth and the duration of response as well as the toxicity are crucial in selecting the rescue regimen. Among a number of possible combinations at relapse, the more effective combinations are IMiD-containing (carfilzomib, LENA, and DEX [KRd] or daratumumab, LENA, and DEX [DRd]) and non-IMiD-containing (carfilzomib and DEX [Kd] or daratumumab, BOR and DEX [DVd]). If the rescue auto-HSCT is performed, post transplant maintenance should be considered. In the event that the transplant is not done, the above treatments are in general until progression.

80.7 Allogenic HSCT in MM

The role of allografting for the treatment of MM remains controversial. The first clinical reports employing MAC regimens proved to be curative for small patient subsets but were associated with an unacceptable high TRM. In the late 1990s, the introduction of minimal intensive conditioning regimens (primarily based on low-dose TBI), which relies on the graft-versus-myeloma (GvM) effect for tumor eradication, drastically reduced TRM, but at the expense of higher disease relapse.

Combining cytoreductive high-dose MEL with an autograft and a subsequent minimal intensity conditioning with an allograft, aimed at inducing GvM, was better tolerated up to the age of 65–70 years old. Before the era of new drugs, seven prospective trials were designed to compare clinical outcomes of auto-HSCT versus tandem autologous-minimal intensity and allo-HSCT in newly diagnosed MM patients. Results were discordant regarding response, OS, and PFS. This may have partly been due to differences in conditioning regimens, GVHD prophylaxis, patient inclusion criteria, and randomization strategies. Thus, comparisons between trials are difficult. However, allografting has steadily been used in Europe in recent years. Sobh et al. recently described use and outcomes of allo-HSCT for MM in Europe between January 1990 and December 2012. A study population of 7333 patients (median age at transplant, 51 years) was divided into 3 groups: allo-HSCT upfront (n = 1924), tandem auto-allo-HSCT (n = 2004), and allo-HSCT as a second-line treatment or beyond (n = 3405). After 2004, 5-year survival probabilities from transplant were 42%, 54%, and 32%, for the three groups, respectively. Unfortunately, only a very minority of MM patients were enrolled in prospective control trials. Remarkable heterogeneity in using allo-HSCT was observed among the different European countries.

80.8 Allogenic HSCT and New Agents

The role of the combination of "new drugs" with GvM has not yet been explored in well-designed prospective studies. In only a Phase II study feasibility of BOR within a RIC and as maintenance post-allografting was evaluated. Conditioning consisted of FLU/MEL/BOR while maintenance treatment of cycles of IV BOR. Sixteen high-risk patients relapsed after an auto-HSCT was prospectively enrolled. Nine/16 (56%) and 5/16 (31%) achieved CR and partial remission. In this heavily pretreated high-risk population, 3-year cumulative incidence of NRM, relapse and OS were 25%, 54%, and 41%, respectively. The latter trial showed the feasibility and efficacy of an intensified conditioning with a "new drug" in poor prognosis patients. Moreover, the concept of maintenance treatment after an allograft was also introduced. A synergy between new drugs and GvM in the relapse setting has recently been described clearly suggesting that allo-HSCT and new drugs are not mutually exclusive.

Whether long-term persistence of MRD negativity may coincide with disease eradication remains a matter of debate though persistent molecular remission of several years may cautiously suggest cure. PCR-based MRD detection represents a powerful predictor of clinical outcomes.

80.9 Indications of allo-HSCT in MM

The role of allo-HSCT in the era of new drugs remains highly controversial, and there are no clear guidelines, despite the relatively high numbers of allo-HSCT yearly performed in Europe. Well-designed prospective trials combining "graft-vs.-myeloma" and new drugs are needed, especially in young high-risk/ultra-high-risk patients whose treatment remains an unmet clinical need.

Key Points

- Auto-HSCT is the preferred treatment approach (standard of care) in young and fit myeloma patients.
- Prior to auto-HCT, patients should receive a BOR-based triplet induction regimen aiming to achieve a deep response.
- High-dose MEL 200 mg/m^2 is the standard conditioning for auto-HSCT in myeloma.
- Patients should receive some form of post auto-HSCT therapy (consolidation and/or maintenance therapy).
- Double auto-HSCT can be considered for high risk myeloma (e.g., patients with a del17p cytogenetic abnormality).
- The role of allo-HSCT is highly controversial in myeloma and should be performed as part of a clinical trial whenever possible.

Recommended References

Attal M, Lauwers-Cances V, Hulin C, et al. Lenalidomide, Bortezomib, and Dexamethasone with Transplantation for Myeloma. N Engl J Med. 2017;376:1311–20.

Bjorkstrand B, Iacobelli S, Hegenbart U, et al. Tandem autologous/reduced-intensity conditioning allogeneic stem-cell transplantation versus autologous transplantation in myeloma: long-term follow-up. J Clin Oncol. 2011;29:3016–22.

Bruno B, Rotta M, Patriarca F, et al. A comparison of allografting with autografting for newly diagnosed myeloma. N Engl J Med. 2007;356:1110–20.

Cavo M, Rajkumar SV, Palumbo A, et al. International Myeloma Working Group consensus approach to the treatment of multiple myeloma patients who are candidates for autologous stem cell transplantation. Blood. 2011;117:6063–73.

Garderet L, Beohou E, Caillot D, et al. Upfront autologous stem cell transplantation for newly diagnosed elderly multiple myeloma patients: a prospective multicenter study. Haematologica. 2016;101:1390–7.

Giralt S, Garderet L, Durie B, et al. American Society of Blood and Marrow Transplantation, European Society of Blood and Marrow Transplantation, Blood and Marrow Transplant Clinical Trials Network, and International Myeloma Working Group Consensus Conference on Salvage Hematopoietic Cell Transplantation in Patients with Relapsed Multiple Myeloma. Biol Blood Marrow Transplant. 2015;21:2039–51.

Harousseau JL, Moreau P. Autologous hematopoietic stem-cell transplantation for multiple myeloma. N Engl J Med. 2009;360:2645–54.

Krishnan A, Pasquini MC, Logan B, et al. Autologous haemopoietic stem-cell transplantation followed by allogeneic or autologous haemopoietic stem-cell transplantation in patients with multiple myeloma (BMT CTN 0102): a phase 3 biological assignment trial. Lancet Oncol. 2011;12:1195–203.

Ladetto M, Ferrero S, Drandi D, et al. Prospective molecular monitoring of minimal residual disease after non-myeloablative allografting in newly diagnosed multiple myeloma. Leukemia. 2015;30:1211–4.

Ludwig H, Durie BG, McCarthy P, et al. IMWG consensus on maintenance therapy in multiple myeloma. Blood. 2012;119:3003–15.

Mateos MV, Zamagni E, Avet-Loiseau H, et al. ESMO Guidelines Committee. Ann Oncol. 2017;28:iv52–61.

McCarthy PL, Holstein SA, Petrucci MT, et al. Lenalidomide Maintenance After Autologous Stem-Cell Transplantation in Newly Diagnosed Multiple Myeloma: A Meta-Analysis. J Clin Oncol. 2017;35:3279–89.

Mohty M, Harousseau JL. Treatment of autologous stem cell transplant-eligible multiple myeloma patients: ten questions and answers. Haematologica. 2014;99:408–16.

Mohty M, Richardson PG, McCarthy PL, Attal M. Consolidation and maintenance therapy for multiple myeloma after autologous transplantation: where do we stand? Bone Marrow Transplant. 2015;50:1024–9.

Moreau P, San Miguel J, Sonneveld P, et al. Multiple myeloma: ESMO Clinical Practice Guidelines for diagnosis, treatment and follow-up. Ann Oncol. 2017;28(suppl_4):iv52–61.

Palumbo A, Cavallo F, Gay F, et al. Autologous transplantation and maintenance therapy in multiple myeloma. N Engl J Med. 2014;371:895–905.

Rosinol L, Oriol A, Teruel AI, et al. Superiority of bortezomib, thalidomide, and dexamethasone (VTD) as induction pretransplantation therapy in multiple myeloma: a randomized phase 3 PETHEMA/GEM study. Blood. 2012;120:1589–96.

Sengsayadeth S, Malard F, Savani BN, et al. Posttransplant maintenance therapy in multiple myeloma: the changing landscape. Blood Cancer J. 2017;7:e545.

Sobh M, Michallet M, Gahrton G, et al. Allogeneic hematopoietic cell transplantation for multiple myeloma in Europe: trends and outcomes over 25 years. A study by the EBMT Chronic Malignancies Working Party. Leukemia. 2016;30:2047–54.

81 Systemic Light Chain Amyloidosis

Monique Minnema and Stefan Schönland

81.1 Definition and Epidemiology

Systemic light chain (AL) amyloidosis is a protein misfolding and deposition disorder with an incidence of 5–12 persons per million per year. Clonal plasma cells or rarely B cells produce immunoglobulin light chains with the potential to misfold. These light chains are deposited as extracellular amyloid fibrils in peripheral tissues and cause morbidity and mortality. Organs most frequently involved are the kidney, heart, liver, autonomic and peripheral nervous system, gastrointestinal tract, and soft tissue.

81.2 Diagnosis

AL amyloidosis should be suspected in any patient with a monoclonal gammopathy and a compatible clinical syndrome such as heart failure with a preserved ejection fraction, nephrotic range proteinuria, unexplained weight loss, peripheral neuropathy, a bleeding diathesis, or carpal tunnel syndrome. Gammopathy work-up should include a serum-free light chain assay, immunofixation of serum and urine, bone marrow cytology, flow cytometry, histology and iFISH, and a full-body scan to exclude bone lesions due to symptomatic MM. AL amyloidosis is diagnosed by histopathology with Congo red staining and the typical apple-green birefringence under polarized light. Screening biopsies such as abdominal fat, rectum, salivary gland, or bone marrow as well as symptomatically involved organs can be utilized. The amyloid subtype has to be further confirmed by immunohistochemistry, immune electron microscopy, or laser microdissection and mass spectrometry.

81.3 Classification

AL amyloidosis can be classified by the origin of the underlying bone marrow disease: a clonal plasma cell or a lymphoid dyscrasia. Plasma cell dyscrasias can further be divided into monoclonal gammopathy, smoldering MM, and symptomatic MM. Finally, IgM-related AL amyloidosis is a specific entity with an underlying lymphocytic, lymphoplasmacytic, or a plasma cellular clone, commonly with cardiac and peripheral nervous system involvement.

M. Minnema
Department of Hematology, UMC Utrecht Cancer Center, Utrecht, The Netherlands

S. Schönland (✉)
Hematology, Oncology and Rheumatology, Medical Department V, University Hospital of Heidelberg, Heidelberg, Germany
e-mail: stefan.schoenland@med.uni-heidelberg.de

E. Carreras et al. (eds.), *The EBMT Handbook*, https://doi.org/10.1007/978-3-030-02278-5_81

81.4 Risk Factors and Prognostic Scores

The underlying bone marrow disease as well as organ damage-related biomarkers can be utilized to stratify patients into risk groups. A bone marrow plasma cell infiltration above 10% (Hwa et al. 2016) and a high difference between involved and uninvolved serum-free light chain (dFLC) are negative prognostic factors (Kumar et al. 2012) for overall survival. Comparable to MM genetic aberrations can be detected on iFISH in plasma cell dyscrasias and be utilized to predict response to specific treatments (e.g., in patients with translocation (11;14) HDM/HSCT is more effective) (Bochtler et al. 2016).

The Mayo clinic first published a staging system utilizing NT-ProBNP and cardiac troponins (cTnI, cTnT) in 2004 which strongly predicted outcome. Median survival for patients in Stages I, II, and III were 26.4, 10.5., and 3.5 months (Dispenzieri et al. 2004a), and for the transplant group Stages I and II median were not reached, and Stage III median was 8.4 months (Dispenzieri et al. 2004b). This staging system was adapted in 2013 by a European cooperative approach and an ultra-high-risk patient group was identified with an NT-proBNP cut-off of 8500 ng/L (Stage IIIb) which must be considered transplant-ineligible (Wechalekar et al. 2013).

For patients with renal involvement, total proteinuria/24 h and estimated glomerular filtration rate (eGFR) can anticipate the risk for terminal renal failure (Palladini et al. 2014).

The depth of response is also a significant prognostic factor as patients achieving an amyloidosis VGPR (dFLC below 40 mg/L) or CR after treatment have a significantly better outcome (Palladini et al. 2012).

81.5 First-Line Treatment

Risk-adapted treatment is preferred since most patients are fragile and do not tolerate standard used dosing regimens (see Table 81.1). Three categories are defined with low-risk patients, transplant eligible, being a minority (≤20%). High-risk patients are defined by Stage IIIb and/or having NYHA class III or IV heart disease. Other factors to consider are age, performance status, eGFR, and systolic blood pressure (Palladini and Merlini 2016). Frequent assessments of hematological response during treatment are needed, and the goal is to achieve a CR or VGPR as a deep hematologic response is closely related to survival. Patients having a hematologic response may gradually achieve an organ response.

Table 81.1 First-line treatment options according to risk status

Risk status	Treatment
Low-risk Stage I	• (± induction treatment) MEL (200 mg/m^2) + auto-HSCT • CYBorD
Intermediate-risk Stages II–IIIa	• MEL-DEX • CYBorD • Bortezomib-MEL-DEX or LENA-MEL-DEX
High-risk Stage IIIb	• Low-dose therapies • Bortezomib weekly monotherapy

CYBorD cyclophosphamide, bortezomib, dexamathasoone

81.6 Second-Line Treatment

There is no randomized trial data to guide treatment at relapse. Patients with a good duration of response who tolerate initial treatment well may be retreated with the same initial regimen. Patients with a poor response are best treated with an alternative agent combination using agents to which the patient has not been exposed, palliation or in a clinical trial tailored to the individual patient in terms of their age, comorbidities, extent of organ involvement, and the patient's wishes. Lenalidomide and pomalidomide can be considered in relapsed disease although data on durability of response are limited (Dispenzieri et al. 2007; Palladini et al. 2017). Toxicity with lenalidomide is a significant issue, and it is recommended to start at a dose of 15 mg daily, with further dose reduction based on glomerular filtration rate (GFR) (Dispenzieri et al. 2007).

81.7 Autologous HSCT

81.7.1 Indication

Eligibility criteria for autologous HSCT are variable depending on the transplanting center. However, the usual eligibility criteria include age ≤70 years, performance status 0–2, NYHA class I or II, absence of significant clinical cardiac involvement (NT pro BNP <5000 ng/L. left ejection fraction ≥45 to 50%), absence of severe orthostatic hypotension (i.e., systolic blood pressure ≥90 mm Hg), and eGFR >40 mL/min. Induction therapy before stem cell mobilization can be given, especially in patients who fulfill (smoldering) myeloma definition criteria, i.e., ≥10% bone marrow plasma cell infiltration.

The correct selection of patients is extremely important since the mortality associated with autologous HCT in AL amyloidosis can be unacceptable high if not done properly. Since the selection criteria also include the cardiac biomarkers, treatment-related mortality has dropped from around 20% to 5%; also see Table 81.2 (Gertz et al. 2013).

81.7.2 Recommended

Stem cell mobilization and leucapheresis can be associated with unusual morbidity, and a syndrome of hypoxia and hypotension has been described both during mobilization with G-CSF and during the leucapheresis procedure itself, probably as a result of a capillary leak syndrome triggered by G-CSF. Therefore, use of reduced doses of G-CSF (such as 10 μg/kg per day for 4–5 days) is recommended. In low-burden disease (i.e., plasma cells <10%), the use of CY mobilization chemotherapy does not seem to be necessary.

Conditioning regimens are based on high-dose MEL. The usual MEL dose is 200 mg/m^2, since lower-dose melphalan is associated with decreased hematological response and PFS and therefore other treatment non-transplant options may be more suitable (Cibeira et al. 2011).

81.7.3 Results

Figure 81.1 shows OS of auto-HSCT until 2010. In Table 81.2 the more recent publications of the last 10 years have been summarized. The use of induction therapy before HSCT has been more frequently applied and seems to demonstrate better hematologic responses than HSCT alone.

81.8 Allogeneic HCT

The largest retrospective analysis on allo-HCT for AL amyloidosis was performed by the EBMT in 2006 (Schönland et al. 2006). Nineteen patients were analyzed. Seven patients received MAC, and eight RIC. 40% of patients died of TRM. Long-term survival and sustained CR were achieved in seven patients and were associated with chronic GVHD in the majority of them. DLI has been successfully performed in a few patients with AL amyloidosis, thereby demonstrating a potent "graft-versus-plasma cell-dyscrasia" effect.

The EBMT initiated a noninterventional prospective study (NIS) for patients with AL amyloidosis undergoing allo-HSCT. Preliminary results have been presented in 2016 with improved overall survival (see Fig. 81.2). Allo-HSCT after RIC can be discussed as a treatment option for relapse after auto-HCT in patients <60 years with preserved organ functions and a HLA-identical donor. It might be a curative treatment for highly selected patients.

Table 81.2 Summary of the outcome of patients with systemic AL amyloidosis undergoing autologous stem cell transplantation, according to the more recent publications

Source	Type	No. of patients	Overall response rate (CR) %	TRM (%)	Overall survival (%)
Landau et al. (2017)	Retrospective	143	CR 43% at 12 months (83 pts only)	5%	Median 10.4 years
Sanchorawala et al. (2015)	Prospective bortezomib-DEX induction	35	ORR 100% CR 63%	8.5%	5 years; 83%
Hazenberg et al. (2015)	Prospective VCR-adriam-DEX induction	69	ORR 46% CR 13%	4%	Median 10 years
Parmar et al. (2014)	Retrospective	80	ORR 75% CR 18.6%	7.5%	10 years, 56%
Huang et al. (2014)	Prospective bortezomib-DEX induction in 28 pts	56	ORR 85.7% and 53.5% CR 67.9% and 35.7% Both at 12 months	3.6%	2 years 95% and 69.4%
D'Souza et al. (2015)	Retrospective	1536	ORR 71% CR 37% (2007–2012 cohort)	5% (2007–2012 cohort)	5 years 77% (2007–2012 cohort)
Cibeira et al. (2011)	Retrospective	421	CR 34%	5.6% (2004–2008 cohort)	Median 6.3 years

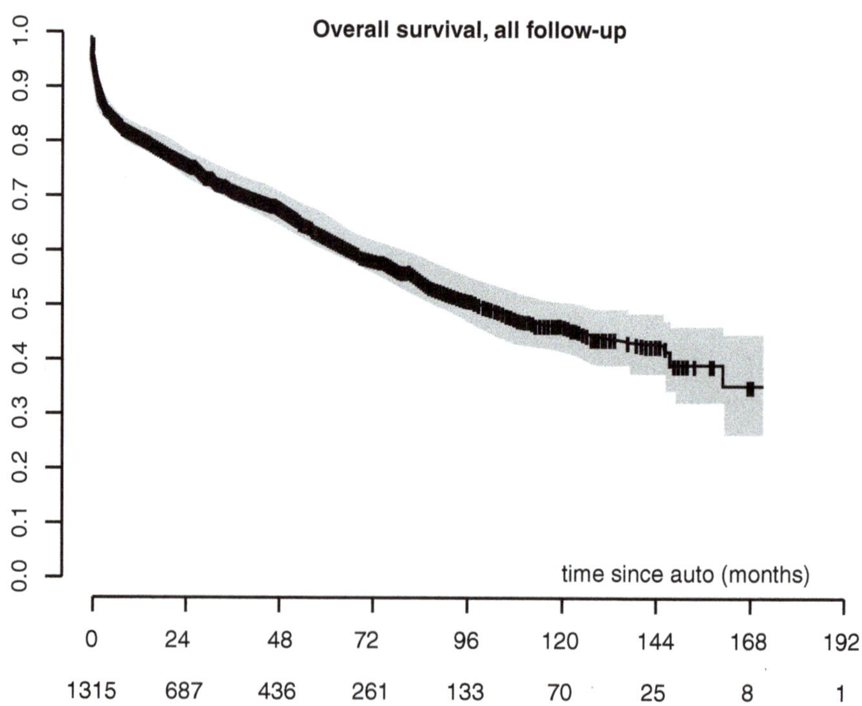

Fig. 81.1 Autologous EBMT data (patients treated until 2010)

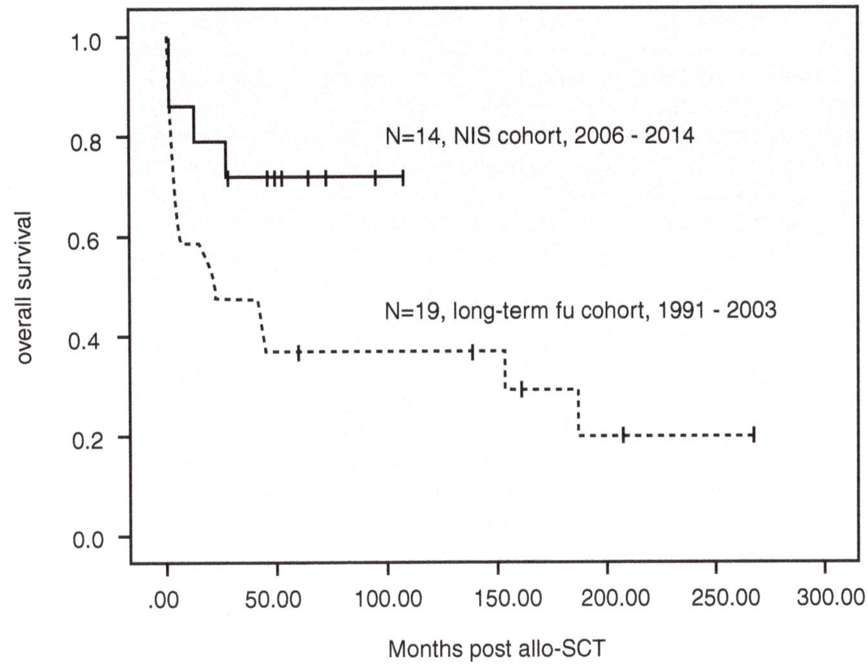

Fig. 81.2 Long-term overall survival after allo-HSCT, an EBMT analysis of patients with AL amyloidosis

Key Points

- AL amyloid therapy is directed against the underlying B cell clone
- Hematological response is the goal of therapy and improves survival
- Intensity of chemotherapy has to be risk adapted
- High-dose chemotherapy with auto-HSCT is the therapy of choice for low-risk patients
- Allo-HSCT might be a curative treatment option for relapse after auto-HCT in younger patients with preserved organ functions and a HLA-identical donor

References

Bochtler T, Hegenbart U, Kunz C, et al. Prognostic impact of cytogenetic aberrations in AL amyloidosis patients after high-dose melphalan: a long-term follow-up study. Blood. 2016;128:594–602.

Cibeira MT, Sanchorawala V, Seldin DC, et al. Outcome of AL amyloidosis after high-dose melphalan and autologous stem cell transplantation: long-term results in a series of 421 patients. Blood. 2011;118:4346–52.

D'Souza A, Dispenzieri A, Wirk B, et al. Improved outcomes after autologous hematopoietic cell transplantation for light chain amyloidosis: a Center for International Blood and Marrow Transplant Research Study. J Clin Oncol. 2015;33:3741–9.

Dispenzieri A, Gertz MA, Kyle RA, et al. Serum cardiac troponins and N-terminal pro-brain natriuretic peptide: a staging system for primary systemic amyloidosis. J Clin Oncol. 2004a;22:3751–7.

Dispenzieri A, Gertz MA, Kyle RA, et al. Prognostication of survival using cardiac troponins and N-terminal pro-brain natriuretic peptide in patients with primary systemic amyloidosis undergoing peripheral blood stem cell transplantation. Blood. 2004b;104:1881–7.

Dispenzieri A, Lacy MQ, Zeldenrust SR, et al. The activity of lenalidomide with or without dexamethasone in patients with primary systemic amyloidosis. Blood. 2007;109:465–70.

Gertz MA, Lacy MQ, Dispenzieri A, et al. Refinement in patient selection to reduce treatment-related mortality from autologous stem cell transplantation in amyloidosis. Bone Marrow Transplant. 2013;48:557–61.

Hazenberg BP, Croockewit A, van der Holt B, Dutch-Belgian Cooperative Trial Group for Hematology Oncology, et al. Extended follow up of high-dose melphalan and autologous stem cell transplantation after vincristine, doxorubicin, dexamethasone induction in amyloid light chain amyloidosis of the prospective phase II HOVON-41 study by the Dutch-Belgian Co-operative Trial Group for Hematology Oncology. Haematologica. 2015;100:677–82.

Huang X, Wang Q, Chen W, et al. Induction therapy with bortezomib and dexamethasone followed by autologous stem cell transplantation versus autologous stem cell transplantation alone in the treatment of renal AL amyloidosis: a randomized controlled trial. BMC Med. 2014;12:2.

Hwa YL, Kumar SK, Gertz MA, et al. Induction therapy pre-autologous stem cell transplantation in immunoglobulin light chain amyloidosis: a retrospective evaluation. Am J Hematol. 2016;91:984–8.

Kumar S, Dispenzieri A, Lacy MQ, et al. Revised prognostic staging system for light chain amyloidosis incorporating cardiac biomarkers and serum free light chain measurements. J Clin Oncol. 2012;30:989–95.

Landau H, Smith M, Landry C, et al. Long-term event-free and overall survival after risk-adapted melphalan and SCT for systemic light chain amyloidosis. Leukemia. 2017;31:136–42.

Palladini G, Dispenzieri A, Gertz MA, et al. New criteria for response to treatment in immunoglobulin light chain amyloidosis based on free light chain measurement and cardiac biomarkers: impact on survival outcomes. J Clin Oncol. 2012;30:4541–9.

Palladini G, Hegenbart U, Milani P, et al. A staging system for renal outcome and early markers of renal response to chemotherapy in AL amyloidosis. Blood. 2014;124:2325–32.

Palladini G, Merlini G. What is new in diagnosis and management of light chain amyloidosis? Blood. 2016;128:159–68.

Palladini G, Milani P, Foli A, et al. A phase 2 trial of pomalidomide and dexamethasone rescue treatment in patients with AL amyloidosis. Blood. 2017;129:2120–3.

Parmar S, Kongtim P, Champlin R, et al. Auto-SCT improves survival in systemic light chain amyloidosis: a retrospective analysis with 14-year follow-up. Bone Marrow Transplant. 2014;49:1036–41.

Sanchorawala V, Brauneis D, Shelton AC, et al. Induction therapy with bortezomib followed by bortezomib-high dose melphalan and stem cell transplantation for light chain amyloidosis: results of a prospective clinical trial. Biol Blood Marrow Transplant. 2015;21:1445–51.

Schönland SO, Lokhorst H, Buzyn A, Chronic Leukemia Working Party, Myeloma Subcommittee of the European Cooperative Group for Blood and Marrow Transplantation, et al. Allogeneic and syngeneic hematopoietic cell transplantation in patients with amyloid light-chain amyloidosis: a report from the European Group for Blood and Marrow Transplantation. Blood. 2006;107:2578–84.

Wechalekar AD, Schonland SO, Kastritis E, et al. A European collaborative study of treatment outcomes in 346 patients with cardiac stage III AL amyloidosis. Blood. 2013;121:3420–7.

POEMS Syndrome and Disease Produced by Other Monoclonal Immunoglobulins

82

Gordon Cook and Montserrat Rovira

82.1 POEMS Syndrome

82.1.1 Introduction

POEMS syndrome (acronym of *p*olyradiculoneuropathy, *o*rganomegaly, *e*ndocrinopathies, *m*onoclonal protein, and dermopathy, *s*kin) is a rare multisystemic disease due to an underlying plasma cell neoplasm. The pathogenesis of the syndrome is not well understood. Other names of the POEMS syndrome that are less frequently used are osteosclerotic myeloma, Takatsuki syndrome, or Crow-Fukase syndrome.

82.1.2 Clinical and Laboratory Manifestations

POEMS predominate in male being the age of maximum incidence (50–60 years).

Characteristic manifestations are:

*P*olyneuropathy: Typically demyelinating. Peripheral, ascending, symmetrical and affecting both sensation and motor function. It is the dominant characteristic.
*O*rganomegaly: Hepatomegaly (50%), splenomegaly, or lymphadenopathy.
*E*ndocrinopathy: Present in 84% of patients: gonadal, thyroid, pituitary, parathyroid, pancreatic, adrenal (in order of frequency, and many times multiple).
*M*onoclonal protein: Almost always λ light chain. Usually Ig A or IgG and ≤3 g/dL. Bone marrow smear <5 to 10% plasma cells.
*S*kin changes: Hyperpigmentation, hypertrichosis, glomeruloid hemangiomata, white nails, plethora, acrocyanosis, flushing.
Other important manifestations are:
— *P*apilledema (in one third of patients)
— *E*xtravascular volume overload
— *S*clerotic bone lesions[a] (95%)
— *T*hrombocytosis (in 54%)
— VEGF elevation[b]
— Castleman disease (in 11–30%)

[a]Radiology and CT/PET can be useful
[b]VEGF = Vascular endothelial growth factor is the cytokine that correlates best with disease activity. The helpful cutoff for plasma and serum VEGF levels for diagnosis are >200 pg/mL (specificity 95%, sensitivity 68%) and >1920 pg/mL (specificity 98%, sensibility 73%), respectively

82.1.3 Diagnosis

Not all the features within the acronym are required to make the diagnosis. There are other relevant features not included in the POEMS acronym also important: PEST

G. Cook
Haematology and Myeloma Studies, Leeds Cancer Centre, St James's University Hospital, Leeds, UK

M. Rovira (✉)
Hematology Department, Hospital Clínic de Barcelona, University of Barcelona, Barcelona, Catalunya, Spain
e-mail: mrovira@clinic.cat

E. Carreras et al. (eds.), *The EBMT Handbook*, https://doi.org/10.1007/978-3-030-02278-5_82

Table 82.1 Criteria for the diagnosis of POEMS syndrome

The diagnosis of POEMS syndrome is confirmed when: — Both mandatory major criteria + — Another of the other three major criteria + — At least one of the minor criteria	
Mandatory major criteria	**Other major criteria**
Polyneuropathy	Castleman disease
Monoclonal immunoglobulin	Sclerotic bone lesions VEGF elevated
Minor criteria	**Other symptoms and signs**
Organomegaly (splenomegaly, hepatomegaly, or lymphadenopathy)	Digital clubbing Weight loss Hyperhidrosis
Extravascular volume overload (edema, pleural effusion, or ascites)	Low vitamin B12 values Diarrhea
Endocrinopathy[a] Skin changes	Pulmonary hypertension/restrictive lung disease
Papilledema Thrombocytosis/erythrocytosis[b]	Thrombosis

Adapted from Dispenzieri (2017)
[a]Hypogonadism is the most frequent, and because of the high prevalence of diabetes mellitus and thyroid abnormalities, these two last abnormalities alone are not sufficient to meet this minor criterion
[b]Anemia and/or thrombocytopenia are rare, unless associated with Castleman disease

(*p*apilledema, *e*xtravascular volume overload, *s*clerotic bone lesions, *t*hrombocytosis/erythrocytosis), elevated VEGF levels, abnormal pulmonary function tests, and a predisposition to thrombosis.

There is a Castleman variant of POEMS syndrome that may be associated with a clonal plasma cell disorder. When Castleman disease variant of POEMS syndrome occurs without evidence of plasma cell disorder, then this entity should be considered separately.

Clinical criteria for POEMS diagnostic are shown in Table 82.1.

82.1.4 Prognosis

Chronic course, median survival of nearly 14 years, rarely progression to multiple myeloma.

The number of POEMS features does not affect survival.

Risk factors associated to better survival are: albumin >3.2 g/dL, achievement of a complete hematological response and younger age. Lower VEGF levels, better response to treatment.

Risk factors associated to shorter survival are: clubbing, extravascular volume overload, respiratory symptoms, papilledema, and coexisting Castleman disease.

Thrombocytosis and high bone marrow infiltration are associated with risk of cerebrovascular accidents.

Patients candidates for radiation therapy have a better overall survival.

82.1.5 Standard Treatment

82.1.5.1 In Case of an Isolated Bone Lesion (or Multiple, But Localized)

Radiotherapy to affected site(s) improves the symptoms of POEMS syndrome and can be curative.

82.1.5.2 Rest of Patients (Disseminated Disease)

- MEL/DEX
- LENA/DEX, THAL/DEX, BOR (these last two agents are of limited use due to the intrinsic risk of peripheral neuropathy), CY/DEX.

- Plasmapheresis, IVIg, IFN-α, tamoxifen, ATRA, bevacizumab (anti-VEGF agent), argatroban, and strontium-89 (mostly single-case reports).
- Attention to supportive care is mandatory (physical therapy, orthotics, etc.).
- Auto-HSCT.

82.1.5.3 Response Criteria

Monitoring the response to treatment in POEMS syndrome is a challenge. Patients must be followed carefully comparing the deficits to baseline. VEGF is an imperfect marker due to discordances between disease activity and response. The size of monoclonal protein is typically small making standard MM response criteria inapplicable. Patients can present clinical benefit without M-protein response therefore a clinical scoring system which can focus on organ-specific response would be useful clinically. So, response criteria for POEMS syndrome could be done as follows: hematological response using a modified amyloid response criteria, VEGF response, CT/PET response, and a simplified organ response (polyneuropathy assessment, pulmonary function tests, and extravascular overload).

82.1.6 Autologous HSCT (Table 82.2)

Table 82.2 Main characteristic of auto-HSCT for POEMS disease treatment

Background	— In MM, another gammopathy, auto-HSCT, has a high rate of responses — In amyloidosis, a disease with similarities to POEMS syndrome with "low tumor" burden, auto-HSCT offers encouraging results
Indication	POEMS syndrome with disseminated disease and: — Good general condition — Without response to standard treatment (MEL + DEX 2–3 months) — With high-risk factors (?)
Conditioning	MEL 140–200 mg/m^2[a]
Stem cell source	PBSC, mobilization with G-CSF ± CY (3 g/m^2)[b,c]
Morbidity	— High rate of engraftment syndrome (up to 50%) (see Chap. 42), important to recognize and treat promptly with PRD. In these cases, higher than expected transfusion need and delayed engraftment — No organ toxicities as observed in amyloidosis
Mortality	As in other auto-HSCT, recently reported 3.3% at 1-year NRM[d]
Response[d,e]	Usually delayed, from 6 months post-auto-HSCT to 24–72 months

[a]With lower dose, inferior responses
[b]Mobilization failure is described, for this reason if there is no response after three courses of MEL + DEX, proceed to mobilization
[c]The incidence of engraftment syndrome can be reduced if mobilization is done with CY + G-CSF
[d]Cook et al. (2017)
[e]In the largest series, 3-year PFS 84% and OS 94%, and 5-year PFS 74% and OS 89%

82.2 Monoclonal Ig Deposition Disease

82.2.1 Introduction

Monoclonal Ig deposition is a clonal plasma cell dyscrasia in which light-chain and/or heavy-chain subunits of Igs form non-fibrillar deposits in various tissues, causing organ dysfunction. Light-chain deposition disease is the most common of these entities.

82.2.2 Clinical Manifestation/Laboratory

Kidney
- Always affected: nephrotic syndrome, hypertension, and rapidly progressing renal insufficiency
- Immunofluorescence shows deposition of light chains along glomerular and tubular basement membranes → nodular glomerulosclerosis
- Deposits are non-fibrillar, almost always composed of κ chain, and do not stain with Congo red dye

Heart and liver
- Less frequently affected: restrictive cardiopathy, myocardial infarction, cholestatic jaundice, hepatic failure

Monoclonal gammopathy
- Electrophoresis, immunofixation of serum and/or urine, serum-free light chain measurement

Table 82.3 Main characteristic of auto-HSCT for monoclonal Ig deposition disease treatment

Background	— As in POEMS syndrome (see Table 82.2)
Indication	— Patients in good general condition and with basic requirements for auto-HSCT — Patients not responding to previous MM-like treatment
Conditioning	Melphalan 140–200 mg/m^2
Stem cell source	PB, mobilization with G-CSF ± CY (3 g/m^2)
Morbidity	Some patients require hemodialysis (HD) before and during the procedure. In that case, MEL should be administered after HD
Mortality	As in other auto-HSCT
Response	In the few cases reported: — Hematological responses are described secondary to the control of the monoclonal gammopathy — It can improve renal function. In selected cases, kidney transplantation could be an option if the patient achieves a CR and remain in HD

82.2.3 Diagnosis

Based on the biopsy of the affected organ (almost always kidney)

82.2.4 Treatment

Controversial, not standard due to the low incidence. Conventional chemotherapy commonly used for MM is unsatisfactory. Possible alternatives are:

- MEL + prednisone
- VAD (vincristine, doxorubicin, DEX)
- THAL/DEX, BOR/DEX
- Auto-HSCT (see Table 82.3)

Recommended References

Batalini F, Econimo L, Quillen K, et al. High-dose melphalan and stem cell transplantation in patients on dialysis due to immunoglobulin light-chain amyloidosis and monoclonal immunoglobulin deposition disease. Biol Blood Marrow Transplant. 2018;24:127–32.

Cook G, Iacobelli S, Van Biezen A, et al. High-dose therapy and autologous stem cell transplantation in patients with POEMS syndrome: a retrospective study of the Chronic Mailnancy Working Party of the European Society for Blood and Marrow Transplantation. Haematologica. 2017;102: 160–7.

D'Souza A, Lacy M, Gertz M, et al. Long-term outcomes after autologous stem cell transplantation for patients with POEMS syndrome: a single-center experience. Blood. 2012;120:56–62.

Dispenzieri A. POEMS syndrome: 2017 update on diagnosis, risk-stratification, and management. Am J Hematol. 2017;92:814–29.

Dispenzieri A, Kyle RA, Lacy MQ, et al. POEMS syndrome: definitions and long-term outcome. Blood. 2003;101:2496–506.

Dispenzieri A, Lacy MQ, Hayman SR, et al. Peripheral blood stem cell transplant for POEMS syndrome is associated with high rates of engraftment syndrome. Eur J Haematol. 2008;80:397–406.

Girnius S, Seldin DC, Quillen K, et al. Long-term outcome of patients with monoclonal IgG deposition disease treated with high-dose melphalan and stem cell transplantation. Bone Marrow Transplant. 2011;46: 161–2.

Hassoun H, Flombaum C, D'Agati VD, et al. High-dose melphalan and auto-SCT in patients with monoclonal Ig deposition disease. Bone Marrow Transplant. 2008;42:1–8.

Jaccard A, Royer B, Bordessoule D, et al. High-dose therapy and autologous blood stem cell transplantation in POEMS syndrome. Blood. 2002;99: 3057–9.

Kourelis TV, Buadi FK, Kumar SK, et al. Long-term outcome of patients with POEMS syndrome: an update of the Mayo Clinic experience. Am J Hematol. 2016;91:585–9.

Li J, Zhang W, Jiao L, et al. Combination of melphalan and dexamethasone for patients with newly diagnosed POEMS syndrome. Blood. 2011a;117: 6445–9.

Li J, Zhou DB, Huang Z, et al. Clinical characteristics and long-term outcome of patients with POEMS syndrome in China. Ann Hematol. 2011b;90: 819–26.

Pozzi C, D'Amico M, Fogazzi GB, et al. Light chain deposition disease with renal involvement: clinical characteristics and prognostic factors. Am J Kidney Dis. 2003;42:1154–63.

Rovira M, Carreras E, Blade J, et al. Dramatic improvement of POEMS syndrome following autologous haematopoietic cell transplantation. Br J Haematol. 2001;115:373–5.

Tovar N, Cibeira MT, Rosiñol L, et al. Bortezomib/dexamethasone followed by stem cell transplantation as front line treatment for light-chain deposition disease. Eur J Haematol. 2012;89(4): 340–4.

83 Follicular Lymphoma

Stephen Robinson

83.1 Introduction

First-line therapy for patients with advanced stage follicular lymphoma (FL) in need of treatment is to administer chemoimmunotherapy followed by maintenance rituximab (RTX). With this approach approximately half of the patients will remain progression-free at 10 years. Both auto-HSCT and allo-HSCT have been employed in the management of patients with FL since the 1980s. However, the roles of both forms of HSCT have continued to evolve as both transplant and non-transplant therapies have been refined. The current indication for auto-HSCT and allo-HSCT are reviewed below.

83.2 Autologous HSCT

83.2.1 Auto-HSCT in First Response

With both the development of auto-HSCT in the 1980s and the realisation that standard-dose chemotherapy was not curative for indolent lymphoma, investigators explored the role of auto-HSCT as a consolidation strategy following first-line therapy. Promising initial studies culminated in the development of several large randomised studies where auto-HSCT was compared with either no further therapy or interferon. Whilst some of these studies demonstrated an improvement in disease control, no overall survival benefit could be demonstrated (Lenz et al. 2004; Ladetto et al. 2008). These observations combined with a growing realisation of the acute and long-term toxicities of auto-HSCT have led to the abandonment of auto-HSCT as a first-line consolidation procedure.

83.2.2 Auto-HSCT for Relapsed FL

To date, the CUP trial has been the only randomised study comparing consolidation with an auto-HSCT (using either purged or unpurged stem cells) with no further therapy in the relapse setting (Schouten et al. 2003). In this trial, 140 patients with relapsed FL were randomised between consolidation with an auto-HSCT (using either purged or unpurged stem cells) or chemotherapy alone. The 2-year PFS for the chemotherapy alone arm was 26% compared with 58% and 55% for those receiving HSCT with either purged or unpurged stem cells, respectively. Further there was an overall survival advantage in favour of the two transplant arms (Schouten et al. 2003).

S. Robinson (✉)
Bristol Cancer Institute, University Hospital's Bristol, Bristol, UK
e-mail: Stephen.Robinson@UHBristol.nhs.uk

E. Carreras et al. (eds.), *The EBMT Handbook*, https://doi.org/10.1007/978-3-030-02278-5_83

More recently the EBMT-LYM-1 study prospectively examined the role of purging and maintenance with Rituximab (RTX) peri-HSCT in RTX naïve patients with relapsed FL (Pettengell et al. 2013). In this study all patients underwent an auto-HSCT, and no benefit could be demonstrated for in vivo purging. However, the study did demonstrate that for patients receiving RTX maintenance, the PFS was in excess of 50%. A number of other studies have also reported long-term follow-up of auto-HSCT in relapsed FL and describe a 10-year PFS ranging between 31 and 50% (Kornacker et al. 2009; Montoto et al. 2007). Taken together these results demonstrate that between 25 and 50% of patients experience prolonged PFS following an auto-HSCT for relapsed FL suggesting that this is a curative procedure for a significant minority of patients.

Although promising it is important to recognise both the acute and long-term toxicities associated with auto-HSCT which continues to limit the application of this therapy. Whilst early TRM may be relatively low in younger patients, there is evidence that for patients over the age of 60, the TRM may be in excess of 10% (Sánchez-Ortega et al. 2016). Given that the median age of patients with relapsing FL is 69 an auto-HSCT will be associated with a significant TRM for the majority of patients. An additional concern is the late risk of developing secondary malignancies including MDS/AML. In a prospective randomised study, patients undergoing an auto-HSCT for FL had a significantly higher rate of both solid malignancies and MDS/AML compared to patients not receiving HSCT (Gyan e al. 2009). Further, in a population-based study of more than 7000 patients undergoing auto-HSCT, the risk of secondary malignancies was 1.4 times greater and the risk of MDS/AML 20.6 times greater than the general population (Bilmon et al. 2014). It is unclear whether the type of conditioning therapy used for an auto-HSCT influences the risk of secondary malignancy and MDS/AML. Evaluation of the bone marrow for clonal haematopoiesis and cytogenetic abnormalities may enable the identification of patients at a greater risk of developing MDS/AML following an auto-HSCT. For these patients alternative relapse therapies may be more suitable.

83.2.3 The Role of Purging, Conditioning Regimen and Maintenance

The BM is infiltrated in approximately 75% of FL patients at diagnosis, and consequently a number of investigators have studied the role of marrow purging in auto-HSCT (Gonzalez-Barca et al. 2000). However, no clear benefit for purging could be demonstrated in prospective studies (Schouten et al. 2003; Pettengell et al. 2013), and there was some evidence that purging resulted in significant additional immune suppression (IS). Consequently, purging remains an experimental procedure in auto-HSCT for FL.

There is a wide variety of different conditioning regimens that may be employed for auto-HSCT in FL but a paucity of randomised trials comparing the efficacy and toxicity of these different regimens. The BEAM (BCNU, VP, Ara-C, MEL) regimen has become the most widely used regimen prior to auto-HSCT in malignant lymphoma and has been adopted in many countries. A number of investigators have looked to improve upon BEAM by including RTX and dexamethasone, substituting BCNU with bendamustine (Visani et al. 2014), or incorporating bortezomib, mitoxantrone or fotemustine. Several groups have also incorporated radioimmunotherapy (RIT) into the conditioning regimen prior to auto-HSCT in NHL. In one small randomised trial comparing Zevalin and BEAM (Z-BEAM) with BEAM in relapsed/refractory B NHL, there was a survival advantage in the Zevalin arm (Shimoni et al. 2012).

Auto-HSCT in FL, Key Points

- Auto-HSCT should not be employed in first response.
- Auto-HSCT should be considered in patients with relapsed disease responding to reinduction therapy.
- Auto-HCT achieves a 5-year PFS of approximately 50% and may be curative in a significant minority of patients.
- There is no proven role for purging strategies.
- Maintenance rituximab for four infusions should be considered post auto-HSCT.

83.3 Allogeneic HSCT

Allo-HSCT offers several advantages over auto-HSCT in FL: the provision of a graft uncontaminated by lymphoma cells or exposed to mutagenic agents and the development of an allogeneic GVL effect. Early studies employed MAC regimens and demonstrated that cure could be achieved in a significant proportion of patients (Peniket et al. 2003; van Besien et al. 2003). In retrospective studies comparing allo- with auto-HSCT, MAC allo-HSCT was associated with a lower relapse rate but a higher TRM and consequently a similar OS. In an attempt to reduce the toxicity of allo-HSCT, RIC allo-HSCT has been developed (Robinson et al. 2002). A number of groups have demonstrated the safety and efficacy of RIC allo-HSCT and demonstrated that this type of transplant may be employed in older patients with significant comorbidities and in those patients who have undergone a prior auto-HSCT. Following a RIC allo-HSCT, the relapse rate is typically below 30%, whether performed as a first transplant procedure (Robinson et al. 2013) or following a previous auto-HSCT (Robinson et al. 2016) and the 5-year PFS rates range from 50 to 85%.

83.3.1 Conditioning Regimen Intensity

It is currently unclear whether a RIC or a MAC allo-HSCT offers superior outcomes in FL. A retrospective registry study demonstrated that the two approaches to allo-HSCT resulted in similar outcomes in the sibling donor setting (3-year OS for the MAC and RIC were 71% and 62% (P = 0.15), respectively) (Hari et al. 2008). However, the EBMT reported that in the unrelated donor setting, RIC allo-HSCT was associated with a lower NRM and significantly longer PFS and OS when compared with MAC allo-HSCT (Avivi et al. 2009). The median age at relapse of FL is 69, and therefore the majority of patients that may be considered for an allo-HSCT will be considered too old for MAC regimens, and many authorities therefore recommend a RIC allo-HSCT for FL. However, in younger patients (<50 years old) and without significant comorbidities, more intensive regimens may also be considered.

83.3.2 Donor Source for Allo-HSCT and TCD

The outcomes of both matched sibling donor (MSD) and MUD allo-HSCT in FL are broadly similar. A recent large retrospective study conducted by the EBMT and the CIBMTR demonstrated that the PFS and OS following MSD and MUD were similar (Sureda et al. 2018). For patients lacking a MSD or MUD, either a cord blood or haploidentical family donor may now be considered. The feasibility of umbilical cord blood (Rodrigues et al. 2009; Brunstein et al. 2009) and haplo-HSCT (with PT-CY) (Dietrich et al. 2016) in NHL (including FL) has been reported. However, the toxicity of both CBT and haplo-HSCT is significant, and it remains to be established whether either type of alternative donor source is superior to MSD and MUD.

TCD of the graft is a well-established method to reduce the incidence of GVHD post-transplant but runs the risk of eliminating allo-reactive T cells that will mediate the GVL effect and consequently result in a higher relapse rate. The risk of relapse may be offset by employing donor lymphocyte infusion (DLI), and with this approach, the 4 years PFS and relapse risk was 76% and 24%, respectively, and the incidence of GVHD was low (Thomson et al. 2010), suggesting that this approach may also be an option for allo-HSCT in FL.

Allo-HSCT for FL, Key Points

- Allo-HSCT should only be considered in patients with relapsed disease.
- Reduced intensity conditioning regimens are most appropriate for patients over the age of 50 or with significant comorbidities.
- Patients under 50 years may be considered for more intensive regimens.
- Matched sibling, matched unrelated, haploidentical and cord blood stem cell sources may be considered.
- T-cell depletion may be employed but should be combined with chimerism directed donor lymphocyte infusions.

83.4 Patient Selection for HSCT in FL

As discussed above HSCT options are no longer considered in first response and are reserved for patients with relapsed disease. However, patients with relapsed FL represent a highly heterogeneous population, and a HSCT will not be appropriate for many patients. Therefore, numerous factors have to be taken into consideration when selecting patients for a HSCT procedure. Patient-related factors such as age, comorbidities, performance status, organ function, the HSCT comorbidity index (HSCT-CI) (Sorror et al. 2005) and patients' personal views will determine if a patient is fit to undergo a transplant and what the likely TRM rate will be. Certain features relating to the patient's lymphoma are prognostic in the relapsed setting, and transplantation should only be considered in patients where the lymphoma is considered to considerably shorten survival. Patients that relapse within 2 years of the first-line therapy (Casulo et al. 2015) and those with high-grade transformation at relapse (Sarkozy et al. 2016) have been shown to have poor survival, and these patients should be considered for a HSCT procedure once adequate disease control has been obtained. Patients with a high FLIPPI score at relapse and those with multiple relapses may also have a poor prognosis, and these patients may also be considered for transplant options. It is important, however, to carefully counsel the patients regarding both the transplant and non-transplant therapies that are currently available of which there are many.

83.5 Auto-HSCT or Allo-HSCT as a First Transplant Procedure

The decision whether to employ either auto- or allo-HSCT in relapsed FL remains challenging. There has been only one prospective randomised study addressing this issue, which was unfortunately closed early due to poor accrual (Tomblyn et al. 2011). An EBMT retrospective comparison demonstrated that the PFS at 5 years was 57% for patients receiving an allo-HSCT compared with 48% for those receiving an auto-HSCT, but overall survival was similar with both types of transplant (Robinson et al. 2013). It is therefore currently not clear which SCT option is superior for relapsed FL, and in the absence of definitive data, the decision regarding an auto- or allo-HSCT needs to be taken on an individual patient basis. Given the excellent results recently reported with auto-HSCT (Pettengell et al. 2013), the relatively low toxicity and the potential for cure a number of authorities now recommend an auto-HSCT as the first transplant of choice and that an allo-HSCT should be reserved for patients relapsing after an auto-HSCT.

83.6 Allo-HSCT in Patients Relapsing After Auto-HSCT

The largest series of patients undergoing a RIC allo-HSCT after the failure of an auto-HSCT was reported by the EBMT. The NRM at 2 years was significant (27%), but the 5-year PFS and OS were 48% and 51%, respectively (Robinson et al. 2016). The duration of response following the allo-HSCT was also significantly longer than after the auto-HSCT illustrating the potential of the allogeneic GVL effect in this disease. This data demonstrates that a RIC allo-HSCT can act as an effective salvage strategy in this setting although the toxicity was significant. There is also a risk that patients may fail to respond to reinduction therapy, and therefore would not be eligible for an allo-HSCT.

Patient Selection Key Points

- Only patients with (a) early relapse or (b) high-grade transformation after first-line therapy or (c) multiple relapses should be considered for HSCT consolidation.
- The superiority of either auto-HSCT or allo-HSCT has not been established.
- Auto-HSCT may cure some patients and is associated with lower toxicity compared to allo-HSCT.

- RIC allo-HSCT may cure patients that relapse after an auto-HSCT.
- Many authorities recommend an auto-HSCT as the first transplant procedure of choice.

83.7 Conclusions

Both auto- and allo-HSCT have an established role in the treatment of relapsed FL, and both forms of transplant can deliver curative therapy to patients with otherwise poor prognosis disease. Patient selection for transplant therapy is critical, and a current understanding of the rapidly evolving field of alternative non-transplant lymphoma therapies is mandatory. The treatment paradigm for FL will change over the coming years as novel agents are incorporated into clinical practice, and the place of these agents relative to transplantation will evolve.

References

Avivi I, Montoto S, Canals C, et al. Matched unrelated donor stem cell transplant in 131 patients with follicular lymphoma: an analysis from the Lymphoma Working Party of the European Group for Blood and Marrow Transplantation. Br J Haematol. 2009;147:719–28.

Bilmon IA, Ashton LJ, Le Marsney RE, et al. Second cancer risk in adults receiving autologous haematopoietic SCT for cancer: a population-based cohort study. Bone Marrow Transplant. 2014;49:691–8.

Brunstein CG, Cantero S, Cao Q, et al. Promising progression-free survival for patients low and intermediate grade lymphoid malignancies after nonmyeloablative umbilical cord blood transplantation. Biol Blood Marrow Transplant. 2009;15:214–22.

Casulo C, Byrtek M, Dawson KL, et al. Early relapse of follicular lymphoma after rituximab plus cyclophosphamide, doxorubicin, vincristine, and prednisone defines patients at high risk for death: an analysis from the National Lympho Care Study. J Clin Oncol. 2015;33:2516–22.

Dietrich S, Finel H, Martinez C, et al. Post-transplant cyclophosphamide-based haplo-identical transplantation as alternative to matched sibling or unrelated donor transplantation for non-Hodgkin lymphoma: a registry study by the European society for blood and marrow transplantation. Leukemia. 2016;30:2086–9.

Gonzalez-Barca E, Fernandez de Sevilla A, Domingo-Claros A, et al. Autologous stem cell transplantation (ASCT) with immunologically purged progenitor cells in patients with advanced stage follicular lymphoma after early partial or complete remission: toxicity, follow-up of minimal residual disease and survival. Bone Marrow Transplant. 2000;26:1051–6.

Gyan E, Foussard C, Bertrand P, et al. High-dose therapy followed by autologous purged stem cell transplantation and doxorubicin-based chemotherapy in patients with advanced follicular lymphoma: a randomized multicenter study by the GOELAMS with final results after a median follow-up of 9 years. Blood. 2009;113(5):995–1001.

Hari P, Carreras J, Zhang MJ, et al. Allogeneic transplants in follicular lymphoma: higher risk of disease progression after reduced-intensity compared to myeloablative conditioning. Biol Blood Marrow Transplant. 2008;14:236–45.

Kornacker M, Stumm J, Pott C, et al. Characteristics of relapse after autologous stem-cell transplantation for follicular lymphoma: a long-term follow-up. Ann Oncol. 2009;20:722–8.

Ladetto M, De Marco F, Benedetti F, et al. Prospective, multicenter randomized GITMO/IIL trial comparing intensive (R-HDS) versus conventional (CHOP-R) chemoimmunotherapy in high-risk follicular lymphoma at diagnosis: the superior disease control of R-HDS does not translate into an overall survival advantage. Blood. 2008;111:4004–13.

Lenz G, Dreyling M, Schiegnitz E, et al. Myeloablative radiochemotherapy followed by autologous stem cell transplantation in first remission prolongs progression-free survival in follicular lymphoma: results of a prospective, randomized trial of the German Low-Grade Lymphoma Study Group. Blood. 2004;104:2667–74.

Montoto S, Canals C, Rohatiner AZS, et al. Long-term follow-up of high-dose treatment with autologous haematopoietic progenitor cell support in 693 patients with follicular lymphoma: an EBMT registry study (LFTU of autoSCT). Leukemia. 2007;21:2324–31.

Peniket AJ, Ruiz de Elvira MC, Taghipour G, et al. An EBMT registry matched study of allogeneic stem cell transplants for lymphoma: allogeneic transplantation is associated with a lower relapse rate but a higher procedure-related mortality rate than autologous transplantation. Bone Marrow Transplant. 2003;31:667–78.

Pettengell R, Schmitz N, Gisselbrecht C, et al. Rituximab purging and/or maintenance in patients undergoing autologous transplantation for relapsed follicular lymphoma: a prospective randomized trial from the lymphoma working party of the European group for blood and marrow transplantation. J Clin Oncol. 2013;31:1624–30.

Robinson SP, Boumendil A, Finel H, et al. Reduced intensity allogeneic stem cell transplantation for follicular lymphoma relapsing after an autologous transplant achieves durable long term disease control. An analysis from the Lymphoma Working Party of the EBMT. Ann Oncol. 2016;27:1088.

Robinson SP, Canals C, Luang JJ, et al. The outcome of reduced intensity allogeneic stem cell transplantation and autologous stem cell transplantation when performed as a first transplant strategy in relapsed follicular lymphoma: an analysis from the Lymphoma Working Party of the EBMT. Bone Marrow Transplant. 2013;48:1409–14.

Robinson SP, Goldstone AH, Mackinnon S, et al. Chemoresistant or aggressive lymphoma predicts for a poor outcome following reduced-intensity allogeneic progenitor cell transplantation: an analysis from the Lymphoma Working Party of the European Group for Blood and Bone Marrow Transplantation. Blood. 2002;100:4310–6.

Rodrigues CA, Sanz G, Brunstein CG, et al. Analysis of risk factors for outcomes after unrelated cord blood transplantation in adults with lymphoid malignancies: a study by the Eurocord-Netcord and lymphoma working party of the European group for blood and marrow transplantation. J Clin Oncol. 2009;27: 256–63.

Sánchez-Ortega I, Basak GW, Beohou E, et al. Autologous hematopoietic cell transplantation in elderly patients aged 65 and older: a retrospective analysis by the complications and quality of life working party of the EBMT. Blood. 2016;128(22):678.

Sarkozy C, Trneny M, Xerri L, et al. Risk factors and outcomes for patients with follicular lymphoma who had histologic transformation after response to first-line immunochemotherapy in the PRIMA trial. J Clin Oncol. 2016;34:2575–82.

Schouten HC, Qian W, Kvaloy S, et al. High-dose therapy improves progression-free survival and survival in relapsed follicular non-Hodgkin's lymphoma: results from the randomized European CUP trial. J Clin Oncol. 2003;21:3918–27.

Shimoni A, Avivi I, Rowe JM, et al. A randomized study comparing yttrium-90 ibritumomab tiuxetan (Zevalin) and high-dose BEAM chemotherapy versus BEAM alone as the conditioning regimen before autologous stem cell transplantation in patients with aggressive lymphoma. Cancer. 2012;118:4706–14.

Sorror ML, Maris MB, Storb R, et al. Hematopoietic cell transplantation (HCT)-specific comorbidity index: a new tool for risk assessment before allogeneic HCT. Blood. 2005;106:2912–9.

Sureda A, Zhang M-J, Dreger P, et al. Allogeneic hematopoietic stem cell transplantation for relapsed follicular lymphoma. A combined analysis on behalf of the Lymphoma Working Party of the EBMT and the Lymphoma Committee of the CIBMTR. Cancer. 2018;124:1733–42.

Thomson KJ, Morris EC, Milligan D, et al. T-cell-depleted reduced-intensity transplantation followed by donor leukocyte infusions to promote graft-versus-lymphoma activity results in excellent long-term survival in patients with multiply relapsed follicular lymphoma. J Clin Oncol. 2010;28(23):3695–700.

Tomblyn MR, Ewell M, Bredeson C, et al. Autologous versus reduced-intensity allogeneic hematopoietic cell transplantation for patients with chemosensitive follicular non-Hodgkin lymphoma beyond first complete response or first partial response. Biol Blood Marrow Transplant. 2011;17:1051–7.

van Besien K, Loberiza FR, Bajorunaite R, et al. Comparison of autologous and allogeneic hematopoietic stem cell transplantation for follicular lymphoma. Blood. 2003;102:3521–9.

Visani G, Stefani PM, Capria S, et al. Bendamustine, etoposide, cytarabine, melphalan, and autologous stem cell rescue produce a 72% 3-year PFS in resistant lymphoma. Blood. 2014;124:3029–31.

84 Chronic Lymphocytic Leukemia

Johannes Schetelig and Peter Dreger

84.1 Introduction

CLL is a rare indication for HSCT since it usually follows an indolent course. Those patients who require treatment have the option of various combinations of chemoimmunotherapy (CIT), several non-cross-resistant pathway inhibitors, and cellular-based immunotherapy.

Three orally available pathway inhibitors with an attractive risk-benefit ratio have been approved for the treatment of CLL in the past 5 years, the Bruton's tyrosine kinase inhibitor ibrutinib, the phosphoinositide 3-kinase inhibitor idelalisib, and the BCL2 inhibitor, venetoclax. Second-generation compounds are under development.

While CAR treatment is still at an early stage of clinical developmental for CLL, already today the sequential use of the available treatment options offers chances for long-term survival. Only a minority of patients shows resistant disease with the current treatment options and requires allo-HSCT.

J. Schetelig (✉)
Medical Clinic I, Department of Hematology, University Hospital Carl Gustav Carus, Technische Universität Dresden, Dresden, Germany
e-mail: johannes.schetelig@uniklinikum-dresden.de

P. Dreger
Abteilung Innere Medizin V, Universitätsklinikum Heidelberg, Heidelberg, Germany

84.2 Principles of Treatment for CLL

The diagnosis of CLL does not justify the start of treatment. This holds true even for relapsing CLL. Criteria which should trigger treatment are, e.g., anemia or thrombocytopenia due to heavy marrow involvement, a lymphocyte doubling time of less than 6 months, severe constitutional symptoms, or bulky lymphadenopathy. Treatment of CLL should be stratified by the *TP53* genotype. Patients with CLL harboring a cytogenetic deletion 17p detected by FISH or karyotyping or with a *TP53* mutation detected by DNA sequencing (combined in this manuscript as *TP53* abnormalities) should not be treated with chemotherapy. While CIT used to be the standard of care for first-line treatment for several decades, this standard is now challenged also in patients with functional *TP53* by the treatment with pathway inhibitors with or without monoclonal B-cell antibodies.

84.3 Results of CLL Treatment with Pathway Inhibitors

Five-year disease control rates in treatment-naive elderly patients on ibrutinib monotherapy have been reported from two phase II trials (5-year PFS of 92% and 100%) (Ahn et al. 2018; O'Brien et al. 2018). Treatment-naive patients with a *TP53* abnormality had a 5-year PFS of 74% (95% CI, 60–92%).

E. Carreras et al. (eds.), *The EBMT Handbook*, https://doi.org/10.1007/978-3-030-02278-5_84

Five-year PFS in relapsed/refractory patients on ibrutinib was 44% (O'Brien et al. 2018). Outcome was worse in patients with a deletion 17p or a *TP53* mutation compared to patients without these abnormalities (O'Brien et al. 2018). In an NIH trial, patients with *TP53* abnormalities had a 5-year PFS of 19% (95% CI, 6–60%) compared to 65% (95% CI, 44–96%) without *TP53* abnormalities (Ahn et al. 2018).

Patients with relapsed/refractory (R/R) CLL with a deletion 17p who received the BCL inhibitor venetoclax had a 2-year PFS of 54% (95% CI: 45%, 62%) (Stilgenbauer et al. 2018). Notably, on venetoclax monotherapy, 20% of patients achieved a CR according to NCI criteria, and 30% reached MRD negativity measured by FACS at cutoff of 10^{-4} CLL cells. Patients who achieved a complete or MRD-negative remission had a very good prognosis despite previously relapsed/refractory CLL with a deletion 17p. Furthermore, venetoclax demonstrated activity in patients who failed on ibrutinib or idelalisib (Jones et al. 2018).

Finally, idelalisib in combination with RTX or ofatumumab has also demonstrated activity in patients with R/R high-risk CLL. For example, the median PFS for patients with del(17p) or *TP53* mutations who had received idelalisib plus ofatumumab was 16 months (95%-CI, 11–19 months) (Jones et al. 2017).

After failure of ibrutinib or idelalisib, sequential treatment with another pathway inhibitor is efficacious (Jones et al. 2017; Coutre et al. 2018; Mato et al. 2016). However, disease control generally is shorter compared to pathway-inhibitor-naïve patients.

84.4 Allogeneic HSCT

The indication for allo-HSCT requires high-risk disease and failure on at least one pathway inhibitor (Dreger et al. 2014). High-risk CLL can be defined clinically by refractory disease or relapse within 2 years after CIT and biologically by *TP53* abnormalities. Information on the IGVH mutation status, IGHV3-21 gene usage, deletion 11q, or complex karyotype adds to biological risk categorization, but only *TP53* abnormalities are broadly accepted for stratified treatment. However, even patients with high-risk disease should have failed at least one pathway inhibitor before being referred for allo-HSCT. Independent of PI exposure, patients with a history of Richter's transformation and patients with a therapy-related myeloid neoplasia have an indication of allo-HSCT.

Available evidence strongly suggests that allo-HSCT is currently the only therapy with curative potential in CLL (van Gelder et al. 2017; Kramer et al. 2017). Many patients reach CR without MRD after allo-HSCT. Allo-HSCT can provide long-term disease control even in patients with an unfavorable biological and clinical risk profile. The timing of allo-HSCT should be individually discussed with the patients by taking into consideration the risk of complications after allo-HSCT and the chances of sequential treatment with pathway inhibitors and or CIT. Standard risk scores like the HCT-CI, the PAM-score, or the EBMT risk score can be used to assess the risk of non-relapse mortality of an individual patient (Schetelig et al. 2017a, b). When assessing the chances of continued conventional treatment, several factors have to be considered:

1. The risk of adverse events during prolonged conventional treatment which affect the eligibility for allo-HSCT
2. The risk of a Richter's transformation
3. The risk of a failed salvage attempt at the next relapse/progression of CLL
4. The risk of worse outcome after allo-HSCT in patients with more resistant CLL

84.4.1 Remission Induction Prior to Start of the Conditioning Regimen

Large prospective and retrospective studies uniformly show that the results of allo-HSCT deteriorate if the disease is not in remission at the time of transplant. Thus, allo-HSCT should be performed in remission of CLL. Different options exist for remission induction and bridging to allo-HSCT. Abundant information exists for CIT prior to allo-HSCT. Data from retrospective registry studies also supports the use of ibrutinib or idelalisib plus RTX for remission induction prior to transplantation (Dreger et al. 2018; Schetelig et al. 2017c). So far, no systematic studies addressed the use of venetoclax prior to allo-HSCT. However, since this drug does not modulate the immune responses, no adverse carry-over effects have to be suspected. As a general rule, the treatment with the highest chance of short-term tumor debulking should be used for remission induction prior to allo-HSCT (van Gelder et al. 2016).

84.4.2 Conditioning Regimens

The crucial therapeutic principle of allo-HSCT in CLL is GVL activity. Evidence for this comes from the observation that even some patients with refractory disease benefit from allo-HSCT. The impact of GVL is reflected by a reduced relapse risk in the presence of cGVHD and the efficacy of immune modulation for the eradication of MRD (Ritgen et al. 2008; Hahn et al. 2015).

Accordingly, long-term disease control can be achieved with a broad range of conditioning regimens. Current evidence does not allow the definition of one standard conditioning regimen for CLL. The most convincing data supporting allo-HSCT in CLL come from studies of NMA conditioning or RIC (Kramer et al. 2017; Schetelig et al. 2017b; Sorror et al. 2008). The choice of conditioning intensity may vary according to the individual situation. In the presence of comorbidity and chemosensitive disease, RIC or NMA conditioning appear to be more appropriate, whereas high-intensity regimens might be preferable in younger patients with good performance status but poorly controlled disease.

84.4.3 Outcome After Allo-HSCT for CLL

Based on a large registry cohort, estimated event-free survival, overall survival, and NRM 10 years after allo-HCT were 28% (95% confidence interval (CI), 25–31), 35% (95% CI, 32–38), and 40% (95% CI, 37–42), respectively (van Gelder et al. 2017). Patients who passed the 5-year landmark EFS ($N = 394$) had a 79% probability (95% CI, 73–85) of surviving the subsequent 5 years without an event. Relapse and NRM contributed equally to late treatment failure. Higher age, lower performance status, unrelated donor type, and unfavorable sex mismatch have an adverse impact on 2-year NRM. Despite the risks of NRM and even late relapse/progression, the prospect of long-term DFS on average in almost one out of three patients remains an argument to consider allo-HCT especially for young patients with high-risk CLL.

84.4.4 Post transplant Minimal Residual Disease Monitoring and Immune Intervention in CLL

In CLL, sensitive MRD quantification (i.e., 1 cell in 10^4 or less) can be obtained by PCR- or flow cytometry-based assays. The decline of the MRD level is often delayed and is closely related to immuno-reconstitution after allo-HSCT. GVL-induced MRD negativity after allo-HSCT is sustained in the majority of patients and is highly predictive of freedom from relapse. MRD monitoring is a valid instrument for the guidance of preemptive immune interventions directed at disease eradication after allo-HSCT, such as the tapering of IS and the use of DLI. The published evidence suggests that CLL is sensitive to timely preemptive immune intervention by modulation of systemic IS (Ritgen et al. 2008; Moreno et al. 2006).

84.5 Summary and Perspectives

Allo-HSCT from MRD or MUD can induce long-term DFS in patients with high-risk CLL. It is a standard treatment option for patients with high-risk CLL who have failed at least one pathway inhibitor. Generally, allo-HSCT should be considered before the disease has advanced to a status of complete refractoriness. At the same time, allo-HSCT should not be recommended for patients who face a higher short-term risk of mortality after transplantation compared to conventional therapy. In the absence of randomized controlled comparisons of these treatment strategies, the outcome of an individual patient has to be predicted based on published data. This requires careful individual assessment of the risk of allo-HSCT versus prolonged conventional treatment. Patients should be referred to a transplant center once their disease proved refractory to at least one pathway inhibitor in order to get consultation with an expert in the field. Finally, all approved drugs for CLL can also be used for the treatment of post transplant relapse, and further improvements of donor selection, patient care, and prevention of complications can be expected; thus, overall outcome after transplantation will continue to improve.

Key Points

Indications for allo-HSCT	• High-risk CLL after failure of pathway inhibitor treatment • CLL in combination with therapy-related MDS • History of Richter's transformation
Remission induction prior to start of conditioning	Patient who receive allo-HSCT in remission enjoy a lower risk of relapse. The most potent option for remission induction should be chosen. This can be any pathway inhibitor or CIT
Donor, graft source, and GVHD-prophylaxis	No disease-specific criteria have to be considered (Michallet et al. 2010; van Gorkom et al. 2018)
Conditioning	Patients should receive either NMA conditioning or alkylator-based RIC. A history of a Richter's transformation or concomitant MDS may justify dose intensification (Schetelig et al. 2017b; Sorror et al. 2008)
MRD monitoring	At least quarterly assessments of MRD by FACS or PCR should be offered after allo-HSCT. Early taper of IS with or without administration of DLI, especially in patients without GVHD but with persistent disease, may result in MRD-negative CR in this group of patients (Ritgen et al. 2008)
Risk factors for non-relapse mortality	• Advanced age • Poor performance status and/or high HCT-CI score • Partially matched as compared to matched donor HSCT
Outcomes	Estimates based on HSCT performed between 2000 and 2010 reported to EBMT registry (van Gelder et al. 2017): 2-year and 5-year NRM, 30% and 36% 2-year and 5-year CI of relapse/progression, 21% and 29% 2-year and 10-year EFS, 49% and 28% 2-year and 10-year OS, 62% and 35%
Relapse after allo-HSCT	Relapse after allo-HSCT may be treated successfully. To current knowledge the history of allo-HSCT does not restrict treatment options for patients with relapsed CLL. Ibrutinib appears to be especially favorable for the treatment of first relapse after transplantation in patients without proven ibrutinib resistance

References

Ahn IE, Farooqui MZH, Tian X, et al. Depth and durability of response to ibrutinib in CLL: 5-year follow-up of a phase II study. Blood. 2018;131:2357–66.

Coutre S, Choi M, Furman RR, et al. Venetoclax for patients with chronic lymphocytic leukemia who progressed during or after idelalisib therapy. Blood. 2018;131:1704–11.

Dreger P, Schetelig J, Andersen N, et al. Managing high-risk CLL during transition to a new treatment era: stem cell transplantation or novel agents? Blood. 2014;124:3841–9.

Dreger P, Michallet M, Bosman P, et al. Ibrutinib for bridging to allogeneic hematopoietic cell transplantation in patients with chronic lymphocytic leukemia or mantle cell lymphoma: a study by the EBMT Chronic Malignancies and Lymphoma Working Parties. Bone Marrow Transplant 2018. https://doi.org/10.1038/s41409-018-0207-4. [Epub ahead of print].

Hahn M, Bottcher S, Dietrich S, et al. Allogeneic hematopoietic stem cell transplantation for poor-risk CLL: dissecting immune-modulating strategies for disease eradication and treatment of relapse. Bone Marrow Transplant. 2015;50:1279–85.

Jones JA, Robak T, Brown JR, et al. Efficacy and safety of idelalisib in combination with ofatumumab for previously treated chronic lymphocytic leukaemia: an open-label, randomised phase 3 trial. Lancet Haematol. 2017;4:e114–26.

Jones JA, Mato AR, Wierda WG, et al. Venetoclax for chronic lymphocytic leukaemia progressing after ibrutinib: an interim analysis of a multicentre, open-label, phase 2 trial. Lancet Oncol. 2018;19:65–75.

Kramer I, Stilgenbauer S, Dietrich S, et al. Allogeneic hematopoietic cell transplantation for high-risk CLL: 10-year follow-up of the GCLLSG CLL3X trial. Blood. 2017;130:1477–80.

Mato AR, Nabhan C, Barr PM, et al. Outcomes of CLL patients treated with sequential kinase inhibitor therapy: a real world experience. Blood. 2016;128:2199–205.

Michallet M, Sobh M, Milligan D, et al. The impact of HLA matching on long-term transplant outcome after allogeneic hematopoietic stem cell transplantation for CLL: a retrospective study from the EBMT registry. Leukemia. 2010;24:1725–31.

Moreno C, Villamor N, Colomer D, et al. Clinical significance of minimal residual disease, as assessed by different techniques, after stem cell transplantation for chronic lymphocytic leukemia. Blood. 2006;107:4563–9.

O'Brien S, Furman RR, Coutre S, et al. Single-agent ibrutinib in treatment-naive and relapsed/refractory chronic lymphocytic leukemia: a 5-year experience. Blood. 2018;131:1910–9.

Ritgen M, Bottcher S, Stilgenbauer S, et al. Quantitative MRD monitoring identifies distinct GVL response patterns after allogeneic stem cell transplantation for chronic lymphocytic leukemia: results from the GCLLSG CLL3X trial. Leukemia. 2008;22:1377–86.

Schetelig J, de Wreede LC, van Gelder M, et al. Risk factors for treatment failure after allogeneic transplantation of patients with CLL: a report from the European Society for Blood and Marrow Transplantation. Bone Marrow Transplant. 2017a;52:552–60.

Schetelig J, Chevallier P, Van Gelder M, et al. Remission status at transplantation and treatment history determine the survival chances of patients after allogeneic hematopoietic stem cell transplantation for chronic lymphocytic leukemia who had received pre-treatment with idelalisib: a report from the EBMT Chronic Malignancies Working Party. Blood. 2017b;130(Suppl 1):4576.

Schetelig J, de Wreede LC, Andersen NS, Moreno C, van Gelder M, Vitek A, et al. Centre characteristics and procedure-related factors have an impact on outcomes of allogeneic transplantation for patients with CLL: a retrospective analysis from the European Society for Blood and Marrow Transplantation (EBMT). Br J Haematol. 2017c;178:521–33.

Sorror ML, Storer BE, Sandmaier BM, et al. Five-year follow-up of patients with advanced chronic lymphocytic leukemia treated with allogeneic hematopoietic cell transplantation after nonmyeloablative conditioning. J Clin Oncol. 2008;26:4912–20.

Stilgenbauer S, Eichhorst B, Schetelig J, et al. Venetoclax for patients with chronic lymphocytic leukemia with 17p deletion: results from the full population of a phase II pivotal trial. J Clin Oncol. 2018;36:1973–80.

van Gelder M, van Oers MH, Alemayehu WG, et al. Efficacy of cisplatin-based immunochemotherapy plus alloSCT in high-risk chronic lymphocytic leukemia: final results of a prospective multicenter phase 2 HOVON study. Bone Marrow Transplant. 2016;51:799–806.

van Gelder M, de Wreede LC, Bornhauser M, et al. Long-term survival of patients with CLL after allogeneic transplantation: a report from the European Society for Blood and Marrow Transplantation. Bone Marrow Transplant. 2017;52:372–80.

van Gorkom G, van Gelder M, Eikema DJ, et al. Outcomes of haploidentical stem cell transplantation for chronic lymphocytic leukemia: a retrospective study on behalf of the chronic malignancies working party of the EBMT. Bone Marrow Transplant. 2018;53:255–63.

Diffuse Large B-Cell Lymphoma

85

Norbert Schmitz, Matthias Stelljes,
and Ali Bazarbachi

85.1 Definition and Epidemiology

Diffuse large B-cell lymphoma (DLBCL) is a neoplasm of morphologically medium to large B-lymphoid cells. The most recent WHO classification of tumors of hematopoietic and lymphoid tissues (Swerdlow et al. 2017) divides DLBCL into DLBCL, NOS with distinct morphological (centroblastic, immunoblastic, anaplastic, rare) and molecular (germinal center B-cell, activated B-cell) subtypes, other lymphomas of large B cells, high-grade B-cell lymphoma (with MYC and BCL2 and/or BCL6 rearrangements or NOS), and B-cell lymphoma, unclassifiable.

With some important exceptions, diagnostic work-up and treatment are identical in all DLBCL subtypes. It is beyond the scope of this article to fully describe the exceptions; we mention the most important differences but otherwise focus on transplantation for patients with relapsed/refractory DLBCL.

DLBCL is the most frequent lymphoma subtype and accounts for approximately one third of newly diagnosed lymphoma cases worldwide. In Europe, the 10-year prevalence of DLBCL is estimated at 43.3 per 100,000 per year (Smith et al. 2015); the age-adjusted incidence rate of DLBCL reported by the US Surveillance, Epidemiology, and End Results (SEER) program is 7.14/100,000 person-years (Howlader et al. 2017). The disease is slightly more frequent in men than in women; it mostly is a disease of the elderly (median patient age beyond 60 years) but can occur also in children and adolescents.

85.2 Diagnosis

The diagnosis is made according to the WHO classification from a sufficiently large surgical specimen or excisional lymph node biopsy; needle biopsies are not recommended. Beyond morphological evaluation by an experienced pathologist, determination of the immunophenotype of the malignant cells (positivity of malignant cells for CD19 and CD20 must be documented because of its therapeutic consequences) and determination of the cell of origin by adequate molecular methods are required (Swerdlow et al. 2017).

N. Schmitz · M. Stelljes
Department of Medicine A, Hematology, Oncology, Pneumonology and Hemostaseology, University Hospital Münster, Münster, Germany

A. Bazarbachi (✉)
Bone Marrow Transplantation Program, Department of Internal Medicine, American University of Beirut Medical Center, Beirut, Lebanon
e-mail: bazarbac@aub.edu.lb

E. Carreras et al. (eds.), *The EBMT Handbook*, https://doi.org/10.1007/978-3-030-02278-5_85

85.3 Classification

The large B-cell lymphomas comprise the morphological and molecular subtypes of DLBCL, NOS, high-grade B-cell lymphomas, and B-cell lymphomas, unclassifiable (see paragraph 1).

The WHO classification describes 12 other (and 1 provisional) lymphomas of large B cells. Among these, primary diffuse large B-cell lymphoma of the CNS (PCNSL), lymphomatoid granulomatosis (LG), primary mediastinal large B-cell lymphoma (PMBCL), and plasmablastic lymphoma not only show significant differences in pathogenesis and clinical manifestation but in most centers are treated different from classical DLBCL. Exact subtyping of diagnostic specimens taking into account their origin (e.g., primary cutaneous DLBCL, leg type; PCNSL; primary effusion lymphoma) is important. In order to fulfill all WHO requirements, the cell of origin (GCB- or ABC-subtype by IHC or gene expression profiling) and the presence/absence of distinct chromosomal translocations (BCL6, BCL2, MYC by FISH testing or IHC) must be determined.

85.4 Risk Factors

The International Prognostic Index (IPI) remains the most important tool in order to estimate the prognosis of patients with DLBCL (Ziepert et al. 2010). The IPI takes into account five factors (age, stage, LDH, performance status, and number of extranodal sites involved). Patients within the low (IPI 0, 1), low-intermediate (IPI 2), high-intermediate (IPI 3), and high-risk group (IPI 4, 5) can expect 3-year overall survival of 91.4%, 80.9%, 65.1%, and 59.0%, respectively, if treated with R-CHOP or one of its variants. Other clinical risk factor models (R-IPI; NCCN-IPI) (Sehn et al. 2007; Zhou et al. 2014, respectively) have been proposed, but advantages over the original IPI seem limited.

85.5 First-Line Treatment

First-line treatment of patients with DLBCL generally consists of RTX at standard dose (375 mg/sqm) in combination with CHOP (CY, DOXO, VCR, PRD) or one of its variants such as ACVBP, CHOEP, or DA-EPOCH chemotherapy. Six cycles of R-CHOP are generally used. However, the cycle number can be reduced to four without jeopardizing treatment outcome in patients with IPI 0. Patients with early disease (IPI 0 and 1) have been treated with abbreviated chemotherapy and involved-field radiotherapy (RT). Recent studies do not support a role for RT in such patients (Lamy et al. 2018). In patients with IPI 2–5, radiotherapy to bulky and extranodal disease is regularly recommended after R-CHOP in some but not in the majority of countries.

Several studies evaluated the role of consolidative high-dose therapy followed by auto-HSCT in the RTX era. The French (Gouill et al. 2007), Italian (Chiappella et al. 2017), and German (Schmitz et al. 2012) studies failed to demonstrate an advantage of auto-HSCT over conventional chemotherapy. The only American study (Stiff et al. 2013) reported an advantage of auto-HSCT in younger patients with high-risk disease (age-adjusted IPI 3); however, this study included patients treated with CHOP only and patients with T-cell lymphoma and as a consequence was underpowered in order to show a significant advantage of auto-HSCT over R-CHOP (Schmitz et al. 2014). In young patients who remain PET positive after two cycles of chemo-immunotherapy, auto-HSCT is performed in some but not in the majority of countries.

Patients with PCNSL or DLBCL with primary involvement of testicles must receive chemotherapy penetrating into the CNS.

More aggressive chemotherapies (CHOEP, DA-EPOCH, or ACVBP) in combination with RTX with or without RT are recommended in patients with PMBCL or plasmablastic lymphoma and in patients with high-intermediate and high-risk disease (Ghielmini et al. 2013; Recher et al. 2011). If patients with DLBCL of ABC subtype or rearrangement of MYC and BCL2 and/or BCL6 (double- or triple-hit lymphoma) should receive more aggressive therapy, therapy remains controversial (Friedberg 2017; Staiger et al. 2017). The same holds true for the value of targeted therapies (ibrutinib, lenalidomide, and others) given in addition to

R-CHOP. Prospective randomized studies addressing these questions have been closed but not published yet.

85.6 Second-Line Treatment

The principles of management of relapsed and refractory DLBCL are shown in Table 85.1. All chemotherapy-based salvage regimens cause hematologic toxicity in many cases necessitating RBC and platelet transfusions. Mucositis, gastrointestinal toxicities, neutropenic fever, and infections are reported in a significant proportion of patients. Nephrotoxicity, hepatotoxicity, and other non-hematologic toxicities are also observed. Failure to mobilize hematopoietic stem cells in 10–20% of cases occurs with all salvage regimens. Efficacy of different salvage options is shown in Table 85.2.

Table 85.1 Management of relapsed or refractory DLBCL

- *New biopsy*: Highly recommended in all patients with R/R DLBCL. Core biopsies acceptable
- *Radiological evaluation*: PET/CT recommended for evaluation of treatment outcome
- *Salvage therapy followed by auto-HSCT* is currently considered *standard of care* for patients with R/R DLBCL. Especially in patients with refractory disease or early relapse (within 12 months from the end of first-line therapy), results are not satisfactory
- *Allo-HSCT* should be considered in younger patients without comorbidities especially in patients with refractory disease or early relapse. Patients relapsing after auto-HSCT are candidates for allo-HSCT
- *CAR T cells* are a valid option whenever available
- *Selection of salvage therapy*: Randomized studies failed to show significant differences in terms of efficacy or toxicity with different salvage regimens. R-DHAP seems superior to R-ICE for patients with a GCB subtype (Thieblemont et al. 2011). Therefore, salvage strategies should take into account individual patient characteristics (age and comorbidities) considering potential cumulative hematologic and non-hematologic toxicity and the possibility of harvesting stem cells. Cardiac, pulmonary, renal, and liver function should be evaluated prior to treatment
- The objective of salvage chemotherapy is to induce a complete or partial response indicating that the tumor remains chemosensitive, this having a major impact on outcome after transplantation. PET negativity after salvage therapy is a surrogate marker of chemosensitivity and predicts patient outcome after auto-HSCT

Table 85.2 Response to salvage regimens

Regimens compared in prospective randomized trials	
R-DHAP (Gisselbrecht et al. 2010)	Dexamethasone, cytarabine, cisplatin ORR 62.8% (44.1%)[a], CR 28% (14.6%)[a]
GDP (Crump et al. 2014)	Gemcitabine, dexamethasone, cisplatin ORR 45.1%, CR 13.8% after 2 cycles
ICE (Gisselbrecht et al. 2010)	Ifosfamide, carboplatin, etoposide ORR 63.5%, CR 24%
Addition of new drugs (lenalidomide, ibrutinib, brentuximab vedotin, polatuzumab, other) to RTX-chemo in order to improve response rates of salvage regimens is not recommended outside clinical trials	

[a]Percentages in brackets from Crump et al. (2014)

85.7 Autologous HSCT

Autologous HSCT is still considered the standard treatment for patients with refractory or relapsed (R/R) DLBCL. In the RTX era, however, the results of salvage therapy followed by auto-HSCT are less convincing than before, and the benefit of auto-HSCT even for those patients achieving PR or CR with salvage chemotherapy and RTX is limited (Crump et al. 2014, 2017). In particular, patients with refractory disease or early relapse pretreated with RTX as part of first-line therapy rarely achieve long-term remissions after auto-HSCT. In the CORAL study, 3-year PFS for such patients was only 23% although those proceeding to auto-HSCT showed 3-year PFS of 39%. Alternative treatment, e.g., allo-HSCT, may be more adequate. EBMT indications (Sureda et al. 2015) for auto-HSCT in DLBCL are shown in Table 85.3. Auto-HSCT is generally not recommended as part of first-line therapy in DLBCL although recent data on PET-guided auto-HSCT are promising (Casasnovas et al. 2017). We discourage auto-HSCT for patients with refractory disease not responding to salvage therapy.

Table 85.3 Indications for auto-HSCT in DLBCL

Disease status	Recommendations
First complete remission	Clinical option Level of evidence I
Sensitive relapse/≥ 2nd complete response	Standard of care Level of evidence I
Refractory disease	Clinical option Level of evidence II

85.7.1 HSC Source

PBSC is used in >90% of auto-HSCT.

85.7.2 Consolidation (High-Dose Therapy)

Consolidation (high-dose therapy) should eliminate malignant cells with minimal impact on organ systems other than hematopoiesis. The choice of the preparative regimen varies and is based on institutional experience rather than evidence. The BEAM regimen typically consisting of BCNU (300 mg/m^2 × 1, day-6), VP (200 mg/m^2, days -5 to -2), Ara-C (200 mg/m^2 bid, days -5 to -2), and MEL (140 mg/kg/day ×1, days -1) is the preferred regimen in EBMT centers.

Acute toxicities of BEAM include severe mucositis, nausea and vomiting, diarrhea, hepatotoxicity, nephrotoxicity, and non-infective pulmonary complications. Late toxicities include pulmonary complications such as chronic interstitial fibrosis and decrease in lung diffusion capacity (21%), infection (30%), metabolic syndrome (17%), cardiovascular complications (12%), secondary tumors (20%), and other toxicities (20%). The most frequent cause of NRM is subsequent malignancy (12-fold increased risk compared with the general population). Late death is also attributed to cardiac toxicity (2%), pulmonary complications (2%), and other treatment-related toxicities (15%).

Other high-dose regimens have been used sometimes because of shortage of MEL or BCNU. Recent publications suggest that the BEAC (CY) and TEAM (TT) regimens show efficacy and toxicity similar to BEAM in most if not all lymphoma subtypes (Robinson et al. 2018; Sellner et al. 2016).

85.7.3 Prognostic Factors

Adverse prognostic factors for auto-HSCT identified in prospective studies include early relapse within 12 months of induction therapy, prior exposure to R, secondary age-adjusted IPI, poor performance status, and involvement of two or more extranodal sites at relapse.

85.7.4 Results of Auto-HSCT[a]

	NRM	OS at 3 years	EFS at 3 years
Gisselbrecht et al. (2012)	1.4%	51% (DHAP)	35% (DHAP)
Crump et al. (2014)	NR	39% (both arms)	26% (both arms)

[a]Results from prospective randomized studies. Differences in OS and EFS may be explained by differing patient characteristics and study design

85.7.5 Consolidation Treatment After Auto-HSCT

There are no data and no recommendation for consolidative therapy after auto-HSCT for DLBCL. In the CORAL study Gisselbrecht et al. (2012), RTX maintenance did not improve outcome.

85.7.6 Tandem Transplantation

No data from the RTX era are available.

85.7.7 Relapse After Auto-HSCT

Patients relapsing after auto-HSCT generally have a poor prognosis. Therapeutic options are limited. Data on new drugs specifically used post auto-HSCT are not available. Results of allo-HSCT after failure of auto-HSCT are reported below. CAR T cells may be a therapeutic option; however, no more than anecdotal data are available.

85.8 Allogeneic HSCT

Allo-HSCT is considered a curative treatment option for patients with DLBCL who relapse or progress after auto-HSCT. The EBMT reported on 101 such patients who had been allografted for DLBCL between 1997 and 2006; 37 patients were transplanted after MAC and 64 patients after RIC (van Kampen et al. 2011). Three-year NRM was 28.2%, relapse rate was 30.1%, PFS was 41.7%, and OS was 53.8% after 3 years. No statistically significant differences were seen between patients transplanted after MAC or RIC or patients transplanted from MRS or MUDs.

The only prospective randomized clinical trial reported so far (Glass et al. 2014) compared GVHD prophylaxis including RTX or not after MAC and allo-HSCT for R/R DLBCL. No significant difference between patients receiving or not receiving RTX in addition to standard MMF and TAC for GVHD prophylaxis was found. OS was 52% for all 82 patients randomized with significant differences between patients transplanted from a MUD or MMUD and patients receiving or not receiving ATG. For patients transplanted from matched family donors or MUD receiving ATG, OS was 64.7%. These data show that allo-HSCT is a valid alternative to any other treatment for patients relapsing after failure from auto-HSCT. Allo-HSCT should also be considered for patients with early relapse after first-line R-CHOP or similar.

85.8.1 Stem Cell Source

PBSC is the preferred stem cell source for allo-HSCT. The use of haploidentical donors has somewhat increased the use of BM in some of the series.

85.8.2 Donor Selection

In recent years, there has been a significant increase in the use of haploidentical donors for allo-HSCT after the introduction of PT-CY. Retrospective analyses from EBMT and CIBMTR (Kanate et al. 2016; Ghosh et al. 2016) suggest that allo-HSCT from HLA-identical family and URD or from haploidentical donors give comparable results. However, no prospective clinical trials comparing haploidentical donors versus HLA-identical siblings and MUD have been published so far.

85.8.3 Conditioning

RIC regimens reduce NRM after transplantation in many indications but also tend to increase RI after transplantation. Because no prospective clinical trials demonstrating the superiority of one conditioning regimen over another have been reported, the question if RIC or MAC should be preferred cannot generally be answered. Aggressive disease not completely responding to salvage therapy and high tumor are situations where MAC should strongly be considered.

85.8.4 Prognostic Factors

The most important adverse prognostic factor that impacts long-term outcome of patients being treated with allo-HSCT is disease status before the treatment. However, unlike the situation with auto-HSCT, also patients not perfectly responding to salvage therapy, e.g., patients with minor response or stable disease, may benefit from allo-HSCT.

85.8.5 The Use of Allo-HSCT in the Era of New Drugs and CAR T Cells

In contrast to the situation for other lymphomas, e.g., Hodgkin's disease, new drugs have not really affected the role and positioning of allo-HSCT in patients relapsing/progressing after auto-HSCT. Lenalidomides, ibrutinib, polatuzumab, or checkpoint inhibitors with or without chemotherapy can be used to bring more patients to transplantation. None of these drugs can substitute for allo-HSCT because remissions are mostly transient, and no cures have been achieved.

CAR T cells (Schuster et al. 2017; Neelapu et al. 2018) are an option for patients failing an autograft for DLBCL. However, results in day-to-day routine are not yet clear, and CAR T cells are not available outside clinical trials.

85.8.6 Results of Allo-HSCT

NRM	OS at 3 years	PFS at 3 years
25–35%	40–60%	30–50%

85.8.7 Disease Relapse After Allo-HSCT

Disease relapse carries a dim prognosis. Beyond DLI, therapeutic options are few, clinical trials should be actively sought, and palliative care is a reality in many cases. Checkpoint inhibitors may be an option with mixed results and risk of GVHD.

85.9 Therapeutic Algorithm Recommended by the Authors (See Fig. 85.1)

85.10 Long-Term Outcomes of Auto- and Allo-HSCT in Patients with R/R DLBCL (See Fig. 85.2)

Key Points

- In the RTX era, auto-HSCT is generally not recommended as part of first-line therapy in DLBCL although recent data on PET-guided auto-HSCT are promising. Auto-HSCT is still the standard of care for those DLBCL patients with chemosensitive first relapse. Results of auto-HSCT might improve with better

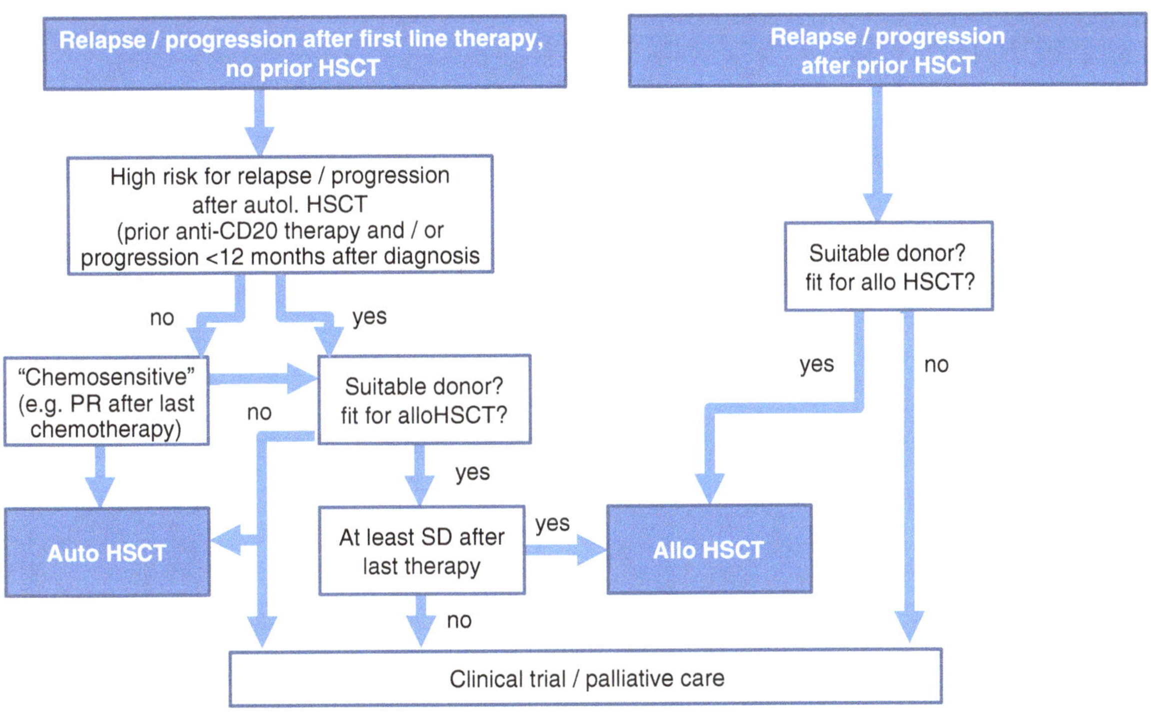

Fig. 85.1 Allogeneic and autologous HSCT in R/R lymphoma: treatment decision

selection of patients (e.g., including PET imaging for patient selection), and improved salvage strategies results.

- Allo-HSCT is the only curative treatment option for patients with refractory disease and those relapsing after auto-HSCT. Patients with early relapse (< 12 months after first-line treatment) should be considered for allo-HSCT. Conditioning should be guided by the individual clinical situation. Haploidentical transplants may substitute for unrelated donor transplants in the near future. New drugs have not really changed the treatment algorithm for DLBCL. The role of CAR T cells is under study.

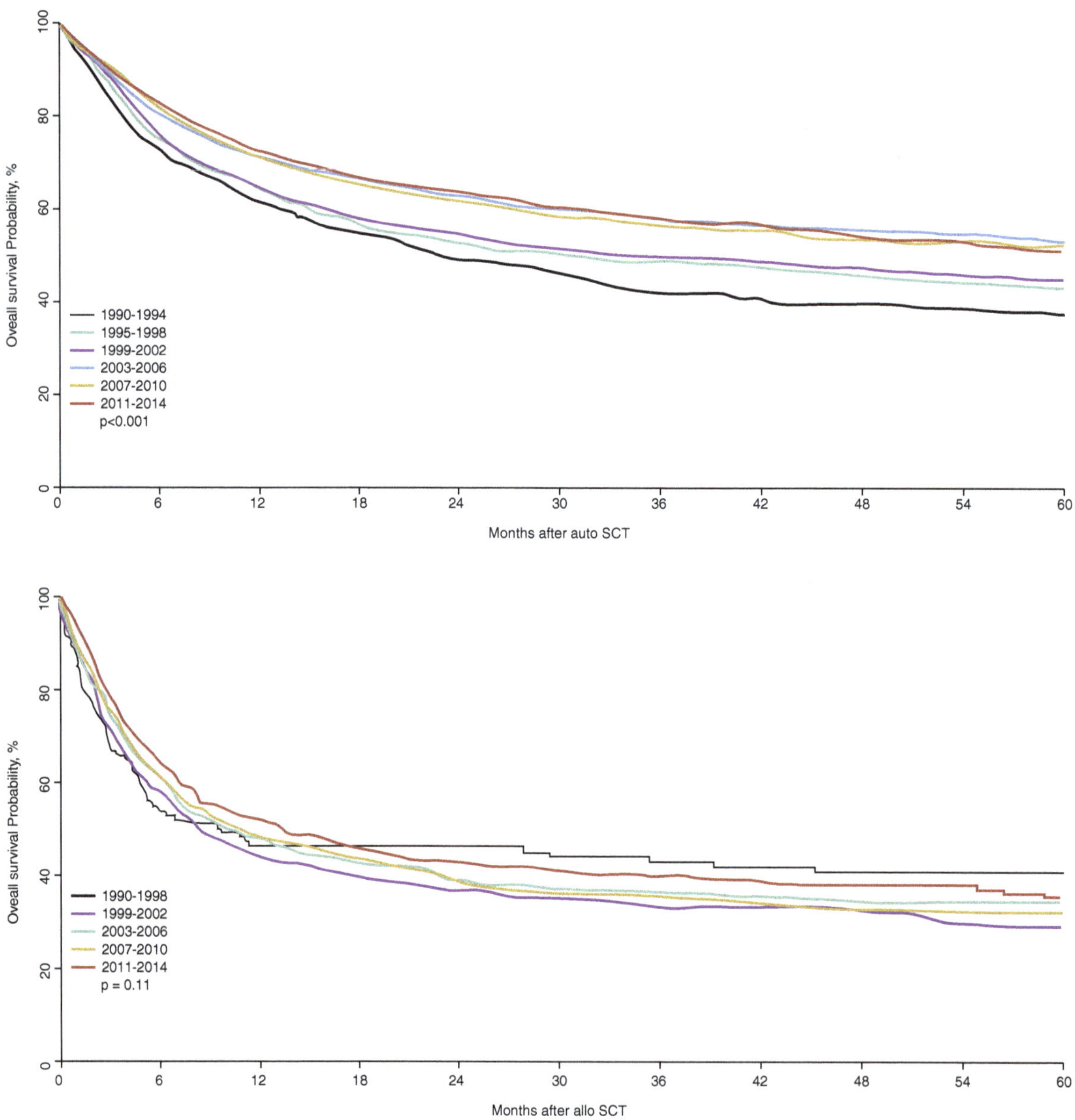

Fig. 85.2 Long-term outcomes of auto- and allo-HSCT in patients with R/R DLBCL (EBMT data base, with permission)

References

Casasnovas RO, Ysebaert L, Thieblemont C, et al. FDG-PET-driven consolidation strategy in diffuse large B-cell lymphoma: final results of a randomized phase 2 study. Blood. 2017;130:1315–26.

Chiappella A, Martelli M, Angelucci E, et al. Rituximab-dose-dense chemotherapy with or without high-dose chemotherapy plus autologous stem-cell transplantation in high-risk diffuse large B-cell lymphoma (DLCL04): final results of a multicentre, open-label, randomised, controlled, phase 3 study. Lancet Oncol. 2017;18:1076–88.

Crump M, Kuruvilla J, Couban S, et al. Randomized comparison of gemcitabine, dexamethasone, and cisplatin versus dexamethasone, cytarabine, and cisplatin chemotherapy before autologous stem-cell transplantation for relapsed and refractory aggressive lymphomas: NCIC-CTG LY.12. J Clin Oncol. 2014;32:3490–6.

Crump M, Neelapu SS, Farooq U, et al. Outcomes in refractory diffuse large B-cell lymphoma: results from the international SCHOLAR-1 study. Blood. 2017;130:1800–8.

Friedberg JW. How I treat double-hit lymphoma. Blood. 2017;130:590–6.

Ghielmini M, Vitolo U, Kimby E, et al. ESMO Guidelines consensus conference on malignant lymphoma 2011 part 1: diffuse large B-cell lymphoma (DLBCL), follicular lymphoma (FL) and chronic lymphocytic leukemia (CLL). Ann Oncol. 2013;24:561–76.

Ghosh N, Karmali R, Rocha V, et al. Reduced-intensity transplantation for lymphomas using haploidentical related donors versus HLA-matched sibling donors: a Center for International Blood and Marrow Transplant Research Analysis. J Clin Oncol. 2016;34:3141–9.

Gisselbrecht C, Glass B, Mounier N, et al. Salvage regimens with autologous transplantation for relapsed large B-cell lymphoma in the rituximab era. J Clin Oncol. 2010;28:4184–90.

Gisselbrecht C, Schmitz N, Mounier N, et al. Rituximab maintenance therapy after autologous stem-cell transplantation in patients with relapsed CD20 (+) diffuse large B-cell lymphoma: final analysis of the collaborative trial in relapsed aggressive lymphoma. J Clin Oncol. 2012;30:4462–9.

Glass B, Hasenkamp J, Wulf G, et al. Rituximab after lymphoma-directed conditioning and allogeneic stem-cell transplantation for relapsed and refractory aggressive non-Hodgkin lymphoma (DSHNHL R3): an open-label, randomised, phase 2 trial. Lancet Oncol. 2014;15:757–66.

Gouill SL, Milpied N, Buzyn A, et al. Allogeneic stem cell transplantation (allo-SCT) in T-cell lymphomas: a French national survey from the Société Française de Greffe de Moelle et de Thérapie Cellulaire (SFGM-TC). J Clin Oncol. 2007;25:8095.

Howlader N, Noone A, Krapcho M, Miller D, et al., editors. SEER cancer statistics review, 1975-2014. Bethesda, MD: National Cancer Institute; 2017.

Kanate AS, Mussetti A, Kharfan-Dabaja MA, et al. Reduced-intensity transplantation for lymphomas using haploidentical related donors vs HLA-matched unrelated donors. Blood. 2016;127:938–47.

Lamy T, Damaj G, Soubeyran P, et al. R-CHOP 14 with or without radiotherapy in nonbulky limited-stage diffuse large B-cell lymphoma. Blood. 2018;131:174–81.

Neelapu SS, Locke FL, Go WY. CAR T-cell therapy in large B-cell lymphoma. N Engl J Med. 2018;378:1065.

Recher C, Coiffier B, Haioun C, et al. Intensified chemotherapy with ACVBP plus rituximab versus standard CHOP plus rituximab for the treatment of diffuse large B-cell lymphoma (LNH03-2B): an open-label randomised phase 3 trial. Lancet. 2011;378:1858–67.

Robinson SP, Boumendil A, Finel H, et al. High-dose therapy with BEAC conditioning compared to BEAM conditioning prior to autologous stem cell transplantation for non-Hodgkin lymphoma: no differences in toxicity or outcome. A matched-control study of the EBMT-Lymphoma Working Party. Bone Marrow Transplant. 2018. https://doi.org/10.1038/s41409-018-0196-3. [Epub ahead of print].

Schmitz N, Nickelsen M, Ziepert M, et al. Conventional chemotherapy (CHOEP-14) with rituximab or high-dose chemotherapy (MegaCHOEP) with rituximab for young, high-risk patients with aggressive B-cell lymphoma: an open-label, randomised, phase 3 trial (DSHNHL 2002-1). Lancet Oncol. 2012;13:1250–9.

Schmitz N, Ziepert M, Vitolo U, et al. The role of myeloablation for lymphoma. N Engl J Med. 2014;370:574–5.

Schuster SJ, Svoboda J, Chong EA, et al. Chimeric antigen receptor T cells in refractory B-cell lymphomas. N Engl J Med. 2017;377:2545–54.

Sehn LH, Berry B, Chhanabhai M, et al. The revised International Prognostic Index (R-IPI) is a better predictor of outcome than the standard IPI for patients with diffuse large B-cell lymphoma treated with R-CHOP. Blood. 2007;109:1857–61.

Sellner L, Boumendil A, Finel H, et al. Thiotepa-based high-dose therapy for autologous stem cell transplantation in lymphoma: a retrospective study from the EBMT. Bone Marrow Transplant. 2016;51:212–8.

Smith A, Crouch S, Lax S, et al. Lymphoma incidence, survival and prevalence 2004-2014: sub-type analyses from the UK's Haematological Malignancy Research Network. Br J Cancer. 2015;112:1575–84.

Staiger AM, Ziepert M, Horn H, et al. Clinical impact of the cell-of-origin classification and the MYC/ BCL2 dual expresser status in diffuse large B-cell lymphoma treated within prospective clinical trials of the German High-Grade Non-Hodgkin's Lymphoma Study Group. J Clin Oncol. 2017;35:2515–26.

Stiff PJ, Unger JM, Cook JR, et al. Autologous transplantation as consolidation for aggressive non-Hodgkin's lymphoma. N Engl J Med. 2013;369:1681–90.

Sureda A, Bader P, Cesaro S, et al. Indications for allo- and auto-SCT for haematological diseases, solid tumours and immune disorders: current practice in Europe, 2015. Bone Marrow Transplant. 2015;50:1037–56.

Swerdlow SH, Campo E, Harris NL et al. WHO classification of tumours of haematopoietic and lymphoid tissues. 4th ed (revised). Lyon: IARC; 2017.

Thieblemont C, Briere J, Mounier N, et al. The germinal center/activated B-cell subclassification has a prognostic impact for response to salvage therapy in relapsed/refractory diffuse large B-cell lymphoma: a bio-CORAL study. J Clin Oncol. 2011;29: 4079–87.

van Kampen RJ, Canals C, Schouten HC, et al. Allogeneic stem-cell transplantation as salvage therapy for patients with diffuse large B-cell non-Hodgkin's lymphoma relapsing after an autologous stem-cell transplantation: an analysis of the European Group for Blood and Marrow Transplantation Registry. J Clin Oncol. 2011;29:1342–8.

Zhou Z, Sehn LH, Rademaker AW, et al. An enhanced International Prognostic Index (NCCN-IPI) for patients with diffuse large B-cell lymphoma treated in the rituximab era. Blood. 2014;123:837–42.

Ziepert M, Hasenclever D, Kuhnt E, et al. Standard International prognostic index remains a valid predictor of outcome for patients with aggressive CD20+ B-cell lymphoma in the rituximab era. J Clin Oncol. 2010;28:2373–80.

86 Mantle Cell Lymphoma

Sascha Dietrich

86.1 Introduction

Mantle cell lymphoma (MCL) is an aggressive B-cell lymphoma, which is characterized by the chromosomal translocation t(11;14)(q13;q32) and overexpression of cyclin D1 in the vast majority of cases. Most patients present with advanced stage disease, often with extra-nodal dissemination, and an unfavourable clinical course. Treatment with conventional chemotherapy resulted in unsatisfactory outcomes and a median survival of less than 3 years after diagnosis of MCL (Zucca et al. 1995).

86.2 Autologous HSCT

During recent years, the prognosis of patients with MCL has improved considerably, and the refinement of dose-intensified approaches such as auto-HSCT has contributed significantly to this development. A prospective randomized trial by the European Mantle Cell Lymphoma Network (EMCLN) has demonstrated the superiority of auto-HSCT consolidation over interferon maintenance (Dreyling et al. 2005) in the pre-RTX era. The introduction of RTX and the addition of high-dose cytarabine (HD-ARAC) to the induction treatment before auto-HSCT have further improved PFS and OS of MCL patients (Geisler et al. 2008). The benefit of high-dose HD-ARAC before auto-HSCT could be confirmed in prospective clinical trial (Hermine et al. 2016). RTX- and HD-ARAC-based induction treatment followed by auto-HSCT is therefore recommended as a first-line treatment standard for young and fit MCL patients (Cheah et al. 2016; Dreyling et al. 2017).

Although a significant proportion of patients with MCL enjoy long-term disease control after auto-HSCT, relapse remains the main cause of treatment failure. The prognosis of patients with MCL recurrence after auto-HSCT appears to be extremely poor, especially if occurring early after transplant (Dietrich et al. 2011; Dietrich et al. 2014a). A proportion of almost 40% of MCL patients relapsing after auto-HSCT were reported to suffer from chemotherapy-refractory disease (Dietrich et al. 2014a) with a high prevalence of clonal TP53 mutations (Halldorsdottir et al. 2011). In order to prevent these refractory courses, treatment strategies, which effectively reduce the risk of relapse after ASCT, are warranted.

Retrospective studies suggested a significantly improved outcome with RTX maintenance subsequent to high-dose chemotherapy and auto-HSCT for patients with MCL (Dietrich et al. 2014b; Graf et al. 2015). The French study group conducted a prospective randomized phase III trial (LyMa trial) that investigated RTX maintenance versus

S. Dietrich (✉)
Department of Hematology, University Hospital of Heidelberg, Heidelberg, Germany
e-mail: sascha.dietrich@med.uni-heidelberg.de

E. Carreras et al. (eds.), *The EBMT Handbook*, https://doi.org/10.1007/978-3-030-02278-5_86

observation after auto-HSCT in previously untreated MCL patients. Final results of the LyMa trial confirmed the superiority of RTX maintenance with regard to PFS and OS (Le Gouill et al. 2017). The beneficial effect of RTX maintenance was observed in both PET-positive and PET-negative patients after induction treatment prior to auto-HSCT (Mei et al. 2017). This finding implies that the benefit of RTX maintenance after auto-HSCT is present for low- and high-risk MCL patients.

86.3 Allogeneic HSCT

In a large EBMT) registry study, which investigated the outcome of MCL patients after first-line auto-HSCT failure, 24% of all MCL patients received a rescue consolidation HSCT. Only a minority of 2% received a second auto-HSCT of whom only one patient experienced a long-term survival. These limited results do not justify a rescue auto-HSCT as reasonable salvage strategy in this situation. In contrast, the majority of patients who received a second HSCT underwent allo-HSCT, and a significant proportion of them achieved a durable remission, translating into a 3-year OS of 43% (Dietrich et al. 2014a). Other registry studies and single-centre experiences report similar results (Cook et al. 2010; Tam et al. 2009; Le Gouill et al. 2012).

Long-term efficacy of RIC allo-HSCT was recently demonstrated in a large cohort of MCL patients (Robinson et al. 2018). The cumulative incidence of relapse was 40% at 5 years, and OS was 40% at 5 years. Patients who developed a chronic GVHD and/or patients who did not receive an in vivo TCD with CAMPATH had a significantly lower relapse rate, suggesting the existence of a graft versus MCL effect. Despite long-term remissions after allo-HSCT, chemo-refractory disease (Robinson et al. 2018) or early relapse after first-line auto-HSCT (Dietrich et al. 2014a) significantly reduced the long-term survival of MCL patients after allo-HSCT. Chemotherapy-free salvage treatments are obvious options for these highly refractory patients. A recent EBMT survey suggested that ibrutinib may improve the perspective of refractory patients scheduled for allo-HSCT (Dreger et al. 2018). It is important to note that there is a small group of relapsed MCL patients who survived longer than 5 years even without allo-HSCT, suggesting a rather indolent disease course in a subset of patients (Dietrich et al. 2014a). Such patients with a low percentage of Ki67-positive tumour cells might not benefit from an allo-HSCT.

Key Points

- First-line auto-HSCT and RTX maintenance is currently challenged against auto-HSCT with ibrutinib maintenance or a transplant-free approach with ibrutinib and chemotherapy in an EMCLN study (TRIANGLE).
- As long as we await these data to redefine the value of auto-HSCT in the ibrutinib era, auto-HSCT and RTX maintenance should be recommended as the standard treatment for transplant-eligible patients with MCL.
- A second auto-HSCT does not appear to be a promising option in patients with MCL failing a first auto-HSCT. For these patients allo-HSCT should be considered.

References

Cheah CY, Seymour JF, Wang ML. Mantle cell lymphoma. J Clin Oncol. 2016;34:1256–69.

Cook G, Smith GM, Kirkland K, et al. Outcome following Reduced-Intensity Allogeneic Stem Cell Transplantation (RIC AlloSCT) for relapsed and refractory mantle cell lymphoma (MCL): a study of the British Society for Blood and Marrow Transplantation. Biol Blood Marrow Transplant. 2010;16:1419–27.

Dietrich S, Tielesch B, Rieger M, et al. Patterns and outcome of relapse after autologous stem cell transplantation for mantle cell lymphoma. Cancer. 2011;117:1901–10.

Dietrich S, Boumendil A, Finel H, et al. Outcome and prognostic factors in patients with mantle-cell lymphoma relapsing after autologous stem-cell transplantation: a retrospective study of the European Group for Blood and Marrow Transplantation (EBMT). Ann Oncol. 2014a;25:1053–8.

Dietrich S, Weidle J, Rieger M, et al. Rituximab maintenance therapy after autologous stem cell transplantation prolongs progression-free survival in patients with mantle cell lymphoma. Leukemia. 2014b;28:708–9.

Dreger P, Michelet M, Bosman P, et al. Ibrutinib for bridging to allogeneic stem cell transplantation (alloHCT) in chronic lymphocytic leukemia (CLL) and mantle cell lymphoma (MCL) is safe and effective update results of a study by the EBMT Chronic Malignancy and the Lymphoma Working Parties, the French Cooperative Group for CLL and the Société Française de Greffe de Moelle et de Therapie Cellulaire (SFGM-TC). Bone Marrow Transplant. 2018. https://doi.org/10.1038/s41409-018-0207-4. [Epub ahead of print].

Dreyling M, Lenz G, Hoster E, et al. Early consolidation by myeloablative radiochemotherapy followed by autologous stem cell transplantation in first remission significantly prolongs progression-free survival in mantle-cell lymphoma: results of a prospective randomized trial of the European MCL Network. Blood. 2005;105:2677–84.

Dreyling M, Campo E, Hermine O, et al. Newly diagnosed and relapsed mantle cell lymphoma: ESMO Clinical Practice Guidelines for diagnosis, treatment and follow-up. Ann Oncol. 2017;28:iv62–71.

Geisler CH, Kolstad A, Laurell A, et al. Long-term progression-free survival of mantle cell lymphoma after intensive front-line immunochemotherapy with in vivo-purged stem cell rescue: a nonrandomized phase 2 multicenter study by the Nordic Lymphoma Group. Blood. 2008;112:2687–93.

Graf SA, Stevenson PA, Holmberg LA, et al. Maintenance rituximab after autologous stem cell transplantation in patients with mantle cell lymphoma. Ann Oncol. 2015;26:2323–8.

Halldorsdottir AM, Lundin A, Murray F, et al. Impact of TP53 mutation and 17p deletion in mantle cell lymphoma. Leukemia. 2011;25:1904–8.

Hermine O, Hoster E, Walewski J, et al. Addition of high-dose cytarabine to immunochemotherapy before autologous stem-cell transplantation in patients aged 65 years or younger with mantle cell lymphoma (MCL Younger): a randomised, open-label, phase 3 trial of the European Mantle Cell Lymphoma Network. Lancet. 2016;388:565–75.

Le Gouill S, Kroger N, Dhedin N, et al. Reduced-intensity conditioning allogeneic stem cell transplantation for relapsed/refractory mantle cell lymphoma: a multicenter experience. Ann Oncol. 2012;23:2695–703.

Le Gouill S, Thieblemont C, Oberic L, et al. Rituximab after autologous stem-cell transplantation in mantle-cell lymphoma. N Engl J Med. 2017;377:1250–60.

Mei MG, Cao TM, Chen L, et al. Long-term results of high-dose therapy and autologous stem cell transplantation for mantle cell lymphoma: effectiveness of maintenance rituximab. Biol Blood Marrow Transplant. 2017;23:1861–9.

Robinson SP, Boumendil A, Finel H, et al. Long-term outcome analysis of reduced-intensity allogeneic stem cell transplantation in patients with mantle cell lymphoma: a retrospective study from the EBMT Lymphoma Working Party. Bone Marrow Transplant. 2018;53:617–24.

Tam CS, Bassett R, Ledesma C, et al. Mature results of the M. D. Anderson Cancer Center risk-adapted transplantation strategy in mantle cell lymphoma. Blood. 2009;113:4144–52.

Zucca E, Roggero E, Pinotti G, et al. Patterns of survival in mantle cell lymphoma. Ann Oncol. 1995;6:257–62.

87 Other T- and B-Aggressive Lymphomas and Lymphomas Associated with HIV

Kai Hübel and Silvia Montoto

87.1 Burkitt Lymphoma (BL)

87.1.1 Definition and Epidemiology

BL accounts for around 2% of all adult NHL with a higher incidence in patients with immunodeficiency and in patients who are HIV positive. There is an endemic pediatric subtype in Equatorial Africa which is strongly associated with EBV. The clinical course of BL usually is highly aggressive with a Ki67 expression of nearly 100% requiring prompt institution of therapy.

87.1.2 Diagnosis

A tissue biopsy/cytology sample is mandatory for the diagnosis. The hallmark of the tumor is the rearrangement of a gene encoding MYC, but the diagnosis requires a combination of morphology, immunophenotype, and genetic analysis.

K. Hübel (✉)
Department I of Internal Medicine, University of Cologne, Cologne, Germany
e-mail: kai.huebel@uni-koeln.de

S. Montoto
Department of Haemato-Oncology, St. Bartholomew's and The Royal London NHS Trust, Queen Mary University of London, London, UK

87.1.3 Risk Factors

Several studies have identified risk factors for poor outcome. Beside older age, advanced stage, and comorbidities, such risk factors are an elevated serum LDH, failure to achieve CR, anemia, CNS involvement, and BM infiltration.

87.1.4 First-Line Treatment

The optimal first-line therapy in BL has not been defined yet. To achieve a fast and stable remission, an intensive regimen combining several compounds is used in most centers. Combinations of RTX, doxorubicin (DOX), alkylators, VCR, and VP with direct therapy to prevent CNS disease are highly active.

The HOVON CODOX-M/IVAC regimen (CY, DOX, VCR, MTX, IFO, Ara-C, and VP) achieved a 2-year EFS of 65% and a 2-year OS of 73% and is very active especially in high-risk patients (Mead et al. 2002).

The B-ALL protocol (MTX, Ara-C, CY, VP, IFO) of the German GMALL study group achieved a CR in 88% of patients, with a 5-year PFS of 71% and a 5-year OS of 80% (Hoelzer et al. 2014). This means that a significant portion of patients have a chance to get cured with first-line therapy.

Recently, using modifications of R-EPOCH (RTX, VP, VCR, CY, DOX), high activity in BL was reported (Roschewski et al. 2017).

E. Carreras et al. (eds.), *The EBMT Handbook*, https://doi.org/10.1007/978-3-030-02278-5_87

87.1.5 Autologous HSCT

There are several studies exploring the role of auto-HSCT in first remission. In a prospective trial, the HOVON group treated 27 patients with 2 cycles of intensive induction followed by BEAM-conditioned auto-HSCT for those patients achieving at least a PR (van Imhoff et al. 2005). The 5-year EFS and OS was 73% and 81%, respectively. In a retrospective analysis of 117 patients receiving auto-HSCT as part of first-line therapy between 1984 and 1994, patients in CR at time of transplant had a 3-year OS of 72% (Sweetenham et al. 1996). In the relapse situation, patients who were chemotherapy-sensitive had a 3-year OS of 37% following auto-HSCT compared to just 7% for those who were chemotherapy resistant (Sweetenham et al. 1996). In summary, auto-HSCT in BL is feasible, but there is no documented advantage compared to standard combination chemotherapy for patients responding sufficiently to first-line treatment. Auto-HSCT may be used to optimize remission in patients with insufficient response or as bridging to allo-HSCT. In the relapse setting, given the intensive regimens usually used as first-line treatment, the difficulty lies in achieving a response good enough to proceed to auto-HSCT and to collect HSC; hence, auto-HSCT is rarely used in BL.

87.1.6 Allogeneic HSCT (Peniket et al. 2003)

Indicated in	CR ≥ 2
Donor	MRS > MUD > MMUD
Conditioning	RIC > MAC
TRM (1 year)	30%
OS (5 year)	30–40%
DFS	35%

87.2 Lymphoblastic Lymphoma (LBL)

87.2.1 Definition and Epidemiology

LBL is an aggressive neoplasm of precursor B cells (B-LBL) or T cells (T-LBL) with features of acute leukemia. It accounts for approximately 2% of all NHL. In adults, around 90% of all LBL are T-LBL.

87.2.2 Diagnosis

The diagnosis is based on a LN biopsy. T-LBL is usually TdT-positive with a variable expression of other T-cell markers (CD7 and CD3 are often positive).

87.2.3 Risk Factors

At this time, no convincing prognostic model for these patients is available. Several studies tried to identify risk factors; the following may be associated with an unfavorable outcome: elevated LDH, BM or CNS involvement, and stage IV disease. The role of MRD in LBL has not been defined yet, but as we learned from acute leukemias and other lymphomas, persisted MRD positivity might be a predictor of poor outcome.

87.2.4 First-Line Treatment

Standard approaches for patients with LBL are adapted to ALL protocols. These regimens contain multiple drugs, such as CY, MTX, VCR, Ara-C, thioguanine, L-asp, VP, nitrosoureas, and anthracyclines. With these protocols, a CR rate of 80% and a DFS of 56% have been reported (Estey et al. 2008).

87.2.5 Autologous HSCT

There are only very few studies evaluating the role of auto-HSCT in LBL. In CR1, the use of auto-HSCT as a consolidation may improve relapse-free survival but has no effect on OS (Sweetenham et al. 2001). In another study in 128 patients with LBL receiving auto-HSCT, RR at 5 years was 56% (Levine et al. 2003). No documented role in more advanced disease >CR1 is reported either. In conclusion, data for auto-HSCT in LBL are too scarce to come to firm conclusions.

87.2.6 Allogeneic HSCT

There is also no established role for allo-HSCT in patients with LBL. Compared to auto-HSCT, allo- HSCT is associated with a higher TRM but lower RR. In 76 patients receiving allo-HSCT, 5-year RR was 34% (Levine et al. 2003). In this retrospective study, there was no significant difference in OS at 1 year and 5 years between auto-HSCT and allo-HSCT. In general, the indication for allo-HSCT should be based on risk factors, remission, and MRD.

87.3 Peripheral T-Cell Lymphomas (PTCLs)

87.3.1 Definition and Epidemiology

PTCLs are a very heterogeneous group of lymphomas originating from the T-cell lineage. They account for approximately 10–15% of all NHL. Because of this low incidence, large randomized studies are difficult to perform.

87.3.2 Diagnosis

The diagnosis, as in any NHL, should be based on a LN biopsy. The differential diagnosis between PTCL and other types of T-NHL is crucial for the outcomes, and in some specific cases, the treatments are very different.

87.3.3 Risk Factors

The IPI is the most commonly used prognostic tool in PTCL. The following factors are associated with worse outcome: age >60 years, ECOG >1, elevated LDH, stages II–IV, and extranodal involvement >1 site. In anaplastic large cell lymphoma (ALCL), the tumors are categorized in ALK+ or ALK- with better prognosis for ALK+ lymphomas.

87.3.4 First-Line Treatment

The primary goal of first-line treatment is to get a deep and continuing remission. Standard regimens are anthracycline-containing combinations like CHOP or CHOEP, achieving a 3-year EFS of 50–70% and a 3-year OS of 75–80% (Schmitz et al. 2010). In the relapse situation, the overall prognosis of PTLC is dismal, and the optimal treatment for these patients has not been defined yet. Relapse patients not able to receive intensive treatment including HSCT may be offered single-agent therapy, e.g., gemcitabine, or in case of CD30 expression, brentuximab vedotin.

87.3.5 Autologous HSCT (Kyriakou et al. 2008; d'Amore et al. 2012; Kewalramani et al. 2006; Wilhelm et al. 2016)

Indicated in	CR1 (IPI > 1), CR ≥ 2
Conditioning	BEAC, BEAM, LEAM, CBV
TRM (1 year)	5–7%
REL (3 years)	40–50%
OS (5 years)	70% (CR1), 50% (CR≥2)
PFS (5 years)	50 % (CR1), 20–35% (CR≥2)

87.3.6 Allogeneic HSCT (Schmitz et al. 2014, 2018; Dodero et al. 2012)

Indicated in	CR ≥ 2, relapse post auto-HSCT
Donor	MRS > MUD > MMUD
Conditioning	RIC > MAC
GVHD prophylaxis	CSA, CSA-MTX, CSA-MMF
Graft failure	<10%
TRM (1 year)	20–25%
REL (3 years)	20–40%
OS (3 years)	40–60%
PFS (3 years)	30–50%

87.4 HIV-Associated Lymphomas

87.4.1 Definition and Epidemiology

Patients infected with HIV have an increased risk of developing NHLs as compared to the general population. The most frequent subtypes are

DLBCL and BL. Both are AIDS-defining illnesses, while HL is one of the non-AIDS-defining malignancies.

87.4.2 Risk Factors

In the era of combined antiretroviral therapy (cART), the risk factors that determine prognosis in patients with HIV-related lymphoma are the same as in the general population and, hence, depend on the subtype of lymphoma, rather than on HIV-related factors.

87.4.3 First-Line Therapy

The optimal therapy for these patients has not been defined yet, but since the availability of cART, the outcome of HIV-lymphoma has considerably improved. The consequent use of cART during therapy is of major importance for successful treatment. In first-line treatment, patients will receive treatment comparable with HIV-negative patients. The indication for HSCT has to be discussed in the relapse situation.

87.4.4 Autologous HSCT (Hübel et al. 2017; Diez-Martin et al. 2009; Balsalobre et al. 2009)

Indicated in	CR ≥ 2; same indications as in the general population with the same type of lymphoma
Conditioning	BEAC, BEAM, LEAM, CBV
TRM (1 year)	5–7%
REL (3 years)	30–40%
OS (5 years)	50–60%
PFS (5 years)	50–60%

87.4.5 Allogeneic HSCT

Experience on the use of allo-HSCT in patients with lymphoma and HIV infection is very limited, and no definitive recommendation can be given at this time. There are some case reports or small retrospective analysis showing that allo-HSCT in HIV-positive patients using MRD, MUD, or CB is feasible, but application of cART and viroimmunological reconstitution is a matter of debate. In a recent report of five HIV-positive patients who underwent allo-HSCT with various hematologic malignancies, there was no TRM or major infections (Mulanovich et al. 2016). HIV virus load remained undetectable with continuous cART. Three patients relapsed 6, 7, and 13 months after transplant, and two were alive and well after 42 and 55 months.

References

Balsalobre P, Diez-Martin JL, Re A, et al. Autologous stem-cell transplantation in patients with HIV-related lymphoma. J Clin Oncol. 2009;27:2192–8.

d'Amore F, Relander T, Lauritzsen GF, et al. Up-front autologous stem-cell transplantation in peripheral T-cell lymphoma: NLG-T-01. J Clin Oncol. 2012;30:3093–9.

Diez-Martin JL, Balsalobre P, Re A, et al. Comparable survival between HIV+ and HIV- non-Hodgkin and Hodgkin lymphoma patients undergoing autologous peripheral blood stem cell transplantation. Blood. 2009;113:6011–4.

Dodero A, Spina F, Narni F, et al. Allogeneic transplantation following a reduced-intensity conditioning regimen in relapsed/refractory peripheral T-cell lymphomas: long-term remissions and response to donor lymphocyte infusions support the role of a graft-versus-lymphoma effect. Leukemia. 2012;26:520–6.

Estey EH, Faderl SH, Kantarjian H. Acute leukemias. Berlin: Springer; 2008. p. 167–76.

Hoelzer D, Walewski J, Dohner H, et al. Improved outcome of adult Burkitt lymphoma/leukemia with rituximab and chemotherapy: report of a large prospective multicenter trial. Blood. 2014;124:3870–9.

Hübel K, Re A, Boumendil A, Finel H, Hentrich M. HIV-associated lymphoma and autologous stem cell transplantation in the rituximab era: a retrospective analysis on indication, outcome and risk factors by the EBMT Lymphoma Working Party. Bone Marrow Transplant. 2017;52(S1):141.

Kewalramani T, Zelenetz AD, Teruya-Feldstein J, et al. Autologous transplantation for relapsed or primary refractory peripheral T-cell lymphoma. Br J Haematol. 2006;134:202–7.

Kyriakou C, Canals C, Goldstone A, et al. High-dose therapy and autologous stem-cell transplantation in angioimmunoblastic lymphoma: complete remission at transplantation is the major determinant of

Outcome-Lymphoma Working Party of the European Group for Blood and Marrow Transplantation. J Clin Oncol. 2008;26:218–24.
Levine JE, Harris RE, Loberiza FR Jr, et al. A comparison of allogeneic and autologous bone marrow transplantation for lymphoblastic lymphoma. Blood. 2003;101:2476–82.
Mead GM, Sydes MR, Walewski J, et al. An international evaluation of CODOX-M and CODOX-M alternating with IVAC in adult Burkitt's lymphoma: results of United Kingdom Lymphoma Group LY06 study. Ann Oncol. 2002;13:1264–74.
Mulanovich VE, Desai PA, Popat UR. Allogeneic stem cell transplantation for HIV-positive patients with hematologic malignancies. AIDS. 2016;30:2653–7.
Peniket AJ, Ruiz de Elvira MC, et al. An EBMT registry matched study of allogeneic stem cell transplants for lymphoma: allogeneic transplantation is associated with a lower relapse rate but a higher procedure-related mortality rate than autologous transplantation. Bone Marrow Transplant. 2003;31:667–78.
Roschewski M, Dunleavy K, Abramson JS, Link BK. Risk-adapted therapy in adults with Burkitt lymphoma: results of NCI 9177, a multicenter prospective phase II study of DA-EPOCH-R. Blood. 2017;130(Suppl 1):188.
Schmitz N, Trumper L, Ziepert M, et al. Treatment and prognosis of mature T-cell and NK-cell lymphoma: an analysis of patients with T-cell lymphoma treated in studies of the German High-Grade Non-Hodgkin Lymphoma Study Group. Blood. 2010;116:3418–25.
Schmitz N, Wu HS, Glass B. Allogeneic transplantation in T-cell lymphomas. Semin Hematol. 2014;51:67–72.
Schmitz N, Lenz G, Stelljes M. Allogeneic hematopoietic stem cell transplantation (HSCT) for T-cell lymphomas. Blood. 2018. https://doi.org/10.1182/blood-2018-01-791335. [Epub ahead of print].
Sweetenham JW, Pearce R, Taghipour G, et al. Adult Burkitt's and Burkitt-like non-Hodgkin's lymphoma—outcome for patients treated with high-dose therapy and autologous stem-cell transplantation in first remission or at relapse: results from the European Group for Blood and Marrow Transplantation. J Clin Oncol. 1996;14:2465–72.
Sweetenham JW, Santini G, Qian W, et al. High-dose therapy and autologous stem-cell transplantation versus conventional-dose consolidation/maintenance therapy as postremission therapy for adult patients with lymphoblastic lymphoma: results of a randomized trial of the European Group for Blood and Marrow Transplantation and the United Kingdom Lymphoma Group. J Clin Oncol. 2001;19:2927–36.
van Imhoff GW, van der Holt B, MacKenzie MA, et al. Short intensive sequential therapy followed by autologous stem cell transplantation in adult Burkitt, Burkitt-like and lymphoblastic lymphoma. Leukemia. 2005;19:945–52.
Wilhelm M, Smetak M, Reimer P, et al. First-line therapy of peripheral T-cell lymphoma: extension and long-term follow-up of a study investigating the role of autologous stem cell transplantation. Blood Cancer J. 2016;6:e452.

88 Classical Hodgkin's Lymphoma

Anna Sureda and Carmen Martínez

88.1 Definition and Epidemiology

HL is a malignancy arising from germinal centre or post-germinal centre B cells. The cancer cells form a minority of the tumour and are surrounded by a reactive inflammatory milieu comprising lymphocytes, eosinophils, neutrophils, histiocytes and plasma cells. These malignant cells can be pathognomonic, multinucleate giant cells or large mononuclear cells and, together, are referred to as Hodgkin and Reed-Sternberg (HRS) cells.

HL accounts for approximately 10% of cases of newly diagnosed lymphoma. The incidence of HL in Europe is 2.2 per 100,000 per year with a mortality rate of 0.7 cases/100,000 a year. The disease is more frequent in men than in women, and peaks in incidence are noted in young adults and in people older than 60 years. Incidence has remained mostly unchanged during the past two decades.

A. Sureda (✉)
Hematology Department and Stem Cell Transplantation Program, Institut Català d'Oncologia – Hospitalet, Barcelona, Catalunya, Spain
e-mail: asureda@iconcologia.net

C. Martínez
HSCT Unit, Department of Hematology, Institute of Hematology and Oncology, Hospital Clínic de Barcelona, Universitat de Barcelona, Barcelona, Spain

88.2 Diagnosis

Pathological diagnosis should be made according to the WHO classification from a sufficiently large surgical specimen or excisional lymph node biopsy to provide enough material for fresh frozen and formalin-fixed samples (Eichenauer et al. 2018).

88.3 Classification

HL is classified as either classical (cHL, defined by the presence of HRS cells) or nodular lymphocyte-predominant (NLPHL). The immunophenotype of the malignant cells in cHL and NLPHL differs significantly and helps to establish the diagnosis. Four subtypes of cHL exist (nodular sclerosis, mixed cellularity, rich in lymphocytes, and lymphocyte depleted), which differ in presentation, sites of involvement, epidemiology and association with EBV. Management, however, is broadly similar in all subtypes. NLPHL has a distinct clinical course, and it only represents less than 5% of the cases of HL.

88.4 Risk Factors

The outlook for patients with early-stage disease (stages I–IIA) is excellent, with OS exceeding 90% in many trials. In advanced-stage disease (IIB, III–IV), OS is 75–90%. Risk factors for patients with early-stage disease are size of

E. Carreras et al. (eds.), *The EBMT Handbook*, https://doi.org/10.1007/978-3-030-02278-5_88

mediastinal mass, age, erythrocyte sedimentation rate, number of nodal areas, B symptoms and mixed cellularity or lymphocyte-depleted histology. Different risk stratification systems combining these factors are defined by the EORTC, GHSG, NCCN and National Cancer Institute of Canada and are currently used in clinical practice. Risk factors for advance stages consist of albumin <4 g/dL, haemoglobin <10.5 g/dL, male, age ≥45 years, stage IV disease, leucocytosis ≥15 x 10^9/L and lymphocytopenia (lymphocyte count less than 8% of white blood cell count and/or lymphocyte count less than 0.6 x 10^9/L) (International Prognosis Score, 1 point per factor) (Eichenauer et al. 2018).

88.5 First-Line Treatment

The treatment of patients with cHL is primarily guided by the clinical stage and prognostic factors of disease. Patients with early-stage disease are usually treated with a combination of chemotherapy (ABVD) plus RTx. The amount of chemotherapy and dose of radiation differ for patients with favourable and unfavourable prognosis of disease. Chemotherapy (ABVD, escalated BEACOPP or Stanford V) is the main treatment for patients with advanced stage, and RTx may be used for selected patients as consolidation (Eichenauer et al. 2018).

88.6 Second-Line Treatment Before Auto-HSCT

The principles of management of relapse or refractory cHL are shown in Table 88.1 (von Tresckow and Moskowitz 2016). All chemotherapy-based salvage regimens are associated with haematologic toxicity. Infection and neutropenic fever are reported in 10–24% of cases. Nephrotoxicity, hepatotoxicity, mucositis and gastrointestinal toxicity are observed in <10%. Haematopoietic stem cell mobilization appears adequate with all regimens. Efficacy of different salvage options is shown in Table 88.2.

Table 88.1 Principles of management of relapse or refractory cHL

New biopsy:
- Mandatory if relapse is ≥12 months after the end of primary treatment in order to exclude alternative diagnoses. Highly recommended for patients with suspected relapse <12 months
- If apparent primary refractory disease, histological confirmation of HL is only recommended if progression is suspected within new sites of disease. Biopsy may not be mandatory in patients with clear radiological progression in sites of primary disease during treatment

Radiological evaluation:
- A whole-body CT scan with contrast dye injection and a PET are recommended for further comparison

Therapy:
- Salvage therapy followed by high-dose chemotherapy and auto-HSCT is currently considered the standard of care for relapsed cHL patients
- No study has compared effectiveness of different salvage regimens
- Salvage strategy should be tailored on an individual basis taking into account the initial therapy given, the risk of adding cumulative non-haematologic toxicity and the possibility of harvesting stem cells
- Cardiac and pulmonary function should be evaluated prior to treatment
- If indicated, reproductive counselling should be proposed prior to treatment
- Objective of salvage chemotherapy: to produce a response (tumour remains chemosensitive), which has a major impact on post-auto-HSCT outcome. Achievement of PET negativity defines chemosensitivity and should be the goal of salvage chemotherapy

Table 88.2 Salvage regimens

Conventional chemotherapy	
DHAP	ORR 89%, CR 21%
ESHAP	ORR 67%, CR 50%
ICE	ORR 88%, CR 67%
Gemcitabine-containing regimens	
• IGEV	ORR 81%, CR 54%
• GVD	ORR 70%, CR 19%
• GDP	ORR 62%, CR 1%
• BeGEV	ORR 83%, CR 73%
No chemotherapy strategies	
Brentuximab vedotin (BV)	Currently approved after failure of at least two prior multiagent chemotherapy regimens in patients who are not auto-HSCT candidates. ORR 50%, CR 12%
Pembrolizumab	Currently approved for the treatment of patients with refractory cHL or who have relapsed after three or more prior lines of therapy. ORR 69%, CR 22%
New drugs in association with chemotherapy[a,b]	
Sequential strategies	
• BV followed by ICE	77%
Combination strategies	
• BV plus bendamustine	74%
• BV plus ESHAP	70%
• BV plus ICE	69%
• BV plus DHAP	90%
• BV plus nivolumab	62%

[a]These combinations are not currently approved for this indication

[b]PET-negative response rate

88.7 Autologous HSCT

Auto-HSCT is currently considered the standard treatment for relapsed/refractory (R/R) cHL patients. Two landmark randomized clinical trials, the British National Lymphoma Investigation (BNLI) in 1993 and the joint German Hodgkin Study Group (GHSG)/EBMT HD-R1 trial in 2002, compared high-dose chemotherapy followed by auto-HSCT versus chemotherapy and showed significant a benefit of auto-HSCT in terms of EFS and FFTF in front of conventional salvage chemotherapy; however, there was no significant OS benefit. EBMT current indications for autologous HSCT in HL are shown in Table 88.3 (Sureda et al. 2015).

Table 88.3 EBMT current indications for autologous HSCT in cHL (Sureda et al. 2015)

Disease status	Recommendations
First complete remission	Generally not recommended Level of evidence I
Sensitive relapse/≥2nd complete response	Standard of care Level of evidence I
Refractory disease	Clinical option Level of evidence II

88.7.1 Stem Cell Source and Conditioning Regimen

Haematopoietic stem cells from mobilized PB are the preferred stem cell source for auto-HSCT.

Although the choice of preparative regimen varies and is typically based on institutional experience, BEAM is the preferred option. Standard BEAM consists of BCNU (300 mg/m^2 ×1, day -6), VP (200 mg/m^2, days -5 to -2), Ara-C (200 mg/m^2 bid, days -5 to -2) and MEL (140 mg/kg/day ×1, days -1). The CY, BCNU and VP (CBV) regimen is also commonly used in North America. The use of TBI-based regimens is not recommended due to the higher risk of developing secondary malignancies.

Late toxicities of BEAM include pulmonary complications (chronic interstitial fibrosis and decrease in lung diffusing capacity, 21%), infection (30%), metabolic syndrome (17%), cardiovascular complications (12%), secondary tumours (20%) and other toxicities (20%). The most frequent cause of NRM is subsequent malignancy (12-fold increased risk compared with the general population).

88.7.2 Prognostic Factors

Adverse prognostic factors for post-auto-HSCT outcome consistent across many reported trials included primary induction failure, initial remission duration of<3 months, relapse within 12 months of induction therapy, extranodal disease, B symptoms, advanced stage at relapse, resistance to salvage chemotherapy and persistent disease at the time of transplant.

88.7.3 Results of Auto-HSCT

Disease status pre-auto-HSCT	NRM (%)	OS at 5 years (%)	PFS at 5 years (%)
Chemosensitive disease	0–18	75	50
Primary refractory disease	0–18	30–36	15–38

88.7.4 Consolidation Treatment After Auto-HSCT

Brentuximab vedotin (BV) is currently the only drug approved for consolidation treatment after auto-HSCT in patients at risk of relapse or progression. This approval was obtained after the results of the phase III AETHERA trial. In this multicentre randomized trial, 329 patients with relapsed or refractory HL were allocated to either consolidation therapy of up to 16 cycles of BV or placebo after auto-HSCT. PFS was significantly longer in patients in the BV group (median PFS 43 months vs. 24 months, $P = 0.0013$). When patients were grouped by the number of risk factors, a higher number led to more notable benefits in the consolidation arm (Moskowitz et al. 2015).

88.8 Tandem Auto-HSCT

Several groups have explored a tandem transplant approach to improve post-transplant outcomes of patients with poor risk factors. These studies showed that tandem auto-HSCT is feasible and associated with a NRM of 0–5%, 5-year OS of 54–84%, and 5-year PFS of 49–55% (Smith et al. 2018). According to these results, risk-adapted tandem auto-HSCT can be considered an option for poor-risk patients, but integration of PET findings and new drugs such as BV and checkpoint inhibitors may help to refine the need for a second auto-HSCT and possibly improve outcomes of these patients.

88.9 Disease Relapse After Auto-HSCT

Patients relapsing following auto-HSCT have an overall poor prognosis with an OS of 30% at 5 years. Early relapse, stage IV, bulky disease, poor performance status and age ≥50 years at auto-HSCT failure have been identified as predictors of poor outcome (Jethava et al. 2017; Kallam and Armitage 2018; Lapo and Blum 2016). Therapeutic options are very heterogeneous (Table 88.4) (Martínez et al. 2013; Hahn et al. 2013).

88.10 Allogeneic HSCT

Allo-HSCT is still considered a curative treatment strategy for patients with cHL who relapse or progress after auto-HSCT (Peggs et al. 2008). Our knowledge on the curative capacity of allo-HSCT relies on the results of several retrospective analyses, some of them registry-based, phase II prospective clinical trials Sureda et al. (2012) that included low number of patients and retrospective analyses that in a donor-versus-no-donor strategy demonstrate that allo-HSCT offers a significant benefit in terms of both PFS and OS. EBMT current indications for allo-HSCT in cHL are shown in Table 88.5.

Table 88.4 Therapeutic options after auto-HSCT relapse

Brentuximab vedotin (Chen et al. 2016)	Currently approved for the treatment of cHL relapsed after auto-HSCT ORR 75%, CR 34% PFS 5.6 months
Nivolumab	Currently approved for the treatment of cHL relapsed after auto-HSCT and BV ORR 69%, CR 16% 1-year OS 92%, median PFS 12–18 months
Pembrolizumab	Currently approved for the treatment of cHL relapsed after auto-HSCT ORR 69%, CR 22% PFS 72% at 6 months
Gemcitabine-based chemotherapy	ORR 69–86%, EFS 10%
Bendamustine	ORR 53–78%, CR 29–33%
Lenalidomide	ORR 19%
Histone deacetylase inhibitors	ORR 4–74%, CR 0–4% 1-year OS 78%
Everolimus	ORR 47%
Second auto-HSCT	NRM 15%, 5-year OS and PFS 30%
Allogeneic transplantation	See Sect. 88.10

Table 88.5 EBMT current indications for allogeneic HSCT in cHL (Sureda et al. 2015)

Disease risk	MSD	MUD	Alternative donors[a]
First remission	GNR Level of evidence III	GNR Level of evidence III	GNR Level of evidence III
CR > 1, previous auto-HSCT: no	Developmental Level of evidence III	Developmental Level of evidence III	GNR Level of evidence III
CRF > 1, previous auto-HSCT: yes	Standard Level of evidence II	Standard Level of evidence II	Clinical option Level of evidence III
Refractory disease	Developmental Level of evidence II	Developmental Level of evidence II	Developmental Level of evidence III

[a]*MMUD* haploidentical donors, CB, *GNR* generally not recommended

88.10.1 Stem Cell Source, Type of Donor and Conditioning Regimen

HSC from mobilized PB are the preferred stem cell source for allo-HSCT. The use of haploidentical donors has increased the use of BM in some of the series. Later studies have demonstrated no significant differences in terms of GVHD incidence with the use of PB in this setting.

In recent years, there has been a significant increase in the use of haploidentical donors with the introduction of the PT-CY approach. The interesting results observed with this type of transplant have already decreased the use of MUD and MRD in the EBMT reporting centres (Gayoso et al. 2016). Retrospectively, registry-based studies from both EBMT and CIBMTR indicate that outcomes of PT-CY-based haplo-HSCT are similar to those of MRD and MUD; cumulative incidence of GVHD seems to be lower with the haploidentical approach and translates into a better PFS-cGVHD in some of the series (Martínez et al. 2017).

More than 50% of the patients with HL treated with allo-HSCT receive a RIC protocol. RIC regimens have demonstrated to significantly reduce NRM after transplantation but also to increase RI after transplant (Sureda et al. 2008). There are no formal prospective clinical trials demonstrating the superiority of a given conditioning protocol in front of the others. Retrospective analysis indicates that low-dose TBI-containing regimens are associated with a higher RI and lower survival than non-TBI-containing protocols.

88.10.2 Prognostic Factors

The most important adverse prognostic factor associated with long-term outcome after allo-HSCT is the disease status before transplant. However, the impact of a PET-negative CR before the procedure is not as straightforward as in the auto-HSCT setting.

88.10.3 The Use of Allo-HSCT in the Era of New Drugs

The role and positioning of allo-HSCT in patient's relapsing/progressing after auto-HSCT are less clear with the introduction of new drugs. Numbers of allo-HSCT for this indication seem to have decreased over the last 2 years.

BV has been used as a bridge to allo-HSCT. There is no evidence of a need of a washout period between the last dose of BV and day 0 of HSCT. The number of BV cycles being given before allo-HSCT is usually between four and six. The use of BV before transplant does not modify post-transplant-related toxicities and might improve results by improving performance status and disease status before allo-HSCT. It might also allow more patients to successfully go through the transplant.

Checkpoint inhibitors (nivolumab, pembrolizumab) before allo-HSCT seem very effective with promising survival results (Dada 2018). However, follow-up is still too short, and it has been suggested that their use could be associated with increase in transplant-related toxicity (SOS/VOD, post-transplant hyperacute febrile syndrome). A retrospective study does not indicate a higher NRM and higher incidence of acute GVHD in patients pretreated with checkpoint inhibitors. There is no clear information on the need of a washout period when using this combined strategy although it seems that nivolumab levels on day 0 do not correlate with incidence of GVHD and NRM.

The final decision of whether to allograft a patient that relapses after auto-HSCT might rely on the risk profile of the underlying disease as well as the transplant-related risk.

88.10.4 Results of Allo-HSCT

Disease status pre-allo-HSCT	NRM (%)	OS at 3 years (%)	PFS at 3 years (%)
Chemosensitive disease	15–20	60–70	40–50
Chemorefractory disease	20–30	40–50	20–30

88.10.5 Disease Relapse After Allo-HSCT

Disease relapse carries out a dim prognosis. Therapeutic options are variable and heterogeneous (Table 88.6), and in some cases, palliative care is the only feasible one.

Table 88.6 Therapeutic options after allo-HSCT relapse

DLI alone	ORR 33–54%
DLI + brentuximab vedotin	ORR 69% (CR 54%/PR 15%), PFS 5.5 months
DLI + bendamustine	ORR 55% (CR 16%/39%), PFS 6 months
Brentuximab vedotin (Gopal et al. 2012)	ORR 50–69% CR 31–38%/PR 37% Median PFS 7–8 months
Nivolumab (Herbaux et al. 2017)	ORR 77–95% CR 42–55%/PR 40–52% 1-year PFS 58%

88.11 Therapeutic Algorithm Recommended by the Authors (Modified from Yethava et al.)

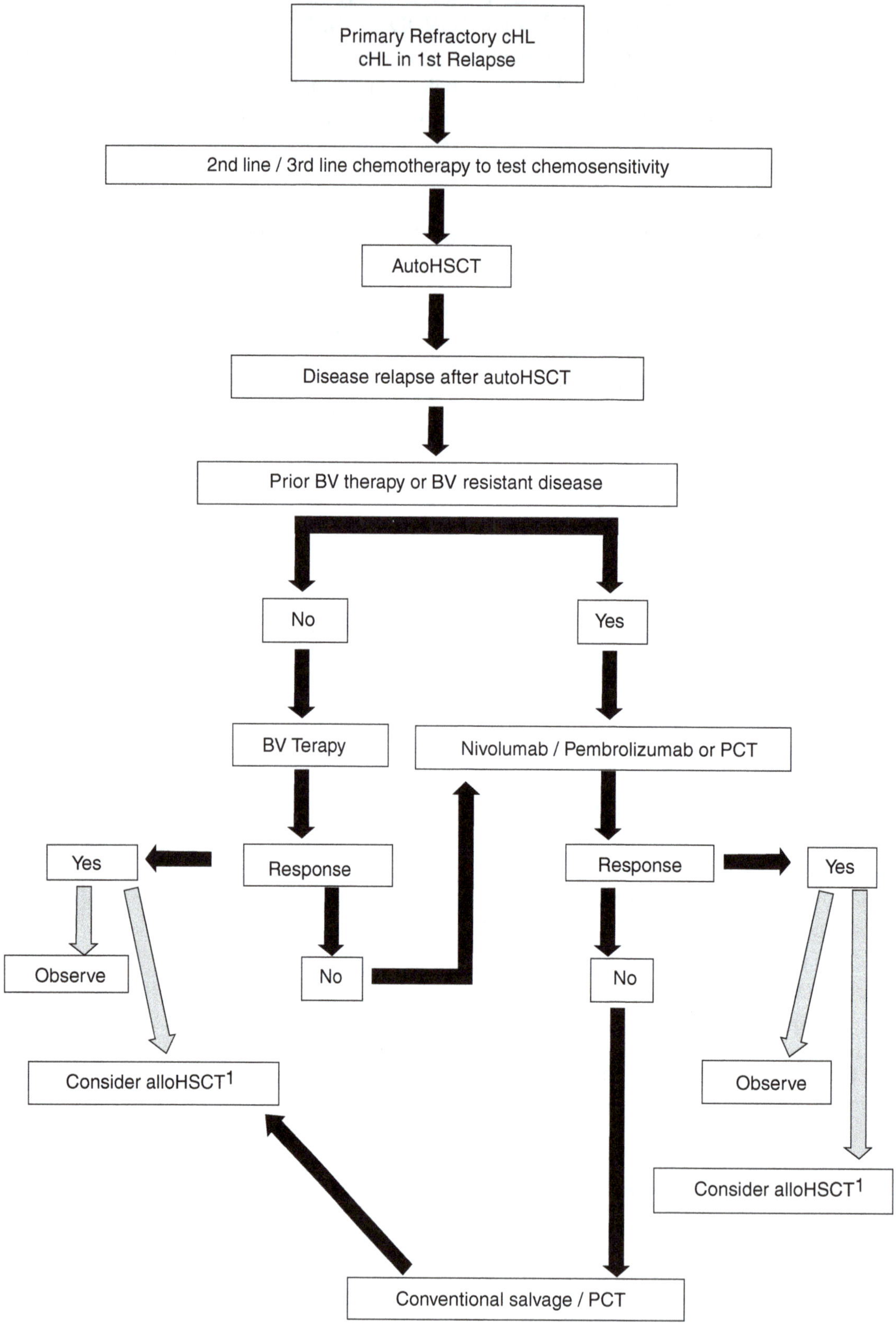

PCT, prospective clinical trials. [1]In young and fit patients with responding disease and an adequate donor available. Grey arrows. Both options can eventually be considered acceptable after a careful balance of adverse prognostic factors of the patient/transplant-related comorbidities/ careful discussion with the patient

88.12 Long-term outcomes of Auto-HSCT and Allo-HSCT in Patients with Relapsed/Refractory cHL (EBMT Database, with Permission)

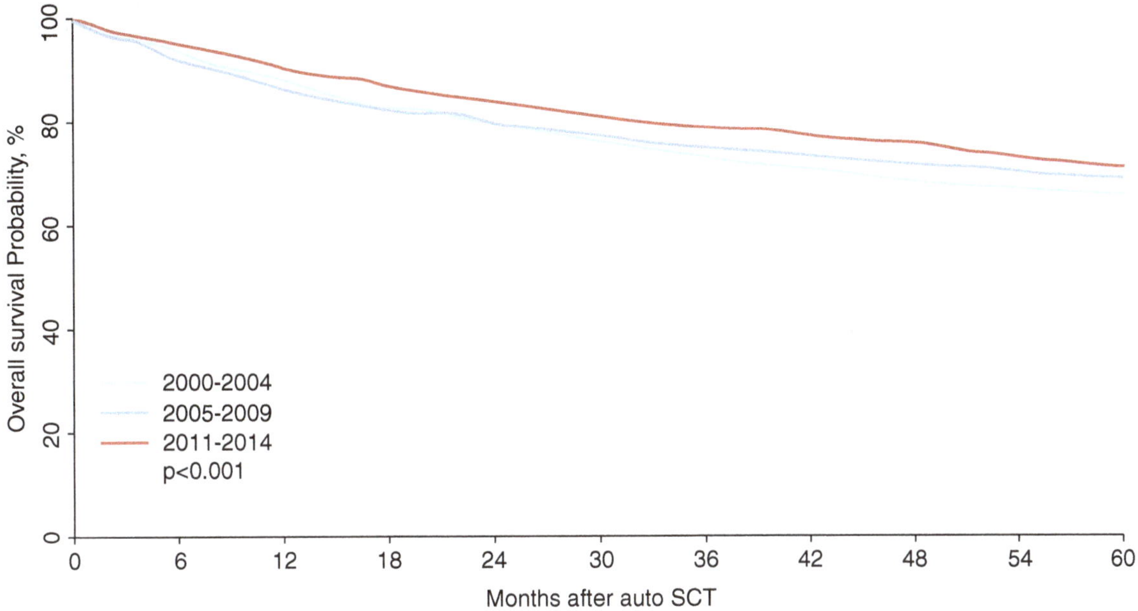

No, at risk										
2000-2004	1699	1469	1322	1217	1118	1047	960	914	857	816
2005-2009	2560	2189	1912	1756	1631	1507	1386	1291	1211	1124
2011-2014	2571	2095	1819	1603	1382	1161	933	763	570	418

OS of auto-HSCT in relapsed/refractory cHL over time

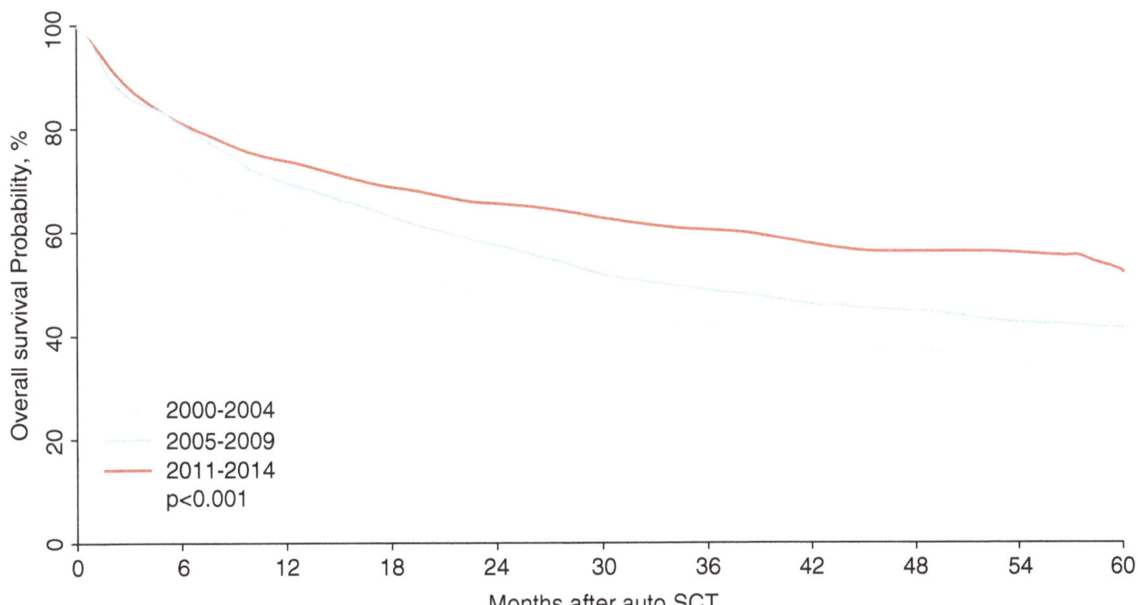

No, at risk										
2000-2004	242	196	175	153	136	127	115	105	94	87
2005-2009	550	447	386	344	297	281	260	238	224	211
2011-2014	729	631	550	477	417	343	271	211	162	104

OS of allo-HSCT in relapsed/refractory cHL over time

Key Points

- Auto-HSCT is still the standard of care for those patients with primary refractory/chemosensitive first relapse. Results of auto-HSCT might improve in the future with better selection of patients, improved results of salvage strategies and consolidation treatment in those patients with high risk of relapse after auto-HSCT.
- Allo-HSCT is the only curative treatment options for those patients relapsing after auto-HSCT. The use of allo-HSCT is being modified by the introduction of haploidentical donors as well as targeted therapies in this setting.

References

Chen R, Gopal AK, Smith SE, et al. Five-year survival and durability results of brentuximab vedotin in patients with relapsed or refractory Hodgkin lymphoma. Blood. 2016;128:1562–6.

Dada R. Program death inhibitors in classical Hodgkin's lymphoma: a comprehensive review. Ann Hematol. 2018;97:555–61.

Eichenauer DA, Engert A, André M, et al. Hodgkin's lymphoma: ESMO Clinical Practice. Guidelines for diagnosis, treatment and follow-up on behalf of the ESMO Guidelines Working Group. Ann Oncol. 2014;25(Suppl 3):iii70–5.

Gayoso J, Balsalobre P, Pascual MJ, et al. Busulfan-based reduced intensity conditioning regimens for haploidentical transplantation in relapsed/refractory Hodgkin lymphoma: Spanish multicenter experience. Bone Marrow Transplant. 2016;51:1307–12.

Gopal AK, Ramchandren R, O'Connor OA, et al. Safety and efficacy of brentuximab vedotin for Hodgkin lymphoma recurring after allogeneic stem cell transplantation. Blood. 2012;120:560–8.

Hahn T, McCarthy PL, Carreras J, et al. Simplified validated prognostic model for progression-free survival after autologous transplantation for Hodgkin lymphoma. Biol Blood Marrow Transplant. 2013;19:1740–4.

Herbaux C, Gauthier J, Brice P, et al. Efficacy and tolerability of nivolumab after allogeneic transplantation for relapsed Hodgkin lymphoma. Blood. 2017;129:2471–8.

Jethava Y, Guru Murthy GS, Hamadani M. Relapse of Hodgkin lymphoma after autologous transplantation: time to rethink treatment? Hematol Oncol Stem Cell Ther. 2017;10:47–56.

Kallam A, Armitage JO. Current and emerging treatment options for a patient with a second relapse of Hodgkin's lymphoma. Expert Rev Hematol. 2018; 22:1–8.

Lapo A, Blum KA. How I treat relapsed classical Hodgkin lymphoma after autologous stem cell transplant. Blood. 2016;127:287–95.

Martínez C, Canals C, Sarina B, et al. Identification of prognostic factors predicting outcome in Hodgkin's lymphoma patients relapsing after autologous stem cell transplantation. Ann Oncol. 2013;24: 2430–4.

Martínez C, Gayoso J, Canals C, et al. Post-transplantation cyclophosphamide-based haploidentical transplantation as alternative to matched sibling or unrelated donor transplantation for Hodgkin lymphoma: a registry study of the Lymphoma Working Party of the European Society for Blood and Marrow Transplantation. J Clin Oncol. 2017;35: 3425–32.

Moskowitz CH, Nademanee A, Masszi T, et al. Brentuximab vedotin as consolidation therapy after autologous stem-cell transplantation in patients with Hodgkin's lymphoma at risk of relapse or progression (AETHERA): a randomised, double-blind, placebo-controlled, phase 3 trial. Lancet. 2015;385: 1853–62.

Peggs KS, Anderlini P, Sureda A. Allogeneic transplantation for Hodgkin lymphoma. Br J Haematol. 2008;143:468–80.

Smith EP, Li H, Friedberg JW, et al. Tandem autologous hematopoietic cell transplantation for patients with primary progressive or recurrent Hodgkin lymphoma: a SWOG and Blood and Marrow Transplant Clinical Trials Network Phase II Trial (SWOG S0410/ BMT CTN 0703). Biol Blood Marrow Transplant. 2018;24:700–7.

Sureda A, Robinson S, Canals C, et al. Reduced-intensity conditioning compared with conventional allogeneic stem-cell transplantation in relapsed or refractory Hodgkin's lymphoma: an analysis from the Lymphoma Working Party of the European Group for Blood and Marrow Transplantation. J Clin Oncol. 2008;26:455–62.

Sureda A, Canals C, Arranz R, et al. Allogeneic stem cell transplantation after reduced intensity conditioning in patients with relapsed or refractory Hodgkin's lymphoma. Results of the HDR-ALLO study - a prospective clinical trial by the Grupo Español de Linfomas/Trasplante de Médula Osea (GEL/TAMO) and the Lymphoma Working Party of the European Group for Blood and Marrow Transplantation. Haematologica. 2012;97:310–7.

Sureda A, Bader P, Cesaro S, et al. Indications for allo- and auto-SCT for haematological diseases, solid tumours and immune disorders: current practice in Europe, 2015. Bone Marrow Transplant. 2015;50:1037–56.

von Tresckow B, Moskowitz CH. Treatment of relapsed and refractory Hodgkin Lymphoma. Semin Hematol. 2016;53:180–5.

Primary Immunodeficiencies

89

Michael Albert, Arjan Lankester, and Andrew Gennery

89.1 Introduction

Primary immunodeficiency (PID) diseases arise from genetic defects that lead to abnormalities in immune cell development or function with a wide spectrum in severity and clinical manifestations. A subgroup of patients with an immunodeficiency present as a medical emergency which is associated with a chronic disabling and life-threatening clinical course. In these cases, allo-HSCT provides a life-saving and curative treatment modality. Replacement of the defective cell lineage by HSCT from healthy allogeneic donors remains the curative approach for these patients. Other management options including enzyme replacement therapy, gene transfer into autologous hematopoietic stem cells, and targeted therapies (see below) may provide an alternative approach to HSCT in specific immune deficiencies.

M. Albert
Pediatric SCT Program, Dr. von Hauner University Children's Hospital, Ludwig-Maximilians Universität, Munich, Germany

A. Lankester
Department of Pediatrics, Stem Cell Transplantation Program, Willem-Alexander Children's Hospital, Leiden University Medical Center, Leiden, The Netherlands

A. Gennery (✉)
Paediatric Immunology + HSCT, Great North Children's Hospital, Newcastle University, Newcastle upon Tyne, UK
e-mail: andrew.gennery@newcastle.ac.uk

89.2 Diseases

For HSCT purposes and thus for this handbook, PID may be broadly categorized into severe combined immunodeficiencies (SCID) and non-SCID. To further subdivide non-SCID, the phenotypic classification as suggested by the International Union of Immunological Societies (IUIS) Inborn Errors of Immunity Committee can be used, which encompasses >300 genetic causes of PID (Table 89.1).

Overall guidelines for HSCT for SCID and non-SCID diseases together with detailed protocols have been produced by the EBMT Inborn Errors Working Party (EBMT IEWP) and can be found online at https://www.ebmt.org/sites/default/files/migration_legacy_files/document/Inborn%20Errors%20Working%20Party%20ESID%20EBMT%20HSCT%20Guidelines%20

Table 89.1 Phenotypic classification of PID as suggested by the International Union of Immunological Societies (IUIS) Inborn Errors of Immunity Committee (Picard et al. 2018)

1. Combined immunodeficiency (CID)
2. CID with associated or syndromic features
3. Predominantly antibody deficiencies
4. Diseases of immune dysregulation
5. Congenital defects of phagocyte number, function, or both
6. Defects in intrinsic and innate immunity
7. Auto-inflammatory disorders
8. Complement deficiencies
9. Phenocopies of PID

E. Carreras et al. (eds.), *The EBMT Handbook*, https://doi.org/10.1007/978-3-030-02278-5_89

2017.pdf. An update of these guidelines is planned for 2018 based on current IEWP studies.

89.3 SCID

The overall frequency of SCID was for a long time estimated to be 1 in 50,000–100,000 live births. However, in recent years newborn screening programs making use of the T-cell receptor excision circles (TREC) technology have demonstrated that the frequency may actually be two- or more-fold higher with clear geographical and ethnic differences (Kwan et al. 2014; Rechavi et al. 2017).

The immunological phenotypes of SCID are shown in Table 89.2 representing monogenic inherited defects in T-, B-, and NK-cell differentiation leading to the absence or inactivity of corresponding mature cells. Over the past two decades, the genetic basis of an increasing number of SCID variants has been identified (Table 89.2) leading to modifications in transplant strategy dependent on the underlying defect particularly in SCID variants caused by defects in DNA repair genes.

In the absence of newborn screening programs, most patients present within the first 3–6 months with unusually severe and recurrent infections or with opportunistic infections, the most common being *Pneumocystis jiroveci pneumonia*. Other common symptoms include diarrhea, dermatitis, and failure to thrive. Survival in SCID patients depends on expeditious T-cell reconstitution, and in the absence of successful HSCT, or in selected cases autologous stem cell gene therapy, most children die usually during the first year of life from overwhelming infection. It is recognized that as many as 50% of SCID patients are engrafted with maternal T-cells but in most instances these cells do not initiate GvHD. Transfusion-associated GvHD, on the other hand, is frequently lethal in SCID, and any patient with a possible diagnosis of SCID should receive irradiated blood products. Bacille Calmette-Guérin (BCG) vaccination can give rise to disseminated BCG-osis in SCID patients and should be avoided at birth if there is any suspicion or family history of immunodeficiency.

Table 89.2 Gene defects typically associated with specific SCID phenotypes

T-B+NK-	T-B+NK+	T-B-NK-	T-B-NK+
IL2RG (SCID-X1)	*IL7R*	*ADA*	*LIG4*
JAK3	*CD3D*	*AK2* (reticular dysgenesis	*RAG1*
	CD3E		*RAG2*
	CD247 (CD3ζ)		*DCLRE1C* (Artemis def.)
	CORO1A		*NHEJ1* (Cernunnos XLF)
	PTPRC (CD45 def.)		*PRKDC* (DNA-PKcs def.)
	FOXN1		

Adapted from Picard et al. (2018)

89.3.1 General Principles in Allo-HSCT for SCID

The Stem CEll Transplant for primary Immune Deficiencies in Europe (SCETIDE) registry has now collected data on SCID transplants comprising 50 years of HSCT experience, and a number of important publications have documented the outcomes and important risk factors (Fischer et al. 1990; Antoine et al. 2003; Gennery et al. 2010). Recently, studies from the North American group have reported similar findings (Pai et al. 2014; Heimall et al. 2017). The major factors influencing outcome reported in these studies include:

1. Preceding comorbidity (particularly infectious complications at HSCT) adversely affecting outcome
2. The type of donor with matched sibling donors having the best outcome[1]

[1] Recent data show that the type of donor and the immunological SCID phenotype have an ever-diminishing influence on outcome.

3. The type of SCID, with T-B- forms of SCID having an inferior outcome (see footnote 1)
4. Age at transplant with patients <3.5 months having a favorable outcome

89.3.2 Matched Sibling Donor HSCT for SCID

During the last decade, the overall survival for MSD HSCT in SCID has improved to over 90%. Somewhat remarkably, sibling donor BM may be infused into SCID recipients without the requirement for conditioning or GvHD prophylaxis. Infusion of sibling BM leads to the rapid development of T- and B-cell function post-HSCT, although usually only T-cells of donor origin develop and myeloid and erythroid cells remain of recipient origin. In T-/B+ SCID, the majority of patients achieve humoral reconstitution despite lack of donor B-cells, whereas following unconditioned HSCT in T-/B- SCID immunoglobulin dependence often persists.

89.3.3 Other Matched Family and URD HSCT for SCID

Overall survival rate following phenotypically matched related as well as URD transplants has steadily improved and is approaching MSD results (Gennery et al. 2010; Pai et al. 2014; Heimall et al. 2017). It is generally considered that the risk of rejection and particularly GvHD is too high for simple infusion of phenotypically matched marrow into SCID patients, so conditioning/GvHD prophylaxis is recommended. In a recent transatlantic study, survival rate in unconditioned URD HSCT was comparable with MSD HSCT, however at the expense of increased acute GvHD and inferior B-cellular immune reconstitution (Dvorak et al. 2014). A variety of conditioning regimes have been used, and current IEWP recommendations include the use of an IV BU/FLU- or TREO/FLU-based protocol (details at http://www.ebmt.org/5WorkingParties/IEWP/wparties-ie5.html). Comparison of survival rates and immune function with these regimens is part of ongoing studies.

89.3.4 HLA-Mismatched Family Donor for SCID

Virtually all children have a haploidentical parental donor, and this is an alternative option especially as the donor is readily available. HLA disparity necessitates rigorous in vitro or in vivo TCD in order to avoid GvHD. Using mobilized PBSC as a preferred stem cell source, most centers employ either CD34-positive selection or CD3-/CD19-negative depletion methods to achieve a 4–5 log TCD achieving a threshold of 1–5 × 10^4/kg $CD3^+$ cells, below which GvHD prophylaxis is not required.

More recently, alternative haploidentical procedures including TCR alpha/beta depletion (Balashov et al. 2015; Shah et al. 2018) and PT-CY have emerged as HSCT options. Although promising survival rates have been reported, longer follow-up in a larger cohort of patients is required to determine the position of these approaches.

Some centers advocate performing transplants without the use of any conditioning, and survival rates of over 80% have been reported (Dvorak et al. 2014). However, the best results are seen in those transplanted at <3.5 months of age and in the absence of active infections. Despite general improvements in survival rate, the best results are still seen in the T^-B^+ subgroup of SCID patients. Even in these cases, B-cell function is only restored in the minority of patients. Conditioning regimes can be used to improve outcome, but the use of MAC regimes in children often <1 year of age is associated with significant comorbidity and leads to survival figures of 50–60%. Individualized approaches making use of therapeutic drug monitoring or antibody-based conditioning strategies may provide novel and less toxic options to improve HSCT outcome in these vulnerable young infants.

89.3.5 Unrelated CBT for SCID

During the last decade, the availability of CBU plus the increased level of HLA matching degree has made CB a suitable alternative source of stem cells (Fernandes et al. 2012). There are some theoretical advantages for the use of cord blood stem cells for SCID, namely, rapid availability, as with haplotype-matched parental donors but with no requirement for TCD; less risk of GvHD compared to adult URD; no medical risk to the donor; and a greater proliferative life span which might be particularly important in such young recipients. Moreover, the usual limitation of cell dose in CBT is usually no issue in infants with SCID. There are also some specific disadvantages including slower engraftment, lack of viral-specific cytotoxic T-cells, and lack of availability of the donor for a boost HSCT.

89.3.6 Omenn's Syndrome

Omenn's syndrome (OS) is characterized by SCID typically associated with the triad of erythroderma, hepatosplenomegaly, and lymphadenopathy. There is a marked eosinophilia and a variable number of autologous, activated, and oligoclonal T lymphocytes (leaky SCID/CID), which infiltrate target organs and are generally poorly responsive to mitogens. Whereas outcomes in HSCT for OS were traditionally more difficult compared the classical SCID, results have improved in recent years (Gennery et al. 2010; Heimall et al. 2017). The overall mortality in these studies was lower than previously reported and was due to early recognition of OS and rapid initiation of treatment with topical/systemic immune suppression with steroids and/or cyclosporin A to control immune dysreactivity before proceeding to HSCT.

89.3.7 HSCT for Radiosensitive SCID

Patients with T-B- SCID due to radiosensitive disorders such as DNA ligase 4 deficiency, Cernunnos deficiency, DNA-PKcs deficiency are increasingly being identified and being considered for HSCT. As many of the conditioning regimens are particularly damaging to DNA, less toxic regimens are required to successfully treat these patients (Slack et al. 2018). No definitive studies are available, but a low-dose FLU/CY regime has been suggested by the EBMT IEWP (http://www.ebmt.org/5WorkingParties/IEWP/wparties-ie5.html).

89.4 Non-SCID Immunodeficiency

From a HSCT viewpoint, the major difference with non-SCID patients in comparison with SCID patients is the requirement for a conditioning regimen to achieve engraftment. It is the goal to establish sufficient long-term donor chimerism in the affected cell lineage. The required degree of donor chimerism for full disease correction varies depending on PID and has not been established for all entities.

Many children with non-SCID PID have significant comorbidities at the time of HSCT. Conventional MAC preparation with BU-/CY-based regimes has historically been associated with significant treatment-related toxicity and TRM. The Inborn Errors Working Party of EBMT has therefore in 2005 published detailed recommendations for conditioning and PID as discussed above. These recommendations include:

1. Replacement of CY with FLU, as the combination of BU/FLU appears to be better tolerated in these patients
2. Adding the option to replace BU with a structural analogue, TREO, which is similarly immuno- and myelosuppressive but causes less hepatic SOS/VOD (Slatter et al. 2018)
3. Establishing RIC to achieve stable engraftment of immunocompetent donor cells with reduced procedure-related morbidity and mortality (Veys 2010)

The latest outcome data for HSCT in non-SCID patients come from Europe (Gennery et al. 2010). In the 2000–2005 period, HSCT using an URD ($n = 124$) gave a 3-year survival rate similar to a genoidentical donor ($n = 73$), 79% for both. Survival was 76% in phenoidentical transplants ($n = 23$) and worse in mismatched related donor transplants ($n = 47$, 46%, $p = 0.016$), in contrast to SCID patients (see above). Ten-year survival was significantly better for patients with WAS, phagocytic, and hemophagocytic disorders than for patients with T-lymphocyte immunodeficiencies (71, 63, 58, 47%, respectively).

Unrelated CB donors appear to also give promising results in non-SCID immunodeficiency with 29/32 (91%) patients surviving CBT matched for 4–6/6 HLA antigens.

The landscape of non-SCID PID and HSCT has dramatically changed over the last decade:

- HSCT outcomes have further improved with 80–90% overall survival and low GVHD rates after MSD or MUD HSCT in almost every non-SCID PID entity (Güngör et al. 2014; Moratto et al. 2011).
- Haplo-HSCT has become a safe alternative, at least in the hands of experienced centers (Balashov et al. 2015; Shah et al. 2018).
- New genetic causes of PID are being described in accelerating frequency thanks to next-generation sequencing techniques.
- The concept of "pure" immunodeficiencies with predisposition to infections has been abandoned with newly described autoimmune, auto-inflammatory conditions or syndromal disorders with immunodeficiency. Many of these diseases can be cured by HSCT, while in syndromal disorders only the hematopoietic portion of the disease can be corrected, which may nevertheless be indicated and result in not just increased survival but also quality of life in selected patients.
- More PID patients are discovered with very mild or atypical phenotypes of well-known PID, and these often hypomorphic genetic variants are especially challenging with respect to timely recognition and management (Notarangelo et al. 2016).
- Especially in these "milder" cases, quality of life is increasingly a factor in HSCT decision making, especially compared to diseases with an immediate indication for HSCT such as SCID (Cole et al. 2013).
- The importance of DFS as compared to OS is increasingly appreciated and addressed in medium- to long-term outcome studies, also in comparison to non-HSCT approaches (Speckmann et al. 2017; Barzaghi et al. 2018).
- Adolescents and young adults with PID are appreciated as candidates for HSCT, and outcomes are encouragingly good (Albert et al. 2018; Fox et al. 2018).
- Patients with DNA double-strand repair disorders can safely undergo HSCT with irradiation-free, reduced-intensity regimens (Slack et al. 2018).

The consequence of all this has been that many more patients with PID are today considered for, referred for, and counselled about HSCT. On the other hand, it has made decision making with respect to HSCT much more difficult. A genetic diagnosis may make the decision to proceed to HSCT easier in patients with severe symptoms, but a genetic diagnosis alone should never be sufficient to indicate HSCT.

89.5 Alternative Therapies

Alternative treatments to HSCT have been developed for specific immunodeficiencies over the last three decades.

89.5.1 Enzyme Replacement Therapy (ERT) for Adenosine Deaminase Deficiency (ADA-SCID)

Enzyme replacement has been used in the treatment of ADA deficiency since 1987 (Chan et al. 2005). PEG-ADA is administered weekly or twice weekly by IM injection and leads to rapid metabolic correction with normalization of metabolic parameters which is then followed by cellular and humoral immune reconstitution. The extent of immune recovery is variable, and a significant number (~50%) remain on Ig replacement. Over a longer time period, patients show a decline in T-cell numbers and remain lymphopenic. Long-term follow-up shows that patients remain clinically well, but a number of cases of EBV-related lymphoma have been reported, suggesting decreased immune surveillance with time. Given the improved outcomes of HSCT in recent times and the availability of gene therapy, ERT may predominantly be considered a bridge to stem cell-based curative therapy.

89.5.2 Gene Therapy for Specific Immune Deficiencies

Autologous stem cell gene therapy (GT) via vector-mediated transfer of healthy copies of an affected gene into autologous CD34⁺ cells has progressed from a highly experimental therapy to the first licensed gene therapy for a PID (ADA-SCID) within the last two decades. One of the major advantages of GT is the elimination of the inherent risk of GVHD connected to any HSCT procedures.

Clinical trials performed with gamma retroviral vectors for ADA-SCID, X-linked SCID (SCID-X1), chronic granulomatous disease (CGD), and Wiskott-Aldrich syndrome (WAS) demonstrated that gene therapy can be an effective treatment option in patients lacking an HLA-identical donor (Hacein-Bey-Abina et al. 2002; Boztug et al. 2010; Stein et al. 2010; Aiuti et al. 2009). However, a high rate of insertional mutagenesis was observed in trials for SCID-X1, WAS, and CGD but not for ADA-SCID (Ott et al. 2006; Hacein-Bey-Abina et al. 2003; Braun et al. 2014). This has prompted the development of safer vectors based on self-inactivating retroviral or lentiviral vectors. Currently, a number of trials are ongoing or concluded for the diseases named above. All share the concept of submyeloablative or lymphodepleting conditioning followed by the infusion of auto-HSCT with added copies of the gene of interest. Promising results were published, especially for ADA-SCID (Cicalese et al. 2016), WAS (Aiuti et al. 2013) and SCID-X1 (Hacein-Bey-Abina et al. 2014). It is expected that gene editing approaches as alternative for gene addition technologies as currently employed will be developed in the next few years and may be employed to correct mature cells in diseases like CD40 ligand deficiency and IPEX Syndrome, as well as HSC.

In theory autologous stem cell gene therapy offers the appealing prospect of avoiding alloimmune reactions such as GVHD or rejection and a lower conditioning-related toxicity compared to allo-HSCT. But its exact role in treatment algorithms still needs to be defined in the absence of comparative studies. Also, logistic, regulatory, and economic hurdles still have to be overcome before its widespread application in the treatment of PID. Nevertheless, it has widened the therapeutic repertoire for patients with some PID. The rapid evolution of novel gene correction approaches promises to lead to even safer and more effective treatment options.

89.5.3 Targeted Therapies

The unravelling of new genetic PID entities, especially those caused by gain-of-function (GOF) variants and their pathophysiology, has for the first time opened the possibility to treat these diseases with highly specific, often small molecule inhibitors, some of which are already approved for other indications. These include but are not limited to abatacept for CTLA4 haploinsufficiency, ruxolitinib for STAT1 GOF, leniolisib for PIK3CD and PIK3R1, etanercept for ADA2 deficiency, and IL-1-targeted therapies (anakinra, rilonacept, and canakinumab) for auto-inflammatory recurrent fever syndromes (Jhamnani and Rosenzweig 2017; Ochs and Petroni 2018). At this point in time, the exact role of these agents in the treatment algorithm of PID is however unclear. Ideally, they could make HSCT unnecessary for some patients. On the other hand, concerns about long-term infection (and lymphoma) risk exist. In any case, in some patients with excessive autoimmunity and/or inflammation, these therapies can be viewed as an ideal bridge to HSCT and considered as a remission induction strategy to control the underlying PID, because they have the ability to bring the patient into the best possible clinical condition for HSCT.

Key Points

- PIDs require a tailored approach to management, and transplant-specific protocols have been developed for these diseases.
- Preceding comorbidity, particularly infectious complications at HSCT and concurrent end-organ damage, adversely affects outcome; for many diseases, transplant at an early age is recommended.
- Alternative therapies instead of, or as a bridge to, transplant are increasingly available to improve patient outcomes.

References

Aiuti A, Cattaneo F, Galimberti S, et al. Gene therapy for immunodeficiency due to adenosine deaminase deficiency. N Engl J Med. 2009;360:447–58.

Aiuti A, Biasco L, Scaramuzza S, et al. Lentiviral hematopoietic stem cell gene therapy in patients with Wiskott-Aldrich syndrome. Science. 2013;341:1233151.

Albert MH, Hauck F, Wiebking V, et al. Allogeneic stem cell transplantation in adolescents and young adults with primary immunodeficiencies. J Allergy Clin Immunol Pract. 2018;6:298–301.

Antoine C, Müller S, Cant A, European Group for Blood and Marrow Transplantation; European Society for Immunodeficiency, et al. Long-term survival and transplantation of haemopoietic stem cells for immunodeficiencies: report of the European experience 1968-99. Lancet. 2003;361:553–60.

Balashov D, Shcherbina A, Maschan M, et al. Single-center experience of unrelated and haploidentical stem cell transplantation with TCRαβ and CD19 depletion in children with primary immunodeficiency syndromes. Biol Blood Marrow Transplant. 2015;21:1955–62.

Barzaghi F, Amaya Hernandez LC, Ambrosi A, et al. IPEX syndrome survivors following different therapeutic strategies: an international multicenter retrospective study. J Allergy Clin Immunol. 2018;141:1036–49.

Boztug K, Schmidt M, Schwarzer A, et al. Stem-cell gene therapy for the Wiskott-Aldrich syndrome. N Engl J Med. 2010;363:1918–27.

Braun CJ, Boztug K, Paruzynski A, et al. Gene therapy for Wiskott-Aldrich syndrome—long-term efficacy and genotoxicity. Sci Transl Med. 2014;6:227ra33.

Chan B, Wara D, Bastian J, et al. Long-term efficacy of enzyme replacement therapy for adenosine deaminase (ADA)-deficient Severe Combined Immunodeficiency (SCID). Clin Immunol. 2005;117:133–43.

Cicalese MP, Ferrua F, Castagnaro L, et al. Update on the safety and efficacy of retroviral gene therapy for immunodeficiency due to adenosine deaminase deficiency. Blood. 2016;128:45–54.

Cole T, McKendrick F, Titman P, et al. Health related quality of life and emotional health in children with chronic granulomatous disease: a comparison of those managed conservatively with those that have undergone haematopoietic stem cell transplant. J Clin Immunol. 2013;33:8–13.

Dvorak CC, Hassan A, Slatter MA, et al. Comparison of outcomes of hematopoietic stem cell transplantation without chemotherapy conditioning by using matched sibling and unrelated donors for treatment of severe combined immunodeficiency. J Allergy Clin Immunol. 2014;134:935–943.e15.

Fernandes JF, Rocha V, Labopin M, et al. Transplantation in patients with SCID: mismatched related stem cells or unrelated cord blood? Blood. 2012;119:2949–55.

Fischer A, Landais P, Friedrich W, et al. European experience of bone-marrow transplantation for severe combined immunodeficiency. Lancet. 1990;336:850–4.

Fox TA, Chakraverty R, Burns S, et al. Successful outcome following allogeneic hematopoietic stem cell transplantation in adults with primary immunodeficiency. Blood. 2018;131:917–31.

Gennery AR, Slatter MA, Grandin L, Inborn Errors Working Party of the European Group for Blood and Marrow Transplantation, European Society for Immunodeficiency, et al. Transplantation of hematopoietic stem cells and long-term survival for primary immunodeficiencies in Europe: entering a new century, do we do better? J Allergy Clin Immunol. 2010;126:602–10.

Güngör T, Albert MH, Teira P, et al. Reduced-intensity conditioning and HLA-matched haemopoietic stem-cell transplantation in patients with chronic granulomatous disease: a prospective multicentre study. Lancet. 2014;838:436–48.

Hacein-Bey-Abina S, Le Deist F, Carlier F, et al. Sustained correction of X-linked severe combined immunodeficiency by ex vivo gene therapy. N Engl J Med. 2002;346:1185–93.

Hacein-Bey-Abina S, von Kalle C, Schmidt M, et al. LMO2-associated clonal T cell proliferation in two patients after gene therapy for SCID-X1. Science. 2003;302:415–9.

Hacein-Bey-Abina S, Pai SY, Gaspar HB, et al. A modified γ-retrovirus vector for X-linked severe combined immunodeficiency. N Engl J Med. 2014;371:1407–17.

Heimall J, Logan BR, Cowan MJ, et al. Immune reconstitution and survival of 100 SCID patients post-hematopoietic cell transplant: a PIDTC natural history study. Blood. 2017;130:2718–27.

Jhamnani RD, Rosenzweig SD. An update on gain-of-function mutations in primary immunodeficiency diseases. Curr Opin Allergy Clin Immunol. 2017;17:391–7.

Kwan A, Abraham RS, Currier R, et al. Newborn screening for severe combined immunodeficiency in 11 screening programs in the United States. JAMA. 2014;312:729–38.

Moratto D, Giliani S, Bonfim C, et al. Long-term outcome and lineage-specific chimerism in 194 patients with Wiskott-Aldrich syndrome treated by hematopoietic cell transplantation in the period 1980-2009: an international collaborative study. Blood. 2011;118:1675–84.

Notarangelo LD, Kim MS, Walter JE, et al. Human RAG mutations: biochemistry and clinical implications. Nat Rev Immunol. 2016;16:234–46.

Ochs HD, Petroni D. From clinical observations and molecular dissection to novel therapeutic strategies for primary immunodeficiency disorders. Am J Med Genet A. 2018;176:784–803.

Ott MG, Schmidt M, Schwarzwaelder K, et al. Correction of X-linked chronic granulomatous disease by gene therapy, augmented by insertional activation of MDS1-EVI1, PRDM16 or SETBP1. Nat Med. 2006;12:401–9.

Pai S-Y, Logan BR, Griffith LM, et al. Transplantation outcomes for severe combined immunodeficiency, 2000–2009. N Engl J Med. 2014;371:434–46.

Picard C, Bobby Gaspar H, Al-Herz W, et al. International Union of Immunological Societies: 2017 primary immunodeficiency diseases committee report on inborn errors of immunity. J Clin Immunol. 2018;38:96–128.

Rechavi E, Lev A, Simon AJ, et al. First Year of Israeli newborn screening for severe combined immunodeficiency—clinical achievements and insights. Front Immunol. 2017;8:1448.

Shah RM, Elfeky R, Nademi Z, et al. T-cell receptor αβ+ and CD19+ cell-depleted haploidentical and mismatched hematopoietic stem cell transplantation in primary immune deficiency. J Allergy Clin Immunol. 2018;141:1417–26.

Slack J, Albert MH, Balashov D, Inborn Errors Working Party of the European Society for Blood and Marrow Transplantation and the European Society for Immunodeficiencies, Stem Cell Transplant for Immunodeficiencies in Europe (SCETIDE), Center for International Blood and Marrow Transplant Research, Primary Immunodeficiency Treatment Consortium, et al. Outcome of haematopoietic stem cell transplantation for DNA-double strand breakage repair disorders. J Allergy Clin Immunol. 2018;141:322–8.

Slatter M, Rao K, Nademi Z, et al. Treosulfan and fludarabine conditioning for haematopoietic stem cell transplantation in children with Primary Immunodeficiency: UK experience. Biol Blood Marrow Transplant. 2018;24:529–36.

Speckmann C, Doerken S, Aiuti A, PCID-study of the Inborn Errors Working Party of the EBMT, et al. A prospective study on the natural history of patients with profound combined immunodeficiency (P-CID): a "first fifty" analysis. J Allergy Clin Immunol. 2017;139:1302–10.

Stein S, Ott MG, Schultze-Strasser S, et al. Genomic instability and myelodysplasia with monosomy 7 consequent to EVI1 activation after gene therapy for chronic granulomatous disease. Nat Med. 2010;16:198–204.

Veys P. Reduced intensity transplantation for primary immunodeficiency disorders. Immunol Allergy Clin N Am. 2010;30:103–24.

Inborn Errors of Metabolism and Osteopetrosis

90

Robert Wynn and Ansgar Schulz

90.1 Inborn Errors of Metabolism

90.1.1 Definition and Epidemiology

Inborn errors of metabolism (IEM) comprise a large group of inherited disease, some of which are due to disordered lysosomal, peroxisomal, or mitochondrial function and only some of which might be improved following HSCT. This review will be limited to the commoner indications reported in HSCT registries and which together account for the most transplanted IEM.

90.1.2 Diagnosis

Timely diagnosis is imperative in IEM since in all such diseases HSCT is better at preventing disease progression than reversing established disease manifestations.

Diagnosis is made in three ways:

- Through early recognition of disease manifestations
- Through screening of presymptomatic individuals within a known affected kindred
- Population screening for disease, such as in the neonatal period

90.1.3 Classification (See Table 90.1)

90.1.4 Risk Factors

Patient performance score at transplant predicts transplant outcome. Patients with an adverse performance score at transplant also have an inferior long-term survival as the transplant fails in advanced disease to prevent disease progression.

R. Wynn (✉)
Blood and Marrow Transplant Unit, Royal Manchester Children's Hospital, University of Manchester, Manchester, UK
e-mail: robert.wynn@cmft.nhs.uk

A. Schulz
Department of Pediatrics, University Medical Center Ulm, Ulm, Germany

E. Carreras et al. (eds.), *The EBMT Handbook*, https://doi.org/10.1007/978-3-030-02278-5_90

Table 90.1 Classification of inborn errors of metabolism

IEM	
Hurler syndrome, MPSIH	Hurler syndrome. This is the most severe phenotype of iduronidase deficiency, a lysosomal storage disorder (LSD) which results in the accumulation of glycosaminoglycans. There is progressive multi-organ dysfunction including psychomotor retardation, severe skeletal disease, life-threatening cardiopulmonary complications, and premature death HSCT prevents early death and attenuates the multi-system disease manifestations as the deficient enzyme is donated by engrafted donor leucocytes to host tissues ("cross-correction")
X-linked adrenoleukodystrophy	In this X-linked disorder, there is accumulation of very long-chain fatty acids in the brain and adrenal glands arising from their defective metabolism by a peroxisomal, membrane protein encoded by the ABCD1 gene Clinical manifestations in genetically affected boys are highly variable, even within a kindred. The principle role of HSCT is to prevent progression of early cerebral ALD, an inflammatory demyelinating disease of childhood that is seen in about 40% of genetically affected individuals HSCT does *not* influence other illness such as adrenal insufficiency or the later myeloneuropathy of the spinal cord
Metachromatic leukodystrophy (MLD)	This is a recessive LSD, and there is accumulation of sulfatides, a myelin component, due to deficiency of the arylsulfatase A enzyme. There is demyelination in the central and peripheral nervous systems, and clinical manifestations are related to residual enzyme activity. In the late infantile disease, the commonest and most severe phenotype, there is progressive neurological dysfunction and early death usually by the age of 4 years HSCT is ineffective in preventing progression of early presenting disease, although it may have a greater impact later, attenuated disease especially when applied early in the course of that illness

90.1.5 Prognostic Index

Not available

90.1.6 First-Line Treatment (Summary)

Multimodality therapies are usual in IEM.

- Residual disease manifestations will require management beyond the HSCT episode. This will include orthopedics, ENT, and speech therapies in lysosomal storage disorders (LSDs), as well as family and educational support in all.
- Pharmacological enzyme replacement therapy (ERT) is used in MPSI but does not correct neurological disease as it does not cross the blood-brain barrier, and alloantibody formation might limit its utility in somatic disease. It is used to improve pre-HSCT performance, but it has *not* been shown to influence transplant outcomes.

90.1.7 Second-Line Treatment (Summary)

See Sect. 90.1.6., above.

90.1.8 Autologous HSCT

Gene-modified auto-HSCT approaches have been shown to improve outcomes in late infantile MLD as the graft delivers more enzyme than possible in a conventional HSCT. Similar approaches have been successful in X-ALD and are likely to be a significant part of the future of HSCT in IEM.

90.1.9 Allogeneic HSCT in MPSIH (Hurler), MLD, and X-ALD (See Table 90.2)

Table 90.2 Main characteristics of allo-HSCT for MPSIH (Hurler), MLD, and X-ALD

Indicated in

MPSIH (Hurler) is a standard indication for HSCT

In MLD, HSCT is usually reserved for later (attenuated) forms of the disease, namely, juvenile and adult forms

In X-ALD, HSCT is indicated in early cerebral inflammatory disease. Ordinarily, a genetically affected individual has serial (annual) MRI scans from early childhood, and HSCT is carried out when there are early MRI changes of demyelination (the MRI changes are scored as a Loes score)

Contraindications

Where MPSIH is diagnosed late then the opportunity for HSCT to meaningfully alter the natural history of the disease might be lost. No hard and fast rules can be applied, but often HSCT is not offered to a child presenting beyond the age of 30 months, but careful multidisciplinary assessment is required

Late infantile MLD is not usually considered for HSCT. Note that such disease—if diagnosed in a timely fashion—has been shown to be markedly improved using an autologous, ex vivo HSC gene therapy approach

Advanced cerebral X-ALD is considered a contraindication to HSCT. Disease will progress through transplant. The MRI scan-derived Loes score might predict those that will benefit most from HSCT

Donor

In LSD, non-carrier MFD > MUD > carrier MFD

In LSD, UCB is frequently preferred to BM, since the post-HSCT chimerism is higher in scuh recipients, and the interval between referral and HSCT is likely shortest (rejection might be higher using UCB)

PB is rarely used as a donor cell source

In X-ALD, MFD > MUD

Haplo-HSCT is rarely indicated in IEM

Conditioning: standard

Engraftment is difficult in IEM. Generally reduced intensity conditioning and ex vivo TCD are associated with high rates of graft loss

MSD/MFD: IV BU (MAC AUC)/FLU (160 mg/m^2)

MUD: IV BU (MAC AUC)/FLU (160 mg/m^2)

Conditioning: reduced toxicity

Occasionally reduced toxicity conditioning might be employed

In somatic IEM, such as Wolman or attenuated MPS: TREO/FLU (160 mg/m^2)/TT (10 mg/kg)

Source of SC

UCB often preferred in LSD

BM rather than PB in MUD donors

No ex vivo TCD as this is shown to contribute to graft loss

GvHD prophylaxis

MSD/MFD: ATG/Campath, CSA + MMF

MUD: ATG/Campath, CSA + MMF

MUC UCB: Proximal ATG, CSA + MMF or CSA + PRD

TRM in MPSIH	*OS in MPSIH*
MSD: < 5% MUD: <10%	Engrafted survival of >80% and overall survival of 90%

MAC AUC doses adjusted to achieve MAC AUC, *MSD* match sibling donor, *MFD* match family donor, *MUD* much unrelated donor, *LSD* lysosomal storage disorder, *EIM* inborn errors of metabolism

90.2 Osteopetrosis

90.2.1 Definition and Epidemiology

Osteopetrosis (OP) is a generic name of a number of rare single gene diseases characterized by sclerosis of the skeleton. At least nine forms are known with different modes of inheritance and severity, which cumulatively have an incidence ~1:100,000. The disease originates from reduced or complete lack of osteoclast function and, as a consequence, impairment of bone resorption

90.2.2 Diagnosis

In addition to the obligate increased bone density of all bones (X-ray), a combination of symptoms can be found in *classical infantile osteopetrosis* after birth. These symptoms include characteristic changes of the head (macrocephalus, frontal bossing, choanal stenosis), vision impairment (due to narrowed foramina), hematological insufficiency (thrombocytopenia, anemia, leukocytosis), hepatosplenomegaly (due to extramedullar hematopoiesis), and hypocalcemia (with secondary hyperparathyroidism). Cave: OP is a genetical and phenotypical heterogenous disease with *atypical presentations* (incomplete and/or delayed onset of symptoms). In these cases, an intensive work-up including spine biopsy and cranial MRI is recommended.

90.2.3 Classification

Osteopetrosis	
Infantile "malignant" autosomal recessive OP (ARO)	Clinical symptoms in infancy, death without HSCT usually in the first decade of life, biallelic mutations in *TCIRG1, CLCN7, SNX10, TNFRSF11A/RANK, and FERMT3/KINDLIN-3;* HSCT indicated, if excluded: – "Neurodegenerative OP" (all *OSTM1* and about half of *CLCN7* cases) – "Extrinsic osteoclast defects" *(TNFSF11/RANKL cases)*
Intermediate osteopetrosis	Clinical symptoms in the first decade, HSCT may be indicated in severe forms with hematological insufficiency and (imminent) visual impairment Specific from: CA2 deficiency (renal tubular acidosis with cerebral calcifications): HSCT is rarely indicated
Benign osteopetrosis (ADO)	M. Albers Schoenberg (monoallelic CLCN7 mutations): HSCT not indicated

90.2.4 Risk Factors

There is an increased risk of pulmonary hypertension (pre and post HSCT) and SOS/VOD (post BMT). The risk of non-engraftment and rejection increases with severity of disease and age.

90.2.5 Prognostic Index

Not available

90.2.6 First-Line Treatment (Summary)

Symptomatic, steroids may be beneficial to improve hematological symptoms

90.2.7 Second-Line Treatment (Summary)

Not available

90.2.8 Autologous HSCT

Preclinical trials for gene-modified auto-HSCT for TCIRG1 defects in preparation.

90.2.9 Allogeneic HSCT (See Table 90.3)

Table 90.3 Main characteristics of allo-HSCT for osteopetrosis

Indicated in	Infantile osteopetrosis: clinical symptoms and exclusion of neurodegenerative and extrinsic osteoclast defect
Contraindications	Neurodegenerative osteopetrosis: symptoms (non-hypocalcemic convulsions/EEC changes, severe progredient developmental delay) and/or biallelic mutations in *OSTM1* and *CLCN7*; cave: only about half of *CLCN7* mutations cause neurodegeneration Osteopetrosis not intrinsic to defects in differentiation or function in osteoclasts: *TNFSF11/RANKL*
Donor	MFD > MUD > haplo (cord blood not recommended)
Conditioning: standard	MSD/MFD: IV BU (MAC AUC)/FLU (160 mg/m^2) MUD: IV BU (MAC AUC)/FLU (160 mg/m^2)/TT (10 mg/kg) Haplo: IV BU (MAC AUC)/FLU (160 mg/m^2)/TT (15 mg/kg)
Conditioning: reduced toxicity	MSD/MFD: TREO/FLU (160 mg/m^2)/TT (10 mg/kg) MUD: TREO/FLU (160 mg/m^2)/TT (10 mg/kg)
Conditioning: post Cy protocol	In patients >10 months of age and haplo donors, an adapted PT-CY protocol should be considered (see updated EBMT guidelines)
Source of SC	Matched donors, PT-CY protocol: T replete BM > PB Haplo (standard protocol): TCD PB
GvHD prophylaxis	MSD/MFD: CSA + MMF (consider ATG or Campath in MFD) MUD: CSA + MMF + ATG (or Campath) Haplo—TCD: ATG (or Campath), consider MMF Haplo—T replete: Campath, PT-CY, TAC (or CSA) + MMF
TRM	MSD/MUD: 10–20% Haplo: ~30 to 40%; cave: high rejection rate (>50%) in pts > 10 months
OS	MSD: ~90% MUD: ~80% Haplo/MMUD: 60–70%

MAC AUC doses adjusted to achieve MAC AUC, *MSD* match sibling donor, *MFD* match family donor, *MUD* much unrelated donor, *MMUD* mismatch unrelated donor

Recommended References

Aldenhoven M, Jones SA, Bonney D, et al. Hematopoietic cell transplantation for mucopolysaccharidosis patients is safe and effective: results after implementation of international guidelines. Biol Blood Marrow Transplant. 2015;21:1106–9.

Biffi A, Montini E, Lorioli L, et al. Lentiviral hematopoietic stem cell gene therapy benefits metachromatic leukodystrophy. Science. 2013;341:1233158.

Boelens JJ, Wynn RF, O'Meara A, et al. Outcomes of hematopoietic stem cell transplantation for Hurler's syndrome in Europe: a risk factor analysis for graft failure. Bone Marrow Transplant. 2007;40:225–33.

Boelens JJ, Prasad VK, Tolar J, et al. Current international perspectives on hematopoietic stem cell transplantation for inherited metabolic disorders. Pediatr Clin N Am. 2010;57:123–45.

Chiesa R, Ruggeri A, Paviglianiti A, et al. Outcomes after unrelated umbilical cord blood transplantation for children with osteopetrosis. Biol Blood Marrow Transplant. 2016;22:1997–2002.

Consensus Guidelines of the EBMT and ESID at: https://esid.org/Working-Parties/Inborn-Errors-Working-Party-IEWP/Resources/UPDATED!-EBMT-ESID-GUIDELINES-FOR-HAEMATOPOIETICSTEM-CELL-TRANSPLANTATION-FOR-PI/Updated-Osteopetrosis-Consensus-Guidelines.

de Vernejoul MC, Schulz A, Kornak U. CLCN7-related osteopetrosis. 2007 Feb 12 [Updated 2013 Jun

20]. In: Pagon RA, Adam MP, Bird TD, et al., editors. GeneReviews™. Seattle, WA: University of Washington; 2013. p. 1993–2013.

Driessen GJ, Gerritsen EJ, Fischer A, et al. Long-term outcome of haematopoietic stem cell transplantation in autosomal recessive osteopetrosis: an EBMT report. Bone Marrow Transplant. 2003;32: 657–63.

Eichler F, Duncan C, Musolino PL, et al. Hematopoietic stem-cell gene therapy for cerebral adrenoleukodystrophy. N Engl J Med. 2017;377: 1630–8.

Prasad VK, Mendizabal A, Parikh SH, et al. Unrelated donor umbilical cord blood transplantation for inherited metabolic disorders in 159 pediatric patients from a single center: influence of cellular composition of the graft on transplantation outcomes. Blood. 2008;112:2979–89.

Shadur B, Zaidman I, NaserEddin A, et al. Successful hematopoietic stem cell transplantation for osteopetrosis using reduced intensity conditioning. Pediatr Blood Cancer. 2018;65:e27010.

Sobacchi C, Schulz A, Coxon FP, et al. Osteopetrosis: genetics, treatment and new insights into osteoclast function. Nat Rev Endocrinol. 2013;9:522–36.

Teti A, Schulz A. Haematopoietic stem cell transplantation in autosomal recessive osteopetrosis. In: Rajendram R, Preedy VR, editors. Stem cells and bone diseases. Vinood Patel Editors. Boca Raton, FL: CRC Press; 2013.

91 Autoimmune Disease

Tobias Alexander, Basil Sharrack, Montserrat Rovira, Dominique Farge, and John A. Snowden

91.1 Introduction

Autoimmune diseases (ADs) are a heterogeneous group of diseases affecting 8–10% of the Western population, which constitute a heavy burden to society and are often debilitating and disabling for affected individuals. Current therapeutic strategies for AD are based on systemic immunosuppression (IS), which ameliorates symptoms and halts progression in the vast majority of patients, but usually require continuous administration and may be associated with long-term side effects and substantial costs. Although introduction of modern biological therapies dramatically improved the treatment landscape in AD, cure remains elusive, and many patients still suffer from progressive disability with shortened life expectancy and comorbidity.

Initially supported by preclinical animal models and 'serendipitous' case reports, auto-HSCT has grown as a promising and feasible treatment option for severe treatment-resistant patients, especially in diseases for which effective therapies are lacking. Allo-HSCT has also been undertaken, although caution related to its intrinsic risks has precluded widespread application.

Following the first international meeting for the use of HSCT in AD in September 1996, the EBMT Autoimmune Diseases Working Party (ADWP) was established in 1997 by Alois Gratwohl, Alberto Marmont, Alan Tyndall and Athanasios Fassas, who developed the registry covering AD indications and produced early guidelines based on consensus opinion (Tyndall and Gratwohl 1997).

T. Alexander (✉)
Department of Rheumatology and Clinical Immunology, Charité – University Medicine Berlin, Berlin, Germany
e-mail: tobias.alexander@charite.de

B. Sharrack
Academic Department of Neuroscience and Sheffield NIHR Translational Neuroscience BRC, Sheffield Teaching Hospitals, NHS Foundation Trust, University of Sheffield, Sheffield, UK

M. Rovira
BMT Unit, Haematology Department, IDIBAPS, Hospital Clinic, Josep Carreras Leukemia Research Institute (IJC), Barcelona, Spain

D. Farge
Unité Clinique de Médecine Interne, Maladies Auto-immunes et Pathologie Vasculaire, UF 04, Hôpital Saint-Louis, EA 3518, AP-HP Assistance Publique des Hôpitaux de Paris, Paris Denis Diderot University, Paris, France

Centre de Référence des Maladies auto-immunes systémiques Rares d'Ile-de-France (site constitutif), Filière FAI2R, Paris, France

J. A. Snowden
Department of Haematology, Sheffield Teaching Hospitals NHS Foundation Trust, Royal Hallamshire Hospital, Sheffield, UK

E. Carreras et al. (eds.), *The EBMT Handbook*, https://doi.org/10.1007/978-3-030-02278-5_91

Subsequently the ADWP built productively on these initial achievements, generating studies from the growing registry and developing relationships with other specialist societies, culminating with successful publication of three randomised controlled trials (van Laar et al. 2014; Mancardi et al. 2015; Hawkey et al. 2015) along with updated guidelines for clinical practice (Snowden et al. 2012) and immune monitoring and biobanking (Alexander et al. 2015).

With the increase in evidence, the guidelines have become more disease specific. A successful collaboration involving significant non-European collaborating partners resulted in the EBMT guidelines for auto-HSCT in systemic sclerosis (Farge et al. 2017). A further collaborative review with the European Crohn's and Colitis Organisation (ECCO), which has recently been published, includes recommendations for patient selection, transplant technique and follow-up of HSCT in patients with Crohn's disease (Snowden et al. 2018). Guidelines for MS and neurological diseases are in preparation.

The current state of the EBMT database in relation to various ADs is summarised in Tables 91.1 and 91.2. At the time of writing, over 2500 patients receiving HSCT for an AD have been reported to the EBMT, the largest international database, with activity reported to other registries adding substantially to the worldwide numbers. The most recent EBMT activity survey identified autoimmune diseases as the fastest growing indication group for HSCT (Passweg et al. 2018). Based on this reported activity, this chapter will cover the main neurological, rheumatological and gastroenterological indications for auto-HSCT, along with reference to the rare AD indications and allogeneic HSCT. More detailed literature can be sourced from recently published reviews (Snowden et al. 2017, 2018; Burt and Farge 2018; Alexander and Hiepe 2017).

Table 91.1 Overview of data reported to the EBMT database (October 2018)

Patients	2725
Transplant procedures	2780
Centres/Countries	267/40
Autografts/Allografts	2605 (94%)/175 (6%)
Median age at transplantation (years)	37 (0.18–76)
Male/Female	39/61%

91.2 HSCT for Multiple Sclerosis (MS)

Since the first case report of using auto-HSCT as a treatment for MS was published in 1995, the EBMT registry has now accumulated over 1000 patients (Table 91.2). This treatment was initially used in patients with advanced progressive disease as a rescue therapy with limited efficacy. More recently, its use in patients with active relapsing MS has been associated with prolonged clinical and MRI responses and, in some cases, significant improvement in disability to a degree rarely seen with other disease-modifying drugs (Muraro et al. 2017). Only one randomised controlled phase II trial of auto-HSCT has been reported in the literature (Mancardi et al. 2015). The bulk of the data has been provided by observational cohort studies in which patients failing to respond to standard disease-modifying drugs were treated with HSCT. Burman et al. identified the four most rigorously conducted cohort studies in which a total of 188 relapsing MS patients received auto-HSCT (Burman et al. 2018). In these studies, PFS was observed in 70–91% of patients at 5 years (where progression is defined as a deterioration of at least 0.5–1 points from baseline in the Expanded Disability Status Scale or EDSS). Furthermore, no evidence of disease activity (NEDA), defined as the absence of clinical relapses, disability progression, and MRI disease activity, was observed in 70–92% of patients at 2 years post-transplantation (Burman et al. 2018; Burt et al. 2015; Atkins et al. 2016; Nash et al. 2017).

The conditioning regimens used in MS vary between treatment centres. The balance of efficacy and acceptable safety profile of 'intermediate intensity' regimens, i.e. either the specific 'BEAM + ATG' regimen or the more generic regimen of CY 200 mg/kg combined with ATG, led to their recommended use in the current

Table 91.2 Distribution of diagnosis in the EBMT database (October 2018)

Multiple sclerosis (MS)	*1285*	*Haematological diseases*	*113*
Connective tissue diseases	*735*	immune thrombocytopenia purpura (ITP)	33
Systemic sclerosis	559	Haemolytic anaemia	27
Systemic lupus erythemathosus	117	Evans syndrome	25
Polymalgia/dermatomyositis	18	Other	28
Sjögren's syndrome	5	*Vasculitis*	*56*
Antiphospholipid syndrome	6	Granulomatosis with polyangiitis (GPA)	14
Other	30	Behcet's disease	11
Arthritis	*186*	Takayasu's arteriitis	2
Rheumatoid arthritis	82	*Microscopic* polyangiitis (MPA)	3
Juvenile chronic arthritis (JIA):		*Polyarteritis nodosa* (PAN)	1
• Systemic JIA	59	*Eosinophilic granulomatosis with polyangiitis* (EGPA) (EGPA)	2
• Other JIA	18	Other	23
• Polyarticular JIA	17	*Other neurological diseases*	*114*
Psoriatic arthritis	3	Chronic inflammatory demyelinating polyneuropathy (CIDP)	52
Other	7	Neuromyelitis optica	26
Inflammatory bowel diseases	*220*	Myasthenia gravis	8
Crohn's disease	182	Other	28
Ulcerative colitis	4	*Insulin dependent diabetes mellitus (IDDM)*	*20*
Other	34	*Other*	*51*

EBMT ADWP guidelines (Snowden et al. 2012). More recent data suggests that 'high-intensity' regimens, incorporating BU, have higher rates of PFS but potentially greater toxicity, including TRM (Atkins et al. 2016). Retrospective registry data suggest that graft purging has no added benefit to the transplant outcome (Snowden et al. 2012).

Currently, auto-HSCT is considered to be most effective in patients with relapsing MS, who are not older than 45 years, have had the illness for less than 10 years, are not very disabled (EDSS ≤6) and have very active disease with evidence of enhancement on their MRI (Muraro et al. 2017). An international randomised controlled phase III trial is currently being conducted to compare auto-HSCT with currently available MDTs (MIST Study, ClinicalTrials.gov Identifier: NCT00273364) and is anticipated to report in full in 2021.

91.3 HSCT for Systemic Sclerosis (SSc)

Over the past 10 years, results from large European prospective observational studies confirmed that SSc patients benefit only marginally from standard immunosuppressive drugs, including CY, with a progressive increase in SSc-specific mortality, predominantly related to cardiac (31%) and pulmonary causes (18%). Indications for auto-HSCT in SSc have increased (Snowden et al. 2018) since three successive randomised trials, namely, ASSIST (Burt et al. 2011), ASTIS (van Laar et al. 2014) and SCOT (Sullivan et al. 2018), have now demonstrated that auto-HSCT is superior to CY for early rapidly progressive SSc in terms of long-term survival as well as improvement of lung function and skin fibrosis.

In addition, patient selection was shown to directly affect transplant outcomes (Farge et al. 2017) with specific concern for cardiac involvement, undetected by echocardiography alone, becoming clinically overt during the transplant procedure, under the stress of fluid overload, CY and ATG administration and sepsis. Current guidelines recommend auto-HSCT for patients with early diffuse SSc with a modified Rodnan skin score ≥15 *plus* major organ involvement in respiratory, cardiovascular or renal systems and treatment should be performed in JACIE-accredited centres where combined expertise from SSc disease specialist and dedicated transplant team can assess and follow patients before, during and after the procedure according to Good Clinical Practice (Snowden et al. 2018). Since toxicity and efficacy arise from individual patient selection and the conditioning regimen, different chemotherapies may account for subtle differences in results, and further studies are warranted to analyse the use of attenuated conditioning regimen, according to cardiac function and risk for renal crises (Burt and Farge 2018).

91.4 HSCT for Systemic Lupus Erythematosus (SLE)

Following the first transplant performed in 1996 by Alberto Marmont and colleagues, several phase I/phase II clinical trials have been reported covering approximately 300 SLE patients worldwide to date (Alexander and Hiepe 2017). The two largest experiences on auto-HSCT for SLE so far come from EBMT data registry (n = 53; mean follow-up, 25 months) and from the single-centre trial by Northwestern University (n = 50; mean follow-up, 29 months), both demonstrating a probability of 5-year DFS of 50% despite discontinuation of chronic IS. Subsequently, a follow-up study from the EBMT registry reported the outcome of auto-HSCT in SLE with various regimens between 2001 and 2008 (n = 28; median follow-up, 38 months; range, 1–110 months) (Alchi et al. 2013). Although PFS in this study was only 29% at 5 years, TRM had gradually improved. In addition, this study indicated that CD34-selection was associated with a significantly reduced relapse incidence.

More recently, reports from two independent Chinese groups, both with 10-year follow-up, demonstrated remarkable clinical responses with PFS of 86% and 68%, respectively, while TRM across both studies was only 2%. Current recommendations suggest HSCT in patients with sustained or relapsed active disease (BILAG category A) remaining steroid dependent after at least 6 months of the best standard therapy (including MMF and CY with or without anti-CD20), with documented evidence of visceral involvement (Snowden et al. 2012). The only controlled study conducted to compare auto-HSCT with currently available MDTs in SLE is currently ongoing in a phase II multicentre trial in Germany (ClinicalTrials.gov Identifier: NCT00750971).

91.5 HSCT for Crohn's Disease (CD)

Despite the major recent progress in the treatment of CD, based around corticosteroids, IS (thiopurines, MTX) and biologic therapies (Ab targeting TNFα, α4β7 integrin or IL-12/IL-23), some patients fail all available therapies. In many cases, surgery may be an option but may lead to short bowel syndrome or to a definitive stoma, which may be unacceptable to patients. With this background, in the past few years, auto-HSCT has emerged as a promising therapy in a subset of patients in whom the disease is refractory to all available therapies, with progressive tissue damage and potentially reduced life expectancy.

Auto-HSCT has been investigated in several studies with encouraging responses, some prolonged, although a progressive incidence of relapse with long-term follow-up is recognised (Burt et al. 2010; Lopez-Garcia et al. 2017). Furthermore, patients regain response to anti-TNF therapy although they had been refractory to this drug class prior to HSCT.

In Europe, the EBMT sponsored ASTIC trial in patients with refractory CD and produced apparently negative results as few patients after auto-HSCT met the stringent primary composite endpoint of clinical remission for 3 months (Hawkey et al. 2015). However, it should not be assumed that this single trial provides the definitive answer to the benefit of auto-HSCT in CD, as the number of patients included was limited and encouraging long-term follow-up of ASTIC trial patients has since been reported (Lindsay et al. 2017). Encouraging results have also been reported by an EBMT retrospective analysis of 82 treatment-resistant patients who were not in the ASTIC trial. In this difficult-to-treat group of patients, around a quarter maintained remission without further medical therapy, and long-term disease control was maintained with reintroduction of salvage therapies in the majority of patients who relapsed. TRM occurred in one patient (Brierley 2018).

Recently, the EBMT ADWP and ECCO (European Crohn's and Colitis Organisation) have published a joint position paper of auto-HSCT in CD, which recommends auto-HSCT ideally in the context of a multicentre clinical trial but on an individual basis may currently be considered for patients with active CD refractory to IS and biological treatments or unacceptable risks of surgical management (Snowden et al. 2018).

91.6 Allogeneic HSCT for Autoimmune Diseases

Autoimmune diseases have also been treated with allo-HSCT from MRD, URD and CB sources. In the last 20 years, the EBMT registry has collated 165 cases, representing just 6% of the total. Because of the higher procedural risks and potential long-term impact on quality of life from late effects, allo-HSCT has been largely restricted to life-threatening AD in paediatric practice with the most common indications in immune cytopenia followed by arthritis (Snowden et al. 2017). In a recent summary of cases in the registry between 1997 and 2015, 105 patients undergoing allo-HSCT were treated with conditioning regimens. The median age was 12 years (range 1–62). Outcome following first allo-HSCT included 3- and 5-year OS of 67% and 64%, PFS 59% and 56% and incidence of relapse 21% and 24%, respectively. Compared with auto-HSCT, NRM is relatively high at 13% at 100 days, although this plateaus at 20% at 3 and 5 years.

In summary, experience in allo-HSCT is limited, but long-term data is supportive of basic biological differences in the responses of AD to allo- and auto-HSCT in terms of the ability to cure. However, with the risks NRM of around 20%, allo-HSCT will remain limited and developmental in its application to AD. With time, allo-HSCT in AD has become safer, perhaps with better patient selection, and activity continues, particularly in the paediatric field. In addition, there has been increasing recognition that the nature of the genetic component of some AD means that allo-HSCT is the only realistic approach for long-term disease control. Thus there is renewed interest in this area, particularly where there is overlap with autoinflammatory and immunodeficiency diseases.

91.7 Other Indications

A variety of other ADs have been treated (Table 91.2). Haematological immune cytopenias have been treated with a mixture of auto-HSCT and allo-HSCT. Type 1 diabetes in early 'honeymoon' phase has been the subject of clinical trials, with some ability to prevent or reduce insulin requirements. Otherwise there is a mixture of rarer neurological, rheumatological and gastroenterological indications for which the registry is essential for developing an evidence base. Cautious recommendations for these rare indications are provided in the EBMT ADWP guidelines (Snowden et al. 2012).

91.8 Mechanisms of Action

HSCT represented an opportunity to gain insights into the aetiology and pathogenesis of AD. Through destroying a dysfunctional autoreactive immune system and rebuilding it with auto-HSCT, it has been possible to demonstrate immune 'rebooting' that can occur through thymic reactivation and re-diversification and other changes in T-cell and B-cell repertoire and regulatory cell function in various disease settings. Allo-HSCT has been less well explored, although there is an element of immune replacement and evidence for a 'graft-versus-autoimmune effect' (Alexander et al. 2016).

91.9 Conclusions and Future Directions

With accumulating evidence and improved outcomes along with recognition that modern biological and other therapies are not universally effective (Snowden et al. 2017), ADs have become the fastest-growing indication for HSCT (Passweg et al. 2018). Initially applied as salvage therapy in patients with poor prognosis, HSCT has emerged as a promising treatment option for AD patients earlier in the treatment algorithm. This is the result of positive results from large phase II and randomised controlled phase III trials and updated guidelines for patient selection and transplant technique (Snowden et al. 2012, 2018; Farge et al. 2017). In 2018, the major indications for HSCT for AD are MS, SSc and CD for which significant subsets of patients still show an unsatisfactory response to both conventional and targeted biologic therapies.

Moving forward, further efforts are needed to drive HSCT into routine clinical care. It is recommended that patients should be treated in experienced and JACIE-accredited transplant centres in a multidisciplinary setting. A future goal is to optimise the conditioning regimens according to disease-specific requirements and to outbalance the intensity to maintain outcomes while minimising toxicity and TRM risk. In addition, comprehensive data reporting, harmonisation and exploitation of existing biobanking infrastructure (Alexander et al. 2015), education at individual centre and network level and health economic evaluations along with evidence-based recommendations will establish the future place of HSCT in the treatment algorithms for various autoimmune and inflammatory diseases.

Acknowledgement The authors thank Manuela Badoglio for helpful assistance with data management.

Key Points

- With accumulating evidence, including randomised controlled trials, AD has become the fastest-growing indication for HSCT.
- Major indications for HSCT in AD include multiple sclerosis (MS), systemic sclerosis (SSc) and Crohn´s disease (CD), where auto-HSCT is now featuring in treatment algorithms.
- Although HSCT for ADs is predominantly autologous, there is renewed interest in allo-HSCT, particularly in ADs with autoinflammatory and immunodeficiency components.
- It is recommended that all patients should be treated in experienced and JACIE-accredited transplant centres with close multidisciplinary collaboration and reporting of data to the EBMT registry.
- Immune reconstitution studies are providing insights into the mechanisms of immune reset following HSCT and disease processes underlying various autoimmune diseases.

References

Alchi B, Jayne D, Labopin M, et al. Autologous haematopoietic stem cell transplantation for systemic lupus erythematosus: data from the European Group for Blood and Marrow Transplantation registry. Lupus. 2013;22:245–53.

Alexander T, Hiepe F. Autologous haematopoietic stem cell transplantation for systemic lupus erythematosus: time ready for a paradigm shift? Clin Exp Rheumatol. 2017;35:359–61.

Alexander T, Bondanza A, Muraro PA, et al. SCT for severe autoimmune diseases: consensus guidelines of the European Society for Blood and Marrow Transplantation for immune monitoring and biobanking. Bone Marrow Transplant. 2015;50:173–80.

Alexander T, Arnold R, Hiepe F, RAIDbruch A. Resetting the immune system with immunoablation and autologous haematopoietic stem cell transplantation in autoimmune diseases. Clin Exp Rheumatol. 2016;34:53–7.

Atkins HL, Bowman M, Allan D, et al. Immunoablation and autologous haemopoietic stem-cell transplantation for aggressive multiple sclerosis: a multicentre single-group phase 2 trial. Lancet. 2016;388:576–85.

Burman J, Tolf A, Hagglund H, Askmark H. Autologous haematopoietic stem cell transplantation for neurological diseases. J Neurol Neurosurg Psychiatry. 2018;89:147–55.

Burt RK, Farge D. Systemic sclerosis: autologous HSCT is efficacious, but can we make it safer? Nat Rev Rheumatol. 2018;14:189–91.

Burt RK, Craig RM, Milanetti F, et al. Autologous nonmyeloablative hematopoietic stem cell transplantation in patients with severe anti-TNF refractory Crohn disease: long-term follow-up. Blood. 2010;116:6123–32.

Burt RK, Shah SJ, Dill K, et al. Autologous nonmyeloablative haemopoietic stem-cell transplantation compared with pulse cyclophosphamide once per month for systemic sclerosis (ASSIST): an open-label, randomised phase 2 trial. Lancet. 2011;378:498–506.

Burt RK, Balabanov R, Han X, et al. Association of non-myeloablative hematopoietic stem cell transplantation with neurological disability in patients with relapsing-remitting multiple sclerosis. JAMA. 2015;313:275–84.

Brierley CK et al, J Crohns Colitis. 2018. https://doi.org/10.1093/ecco-jcc/jjy069.

Farge D, Burt RK, Oliveira MC, et al. Cardiopulmonary assessment of patients with systemic sclerosis for hematopoietic stem cell transplantation: recommendations from the European Society for Blood and Marrow Transplantation Autoimmune Diseases Working Party and collaborating partners. Bone Marrow Transplant. 2017;52:1495–503.

Hawkey CJ, Allez M, Clark MM, et al. Autologous hematopoetic stem cell transplantation for refractory Crohn disease: a randomized clinical trial. JAMA. 2015;314:2524–34.

Lindsay JO, Allez M, Clark M, et al. Autologous stem-cell transplantation in treatment-refractory Crohn's disease: an analysis of pooled data from the ASTIC trial. Lancet Gastroenterol Hepatol. 2017;2:399–406.

Lopez-Garcia A, Rovira M, Jauregui-Amezaga A, et al. Autologous hematopoietic stem cell transplantation for refractory Crohn's disease: efficacy in a single-centre cohort. J Crohns Colitis. 2017;11:1161–8.

Mancardi GL, Sormani MP, Gualandi F, et al. Autologous hematopoietic stem cell transplantation in multiple sclerosis: a phase II trial. Neurology. 2015;84:981–8.

Muraro PA, Pasquini M, Atkins HL, et al. Long-term outcomes after autologous hematopoietic stem cell transplantation for multiple sclerosis. JAMA Neurol. 2017;74:459–69.

Nash RA, Hutton GJ, Racke MK, et al. High-dose immunosuppressive therapy and autologous HCT for relapsing-remitting MS. Neurology. 2017;88:842–52.

Passweg JR, Baldomero H, BAIDer P, et al. Is the use of unrelated donor transplantation leveling off in Europe? The 2016 European Society for Blood and Marrow Transplant activity survey report. Bone Marrow Transplant. 2018. https://doi.org/10.1038/s41409-018-0153-1. [Epub aheAID of print].

Snowden JA, Saccardi R, Allez M, et al. Haematopoietic SCT in severe autoimmune diseases: updated guidelines of the European Group for Blood and Marrow Transplantation. Bone Marrow Transplant. 2012;47:770–90.

Snowden JA, Badoglio M, Labopin M, et al. Evolution, trends, outcomes, and economics of hematopoietic stem cell transplantation in severe autoimmune diseases. Blood Adv. 2017;1:2742–55.

Snowden JA, Panes J, Alexander T, et al. Autologous haematopoietic stem cell transplantation (AHSCT) in severe Crohn's disease: a review on behalf of ECCO and EBMT. J Crohns Colitis. 2018;12:476–88.

Sullivan KM, Goldmuntz EA, Keyes-Elstein L, et al. Myeloablative autologous stem-cell transplantation for severe scleroderma. N Engl J Med. 2018;378:35–47.

Tyndall A, Gratwohl A. Blood and marrow stem cell transplants in auto-immune disease: a consensus report written on behalf of the European League against Rheumatism (EULAR) and the European Group for Blood and Marrow Transplantation (EBMT). Bone Marrow Transplant. 1997;19:643–5.

van Laar JM, Farge D, Sont JK, et al. Autologous hematopoietic stem cell transplantation vs intravenous pulse cyclophosphamide in diffuse cutaneous systemic sclerosis: a randomized clinical trial. JAMA. 2014;311:2490–8.

Solid Tumours

92

Ruth Ladenstein, Evgenia Glogova, and Francesco Lanza

92.1 Introduction

In the absence of randomized prospective trials, the EBMT registry remains an important source to survey indications, outcome and clinical risk factors in patients with solid tumours treated by auto- and allo-HSCT. In early 2018, the EBMT registry includes 57,888 transplant procedures in 42,106 patients, with a slight prevalence in adults compared with children (58% vs. 42%). Auto-HSCT represents 97% of the total HSCT, whereas allo-HSCT was used in 3% of the procedures. Multiple transplants were performed in 1/3 of the cases (Table 92.1). More than 10,000 transplants were performed in the last 5 years (Passweg et al. 2018). Figures 92.1 and 92.2 compare activity and indications between adults and children.

Table 92.1 EBMT registry on HSCT for solid tumours (data updated on January 2018)

Solid tumour registry	*57,025*	
Patients	*40,593*	
Adults/pediatric (%)	*58/42*	
Male/female (%)	*48/52*	
Auto/allo (%)	*97/3*	
Nb of HSCT	*Auto (n = 55,240)*	*Allo (n = 1755)*
First HSCT	*40,412*	*1173*
Second HSCT	10,144	440
Third HSCT	3589	100
Fourth HSCT	651	27
≥ Fifth HSCT	194	9
Median follow up (year < 2016)	*2.4 (<1 to 35)*	*1.95 (<1 to 31)*

92.2 Solid Tumours in Children and Adolescents

Ruth Ladenstein and Evgenia Glogova

92.2.1 Introduction

The EBMT registry remains an important source to survey indications, outcome and clinical risk factors in children and adolescents with solid tumours treated by high-dose therapy (HDT) and HSCT.

R. Ladenstein (✉)
Studies and Statistics for Integrated Research and Projects, St. Anna Children's Hospital, Department of Paediatrics and Children's Cancer Research Institute (CCRI), Medical University of Vienna, Vienna, Austria
e-mail: ruth.ladenstein@ccri.at

E. Glogova
Studies and Statistics for Integrated Research and Projects, St. Anna Kinderkrebsforschung e.V., Vienna, Austria

F. Lanza
Hematology and HSCT Unit, Department of Onco-Hematology, Hospital S. Maria delle Croci, Ravenna, Italy

E. Carreras et al. (eds.), *The EBMT Handbook*, https://doi.org/10.1007/978-3-030-02278-5_92

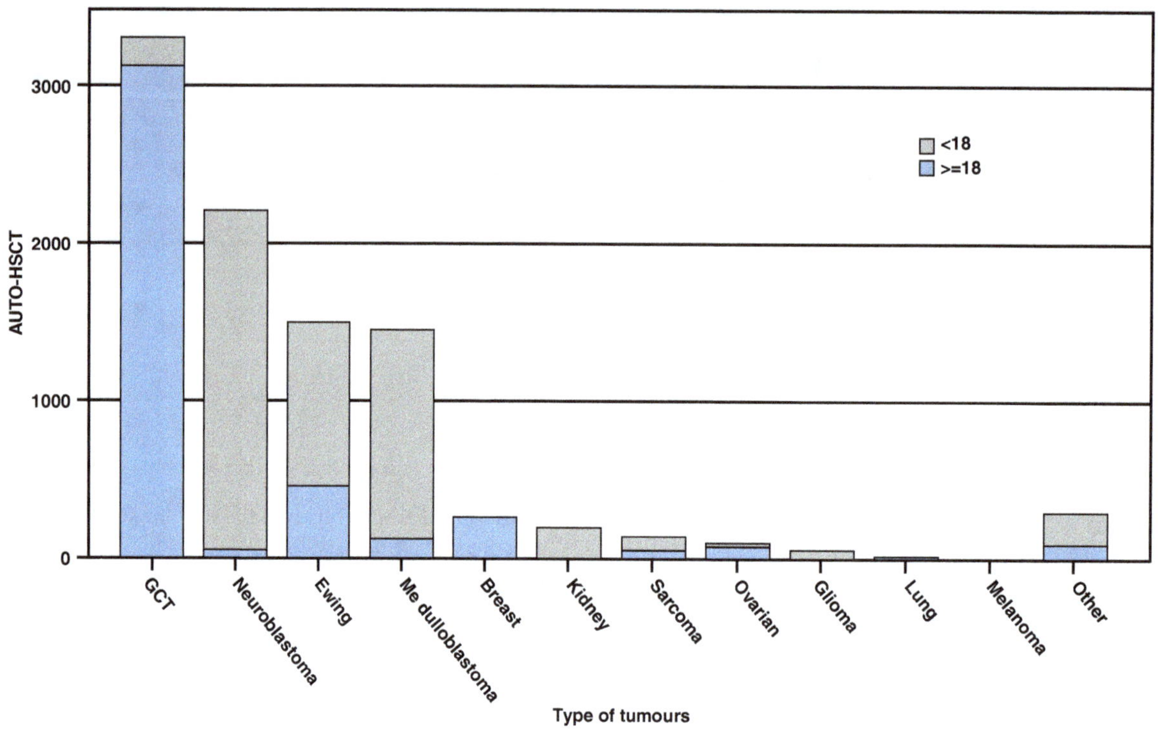

Fig. 92.1 EBMT registry on auto-HSCT for solid tumours in the period 2012–2017 (n = 9519). Adults vs. paediatric HSCT is shown (January 2018)

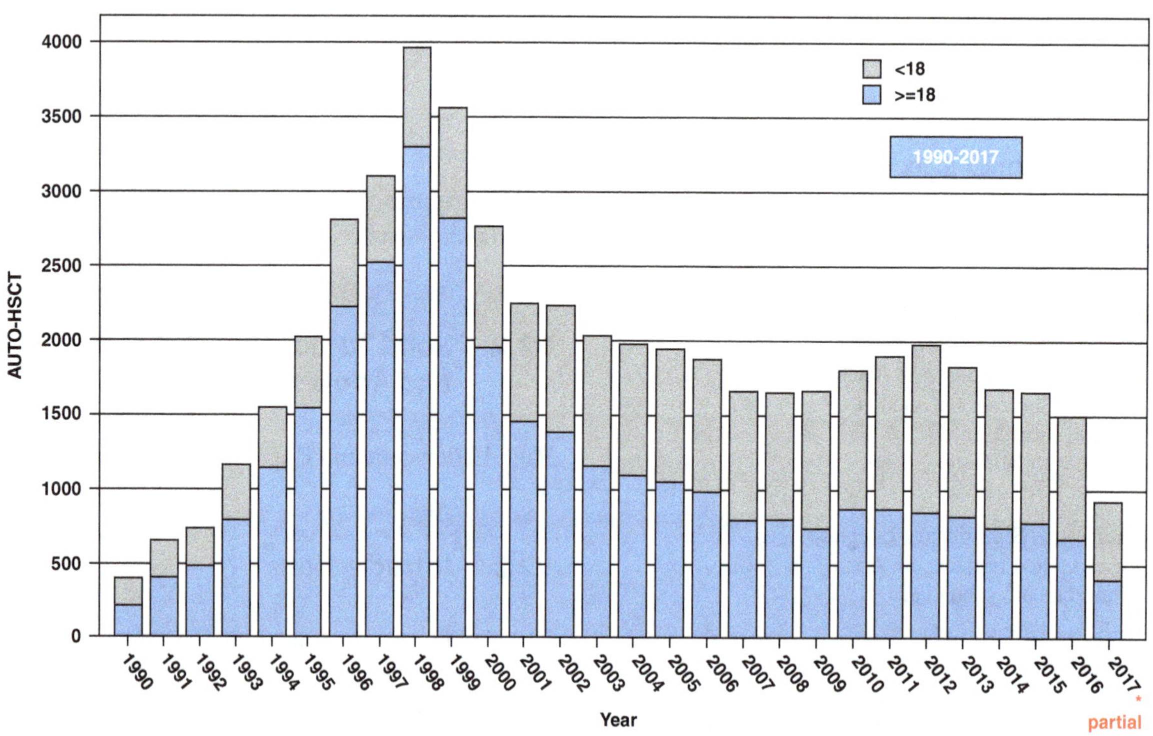

Fig. 92.2 EBMT registry showing numbers of auto-HSCT for solid tumour indication over the years: 1990/2017 in both adults and children

In view of evolving diagnostic and therapeutic strategies, the definition of high risk needs careful consideration. To date evidence for HDT/HSCT from prospective randomized trials is still limited to high-risk neuroblastoma and Ewing sarcoma (Matthay et al. 2009; Whelan 2018).

92.2.2 2018 EBMT Data on HSCT for Solid Tumours in Children and Adolescents

In 2018 the EBMT database contained information on 17,159 transplants in young people with solid tumours. Their median age is 5.2 years (0.1–18.0); 58% are male. Auto-HSCT is the most frequent procedure with 14,135 transplants performed, whereas only 446 allo-HSCTs are registered. Data was gathered in 43 countries and reported by 390 centres. The first HSCT was autologous in 16,814 patients and allogeneic in 345 patients. Table 92.2 summarizes the outcomes with auto-HSCT for the most frequent indications for 13,838 with adequate event information in the EBMT database.

92.2.2.1 General Lessons from EBMT Data

The experience of more than 17,000 HSCT procedures in the paediatric age group over 35 years conveys a number of important messages:

Transplant-related mortality. TRM markedly decreased over time and is related with the HDT regimen (i.e. elimination of TBI) and most importantly use of peripheral stem cells. TRM rates associated to auto-HSCT dropped to under 5% after 1992 and is since 2012 only 1%.

Total body irradiation. TBI showed no advantage in any of the solid tumour indications and should thus be avoided in children with solid tumours in view of late effects.

Remission status. First-line high-risk patients perform significantly better than after relapse. Response to induction treatments prior to HDT/HSCT is critical in all indications. A short summary is:

CR > VGPR/PR > SR/MR > NR (SD) > RR/UR
[*CR* complete response, *VGPR* very good partial response, *PR* partial response (>50%), *SR* sensitive relapse = >50% response, *MR* minor response (<50%), *NR* no response, *SD* stable disease, *RR/UR* resistant or untreated relapse (<50% response)]

Patients in good response to first-line treatment (CR/VGPR/PR) and sensitive relapse (SR) are good indications for most high-risk solid tumour patients, while patients with stable disease or minor response (<50%) (SD/MR) should only be considered for well-defined phase I/phase II trials. Patients with no response (NR) or tumour progression or resistant relapse (RR) have a very short life expectancy even after HDT/HSCT and thus should not be considered.

Age (see Table 92.3). Age plays a crucial role for outcome predictions. Adolescent age is generally associated with inferior outcome. While age <10 years is a favourable factor in sarcomas (Ewing tumours and rhabdomyosar-

Table 92.2 EBMT database outcomes after HDT/ASCT in paediatric solid tumours

	All patients			First line patients		Relapsed patients		
Diagnoses	Patients	5-years pSU	5-years pEFS	Patients	5-years pEFS	Patients	5-years pEFS	*p*-value[a]
Neuroblastoma	7303	0.44 ± 0.01	0.36 ± 0.01	5993	0.37 ± 0.01	432	0.25 ± 0.02	<0.001
Ewing tumors	2886	0.47 ± 0.01	0.40 ± 0.01	2101	0.44 ± 0.01	483	0.29 ± 0.02	<0.001
Wilms tumors	601	0.55 ± 0.02	0.51 ± 0.02	208	0.52 ± 0.04	345	0.53 ± 0.03	0.567
Soft tissue sa.	1097	0.29 ± 0.02	0.24 ± 0.01	673	0.26 ± 0.02	260	0.20 ± 0.03	0.003
Brain tumors	2733	0.45 ± 0.01	0.39 ± 0.01	2020	0.43 ± 0.01	444	0.22 ± 0.02	<0.001
Germ cell tu.	529	0.59 ± 0.03	0.49 ± 0.02	270	0.50 ± 0.03	201	0.44 ± 0.04	0.083
Retinoblastomas	162	0.64 ± 0.04	0.59 ± 0.04	98	0.64 ± 0.05	53	0.50 ± 0.07	0.099
Kidney tumors	73	0.49 ± 0.07	0.48 ± 0.07	30	0.51 ± 0.10	30	0.48 ± 0.10	0.615
Osteosarcomas	290	0.28 ± 0.03	0.24 ± 0.03	129	0.34 ± 0.05	128	0.13 ± 0.03	<0.001
Miscellaneous	784	0.40 ± 0.02	0.33 ± 0.02	511	0.34 ± 0.02	146	0.21 ± 0.04	0.057

[a]Log-rank test: first line versus relapse patients

Table 92.3 EBMT database outcomes after HDT/ASCT in paediatric solid tumours according to patient age

		Age ≤ 5 years		5 < age ≤ 10 years		10 < age ≤ 18 years		
Diagnoses	Patients	Patients	5-years pEFS	Patients	5-years pEFS	Patients	5-years pEFS	*p*-value
Neuroblastoma	7303	5267	0.41 ± 0.01	1742	0.26 ± 0.01	361	0.18 ± 0.03	<0.001
Ewing tumors	2886	388	0.38 ± 0.03	622	0.47 ± 0.02	1913	0.39 ± 0.01	0.001
Wilms tumors	601	201	0.57 ± 0.04	318	0.49 ± 0.03	96	0.43 ± 0.06	0.173
Soft tissue sa.	1097	286	0.30 ± 0.03	287	0.29 ± 0.03	453	0.17 ± 0.02	<0.001
Brain tumors	2733	1243	0.44 ± 0.02	799	0.37 ± 0.02	751	0.33 ± 0.02	0.039
Germ cell tu.	529	165	0.52 ± 0.04	47	0.41 ± 0.08	328	0.49 ± 0.03	0.273
Retinoblastomas	162	132	0.58 ± 0.05	26	0.69 ± 0.10	10	0.50 ± 0.18	0.727
Kidney tumors	73	33	0.51 ± 0.10	22	0.53 ± 0.11	12	0.36 ± 0.15	0.631
Osteosarcomas	290	4	0.75 ± 0.22	35	0.29 ± 0.08	248	0.22 ± 0.03	0.260
Miscellaneous	784	342	0.40 ± 0.03	145	0.23 ± 0.05	302	0.29 ± 0.03	0.016

coma), neuroblastoma has an earlier cut-off at 5 years. Patients with neuroblastoma ≤18 months at diagnosis need biological profiling and are only eligible with high-risk biological features, in particular MYCN amplification (Canete et al. 2009).

Double HSCT approaches. The EBMT data on repetitive HDT/HSCT approaches shows no advantage over single HDT/HSCT. However, the elective selection of particular poor-prognosis patients in phase II settings is a likely bias. Recent data from a randomized trial in neuroblastoma emerged with superiority for the tandem strategy for high-risk neuroblastoma front-line patients (Park et al. 2016).

Busulfan-melphalan. This HDT combination is the only one in the EBMT database resulting in significantly improved survival rates in neuroblastoma and Ewing tumours.

Allo-HSCT. No advantage for allo-HSCT can be detected in the EBMT data for any paediatric solid tumour indication. The potential bias of negative selection of particular poor-prognosis patients needs to be considered.

92.2.3 Neuroblastoma

High-risk neuroblastoma (NBL) is defined by widespread disease >18 months, including any stage and age in the presence of MYCN oncogene amplification (Cohn et al. 2009; Moroz et al. 2011). In 2018 standard treatments include multicycle induction, extensive surgery to the primary tumour site, HDT/auto-HSCT, at least local radiotherapy and maintenance with 13-cis retinoid acid, ideally with ch14.18 antibody-based immunotherapy in addition (Park et al. 2016; Yu et al. 2010; Ladenstein et al. 2017, 2018).

Age <18 months is an important prognostic discriminator (Cohn et al. 2009; Moroz et al. 2011). The European high-risk NBL study (HR-NBL-1/SIOPEN) randomized BU/MEL and CEM (CBP, VP, MEL) after an adequate response to COJEC induction. BU/MEL HDT resulted in a better EFS and OS with fewer severe adverse events than CEM reporting a 3-year EFS of 50% (95% CI 45–56) for BU/MEL versus 38% (32–43) for CEM prior immunotherapy was available for all trial patients in Europe (Ladenstein et al. 2017).

After decades of dose escalation being explored by many teams, the randomized results of the ANBL0532 COG as presented at ASCO 2016 finally found superiority for double HDT/HSCT [1st HDT, CY and TT; 2nd HDT, CBP, VP and MEL (with reduced doses of single HDT CEM) vs. single HDT (CEM)/auto-HSCT (Park et al. 2016)]. The 3-year EFS and OS were significantly higher for tandem transplant patients (73.2%; 85.6%) in comparison with the single transplant arm (55.5%; 75.8%). Anti-GD2 antibody-based immunotherapy was beneficial for both arms (Yu et al. 2010).

Targeted therapies, in particular iodine-131-metaiodobenzylguanidine (mIBG) therapy with and without chemotherapy and/or HDT followed by HSCT, have generated increasing interest (Lee et al. 2017; Johnson et al. 2011).

Further HDT tandem approaches with or without mIBG are currently explored by the COG as well as SIOPEN in planned randomized trials. Published mIBG treatments refer to tandem mIBG in rapid sequence, to mIBG as component of HDT (CEM or BU/MEL) and mIBG combination therapies. They vary in dose, single vs. tandem schedules applied and various combinations with chemotherapy (topotecan or irinotecan and VCR) or radiation sensitizers (i.e. vorinostat increasing mIBG uptake).

In relapse patients the EBMT data (Ladenstein et al. 1993) showed a benefit from salvage HDT/HSCT in responding patients relapsing after 12 months from diagnosis and without a previous HDT.

Allo-HSCT as immunotherapy received special attention after introduction of RIC and NMA transplants. Some reports highlight a graft-versus-tumour (GvT) effect with adopted allo-HSCT approaches, while the EBMT data shows no benefit with classical allo-HSCT (Ladenstein et al. 1994). Research on experimental approaches to allogeneic HSCT is ongoing. Haplo-HSCT is a feasible option in very high-risk R/R patients capable to induce long-term remission in some with tolerable side effects allowing addition of post-transplant immune adoptive strategies (Illhardt et al. 2018).

92.2.3.1 EBMT Data (See Tables 92.2 and 92.3)

Median age of 7672 patients is 3.7 years (7,504 auto-HSCT, 168 allo-HSCT). EBMT registry data pointed at an early stage to the superiority of the BU/MEL HDT (Ladenstein et al. 2017). A multivariate analysis of the EBMT data found significantly better EFS associated with age <2 years at ASCT ($p < 0.0001$), a good remission status (≥PR) before HDT/HSCT ($p < 0.0001$), use of PBSC ($p = 0.014$), ASCT (vs. allo-HSCT) ($p = 0.031$), as well as with the BU/MEL combination for HDT ($p < 0.01$) (Ladenstein et al. 2008).

92.2.3.2 Indications 2018

Standard indications include first-line high-risk NBL >18 months at diagnosis with widespread metastatic disease or those of any age with MYCN amplified tumours with INSS stages 2–4. Any responding metastatic relapse in patients >18 months and any MYCN amplified tumour without prior HDT/HSCT are good indications. Any other indication is reserved for well-designed experimental phase I/phase II trials. Children <18 months need to be evaluated for a high-risk biological risk profile prior to being considered for HDT/auto-HSCT (Canete et al. 2009; Moroz et al. 2011; Cohn et al. 2009).

92.2.4 Ewing Tumours

A number of publications proposed a potential role of HDT/HSCT in Ewing tumours (Ladenstein et al. 2010; Luksch et al. 2012) during primary treatments for patients with multifocal bone or BM metastases, whereas indications for those with lung metastases is more questionable (Burdach and Jürgens 2002). Some publications found BU/MEL HDT more active in comparison to other HDT regimes (Tenneti et al. 2018). TBI was investigated (Burdach and Jürgens 2002) without any clear benefit but high toxicity and mortality.

The Euro-EWING 99 study group (Ladenstein et al. 2010) published the largest population of HSCT on primary disseminated multifocal Ewing sarcomas (PDMES) with 281 patients receiving BU/MEL HDT/auto-HSCT after VIDE (VCR, IFO, DOX, VP) induction. The 3-year EFS and OS were 27 ± 3% and 34 ± 4% and were 45% for patients ≤14 years. Patients ≥14 years (HR = 1.6), with a primary tumour volume >200 mL (HR = 1.8), more than one bone metastatic site (HR = 2.0), BM metastases (HR = 1.6) and additional lung metastases (HR = 1.5), carry an increased risk at diagnosis. A score based on these factors identified patients with an EFS rate of 50% for scores ≤3 (82 patients), 25% for a score >3 and ≤5 (102 patients) and 10% for score ≥5 (70 patients; $p < 0.0001$).

In 2018 the Euro-EWING 99 study group published the results of the randomized comparison of BU/MEL over standard chemotherapy with VAI (7 courses) which was offered to patients if aged <50 with poor histologic response (≥10% viable cells) after VIDE induction (6 courses) or large tumour volume at diagnosis (≥200 mL). The risk of event was significantly decreased by BU/MEL compared to VAI (VCR, actinomycin, IFO) (HR = 0.64, 95% CI = 0.43–0.95; $p = 0.026$); 3- and 8-year EFS were, respectively, 69.0% (60.2–76.6%) versus 56.1% (47.6–65.4%) and 60.7% (51.1–69.6%) versus 47.1% (37.7–56.8%). OS results also favoured BU/MEL. For this group of patients, BU/MEL is now a standard of care (Whelan 2018).

Tandem HDT and allo-HSCT were part of the EICESS92 and Meta-EICESS protocols yielding long-term DFS in patients with advanced Ewing tumours (Burdach and Jürgens 2002).

Patients suffering a relapse generally have a poor prognosis with conventional chemotherapy. The role of HDT/auto-HSCT still awaits clarification in randomized controlled studies (Tenneti et al. 2018; Ferrari et al. 2015). A GvT or improved survival following allo-HSCT effect was highlighted in some reports, but a retrospective review (Thiel et al. 2011) could not identify benefits with either RIC or MAC or with either HLA-matched or HLA-mismatched grafts.

92.2.4.1 **EBMT Data** (See Tables 92.2 and 92.3)

The median age of 3019 (2970 autologous, 49 allogeneic) evaluable Ewing tumour patients is 12.5 years with 2161 patients who received HDT during primary treatment and 498 after relapse (disease status not specified in 360). BU/MEL HDT achieved better results in first-line settings, while TBI clearly was associated with poorer outcomes. Multivariate analysis of the EBMT data showed increased risks for patients >14 years, a remission status less than CR1, PR or CR2, BM as stem cell source and HDT other than BU/MEL.

92.2.4.2 Indications 2018

BU/MEL HDT for patients with a poor histological response after induction and/or a tumour volume ≥200 mL is now standard of care. Patients with primary metastatic disease at sites other than the lungs and a low-risk score may be considered good candidates in the absence of a controlled trial. Any metastatic relapse without prior HDT may be considered for controlled phase II HDT protocols.

92.2.5 Soft Tissue Sarcoma (STS)

Rhabdomyosarcoma (RMS) is the most common STS of childhood. A multivariate analysis of 269 patients with metastatic RMS found age (>10 years, $p < 0.0001$) and bone/BM involvement ($p < 0.019$) to be the most important predictors for fatal outcome (Thiel et al. 2013). In STS dose escalation with auto-HSCT produced only short-lived remissions with generally disappointing outcome data unless patients were chemosensitive and receiving HDT as consolidation in CR (Admiraal et al. 2010). Results of a recent review do not justify the use of HDC/HSCT as standard therapy for children with metastatic RMS (Admiraal et al. 2010).

A systematic review of HDT/auto-HSCT in locally advanced or metastatic non-rhabdomyosarcoma soft tissue sarcoma (NRSTS) was undertaken and evaluated 294 patients with 19 different subtypes of malignant NRSTS in 62 studies covering an age span between 10 and 46 years. This analysis found no advantage for HDT over standard chemotherapy (Peinemann and Labeit 2014).

The use of allo-HSCT in patients with advanced RMS is still experimental. No patients with residual disease before allo-SCT were converted to CR. In a subset of patients, it may constitute a valuable approach for consolidating CR, but this awaits prospective validation (Thiel et al. 2013).

92.2.5.1 **EBMT Data** (See Tables 92.2 and 92.3)

The median age of 1116 evaluable patients (1035 autologous, 81 allogeneic) is 9 years with 718 receiving HDT during primary treatment and 275 after relapse (disease status not specified in 123 patients).

92.2.5.2 Indications 2018

Currently there is no evidence-based standard indication for HDT/HSCT in STS.

92.2.6 Brain Tumours

Paediatric embryonal brain tumour patients treated with craniospinal irradiation (CSI) are at risk for adverse effects, with greater severity in younger patients. Two publications in 2017 refer to this situation. Outcomes of CSI vs. HDT/auto-HSCT and delayed CSI were compared in 201 newly diagnosed patients [medulloblastoma (72%), supratentorial primitive neuroectodermal tumour (sPNET; 18%) or pineoblastoma (10%)]. Outcomes with adjuvant HD/HSCT followed by delayed CSI are comparable to upfront CSI for young paediatric embryonal brain tumour patients, but benefits regarding neurocognitive outcomes await future assessment (Raleigh et al. 2017).

The second report summarizing HDT/HSCT (29 with 3 tandem transplants and 15 with 2 tandem transplants) as irradiation-avoiding or irradiation-minimizing approach reported encouraging irradiation-free survival in children with newly diagnosed malignant brain tumours [medulloblastoma/primitive neuroectodermal tumour (21 patients), atypical teratoid/rhabdoid tumour (8), high-grade glioma (5), malignant germ cell tumour (4), ependymoma (3) and choroid plexus carcinoma (3)] (Guerra et al. 2017). The PFS and OS for newly diagnosed patients were 68.9 ± 9.9% and 73.5 ± 9.3%, while it was only 11.8 ± 9.8% ($p < 0.001$) and 15.1 ± 12.3% ($p = 0.0231$) at relapse, respectively.

The Children's Cancer Group 99703 study assessed 92 patients receiving 3 consolidation cycles of HDT (TT and CBP) and auto-HSCT after biopsy/resection and 3 conventional-dose chemotherapy cycles. Response rates to induction and consolidation were high in patients with residual tumour with 73.3% and 66.7%, respectively, resulting in 5-year EFS and OS of 43.9 ± 5.2% and 63.6 ± 5%. Gross total resection versus less than gross total resection was the only significant outcome comparison (Cohen et al. 2015).

The HIT97 national trial tested a stratified relapse protocol using either intensive chemotherapy, potentially high dose, or oral chemotherapy. Adding HDT in patients who responded to the initial courses of chemotherapy did not improve survival. Patients with relapsed cerebral PNET responding to conventional chemotherapy did not profit from HDT (Bode et al. 2014).

92.2.6.1 EBMT Data (See Tables 92.2 and 92.3)

The median age for 2818 evaluable brain tumour patients (2809 autologous, 9 allogeneic) is 6 years with 2039 receiving HDT during primary treatments and 442 after relapse (disease status not specified in 337).

Medulloblastoma is the leading indication with 69% followed by astrocytoma (7%), glioblastoma (7%), ependymoma (6%) and other non-specified CNS tumours (11%). Medulloblastoma patients' outcome is better when submitted to HDT/SCT in first remission and if younger <3 years. A more detailed analysis by various brain tumours histologies and distinct risk factors is not possible in the current dataset.

92.2.6.2 Indications 2018

Patients with high-risk medulloblastoma (primary metastases/relapse) of any age older than 3 years are eligible for HDT/HSCT in combination with radiation, while in infants HDT/HSCT is used with the aim of reducing (volumes and doses) or avoiding radiation (Finlay and Massimino 2010).

Metastatic PNETs at diagnosis or with additional high-risk features such as incomplete resection or young age (younger than 3 or 5 years) as well as infants and young children (<4 years) with malignant brain tumours are further indications. Very controversial indications include high-grade glioma. Currently there is little or no indication for HDT/HSCT in ependymoma, brain stem glioma or pineoblastoma. More investigations are required to define the optimal HDT for each tumour type. Most groups use similar HDT regimens, i.e. BU/TT (SFOP, Spain), VP/TT/CBDCA (US/CCG, Germany, Spain) or a tandem approach Vp16/CBDCA - TTP/L-PAM (Italy).

92.2.7 Wilms' Tumour (WT)

Pooling data of 19 publications (5 HDT, 6 NoHDT, 8 both), an advantage to HDT with a hazard ratio (HR) of 0.87 for EFS and 0.94 for OS was observed. Further analyses of risk groups, defined by treatment and/or histology prior to first relapse, suggested a HR for EFS of 0.90 for those of high- and 0.50 for the very high-risk patients. However, a great uncertainty persists in the absence of randomized trials concerning the role of HDT following relapse after treatment for WT (Ha et al. 2013).

The CIBMTR retrospective analysis on 253 relapsed WT receiving HDT/auto-HSCT reports 5-year EFS and OS rates of 36% (95% CI, 29–43%) and 45% (95% CI, 38–51%), respectively. Outcomes are similar to those reported in the literature. So far attempts to conduct a randomized trial comparing maintenance chemotherapy with consolidation versus HDT/auto-HSCT have failed in this indication (Malogolowkin et al. 2017).

92.2.7.1 EBMT Data (See Tables 92.2 and 92.3)

The median age in 625 patients with auto-HSCT (212 HDT during primary treatment; 348 after relapse) is 6 years. Reported superior results for patients receiving MEL alone may be correlated to the favourable response status prior HDT: 76% in CR1 and 64% in CR2.

92.2.7.2 Indications 2018

Experience of the SIOP, GPOH, NWTS, MRC and respective national groups over the last 20 years found the probability of cure of 30% at best in the presence of adverse prognostic factors. High-risk factors are unfavourable histology and metastatic disease (Presson et al. 2010) and are after relapse again unfavourable histology and one of the following criteria: extra-pulmonary relapse or abdominal relapse after radiation, stage IV, more than two drugs in the first-line regimen or relapse within 1 year. HDT is indicated if a response to second-line treatment is achieved.

92.2.8 Germ Cell Tumours

CNS germ cell tumours (GCTs) can be divided into major groups including germinomas (having a superior prognosis) and non-germinomatous GCTs (NGGCTs), with teratomas often considered a separate category- and represent approximately 3% of primary paediatric brain tumours. NGGCTs are less radiosensitive, but adjuvant chemotherapy improved survival.

CNS GCT relapses commonly occur at the primary tumour site, and in about 30% there is concomitant leptomeningeal spread. Salvage therapies include additional surgery, focal or CSI and HDT/auto-HSCT. For pure germinoma patients previously receiving radiation therapy, HDT/auto-HSCT is often recommended. HDT/HSCT showed curative potential for some relapsed systemic NGGCTs, in particular for those achieving a CR to chemotherapy (Echevarria et al. 2008).

The management of intracranial GCTs is complex because of varied clinical presentations, tumour sites, treatments and outcomes and the need for multidisciplinary input.

In an international Delphi approach, key areas of consensus were defined to guide and streamline clinical management of patients with intracranial germ cell tumours (Murray et al. 2015).

92.2.8.1 EBMT Data (See Tables 92.2 and 92.3)

The median age of 553 patients with HDT/ASCT (270 during primary treatment, 211 after relapse, disease status not reported in 72) registered as GCT and considered high risk is 13 years. However, differentiation of subgroups is poor.

92.2.8.2 Indications 2018

As paediatric patients with extracranial GCTs may expect an excellent outcome with conventional chemotherapy approaches, there is no standard indication for HDT/ASCT.

High-risk patients with extracranial GCTs are initial nonresponders or poor responders (no local control achieved) and patients after relapse failing to achieve second CR. In high-risk CNS GCT patients <18 years, the following criteria for HDT may be adopted: recurrent CNS GCT when biological remission is achieved prior to HDC and insufficient response to primary chemotherapy.

92.2.9 Osteosarcoma

Even in responding high-risk patients treated with HDT/HSCT in first or second remission, the length of remission is short, and relapse occurs early after HDT. High-risk features include poor histological response or nonresponse of the primary tumour at the time of definitive surgery, inoperable, axial tumours (large volume), primary dissemination or relapse other than isolated, late lung metastases.

The French Society of Paediatric Oncology (SFCE) explored HDT with high-dose TT and auto-HSCT in 45 children with relapsed osteosarcoma (median age 15.9 years) after initial progression of metastatic disease (2), first relapse (26) and second or third relapse (17). Three-year OS was 40% and 3-year PFS 24%. A randomized study for recurrent osteosarcoma between standard salvage chemotherapy and high-dose TT with auto-HSCT is ongoing (Marec-Berard et al. 2014).

Earlier reports did not encourage HDT regimens (Sauerbrey et al. 2001) and included MEL and VP, with additional CBP by the Cooperative Osteosarcoma Study Group, or two courses of high-dose VP and CBP by the Italian Sarcoma Group (Boye et al. 2014; Fagioli et al. 2002).

92.2.9.1 EBMT Data (See Tables 92.2 and 92.3)

The median age in 294 evaluable patients (134 HDT during primary treatment; 130 after relapse, disease status not specified in 30; 288 autologous, only 6 allogeneic) is 14.3 years.

92.2.9.2 Indications 2018

There is no standard indication for HSCT based on published results or EBMT data.

92.2.10 Retinoblastoma

There is one systematic review on HDT/auto-HSCT based on 15 studies and a total of 101 patients (Jaradat et al. 2012). Following treatment for metastatic and relapsed disease, 44 of 77 patients (57.1%) were alive with no evidence of disease at the time of follow-up. However, a higher rate of local relapse developed in patients with CNS metastases (73.1%), which dropped to 47.1% in patients who received thiotepa. In patients with trilateral or bilateral advanced retinoblastoma, five of seven (71.4%) with reported outcome data as well as patients with tumour at the surgical margin of the optic nerve and/or extrascleral extension, six of seven patients (85.7%) were alive without evidence of disease at last follow-up. Durable tumour control was achieved in patients with non-CNS metastases, trilateral or bilateral advanced retinoblastoma, and with tumour at the surgical margin of the optic nerve and/or extrascleral extension. Patients with CNS metastases require TT to improve tumour control (Dunkel et al. 2010).

Advocated HDT/auto-HSCT approaches are CARBOPEC (CBP, VP, CY) (Jaradat et al. 2012), but for CNS-positive patients, TT or BU was introduced. Other groups used combinations including MEL and CBDCA and/or VP for metastatic retinoblastoma and reported promising survival results for patients without CNS involvement.

92.2.10.1 EBMT Data (See Tables 92.2 and 92.3)

The median age for 170 evaluable patients (99 during primary treatment (40% with localized/regional disease; 60% with metastatic disease); 54 after relapse; 17 disease status not specified; 169 autologous, 1 allogeneic) is 3.5 years.

92.2.10.2 Indications 2018

Future trials should take the following high-risk factors into consideration: involvement of the cut end or subarachnoidal space of the optic nerve after enucleation, orbital involvement and distant metastatic disease and CNS disease.

Key Points

- In neuroblastoma and Ewing sarcoma, there is clear evidence for the advantage of HDT/auto-HSCT with an increasing interest in tandem transplants.
- In other paediatric solid tumour, indication still lacks randomized trials, and indications are based on observational studies, case reports and EBMT database only.

92.3 Solid Tumours in Adults

Francesco Lanza

92.3.1 Auto-HSCT

Supported by a strong rationale from laboratory studies and apparently "convincing" results of early phase II studies, in the 1990s auto-HSCT was uncritically adopted as a potentially curative option for solid tumours. For this reason, randomized trials comparing high-dose therapy with conventional control arm were difficult to conduct. As a result, the number and size of clinical studies initiated (and often abandoned before completion) to prove or disprove its value were largely insufficient. Nowadays, after 25 years of clinical research and thousands of patients receiving auto-HSCT, the benefit of autotransplant in solid tumours, with the possible exception of selected patients with breast cancer (BC) and germ cell tumours (GCTs), is still unsettled (Fig. 92.1) (Sureda et al. 2015).

92.3.1.1 Breast Cancer (BC)

The role of auto-HSCT for primary breast cancer at high risk of recurrence (at least four involved axillary lymph nodes) has been assessed by several randomized trials, recently evaluated by a meta-analysis of individual patient data (Berry et al. 2011; Pedrazzoli et al. 2015). Overall, it was shown that auto-HSCT prolonged DFS when used as adjuvant therapy and showed a benefit on BC-specific survival and OS in selected cohorts of patients (Nitz et al. 2005; Pedrazzoli et al. 2015).

Whether auto-HSCT has benefit in the context of contemporary taxane-based regimens and targeted therapies is largely unknown. Seven phase III studies have been published in peer-reviewed journals. Most of these trials showed improved PFS in the auto-HSCT arm but only one OS advantage. Six randomized trials, including 866 metastatic breast cancer (MBC) patients, have been analysed in the parallel meta-analysis of individual patient data (Berry et al. 2011) showing a significant improvement in PFS but no improvement in OS.

Overall, based on the randomized studies so far, meta-analyses and retrospective studies, auto-HSCT may still represent a therapeutic option for younger patients harbouring HER2-negative tumours and having gross involvement of axillary nodes (adjuvant setting) or highly chemosensitive disease (advanced setting) (Martino et al. 2016).

92.3.1.2 Germ Cell Tumours (GCTs)

Auto-HSCT is not recommended as first-line therapy in GCT. In relapsed GCT high-dose therapy is considered a therapeutic option, especially when poor prognostic factors are present (Lorch et al. 2011; Necchi et al. 2015; De Giorgi et al. 2017a; b). A randomized study (Tiger study) comparing conventional-dose therapy with high-dose therapy is ongoing. Auto-HSCT is a standard of care for patients that are (primary) refractory to platinum-based chemotherapy or for those with a second or further relapse (Necchi et al. 2015). Multiple intensified cycles with CBP/VP are recommended as the standard HDT for GCT also due to concerns that using a three-drug regimen would require dose reductions of the two most active drugs in this disease.

Furthermore, auto-HSCT can be safely administered in high-risk patients older than 45 years. However, since the prognosis is poorer for older patients with non-seminoma histology, a comprehensive risk-benefit evaluation should include co-morbidities and the patient's risk category.

The assessment of a large series of EBMT centres, including 46 cases with pure seminoma, seems to support the notion that auto-HSCT may represent a valuable therapeutic option after standard-dose chemotherapy failure in this patient category (Necchi et al. 2017).

EBMT conducted a retrospective analysis on 29 patients with refractory gestational trophoblastic neoplasia (GTN) treated with auto-HSCT. Data showed that HDT based on CBP seems to be active in this heavily pretreated patient population and that auto-HSCT represents a possible option for patients with refractory GNT (Necchi et al. 2016).

The role of auto-HSCT in mediastinal non-seminoma (MnS) GCT disease category is under evaluation. Data from EBMT confirmed that the

MnS was characterized by the poorest outcome with 5-year OS ranging from 40% to 45%. The use of auto-HSCT as both early intensification and at disease recurrence proved to be effective, given upfront, and may produce a 15–20% absolute improvement in survival compared with standard-dose CT.

92.3.1.3 Soft Tissue Sarcoma (STS)

STS accounts for about 1% of adult cancers. Based on the observation of a dose-response correlation for some drugs used in STS, e.g. DOX and IFO, HDT with auto-HSCT has been investigated in some, mostly non-randomized phase II trials. Most of these trials found few patients to possibly benefit from auto-HSCT but, owing to the small patient numbers of each of the included histologic subgroups, could not establish robust markers for identifying these patients. A recent meta-analysis on this subject found no evidence for a benefit of auto-HSCT but, again, did not sufficiently report on outcomes in the different histologic subgroups. However, taking into account that the current WHO classification differentiates more than 50 histological subtypes of STS, it might be hypothesized that clinical response to auto-HSCT may vary significantly from different histological varieties.

92.3.1.4 Other Solid Tumours

Data from randomized phase III studies comparing HDT vs. conventional-dose chemotherapy for first-line treatment of advanced ovarian cancer and limited or extensive small cell lung cancer have shown no statistically significant difference in PFS or OS. Limitations due to study design, difficulty in recruitment and toxicity may have accounted for the lack of favourable results that were expected based on previous phase II and retrospective analyses of such highly chemosensitive diseases.

In other chemosensitive histologies, including sarcomas and CNS tumours, data regarding auto-HSCT in adult patients are limited, again based on clinical trials without randomization and retrospective analyses. For this reason, auto-HSCT cannot be recommended as standard of care. High-dose therapy can be regarded as a potential clinical option in selected patients with Ewing's sarcoma and medulloblastoma.

92.3.2 Allo-HSCT

Immune therapy for cancer is being pursued with extraordinary interest by researchers all over the world, given the recent scientific acquisitions on immune mechanisms that control cancer and the introduction in the marketplace of checkpoint inhibitor molecules, such as nivolumab/pembrolizumab (PD-1/PDL-1 inhibitors), ipilimumab (anti-CTLA4), etc. The paradigm for immune therapy of cancer is allo-HSCT, whose therapeutic effect is carried out by immunocompetent T cells of the donor, an effect known as GvT or graft-versus-tumour effect. Several studies of allo-HSCT in selected solid tumours, namely, renal cell cancer (RCC), ovarian cancer, BC, colorectal cancer and others, with some evidence of GvT and occurrence of transplant-related toxicities, mostly GvHD have been reported. In RCC, a long-term survival effect in a fraction (20%) of patients was documented. Since 2004, when molecularly targeted drugs were introduced into the clinic for renal cell cancer, patient referral for transplant dropped precipitously, and transplant rate evaluation for solid tumours from 2009 was limited to a few patients in Europe.

A recent survey provided a picture of the status of allo-HSCT for solid tumours in EBMT centres (Bregni et al. 2016). In contrast to our expectations, allo-HSCT for solid tumour indications has not been abandoned, even if its use has been markedly reduced. Based on these findings, allograft for solid tumours as adoptive immunotherapy is still being used in EBMT centres, in a few institutions and in a few selected indications, thus confirming the willingness of several centres to share data, adopt common protocols and continue to use this strategy in highly selected cases.

92.3.2.1 Renal Cell Cancer

There is no clinical experience of allografting in RCC, that is, TKI and mTOR refractory; nowadays, allo-HSCT should be considered only in the context of prospective studies.

92.3.2.2 Soft Tissues Sarcomas

The use of allo-HSCT has been investigated in paediatric sarcoma and rhabdomyosarcoma. Original data on allo-HSCT in adult STS is rare and stems from small case series (Sureda et al. 2015). In 2007, a retrospective study of the EBMT investigated the use of reduced-conditioning allo-HSCT in 14 STS patients. The authors concluded that an immune-mediated effect might have contributed to tumour control in some patients. Interestingly, the low number of patients examined did not permit a histotype-stratified analysis.

Key Points

- The benefit of auto-HSCT in solid tumours of the adults, with the possible exception of selected patients with breast cancer and germ cell tumours, is still unsettled.
- Despite the great potential, cell therapy programmes for cancer control still have a marginal role in the management of patients with solid tumours. This issue should be regarded as a priority for medical oncology and cell therapy/transplantation societies, also in view of the recent development of immune checkpoint inhibitors that represent a major breakthrough in cancer treatment and may well be incorporated in cell therapy programmes.
- The story of HSCT in solid tumours demonstrates the importance of adopting an internationally co-ordinated approach to the investigation of this treatment modality. There needs to be an increased emphasis on prospective trials that are statistically robust and have well-defined criteria for patient selection. Only these will be able to demonstrate whether HSCT, alone or incorporated into programmes with novel therapeutic modalities, is worthwhile in patients for whom conventional treatments have often limited impact on survival.

References

Admiraal R, van der Paardt M, Kobes J, et al. High-dose chemotherapy for children and young adults with stage IV rhabdomyosarcoma. Cochrane Database Syst Rev. 2010;12:CD006669.

Berry DA, Ueno NT, Johnson MM, et al. High dose chemotherapy with autologous stem cell support versus standard-dose chemotherapy: overview of individual patient data from 15 randomized adjuvant therapy breast cancer trials. J Clin Oncol. 2011;29:3214–23.

Bode U, Zimmermann M, Moser O, et al. Treatment of recurrent primitive neuroectodermal tumors (PNET) in children and adolescents with high-dose chemotherapy (HDC) and stem cell support: results of the HITREZ 97 multicentre trial. J Neuro-Oncol. 2014;120:635–42.

Boye K, Del Prever AB, Eriksson M, et al. High-dose chemotherapy with stem cell rescue in the primary treatment of metastatic and pelvic osteosarcoma: final results of the ISG/SSG II study. Pediatr Blood Cancer. 2014;61:840–5.

Bregni M, Badoglio M, Pedrazzoli P, Lanza F. Is allogeneic transplant for solid tumors still alive? Bone Marrow Transplant. 2016;51:751–2.

Burdach S, Jürgens H. High-dose chemoradiotherapy (HDC) in the Ewing family of tumors (EFT). Crit Rev Oncol Hematol. 2002;41:169–89.

Canete A, Gerrard M, Rubie H, et al. Poor survival for infants with MYCN-amplified metastatic neuroblastoma despite intensified treatment: the International Society of Paediatric Oncology European Neuroblastoma Experience. J Clin Oncol. 2009;27(7):1014–9.

Cohen BH, Geyer JR, Miller DC, et al. Pilot study of intensive chemotherapy with peripheral hematopoietic cell support for children less than 3 years of age with malignant brain tumors, the CCG-99703 phase I/II study. A report from the Children's Oncology Group. Pediatr Neurol. 2015;53:31–46.

Cohn SL, Pearson ADJ, London WB, et al. The International Neuroblastoma Risk Group (INRG) classification system: an INRG task force report. J Clin Oncol. 2009;27:289–97.

De Giorgi U, Nicolas-Virelizier E, Badoglio M, et al. High-dose chemotherapy for adult-type ovarian granulosa cell tumors: a retrospective study of the European Society for Blood and Marrow Transplantation. Int J Gynecol Cancer. 2017a;27:248–51.

De Giorgi U, Richard S, Badoglio M, et al. Salvage high-dose chemotherapy in female patients with relapsed/refractory germ-cell tumors: a retrospective analysis of the European Group for Blood and Marrow Transplantation (EBMT). Ann Oncol. 2017b;28:1910–6.

Dunkel IJ, Chan HSL, Jubran R, et al. High-dose chemotherapy with autologous hematopoietic stem cell rescue for stage 4B retinoblastoma. Pediatr Blood Cancer. 2010;55:149–52.

Echevarria ME, Fangusaro J, Goldman S. Pediatric central nervous system germ cell tumors: a review. Oncologist. 2008;13:690–9.

Fagioli F, Aglietta M, Tienghi A, et al. High-dose chemotherapy in the treatment of relapsed osteosarcoma: an Italian Sarcoma Group Study. J Clin Oncol. 2002;50:2150–6.

Ferrari S, Luksch R, Hall KS, et al. Post-relapse survival in patients with Ewing sarcoma. Pediatr Blood Cancer. 2015;62:994–9.

Finlay JL, Massimino M. A consensus and state-of-the-art workshop: marrow ablative chemotherapy with hematopoietic cell rescue for malignant brain tumors of childhood and adolescence. Pediatr Blood Cancer. 2010;54:634.

Guerra JA, Dhall G, Marachelian A, et al. Marrow-ablative chemotherapy followed by tandem autologous hematopoietic cell transplantation in pediatric patients with malignant brain tumors. Bone Marrow Transplant. 2017;52:1543–8.

Ha TC, Spreafico F, Graf N, et al. An international strategy to determine the role of high dose therapy in recurrent Wilms' tumour. Eur J Cancer. 2013;49:194–210.

Illhardt T, Toporski J, Feuchtinger T, et al. Haploidentical stem cell transplantation for refractory/relapsed neuroblastoma. Biol Blood Marrow Transplant. 2018;24:1005–12.

Jaradat I, Mubiden R, Salem A, et al. High-dose chemotherapy followed by stem cell transplantation in the management of retinoblastoma: a systematic review. Hematol Oncol Stem Cell Ther. 2012;5: 107–17.

Johnson K, McGlynn B, Saggio J, et al. Safety and efficacy of tandem 131I-metaiodobenzylguanidine infusions in relapsed/refractory neuroblastoma. Pediatr Blood Cancer. 2011;57:1124–9.

Ladenstein R, Lasset C, Hartmann O, et al. Impact of megatherapy on survival after relapse from stage 4 neuroblastoma in patients over 1 year of age at diagnosis: a report from the European Group for Bone Marrow Transplantation. J Clin Oncol. 1993;11:2330–41.

Ladenstein R, Lasset C, Hartmann O, et al. Comparison of auto versus allografting as consolidation of primary treatments in advanced neuroblastoma over one year of age at diagnosis: report from the European Group for Bone Marrow Transplantation. Bone Marrow Transplant. 1994;14:37–46.

Ladenstein R, Pötschger U, Hartman O, Pearson AD, Klingebiel T, Castel V, Yaniv I, Demirer T, Dini G, EBMT Paediatric Working Party. 28 years of high-dose therapy and SCT for neuroblastoma in Europe: lessons from more than 4000 procedures. Bone Marrow Transplant. 2008;41(Suppl 2):S118–27. https://doi.org/10.1038/bmt.2008.69.

Ladenstein R, Pötschger U, Le Deley MC, et al. Primary disseminated multifocal Ewing sarcoma: results of the Euro-EWING 99 trial. J Clin Oncol. 2010;28:3284–91.

Ladenstein R, Pötschger U, Pearson ADJ, et al. Busulfan and melphalan versus carboplatin, etoposide, and melphalan as high-dose chemotherapy for high-risk neuroblastoma (HR-NBL1/SIOPEN): an international, randomised, multi-arm, open-label, phase 3 trial. Lancet Oncol. 2017;18:500–14.

Ladenstein R, Pötschger U, Valteau-Couanet D, et al. Interleukin 2 with anti-GD2 antibody ch14.18/CHO (dinutuximab beta) in patients with high-risk neuroblastoma (HR-NBL1/SIOPEN): a multicentre, randomised, phase 3 trial. Lancet Oncol. 2018. https://doi.org/10.1016/1470-2045(18)30578-3

Lee JW, Lee S, Cho HW, et al. Incorporation of high-dose 131I-metaiodobenzylguanidine treatment into tandem high-dose chemotherapy and autologous stem cell transplantation for high-risk neuroblastoma: results of the SMC NB-2009 study. J Hematol Oncol. 2017;10:108.

Lorch A, Bascoul-Mollevi C, Kramar A, et al. Conventional-dose versus high-dose chemotherapy as first salvage treatment in male patients with metastatic germ cell tumors: evidence from a large international database. J Clin Oncol. 2011;29:2178–84.

Luksch R, Tienghi A, Hall KS, et al. Primary metastatic Ewing's family tumors: results of the Italian Sarcoma Group and Scandinavian Sarcoma Group ISG/SSG IV Study including myeloablative chemotherapy and total-lung irradiation. Ann Oncol. 2012;23:2970–6.

Malogolowkin MH, Hemmer MT, Le-Rademacher J, et al. Outcomes following autologous hematopoietic stem cell transplant for patients with relapsed Wilms' tumor: a CIBMTR retrospective analysis. Bone Marrow Transplant. 2017;52:1549–55.

Marec-Berard P, Segura-Ferlay C, Tabone MD, et al. High dose thiotepa in patients with relapsed or refractory osteosarcomas: experience of the SFCE Group. Sarcoma. 2014;2014:475067.

Martino M, Lanza F, Pavesi L, et al. High-dose chemotherapy and autologous hematopoietic stem cell transplantation as adjuvant treatment in high-risk breast cancer: data from the European Group for Blood and Marrow Transplantation Registry. Biol Blood Marrow Transplant. 2016;22:475–81.

Matthay KK, Reynolds CP, Seeger RC, et al. Long-term results for children with high-risk neuroblastoma treated on a randomized trial of myeloablative therapy followed by 13-cis-retinoic acid: a children's oncology group study. J Clin Oncol. 2009;27:1007–13.

Moroz V, Machin D, Faldum A, et al. Changes over three decades in outcome and the prognostic influence of age-at-diagnosis in young patients with neuroblastoma: a report from the International Neuroblastoma Risk Group Project. Eur J Cancer. 2011;47:561–71.

Murray MJ, Bartels U, Nishikawa R, et al. Consensus on the management of intracranial germ-cell tumours. Lancet Oncol. 2015;19:e470–7.

Necchi A, Lanza F, Rosti G, European Society for Blood and Marrow Transplantation, Solid Tumors Working Party (EBMT-STWP) and the Italian Germ Cell Cancer Group (IGG), et al. High-dose chemotherapy for germ cell tumors: do we have a model? Expert Opin Biol Ther. 2015;15:33–44.

Necchi A, Miceli R, Bregni M, et al. Prognostic impact of progression to induction chemotherapy and prior paclitaxel therapy in patients with germ cell tumors receiving salvage high-dose chemotherapy in the last 10 years: a study of the European Society for Blood and Marrow Transplantation Solid Tumors Working Party. Bone Marrow Transplant. 2016;51:384–90.

Necchi A, Lo Vullo, Bregni M·et al. Salvage high-dose chemotherapy for relapsed pure seminoma in the last 10 years: results from the European Society for Blood and Marrow Transplantation series 2002-2012. Clin Genitourin Cancer 2017; 15: 163-167.

Nitz UA, Mohrmann S, Fischer J, et al. Comparison of rapidly cycled tandem high-dose chemotherapy plus peripheral-blood stem-cell support versus dose-dense conventional chemotherapy for adjuvant treatment of high-risk breast cancer: results of a multicentre phase III trial. Lancet. 2005;366:1935–44.

Park JR, Kreissman SG, London WB, et al. A phase III randomized clinical trial (RCT) of tandem myeloablative autologous stem cell transplant (ASCT) using peripheral blood stem cell (PBSC) as consolidation therapy for high-risk neuroblastoma (HR-NB): a Children's Oncology Group (COG) study. J Clin Oncol. 2016;34(18_Suppl):LBA3. https://doi.org/10.1200/JCO.2016.34.18_suppl.LBA3.

Passweg JR, Baldomero H, Bader P, et al. Is the use of unrelated donor transplantation leveling off in Europe? The 2016 European Society for Blood and Marrow Transplant activity survey report. Bone Marrow Transplant. 2018. https://doi.org/10.1038/s41409-018-0153-1.

Pedrazzoli P, Martino M, Delfanti S, et al. High-dose chemotherapy with autologous hematopoietic stem cell transplantation in high-risk breast cancer patients. J Natl Cancer Inst. 2015;51:70–5.

Peinemann F, Labeit AM. Autologous haematopoietic stem cell transplantation following high-dose chemotherapy for non-rhabdomyosarcoma soft tissue sarcomas: a Cochrane systematic review. BMJ Open. 2014;4:e005033.

Presson A, Moore TB, Kempert P. Efficacy of high-dose chemotherapy and autologous stem cell transplant for recurrent Wilms' tumor: a meta-analysis. J Pediatr Hematol Oncol. 2010;32:454–61.

Raleigh DR, Tomlin B, Buono BD, et al. Survival after chemotherapy and stem cell transplant followed by delayed craniospinal irradiation is comparable to upfront craniospinal irradiation in pediatric embryonal brain tumor patients. J Neuro-Oncol. 2017;131:359–68.

Sauerbrey A, Bielack S, Kempf-Bielack B, et al. High-dose chemotherapy (HDC) and autologous hematopoietic stem cell transplantation (ASCT) as salvage therapy for relapsed osteosarcoma. Bone Marrow Transplant. 2001;27:933–7.

Sureda A, Bader P, Cesaro S, et al. Indications for allo and auto-SCT for haematological diseases, solid tumors, and immune disorders: current practice in Europe 2015. Bone Marrow Transplant. 2015;50:1037–56.

Tenneti P, Zahid U, Sagar F, et al. Role of high-dose chemotherapy and autologous stem cell transplantation for relapsed Ewing's sarcoma: a case report with focused review of literature. Cureus. 2018;10:e2581.

Thiel U, Wawer A, Wolf P, et al. No improvement of survival with reduced- versus high-intensity conditioning for allogeneic stem cell transplants in Ewing tumor patients. Ann Oncol. 2011;22:1614–21.

Thiel U, Koscielniak E, Blaeschke F, et al. Allogeneic stem cell transplantation for patients with advanced rhabdomyosarcoma: a retrospective assessment. Br J Cancer. 2013;109:2523–32.

Whelan J, Le Deley MC, Dirksen U, Euro-E.W.I.N.G.99 and EWING-2008 Investigators, et al. High-dose chemotherapy and blood autologous stem-cell rescue compared with standard chemotherapy in localized high-risk ewing sarcoma: results of Euro-E.W.I.N.G.99 and Ewing-2008. J Clin Oncol. 2018. https://doi.org/10.1200/JCO.2018.78.2516

Yu AL, Gilman AL, Ozkaynak MF, et al. Anti-GD2 antibody with GM-CSF, interleukin-2, and isotretinoin for neuroblastoma. N Engl J Med. 2010;63:1324–34.

Appendix: EBMT Registry

Carmen Ruiz de Elvira
and Shelley Hewerdine

Introduction

The EBMT maintains a Registry which encompasses all HSCT procedures for all indications. It also stores immunosuppressive treatments for bone marrow failure syndromes (i.e., aplastic anaemias), cell therapy treatments other than HSCT and donor information pertaining to collection and donor follow-up.

Content of the Registry

The clinical content of the EBMT Registry is decided by EBMT researchers through the Working Parties (WP). All requests have to be endorsed by the relevant WP Chair and must be accompanied by adequate definitions of the new data items. The final structure, format and clinical definitions of the data collection forms are supported by EBMT staff and important stakeholders of the Registry. This is done through recognised structures such as the Registry Committee, the Definitions Group and the Data Registries Group. For more details on these groups, please refer to the EBMT website. Final decisions are made by the Scientific Council and the Board of the Association.

C. R. de Elvira (✉) · S. Hewerdine
EBMT, London, UK
e-mail: carmen.ruiz@ebmt.org

Data Collection Forms

The EBMT has four main types of Data Collection Form which are implemented in the Registry IT system. For reference you can download data forms from the Data Management pages of the EBMT website:

MED A for HSCT	Minimum Essential Data. All EBMT member centres that perform transplants need to submit MED A for every HSCT to retain full membership. Transplant centres that do not report for 2 years or more will be demoted to associate members until they resume reporting
MED B for HSCT	Contains more data than MED A and is optimal for studies. Includes all items from the above MED A form
MED A for Cell Therapy	Contains the minimum essential data for this type of treatment
Donor Outcome	Minimum essential data to follow stem cell donors

IT System

At the time of writing the EBMT Registry is using ProMISe software designed by Ronald Brand, who worked as a Professor of Biostatistics at LUMC in the Netherlands prior to his retirement in 2017. The data is stored in an SQL server database based in the same location. During 2018, the EBMT Registry is continuing with an upgrade project and intends to switch to an electronic data capture system named MACRO, part

E. Carreras et al. (eds.), *The EBMT Handbook*, https://doi.org/10.1007/978-3-030-02278-5

of the company Elsevier. Again, this will be a hosted environment and the server will abide by all standards in safety and security, and any other data protection standards required by the EU GDPR, that has become law in May 2018.

IT Security

The IT system uses all reasonable, appropriate, practical and effective security measures to protect our important processes and assets. The system utilises NEN7510 (2011) with the ISO27001 internal foundation as a framework for guiding our approach to managing security. The system provider continually reviews its use of security measures to improve the way in which we protect our systems, and the data entrusted to us.

Data Protection

The EBMT Registry follows EU directives regarding data protection. It is the responsibility of the EBMT to ensure that centres and donor registries are aware of this. The EBMT requests that all centres outside the EU sign an EU Regulations Statement declaring they will follow EU regulations regarding data safety. The most up-to-date information on EBMT data protection can be found on the Data Management pages of the EBMT website, in particular the full *Registry Function* document. As the Registry Office is located in London, the database has been registered with the Information Commissioner's Office in the United Kingdom.

All EBMT centres must obtain informed consent from their patients and/or donors before the data can be submitted to the EBMT. Data is semi-anonymised: we store date of birth and usually the patient initials; never full names. Emailing, downloading or transferring EBMT data containing even semi-anonymous identifiers is NOT allowed, unless strong password protection or an EBMT approved secure server is used. In the unlikely cases of patients refusing consent to their data being stored, then fully anonymous, bare minimum data can be registered, purely to include these transplants in the centre counts.

Registry Function

The main function of the Registry is to collect pertinent and good quality clinical data. The main use of these data is clinical research, but it will also be used to support the mission of the EBMT in aspects such as the inspection, auditing and accreditation of transplant centres.

EBMT led studies is the single most important use of the Registry data. The EBMT registry can use all the data submitted to them. It is understood that data submitted to the EBMT can be used for research and published by the EBMT WP as long as the existing *Guidelines for the Conduct of Registry Studies using the EBMT Registry Database* and the *Authorship guidelines for EBMT publications* are followed. Both documents are mandatory reading for any WP investigator wishing to perform a registry study. Although the EBMT Registry Office has the primary responsibility for cleaning, and updating the data, the EBMT study coordinators contribute to this for specific studies.

Registry Stakeholders

Centres

Member centres use the Registry to store their own data while simultaneously making it available to the EBMT. Each EBMT member can be considered as the main owner of their data, although it is understood that the ultimate owner is the patient. Members submitting data can use their own data for their own purposes without having to require permission or notify the EBMT. Members have access to their own data at all times and can actively block access to selected patients by other authorised users. Member centres can also obtain aggregate anonymised data of the entire Registry, where neither the patient nor the centre is identifiable.

National Registries for HSCT

National registries operating in some countries, usually under the umbrella of a medical association, have become part of the EBMT data flow by mutual consent and are using the same central database. These national registries use their data for their own purposes, which may encompass national requirements for registration of transplants, research, demographics, etc. Where these registries exist, the responsibility of the EBMT Registry for data management may be partially devolved to them. That said, EBMT centres belonging to a National Registry have as much access to the EBMT Registry staff and services as any other centre member. We enjoy a close collaboration with a number of national societies and a list of partners can be found on the EBMT website.

Government Agencies

Registry data may be accessed by public agencies in one of two ways: (1) they can request direct access to data submitted by centres in their country. As with any other type of access, centres need to make the request to the Registry for their data to be accessed directly by these agencies. (2) National registries may collaborate with public agencies providing them with data extracted from the EBMT Registry.

Donor Registries

Donor Registries can use the EBMT Registry to store their own data while simultaneously making it available to the EBMT. Donor Registries submitting donor data can use their own data for their own purposes without having to require permission or notify the EBMT. Donor Registries have access to their own data at all times.

Donor registries may also request access to the Registry in order to follow the donors or the patients that have received donations from them. In the latter case, the centre has to give permission for the donor registry to be able to see selected patient data.

Study Groups

Groups of centres can set up studies and use the EBMT Registry as their database. The study group requests explicit permission from the Principal Investigator of each centre involved and forwards these to the EBMT. All centres must be members of the EBMT. Permission templates are available.

International Research Organisations

Centres that submit data to other organisations can request the EBMT to provide data access to these organisations, so they do not have to do double reporting. In these cases, the EBMT can set up "virtual registries" that replicate the scope of the organisation and provide access to a data manager of this organisation to access the permitted data. Such requests have to be submitted explicitly by the Principal Investigator of the involved centre. All centres must be members of the EBMT. Permission templates are available.

Corporate Sponsors

Corporate members can obtain aggregate anonymised data as part of their contract, where neither the patient nor the centre is identifiable. Sponsors cannot obtain outcome data. To safeguard centre anonymity, all countries with less than ten member centres appear under the label of "Other".

Access to the Registry

All individuals must submit an Access request for internet access to the data. Accepted signatories are:

- Principal investigator of a transplant centre (centre's data only) or donor registry (donor registry's data only)
- Working Party chair (for access to data within the remit of that WP)

- The President of the EBMT (for data within the remit of an EBMT Committee)
- Director of an institution or study group with which we have a partnership. In this case, the partner must also submit a signed form from every centre involved granting access of their data to that institution or study group.
- Registry head for EBMT Registry staff

Individuals who by the nature of their work have direct access to the EBMT Registry databases (IT system/server managers) have no access rights to the data and would be in breach of contract if they manipulate it.

Some individuals work in multiple roles and it is possible to request multiple user roles and rights, as long as the above procedures are followed.

Types of Access

Users of the Registry system can access their own data in which case they can request permission to do any of the following:

- Data entry*
- Lists of patient data*
- Data download*
- Tables with aggregated data (frequencies and cross tabulations)

The types of access marked with (*) are restricted since they may include identification of the patients. This type of access can only be requested by an accepted signatory for a set of nominated individuals. The access provided is personal and cannot be transferred to other individuals, not even within the same centre. The Central Registry Office reserves the right to cancel access without warning if it is felt that patient confidentiality might be at risk.

The unrestricted access, tables with aggregated data, is available to all members and sponsors. This statistical function does not allow patients or centres to be identified. Transplant centres who are members can access statistics of the entire registry as part of their database access. Aggregated data requests from other recognised groups should be made to the Central Registry Office.

Data Flow

For MED A or B for HSCT, the first registration must be submitted on the day of transplant (day 0) or within a week of day 0. An update should be submitted when 100 days have elapsed from the date of transplant, or when the patient dies, whichever comes first. Regular annual follow-up data must be submitted for all patients from then onwards.

For MED A for cell therapy (without HSCT), the first registration must be submitted on the day of infusion (day 0) or within a week of day 0. An update should be submitted every 6 months.

For more detailed and up-to-date information, see document *Submitting data to the EBMT*

The data can reach the Registry through two channels:

(a) Direct data entry by a centre. This is the preferred and most common method.
(b) Direct data entry by a small number of national registries on behalf of specific centres that submit paper forms to them.

Centres can enter the data directly (option a), or fill in the MED A or MED B paper forms and send it to their national registry if available (option b).

When the data is entered directly by the centre into the EBMT database, this ensures immediate access by the EBMT and authorised users to the centre's data. This is the preferred method. Centres who use this system may be approached by the national registry, if they belong to one, or by the EBMT registry with requests for data corrections or clarifications. All centres can request to view their data, even if it has been entered by a National Registry on their behalf.

Support

The Registry has a small team of staff based in London who work on the database structure, form design, data quality, user support and documentation. Contact details can be found on the EBMT website.

www.ingramcontent.com/pod-product-compliance
Lightning Source LLC
LaVergne TN
LVHW062152200926
848484LV00007B/1901